Clinical Hematology

Clinical Hematology
Principles, Procedures, Correlations

Second Edition

EDITED BY

E. Anne Stiene-Martin, PhD, MT(ASCP)

Professor and Director
Division of Clinical Laboratory Sciences
Department of Clinical Sciences
College of Allied Health Professions
University of Kentucky
Lexington, Kentucky

Cheryl A. Lotspeich-Steininger, MS, MBA, MT(ASCP), CLS(NCA)

Formerly Assistant Professor
Department of Clinical Laboratory Sciences
School of Allied Health Sciences
Program in Medical Technology
The University of Texas–Houston Health Science Center
Houston, Texas

John A. Koepke, MD

Emeritus Professor of Pathology
Department of Pathology
Duke University Medical Center
Durham, North Carolina

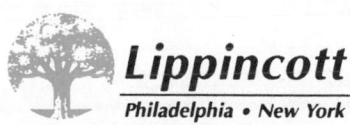

Lippincott
Philadelphia • New York

Acquisitions Editor: Lawrence McGrew
Editorial Assistant: Holly Chapman
Project Editors: Susan Deitch
 Roberta Spivek
Production Manager: Helen Ewan
Production Coordinator: Patricia McCloskey
Design Coordinator: Nicholas Rook

Second Edition

9   8   7   6   5   4   3   2

Library of Congress Cataloging-in-Publications Data

Clinical Hematology : principles, procedures, correlations / edited by
 E. Anne Stiene-Martin, Cheryl A. Lotspeich-Steininger, John A.
 Koepke. — 2nd ed.
     p.   cm.
   Includes bibliographical references and index.
   ISBN 0-397-55321-8
   1. Hematology.   2. Blood—Examination.   I. Stiene-Martin, E.
 Anne.   II. Lotspeich-Steininger, Cheryl A.   III. Koepke, John A.,
 1929-   .
   [DNLM: 1. Hematologic Diseases.   WH 120 C641 1998]
 RB45.C57   1998
 616.1'5—dc21
 DNLM/DLC
 for Library of Congress   97-17765
                                                                CIP

Care has been taken to confirm the accuracy of the information presented and to describe generally accepted practices. However, the authors, editors, and publisher are not responsible for errors or omissions or for any consequences from application of the information in this book and make no warranty, express or implied, with respect to the contents of the publication.

The authors, editors and publisher have exerted every effort to ensure that drug selection and dosage set forth in this text are in accordance with current recommendations and practice at the time of publication. However, in view of ongoing research, changes in government regulations, and the constant flow of information relating to drug therapy and drug reactions, the reader is urged to check the package insert for each drug for any change in indications and dosage and for added warnings and precautions. This is particularly important when the recommended agent is a new or infrequently employed drug.

Some drugs and medical devices presented in this publication have Food and Drug Administration (FDA) clearance for limited use in restricted research settings. It is the responsibility of the health care provider to ascertain the FDA status of each drug or device planned for use in their clinical practice.

To my husband Ken for his understanding and support throughout, and to all former and present students who have given so many good suggestions and ideas over the years on how better to teach the subject of hematology.

E.A.S.M.

To my husband John and my daughter Katherine for their patience and support during this endeavor, and to all of my family for their constant love and understanding.

C.A.L.S.

To those many laboratory professionals, friends, and coworkers who have worked so diligently to advance laboratory hematology.

J.A.K.

Contributors

F. Sue Allison, MA, MT(ASCP), CLS(NCA)
Associate Professor of Medical Technology
Biological Sciences
The University of Alabama
Tuscaloosa, Alabama

Joyce A. Behrens, MS, MT(ASCP)
Assistant Professor
University of Washington
Department of Laboratory Medicine
Division of Medical Technology
University of Washington Medical Center
Seattle, Washington

Ann Bell, MS, SH(ASCP), CLSpH(NCA)
Assistant Professor of Medicine
Professor of Clinical Laboratory Science
The University of Tennessee, Memphis
The Health Science Center
Division of Hematology/Oncology
Department of Medicine
Memphis, Tennessee

Cheryl S. Cook, BS, MT(ASCP)
Supervisor
Coagulation Department
Riverside Methodist Hospital
Columbus, Ohio

Gerald L. Davis, MT(ASCP), PhD
Professor of Physiology
Michigan State University
East Lansing, Michigan

Mary Ann Dotson, BS, CLS(NCA), MT(ASCP)
Analytical Specialist—Hematology
Department of Pathology—Clinical Laboratories
Duke University Medical Center
Durham, North Carolina

Rita C. East, MS, MT(ASCP)
Medical Technologist
Hematology/Oncology Section, Medical Service
Veterans Affairs Medical Center
Lexington, Kentucky

Gordon E. Ens, BA, MT(ASCP)
Laboratory Director
Colorado Coagulation Consultants, Inc.
Aurora, Colorado
Associate Editor
Clinical Hemostasis Review
Tucson, Arizona

Valerie J. Evans
Laboratory Director
Department of Clinical Pathology
University of Arizona
Tucson, Arizona

Angela B. Foley, BS, MS, MT(ASCP), CLS(NCA)
Associate Professor of Clinical Medical Technology
Department of Medical Technology
Louisiana State University School of Allied Health
    Professions
New Orleans, Louisiana

Joy Jarvis Gall, BHS, MT(ASCP)SH
Senior Technologist/Clinical Faculty
Department of Pathology/Hematology
University of Kentucky Medical Center
Lexington, Kentucky

Vincent Salvatore Galliocchio, BA, MS, PhD,
MT(ASCP)
Associate Dean, Professor of Clinical Sciences and Internal
    Medicine
Department of Clinical Sciences and Internal Medicine
Chandler Medical Center, University of Kentucky
Lexington, Kentucky

Virginia Haight, BS
Hematology Manager
Department of Pathology
Lawrence Memorial Hospital
New London, Connecticut

Dianne M. Hansen, BA, MT(ASCP)
Education Specialist
Partners in Home Care, Inc.
Missoula, Montana

Barbara J. Helbert, MT(ASCP)
Formerly Supervisor
Scott & White Clinic and Hospital
Temple, Texas

Ruth Ann Henriksen, PhD
Associate Professor
Medicine
East Carolina University School of Medicine
Greenville, North Carolina

Anne S. Hobson, MA, MT(ASCP)SH
Formerly Technical Director of Hematology
University of Virginia Medical Center
Clinical Laboratories
Charlottesville, Virginia

Muriel I. Jobe, BS, MT(ASCP)SH, CLS(NCA)
Formerly Supervisor
Hematology Laboratories
St. Louis University Hospital
St. Louis, Missouri

Dona D. Knapp, PhD, MT(ASCP), CLS(NCA)
Professor
Director of Medical Technology
The University of South Dakota Medical School
Department of Laboratory Medicine
Vermillion, South Dakota

John A. Koepke, MD
Emeritus Professor of Pathology and Associate Professor
    of Medicine
Department of Pathology
Duke University Medical Center
Durham, North Carolina

William Koss, MD
Director, Clinical Pathology
Scott & White Clinic and Memorial Hospital
Associate Professor of Pathology
Texas A&M University Health Science Center
College of Medicine
Temple, Texas

Louann W. Lawrence, DrPH, CLSpH(NCA), MT(ASCP)SH
Associate Professor and Department Head
Department of Medical Technology
Louisiana State University Medical Center
New Orleans, Louisiana

Susan J. Leclair, MS, CLS(NCA)
Professor of Medical Laboratory Science
Department of Medical Laboratory Science
University of Massachusetts Dartmouth
Dartmouth, Massachusetts

Karen G. Lofsness, MS, CLSpH
Associate Professor
Division of Medical Technology
Department of Laboratory Medicine and Pathology
University of Minnesota
Minneapolis, Minnesota

Cheryl A. Lotspeich-Steininger, MS, MBA, MT(ASCP), CLS(NCA)
Formerly Assistant Professor
Department of Clinical Laboratory Sciences
School of Allied Health Sciences
Program in Medical Technology
The University of Texas–Houston Health Science Center
Houston, Texas

Jeffrey Louie, BS Medical Technology, MT(ASCP)
Chief Technologist
USC Clinical Laboratories—Flow Cytometry Section
University of Southern California
Los Angeles, California

Lois Lucas, BS, MT(ASCP)
Chief Medical Technologist, Section of Hematopathology
Division of Laboratory Medicine
The University of Texas MD Anderson Cancer Center
Houston, Texas

F. Bernhard Ludvigsen, PhD
Adjunct Associate Professor
Medical Technology
University of South Alabama
Mobile, Alabama

Lynne H. Lyons, MS, MT(ASCP)
Senior Clinical Technologist
Department of Pathology
Stem Cell Processing Laboratory
University of Kentucky Medical Center
Lexington, Kentucky

Charles E. Manner, MD
Formerly Assistant Professor
Health Science Center at Houston
School of Medicine, Department of Internal Medicine
Division of Hematology–Oncology
The University of Texas
Houston, Texas

Sherry Martin, MEd, MT(ASCP)SC
Administrative Director of Educational Programs
Division of Laboratory Medicine
The University of Texas MD Anderson Cancer Center
Houston, Texas

Jennifer K. Morrow, BS, MS, PhD
Formerly Director of Molecular Diagnostic Laboratory
Department of Pathology
University of Kentucky
Director and General Manager of Laboratory Sciences
Equine Biodiagnostics, Inc.
Lexington, Kentucky

Kathleen M. Mugan, MEd, MT(ASCP)SH
Instructor
University of Arkansas for Medical Sciences
Department of Medical Technology
Little Rock, Arkansas

Loretta Nemchik, MS, MT(ASCP)SH
Hematology Coordinator
Laboratory Science Programs
Allegheny University of the Health Sciences
Philadelphia, Pennsylvania

Raymond L. Olesinski, PhD, MT/PBT(ASCP)SH,
CLS(NCA)
Director, Division of Technology & Information Services
Assistant Professor, Clinical Laboratory Sciences
Center for Rural Health
University of Kentucky
Hazard, Kentucky

John W. Parker, BS, MD
Professor of Pathology
Department of Pathology
University of Southern California School of Medicine
Los Angeles, California

Irma T. Pereira, MT(ASCP)SH
Clinical Hematology Specialist
Clinical Hematology
Adjunct Lecturer in Hematology
Department of Medicine
Stanford University Hospital
Stanford, California

Powers Peterson, MD
Professor of Pathology and Laboratory Medicine
Associate Director of Clinical Laboratories
Director of Hematology
Allegheny University of the Health Sciences
Philadelphia, Pennsylvania

Robert V. Pierre, MD
Chief, Clinical Hematology Laboratories
Department of Pathology
University of Southern Carolina
Los Angeles, California

Edward S. Rappaport, MD
Director of Hematopathology
Scott & White Clinic and Hospital
Temple, Texas

Tina M. Riedinger, BS, MT(ASCP)SH
General Supervisor
Pathology–Hematology/Oncology Laboratory
Indiana University Medical Center
Indianapolis, Indiana

Robert Rifkin, MD, FACP
Director, Blood and Marrow Transplant Program
Columbia–Presbyterian/St. Luke's Medical Center
Denver, Colorado

Bernadette F. Rodak, MS, CLSpH(NCA),
MT(ASCP)SH
Assistant Professor
Medical Technology Program
Indiana University–Purdue University at Indianapolis
Indianapolis, Indiana

Robbi Safko, AS
Medical Laboratory Supervisor/Hemoglobinopathies
    Supervisor
Division of Laboratory Sciences
North Carolina Department of Environment, Health &
    Natural Resources
Raleigh, North Carolina

Margaret C. Schmidt, EdD, CLS(NCA),
CLSpH(NCA)
Assistant Clinical Professor of Pathology
Director, Education Service
Pathology/Clinical Laboratories
Duke University Medical Center
Durham, North Carolina

Marian Schwabbauer, PhD
Program Director
Clinical Laboratory Sciences Program
University of Iowa
Iowa City, Iowa

Jean Shafer, MA, MT(ASCP)
Associate Professor of Medicine and Pathology
University of Rochester School of Medicine and Dentistry
Department of Medicine
Hematology Unit
Rochester, New York

Catherine Sherry, SC, MS, MPS, MT(ASCP)
Administrative Director
Department of Laboratories/Pathology
Saint Vincent's Hospital and Medical Center
New York, New York

Jamie Siegel, MD
Assistant Professor
Pathology and Laboratory Medicine
Director of Coagulation
Allegheny University of the Health Sciences
Philadelphia, Pennsylvania

Barbara A. Smith Michael, MS, JD, MT(ASCP)
Formerly Assistant Professor
Department of Clinical Laboratory Sciences
School of Allied Health Sciences
Program in Medical Technology
The University of Texas–Houston Health Science Center
Houston, Texas

Sandra R. Sommer, PhD, MT(ASCP)SH
Associate Professor
Clinical Laboratory Sciences
Virginia Commonwealth University
Richmond, Virginia

Ella M. Spanjers, BS, MT(ASCP), CLS(NCA)
Formerly Laboratory Manager
Special Hematology Laboratory
Department of Laboratory Medicine and Pathology
University of Minnesota Hospitals
Minneapolis, Minnesota

E. Anne Stiene-Martin, PhD
Professor and Director
Division of Clinical Laboratory Sciences
Department of Clinical Sciences
University of Kentucky
Lexington, Kentucky

Joan C. Terrell, BA, MA, MT(ASCP)
Formerly Instructor in Hematology
The University of Texas
Health Science Center at Houston
School of Allied Health Sciences
Program in Medical Technology
Houston, Texas

Martha T. Thomas, MS, MT(ASCP), CLS(NCA)
Professor Emeritus
Michigan State University
Medical Technology Program
East Lansing, Michigan

Robert A. Van Dyne, MBA, MT(ASCP)SH
Analytical Supervisor, Clinical Coagulation Laboratory
Department of Pathology
Duke University Medical Center
Durham, North Carolina

Gary Van Zant, PhD
Professor
Medicine
University of Kentucky Medical Center
Lexington, Kentucky

J. Lynne Williams, PhD, MT(ASCP)
Professor
Medical Laboratory Sciences
Oakland University
Rochester, Michigan

Foreword

When the editors asked me to contribute a chapter to this book, I was very pleased to be included in this select group of hematology practitioners and educators from across the United States. When they asked me to write this Foreword, I was delighted to be able to explain why I was eager to be included and to contribute to this text. Why indeed, in this day and age of global communication and easily updated sources of information on the Internet, would I choose to write a book chapter?

Several reasons come to mind. As a student, I did not particularly enjoy hematology. I found the subjectivity of morphology confusing. I almost certainly would have benefited from color plates such as those included in this edition. It was difficult for me, a global learner, to pull together in any meaningful way what seemed to be disjointed subtopics.

Sure enough, my first job was in hematology, which I considered to be one of my weaker areas. But the longer I worked in hematology and the better I understood it, the more I enjoyed it. The more I learned, the more exciting hematology became. These then, are the goals of this text: to help students learn more than just the facts; to give students enough background and history so that the field makes sense; and to give them enough understanding of related and developing areas so that they not only find hematology interesting and enjoyable, but challenging and exciting enough to continue learning about new discoveries and new techniques after they graduate.

Once I gained the essential knowledge base, I found hematology more stimulating than any other area of the laboratory. Hematology has always incorporated leading-edge technology to help decipher and treat troubling diseases, both those that have long plagued humankind and those newly emergent. There is also something mystical about the study of living cells—cells that contain the essence of the person, ill or healthy, from whom they were taken; cells that still harbor so many important secrets, even today. Hematology literally means "the study of the formed elements (cells) of the blood." These cells hold the key to life itself. To understand cells and their possibilities, we must approach them with the sense of wonder and mystery that permeates this text.

Hematology has evolved greatly during my laboratory career. As a student, I learned to use a hematocytometer to do manual cell counts. I ran a Coulter™ Model A® and the very first Technicon™® instruments. Now, fourth-generation instruments that utilize principles and techniques drawn from a variety of disciplines are commonplace in the hematology laboratory. Today, morphologists work productively alongside engineers. Yesterday, we worked to produce timely, accurate, and precise data. Now hematologists increasingly hand that task over to technology and engineers, while they strive to interpret and to convert these data into useful information that will make difficult diagnostic and treatment decisions easier and clearer.

Hematologists must now produce much more than data; they are asked to provide information that will improve the diagnosis, management, and treatment of disease. To do that, one must understand the possibilities that lie with the chosen technology, and even more important, one must understand the limits of that technology. Thus hematologists must also possess a working knowledge of chemistry, cellular biology, immunology, histology, molecular pathology, hemostasis, and body fluids—just to mention a few of the related areas of study covered, when appropriate, in this text. New chapters in this edition describe the ongoing integration of developing fields such as oncology and molecular pathology into hematology, and help clarify what once seemed to be inexplicable overlaps and gaps between areas.

This book will help students integrate what they have learned and will continue to learn in many areas. Good texts are essential tools to prepare students and practitioners to become knowledgeable and adept health professionals. As a hematology educator, I long rued the lack of a definitive hematology text that would bridge the chasm between the lofty texts written for specialists by specialists and those that, while very useful in the laboratory, are basically technical procedure manuals. I believe that this book can be that bridge, presenting the requisite theory in a simple, yet scholarly fashion, and integrating it with the principles and procedures that comprise good, current laboratory practice for students, researchers, and practitioners.

In education, the questions are often considered to be more important than the answers. However, the answers are still crucial, for when they are informative and well-phrased, they frequently lead to more, and even more important, questions. These are the sorts of answers that students will find within this book's covers—answers that lead to novel questions, fresh ways to integrate information, and new discoveries. We need those questions in hematology to structure and advance the acquisition of new knowledge, useful technology, and better treatments for diseases. Patients will survive previously incurable hematologic diseases because of readers' persistent searches for new ways to provide the best possible patient care. Many patients will live longer, higher quality lives than individuals with the same dyscrasias just a decade ago because of students' continuing quests for more knowledge and understanding.

Finally, I found it personally rewarding to help produce a book in concert with authors and editors who understand their topics well enough to be able to carefully and thoroughly explain them in simple and concise, yet clear and unique, ways. They are master teachers who unabashedly love hematology and unraveling its mysteries to others. Their passion shines through and brings their words to life for the reader. As Mark Twain once explained, "Words are only painted fire; a book is the fire itself." It is our desire that the fire within this book will indirectly bring healing and hope to many who suffer from hematological diseases.

Marian Schwabbauer, PhD
University of Iowa

Preface

As the editors of *Clinical Hematology—Principles, Procedures, Correlations*, we have been very gratified by the positive response to the first edition of the text. It has been used in both graduate and undergraduate CLS (MT) programs as well as in pathology residency programs. It has also been used as a reference in numerous CLT (MLT) programs and in working hematology laboratories.

When this text was first proposed, we wanted to develop a textbook that would contain many of the "tricks of the trade" that have been presented at professional seminars and workshops but not published in a textbook. The contributors have helped us to meet this challenge. We strongly believe that a major advantage of this text is that it is written by clinical laboratory scientists (medical technologists) with a wide range of expertise. We have endeavored to provide students and practitioners with valuable information regarding the various disease states and the clinical laboratory procedures for their diagnosis. We have paid special attention to the sources of technical and physiologic error in procedures and their possible solutions in extensive "Comments and Sources of Error" sections. Procedures are not always delineated step-by-step because this information is available in original references, laboratory manuals, or commercial package inserts.

Several additions and changes have been made in this second edition in an attempt to present the most up-to-date information in the field of clinical hematology and hemostasis and to improve its value to students and educators. In the area of content, we have combined some chapters to make room for new concepts and techniques that are being introduced in some hematology laboratories. These include methods used to harvest stem cells for bone marrow transplantation, an expanded chapter on flow cytometry, and a brief introduction to molecular biological techniques and their impact on the diagnosis and monitoring of hematologic disorders. In addition, we have added more color plates to the text, bringing their number to well over 100.

Several pedagogic enhancements have also been made, including the addition of educational objectives and review questions for each chapter, more case studies, and an extensive glossary of significant words and acronyms in the fields of hematology and hemostasis. Answers to the case study and chapter review questions are found in appendices at the end of the text.

We look forward to receiving comments and suggestions from interested readers, and hope that those of you who suggested improvements for the first edition will recognize the fruits of your efforts.

E. Anne Stiene-Martin, PhD, MT(ASCP)

Cheryl A. Lotspeich-Steininger, MS, MBA, MT(ASCP), CLS(NCA)

John A. Koepke, MD

Acknowledgements

The editors are very grateful to the 54 contributors for sharing their knowledge and insight in this textbook, and for their cooperation, patience, and endurance during the lengthy writing and editing process. Each contributor was selected based on his or her expertise in hematology or hematosis. As evidenced by the contributor list, the vast majority are laboratory scientists who are actively engaged in the practice of laboratory hematology or hemostasis, or in education related to these fields. Six are medical doctors who, like the other contributors and the editors, have a keen interest in the education of clinical laboratory scientists and others studying clinical hematology and hemostasis.

We are also grateful to the staff at Lippincott-Raven Publishers who have worked diligently with us during this lengthy and complex project to make this textbook a reality. We wish to extend our personal thanks to Lawrence McGrew, Holly Chapman, Kathy Lyons, Stephanie Harold, and Andrew Allen, all of whom worked with us directly to assist with every aspect of this publication. We are most appreciative of them and of everyone who contributed to this endeavor.

Contents

PART I

Introduction to Hematology

CHAPTER 1

Introduction to Clinical Hematology and Safety in the Hematology Laboratory

E. Anne Stiene-Martin

History of Clinical Hematology

Basic Terminology

Safety in the Clinical Hematology Laboratory
Biologic Hazards

Chemical Hazards
Electrical Hazards
Mechanical Hazards
Fire Hazards

Case Studies 1-1 and 1-2

Objectives

1. Describe how Greek and Latin prefixes and suffixes can be combined to form hematologic terms.
2. List at least eight rules for the handling of biologically hazardous materials.
3. Describe the purpose and uses of MSD sheets and NFPA labels.
4. Describe at least one electrical, one mechanical, and one fire hazard in the hematology laboratory and how each may be avoided.

This chapter will provide a brief background on the development of clinical hematology, an introduction to hematologic vocabulary in terms of common prefixes and suffixes used to form the medical terms in this discipline, and a discussion of the principal laboratory safety rules as related to hematology.

An understanding of safety rules is an absolute necessity before beginning work in any laboratory. Safe laboratory practice ensures the well-being of laboratory personnel as well as those who enter the laboratory for consultation and those responsible for cleaning the laboratory and discarding hazardous waste.

The intent of this chapter is not to be all-inclusive but to stress the safety hazards that are of particular concern in the hematology and hemostasis laboratories. These hazards may be classified as biologic, chemical, electrical, mechanical, and thermal (fire).

HISTORY OF CLINICAL HEMATOLOGY

Clinical hematology has a relatively short history in that until the 1920s, the study of diseases related to alterations in blood cell number or appearance was a branch of clinical medicine and pathology.[8] In the last 70 years, however, the science of clinical hematology has grown enormously and now is concerned with the study of normal and abnormal development, physiology, function, reaction to disease, and death or destruction of the formed elements (cells and platelets) of blood. Additionally, because of a variety of factors, the modern hematology laboratory frequently encompasses the study of hemostatic mechanisms, hemorrhagic disease, and thrombosis.

Unlike other subdivisions of the clinical laboratory, hematology does not have a single basic science as its foundation. Clinical chemistry is founded on the basic chemical sciences (inorganic, organic, analytical, biologic). Clinical bacteriology is likewise based on microbiology, and immunohematology (blood banking) depends largely on the basic science of immunology. Clinical hematology, on the other hand, draws from a wide range of basic sciences including biochemistry, cell biology, cytology, genetics, histology, immunology, pathology, oncology, physiology, and even, to some extent, radiation physics (nuclear medicine).

The clinical hematology laboratory has evolved over the past half century from a place where small aliquots of blood cell suspensions were measured, counted, and examined visually with the aid of stains and microscopes, to the present where larger, statistically sound aliquots of blood cell suspensions are analyzed by multiparameter, automated instruments. For example, a manual leukocyte count performed with a hemocytometer and microscope routinely samples only 0.02 μL of blood, whereas some automated counters today sample at least one full μL of blood. Today's analyses are based on cellular resistance to electrical current, the manner in which cells deflect a light beam, their ability to bind or incorporate dyes, their functions, or the ability of their surface receptors to bind marker ligands. Automation in the modern hematology laboratory has increased precision (or decreased variability) as well as accuracy (or decreased bias) in the identification, classification, and counting of cells; and it has decreased to a considerable extent the labor-intensive aspects of cell analysis.

Laboratory investigation of hemostasis has also matured considerably. Forty years ago there were only a few routine determinations for evaluating the hemostatic mechanism: the platelet count, bleeding time, whole-blood clotting time, and the prothrombin time (which, before commercial preparations of thromboplastin were available, required the tedious preparation of homemade thromboplastin from rabbit brain extracts). Today, with commercially available reagents, automation has improved the precision and accuracy of coagulation testing. Coagulation enzymes are no longer regarded as mysterious and magical but can be evaluated functionally by use of synthetic molecules that act as substrates for the enzymes. The number of tests has grown exponentially, to the point where many hemostasis laboratories have become independent sections of the clinical laboratory.

The extent of services provided by the modern clinical hematology laboratory differs considerably from one institution to another. Services that may be offered can be categorized as listed in Table 1-1. To perform these services adequately, the student laboratorian will find it necessary to learn normal blood cell physiology and common pathologic alterations of the hematologic mechanism. The principles and procedures of both routine and special hematology tests must be studied, and a thorough understanding of the sources of error in each test must be gained to ensure that valid results are generated for the benefit of the patient. In addition to learning hematologic theory and techniques, it is important to understand the operation of the instruments used in the clinical hematology laboratory. These topics are addressed in subsequent chapters.

TABLE 1-1
Primary Services Offered by the Hematology and Hemostasis Laboratory

Specimen collection and preparation for examination

Quantitative manual and instrumental measurements of cells

Measurements of cell volumes

Evaluation of cellular contents and components

Cellular identification according to various criteria:
　　Morphologic
　　Cytochemical markers
　　Cell surface markers

Identification of reative or neoplastic alterations in cell populations

Evaluation of leukocyte, erythrocyte, and platelet function

Evaluation of cellular development and formation (bone marrow)

Evaluation of hemostatic function

BASIC TERMINOLOGY IN HEMATOLOGY

Learning will be aided by an understanding of common terminology used in hematology and of the origin of some of these terms. Like any other science, hematology has a distinct vocabulary. A clinical chemist once observed, "The problem with hematology is that all words begin with *m*"—a humorous exaggeration that underscores the need to have a working knowledge of the common terms.

Most hematology terms used in this text are defined as they are introduced, and a glossary of common terms has been provided. Nevertheless, it may be helpful to know the meanings of several prefixes and suffixes generally derived from Greek and Latin that are commonly used in hematologic vocabulary. For example, most people will recognize the suffix "cyte" as meaning cell and the prefix "micro" as meaning small. These two words form the term *microcyte*, which means small cell. This word is used most often in hematology to refer specifically to small erythrocytes (red cells). Table 1-2 is a list of commonly used prefixes, and Table 1-3 provides commonly used suffixes. Table 1-4 demonstrates how prefixes and suffixes may be combined to form hematologic terms.

SAFETY IN THE CLINICAL HEMATOLOGY LABORATORY
Biologic Hazards

DEFINITION

Blood, urine, feces, spinal fluid, and all other body fluids present biologic safety hazards because they may contain highly infectious and potentially lethal organisms. Extreme caution should be used in collecting, handling, and processing all body fluids. These materials are referred to collectively as "biohazards."

TABLE 1-2
Common Prefixes from Greek and Latin Used in the Vocabulary of Hematology

Prefix	Meaning
a-/an-	Lack, without, absent, decreased
aniso-	Unequal, dissimilar
cyt-	Cell
dys-	Abnormal, difficult, bad
erythro-	Red
ferr-	Iron
hemo- (hemato-)	Pertaining to blood
hypo-	Beneath, under, deficient, decreased
hyper-	Above, beyond, extreme
iso-	Equal, alike, same
leuk(o)-	White
macro-	Large, long
mega-	Large, giant
meta-	(1) After, next; (2) change
micro-	Small
myel(o)-	(1) From bone marrow; (2) spinal cord
pan-	All, overall, all-inclusive
phleb-	Vein
phago-	Eat, ingest
poikilo-	Varied, irregular
poly-	Many
schis-	Split
scler-	Hard
splen-	Spleen
thromb(o)-	Clot, thrombus
xanth-	Yellow

TABLE 1-3
Common Suffixes from Greek and Latin Used in the Vocabulary of Hematology

Suffix	Meaning
-cyte	Cell
-emia	Blood
-itis	Inflammation
-lysis	Destruction or dissolving
-oma	Swelling, tumor
-opathy	Disease
-osis	(1) Abnormal increase; (2) disease
-penia	Deficiency, decreased
-phil(ic)	Attracted to, affinity for
-plasia (plastic)	Cell production or repair
-poiesis	Cell production, formation, and development
-poietin	Stimulates production

TABLE 1-4
Examples of Hematologic Terms Formed by Combining Prefixes and Suffixes

Prefix-Suffix Combination	Hematologic Term	Interpretation
an + iso + cyte + osis	= anisocytosis	Abnormal (osis) lack (an) of equality (iso) among cells (cyte): variation in cell size
a + plasia	= aplasia	Absent (a) cell production (plasia)
an + emia	= anemia	Decreased (an) blood (emia)
dys + myelo + poiesis	= dysmyelopoiesis	Abnormal (dys) development (poiesis) of marrow cells (myelo)
pan + myel(o) + osis	= panmyelosis	An abnormal increase (osis) in all (pan) marrow cells (myel)

SAFE HANDLING OF BIOHAZARDS

Biohazards probably cause the greatest concern of all the hazards in the hematology laboratory because a primary function is the collection, analysis, and safe disposal of blood. Blood may contain many highly infectious agents, including the viral agents that cause infectious hepatitis and acquired immune deficiency syndrome (AIDS). Because the infectious agent may be present in the specimen long before the patient shows any signs or symptoms of disease, *all biologic specimens, regardless of source, should be considered biohazardous.* The next chapter on specimen collection will address the precautions that should be taken while collecting blood specimens. The Occupational Safety and Health Administration (OSHA) has published rules that specifically address this subject.[1] In addition, the National Committee for Clinical Laboratory Standards (NCCLS) has published guidelines relative to the safe handling of biohazardous materials.[4] All laboratory workers should be familiar with both of these documents.

The following general rules should be strictly followed in the laboratory:

1. **Personal protective equipment (PPE) must be worn when handling biologic specimens.** PPE includes gloves, laboratory coats of non-permeable material that are long sleeved and have tight-fitting cuffs, protective free-standing shields or face shields, and shoes that are not permeable to liquids. A laboratory coat that is worn while handling specimens may be contaminated with hazardous specimen droplets. Frequent laundering is mandatory unless the clothing is disposable, and laboratory coats should never be worn outside of the laboratory. Gloves are an absolute necessity in all laboratories to prevent skin contamination with infectious agents. Latex, vinyl, or polyethylene gloves all provide adequate protection. However,

gloves present a problem in hematology. They usually are packaged by the manufacturer with a liberal amount of powder or starch to make them easier to put on. If these particles of powder get into the specimen or a specimen dilution, they may be counted as cells, causing a falsely elevated count. One possible solution is to use special "powder-free" gloves when preparing specimens for cell counting and during the operation of cell counters. Otherwise, once the gloves are put on, they may be wiped with a dry, lint-free towel to remove powder from the outside. Rinsing gloves with water or any other liquid is no longer considered an acceptable practice because the gloves' barrier may be compromised.

2. **Areas or equipment used by personnel who are not gloved should not be touched with contaminated gloves.** Nothing that personnel who are not gloved may touch, such as the telephone or door knob, should ever be touched with contaminated gloves. When gloves become contaminated, they should be discarded and a clean pair put on. Gloves must be removed aseptically to prevent hand contamination. As long as the hands are not contaminated, hand washing between glove changes is not required.[1] Some equipment, such as computer keyboards and certain telephones, may be specially labeled as biohazardous, to be used only with gloved hands.

3. **Wash hands immediately if they become contaminated.** Always wash hands after removing gloves when work is completed and before leaving the laboratory. Handwashing facilities should be separate from those used for washing equipment or for waste disposal. Hands must be washed before eating, drinking, smoking, applying makeup, handling contact lenses, and before and after using lavatory facilities. They must also be washed before hand contact with mucous membranes, eyes, or breaks in the skin. Washing with soap and water is recommended. Hand towelettes and cleansing foams are not recommended except in field conditions where water is not available. No additional benefit has been established for washing with antiseptic soaps or antiseptics.[3]

4. **Do not remove specimen tube stoppers until necessary.**
   A. Tube centrifugation should be performed with stoppers in place to prevent contamination with aerosols.
   B. Stoppers should be covered with absorbent material such as gauze before removing them to prevent spraying of the specimen.
   C. Devices are available in some counters that obtain an aliquot of blood specimen by piercing the stopper, thus avoiding stopper removal. Devices are also available for obtaining a drop of blood to make a blood film.
   D. A clear Plexiglas shield between laboratorian and blood sample being manipulated has been used successfully in many laboratories.

5. **Mouth pipetting is strictly prohibited.** There are numerous types of safety devices on the market for pipetting and measuring blood as well as other hazardous substances.

6. **Replace clay slabs for microhematocrit tube sealing frequently.**[3] (See Chapter 9 for a discussion of the microhematocrit determination). The clay slabs used in this procedure often become contaminated with blood. Therefore, they should be treated as biohazards and should not be recycled (*i.e.*, reformed to extend their life). Rather, they should be replaced at appropriate intervals.

7. **Decontaminate sedimentation tube racks regularly.** Chapter 9 describes the erythrocyte sedimentation rate. The racks used in this test are prone to contamination with whole blood and should be decontaminated immediately if a leak occurs.

8. **Unfixed or unstained slides should be considered infectious.** They should be discarded in clearly marked biohazard containers with appropriate labeling that the contents include glass.

9. **Do not handle needles.** Accidental needle sticks are one of the most common accidents that can transmit infectious diseases. Needles should be disposed of, without recapping, bending, or cutting, in rigid puncture-resistant containers clearly marked as biohazardous. These containers should be carried in the collection tray. Disposable needles that attach to adapters for use with evacuated tubes can be removed from the adapter without touching the needle with the aid of special devices. Inexpensive disposable single-use adapters are available. One-handed needle removal techniques are described by NCCLS[3] if needle removal from the adapter is absolutely necessary.

10. **Obtain immediate treatment for accidental and inappropriate contact with biohazards.** Any such contact (*e.g.*, contamination of skin cuts or needle punctures of skin) must be reported immediately to the supervisor so that appropriate prophylactic precautions may be taken.

11. **Properly dispose of contaminated laboratory supplies.** All laboratory supplies, such as gauze, tissues, work mats, or Pasteur pipettes, that come in contact with patient specimens must be disposed of properly as biohazardous waste. All contaminated supplies should be incinerated or autoclaved prior to being discarded. Nondisposable items used to measure or dilute blood should be disinfected using a solution such as a 1:100 dilution of household bleach before being washed with glassware detergent.

12. **Disinfect and clean biohazardous spills immediately.** Decontaminate all surfaces and devices wherever biologic materials are handled at completion of work. All spills should be cleaned immediately with appropriate disinfectant solutions, and materials used to wipe up spills should be disposed of as potentially biohazardous. NCCLS recommends the steps listed in Table 1-5 for spill decontamination.[4] Table 1-6 lists the dilutions of household bleach that may be used for decontamination. For example, a 1:10 dilution may be required if the contaminated surface is porous and cannot be cleaned adequately before disinfection. For hard, smooth surfaces that can be decontaminated adequately, disinfection with a 1:100 dilution of bleach may be sufficient. Time of exposure to diluted bleach may be brief; a 1:100 dilution inactivates hepatitis B

TABLE 1-5
Appropriate Steps for Decontamination and Disinfection of Spills Involving Biohazardous Materials

1. Put on heavyweight puncture-resistant utility gloves, a gown, and, if necessary, water-impermeable shoes.
2. Remove any sharp broken objects without touching them by using rigid sheets of cardboard to scrape them up. Discard cardboard with broken objects in puncture-resistant biohazard container.
3. Absorb the spill with disposable absorbent material (e.g., paper towels, gauze pads, or tissue paper wipes). Dispose of contaminated materials in biohazardous waste.
4. Clean spill site of all visible spilled material using any aqueous household detergent. This dilutes spilled material, lyses erythrocytes, and removes proteins.
5. Disinfect spill site using intermediate- to high-level hospital disinfectant such as a dilution of household bleach (see Table 1-2). Flood spill site or wipe down with disposable towels soaked in disinfectant to make site glistening wet. Phenolic disinfectants are acceptable for use on laboratory instruments, floors, or countertops.
6. Absorb disinfectant with disposable material or allow disinfectant to dry.
7. Rinse spill site with water to remove odors. Dry spill site to prevent slipping.
8. Dispose of all contaminated materials used in cleaning process in a biohazard container.

Adapted from National Committee for Clinical Laboratory Standards: Protection of Laboratory Workers from Infectious Disease Transmitted by Blood, Body Fluids, and Tissue: Tentative Guideline M29-T, vol 9, no 1. Villanova, PA, NCCLS, 1989, with permission.

---

virus (HBV) in 10 minutes and human immunodeficiency virus (HIV) in 2 minutes.[4]

Note that some metals may be corroded by bleach; therefore, alternative disinfectants must be considered, such as iodophors registered as hard-surface disinfectants (iodophors labeled as antiseptics should not be used) or phenolic disinfectants.[4]

Large spills of infectious agents should first be flooded and mixed with a concentrated disinfectant such as 1% (1:5 dilution) bleach and then allowed to stand for 20 minutes before being decontaminated. Likewise, biohazardous waste generated by automated cell counters should be chemically decontaminated.[5] There are generally well-defined institutional and community standards for disposal of biohazardous waste.

Chemical Hazards

DEFINITION
A hazardous chemical is one for which there is statistically significant evidence based on at least one study conducted in accordance with established scientific principles that acute or chronic health effects may occur in exposed employees.[2] Solid, liquid, or gaseous chemicals may be hazardous if transported, handled, stored, or dispensed inappropriately. Chemicals may have toxic, flammable, or carcinogenic properties.

SAFE HANDLING OF CHEMICALS
Federal law requires that all laboratories that use hazardous chemicals implement a "chemical hygiene plan."[2] Such a plan should include the following:

1. **Written procedures** that delineate proper engineering controls and personal protective equipment to be used when handling specific chemicals and proper disposal of such chemicals.
2. **An ongoing program that ensures that fume hoods and other engineering controls are functioning properly.**
3. **Specified training requirements for all employees.**
4. **Designation of a Chemical Hygiene Officer.**

For example, toxic or corrosive chemicals may adversely affect one or more body systems and should be labeled as to toxicity and reactivity, and whether protective equipment should be used. National Fire Protection Association (NFPA) labels are commonly used for this purpose. Flammable or explosive chemicals should be stored in a safety cabinet designed for such chemicals.

Carcinogenic chemicals are those capable of causing mutations in body cells that may lead to the development of cancer. A few reagents in hematology are

TABLE 1-6
*Dilutions of Household Bleach Used for Decontamination of Biohazard Spills**

Volume of Bleach (Part)	Volume of Water (Part)	Dilution Ratio	Sodium Hypochlorite (%)	Available Chlorine (mg/l)
Undiluted	0	1/1	5.25	50,000
1	9	1/10	0.5	5,000
1	99	1/100	0.05	500

* All dilutions should be made up daily with tap water to prevent loss of germicidal action during storage.
From National Committee for Clinical Laboratory Standards: Protection of Laboratory Workers from Infectious Disease Transmitted by Blood, Body Fluids, and Tissue: Tentative Guideline M29-T, vol 9, no 1. Villanova, PA, NCCLS, 1989, with permission.

considered carcinogenic. These include some chemicals used in cytochemistry (Chap. 29) and certain chemicals used in the identification of variant hemoglobins (Chap. 14). Gloves and sometimes masks must be worn when performing such procedures when no alternative reagent is available. When possible, substitute reagents are recommended.

Safety glasses should be used when working with acid or alkaline solutions to avoid chemical burns in the eyes. Mouth pipetting is not permissible. Bottles or flasks of chemicals should be carried with both hands by securely grasping the body of the container rather than the neck.

When preparing a reagent requiring the mixing of concentrated acid and water, the acid should be added very slowly to the water. *Never add water to concentrated acid.* Mixing of acid with water should be performed in a deep sink so that the area may be immediately flooded with water if necessary.

In addition to NFPA labels, all reagents must be properly labeled with the name and concentration of the reagent, the initials of the person who prepared the reagent, and the date on which the reagent was prepared. Any special storage requirements and the expiration date should be included.

Federal law requires that all employees be informed on methods for detecting the presence or release of a hazardous chemical; the physical and health hazards of the chemicals, their proper disposal, the work practices, personal protective equipment, and emergency procedures to be followed for self-protection; and procedures to follow for medical consultation and examination.[2] The manufacturer's Material Safety Data Sheets (MSDS) will generally contain much of the above information. Employee training must be performed at regular intervals and be documented.

Electrical Hazards

DEFINITION

Electrical hazards are caused by inappropriate use or maintenance of electrical instruments or equipment that can cause electrical shock, burns, or a fire or explosion.

SAFE USE OF ELECTRICAL EQUIPMENT

Proper equipment maintenance is mandatory for its safe use in the laboratory.[6] This maintenance includes immediate replacement of frayed wires or electrical connections. In the hematology laboratory the electrical connections of microscopes, automated cell counters, spectrophotometers, centrifuges, and any other equipment should be inspected regularly. All equipment must be grounded by a three-pronged plug according to federal regulations stipulated by the Occupational Safety and Health Act (OSHA) of 1970. The NCCLS strongly opposes the use of extension cords for any laboratory equipment.[6]

Electrical equipment should never be operated with wet hands.

Mechanical Hazards

DEFINITION

Mechanical hazards may result from improper use, storage, or disposal of glassware, sharp instruments, compressed gases, or equipment.

SAFE HANDLING OF MECHANICAL DEVICES

Glassware must be treated carefully to avoid breakage that could cause injury or infection. Glass and sharp objects such as glass slides, microcapillary pipettes, Pasteur pipettes, or needles that are contaminated with biologic specimens should be disposed of in puncture-proof containers to avoid injury to either laboratory personnel or those responsible for discarding hazardous waste.

Sharp instruments should be stored and used carefully to avoid skin puncture or cuts. See rule 9 (listed earlier) for handling biohazardous material for safe handling of needles.

Compressed gases are not used routinely in the hematology laboratory. Whenever they are used, strict guidelines for their handling and storage should be observed because of the dangers of explosion, mechanical injury, and fire. These guidelines are outlined elsewhere.[2]

Safe handling of equipment dictates that the laboratorian be instructed by a knowledgeable colleague or by carefully reading the manufacturer's instruction manual before operating any equipment. In the hematology laboratory, for example, centrifuges may be a source of injury if sample tubes are not balanced or if the lid is raised before the centrifuge rotor has stopped. Long hair should always be tied back to avoid catching in an instrument, which could result in serious injury.

Fire Hazards

DEFINITION

Fire or thermal hazards may result from the improper use or storage of either cryogenic substances (those stored at very low temperatures such as in liquid nitrogen) or substances capable of combustion (igniting into flames). Fires can obviously cause burns, and skin contact with cryogenic substances has essentially the same effect—it causes a thermal burn. Cryogenic and combustible substances may cause a fire, explosion, or asphyxiation.

FIRE SAFETY

Prevention is the easiest way to deal with fire hazard. A fire extinguisher must be easily accessible from anywhere in the laboratory. A dry chemical extinguisher is popular because of its versatility. It can be used on many types of fires. A safety shower should also be available in case clothing catches fire or a laboratorian is exposed to a large chemical spill. A fire blanket for smothering small fires should be readily available.

The NFPA[7] and OSHA publish standards on fire prevention that are useful in planning a good fire prevention and containment program.

TABLE 1-7
Cardinal Safety Rules of the Clinical Laboratory

Good Personal Habits

Wear proper attire and protective clothing; do not wear protective clothing outside laboratory.

Tie back long hair.

Do not eat, drink, or smoke in the work area.

Wear gloves when working with biologic specimens or hazardous chemicals.

Never pipet by mouth.

Do not put any objects in mouth (e.g., pens or pencils).

Wash hands frequently.

Keep hands away from mouth, nose, eyes, and any other mucous membranes.

Good Housekeeping Practices

Keep work areas free of chemicals and dirty glassware.

Store chemicals properly.

Label reagents and solutions.

Post warning signs.

Good Laboratory Technique

Be careful when transferring chemicals from container to container and always add acid to water slowly.

Do not operate new or unfamiliar equipment until you are trained and authorized.

Read all labels and instructions carefully.

Use the personal safety equipment that is provided.

For the safe handling, use, and disposal of chemicals, learn their properties and hazards.

Learn emergency procedures and become familiar with the location of fire exits, fire extinguishers, fire blankets, and eyewash stations.

Adapted from Michael BS, Chantly PDJ: Laboratory safety. In Bishop ML, Duben–Von Laufen JL, Fody EP (eds): Clinical Chemistry—Principles, Procedures, Correlations. Philadelphia, JB Lippincott, 1985, with permission.

Cryogenic substances are not routinely used in the clinical hematology laboratory; they have specific safety requirements for their use and storage, which are explained elsewhere.[2]

CHAPTER SUMMARY

Clinical hematology is a unique science founded on several distinct basic sciences. The student of hematology is challenged with the need to learn a wide variety of physical and biologic concepts. A large number of terms in the hematologic vocabulary are based on Greek and Latin roots. A knowledge of these roots will greatly enhance the student's understanding of the subject. The primary concern of any laboratory is the safety of its employees. Table 1-7 provides a summary of the cardinal rules of laboratory safety. Observance of these rules and those discussed in detail in the sections above is in the best interest of each laboratorian as well as of those who enter the laboratory for business or custodial services.

Case Study 1-1

A laboratory employee, carrying a rack of blood tubes to the multiparameter cell counter, trips and falls. Several of the tubes cracked and two were broken outright, spilling blood on the floor and on the laboratory coat of the individual who fell.
1. How would you proceed to decontaminate?
2. What can be done about the tubes that are cracked?

Case Study 1-2

A technologist is coverslipping some blood films in the fume hood using xylene as the solvent. After a few minutes, she complains of the smell.
1. What appears to be the immediate problem and what should be done?

Review Questions

1-1. The removal of specimen tube stoppers

    A. should occur just prior to centrifugation.

    B. should not generate an aerosol of the specimen.

    C. must never be done in the laboratory.

    D. both A and B are correct.

1-2. A 1:100 dilution of bleach will inactivate the hepatitis B virus in

    A. 2 minutes.

    B. 5 minutes.

    C. 10 minutes.

    D. 20 minutes.

1-3. When preparing a reagent requiring the mixture of water and concentrated acid,

    A. measure the water first and then add the acid slowly.

    B. measure the acid first and then add the water slowly.

    C. the mixing is best performed on a solid flat surface such as a laboratory bench.

    D. None of the above.

1-4. How many extension cords is (are) considered acceptable between an instrument and the wall plug?

    A. None

    B. One

    C. Two

    D. Three

References

1. Department of Labor, Occupational Safety and Health Administration: Occupational exposure to blood-borne pathogens; final rule (29 CFR 1910.1030) Federal Register, *December 6, 1991*
2. Department of Labor, Occupational Safety and Health Administration: Occupational exposures to hazardous chemicals in laboratories: Standard (29 CFR 1910.1450). Federal Register, *January 31, 1990*
3. National Committee for Clinical Laboratory Standards: Protection of Laboratory Workers from Instrument Biohazards; Proposed Guideline 117-P. Villanova, PA, NCCLS, 1991
4. National Committee for Clinical Laboratory Standards: Protection of Laboratory Workers from Infectious Disease Transmitted by Blood, Body Fluids, and Tissue, 2nd ed; Tentative Guideline M29-T2. Villanova, PA, NCCLS, 1991
5. National Committee for Clinical Laboratory Standards: Clinical Laboratory Waste Management; Approved Guideline GP5-A. Villanova, PA, NCCLS, 1993
6. National Committee for Clinical Laboratory Standards: Power Requirements for Clinical Laboratory Instruments and for Laboratory Power Sources: Approved Standard 15-A. Villanova, PA, NCCLS, 1980
7. National Fire Protection Association: Fire Protection for Laboratories Using Chemicals, NFPA-45. Batterymarch Park, Quincy, MA, NFPA, 1982

8. Wintrobe MM: Hematology: The Blossoming of a Science, p 1. Philadelphia, Lea and Febiger, 1985

Suggested Readings

Brown JW, Blackwell H: Complying with the new OSHA regs, Part 1: Teaching your staff about biosafety. MLO 24:24 (1992) Part 2: Safety protocols no lab can ignore. MLO 24:27, 1992. Part 3: Compiling employee safety records that will satisfy OSHA. MLO 24:45, 1992

Centers for Disease Control: Recommendations for prevention of HIV transmission in health-care settings. Morbidity and Mortality Weekly Report Supplement 36(2S):1S, 1987

Hawk WA, Hoeltge GA: Safety in the medical laboratory. Clin Lab Med 3:467, 1983

Kennedy DA: Blood samples and reagents: hazards and risks. In Lewis SM, Koepke JA (eds): Hematology Laboratory Management and Practice. Oxford, UK, Butterworth-Heinemann Ltd, 1995

Vlahov D, Polk BF: Transmission of human immunodeficiency virus within the health-care setting. Occup Med State Art Rev 2:429, 1987

CHAPTER 2

Specimen Collection for Hematology and Hemostasis

Raymond L. Olesinski

Objectives

1. Explain the quality assurance considerations associated with blood specimen collection by venipuncture, by skin puncture, and from indwelling catheters for hematology and hemostasis testing.
2. Describe the precautions required during blood specimen processing and handling to ensure valid hematology and hemostasis test results.

Proper blood specimen collection is the first step in ensuring accurate and reliable results from clinical laboratory testing. This chapter focuses on those aspects of blood specimen collection that affect the validity of results in hematology and hemostasis testing. Blood specimens may be obtained for hematologic tests either by venipuncture, by skin (capillary) puncture, or from indwelling catheters; the quality assurance considerations of each of these methods will be discussed. It is beyond the scope of this chapter to provide complete details on the procedures for routine venipunctures and skin punctures or on the safety, professional, and ethical issues related to phlebotomy. For details on these procedures, the reader is directed to a series of references.[8,18,23,24,28] Regardless of the method used, specimen collection requires knowledge of the necessary equipment and supplies and technical skills, strict attention to patient and specimen identification, awareness of and adherence to institutional safety requirements, and proper specimen transport and processing techniques.

Blood specimen collection, or phlebotomy, is a skill practiced by many members of the health care team including phlebotomists, clinical laboratory technicians and scientists, physicians, and nurses. The term *phlebotomist* will be used throughout this chapter to apply to any individual with blood specimen collection responsibilities.

Universal precautions should be followed when collecting and processing all blood specimens. All phlebotomists should be familiar with these precautions and adhere to them strictly.

SPECIMEN COLLECTION BY VENIPUNCTURE

The most common technique used to obtain a blood specimen is venipuncture. This section includes a discussion of the equipment and anticoagulants used in venipuncture, the procedure, and quality assurance considerations.

Equipment

EVACUATED TUBE COLLECTION SYSTEM

Routine collection of most blood specimens is accomplished using an evacuated tube collection system, which consists of an evacuated glass or plastic collection tube, a needle which is pointed and beveled at both ends, and a needle holder (see Fig. 2-1). The tubes are evacuated (contain no air) so that when their rubber stoppers are pierced, blood is automatically drawn into the tube. Several sizes of evacuated tubes are available, and holders come in different sizes to match the diameter of the tubes used. In most laboratories, 5- or 7-mL evacuated tubes are used for adult specimen collection. However, tubes of the size used commonly for pediatric patients (2–3 mL) usually contain enough blood or serum to meet most requirements for testing and would reduce the amount of blood drawn from adults by 40% to 45% if they were used for adult patients.[35]

Tubes may be additive-free or contain additives that serve as anticoagulants, preservatives, coagulation enhancers, or as facilitators in the separation of cells from serum or plasma. The specific additive in the tube is indicated by the color of the rubber stopper (see Table 2-1). Tube label information should be checked in situations in which tubes with the same stopper color may contain

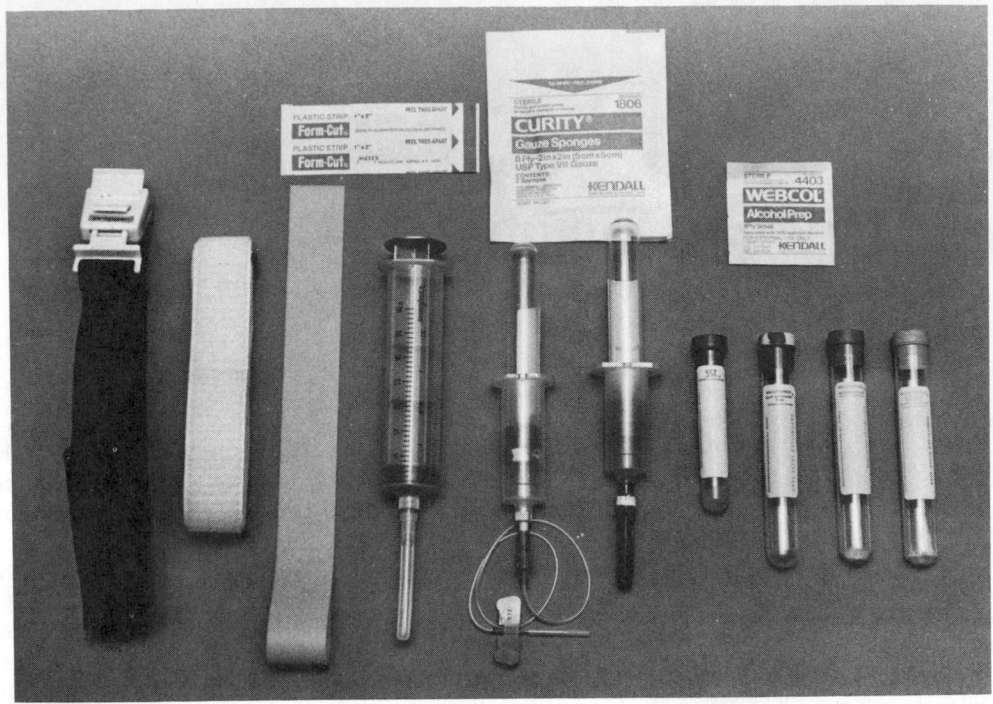

FIGURE 2-1. Venipuncture supplies. (*Bottom, left to right*) Tourniquets: Seraket, Velcro, and rubber tubing; syringe with Luer-Lock needle; evacuated tube holder with Luer adapter connecting butterfly set; tube holder with evacuated tube and multisample needle; other evacuated tubes. (*Top*) Adhesive bandage, gauze sponge, alcohol preparation pad. (From Lotspeich CA: Specimen collection and processing. In Bishop ML, Duben-Von Laufen JL, Fody ET (eds): Clinical Chemistry—Principles, Procedures, Correlations. Philadelphia, JB Lippincott, 1986, with permission. Photograph by J Bradley Perkins.)

TABLE 2-1
Specimen Type and Collection Tubes

Specimen Type	Color Code	Additive	Type of Additive	Department
CLOTTED SPECIMEN				
Serum	Red	None		Chemistry
				Serology
		Sterile		Blood bank
	Red/yellow	Glass particles	Clot activator	Chemistry
	Black/yellow	Thrombin		
	Red/gray	Thixotropic gel	Clot activator	Chemistry
	Rose	Thixotropic gel	Clot activator	Chemistry
	Navy	None		Special chemistry
ANTICOAGULATED SPECIMEN				
Plasma	Light blue	Sodium citrate	Anticoagulant	Coagulation
	Gray	Sodium fluoride	Anticoagulant	Chemistry
	Green	Lithium heparin	Anticoagulant	Chemistry
		Sodium heparin	Anticoagulant	
	Navy	Sodium heparin	Anticoagulant	Special chemistry
	Lavender	Ethylenediamine-tetraacetate (EDTA)	Anticoagulant	Special chemistry
Whole Blood	Lavender	EDTA	Anticoagulant	Hematology
	Green	Sodium heparin	Anticoagulant	Hematology
	Yellow	Sodium polyanethole sulfonate (SPS)	Anticoagulant	Microbiology
		Acid citrate dextrose (ACD)	Cell preservative	Blood bank

McCall RE, Tankersley CM: Phlebotomy Essentials, p 118. Philadelphia, JB Lippincott, 1993.

different additives. Evacuated tubes should not be used after their indicated expiration date because they may have lost vacuum or additive effectiveness.[22] Tubes for special procedures are also available (*e.g.*, special tubes for Westergren sedimentation rate determination; Chap. 9).

SYRINGE METHOD

Blood specimen collection using syringes involves the use of plastic or glass syringes and needles manufactured specifically for use with syringes. Glass syringes should be avoided because coagulation is initiated when blood contacts untreated glass surfaces. The use of a syringe allows the phlebotomist to control the amount of pressure required to remove blood from a vein. This is especially helpful in difficult to draw patients or pediatric patients or in cases when small veins must be used.

The smallest size syringe should be used for the blood specimen volume necessary to avoid excessive pressure. Besides collapsing veins, excessive pressure may cause hemolysis, resulting in an unacceptable blood specimen. For pediatric collection, a 3-mL or tuberculin syringe may be used.

NEEDLES

The selection of needle size depends on the size and depth of the patient's vein and the amount of blood to be drawn. Needles are designated by gauge number, which refers to the inside diameter, or bore, of the needle and length. For example, a 21G1 needle has a gauge number of 21 and is 1 inch in length from the tip of the needle to its insertion into the syringe hub. The higher the gauge, the smaller the diameter. Needles that are 19 to 23 gauge are commonly used for routine venipunctures; 20- to 22-gauge needles are most commonly used for adults, whereas 23-gauge needles may be used for pediatric or difficult veins.[24] Use of higher gauge needles has been reported as a cause of hemolysis during venipuncture. Hemolyzed specimens are unacceptable for hematology and most other laboratory tests.[34]

The needle length chosen is an individual preference. The most commonly used lengths are 1 and 1.5 inches. Shorter needles are easier to control and cause less patient anxiety. For the evacuated tube system, needles are available for single and multi-sample collection. A multi-sample needle should be used if more than one tube of blood needs to be collected to prevent leakage of blood into the needle holder during tube changes. Single-sample needles or butterfly (winged infusion set) needles are manufactured specifically for syringes. Adapters are also available that allow butterfly needles to be used with standard evacuated collection tubes and holders (see Figs. 2-1 and 2-2). This arrangement improves control during difficult venipunctures and permits the direct filling of collection tubes.

Anticoagulants

When blood is collected in glass tubes without additives, coagulation normally takes place and serum may be separated from blood cells by subsequent centrifugation. However, some laboratory tests, including those per-

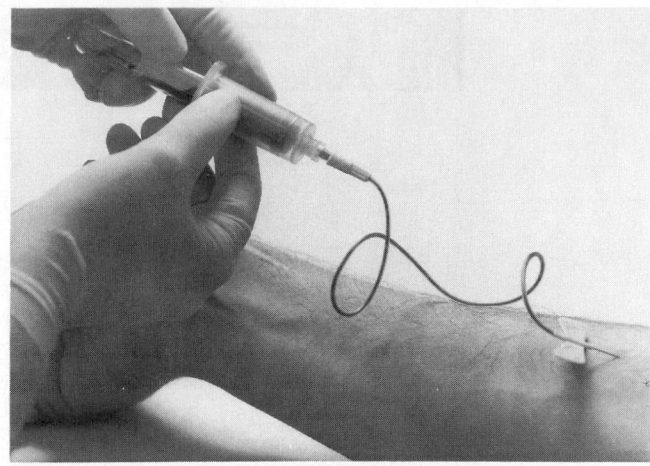

FIGURE 2-2. Blood collection by modified evacuated system using a Luer adapter to attach the tube holder to a butterfly set. (From Oxford BS, Dovenbarger S: Specimen collection and processing. In Bishop ML, Duben-Engelkirk JL, Fody ET (eds): Clinical Chemistry—Principles, Procedures, Correlations, 3rd ed. Philadelphia, JB Lippincott, 1996, with permission.)

formed in hematology, require whole blood or plasma, in which case an anticoagulant must be mixed immediately with the blood to prevent coagulation. The most commonly used anticoagulants for hematologic procedures are ethylenediaminetetraacetic acid (EDTA), sodium citrate, and heparin. An appropriate concentration of the anticoagulant for the volume of blood drawn is critical, and significant errors may result if the ratio of blood to anticoagulant is not correct.

ETHYLENEDIAMINETETRAACETIC ACID (EDTA)

The potassium salt of EDTA is the most commonly used anticoagulant in hematology. Blood coagulation is inhibited by the chelation or binding of calcium ions. The optimal anticoagulant concentration is 1.5 mg/mL of blood (see Table 2-2). This quantity has no adverse effects on routine cell counts and preserves cellular morphology when blood films are made within 2 hours of collection.

It should be noted that there may be tubes on the market with a lower, unacceptable EDTA concentration. On the other hand, excessive EDTA induces red blood cell (RBC) shrinkage, causing the hematocrit value and erythrocyte sedimentation rate to be falsely decreased. EDTA prevents platelet aggregation and is therefore the preferred anticoagulant for platelet counts. It is not a satisfactory anticoagulant for coagulation testing because it inhibits the fibrinogen-thrombin reaction and factor V is not stable in its presence.

SODIUM CITRATE

The anticoagulant of choice for most hemostasis testing is trisodium citrate. Citrated plasma preserves the labile clotting factors V and VIII better than other anticoagulants, and it is the most satisfactory anticoagulant for platelet aggregation studies. Citrated plasma specimens also are more sensitive to the effects of heparin and are

TABLE 2-2
EDTA Vacuum Collection Tubes for Hematology Specimens*

Tube			EDTA Anticoagulant	
Draw Volume	Size (mm)	Form	mg/Tube	Final Concentration (mg/mL)
2	10.25 × 47–50	K$_2$ (spray dried)	3.6	1.8
3	10.25 × 64–65	K$_2$ (spray dried)	5.4	1.8
4	10.25 × 82	K$_2$ (spray dried)	7.2	1.8
2	10.25 × 47–50	K$_3$ (7.5% liquid)	3.0	1.5
3	10.25 × 64–65	K$_3$ (7.5% liquid)	3.75	1.25 (too low)
3.5	16 × 75	K$_3$ (15% liquid)	5.25	1.5
7	13 × 100	K$_3$ (15% liquid)	10.5	1.5
10	16 × 100	K$_3$ (15% liquid)	15.0	1.5

* As marketed by Becton-Dickinson Vacutainer Systems, Rutherford, NJ 07070; Terumo Medical Corp., Elkton, MD 21921; or Jelco Laboratories; Raritan, NJ 08869. Other tubes are available that are not listed.

therefore preferred for tests to monitor heparin therapy.[31] In the past, both sodium citrate and sodium oxalate were used as anticoagulants for hemostasis testing. Both inhibit coagulation by binding ionized calcium, but when oxalated plasma is recalcified in the test system, insoluble complexes or precipitates are formed that may interfere with endpoint detection by instruments that measure changes in optical density. For this reason sodium oxalate is not recommended for hemostasis testing.[5]

Sodium citrate is available in concentrations of 3.2% (0.109 M) or 3.8% (0.129 M) in evacuated collection tubes. The ratio of blood to citrate anticoagulant is critical for valid coagulation test results. The standard ratio is nine parts of blood to one part of anticoagulant (9:1). This ratio is satisfactory for specimens with relatively normal hematocrits. However, if the hematocrit value exceeds 0.55 L/L (*i.e.*, low plasma volume), or if there is incomplete filling of the collection tube, the relatively increased amount of unbound citrate in the citrate-plasma mixture causes a false prolongation of clotting times, particularly for the prothrombin time (PT) and partial thromboplastin time (PTT) tests.[21] This occurs because the standard amount of calcium used to recalcify plasma in these procedures is not adequate to inactivate excessive unbound citrate in addition to initiating clotting of the specimen.[10]

HEPARIN

Heparin is an acid mucopolysaccharide that acts with antithrombin III and inhibits the reactions of all serine proteases of coagulation. The optimal concentration is 15 to 20 U/mL of blood. Heparin is not satisfactory for blood film preparation because it causes morphologic distortion of platelets and leukocytes. In addition, a bluish coloration in the background of blood films stained with a Romanowsky stain will occur because of its pH.[14]

Heparin is the anticoagulant of choice for the osmotic fragility test if defibrinated blood is not used and for the platelet retention test.[3] However, heparinized blood should never be used for coagulation studies because of heparin's inhibitory effect on thrombin. Heparin may also cause errors in automated cell counting. For example, platelets from some individuals will agglutinate in the presence of heparin.

Venipuncture—Quality Assurance Considerations

DIETARY RESTRICTIONS

Fasting is not required for routine hematology procedures; however, it should be noted that blood films made from blood taken from a person shortly after he or she has had a fatty meal will have small holes throughout the film caused by chylomicrons.

PATIENT REASSURANCE

Phlebotomy procedures induce stress and anxiety in many patients, which can alter certain laboratory test values including elevation of the white blood cell (WBC) count.[8] Phlebotomists therefore should attempt to relieve such apprehension by communicating with patients in a calm, professional, and reassuring manner. Patient confidence may be gained by soliciting cooperation whenever possible. Patients should be reassured that although the puncture itself may be slightly painful, it will be over quickly.

PATIENT POSITION

Patient position should be noted on the requisition because blood count values may vary depending on whether the patient is sitting up or lying down. For example, the hematocrit can decrease an average of 8% because of hemodilution when a patient is lying down.[15,40] Conversely, when a patient gets out of bed, hemoconcentration occurs. This same type of variation occurs with WBC counts.[37,43]

SITE SELECTION

In general the veins of the antecubital fossa will be used for routine venipunctures. When selecting the site, several factors should be considered. Areas with hematomas, burns, scars, or edema should be avoided. Collection from veins in an arm on the side where a mastectomy was performed is contraindicated because of possible lymphostasis.

If a patient is receiving an intravenous (IV) infusion, specimens should be drawn from the opposite arm. Certain situations may preclude collection from the opposite arm. Under these circumstances, blood should be drawn below the IV site from a vein other than the one with the IV line and after the IV fluids have been stopped for 2 minutes.[24,34] Stoppage of the IV should only be done by the patient's nurse or physician. Five mL of blood should be collected and discarded before specimen collection to avoid potential sample dilution with IV fluid. Evidence indicates that acceptable blood specimens for hematologic and serum biochemical profiles for all analytes except glucose and phosphorus may be drawn below the IV line during infusion or from the IV needle once the IV infusion has been stopped for 2 minutes and a small amount of blood is first discarded.[23,42] In all cases when collecting specimens from below IV sites, the phlebotomist should adhere to the procedure recommended by the individual laboratory. The site from which the specimen was taken should be noted on the test requisition form.

Veins that are difficult to locate can be made more prominent by gently massaging the arm from wrist to elbow and warming or tapping the puncture site.[24] Vigorous hand pumping by the patient, however, may result in hemoconcentration and should be avoided.

TOURNIQUET APPLICATION

Several forms of tourniquets are available. The most commonly used is a pliable piece of flat latex. Velcro tourniquets, the Seraket, and blood pressure cuffs are additional types. The Seraket (Propper Manufacturing Company, Inc., Long Island, NY) is made of cloth, and is secured using a seat belt–like apparatus (Fig. 2-1). This allows the phlebotomist to partially release venous pressure, preventing hemoconcentration, without removing the tourniquet from the patient's arm. The tourniquet may easily be retightened if necessary.

Tourniquets should never be left on for longer than 1 minute because prolonged application may cause hemoconcentration and increased fibrinolytic activity.[31,33] If the tourniquet is left on the arm for longer than 1 minute when locating a vein, it should be removed and reapplied after 2 minutes have elapsed.[24] To avoid prolonged application, reapply the tourniquet only after the site has been cleansed and just prior to insertion of the needle. During collection the tourniquet should be removed as soon as possible after an adequate flow of blood into the collection device has been established.

CLEANSING THE VENIPUNCTURE SITE

The venipuncture site must be cleansed thoroughly with a commercial alcohol prep pad or a cotton ball or gauze pad soaked in 70% isopropanol. Dry the area with sterile gauze or allow it to air dry. Residual alcohol at the venipuncture site, aside from being painful to the patient, may cause hemolysis.

SPECIMEN COLLECTION

Normally evacuated collection tubes will not fill totally, so a small unfilled portion remains. However, tubes should be filled as much as their vacuum allows to avoid improper ratios of blood to additives. Evacuated tubes containing anticoagulant or other additives must be mixed immediately (especially if K_2EDTA is used) after removal from the holder or after filling by syringe by gentle inversion 5 to 10 times.[24] If multiple tubes are collected, one tube can be mixed while another is filling with blood. Do not mix or shake vigorously because hemolysis may result.

When collecting multiple tubes, it is important to do so in the correct order. The following order is recommended:

1. Sterile blood culture tubes
2. Nonadditive tubes
3. Tubes containing anticoagulants (collecting citrated specimens first followed by heparin, EDTA, and oxalate/fluoride)[24]

Studies have suggested that the order of draw of multiple additive tubes is important because the additive in one tube may contaminate the specimen collected into the subsequent additive tube.[4] The sources of error in venipunctures are summarized in Table 2-3.

PERFORMANCE OF THE VENIPUNCTURE BY THE SYRINGE METHOD

When using a syringe the same basic considerations as for the evacuated tube method apply. However, blood must be transferred from the syringe to appropriate evacuated tubes. For non-hemostasis testing the needle of the syringe is carefully inserted through the tube stopper, allowing the vacuum to draw blood slowly into the tube.[34]

TABLE 2-3
Sources of Error in Venipuncture

Errors in Venipuncture Preparation
    Improper patient identification
    Failure to check patient adherence to dietary restrictions
    Failure to calm patient prior to blood collection
    Use of improper equipment and supplies
    Inappropriate method of blood collection

Errors in Venipuncture Procedure
    Failure to dry the site completely after cleansing with alcohol
    Inserting needle bevel side down
    Use of needle that is too small, causing hemolysis of specimen
    Venipuncture in an unacceptable area (*e.g.,* above an IV line)
    Prolonged tourniquet application
    Wrong order of tube draw
    Failure to mix blood collected in additive-containing tubes immediately
    Pulling back on syringe plunger too forcefully
    Failure to release tourniquet prior to needle withdrawal

Errors after Venipuncture Completion
    Failure to apply pressure immediately to venipuncture site
    Vigorous shaking of anticoagulated blood specimens
    Forcing blood through a syringe needle into tube
    Mislabeling of tubes
    Failure to label appropriate specimens with infectious disease precaution
    Failure to put date, time, and initials on requisition
    Slow transport of specimens to laboratory

Blood must not be forced through the syringe needle because this may cause hemolysis. If non-evacuated tubes are used, the syringe needle and tube cap are removed and the blood is allowed to flow slowly down the side of the tube. Because there is a potential for activation of coagulation in the syringe, the order of filling evacuated tubes after a syringe collection is different from that followed when filling tubes directly using a needle and holder. In the latter case, blood culture collection devices are filled first followed by anticoagulant-containing tubes in the order listed above. Finally, fill any non–anticoagulant-containing tubes that will be processed for serum collection.

SPECIMEN COLLECTION BY CAPILLARY PUNCTURE

Capillary Puncture—Quality Assurance Considerations

Venous blood is preferred to skin or capillary puncture specimens for most hematologic tests. However, there are several situations in which skin puncture should be used to obtain the blood specimen. Infants, particularly newborns, have a much smaller blood volume than adults; drawing blood by routine venipuncture on a daily basis can quickly result in hospital-induced anemia. Skin puncture is also a much safer means of blood collection. Venipuncture is often difficult and even dangerous when performed on very small children and infants.[2,9,19,23] For adults, skin puncture may be required because of obesity, burns, or extremely small or severely damaged veins, or when IV fluid is flowing into the only accessible veins. Skin puncture is also used to save the veins of patients receiving chemotherapy and in the elderly when possible.

Blood collected by skin puncture is a mixture of capillary, venous, and arterial blood and also contains interstitial and intracellular fluids. Therefore, the laboratory values obtained may be different from those obtained on venous specimens.[9] For example, the erythrocyte count, hematocrit, hemoglobin, and platelet count are lower in skin puncture blood than in venous blood.[3] Therefore, collection of specimens by skin puncture should be noted on the requisition. Refer to standard references for the exact procedure.[8,18,23,27,28]

Sources of Error

Hemolyzed specimens are a common source of error, especially in blood specimens obtained from skin puncture of infants.[20] Infants' erythrocytes are more fragile than those of adults, and their hematocrit values are much higher; therefore, the risk of hemolysis is somewhat greater.[20] Other important sources of error include failure to dry the site completely after cleansing with alcohol, excessively deep skin puncture, failure to wipe away the first drop of blood, vigorous massaging or milking of area causing hemolysis, and accidental capturing of air bubbles in capillary tubes or Unopette (Becton Dickinson, Rutherford, NJ) pipettes used for the collection of exact specimen amounts (e.g., for platelet counting).

Skin punctures must be performed properly to ensure an adequate flow of blood for collection of the necessary specimen volume. Excessive squeezing can dilute the specimen, with tissue fluids resulting in invalid test results. Also care should be taken to use a lancet no longer than 2.4 mm for infant heel punctures to avoid the risk of osteomyelitis.[23]

A number of devices are currently available that allow larger quantities of capillary blood to be collected than can be conveniently collected in capillary tubes or Unopettes; these include the Microtainer and Microvette (Becton Dickinson, Rutherford, NJ), Capiject (Terumo TMG, Somerset, NJ), and Samplette (Sherwood Medical, St. Louis, MO). These devices may be additive-free or contain additives similar to evacuated collection tubes. When using these devices it is important to follow the manufacturer's directions precisely as to maximum and minimum allowable fill volumes and mixing. If these instructions are not followed, test results are likely to be altered because of an improper ratio of additive to specimen or ineffective anticoagulation.

The order of draw is also important when collecting specimens by skin puncture. Specimens for manual platelet counts should be collected first. Peripheral blood films may be made next, if required, followed by the filling of any anticoagulant-containing devices. EDTA anticoagulated tubes should be filled first, followed by other anticoagulant-containing tubes. Containers that will be processed for serum collection should be filled last.[23]

SPECIMEN COLLECTION FROM INDWELLING CATHETERS

Most phlebotomists do not collect blood specimens from an indwelling catheter. However, the phlebotomist should be aware of the special demands for such collections in order to help other members of the health care team provide the laboratory with suitable specimens. Generally, a specific volume of blood must be discarded (discard volume) prior to filling the specimen tubes.

Studies have indicated significant alterations in hematology test results when the discard volume is less than the optimal amount recommended. Hematocrits were significantly higher and WBC counts lower when the discard volume was less than four times the catheter dead space volume.[36] In another study PTT results were inversely proportional to the discard volume removed from heparinized arterial lines.[38]

The discard volume is dependent on the length and diameter of the catheter. Collecting blood from an indwelling catheter for hemostasis specimens is not recommended. However, if it is unavoidable, it may be necessary to discard as much as 30 mL, especially if the thrombin clotting time (Chap. 49) is to be determined.

SPECIMEN COLLECTION FOR COAGULATION TESTING

Quality Assurance Considerations

This section focuses on the aspects of phlebotomy that specifically apply to obtaining and processing blood specimens for hemostasis.

A nontraumatic venipuncture is the goal any time a blood specimen is collected, but it is essential to obtain valid results from hemostasis testing. A prime concern is the elimination of premature activation of the coagulation process before the specimen can be evaluated in the test procedures. The causes of such activation include contamination of the specimen with tissue thromboplastin, contact with the surface of an inappropriate specimen container, improper temperature, and hemolysis.

Tissue thromboplastin is a potent clot-activating substance found in fluids that escape from injured cells and tissue spaces. When tissues are traumatized or blood vessels are disrupted or cut, this substance activates the extrinsic coagulation pathway (Chap. 47) and causes erroneous test results. Even slight contamination with tissue thromboplastin is enough to affect the results. Hemolysis is the release of hemoglobin from ruptured red cells into the plasma. Hemolyzed red cells act like tissue thromboplastin to activate plasma clotting factors. When hemolysis occurs in the blood, technical problems with the collection process are usually the cause (see Table 2-4).

The effect of glass surfaces on hemostasis is well known. The contact factors (prekallikrein [Fletcher], XII, and XI) are activated prematurely by contact with glass, causing a shortening of coagulation times of tests used to assess both the intrinsic and the extrinsic coagulation pathway. The recommended materials for collecting, transporting, and storing blood specimens for hemostasis testing are plastic, polystyrene, or silicone-coated glass.

A poor venipuncture can cause erroneous test results. The fact that blood obtained by defective collection techniques often is satisfactory for biochemical or cytologic studies may cause phlebotomists to believe that the same applies to studies for blood coagulation. Ideally, a person familiar with coagulation tests should obtain the blood for clotting studies, or a member of the coagulation laboratory should supervise its collection. Another option would be to draw such blood separately rather than as part of a large collection for other tests. Because these approaches are often impractical, it is acceptable for specimens for coagulation testing to be drawn by well-trained personnel and as a part of a group of specimens as long as specific standards and guidelines for such collections are followed.[21,24,25]

It is recommended that capillary blood be avoided for traditional methods of coagulation testing.[6,29] Sometimes, however, only capillary blood can be obtained from a patient. The PT test done on such blood probably is reliable provided the specimen is obtained rapidly and anticoagulated immediately. Recent advances in bedside testing devices allow the use of skin puncture specimens for coagulation testing.[13] When using these devices, the manufacturer's directions should be followed precisely.

Venous occlusion or stasis can occur during specimen collection if the tourniquet is applied too tightly or for an extended period of time (more than 1 minute). When arterial flow or venous return is interrupted, there is activation of the fibrinolytic system and clotting factors.[31] To minimize such stasis and the hemoconcentration that also develops, the tourniquet should be released as soon as the vein is entered and blood begins flowing into the collection device.

Equipment

Many types of tourniquets can be used, but because increased stasis is the concern, the Seraket tourniquet (see above and Fig. 2-1) or a similar type of device is recommended.

The use of the appropriate needle size is important. Small-gauge needles are more likely to cause hemolysis. When collecting blood for coagulation tests, the 20-gauge needle is most commonly used, but when more than 20 mL of blood is to be drawn, a 19-gauge needle may be preferred. For pediatric patients or those with small veins, a smaller size (21 gauge) might be selected. Needles should be of the disposable type and coated with polymeric silicone. These needles make skin penetration and vein entry smooth with minimal pain, trauma, or activation of coagulation factors.

Specimens for coagulation tests should be collected in silicone-coated evacuated tubes or plastic syringes to minimize the effect of contact coagulation activation. Silicone-coated evacuated tubes containing the anticoagulant trisodium citrate may be used whenever citrated plasma is required.[31]

Specimen Collection

A clean rapid venipuncture prevents tissue thromboplastin or air from entering the specimen. If there is any difficulty in performing the venipuncture, the attempt should be aborted, a new site should be chosen, and fresh blood-drawing equipment should be used. For common coagulation tests such as the PT and PTT tests, routine evacuated tube collection is satisfactory so long as contamination with tissue fluids is avoided. Blood for coagulation testing should never be the first tube collected because tissue thromboplastin from the initial puncture may contaminate the specimen and invalidate the coagulation results. If only coagulation tests are ordered, the "two-syringe technique" described below is recommended.

TWO-SYRINGE TECHNIQUE

The two-syringe method of blood collection minimizes the introduction of tissue thromboplastin to the specimen. The term refers to the practice of drawing a small amount

---

TABLE 2-4
Technical Errors That May Cause Hemolysis

Excessive stasis through prolonged application of the tourniquet

Moisture or contamination in the needle, syringe, or blood container

Using needles with too small a bore

Frothing of sample due to entry of air

Expelling blood from the syringe through the needle

Excessive and vigorous mixing of blood with the anticoagulant

of blood into a syringe or evacuated tube and then changing to a second syringe or the evacuated tube specified for the coagulation test to be performed. This rinses the needle of any tissue fluid that may have been introduced during the venipuncture.

The butterfly needle is recommended instead of the standard disposable needle because the use of the butterfly needle is less likely to result in accidental removal of the needle from the vein while switching collection devices. Use of the butterfly needle is also recommended when blood must be drawn directly into syringes containing an anticoagulant or some other toxic solution, such as the formalin used in some procedures to evaluate platelet hyperactivity. The long connecting tubing prevents accidental infusion of such a solution into the vein, facilitates the procedure, and diminishes the possibility of accidental needle puncture for the phlebotomist.

Procedure Using Evacuated Tubes. For coagulation specimens, the evacuated system of collecting blood is preferable to syringes because blood goes directly from the vein into the tube and is immediately mixed with anticoagulant, thus reducing the likelihood of clotted specimens (Fig. 2-2).[32] This is an important factor when collecting blood for hemostatic workups that include the evaluation of platelets and clotting factors and require as much as 30 to 50 mL of blood. If specimens for other than hemostasis testing are required, the recommended order of draw for evacuated tubes discussed earlier should be followed.

A multiple-sample Luer adapter (Fig. 2-1) should be used. After the needle enters the vein, the tourniquet is released and the system cleansed of tissue thromboplastin by drawing 5 mL of blood into a non-additive evacuated tube. This blood may be used for other tests requiring serum, or it may be discarded. Specimens for tests requiring citrated plasma are drawn next. If platelet function tests are ordered, while the needle is still in the vein, the tubing is pinched to stop blood flow, the needle holder and Luer adapter are removed from the butterfly tubing adapter, and a plastic syringe is attached. Blood is drawn into this syringe and dispensed into appropriate tubes.

Procedure Using Syringes. When a specimen is being drawn directly into a syringe, the tourniquet is released and approximately 5 mL of blood is withdrawn into the first syringe after the vein is entered. Before syringes are switched, sterile gauze is placed beneath the hub of the needle to absorb any blood that might escape. With the needle in the vein, the first syringe is carefully detached from the needle and replaced with the second syringe. Blood for coagulation testing is drawn into this syringe and transferred without delay into the appropriate tubes. To avoid air bubbles and frothing of the specimen, the needle should be securely fitted on the syringe. When blood is being aspirated with a syringe, the plunger should be withdrawn at a rate equal to the flow of blood. If the rate is in excess of that needed to aspirate the blood, air bubbles will enter the syringe and cause hemolysis.[39] Forced aspiration may also cause the vein to collapse and result in a sudden release of gases from RBCs, also resulting in hemolysis.[7] Because there is a risk of blood

splatter using this technique, a face shield is recommended.

Transferring and Mixing Specimens. To avoid frothing and hemolysis of the specimen, blood should not be expelled through the needle. Immediately after the venipuncture is completed, the needle should be safely and carefully removed from the syringe. Blood is slowly expelled into the collection tubes by allowing it to run down the side of the tube.[34] Specimens transferred into tubes containing anticoagulants should be stoppered and thoroughly mixed by gently inverting the tubes 5 to 10 times. Blood drawn directly into evacuated tubes is partially mixed with the anticoagulant when the blood enters the tube, but to ensure that mixing is thorough, the tubes should be inverted gently 5 to 10 times immediately after removal from the needle holder.

Processing and Storing Hemostasis Specimens

Changes that occur once blood is collected range from surface activation of coagulation (which results in shortened clotting times) to increased lability of factors V and VIII (which may lengthen clotting times). Such changes become significant sources of errors in testing if measures are not taken to minimize and control them when processing and storing specimens.

EFFECT OF pH

Changes in the pH of specimens, mediated by the loss of carbon dioxide, can affect results by causing prolongation of clotting times. As carbon dioxide is lost, the pH of the specimen increases. The buffered citrate solution contained in evacuated tubes protects specimens against such loss for a period of time. Also, red cells have a buffering effect that helps stabilize the pH of blood specimens. To maintain this effect, specimens should remain in unopened tubes if testing is not done immediately. Normal specimens collected in evacuated tubes and stored unopened at room temperature for as long as 6 hours show no significant changes in PT or PTT results.[16]

EFFECT OF TEMPERATURE

If specimens are left at room temperature for an extended time (greater than 6 hours), factors V and VIII are likely to deteriorate. On the other hand, factors VII and XI tend to be prematurely activated at refrigerator temperatures (4°C).[26] However, for common coagulation tests such as the PT, specimens are quite stable for up to 12 hours if collected in buffered sodium citrate.[30]

CENTRIFUGATION

For most coagulation testing, platelet-poor plasma (PPP) is required. PPP is prepared by centrifuging anticoagulated blood at 2000 × g for 10 minutes. Plasma should be removed immediately with a plastic or silicon-coated pipette and stored in a stoppered plastic or silicon-coated tube. Only the upper three-fourths of the plasma layer should be aspirated. For some special tests, centrifugation of the specimen at a temperature of 2° to 4°C is advisable.

For this process, a refrigerated centrifuge or a small centrifuge placed in a refrigerator is required.

The buffering effect of red cells is lost once the specimen is centrifuged and the plasma is exposed to air.[1,41] Testing should be done immediately on centrifuged specimens, or the plasma should be stored at 4°C for a time not to exceed 2 hours.

FROZEN SPECIMENS

Specimens should not be frozen if testing can be done within 2 hours after collection. If freezing is necessary, it should be done rapidly at −20°C or lower. Slow freezing causes ice particles to form that may denature the clotting proteins.[17] If frozen properly, fibrinogen is stable for at least 4 hours after thawing and survives refreezing and thawing.[12]

SPECIMEN PREPARATION FOR PLATELET FUNCTION TESTING

Collection

Hemolysis should be avoided at all times because red cells contain adenosine diphosphate (ADP), which, if released into the plasma, may prematurely activate platelets. The pH of the specimen is critical and is best controlled with buffered sodium citrate anticoagulant.

Centrifugation

Specimens collected for platelet function studies (Chap. 56) should be processed immediately. To prepare platelet-rich plasma (PRP), the anticoagulated specimen is centrifuged at 60 to 100 × g for 10 minutes at room temperature. The plasma is removed immediately with a plastic or silicon-coated pipette and transferred to stoppered plastic or silicon-coated test tubes. Red cell contamination should be avoided by removing only as much PRP as necessary from the upper portion of the specimen. Platelet aggregation studies also require PPP. This is obtained by recentrifuging the remaining specimen.

For some platelet function tests, such as beta-thromboglobulin (βTG) and platelet factor 4 (PF4), the specimens should be centrifuged at 2° to 4°C.

Influence of Time

Platelets are stable and most responsive between 30 minutes and 3 hours after blood is drawn.[11] Thereafter, platelet function diminishes significantly and test results are unreliable. The response of platelets to various aggregating agents is different and varies as a function of time. Ristocetin aggregation testing should be done immediately after the specimen is processed, because the response of platelets to Ristocetin decreases as the pH of the plasma changes. On the other hand, aggregation with epinephrine should be performed last because the response of platelets to this agent continues to increase with time. Consistent or maximum aggregation with epinephrine is reached after PRP has been at room temperature for about 60 minutes.

Influence of Temperature

The storage temperature of PRP prepared for platelet function studies has a significant influence on the rate and degree of platelet response in the tests. Platelets prepared for aggregation studies and stored at room temperature are more sensitive to various aggregating agents than platelets stored at 37°C. The storage of platelets at low temperatures (0°–4°C) increases the tendency of platelets to aggregate spontaneously.[44] Because of the variability of platelet activity at these temperatures, specimens collected and prepared for platelet function studies, particularly platelet aggregation, should remain at room temperature until testing.

DEFIBRINATED SPECIMENS

Certain hematology tests, such as osmotic fragility (Chap.17), autohemolysis (Chap.17), and the acid serum test (Chap.19), require a defibrinated specimen. Defibrination involves the removal of fibrin from a whole blood specimen. The phlebotomist must prepare the defibrinated specimen at the patient's bedside before blood is allowed to clot. Immediately after venipuncture using a syringe, whole blood is gently added to an Erlenmeyer flask containing glass beads or paper clips. After gauze or cotton is placed in the top of the flask to prevent specimen contamination, the flask is rotated for about 10 minutes until the beads (or clips) are covered with fibrin and no longer make a rattling noise. For some tests a sterile flask and beads are required.

CHAPTER SUMMARY

In order to ensure the validity of test results from hematology and hemostasis testing, phlebotomists need to be aware of how the steps involved in venipuncture and skin puncture can affect test results. Phlebotomists must be able to select the best methods of collection and the most appropriate equipment for the specimen required and the patient's characteristics. Errors resulting from failure to adhere to accepted standards of phlebotomy and specimen handling and transport can result in altered cell counts, activity, or morphology. Such errors can also alter the hematocrit, cause hemolysis, and either inhibit or prematurely activate hemostasis.

Case Study 2-1

A 93-year-old female homebound patient had a skin puncture specimen collected for a CBC in an EDTA anticoagulated Microtainer. The specimen volume was within that required for the collection device. A hemoglobin and hematocrit performed on the specimen were as follows: Hb 9.1 g/dL and Hct 0.26 L/L. The tests were repeated on the same specimen with similar results. The patient was admitted to a hospital that evening for further evaluation and treatment of the anemia. The admission CBC revealed a Hb of 11.4 g/dL and Hct of 0.34 L/L. A subsequent specimen taken 4 hours later produced similar results, and the patient was discharged untreated the following morning.

1. Assuming that the patient was never anemic and that the instrumentation used to obtain the initial CBC results was working properly, what might have produced the erroneous result?

2. What could have been done from a phlebotomy quality assurance perspective to avoid the unnecessary hospitalization?

Case Study 2-2

A 56-year-old male patient with a history of thrombotic episodes was on oral anticoagulant therapy. The effectiveness of the therapy was assessed by weekly PTs. The patient consistently had a PT between 18 and 20 seconds. However, on the most recent assessment, the patient's PT was 11.2 seconds. After questioning the patient, his physician had no reason to believe that the patient had not adhered to his treatment regimen. Later that same day the PT was repeated with a result of 19.6 seconds. It was discovered that two different phlebotomists had collected the specimens.

1. Assuming that there were no technical errors involved during PT testing, what situation might have led to the apparently erroneous PT result of 11.2 seconds?
2. How could this situation be avoided in the future?

Review Questions

2-1. A patient's hematocrit from a morning specimen was 0.35 L/L; later that afternoon it was 0.40 L/L. Both specimens were collected in EDTA evacuated tubes. Assuming that there should not have been any significant change in the hematocrit, what is one possible explanation for the discrepancy?

A. The correct order of draw was not followed.
B. The tourniquet was applied too long during the first collection.
C. The tourniquet was applied too long during the second collection.
D. An improper anticoagulant was used.

2-2. A physician orders a PT on a known polycythemic patient with a hematocrit of 0.58 L/L. To ensure proper specimen collection, the phelebotomist should

A. eliminate the discard tube.
B. adjust the anticoagulant to blood ratio appropriately.
C. do nothing; this situation will present no problem if blood is collected in a standard sodium citrate evacuated tube.
D. collect the blood in an oxalated tube.

2-3. A heel puncture was performed on a neonate to obtain specimens for chemistry testing and a CBC. Non-additive and EDTA Microtainers were used. The EDTA specimen for the CBC could not be aspirated by the hematology analyzer due to clotting. This may have been caused by

A. collecting the non-additive specimen before the EDTA specimen.
B. collecting the EDTA specimen before the additive specimen.
C. removing the first drop of blood prior to collecting the specimen.
D. using a lancet 2.2 mm in length.

References

1. Bandi ZL: Estimation, prevention and quality control of carbon dioxide loss during aerobic sample processing. Clin Chem 27:1676, 1981
2. Blumenfeld TA: Infant blood collection and chemical analysis. Diagn Med 1:58, 1978
3. Brown BA: Hematology: Principles and Procedures, 6th ed. Philadelphia, Lea & Febiger, 1993
4. Calam RR, Cooper MH: Recommended "order of draw" for collecting blood specimens into additive-containing tubes. Clin Chem 28:1399, 1982
5. Corriveau DM: Chemical assessment of coagulation. In Bishop ML, Duben-Von Laufen JL, Fody EP (eds): Clinical Chemistry: Principles, Procedures, Correlations, p 512. Philadelphia, JB Lippincott, 1985
6. Dacie JV: Practical Haematology, 5th ed, p 326. London, Churchill Livingstone, 1975
7. Diggs LW: Hematological techniques. In Miller SE (ed): A Textbook of Clinical Pathology, 8th ed, p 3. Baltimore, Williams & Wilkins, 1971
8. Garza D, Becan–McBride K: Phlebotomy Handbook, 3rd ed. Norwalk, Appleton-Century-Crofts, 1993
9. Hammond KB: Blood specimen collection from infants by skin puncture. Lab Med 11:9, 1980
10. Hardisty RM, Ingram GIC: Bleeding Disorders: Investigation and Management, p 162. Oxford, Blackwell Scientific Publications, 1965
11. Harms CS: Routine laboratory procedures. In Triplett DA (ed): Platelet Function: Laboratory Evaluation and Clinical Application, p 214. Chicago, American Society of Clinical Pathologists, 1978
12. Hoffman M, Koepke JA, Widman FK: Fibrinogen content of low volume cryoprecipitate. Transfusion 27:356, 1987
13. Jones BA: Testing at the patient's bedside. Clin Lab Med 14:473, 1994
14. Kjeldsberg CR: Principles of hematologic examination. In Lee GR, Bithell TC, Foerster J et al (eds): Wintrobe's Clinical Hematology, 9th ed, p 7. Philadelphia, Lea & Febiger, 1993
15. Koepke JA: Specimen collection—cellular hematology. In Koepke JA (ed): Laboratory Hematology, vol 1, p 821. New York, Churchill Livingstone, 1984
16. Koepke JA, Rodgers JL, Ollivier MJ: Pre-instrumental variables in coagulation testing. Am J Clin Pathol 64:591, 1975
17. Lenahan JG, Smith K: Hemostasis, 16th ed, p 13. Morris Plains, NJ, General Diagnostics, 1982
18. McCall RE, Tankersley CM: Phlebotomy Essentials. Philadelphia, JB Lippincott, 1993
19. Meites S, Levitt MJ: Skin-puncture and blood-collecting techniques for infants. Clin Chem 25:183, 1979
20. Meites S, Lin SS, Thompson C: Studies on the quality of specimens obtained by skin puncture of children 1. Tendency to hemolysis, and hemoglobin and tissue fluid as contaminants. Clin Chem 27:875, 1981
21. National Committee for Clinical Laboratory Standards: Collection, transport, and processing of blood specimens for coagulation testing and performance of coagulation assays—2nd ed; Approved Guideline Document H21-A2. Villanova, PA, NCCLS, 1991
22. National Committee for Clinical Laboratory Standards: Evacuated tubes for blood specimen collection—3rd ed; Approved Standard Document H1-A3. Villanova, PA, NCCLS, 1991
23. National Committee for Clinical Laboratory Standards: Procedures for the collection of diagnostic blood specimens by skin puncture—3rd ed; Approved Standard Document H4-A3. Villanova, PA, NCCLS, 1991
24. National Committee for Clinical Laboratory Standards: Procedures for the collection of diagnostic blood specimens by venipuncture—3rd ed; Approved Standard Document H3-A3. Villanova, PA, NCCLS, 1991
25. National Committee for Clinical Laboratory Standards: Procedures for the handling and processing of blood specimens; Approved Guideline Document H18-A. Villanova, PA, NCCLS, 1990
26. Palmer RN, Gralnick HR: Cold induced contact activation of the prothrombin time in whole blood.. Blood 59:38, 1981

27. Pendergraph GE: Handbook of Phlebotomy, 3rd ed. Philadelphia, Lea & Febiger, 1992

28. Phelan S: Phlebotomy Techniques. Chicago, American Society of Clinical Pathologists, 1993

29. Raphael SS: Lynch's Medical Laboratory Technology, 4th ed, p 734. Philadelphia, WB Saunders, 1983

30. Simmons A, Paulo MA: Prothrombin time stability and precision using buffered sodium citrate. Lab Medica 10(b):22, 1993

31. Sirridge MS, Shannon R: Laboratory Evaluation of Hemostasis and Thrombosis, 3rd ed, pp 58, 60, 170. Philadelphia, Lea & Febiger, 1983

32. Slockbower JM: Blood drawing techniques. In Seligson D, Schmidt RM (eds): Handbook Series in Clinical Laboratory Science, p 22. Boca Raton, CRC Press, 1979

33. Slockbower JM: Venipuncture procedures. Lab Med 10:74, 1979

34. Slockbower JM, Blumenfeld TA: Collection and Handling of Laboratory Specimens: A Practical Guide. Philadelphia, JB Lippincott, 1983

35. Smoller BR, Kruskall MS: Phlebotomy for diagnostic laboratory tests in adults: Pattern of use and effect on transfusion requirements. N Engl J Med 314:1233, 1986

36. Soong WJ, Hwang B: Contamination errors when sampling blood from an arterial line. Clin Pediatr 32(8):501, 1993

37. Statland BE, Winkel P, Harris SC et al: Evaluation of biologic sources of variation of leukocyte counts and other hematologic quantities using very precise automated analyzers. Am J Clin Pathol 69:48, 1978

38. Templin K, Shively M, Riley J: Accuracy of drawing coagulation samples from heparinized arterial lines. Am J Crit Care 2(1):88, 1993

39. Tocantins LM: Processing of blood, preparation of glassware and reagents. In Tocantins LM, Kazal LA (eds): Blood Coagulation, Hemorrhage and Thrombosis, p 3. New York, Grune & Stratton, 1964

40. Tombridge TL: Effect of posture on hematology results. Am J Clin Pathol 49:491, 1968

41. Triplett DA, Smith C: Routine testing in the coagulation laboratory. In Triplett DA (ed): Laboratory Evaluation of Coagulation. Chicago, American Society of Clinical Pathologists, 1982

42. Watson KR, O'Kell RT, Joyce JT: Data regarding blood drawing sites in patients receiving intravenous fluids. Am J Clin Pathol 79:119, 1983

43. Winkel P, Statland PE, Saunders A et al: Within-day physiologic variation of the concentration of leukocyte types in healthy subjects as assayed by two automated leukocyte differential analyzers. Am J Clin Pathol 75:693, 1981

44. Zucker MB, Borrelli J: Reversible alterations in platelet morphology produced by anticoagulants and by cold. Blood 9:602, 1954

CHAPTER 3

Preparation of Blood Films for Examination

Jean A. Shafer

Objectives

1. Describe two manual methods for making a blood film, and give the advantages and disadvantages of each.
2. Describe at least two different ways a buffy coat preparation can be made, and discuss reasons why a buffy coat preparation might be preferred over a blood film.
3. Discuss the principle of Romanowsky staining, and describe at least two manual and two automated methods for staining a blood film.
4. Discuss the problems caused by artifacts that occur commonly in blood film preparation and staining, and describe how to troubleshoot the problems.

MANUAL BLOOD FILM PREPARATION

Coverslip Method

Innate difficulties in the spreading of a drop of blood between two glass coverslips have prevented the coverslip method from being popular for routine peripheral blood films. However, the technique is used extensively for bone marrow preparations.

ADVANTAGES AND DISADVANTAGES

The one significant advantage of the coverslip preparation is its superior leukocyte distribution. In other words, a leukocyte differential count (Chap. 24) performed on a coverslip preparation is less likely to contain errors caused by poor distribution.

The disadvantages are several. One is the difficulty in learning the technique. Second, to ensure an even distribution of blood, coverslips must be manually cleaned of dirt, dust, grease, and fingerprints just prior to use. Third, because of the difficulty in labeling, transporting, and staining the small and easily broken glass coverslips, they must be mounted on glass 3 × 1-inch slides for microscopic examination. The use of mounting media prevents immediate storage. Fourth, the two coverslips used to make the films in this method must be kept matched for estimating platelet numbers, because platelets may be unevenly distributed between the two coverslips. Finally, there are no specific areas to examine for unusual cells.

TECHNIQUE

1. Hold a clean No. 1.5 coverslip (22 × 22 mm) at two adjacent corners between the thumb and index finger of one hand (see Fig. 3-1A).
2. Place a small drop of blood (approximately 2 mm in diameter) in the center of the top surface of the coverslip. Place another clean coverslip on top in a crisscross direction so that the two coverslips resemble an eight-pointed star (Fig. 3-1B and C). *Note:* If using finger-stick (capillary) blood, wipe away the first drop that emerges from the puncture and touch the undersurface of the coverslip to a fresh drop. Avoid touching the skin. Place this coverslip on top of another clean coverslip to form an eight-pointed star, as described above.
3. The drop of blood should begin to spread in all directions by capillary action. When its spread is almost complete, pull the two coverslips apart with a smooth, lateral, parallel sliding movement (Fig. 3-1D).
4. Keep coverslip pairs matched, and air dry them rapidly.
5. After staining, air dry and mount with the blood-film side down on a 3 × 1-inch glass slide. Label the slide.

A modification of the coverslip method is the substitution of two 3 × 1-inch glass slides for the coverslips. The top slide is placed directly over the slide containing a drop of blood in its center, with one end extending slightly (see Fig. 3-2). The advantages of this modification are the larger examination area, the use of slides that are not as breakable as coverslips, and ease of labeling of the blood films.

TROUBLESHOOTING

1. Assess the size of the drop of blood. Too large a drop may result in too thick a spread. Too small a drop may produce a thin spread or too small an examination area.
2. Timing and speed of coverslip separation is important.

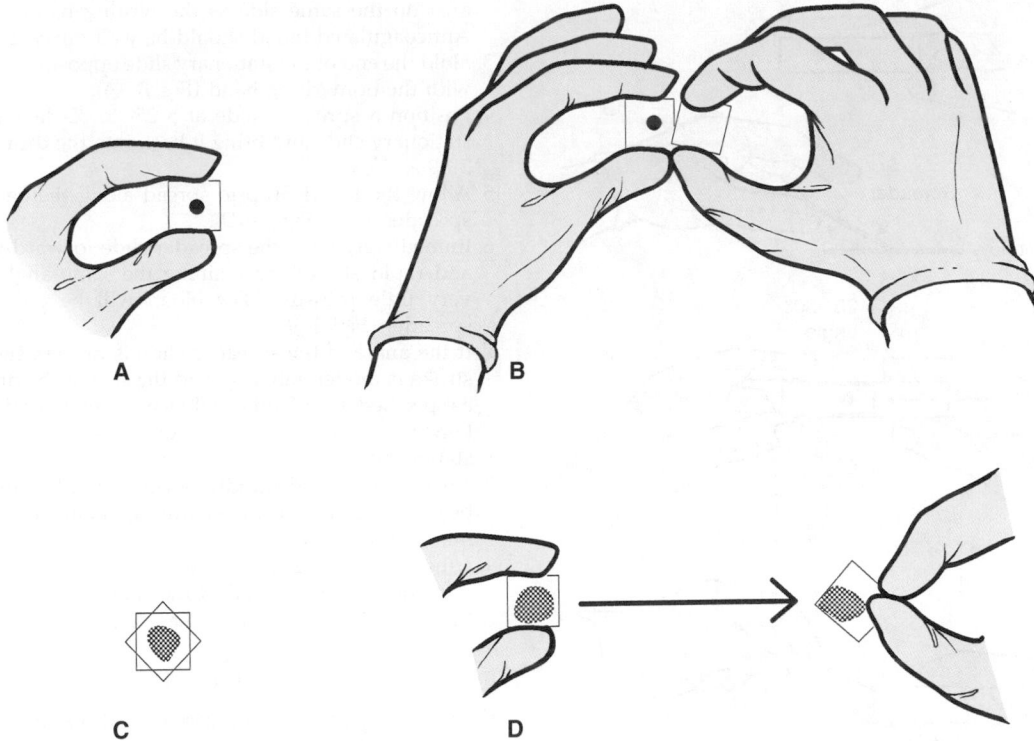

FIGURE 3-1. Coverslip blood film preparation. (**A**) A drop of blood is placed on a clean 22-mm-square coverslip. (**B**) A second coverslip is placed on top so that the two form (**C**) an eight-point star. (**D**) The two coverslips are pulled apart with a smooth, lateral, parallel sliding motion.

Pulling the coverslips apart prematurely or too rapidly may create a thick or uneven spread. Delay in their separation may cause the coverslips to become stuck to each other, the platelets to clump, or the leukocytes to distribute unevenly.

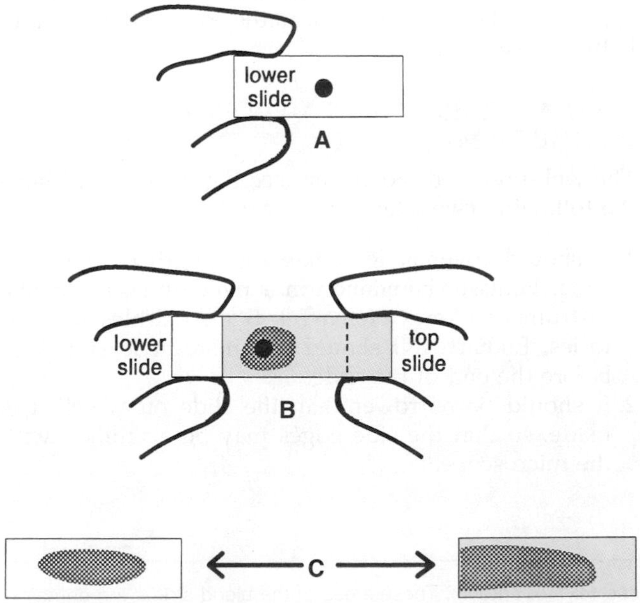

FIGURE 3-2. Modification of the coverslip blood film technique using 3 × 1-inch slides. (**A**) A drop of blood is placed in the center of the lower slide. (**B**) The top slide is placed on the blood drop so that the ends of the two slides overlap slightly. (**C**) The two slides are pulled apart in a smooth, parallel motion.

3. Separation movement must be smooth. A jerky pulling movement or a variation in the horizontal level will cause uneven distribution of the cellular elements.
4. Assess the staining quality. The small surface area of coverslips makes it difficult to mix stain and buffer adequately, as well as to wash off the stain solution.

Wedge Technique

Variations of the wedge technique are the most widely used for blood film preparation. The product may be termed a wedge, spreader-slide, or push blood film.

ADVANTAGES AND DISADVANTAGES

There are several advantages to the wedge technique, including the fact that the technique is easier to master; commercially "precleaned" slides are generally adequate, although an occasional lot or batch may require further cleaning; the slides are not easily broken; labeling, transporting, and staining are easier; a coverslip is not necessary, and blood films can be put in storage immediately; the combination of the above assets makes this the least expensive type of preparation; and the tendency of larger cells to settle at the edges and the feathered end of the film makes it easier to find abnormal cells.

A major disadvantage of the wedge technique is that there is inherently poor distribution of nucleated cells. Neutrophils and monocytes have a greater tendency to appear in the feathered end of the preparation rather than in the examination area. This may lead to artifactually increased lymphocyte and decreased neutrophil and

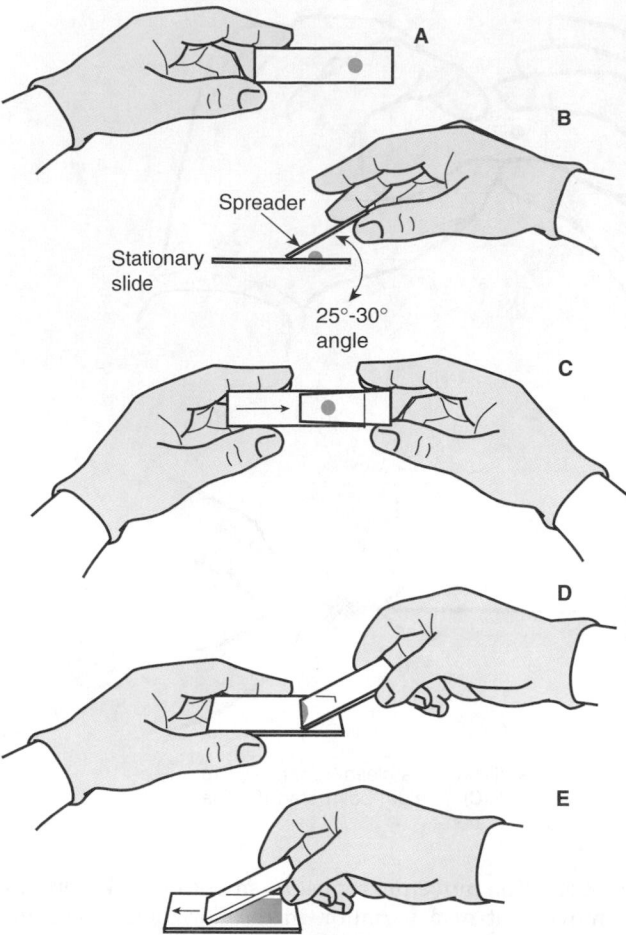

FIGURE 3-3. Wedge-type blood film preparation. (**A**) A drop of blood is placed near one end of a clean 3 × 1-inch (stationary) glass slide. (**B**) A spreader slide is positioned at a 25 to 35° angle in front of the drop of blood. (**C**) The spreader slide is backed into the drop of blood. (**D**) The drop of blood is allowed to spread evenly along the edge of the spreader slide. (**E**) The spreader slide is pushed forward with a smooth, rapid stroke.

monocyte counts when performing a leukocyte differential count.

Another disadvantage is that there is greater trauma to the cells during the making of the blood film. This may lead to large numbers of "smudged" or "basket" cells (ruptured leukocytes), especially in lymphoproliferative disorders.

TECHNIQUE

1. Place a clean 3 × 1-inch glass slide on a flat surface (stationary slide).
2. Transfer a drop of blood approximately 2 to 3 mm in diameter to the stationary slide about ¼-inch from the end or frosted

area on the same side as the writing hand (see Fig. 3-3*A*). Anticoagulated blood should be well mixed before transfer.
3. Hold the end of the stationary slide opposite the drop of blood with the nonwriting hand (Fig. 3-3*A*).
4. Position a spreader slide at a 25- to 35-degree angle to the stationary slide and bring it back into the drop of blood (Fig. 3-3*B* and *C*).
5. Allow the blood drop to spread along the back edge of the spreader slide (Fig. 3-3*D*).
6. Immediately push the spreader slide forward with a smooth and rapid stroke, maintaining the same angle and exerting very little pressure. The blood will be pulled behind the spreader (Fig. 3-3*E*).
7. If the angle of the spreader slide is proper, the speed of the stroke is moderately fast, and the size of the drop of blood is as specified, the blood should feather into nothing somewhere between one-half and three-quarters of the way along the stationary slide.
8. Air dry the blood rapidly but thoroughly (several minutes) before staining. This can be done manually or with an electric fan or cool air blower.
9. Labeling with patient name, log number, and date may be done on the frosted end of the slide or in the thicker end of the blood film itself after it has dried.

THE SPREADER SLIDE

Certain properties of the spreader slide affect the distribution of the leukocytes and consequently the accuracy of the differential count.[9,18,29,48,53] This slide should be narrower than the glass slide on which the blood film will be deposited (stationary slide). The spreading edge should be clean, smooth, polished, and thin, with no chips or scratches. A few companies manufacture beveled-edge microscope slides that meet these specifications.

An excellent spreader is a hemocytometer cover glass (20 × 26 × 0.4–0.6 mm). The 20-mm edge is the spreader edge. The cover glass may be held by a straight artery clamp, one prong of which is enclosed in rubber tubing to prevent slipping.[52] A disadvantage of this type of spreader is the necessity to clean the edge of the spreader between patients.

CHARACTERISTICS OF A PROPER WEDGE FILM

The well-prepared blood film (see Fig. 3-4) should have the following characteristics:

1. It should cover at least half the length of the glass slide. Films to be stained in a platen-type automatic instrument (Ames Hema-Tek Stainer, Miles Laboratories, Elkhart, IN) should terminate at least ½-inch before the end of the slide.
2. It should be narrower than the slide on which it is made, so that the side edges may be examined with the microscope.[41]

FIGURE 3-4. A good blood smear (see text for criteria). These areas of the blood smear are demarcated on low power (*right row*) and high power (*left row*). (**A**) Feather edge (tail)—blood film is too thin for examination. Note distribution of red cells and the fact that they have no central pallor. (**B**) Examination area. Note cell distribution, the fact that some red cell overlapping occurs, and central pallor of the red cells. (**C**) Body of smear—blood film is too thick for examination. Note that all red cells are overlapped and that leukocytes are smaller and appear thicker.

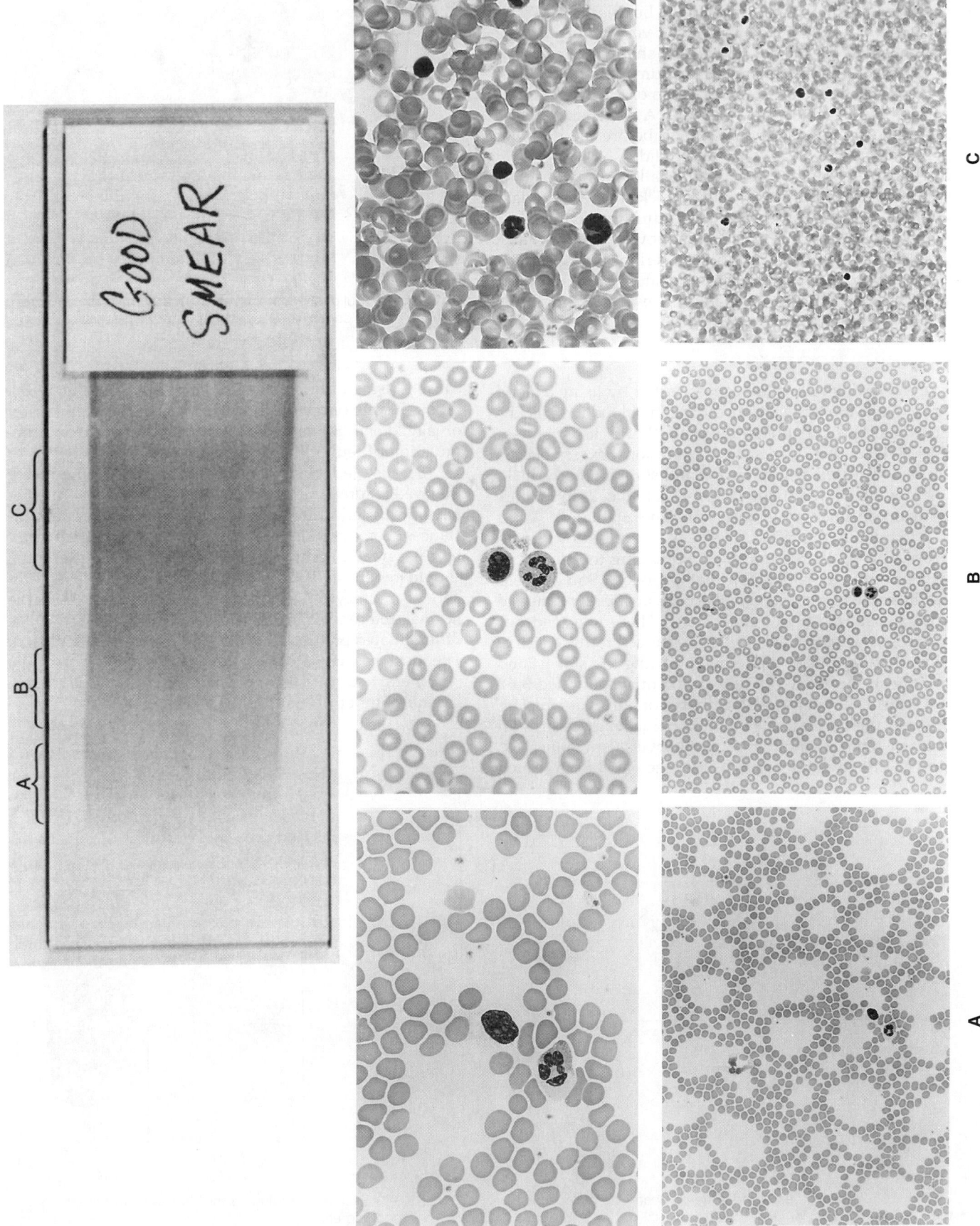

3. A homogeneous spread should be displayed with a gradual transition from thick to thin areas and with no waves, streaks, troughs, holes, or bubbles.

4. It should terminate in a straight or very slightly curved feathered end (see Fig. 3-5). Bullet-shaped preparations (Fig. 3-5) tend to have higher accumulations of leukocytes along the side and tail edges of the film than the straight-ended film (see Fig. 3-6). A bullet-shaped end results from spreading the blood before the drop has spread fully along the spreader slide.[53]

5. The film should be thin enough to allow proper fixation during the staining procedure. Thick areas appear dark green or gray or are washed off during staining.

6. It should contain at least 10 low-power fields in which 50% of the erythrocytes do not overlap. The remainder may overlap slightly (doublets and triplets). Single erythrocytes should have a well preserved central pale area (Fig. 3-4B).

TROUBLESHOOTING

Extremely thick films are caused either by using a blood drop that is too large, by spreading the blood too quickly, or by using a spreader-slide angle that is too high (see Figs. 3-4C and 3-7). In such preparations, excess plasma causes nucleated cells to shrink and stain intensely, making identification difficult (Fig. 3-4C). Red cells form more rouleaux in thick areas and cannot be evaluated.

Extremely thin films (Fig. 3-7) are caused by using a drop of blood that is too small, spreading too slowly, or using a spreader-slide angle that is too low. Smudge cells are increased, and red cells become artificially spheroid with a distorted shape (Fig. 3-4A). There is a tendency for more nucleated cells to be carried out to the edges of films that have been made by spreading too slowly, and this affects the accuracy of the differential count (Fig. 3-6).

A gritty appearance of feathered or tail areas indicates an accumulation of nucleated cells, which may be attributable to a large number of leukocytes, spreading too slowly, or to a delay in spreading (see Fig. 3-8). A related cause is using only a part of the drop of blood (Fig. 3-8B). A rough edge or dirty spreader may also produce a gritty or jagged end. Some anticoagulants may lead to an accumulation of leukocytes at the feathered end.[13]

Because leukocytes may be poorly distributed with the wedge preparation, many hematology laboratories have instituted rules to govern procedures in certain instances. For example, if the leukocyte differential count reveals greater than 40% lymphocytes, the differential should be repeated on another slide. Likewise, if the numbers of monocytes, eosinophils, or basophils exceed the normal reference ranges, a second 100 cells are to be differentiated on the same slide and the average reported. The most efficient check is a low-power inspection of the peripheral (side and feathered end) areas for a disproportionate number of neutrophils.

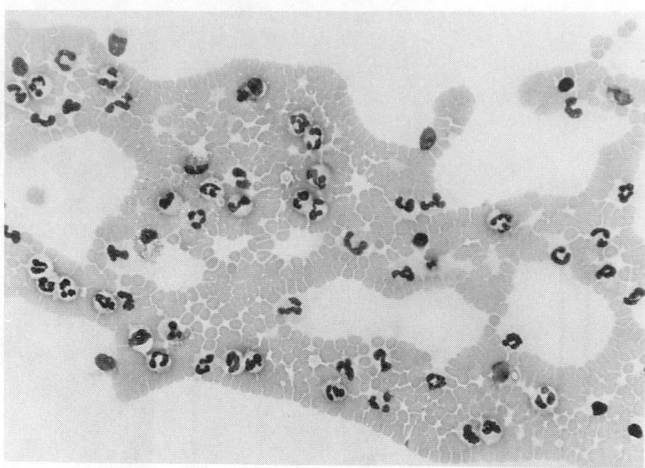

FIGURE 3-6. Bullet-shaped film results in accumulation of leukocytes along the edges.

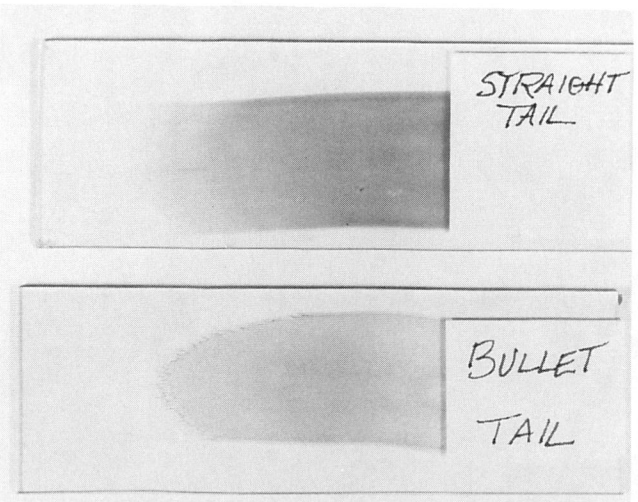

FIGURE 3-5. Straight feathered edge compared to bullet edge or tail.

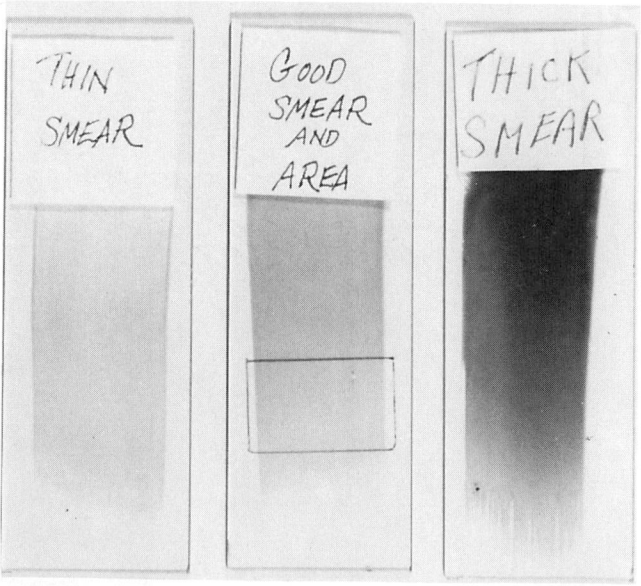

FIGURE 3-7. Excessively thin and thick smears are compared with a "good" smear.

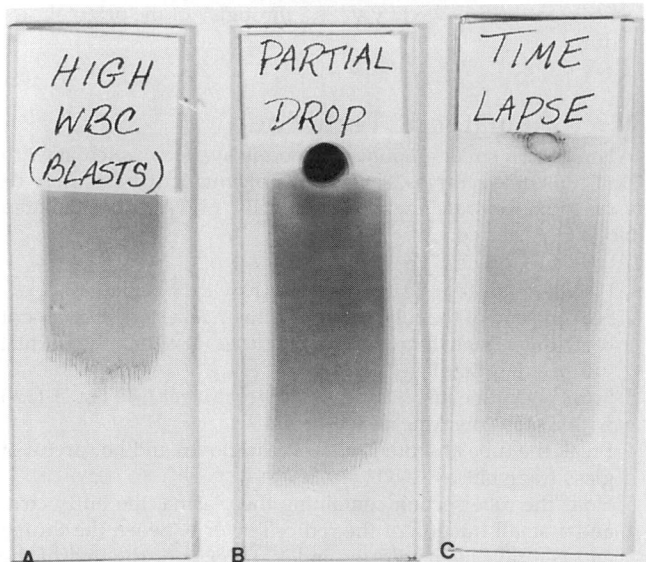

FIGURE 3-8. Causes of streaks in feathered edge. (**A**) Extremely high leukocyte count with blast forms. (**B**) Picking up only part of the blood drop. (**C**) Allowing too much time to elapse between placing blood on slide and spreading.

AUTOMATED BLOOD FILMS

Automatic methods for blood film preparations have been introduced by several manufacturers over the years. At present, the only one remaining on the market is the Autoprep (Barret Healthcare Corporation, Tucker, GA). This is a portable semiautomatic instrument that simulates the manual spreader-type technique (see Fig. 3-9).

It contains two spreader blades mounted at a set angle that are moved mechanically along the length of a 3 × 1-inch glass slide containing a drop of blood. The operator must place the slides in the machine, place a drop of blood on each slide, and press a lever to initiate the spreader's movement. The speed can be varied according to the hematocrit. The advantages and disadvantages of this automated wedge film are the same as those of manual wedge preparation with the added advantage of more consistency between blood films.

Other automated instruments that have been introduced are based on the centrifugal technique (utilizing centrifugation to spread a monolayer of whole blood on a 3 × 1-inch glass slide).

BUFFY COAT PREPARATION

Nucleated cells and platelets will layer above red cells during centrifugation (see Fig. 3-10). This fraction of nucleated cells is referred to as the "buffy coat" because of its buff or tan color. A white top layer usually represents platelets accumulated above the nucleated cells. The buffy coat can be removed, mixed, and used to prepare blood films.

The buffy coat preparation is a simple procedure that often provides diagnostic information and may reduce or eliminate the need for more complex, costly, and time-consuming tests. A buffy coat preparation may be indicated for detecting the presence of the following:

Reactive, immature, or abnormal cells (*e.g.,* rare blasts or mast cells[7]) that are present in small numbers, especially with pancytopenic samples

Megaloblastic nucleated red cells or an increased number

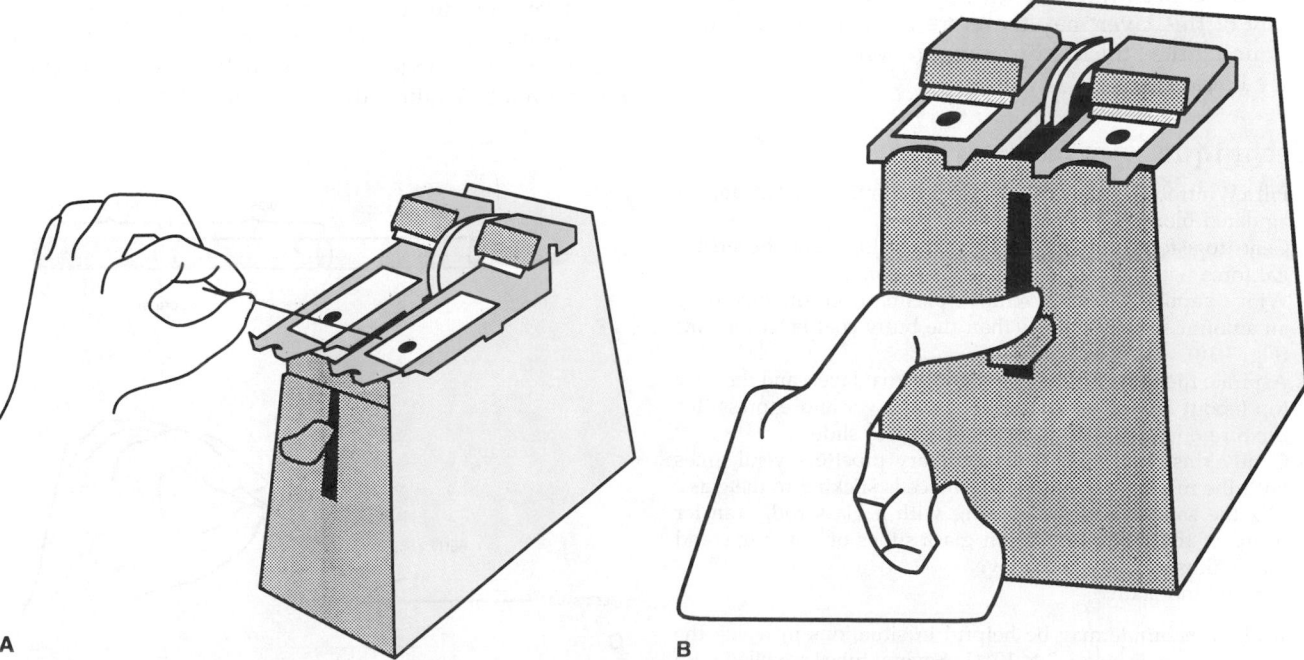

FIGURE 3-9. Automated wedge-type smear. (**A**) A drop of blood is placed at a specific spot on each of two slides. (**B**) By pressing a lever, the wedges are advanced, placed into the blood drops, and pulled back to spread the blood.

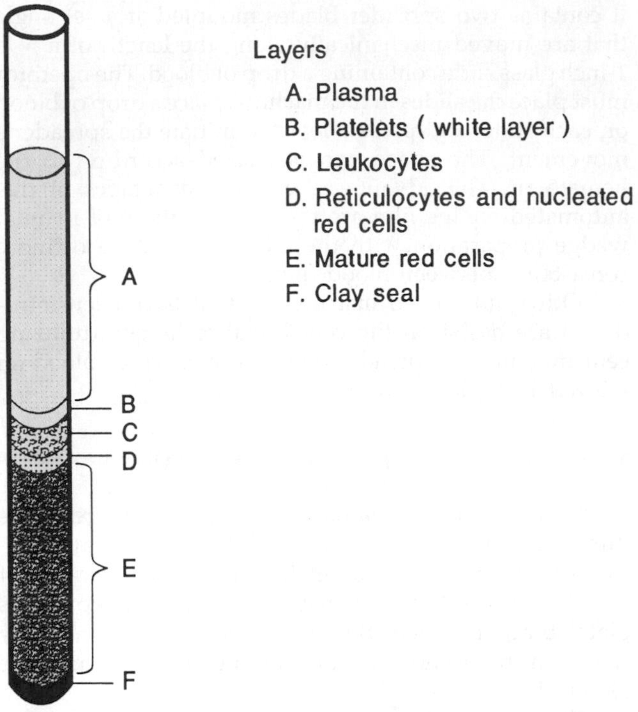

Layers

   A. Plasma

   B. Platelets (white layer)

   C. Leukocytes

   D. Reticulocytes and nucleated
      red cells

   E. Mature red cells

   F. Clay seal

FIGURE 3-10. Layers of blood components after centrifugation.

of hypersegmented neutrophils in megaloblastic anemias
Abnormal plasma cells
Tumor cells circulating in the blood
Bacteria or parasites[6]

For example, mature red cells containing malarial parasites are concentrated at the top of the red cell layer. Study of this layer may therefore be more fruitful than examining the "thick drop" preparation described in the early literature.

Technique

1. Fill a Wintrobe hematocrit tube with well-mixed EDTA-anticoagulated blood.
2. Centrifuge for 6 minutes at 1000 × g. The low relative centrifugal force will not cause cellular distortion.
3. With a capillary pipette, remove plasma from the tube until an amount slightly greater than the buffy coat layer remains (Fig. 3-10).
4. Aspirate the remaining plasma, buffy coat layer, and the very top (about 1%) of the mature red cell layer and express this mixture onto a watch glass or clean glass slide.
5. Gently rinse the bore of the capillary pipette several times with the mixture to remove all the cells sticking to the glass.
6. Mix the sample well by stirring with a glass rod. Transfer drops of the mixture to clean glass slides or coverslips and make films as described above.
7. Air dry and stain.

A *double concentrate* may be helpful in situations in which the leukocyte count is below 3×10^9/L. Several tubes are filled with the specimen and centrifuged as above. Two-thirds of the plasma is discarded from each. The remaining plasma, the buffy coat, and ¼-inch of the red cell layer is removed from all tubes, mixed thoroughly, and placed in another tube for a second

centrifugation followed by steps 3 through 7 of the original procedure.

Microhematocrit Technique

When only a small amount of blood is available, such as with skin puncture samples, several microhematocrit tubes may be used to concentrate the nucleated cells. EDTA anticoagulated blood is preferred.

1. Fill the tubes to at least three-fourths with blood.
2. Seal one end of the tubes and place them in a microhematocrit centrifuge. Centrifuge for 2 to 3 minutes (less than the normal full-packing time).
3. Score each tube just *below* the buffy coat layer (see Fig. 3-11A) with a glass marking pencil or file.
4. Break the tube at scored mark. Wear gloves and be careful of glass fragments.
5. Hold the tube section containing the plasma, the buffy coat, and a small fraction of the red cell layer between the thumb and central finger with the index finger over the end of the tube to control fluid flow. A smallpox vaccination bulb may be used to control fluid flow.
6. Touch the tube to a clean glass slide and allow the red cells, buffy coat and a small amount of the plasma to flow onto the slide (Fig. 3-11B). Mix thoroughly and make a wedge film. Air dry, stain, and examine. Repeat for each capillary tube.

If the microhematocrit tube contains heparin anticoagulant, there will be a tendency for white cell and platelet agglutination, a more intense blue–purple staining quality of the white cells, and an orange–red coloration of the red cells.

Evaluation of a Buffy Coat Preparation

The well-made buffy coat preparation should be representative of the general population of nucleated cells in a blood sample. However, because of the manipulations of the specimen and centrifugation, an accurate differential count cannot be made. Likewise, mature red cell morphology cannot be evaluated, and platelets cannot be quanti-

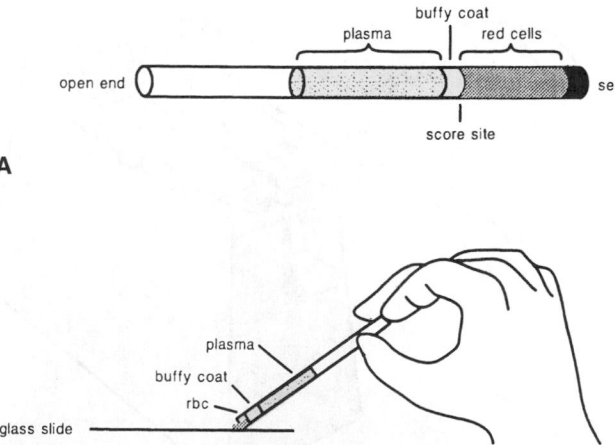

FIGURE 3-11. Microhematocrit technique for buffy coat preparation. (**A**) After centrifugation, the capillary tube is scored just below the buffy coat layer. (**B**) Remaining red cells, buffy coat, and a small amount of plasma are gently expressed onto a clean glass slide. They are mixed and spread.

tated. A report of the buffy coat preparation should include a description of the predominant populations of leukocytes and notation of the presence of any immature or abnormal nucleated cells, nuclei, or extraneous cellular findings. In cases of leukopenia or even with a normal leukocyte count, a few minutes of careful examination of a buffy coat preparation allows one to review many times the number of nucleated cells seen in a routine examination of a blood film, and abnormalities are more likely to be discovered. When examining an ordinary wedge film, it is advantageous to carefully observe the side edges and the feathered end, because immature and abnormal leukocytes and nucleated red cells may collect in these areas.

Rare immature neutrophilic cells (metamyelocytes and myelocytes) and megakaryocytic nuclear fragments[14] may be found in a buffy coat preparation of a healthy individual. Monocytes often are concentrated selectively, and large clusters of monocytes may be found on buffy coat preparations. Nucleated red cells are not present in normal adults.

In addition, if the blood specimen anticoagulated with EDTA is at least 1 hour old, morphologic distortions may be more pronounced on buffy coat preparations than on direct blood films. Smudge cells and necrotic (dead) cells may be more numerous.

Cytocentrifuged Buffy Coat

The cytocentrifuge[1,50] has been used primarily to concentrate nucleated cells in body fluid specimens, although there are at least two reports of its use for buffy coat preparations.[12,15] Some laboratories are experimenting with the methodologies, but no evaluations have been published. One procedure[12] includes one or two concentrations using a Wintrobe tube as described above, the addition of normal (0.85%) saline and 22% bovine albumin to the concentrated buffy coat, and cytocentrifugation (Chap. 30). A balance between too much saline (too dilute) and too much albumin (dark cells with artifactual pseudopods) must be worked out for each sample. Another unpublished experimental technique entails incubation with erythrocyte-lysing agents before cytocentrifugation. As with the body fluid cytocentrifuged preparations, morphologic distortions (nuclear indentations and segmentation, localized or prominent cytoplasmic granulation, vacuolization) are introduced. Buffy coat cytocentrifuge methods will undoubtedly become refined in the future.

ARTIFACTS OF BLOOD FILM PREPARATION

Most blood films are prepared from EDTA-anticoagulated samples. Assuming proper anticoagulant to blood ratios, cellular morphology in fresh samples is well preserved.[45] Normal cells continue to demonstrate satisfactory morphology for at least 5 hours.[19,27] However, reactive and pathologic cells may assume changes within an hour that render them difficult to identify with certainty.[49] Storage at room temperature may accelerate these changes.[27]

Monocytes demonstrate immediate alteration in EDTA samples. Vacuolization is usual (see Fig. 3-12). Reactive (variant) lymphocytes quickly develop vacuolated (Swiss cheese) cytoplasm and convoluted or clover leaf nuclei (Fig. 3-12*E* and *F*) similar to pathologic blast cells (Fig. 3-12*C*). Toxic neutrophils may become vacuolated (autophagocytosis). Necrobiotic or dead leukocytes (Fig. 3-12*D*) are more frequent if there is a delay in making the blood film, especially in samples containing reactive and pathologic cells, and it is important not to mistake them for nucleated red cells. Red–purple cytoplasmic granulation in neutrophils is helpful in making the distinction. Some necrobiotic cells have multiple round nuclear fragments or prominent vacuoles.

Normal erythrocytes retain their size, color, and shape for at least 6 hours, after which a few may take on a spiculated or crenated appearance. In day-old blood, crenated red cells are frequent, and spherocytes are conspicuous (Fig. 3-12*A*). Abnormal erythrocytes may begin to manifest a spiculated appearance within an hour of blood collection, and within 2 to 4 hours this change may be significant. Coarse basophilic stippling and Döhle bodies may disappear on standing in EDTA-anticoagulated blood.[4]

Platelet distribution, size, and granules are affected by EDTA. Platelets are more uniformly distributed on an EDTA blood film than on one made from capillary (skin puncture) or needle point blood. However, platelets tend to swell and become spherical, and their granules spread, with consequent lighter staining than is usual on capillary blood films. Platelet autoagglutinins have been reported to cause platelet clumping in the presence of EDTA.[20,30,51] Satellitism, the tendency for platelets to adhere to neutrophils in EDTA (see Fig. 3-13),[3,21,43] is falsely interpreted as thrombocytopenia by particle counters and can be recognized only by visual film evaluation.

Wedge-type films prepared from day-old EDTA-anticoagulated blood will show distribution defects, with many nucleated cells being carried to the feathered or tail area (see Fig. 3-14). It is not possible to evaluate such samples accurately.

Slow air drying of a freshly prepared blood film can cause drying or moisture red-cell artifact, a hairy appearance of the cytoplasm of normal lymphocytes,[42] and shrinkage of normal leukocytes. Drying artifact may render red cells falsely hypochromic; however, the sharp rather than gradual transition between the hemoglobinized rim and the clear center is helpful in identifying this artifact (see Fig. 3-15). Sometimes the periphery of the cell has a crenated or moth-eaten appearance. This drying artifact may have any of several causes:

Severe anemia, in which excessive amounts of plasma cause poor drying, regardless of the technique
Preparing the blood film in a humid environment
An inadequate fixation period; may be avoided by pre-fixing the smears
Water contamination of the fixative or staining solution[5]
Excess buffer in the stain solution

The area of the blood film may affect leukocyte morphology. In thin areas a glass effect enhances their spreading.

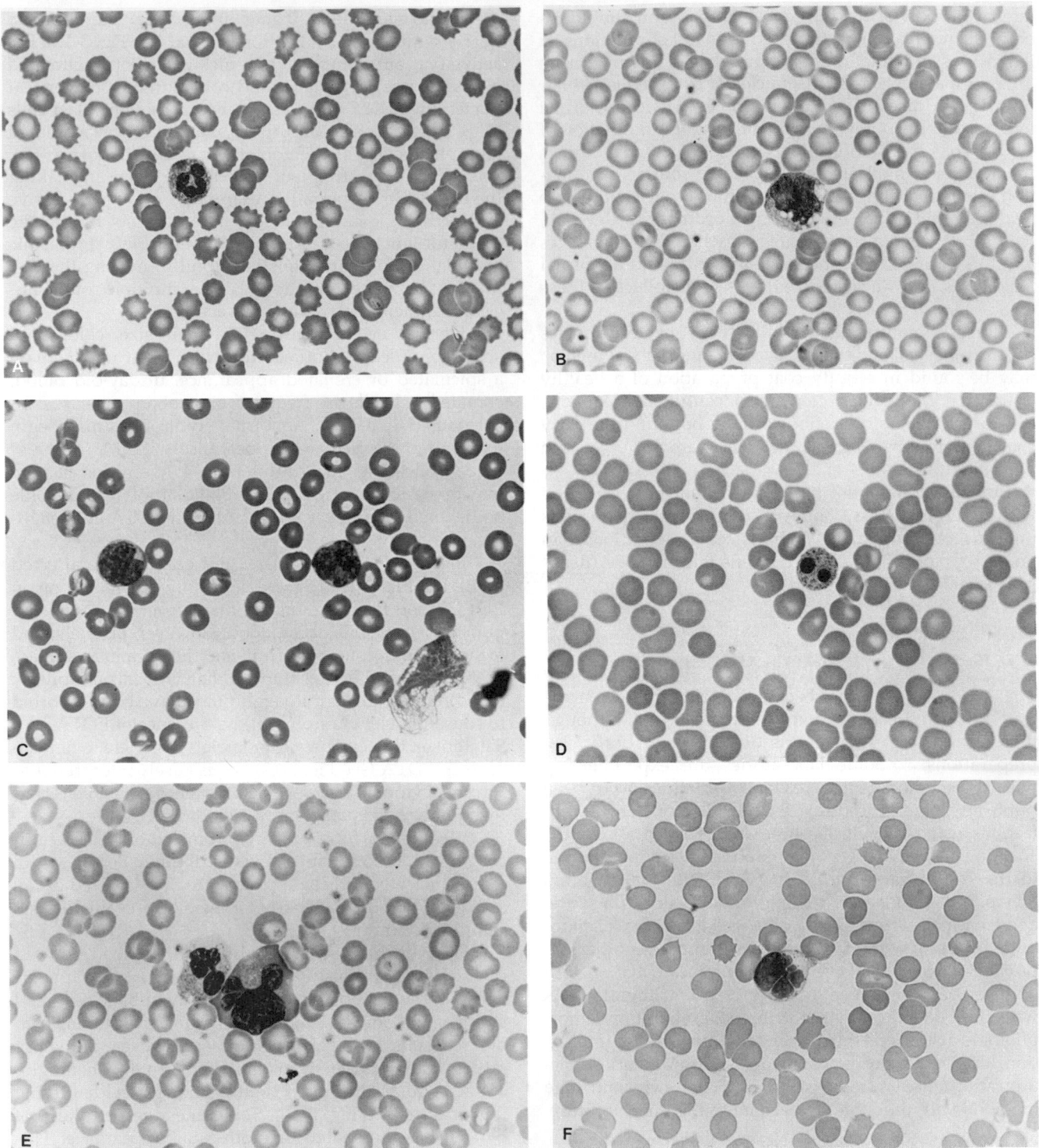

FIGURE 3-12. Morphologic alterations resulting from storage of blood in EDTA. **(A)** Red cells crenate after 6 hours. **(B)** Monocytes vacuolate within a few minutes. **(C)** Blast forms may acquire highly contorted nuclei. **(D)** Cells may die (necrotic neutrophils) after a few hours. **(E)** Variant (atypical) lymphocytes may become vacuolated. **(F)** Their nuclei may become contorted so that they might resemble blasts as depicted in C.

In thick areas increased plasma causes shrinkage, and leukocytes remain three-dimensional with less cytoplasm.[8,49]

Even in a well-prepared wedge-type blood film, a few disintegrated or "smudge" cells will be found (see Color Plate 37-1). Smudge cells represent leukocytes rup-

tured during preparation of the blood film. Because these smudge cells were intact before blood film preparation, their counterparts were included as leukocytes in the automated cell count. When the smudge cell number is noticeably increased (more than 20 per 100 leukocytes), they should be reported in the manual leukocyte differen-

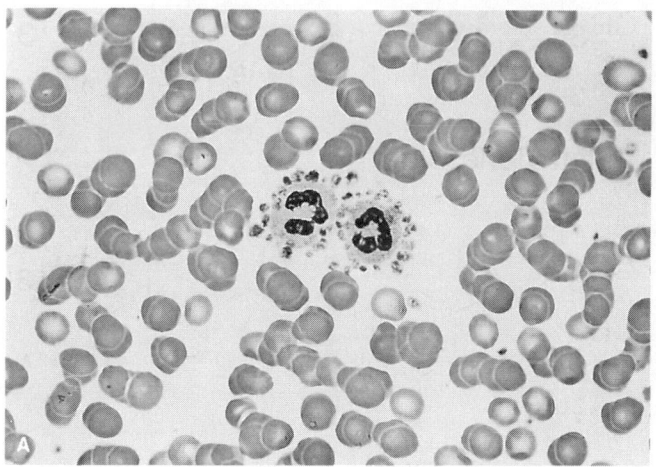
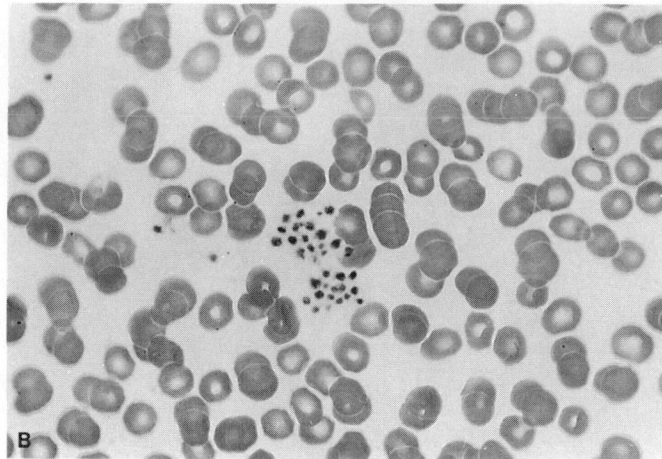

FIGURE 3-13. Artifacts of platelet on blood films. (**A**) Satellitism. (**B**) Clumping.

tial count as the number per 100 leukocytes. The addition of one drop of 22% albumin to five drops of whole blood before blood film preparation reduces the number of smudge cells.[11] Ruptured granulocytes often are surrounded by scattered granules, making their identification possible. Ruptured lymphocytes generally show only a smudged, amorphous nucleus with the cytoplasm dissolved in the background plasma. Nuclear remnants having an expanded, loosely woven network appearance are sometimes called "basket cells." Immature damaged cells may retain a blue-staining nucleolus.

STAINING THE BLOOD FILM
Romanowsky Stains

Romanowsky stains are composed of methylene blue, oxidative products of methylene blue (azures; see Fig. 3-16), and eosin dyes. Wright or Wright-Giemsa polychrome stains have been the most commonly used modifications of Romanowsky stains in the United States. Other types that are more popular elsewhere are the Leishman, May–Grünwald, and Jenner stains, all named for their developers. Modifications differ in the ratios of dye components and the manufacturing methods used to oxidize the methylene blue.* Romanowsky stains may be used in combination with Giemsa, which contains azure dyes, to intensify nuclear features or azurophilic and toxic granulation. Alone, Giemsa is inadequate for staining red cells, platelets, and leukocyte cytoplasm.

Cells must first be fixed to the slide with chemically pure, acetone-free methanol alone or in solution with the dye; no staining occurs during this step. After fixation, addition of a buffer solution changes the pH of the solution and ionizes the reactants to initiate the pH-dependent staining process. In general the acidic cellular elements such as nucleoproteins, nucleic acids, and certain cytoplasmic proteins react with the basic dyes, methylene blue and its oxidation products and stain variations of blue. The term *basophilic* is used for these acidic elements and

---

* *For information, see references 25, 26, 28, 31–33, 36, 37, 39, 44, 46, 47, and 57.*

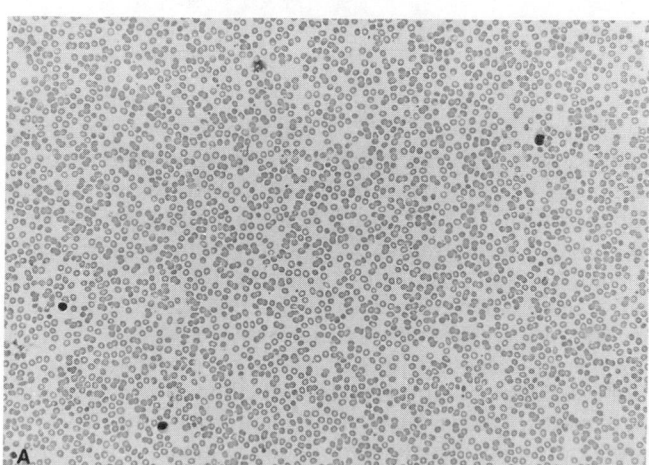
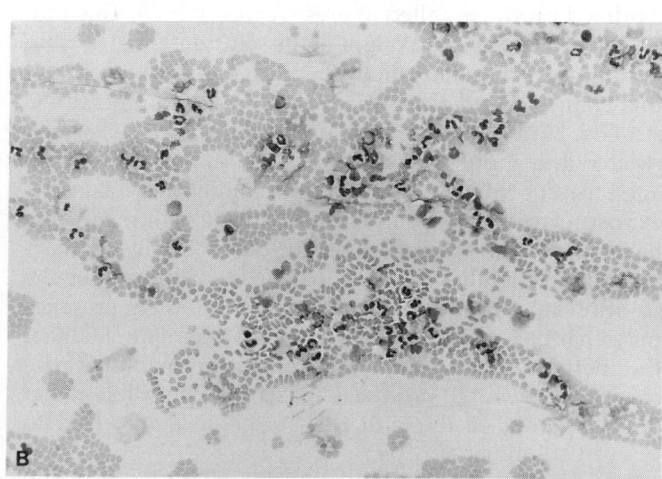

FIGURE 3-14. Day-old specimen with increased leukocyte count. (**A**) Examination area. Note that there are only three intact leukocytes and one broken leukocyte. (**B**) Feather edge. Note excessive accumulation of cells. Poor distribution such as this could lead to falsely low leukocyte estimates and to falsely high lymphocyte percentages in a differential count.

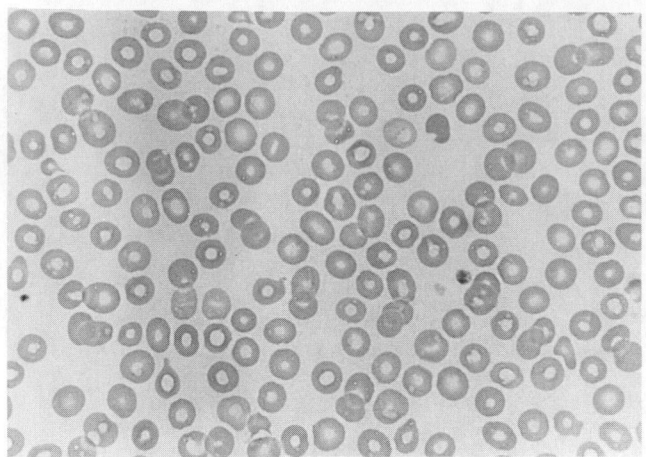

FIGURE 3-15. Red cells show drying artifact.

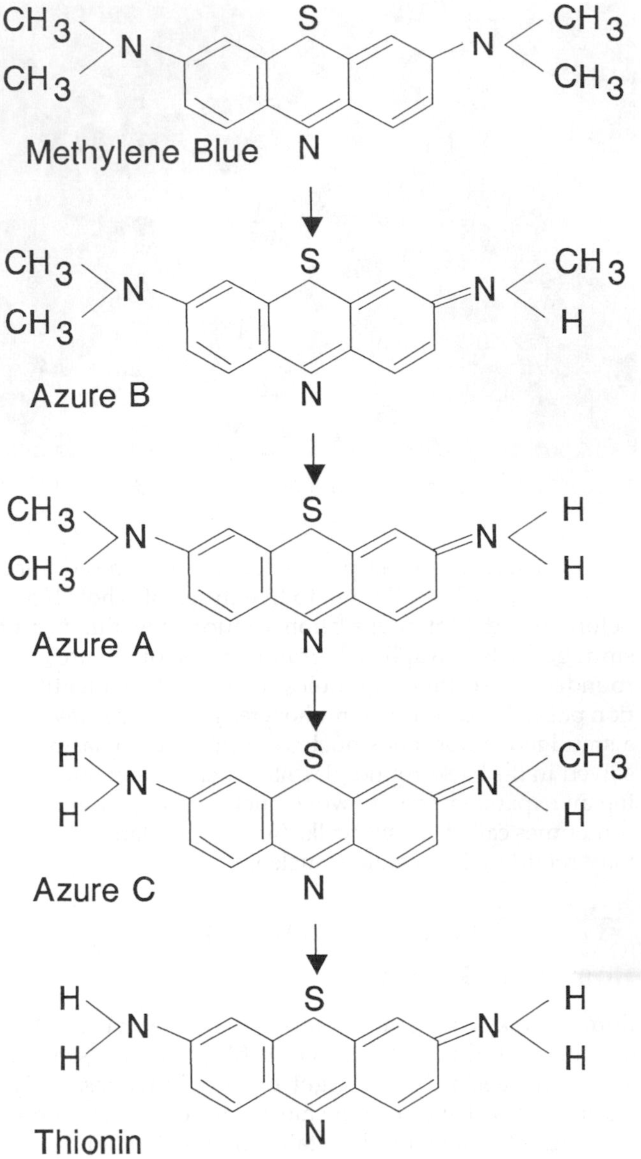

denotes their affinity or "love" (Greek, *philic*) for basic dyes. Basic cellular elements such as hemoglobin molecules in red cells and some cytoplasmic constituents in leukocytes react with the acidic dye eosin, and stain a variation of orange–red. They may be called *acidophilic* or *eosinophilic*.

The term *neutrophil* was coined to denote that cell's neutral staining characteristics between vivid acidic (red) and basic (blue) colors. Some cellular organelles display blended shades of color, such as purple, representing combinations of acidic and basic molecular groups. Azures (Fig. 3-16) produce red–purple staining and are important for their ability to color primary or nonspecific granules in most myeloid cells, hence the term *azurophilic granules*.

Romanowsky dyes have always been capricious. In the past, the best test for the quality of each stain lot was a trial run with different buffers and timings. Recent sophisticated analytical methods permit more exacting analysis of the constituent dye elements. As shown in Figure 3-16, demethylation (removal of −CH₃ groups) of methylene blue in alcoholic solution produces various oxidized products called azures (A through C). This process continues as the Wright stain solution ages, causing variation in the stain quality. Refrigeration will inhibit this change,[10] and some manufacturers recommend 4°C storage. However, other blends of stains may be harmed by cold and should be stored at room temperature. Package inserts provide storage recommendations. Likewise, exposure to winter temperature during shipment may have adverse effects on stain solutions.[2,23] Some manufacturers add metallic elements to act as stabilizers for the solution to extend its shelf life,[16,23,32] but their presence may change the stain quality. The replacement of 50% of the methanol by glycerol will retard the oxidative process[24–26]; however, it produces a viscous stain solution that does not mix easily with the buffer and may lead to uneven staining.

Research on the "Romanowsky–Giemsa effect" by several investigators has provided an empiric basis for standardization of the Romanowsky-type stains. Methylene blue's prime function is to provide its oxidative prod-

FIGURE 3-16. Oxidation of methylene blue and the sequential oxidation products.

ucts, the azures. Azure B is superior to the other azure stains. New polychrome stains composed of measured amounts of pure azure B and eosin Y have been developed.[22,34,35,37,38,40,55,56] Because oxidation is complete in these solutions and extraneous dyes and elements are eliminated, standardized stain quality is achieved. Despite the advances in manufacturing and testing, it is still advisable to test every new stain solution.

Several fast or "quickie" stains have been developed for use in stat situations and small laboratories. Although adequate for assessing normal cell morphology, they generally are unsatisfactory for the evaluation of abnormal cells. The fixation period is short, which causes poor penetration of the stain, and the short stain exposure may produce unusual color tones. In addition, there is much variability from film to film.

Manual Staining Methods

Two types of manual methods are common: rack and dip.

RACK METHOD

The rack method uses rods overlying a sink or dish that hold glass slides in a horizontal position during staining (see Fig. 3-17*A*). Small rubber corks set inside a dish can be used when staining coverslip preparations (Fig. 3-17*B*).

Technique

1. Films should be air dried for several minutes.
2. Wright stain solution is spread over the slide with a dropping bottle or pipette until the top surface is flooded. The edges of the slide should not touch other slides to prevent stain runoff. Fixation of the cells to the slide takes place because of the alcoholic base of the stain solution. A *minimum* of 1 minute is required for proper fixation assuming a thin film with normal or a decreased cell count. Specimens with greatly elevated leukocyte counts or bone marrow preparations require longer fixation times.
3. An equal amount of dilute phosphate buffer is added to each slide. The pH of the buffer will affect the quality of staining, the optimum being between pH 6.4 and 6.8. The buffer–stain solution is mixed gently by blowing on it. A greenish metallic sheen indicates the proper stain : buffer ratio. Stain for 4 to 6 minutes (depending on laboratory preference and experience with that particular stain).
4. The staining mixture is flushed thoroughly from the slide with a stream of distilled or deionized water until all stain is removed. Do not overwash. The pH of the wash water must be neutral to avoid changing the coloration of the stain.
5. The stain residue is cleaned off the back of the slide with laboratory tissue or gauze, and the specimen is air dried.

Although most laboratories buy commercially prepared Wright stain solution, it can be prepared manually by mixing 1 g of biologically certified Wright powder per 500 mL of chemically pure, acetone-free methanol. The stain is incubated for 1 week at 37°C and then at room or refrigerator temperature. Incubation can be shortened

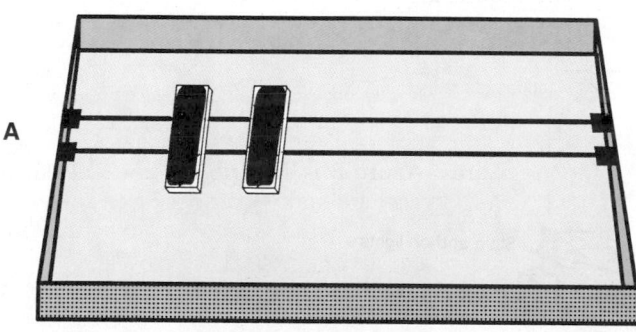

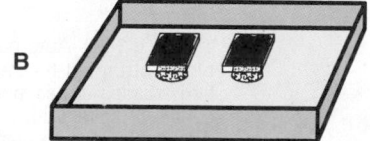

FIGURE 3-17. Rack method for manual staining of blood films. (**A**) Parallel rods accommodate 3 × 1-inch glass slides. (**B**) Rubber corks are used for staining coverslip preparations.

considerably by adding 0.1 g of Giemsa powder per 500 mL of stain. Polyethylene bottles may be more stable than glass for stain storage. Aging may cause lighter, less intense staining of cells, although the color balance generally remains the same. The stain should be filtered prior to use.

Buffer solutions may be made by dissolving commercially prepared buffer salts or tablets in distilled or deionized water. They may also be prepared by combining monobasic potassium phosphate and dibasic sodium phosphate in distilled water according to the desired pH. Specific directions for making phosphate buffers are available in various chemistry manuals. The final solution pH should be checked with a pH meter.

The rack method is very cost effective for a small number of slides because it uses a minimum of stain solution per slide. One or several slides may be stained simultaneously. The disadvantages of the rack method include vulnerability to precipitate (blue–black granules or filaments on the blood film), the time involved, and the inconsistency in staining quality related to variances in the amounts of stain and buffer per slide and the timing per step.

DIP (INCUBATION) METHOD

Several dishes (large enough to contain a portable slide holder and an adequate amount of solution to cover the slides) are required. A method developed by this author has proven to be very satisfactory and reliable for more than 15 years.

Technique

1. The blood films are fixed for 1 to 2 minutes in a dish with anhydrous, chemically pure methanol. The basket holding the slides should be completely dry to avoid water contamination.
2. The slides are transferred to a dish containing undiluted Wright stain for 4 minutes.
3. The slides are transferred to another dish with 75 mL of Wright stain and 325 mL of buffer (pH 6.4) for 4 minutes.
4. The blood films are then transferred to a dish with 20 to 25 mL of Giemsa solution and 200 mL of deionized water for 4 minutes.
5. The slides are rinsed briefly in two dishes of distilled water and air dried.

The advantages of this method are greater consistency in staining quality, better penetration of the stain with more vivid colors and less precipitate, cost effectiveness for a large number of slides, and effective adaptability to an automated dip method. The disadvantages are the time necessary to prepare the stain solutions and transfer the slides from dish to dish and the limited stability (4 hours maximum) of the Wright-buffer and Giemsa stain solutions, making the method expensive for small numbers of films.

Automated Staining Methods

PLATEN TYPE

The Ames Hema-Tek Slide Stainer[1] represents the platen type of stainer. Glass slides are placed on a platen with the blood film side down and moved by a spiral conveyer through a polychrome methylene blue–eosin solution, a buffer solution, and a rinse solution, each of which is delivered from commercially prepared reagent packs through pump tubing (see Fig. 3-18).

CAROUSEL TYPE

Another instrument is the Aerospray Hematology Slide Stainer (Wescor, Inc., Logan, UT).[54] This instrument sprays a measured amount of stain reagents onto the blood films as they are transported in a rotating carousel. Details of its operation are available from the manufacturer.

The advantages of the platen and automated carousel stainers include the following:

They are time saving. Once the slides are loaded into the instrument, the operator can walk away, and staining time is less than 10 minutes.

Stain quality is consistent from film to film.

Since small amounts of stain reagents are used compared with other staining techniques, the cost is lower.

Stat films may be added and stained at any time with the Hema-Tek Slide Stainer.

The disadvantages include the following:

High maintenance is required. The platen must be kept clean to prevent precipitation of the dyes onto blood films. Tubing must be checked daily for precipitate and changed at least every 3 months.

The short fixation time often necessitates prefixation of films in methanol, especially when leukocyte counts are markedly increased.

Stain reagents must be purchased and may be more expensive than "home-made." They are also subject to problems caused by shipping conditions such as freezing or heat that may affect the quality of staining.[2,10] In addition the manufacturing process is not reproducible from lot to lot, creating variances in color tones and the propensity for dye precipitation.

The instruments are not versatile relative to modifying the amount of stain delivered, the pH of the buffer, and the rinse and the timing for each step.

Incorporation of Giemsa stain to enhance coloration of the nucleus and granules is not possible unless a package with Giemsa is purchased. Toxic and basophilic granules may not be stained if Giemsa is not added to the stain system.

Slides must be completely clean and not warped to obtain even staining on the platen-type instrument.

The Aerospray instrument uses stain solutions for a full carousel (12 slides) regardless of the the number of slides present, which reduces its cost effectiveness.

Stat films cannot be introduced into the Aerospray's carousel once it has begun the staining cycle.

DIP-TYPE INSTRUMENTS

Several automated instruments use dip or immersion staining techniques similar to those of traditional histology staining. Batches of films are moved from dish to dish at programmed time intervals (see Fig. 3-19). The advantages include the following:

Walk-away instruments conserve operator time.

There is more versatility in the type and number of staining solutions, time per step, pH of the buffer and rinse solutions, and the ability to make stain reagents rather than purchasing them.

If staining solutions are replaced regularly, quality of the staining is standardized.

Stain penetration is better and coloration of cellular elements is more intense, especially if Giemsa is added.

There is less chance of precipitate than on platen-type stainers.

The disadvantages of dip-type instruments include the following:

Staining of slides is lengthier than on platen-type instruments.

More time is required for preparing stain solutions daily or twice daily, since stains have a limited working time.

More expense is incurred, since large amounts of stain are required.

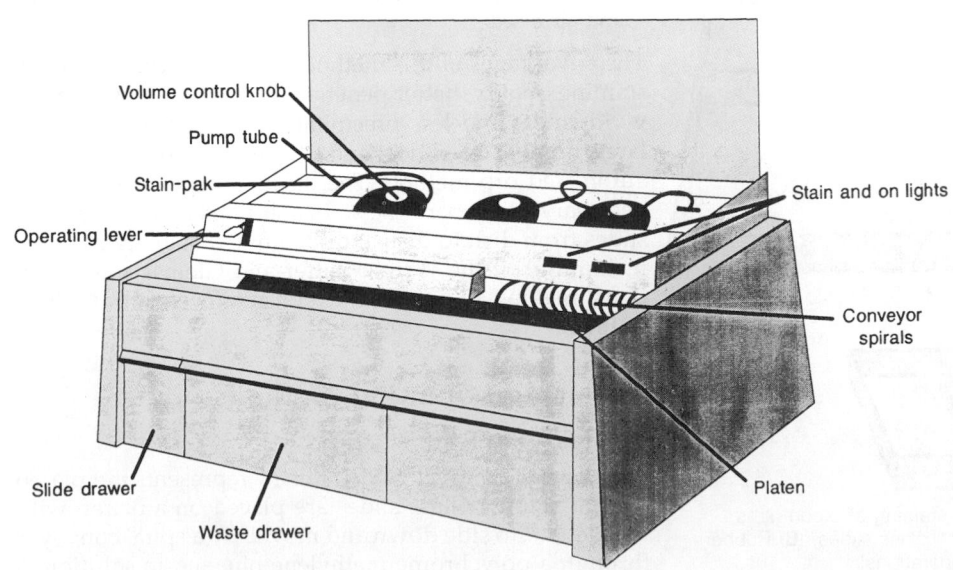

Volume control knob

Pump tube

Stain-pak

Operating lever

Stain and on lights

Conveyor spirals

Slide drawer

Waste drawer

Platen

FIGURE 3-18. Automated, platen-type instrument for staining blood films. Slides are advanced by a conveyor spiral with the blood film side down along a platen. Stain, buffer, and rinse water are pumped up into the space between the blood film and platen.

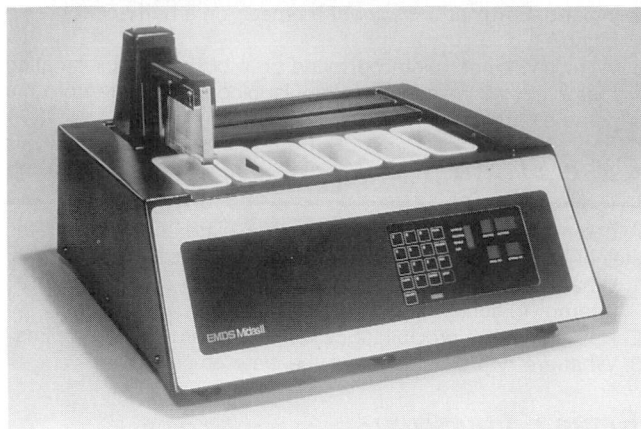

FIGURE 3-19. The Midas II stainer, an automated stainer that uses the dip technique. (Courtesy of EM Diagnostic Systems, Inc, Gibbstown, NJ; Subsidiary of E Merck, Darmstadt, Germany.)

The instruments are unable to accept additional slides (*e.g.*, stats) if a staining cycle has begun.

Criteria for a Good Stain

The well-stained film should be reddish-brown. Microscopically, erythrocytes should be salmon pink, leukocyte nuclei should be purple–blue (depending on maturation), and platelets should have purple–blue to lilac cytoplasm containing red–purple granules. Additional criteria include distinct orange granules in eosinophils (an excellent stain pH indicator), pinkish-tan cytoplasm in neutrophils, and gray, ground-glass cytoplasm with many tiny red–purple granules in monocytes. Causes for deviations in color (the "red and blue stains") are listed in Table 3-1.

TABLE 3-1
Causes of Color Deviations

"Red Stain"

Too acid a buffer or stain solution (pH below 6.4)
Excess buffer for stain solution
Insufficient staining time
Excessive washing
Very thin smear
Contaminants (*e.g.*, chlorine) in wash water
Exposure of buffer or stain solution to acid fumes
Old stain in which methanol has oxidized to fumaric acid

"Blue Stain"

Too alkaline a buffer or stain solution (pH above 6.8)
Too little buffer for stain solution
Excessive staining time
Inadequate washing
Short drying period
Wash water too alkaline
Thick smears
Old smear (dried plasma produces blue background)
Protein abnormality (*e.g.*, multiple myeloma)
Heparin blood sample
Very high leukocyte count with many blasts
Low hematocrit

TROUBLESHOOTING STAIN PROBLEMS

Despite the advances in our knowledge of the action of Romanowsky-type stains and progress in their standardization, staining problems still occur. A few general hints to correct the more general problems are discussed below.

Fixation

Inadequate fixation may result in the blood film being washed off the slide, indistinct nuclear detail, or poor staining of granules, especially in basophils. In addition, water contamination of the fixative may lead to the drying artifact.[5]

Freshly prepared films should be air dried for at least 5 minutes to prevent drying artifact. Glass slides should be clean and clear before use. A haze on the slide may represent material that will interfere with proper fixation or disturb the acid–base balance needed for good-quality staining.

Methanol should be anhydrous and chemically pure, and kept tightly stoppered away from moisture or chemical fumes. Moisture contamination of the Wright stain dissolved in the methanol may create problems. All staining dishes containing alcohol or alcoholic solutions should be kept covered to prevent evaporation and contamination and should be changed as necessary.

The fixation period should be a minimum of 1 minute.

Staining

Stain–buffer solutions have a limited working time, only a few hours. This becomes important in the dip methods. Some laboratories use interval timers to remind them to change the stain–buffer solution.

Tap water is *never* acceptable as a substitute for the buffer because it frequently is too alkaline or too acidic (depending on locale) and because it may contain chlorine. Distilled water often is unreliable because of contaminants in the system, and distilled or deionized water may absorb CO_2 on standing and become too acidic.[17]

For best results, use a staining time at least twice the fixation period.

For the rack method, the amount of buffer should be equal to or slightly greater than the amount of stain solution. Buffer and stain should be well mixed for uniform staining.

Rinse or Wash

Distilled water or a buffered rinse water should be used to wash off the stain. Too vigorous or prolonged washing may dislodge cells from films that were not adequately fixed or cause nuclear clumping or a lightly stained film.

Underwashing may result in a blue film or precipitate.

Drying

Air drying is most satisfactory. Forced rapid drying may alter the color intensities by shortening the exposure time to the wash water, because the red spectrum of colors continues to develop as long as the cellular elements are wet.

Stain Precipitate

Multiple blue–black granules or filamentous material overlying cellular and noncellular areas on the blood film have several possible causes:

Precipitated stain powder may be in the stain solution. Filtration should remove this material.

A dirty or scratched platen with accumulated dried stain, precipitate in the stain pack, or too little stain pumped onto the film will result in precipitate. Stain complexes may also precipitate within the instrument tubing. Replacement of tubing at regular intervals will alleviate this problem.

When using the rack method, evaporation or uneven spread of stain solution will result in precipitate on the slide. This may be caused by insufficient stain, unevenness of the rods on which the slides are placed, or placement of slides too close together, causing stain runoff.

The slides may be dirty.

Precipitate may be removed in either of the following ways. Redissolve the precipitate with additional stain by covering the film with Wright stain for 5 to 10 seconds and flushing with distilled or deionized water. Or, dip the slide three or four times in a solution of 30% ethanol in distilled water and air dry.

CHAPTER SUMMARY

Most hematology laboratories in this country produce blood films using manual techniques. Of the two available manual techniques the wedge or spreader-slide is more popular. At the time of this writing only the Autoprep is available for purchase for automating the blood film technique, and it possesses the advantages and disadvantages of the manual wedge preparation. The chief inherent error of the wedge-type preparation (both manual and automated) is poor distribution of leukocytes, which is directly related to the speed and thinness of the preparation.

A poorly made or poorly stained blood film, whether prepared manually or by automated instruments, is useless. It may, in fact, be the source of grave errors in diagnosis, patient monitoring, and quality control. A properly made and stained blood film requires skill and practice. This chapter has described the proper procedures and techniques and has discussed the problems and their solutions.

Case Study 3-1

A 53-year-old female presented to her physician with symptoms of anemia. Laboratory data included a leukocyte count of 1.8×10^9/L; erythrocyte count of 2.61×10^{12}/L; hemoglobin 11.6 g/dL; hematocrit 0.32 L/L; MCV 122 fL; MCH 44 pg; MCHC 36g/dL; RDW 22%; and, platelet count 155×10^9/L.

The physician suspected megaloblastic anemia and wanted to know if megaloblastic red cell precursors or hypersegmented neutrophils were present.

1. What is the best blood preparation for answering the physician's question?

2. What determinations *cannot* be made on a buffy coat preparation?

3. What cell types might be found on a buffy coat preparation that might not be seen on a regular blood film made from the same sample?

Case Study 3-2

A batch of blood films stained with a platen-type automated stainer are found to have excessive precipitate.

1. What maintenance procedures should be performed in an attempt to solve the problem?

2. How might the precipitate be removed from the blood films?

3. What are two advantages of the platen-type stainer?

Review Questions

3-1. The coverslip method for making blood films has the following advantage(s):

A. ease of storage
B. superior leukocyte distribution
C. specific area to look for unusual cells
D. all of the above

3-2. When making a blood film using the spreader-slide technique, a thinner film can be obtained by

A. increasing the angle of the spreader slide.
B. using a larger drop of blood.
C. spreading the blood at a slower speed.
D. all of the above.

3-3. An accumulation of leukocytes in the feathered end of a wedge-type blood film could be due to

A. the anticoagulant.
B. spreading the blood too slowly.
C. spreading only part of the blood drop.
D. all of the above.

3-4. The two leukocyte types that are most vulnerable to a delay in making a blood film after the blood has been collected into an EDTA tube are

A. neutrophils and lymphocytes.
B. eosinophils and basophils.
C. lymphocytes and monocytes.
D. neutrophils and eosinophils.

3-5. A basket cell is a type of

A. monocyte.
B. poorly stained red cell.
C. platelet.
D. damaged leukocyte.

3-6. Giemsa is added to Wright stain in order to increase the concentration of

A. methylene blue.
B. acid dyes.
C. azures.
D. eosin.

References

1. Ames Division, Miles Laboratories, Elkhart, IN 46515
2. Baer DM: Slide stainer problems. Med Lab Observ, August 1986
3. Bauer HM: *In vitro* platelet–neutrophil adherence. Am J Clin Pathol 63:824, 1975
4. Ben-Bassat I, Brok-Simoni F, Kende G et al: A family with red cell pyrimidine 5-nucleotidase deficiency. Blood 47:919, 1976

5. Bettigole RE: Red cell staining artifacts and how to avoid them. N Engl J Med 271:1156, 1964

6. Bose R, Jorgensen WK, Dalgesh RJ et al: Current state and future trends in the diagnosis of babesiosis. Vet Parasitol 57:61 1995

7. Cayatte SM, McManus PM, Miller WH Jr et al: Identification of mast cells in buffy coat preparations from dogs with inflammatory skin diseases. J Am Vet Med Assoc 206:325, 1995

8. Cuadra M: The spreading of leukocytes released from their liquid environment. Blut 37:95, 1978

9. Dacie JV, Lewis SM: Practical Haematology, 7th ed. New York, Churchill Livingstone, 1991

10. Dean WW, Stastny M, Lubrano GJ: The degradation of Romanowsky-type blood stains in methanol. Stain Technol 52:35, 1977

11. Densmore CM: Eliminating disintegrated cells on hematologic smears. Lab Med 12:640, 1981

12. DeNunzio J: Preparation of buffy coats from blood samples with extremely low white cell counts. Lab Med 16:497, 1985

13. Deol I, Hernandez AM, Pierre RV: Ethylenediamine tetraacetic acid-associated leukoagglutination. Am J Clin Pathol 103:338, 1995

14. Efrati P, Rosenszajn L: The morphology of buffy coat in normal human adults. Blood 16:1012, 1960

15. Garnet RF, Atkinson BF, Bonner H et al: Rapid screening for lupus erythematosus cells using cytocentrifuge-prepared buffy coat monolayers. Am J Clin Pathol 67:537, 1977

16. Gilliland JHW, Dean WW, Stastny M et al: Stabilized Romanowsky blood stain. Stain Technol 54:141, 1979

17. Green FJ: Getting more uniform results from biological stains. Lab Manage, Nov 1969

18. Gyllensward C: Some sources of error at differential count of white corpuscles in blood-stained smears. Acta Paediatr (suppl II) 8:1, 1929

19. Kennedy JB, Machara KT, Baker AM: Cell and platelet stability in disodium and trisodium EDTA. Am J Med Technol 47:89, 1981

20. Kjeldsberg CR, Hershgold EJ: Spurious thrombocytopenia. JAMA 227:628, 1974

21. Kjeldsberg CR, Swanson J: Platelet satellitism. Blood 43:831, 1974

22. Lapen D: A standardized differential stain for hematology. Cytometry 2:309, 1982

23. Liao JC, Ponzo JL, Patel C: Improved stability of methanolic Wright's stain with additive reagents. Stain Technol 56:251, 1981

24. Lillie RD: Blood and malaria parasite staining with eosin azure methylene blue methods. Am J Public Health 33:948 1943

25. Lillie RD: Factors influencing the Romanowsky staining of blood films and the role of methylene violet. J Lab Clin Med 29:1181, 1944

26. Lillie RD: The deterioration of Romanowsky stain solutions in various organic solvents. Publ Health Rep (suppl) 178:1, 1944

27. Lloyd E: The deterioration of leukocyte morphology with time: Its effect on the differential count. Lab Perspect 1:13, 1982

28. Lubrano GJ, Dean WW, Heinsohn HG et al: The analysis of some commercial dyes and Romanowsky stains by high performance liquid chromatography. Stain Technol 52:13, 1977

29. MacGregor RGS, Richards W, Loh GL: The differential leukocyte count. J Pathol Bacteriol 51:337, 1940

30. Manthorpe R, Kofod B, Wiik A et al: Pseudothrombocytopenia: *In vitro* studies on the underlying mechanisms. Scand J Haematol 26:385, 1981

31. Marshall PN, Lewis SM: Batch variations in commercial dyes employed for Romanowsky-type staining: A thin layer chromatographic study. Stain Technol 49:351, 1974

32. Marshall PN, Lewis SM: Metal contaminants in commercial thiazine dyes. Stain Technol 50:143, 1975

33. Marshall PN, Bentley SA, Lewis SM: An evaluation of some commercial Romanowsky stains. J Clin Pathol 28:680, 1975

34. Marshall PN, Bentley SA, Lewis SM: A standardized Romanowsky stain prepared from purified dyes. J Clin Pathol 28:920, 1975

35. Marshall PN: Methylene blue–azure B–eosin as a substitute for May Grünwald–Giemsa and Jenner–Giemsa stains. Microsc Acta 79:153, 1977

36. Marshall PN: Romanowsky-type stains in haematology. Histochem J 10:1, 1978

37. Marshall PN, Bentley SA, Lewis SM: Standardization of Romanowsky stains: The relationship between stain composition and performance. Scand J Haematol 20:206, 1978

38. Marshall PN, Bentley SA, Lewis SM: Staining properties and stability of a standardized Romanowsky stain. J Clin Pathol 31:280, 1978

39. Marshall PN: Romanowsky staining: State of the art and "ideal" techniques. In Koepke JA (ed): Differential Leukocyte Counting. Skokie, IL, College of American Pathologists, 1979

40. Marshall PN, Galbraith WG, Navarro EF et al: Microspectrophotometric studies of Romanowsky stained blood cells. J Microscopy 124:197, 1981

41. National Committee for Clinical Laboratory Standards: Reference Leukocyte Differential Count (Proportional) and Evaluation of Instrumental Methods; Approved Guideline. H-20. Villanova, PA, NCCLS, 1992

42. Nguyen DT, Moskowitz FB, Diamond LW: Potential diagnostic pitfalls caused by blood film artifacts in prolymphocytic leukaemia. Observations in two cases. Br J Biomed Sci 51:371, 1994

43. Payne CM: Platelet satellitism: An ultrastructural study. Am J Pathol 103:116, 1981

44. Power KT: The Romanowsky stains: A review. Am J Med Technol 48:519, 1982

45. Robertson GW, Maxwell MH: Importance of optimal mixtures of EDTA anticoagulant: Blood for the preparation of well stained avian blood smears. Br Poult Sci 34:615, 1993

46. Roe MA, Lillie RD, Wilcox A: American azures in the preparation of satisfactory Giemsa stains for malarial parasites. Public Health Rep 55:1272, 1940

47. Scott BE, French RW: Standardization of biological stains. Military Surg 55:229, 1924

48. Shafer JA, Stein BL: Blood smear observations: Workshop manual. New York, University of Rochester, 1975

49. Shafer JA: Artifactual alterations in phagocytes in the blood smear. Am J Med Technol 48:507, 1982

50. Shandon Inc, Pittsburgh, PA 15275

51. Shreiner DP, Bell WR: Pseudothrombocytopenia: Manifestation of a new type of platelet agglutinin. Blood 42:541, 1973

52. Stein BL, Shafer JA: A blood smear pusher. ESAMT Technol J 8:11, 1962

53. Stiene–Martin EA: Causes for poor leukocyte distribution in manual spreader-slide blood films. Am J Med Technol 46:624, 1980

54. Wescor, Inc, 459 South Main Street, Logan, UT 84321

55. Wittekind DH, Kretschmer V, Sohmer I: Azure B–eosin Y stain as the standard Romanowsky–Giemsa stain. Br J Haematol 51:391, 1982

56. Wittekind DH: On the nature of Romanowsky–Giemsa staining and its signficance for cytochemistry and histochemistry: An overall view. Histochem J 15:1029, 1983

57. Woronzoff-Dashkoff KP: The Erlich–Chenzinsky–Plehn–Malachowski–Romanowsky–Nocht–Jenner–May–Grünwald–Leishman–Reuter–Wright–Giemsa–Lillie–Roe–Wilcox stain. The mystery unfolds. Clin Lab Med 13:759, 1993

CHAPTER 4

Basic Microscopy in Hematology

Barbara A. Smith Michael
Sherry Martin
Lois Lucas

Objectives

1. Identify the components of the compound light microscope and describe their function.
2. Compare brightfield, oil immersion, phase contrast, and fluorescence microscopy with respect to principles, applications, and equipment.
3. Describe the steps required to achieve optimum contrast and resolution for the maximum definition of specimen details and perform the Koehler illumination procedure.

There are three basic requirements for accurate identification and enumeration of blood cells and recognition of cellular changes that reflect disease processes: properly collected and processed specimens; an experienced morphologist/hematologist; and a quality optical microscope system that is adjusted and maintained for optimum performance. Adjustment of the microscope's illumination system for optimum specimen contrast and resolution is a prerequisite for accurate image recognition and is crucial when using oil immersion microscopy. To fully utilize the analytical capability of the light microscope, the technologist must have a basic knowledge of the principles of image formation and of microscope components, their function, and correct operation. Unfortunately, "microscope illiteracy" is common.

IMAGE FORMATION IN LIGHT MICROSCOPY— THE ESSENTIALS

Light

THE NATURE OF LIGHT

Light, which is the raw material of light microscopy, is a form of radiant energy. Although it is possible to describe some of light's properties and effects on matter, its true nature is still unclear. If a beam of white light, a mixture of all colors, is passed through a prism or lens, it is split into its component colors. These colors, which can be seen by the eye, comprise the visible spectrum or the wavelengths between 400 and 750 nm.

Light, which is proposed to travel in a manner analogous to waves, can be described by properties such as wavelength, frequency, amplitude, and phase. We can represent a light wave mathematically by a sine curve. *Wavelength*, the distance between corresponding points on adjacent waves, determines what the eye perceives as color. *Frequency*, the number of vibrations or cycles per second of a given light wave, is closely related to wavelength: the shorter the wavelength, the higher the frequency and the greater the amount of radiant energy. Differences in frequency also register on the eye as differences in color. *Amplitude*, the vertical displacement of a wave from the optical axis or equilibrium position, determines the intensity or brightness of an object as it is seen by the eye. *Phase* refers to the point or stage to which a wave has progressed. Waves are "in phase" when the peaks of one wave coincide in position to the peaks of another wave. Phase shifts occur when one light wave is delayed during its travels in relation to another wave. However, the human eye cannot distinguish waves that differ only in phase unless some optical mechanism converts these differences into changes in intensity or color. These topics are discussed in detail in the referenced publications.[1,3]

LIGHT AND IMAGE-FORMING PHENOMENA

Light rays that pass from an optically less dense to an optically more dense medium (*e.g.*, from air to inside a microscope lens) are changed in speed and direction. The optical density of a medium is indicated by its refractive index (RI) or the ratio of the speed of light in air to its speed in the different medium.

Absorption, refraction, diffraction, and interference are some phenomena (effects) which play an important role in the creation of a microscope image. *Absorption* is the reduction in the intensity of light as it is transmitted through a structure. *Refraction* is the change in direction or bending of light rays. *Diffraction* is a deflection of light rays at the interface between small details of the specimen which have different absorption or refraction properties. *Interference* is the effect that two or more light rays from the same source have on one another.

Optical Lens Systems

TYPES OF LENSES

A lens is an optical element composed of glass or other transparent material that is ground and polished to a specific shape.[3,4,6,7,10,13] Eyepieces, objectives, and condensers—the optical components of the microscope—are constructed of lenses in combinations. There are two basic lens types: (1) positive, convex lenses, which cause light rays passing through them to converge or collect to form an image; and (2) negative, concave lenses, which cause parallel light rays to diverge or separate to form an image. Thus, lenses change the direction of entering light rays and also enlarge or reduce the size of a specimen image.

RELATIONSHIP OF RESOLUTION AND NUMERICAL APERTURE

Resolution is the ability of a lens to delineate detail in a specimen. Resolution (R) is determined by two factors: (1) the numerical aperture (NA) or performance rating of a lens for gathering light and (2) the wavelength (λ) of the illuminating light. The relationship of NA and λ to R can be expressed mathematically as:

$$R = \frac{1.2\lambda}{2NA}$$

Resolution is expressed in micrometers (μm) as the smallest distance between two structural elements that can still be visually distinguished from each other rather than seen as only one blurred element. Thus, the smaller the R value, the greater the resolution.

From the equation, it can be inferred that the highest resolution (smallest R value) can be obtained by using short wavelength (*e.g.*, ultraviolet) light. However, in optical light microscopy the effect of wavelength on resolution is not very significant, because a mixture of white light in the visible spectrum between 400 and 700 nanometers (nm) is the primary source of illumination. Therefore, the NA of the objective lens used is of critical importance in determining R. From the equation it is apparent that the higher the NA rating, the smaller the R value and thus the greater the resolution.

When calculating R, the wavelength used is that for green light (550 nm = 0.55 μm), which is the midpoint of the visible spectrum. Note that the same units must be used for R and wavelength. Since R is usually expressed in μm, λ = 0.55 μm is used in the equation. For example, the R value for an objective lens with an NA of 1.25 μm can be calculated as:

$$\frac{1.2 \times 0.55 \,\mu m}{2 \times 1.25 \,\mu m} = 0.26 \,\mu m$$

which means that the lens has the ability to distinguish structural elements as close as 0.26 μm apart (Table 4-1).

NA can also be expressed mathematically as n sine μ. That is, NA is the product of n (the refractive index of the medium in the space between the specimen object and the front lens of the objective) and sine μ (the sine of half the angle of aperture or the cone of light admitted by the lens).

Dry, non-immersion objective lenses are designed to work with air in the "object space" and therefore cannot have a NA greater than 1.00, the refractive index of air. Immersion objectives, which are used for most hematologic observations, must always have an immersion medium (oil) in the space between the objective and the specimen slide. If an air space exists, the NA of the immersion lens is reduced to no more than 1.00, and the effective NA and full resolving power of the objective cannot be achieved (Fig. 4-1). Note that condensers also have NA ratings that indicate light-concentrating ability and should be matched with the objectives used.

LENS ABERRATIONS AND CORRECTION

Aberrations are optical system defects that degrade image quality (*i.e.*, brilliance, contrast, and sharpness). In microscopy there are three important types of defects. *Chromatic aberrations* result in undesired color fringes and poor image definition. *Spherical aberrations* result in poor image definition and loss of contrast. *Field curvature aberrations*

TABLE 4-1
Characteristics of Typical Objective Lenses

Type of Lens	Resolving Power (μm)	Numerical Aperture (NA)	Magnifying Power ($\times$)	Working Distance (mm)
Low power	1.1	0.30	10	9.22
High dry	0.47	0.70	40	0.61
Oil immersion	0.26	1.25	100	0.16

These figures are only approximate; objective lenses of different correction, types, and manufacturers are not identical.

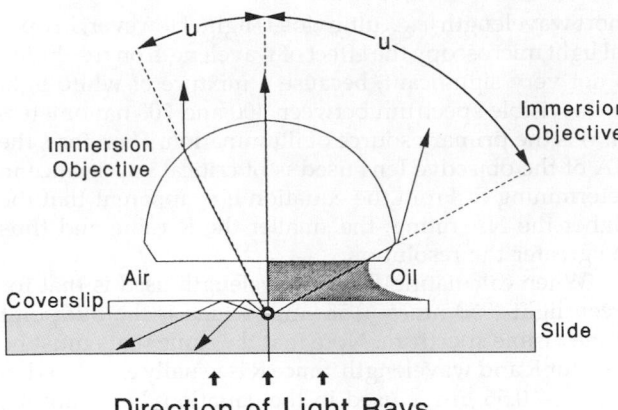

FIGURE 4-1. Principle of oil immersion microscopy. Note gain in numerical aperture and increase in cone of light admitted by lens when oil is used with an immersion objective. (Modified from Mollring FK: Microscopy from the Very Beginning. Thornwood, NY, Carl Zeiss, Inc. 1979, with permission.)

result in a "curved" image of a flat specimen and create an out-of-focus edge while the center of the field is in focus, or *vice versa*.

Correction or minimization of lens defects is achieved by using carefully selected combinations of lens shapes and different types of glass. Achromats, the most common and least expensive type of objectives, partially correct for chromatic and spherical aberrations and are suitable for routine observations. Apochromats, required for critical microscopy and photomicrography, have superior chromatic correction (three-color) and spherical (two-color) correction. Semiapochromats have intermediate correction. Like objectives, condensers are also available with different degrees of optical correction and NA.

Field curvature is a serious problem, particularly in photomicrography. Therefore, plan or flatfield lenses are recommended. In addition, the optimal correction of objective lenses is achieved when they are used with matched or compensating eyepieces. Refer to Figure 4-2 for objective indicators.

THE COMPOUND LIGHT MICROSCOPE

Principle

The compound light microscope is basically two sets of lenses mounted in tandem with one magnifying the image produced by the other and the final enlarged image appearing inverted and laterally reversed.[3,10,13] The objective lens projects an intermediate enlarged image of the specimen inside the focal length of the eyepiece which, in turn, projects a further enlarged image of the object that appears to be located 250 mm from the eye at the level of the specimen stage. This is termed the *virtual* or "mind's eye" image, because it cannot be focused on a screen (see Fig. 4-3).

Basic Components and Function

The basic components of a standard light microscope include eyepieces, binocular eyepiece tube, objectives attached to a revolving nosepiece, mechanical stage, substage condenser, illumination system and base (see Figs. 4-2 and 4-4).[3,6,10,13]

Improvements in optics and ergonomic design have resulted in more user-friendly instruments. Some microscopes feature armrests and a tilting binocular head, which can be adjusted to the viewing angle most comfortable for the individual user.

Magnification

Magnification is the visual enlargement of a specimen image by an optical instrument and is expressed in terms of diameters, power, times, or ×.[4,6,7,10,13] In the compound light microscope the total magnification of an objective/

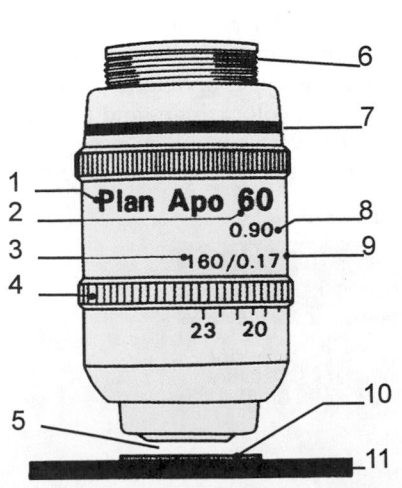

1. Objective type
2. Magnification
3. Mechanical tube length
4. Cover-glass-correction ring (on special objectives)
5. Working distance
6. Screw thread
7. Color code (objective magnification)
8. Numerical aperature (N.A.)
9. Specified cover glass thickness
10. Cover glass
11. Specimen slide
12. Special application marking
13. Immersion objective
14. Immersion marking
15. Immersion oil

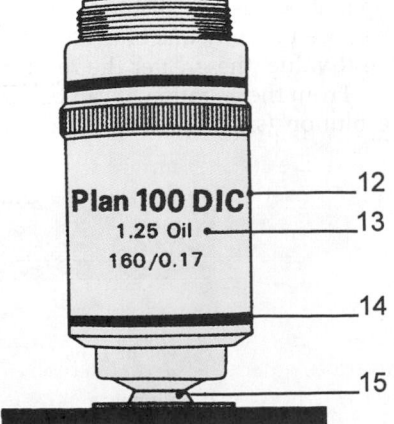

FIGURE 4-2. Objective lens indicators. Letters, numbers, symbols, and color codes inscribed on the lens barrel provide important information for the user. Eyepieces and condensers are similarly marked. (Courtesy of Nikon Inc Instrument Group, Melville, NY.)

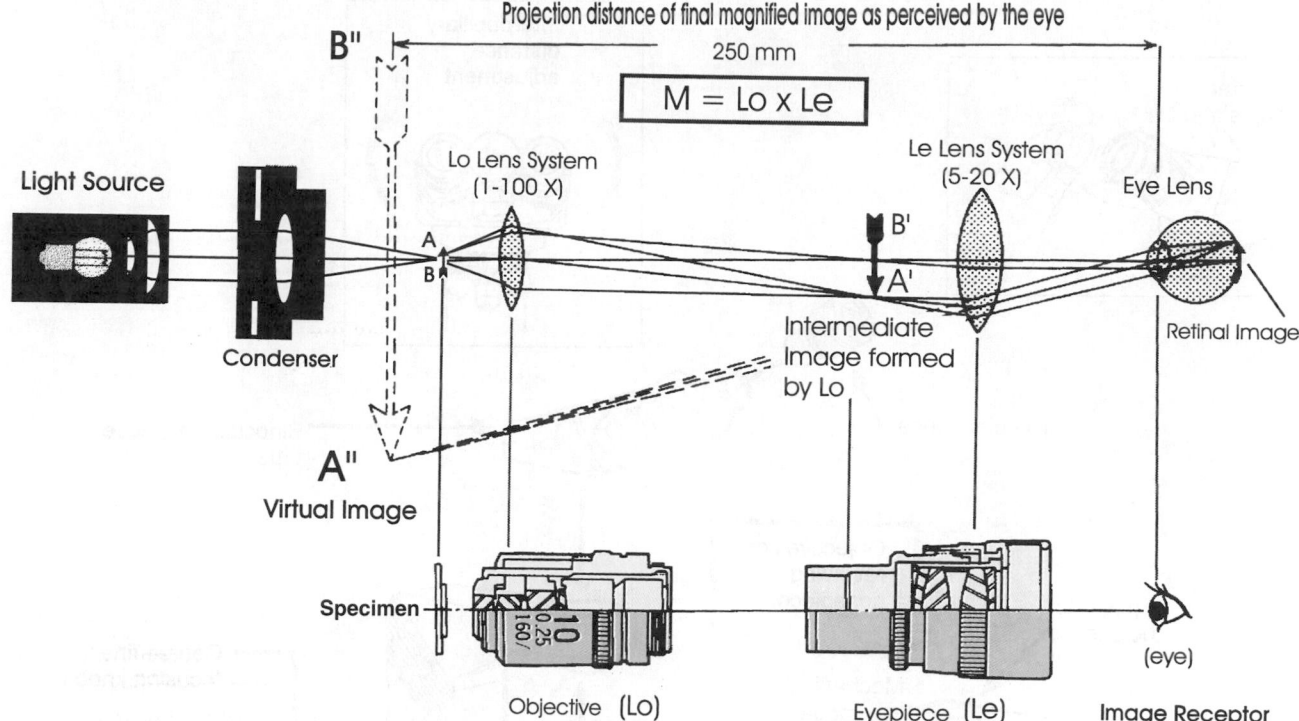

Projection distance of final magnified image as perceived by the eye

250 mm

$$M = Lo \times Le$$

B"

A"

Virtual Image

Light Source

Condenser

Lo Lens System
(1-100 X)

A
B

Intermediate
Image formed
by Lo

Le Lens System
(5-20 X)

B'
A'

Eye Lens

Retinal Image

Specimen

10
0.25
160/

Objective (Lo)

Eyepiece (Le)

(eye)

Image Receptor

FIGURE 4-3. Formation of the magnified image in the compound light microscope. (Modified and redrawn, courtesy of Nikon Inc Instrument Group, Melville, NY.)

eyepiece combination equals the product of the magnifying power of the objective lens and that of the eyepiece. If applicable, auxiliary optics and tube factors must also be taken into account when calculating total magnification.

Relationship of Microscope Optical Parameters

Magnification, working distance, field diameter, depth of focus, and field brightness are interdependent.[6,13] *Working distance,* which decreases with increasing magnification, is the depth of space in millimeters between the top surface of the specimen slide and the front surface of the objective lens (Table 4-1, Fig. 4-2). It is an important factor, particularly when using high-power objectives that have limited free working distances. With these objectives the optics or specimen can easily be damaged. This is why they usually have a spring-loaded front element that allows the lens to retract inside its housing if it comes into contact with a stationary surface.

Field diameter or *field of view* is the area of specimen that can be seen. It decreases with increasing magnification. Higher-power objectives thus show a smaller specimen area, but resolve more detail than lower-power objectives. The actual diameter of the field of view in millimeters can be calculated by dividing the field number of the eyepieces by the objective magnification; check the manufacturer's technical specifications for the eyepiece field number. This calculation is important if different microscopes with different field diameters are used for cell count estimates on peripheral blood films in the same

laboratory. A correction factor must then be used to maintain consistency when reporting results.

Increasing magnification not only reduces the field of view but also reduces the *depth of focus,* or the distance throughout which all parts of the specimen image are clearly in focus simultaneously. Also, with increasing magnification a greater amount of light is required to illuminate the field.

EXAMPLE CALCULATION OF FIELD DIAMETER AND CORRECTION FACTOR

For example, assume two different microscopes are used for leukocyte and platelet count estimates in the hematology laboratory:

Microscope A: objective: 100×
        eyepiece field number: 18
        field of view diameter 18/100 = 0.18 mm
Microscope B: objective: 100×
        eyepiece field number: 20
        field of view diameter 20/100 = 0.20 mm

In the example, the field diameter of microscope A is 0.18 mm and microscope B, 0.20 mm. To calculate the correction factor, compare the largest field of view with the smallest, and assume that the smallest field of view equals 100%. A ratio and proportion should be set up to solve for the correction factor:

$$0.18 : 100 = 0.20 : x$$

The correction factor (x) equals 90% or 0.90. In this example all cell count estimates performed on microscope B must be multiplied by the correction factor 0.90 to adjust the counts to match those of microscope A.

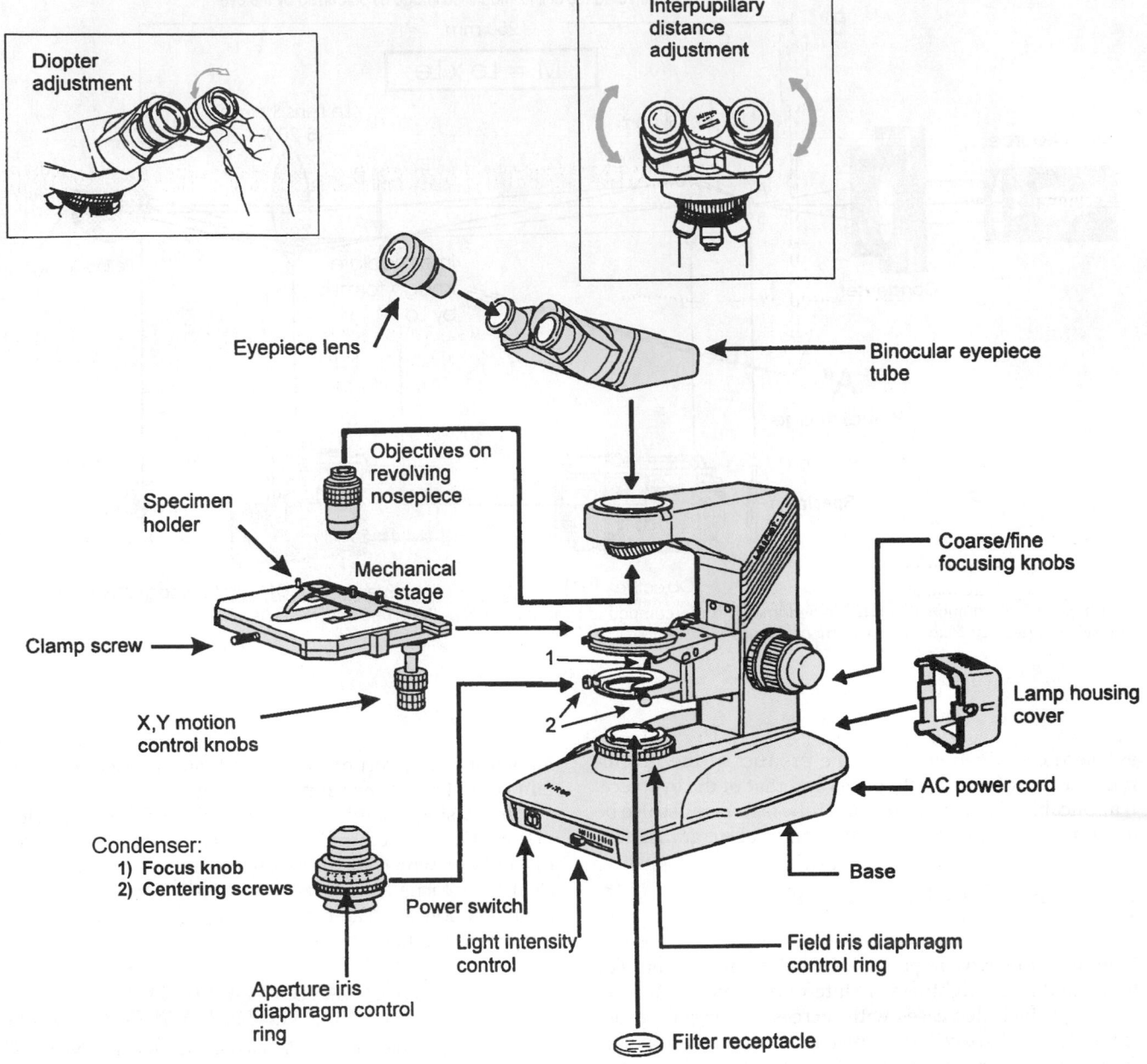

Diopter adjustment

Interpupillary distance adjustment

Eyepiece lens

Binocular eyepiece tube

Objectives on revolving nosepiece

Specimen holder

Coarse/fine focusing knobs

Mechanical stage

Clamp screw

1

Lamp housing cover

X,Y motion control knobs

2

AC power cord

Condenser:
1) Focus knob
2) Centering screws

Base

Power switch

Light intensity control

Field iris diaphragm control ring

Aperture iris diaphragm control ring

Filter receptacle

FIGURE 4-4. Basic components of a compound light microscope. (Adapted and modified, courtesy of Nikon Inc Instrument Group, Melville, NY.)

Optimizing the Specimen Image: Koehler Illumination

PRINCIPLE

Koehler illumination ensures optimum contrast and resolution for the maximum definition of specimen details by precisely focusing and centering the light path and spreading the light uniformly over the field of view.[3,4,6,7,10,11,13] Whereas final specimen image definition is ultimately limited by the quality and maintenance of the optics, obtaining the best possible image depends on the microscopist's control of illumination.

PRACTICE TIPS

The Koehler procedure must be performed before using the microscope, but with practice the procedure takes less than 20 seconds. Table 4-2 lists the basic steps for the procedure. Ideally it should be repeated when objectives are changed from one magnification to another, because objectives have different fields of view and require different illumination apertures depending on the magnifying power and NA. This is particularly important for critical microscopy and photomicrography.

Remember to adjust light intensity only with the brightness control, never by adjusting the field or substage condenser aperture diaphragm. Once these apertures are set during the Koehler illumination procedure, they should not be changed unless the objectives or operator are changed.

TABLE 4-2
Basic Steps of Koehler Illumination

1. Turn on microscope and adjust light intensity.

2. Switch to 10× objective, place specimen on stage, and focus using focus control knobs.

3. Close condenser aperture iris diaphragm and raise substage condenser with height adjustment knob to the top "stop." (Condenser aperture diaphragm controls angle of illumination and thus amount of light to objective lens.)

4. Close field iris diaphragm with field diaphragm control. (Field diaphragm limits area of illumination to image field.)

5. Move substage condenser until image of field diaphragm is in sharp focus. Refocus specimen image using focus control knobs if necessary.

6. Center field diaphragm image by adjusting condenser or field diaphragm centering screws; this depends on microscope type or model, and some microscopes have a preset light source and field diameter and do not have centering controls.

7. Enlarge field diaphragm image until it is just outside field of view and entire observation area is illuminated.

8. Remove one eyepiece; open and close substage condenser aperture diaphragm while looking down eyepiece tube and observe circular beam of light.

9. Adjust aperture diaphragm with aperture control until light beam fills approximately 75% of field.

10. Replace eyepiece.

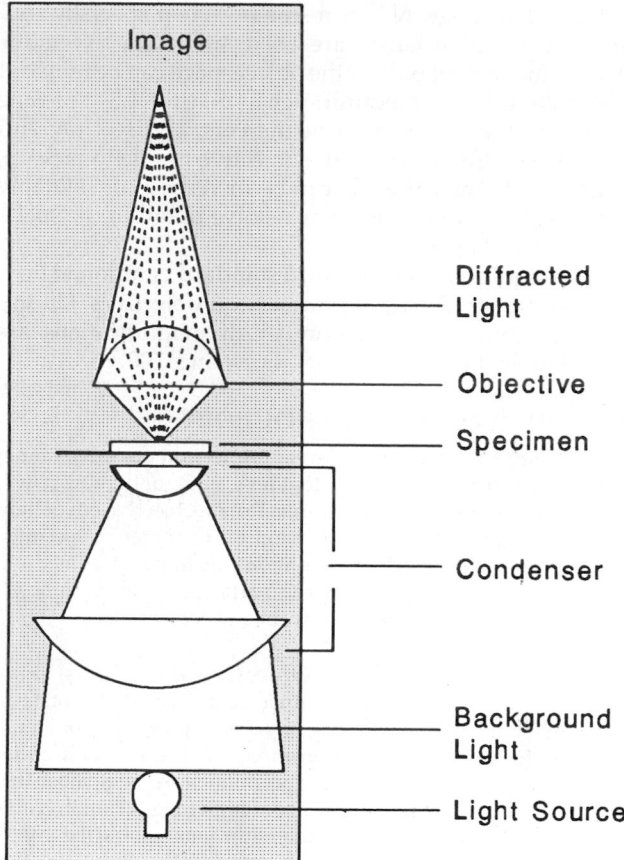

FIGURE 4-5. Image formation in brightfield microscopy.

TYPES OF LIGHT MICROSCOPY

Brightfield Microscopy

APPLICATION, PRINCIPLE AND EQUIPMENT

Brightfield microscopy is the cornerstone of diagnostic hematology and the most common type of microscopy used in the clinical laboratory.[6,10,11,13] In hematology, brightfield microscopy is used primarily to examine stained blood films.

Brightfield microscopy is a method of examining specimens using transmitted light in which structural details of the object appear darker than the illuminated field of view (Fig. 4-5). The substage condenser directs and focuses light from the illumination source onto the specimen positioned on the mechanical stage. The specimen modifies the light rays that illuminate it: absorption, refraction, and diffraction are the three dominant effects. The background light from the light source, the illuminated area which one sees through the microscope without a specimen present, and the diffracted light from the specimen then combine to produce the specimen image.

Specimens must be stained to enhance selective absorption and contrast to reveal the details and information in the specimen image. Since different parts of a specimen are able to absorb light to varying degrees, we see structural details as differences in amplitude or light intensity (brightness). Thus, brightfield microscopy depends on "amplitude modulation" to make the specimen visible.

The equipment consists of a standard compound light microscope and a brightfield or transmitted light condenser. The usual objectives used are 10×, 40×, and 100×. Achromat lenses are suitable for routine observations; however, plan achromats, which also provide flatness of field, are recommended.

PRACTICE TIPS

Low power (10×) is used to identify the cells or area to be examined. Medium high-dry (40×) and high power (100×) objectives are used for the identification and enumeration of normal and abnormal cellular constituents and diagnosis of disease. Most high numerical aperture dry objectives (NA > 0.65) are designed for use with a cover glass (0.17 mm thick) to prevent deterioration in resolving power and contrast. To avoid these problems many manufacturers offer no-cover-glass objectives for use with uncovered smears. There are also long-working-distance objectives for applications requiring the use of special chambers, thick slides, and other unusual situations.

Oil Immersion Microscopy

APPLICATION, PRINCIPLE, AND EQUIPMENT

Oil immersion microscopy is used extensively in hematology to observe erythrocyte morphology, estimate platelet counts, and differentiate leukocytes.[1,3,6,10,11]

To review, the objective lens accepts illumination from an area of the specimen to produce an image and the measure of the aperture of light an objective can collect is dependent on its NA or n sine μ. When specially constructed objective lenses are used, air (refractive index [n] = 1) in the light path of the object space can be replaced with an immersion medium such as oil (n = 1.5–1.6). Sine μ, sine of the angle between the central direct ray and the greatest diffracted ray the objective is able to pick up, is increased. Thus, the NA can be increased considerably and the ability to delineate or resolve detail in the specimen image (Fig. 4-1).

The equipment consists of a standard compound light microscope fitted with oil immersion objectives. Oil immersion objectives of a number of magnifications are available, including 40×, 50×, 60×, and 100×.

THE OIL IMMERSION PROCEDURE

Focus Under Low Power. An oil immersion objective cannot be focused just by switching to that lens. First, under low power (10×), focus and select viewing area. Rotate objective out of light path, and place a drop of immersion oil in center of specimen above beam of light. (Refractive index of immersion medium should match that required by the particular immersion objective; check microscope manufacturer's specifications.)

Switch to Oil Immersion Objective and Adjust Fine Focus. Watching from side of microscope, carefully rotate to oil immersion lens. Do not drag any dry objectives through oil. As oil objective is clicked into position, make sure it only glides into oil and does not break the specimen slide; remember that there is minimum working distance at high magnification (Table 4-1, Fig. 4-2). Note that the immersion lens should be gently rotated into place rather than lowered into oil by the fine adjustment knob to avoid trapping troublesome air bubbles between slide and objective. If air bubbles are suspected, remove the eyepiece and look down the tube toward the objective lens to check. Finally focus carefully using fine adjustment knob only.

Adjust Field Diaphragm Image and Light Intensity. Recenter and focus field diaphragm image if necessary, using the condenser focus control. Enlarge field diaphragm image just outside field of view. Remove one eyepiece and look down

eyepiece tube; adjust condenser aperture iris diaphragm control ring to light three-fourths of the field of view. Replace eyepiece. Adjust light intensity control; more light is required at high magnification.

Examine Specimen and Clean Oil Immersion Objective. When observation is complete, rotate lens from the oil and clean excess oil from both lens and specimen slide. (Check microscope instruction manual for recommended procedure.)

USE OF AN OIL IMMERSION CONDENSER

In high-precision microscopy and photomicrography, if the NA of the objective is greater than 1.00, use of an oil immersion condenser is recommended. In this case, oil is also applied to the front lens of the condenser and the condenser is raised until contact with the undersurface of the specimen slide is made to form a homogeneous oil immersion system. However, under no circumstance should non-immersion objectives and condensers be used with oil. This may cause permanent damage. Note that special high-magnification dry objectives (60× and 100×) are available which eliminate the use of oil.

Phase Contrast Microscopy

APPLICATION, PRINCIPLE, AND EQUIPMENT

In hematology, phase contrast is used to perform manual platelet counts in situations in which the electronic count may be inaccurate.[1,4,6,7,12,13]

Phase contrast is an optical contrast enhancement technique that allows examination of unstained, transparent specimens that are invisible under brightfield microscopy because they cannot absorb light. This is accomplished by converting slight differences in thickness and refractive index *(phase differences)* in the object into intensity or brightness differences that are detectable by the human eye.

Contrast is obtained by conditioning the input light and modifying the output light. The condenser with a phase annular ring controls the input illumination (see Fig. 4-6). A phase-changing plate (ring) in the objective

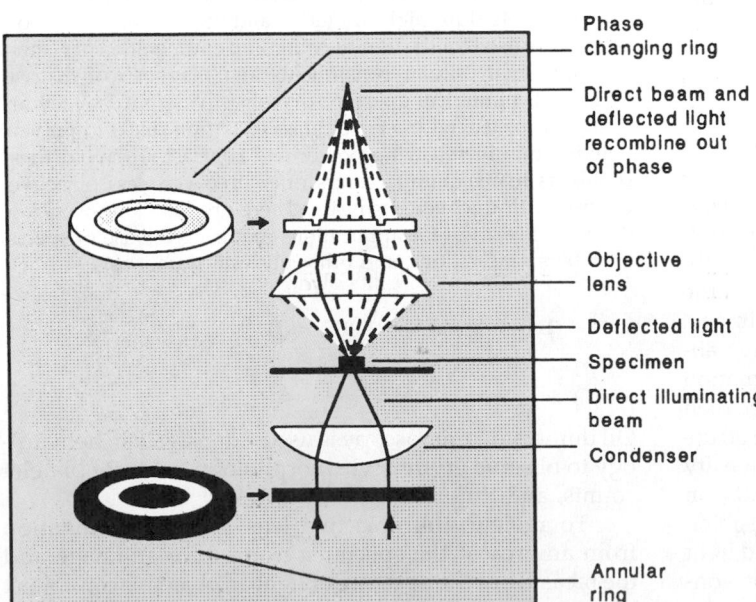

Phase
changing ring

Direct beam and
deflected light
recombine out
of phase

Objective
lens

Deflected light

Specimen

Direct illuminating
beam

Condenser

Annular
ring

FIGURE 4-6. Image formation in phase contrast microscopy. (From Special Contrast Enhancement Techniques—Transmitted Light Microscopy, Cambridge, MA, Polaroid Corporation, 1981, with permission.)

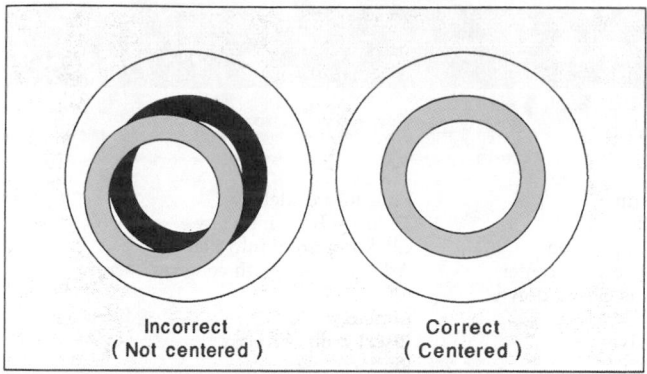

FIGURE 4-7. Quality control in phase microscopy. A centering telescope must be used for verification that the annular ring in the condenser and the phase-changing ring in the objective are coincident (aligned). The rings will appear either not centered (**left**) or centered (**right**). The rings must be exactly centered.

creates a uniform phase change that increases the differences between the background light and the deflected light from the specimen and collects the light resulting from interaction of the specimen and the input light. The input and output light interfere when they recombine at the eyepiece, which changes intensity and enhances image contrast. Depending on the type of phase optics used, the specimen appears brighter (bright contrast) or darker (dark contrast) than the surrounding area.

The equipment consists of a standard compound light microscope with special accessories: a phase condenser and phase objectives. Note that the revolving disk in the phase condenser contains an annular ring to match the phase-changing ring in each phase objective lens. A centering telescope is used to verify that the annular ring in the condenser and the phase-changing ring in the objective are coincident or aligned (Fig. 4-7).

PRACTICE TIPS

Many precautions must be taken in phase contrast microscopy. For example, debris may result in misleading data (*e.g.*, dust may be counted as platelets, resulting in a falsely elevated plate-

let count). Also the "halo effect," which is an optical artifact characteristic of phase contrast, may conceal useful data. The exact centering of the annular ring in the condenser and phase-changing ring in the matched objective is critical for achieving the desired contrast effect. Therefore, alignment must be checked routinely. In critical microscopy and photomicrography the centering must be checked at each magnification used. Even a slightly off-center placement can result in an image of lower contrast and a shadowing effect that can cause inaccurate cell counts.

Fluorescence Microscopy

APPLICATION AND PRINCIPLE

In hematology fluorescence microscopy is used primarily in antinuclear antibody (ANA; Chap. 24) and T- and B-cell studies (Chap. 23).[2,4,7,9,13]

Fluorescence describes the absorption of light energy of a certain wavelength (*e.g.*, blue light) followed by emission of light of a longer wavelength (*e.g.*, yellow light) (Fig. 4-8). There are three basic observation methods: autofluorescence when the object itself is fluorescent; induced fluorescence when the specimen is stained with a fluorochrome or chemical dye; and the fluorescence antibody technique based on immunologic staining. Information on equipment may be obtained from the above references.

TROUBLESHOOTING PROBLEMS AND QUALITY CONTROL/ PREVENTIVE MAINTENANCE IN LIGHT MICROSCOPY

Although a microscope is not difficult to operate, occasionally there are problems–electrical, mechanical, or optical.[1,8,13] Table 4-3 lists some common problems with their probable causes and corrective actions.

The microscope is a precision optical instrument. Whereas more complex instruments in the clinical laboratory often receive scheduled quality control and preventive maintenance, the microscope often receives little or

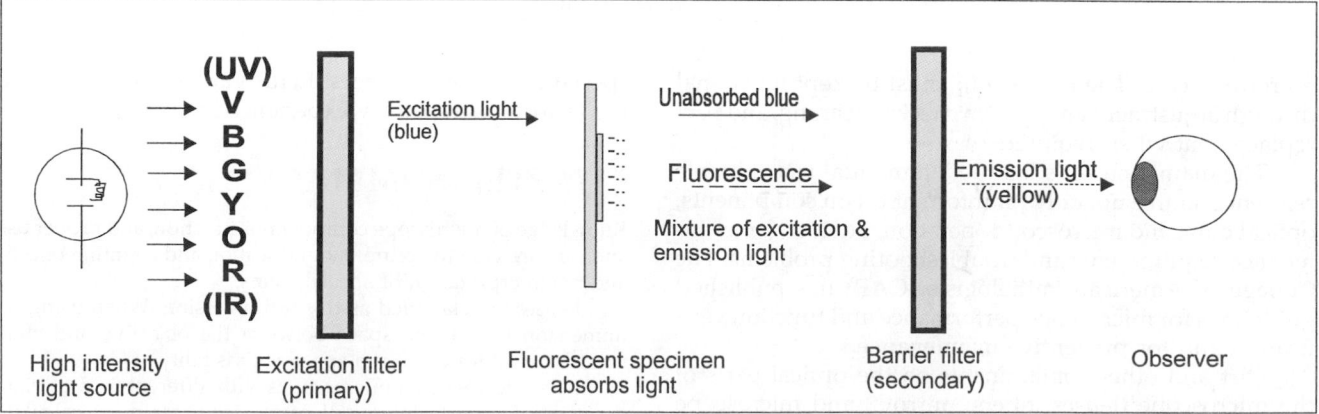

FIGURE 4-8. Principle and basic components of a fluorescence microscope. Selection of the filter combination depends on the fluorochrome used; in this illustration, fluorescein isothiocyanate (FITC). UV—ultraviolet; V—violet; B—blue; G—green; Y—yellow; O—orange; R—red; IR—infrared. From UV to IR, wavelength of light increases.

TABLE 4-3
Troubleshooting in Light Microscopy

Problem	Probable Cause	Corrective Action
LIGHTING		
No light	Microscope not plugged in	Plug into outlet
	Brightness control dial turned off	Turn up light intensity
	Objective not clicked into position	Click objective into place
	Condenser image completely off center when field diaphragm is closed down	Adjust image with centering screws
	Bulb burned out	Replace bulb
	Bulb not inserted properly	Insert bulb correctly
	Fuse blown	Replace fuse
	Fuse not inserted properly	Insert fuse correctly
	No power from wall outlet	Test or try different outlet
Insufficient light	Brightness control dial set too low	Increase brightness
	Condenser diaphragm closed	Open condenser diaphragm
	Substage condenser lowered too far (not correctly focused)	Adjust height of substage condenser as per Koehler method
Flickering	Loose power connection	Plug in microscope or try another wall outlet
	Corrosion on bulb pins	Clean pins on bulb
	Defective bulb socket	Replace socket
	Bulb not inserted properly	Insert bulb correctly
	Situation not covered above	Call for repair
Too bright	Light turned up too high	Adjust brightness
FOCUSING		
Won't focus on 40× or higher magnification	Specimen slide upside down	Turn glass slide over so that the specimen faces up
Nonparfocal (not focused when objective changed)	Objective has come partially unscrewed	Tighten objective
MISCELLANEOUS		
Eyestrain	Illumination of field too intense	Reduce light intensity
	Eyepieces not focused for each eye	Adjust to correct
Floating spots	"Debris" in the vitreous humor of the retina noticeable at high magnifications	Taking a break and resting will often help
Field diaphragm noncenterable	Substage condenser seated improperly in condenser carrier	Loosen condenser centering screws and reseat condenser
Bubbles or dark wave pass across the field of view when using immersion oil	Air bubbles in oil: contact between oil immersion objective and oil "broken"	Clean slide and/or add more oil

Courtesy of Nikon Inc. Instrument Division, Melville, NY. and Health Sciences Consortium, Chapel Hill, NC.

no routine care. The microscope must be kept functional through adjustment and system checks, cleaning, and part replacement when required.[1,5,10,13]

The manufacturer's instruction manual is a valuable reference source not only for information on components, optical data, and microscope operation, but also for maintenance requirements and troubleshooting problems. The College of American Pathologists (CAP) has published guidelines for microscope performance and function verification and for preventive maintenance.[5]

Dirt and other contaminants on the optical parts of the microscope (lenses, filters, mirrors, and microscope frame) are a frequent problem. External surfaces can be cleaned by the user with appropriate care. However, eyepieces, objectives, and condensers must never be dismantled for cleaning. Correct reassembly is only possible with special adjustment devices. Return any damaged part to the factory for repair by experienced personnel.

CHAPTER SUMMARY

Knowledge of microscope components, function, and proper use and care are vital to accurate identification and counting of cells and the interpretation of special stains.

Lenses are classified as dry or immersion. When using oil immersion lenses, the space between the objective and slide must have oil for optimum specimen visibility.

Laboratories using microscopes with different field-of-view diameters for performing cell count estimates must calculate a correction factor to use in adjusting the counts to maintain consistency in results.

Brightfield microscopy is the most frequently used type of microscopy in hematology. Koehler illumination must be used to ensure optimum specimen contrast and resolution for accurate cell identification. The proper technique for oil immersion examination must be mastered because cell identification requires it.

Phase contrast microscopy is used to perform manual platelet counts when automated counts are unreliable. For accurate counts the microscope must be checked periodically to ensure that it is "in phase." Fluorescence microscopy is used primarily in antinuclear antibody (ANA) and T- and B-cell studies.

Case Study 4-1

After focusing on a cell with a suspected Auer rod using a 10× eyepiece and 10× objective, a nightshift technologist could not adjust the microscope to focus on 40× or higher magnification. What should be done to solve this problem?

Case Study 4-2

A specimen image did not show the detail in some lymphoma cells that a technologist had expected to see. In fact, he noticed that the light was darker toward the lower right side of the slide than it was on the left. What should be done to improve the specimen image?

Case Study 4-3

A request for a stat peripheral blood count was received for a patient who was undergoing therapy for cancer. The platelet count was low, and the technologist was having difficulty seeing the platelets using phase contrast microscopy due to a "halo effect." What should be done to correct the situation?

Case Study 4-4

A technologist could not make a bubble on a slide go away. It kept "following" wherever the technologist moved on the slide. What should be done to solve the bubble problem?

Review Questions

4-1. The total magnification when a 40× objective and 10× eyepiece is used is

A. 400×.
B. 40×.
C. 4×.
D. 0.4×.

4-2. The resolution (R) of a lens refers to its

A. ability to delineate detail in a specimen.
B. magnification of the specimen image.
C. performance rating for gathering light.
D. field-of-view diameter.

4-3. The type of microscopy recommended for a manual platelet count is

A. fluorescence.
B. phase.

C. brightfield.
D. oil immersion.

For the following questions, use the following format to answer:
A. 1, 3
B. 2, 4
C. 1, 2, and 3
D. 4 only
E. All are correct

4-4. When work is begun on a microscope, the Koehler illumination procedure must be performed because it allows for

1. increased specimen image resolution.
2. uniform illumination over the entire field of view.
3. optimum specimen contrast by precise light path control.
4. increased specimen magnification.

4-5. Immersion oil must be used with immersion objectives because oil causes a(n)

1. increase in the cone of light admitted by the lens.
2. decrease in image resolution.
3. gain in numerical aperture.
4. increase in the working distance between the specimen and lens.

References

1. Abramowitz M: Contrast Methods in Microscopy—Transmitted light. Lake Success, NY, Olympus Corporation, 1987
2. Abramowitz M: Fluorescence Microscopy—The Essentials. Lake Success, NY, Olympus America Inc, 1993
3. Abramowitz M: Microscope Basics and Beyond. Lake Success, NY, Olympus Corporation, 1985
4. Benford JR: The Theory of the Microscope. Deerfield, IL, Leica Inc, 1991
5. College of American Pathologists: Laboratory Instrument Evaluation, Verification and Maintenance Manual, 4th ed, p 97. Skokie, IL, College of American Pathologists, 1989, reprinted 9/91
6. Delly JG: Photography Through the Microscope, 9th ed. Rochester, NY, Eastman Kodak Company, 1988
7. Kapitza HG: Microscopy from the Very Beginning. Thornwood, NY, Carl Zeiss, Inc, 1994
8. Michael BS, Lotspeich CA, Tryon CT: Introduction to the Microscope—Operation and Preventive Maintenance Using the Nikon Labophot. Guidebook accompanying a color videotape. Chapel Hill, NC, Health Sciences Consortium, 1985
9. Nikon: Fluorescence Microscopes—Technical Bulletin. Melville, NY, Nikon Inc Instrument Group
10. Nikon: How to Use a Microscope and Take a Photomicrograph. Melville, NY, Nikon Inc Instrument Group
11. Nikon: Instruction Manual for the Labophot-2 Clinical Microscope. Melville, NY, Nikon Inc Instrument Group
12. Polaroid: Special Contrast Enhancement Techniques—Transmitted Light Microscopy. Cambridge, MA, Polaroid Corporation, 1981
13. Richardson JH: Handbook for the Light Microscope—A User's Guide. Park Ridge, NJ, Noyes Publications, 1991

Hematopoiesis and Review of Genetics

Vincent S. Gallicchio

Objectives

1. Describe the ontogeny of hematopoiesis from the yolk sac to bone marrow (medullary) hematopoiesis.
2. Describe the anatomy of bone marrow and the location of hematopoiesis in relation to the venous sinuses.
3. Discuss the theories of hematopoiesis to include a discussion of the totipotential stem cell, committed stem cells, progenitor cells, and precursor cells.
4. Describe how hematopoiesis is regulated by means of growth factors.
5. Briefly summarize the steps involved in meiosis and mitosis and how they differ.
6. Describe the genetic code and how it operates to develop genetic characteristics.
7. Discuss how genetic traits or characteristics are passed on from parent to child. Include the concepts of homozygosity and heterozygosity, dominant and recessive, autosomal and sex-linked.
8. Describe how a karyotype is developed and how it is used.

HEMATOPOIETIC SYSTEM DEVELOPMENT

Blood cell production (hematopoiesis) encompasses cellular proliferation, differentiation, morphogenesis, functional maturation, and death. Cellular differentiation is an orderly process involving structural and functional changes for which regulatory mechanisms are not well understood. Figure 5-1 provides a summary of the embryonic and fetal hematopoietic developmental process. The discussion below outlines three developmental periods.

Mesoblastic Development

Hematopoiesis begins during embryonic development in the blood islands of the yolk sac. The blood islands are first detectable at approximately 19 to 20 days of gestation, and their appearance marks the beginning of the mesoblastic period of hematopoiesis. Most likely, blood islands develop from the mesodermal extraembryonic layer of the yolk sac. These blood islands remain active only through the 8th to 12th week of gestation and are primarily responsible for red cell production (erythropoiesis). Immature red cells or erythroblasts produced by the yolk sac are unique in their morphology as well as the type of hemoglobin they produce, and they generally are not found after the third month of gestation. Primitive erythroblasts of the yolk sac are large and do not extrude their nucleus. The globin chains produced by primitive erythroblasts include epsilon (ε) and zeta (ζ), which are required for production of three embryonic types of hemoglobin, Gower I, Gower II, and Portland (Chaps. 7 and 14). Erythroblasts of the later definitive series are smaller than the primitive series but still larger than the cells found in adults.

Hepatic Period

Definitive morphologic hematopoiesis begins in the liver during the fifth to sixth week of gestation and marks the beginning of hepatic hematopoiesis. The liver is the primary site of blood cell development between the 10th and 30th weeks of gestation and remains active until the first or second week after birth. At first the fetal liver is primarily an erythroid organ and produces red cells containing fetal hemoglobin (two alpha and two gamma globin chains) that is distinguishable from the embryonic hemoglobins. Because liver hematopoiesis is intravascular, infants normally have a few circulating nucleated red cells. The production of granulocytes and lymphocytes is minimal in the fetal liver. During the hepatic period, the spleen, thymus, and lymph nodes also become active in blood cell production. These other sites, except for the thymus, continue to produce lymphocytes throughout life.

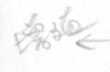

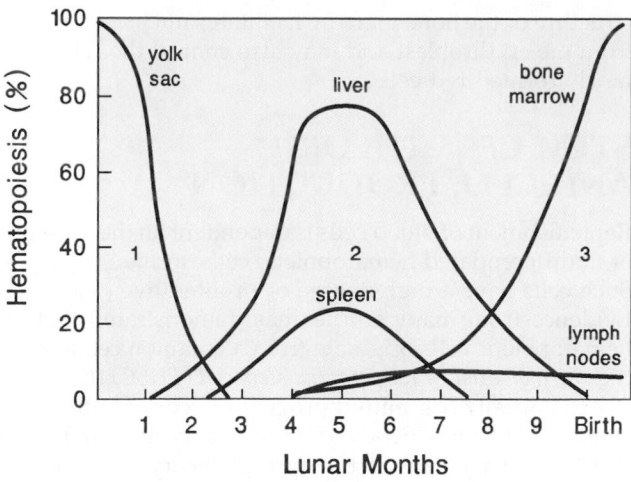

FIGURE 5-1. Sites of prenatal hematopoiesis: (1) mesoblastic, (2) hepatic, (3) myeloid.

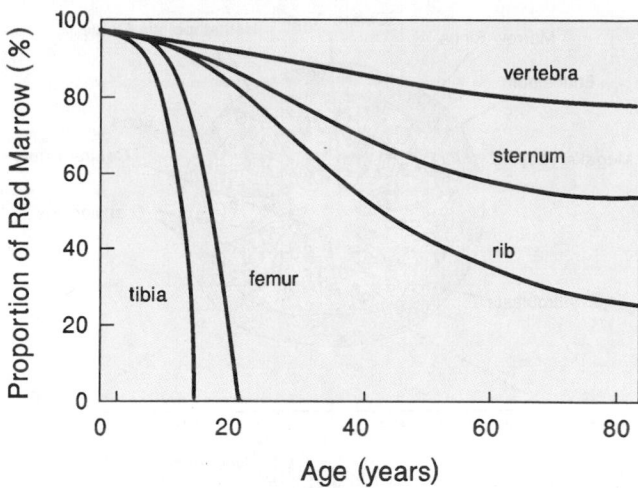

FIGURE 5-2. Sites of postnatal hematopoiesis.

Hepatic as well as splenic hematopoiesis may occur in the adult. When this happens, it is referred to as *extramedullary hematopoiesis (i.e.,* blood cell production outside the bone marrow). When bone marrow is called upon to produce increased numbers of blood cells, there is frequently a sufficient amount of reserve marrow space to accommodate the demand. However, there are instances in which bone marrow fails to produce blood cells normally leading to extramedullary production. Other terms for this phenomenon are *ectopic hematopoiesis* and *myeloid metaplasia.*

Myeloid Period

During the fifth month of gestation, bone cavities begin to form, and bone marrow begins to become the main site of blood cell production. This marks the beginning of the myeloid period. During this time hemoglobin A_1 (HbA_1), consisting of two alpha and two beta globin chains, begins to appear and gradually increases in concentration (Chap. 7).

After the first 3 weeks postpartum, the bone marrow becomes the only normal site of blood cell production and remains so throughout life. During the first few years of life, a delicate balance exists between developing bone marrow space and the infant's need for blood cells. Consequently, the hematopoietic capability of both the liver and spleen remains available. During the fourth year of life, the rate of bone marrow growth exceeds the need of blood cells, resulting in active marrow sites being replaced with areas of fatty reserve.[46] Fat continues to replace hematopoietic (red) marrow of long bones until the age of 18 years, when the only active hematopoietic sites are in the pelvis, vertebrae, ribs, sternum, skull, and proximal extremities of the long bones (Fig. 5-2). If necessary, fatty marrow (yellow marrow) may be reactivated for hematopoiesis in a relatively short time. Normally, however, there is a gradual increase in marrow fatty tissue throughout life. Approximately one quarter of a child's marrow is fat. A young adult may have up to 50% fat, whereas

the hematopoietic marrow of an elderly individual may have as much as 60% to 70% fat.

BONE MARROW VOLUME AND ANATOMY

The volume of bone marrow increases from 1.5% of body weight at birth to about 4.5% in the adult. Blood volume, on the other hand, decreases from 8% of total body weight at birth to 7% in the adult.

Anatomically, bone marrow consists of a pattern of vessels and nerves, differentiated and undifferentiated hematopoietic cells, reticuloendothelial cells, and fatty tissue, all of which are encased by the endosteum (a membrane lining the marrow cavity of bone). The vascular system consists of a network of arterioles that empty into a complex system of venous sinusoids (or sinuses), which drain into a central collecting vein (Fig. 5-3).

The venous sinusoids are lined by an endothelial layer supported by intermittent fat cells and adventitial cells (Fig. 5-4). The endothelium is a complete layer of cells attached to one another at their edges and is usually one cell thick. A basement membrane is present but markedly deficient, irregular in thickness, and absent from large stretches of the sinusoidal wall, especially in areas where cells are in direct passage. Adventitial cells of the sinus walls are phagocytic and form the outer portion of the sinus walls. They are classified as reticular cells—a form of connective tissue. The endothelial cell, basement membrane, and the adventitial cell form what is sometimes referred to as the *trilaminar sinus wall.* Apertures are areas within endothelial cells through which hematopoietic cells pass rather than through intracellular gaps.

Primary blood cell formation occurs outside the sinusoids in the hematopoietic cords, which have an intimate relation with the sinuses. Mature cells are capable of deforming to enable them to pass through narrow sieve-like apertures in the endothelial vascular lining and enter the bone marrow sinuses and circulation (Fig. 5-3). This

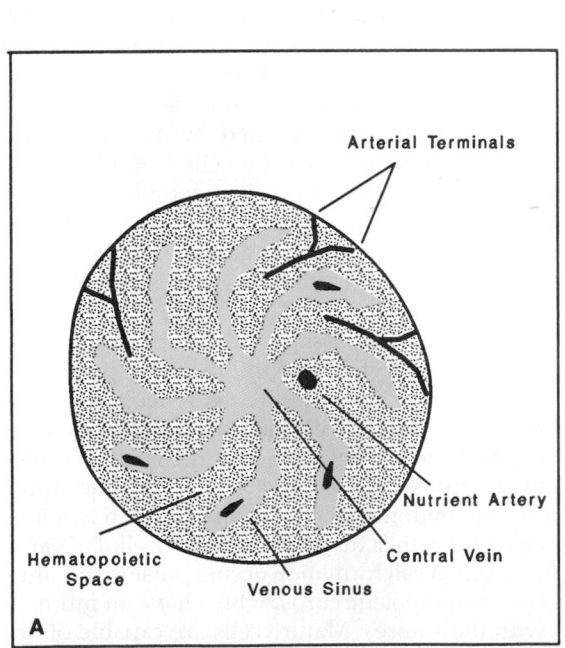

FIGURE 5-3. Cross-section of bone with active marrow.

structure of the bone marrow facilitates nuclear extrusion from the erythroblast and may also control the release of newly formed red cells.

STEM CELL THEORIES AND CELL PRODUCTION

Replenishment of blood cells is dependent on the presence of undifferentiated hematopoietic cells, termed *stem cells*. Such cells have a high degree of proliferative capability. Evidence from many studies has demonstrated that all hematopoietic cells originate from a common cell termed the *pluripotential* or *totipotential stem cell (THSC)* that gives rise to partially committed progenitor cells of both a myeloid (*CFU-S* or *CFU-GEMM*) and a lymphoid nature (CFU-L).[23] This leads to the current theory of stem cells and their progenitors (Fig. 5-5). The opposing concepts of self-renewal and of differentiation are central to the description of the stem cell; indeed, the potential to manifest these two developmental options is the only rigorous criterion used in defining what constitutes a true stem cell. Consequently, in studying stem cells, one of the most important questions to consider is how the critical decision of whether to self-renew or differentiate is made. It has been determined that both the environment of the stem cell and extrinsic signals (*e.g.*, cytokines) determine the outcome of the self-renewal decision. In other words, stem cells are not intrinsically committed to a particular

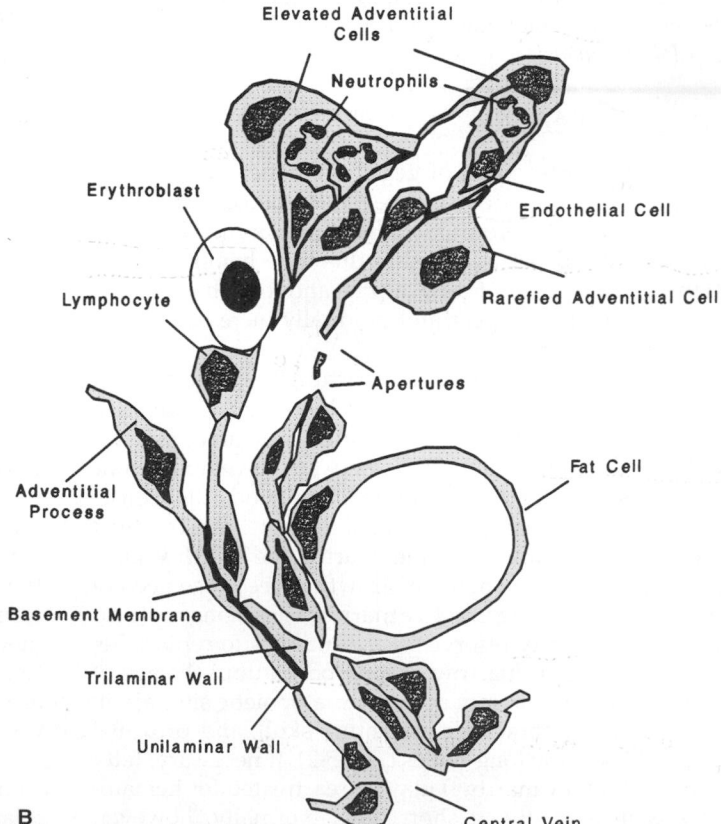

FIGURE 5-4. Anatomy of a bone marrow sinus. (**A**) Anatomy of the marrow as a cross-section of a marrow sinus into which various cell types pass through the endothelial cell network on their way to the circulation. (**B**) View of the sinus down the central vein.

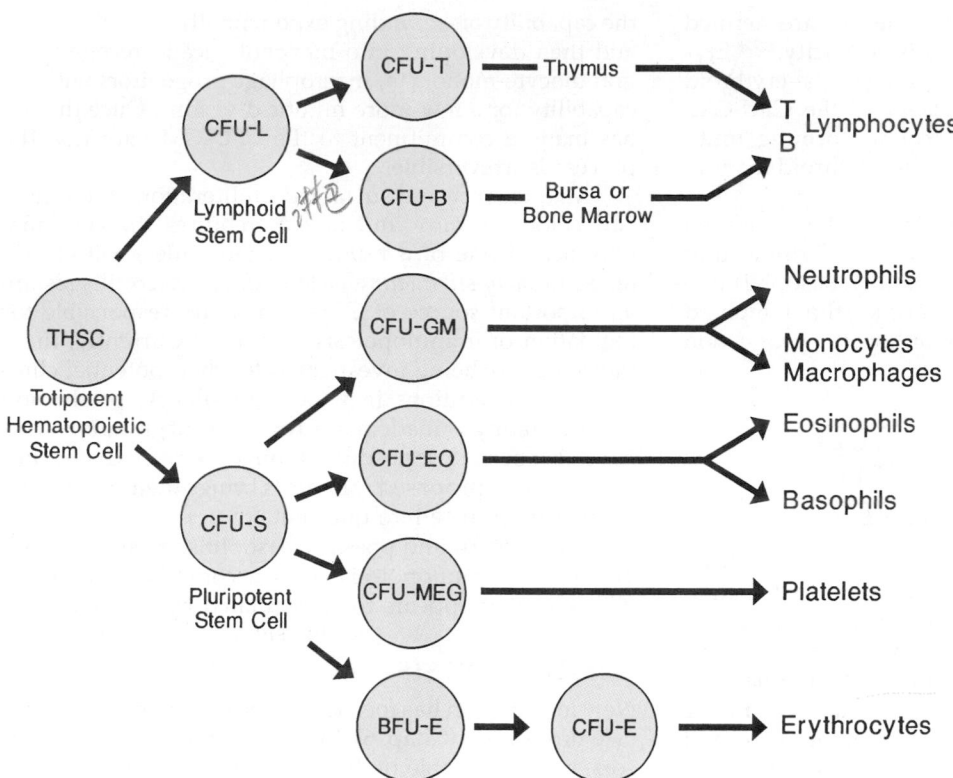

developmental fate; rather, their environment mediates the differentiation decision.

Pluripotential Stem Cells

A quantitative assay for pluripotential hematopoietic stem cells was developed using mice in 1961.[44] Colony-forming unit–spleen (CFU-S) is one term applied to this stem cell, which morphologically may resemble a lymphocyte.[3,9] The term was derived from the observation that bone marrow stem cells, after injection into lethally irradiated mice that are genetically identical (syngeneic), form colonies of regenerating hematopoietic cells located in the recipient's spleen. After 9 to 12 days, the CFU-S colonies consist of lineage-specific cells of erythroid, myeloid, and megakaryocyte lineage. The analogous cell in humans, based on cell surface antigenic recognition, has been termed the $CD34^+33^-$ cell.[33,35,36]

Stem cells have an extensive self-maintenance capability that does not appear to decline with age. The cell appears to proceed slowly through the cell cycle (see Fig. 5-6) with 1-week transit time, spending most of the time in the portion of the mitotic cycle known as G_0.[2,23] Some cells move continuously around the cell cycle, whereas others leave the cycle temporarily to enter the limbo or resting state (G_0). A long G_0 phase allows time for DNA repair.[7] Other cells leave the cycle and die without dividing again. The population of pluripotential stem cells, often referred to as the stem cell pool, provides adequate numbers for differentiation into the various cell lines at different rates depending on the demand and the amount of stem cells in reserve.

Committed Stem Cells

The CFU-S or CFU-GEMM and the CFU-L give rise to descendants that eventually become restricted to a specific line of development. Under appropriate conditions, stem cells continue their differentiation along a specific pathway, thereby losing their potential to develop along other cell lines. This loss of potential is termed *commitment*. Descendants of stem cells committed to the granulocyte

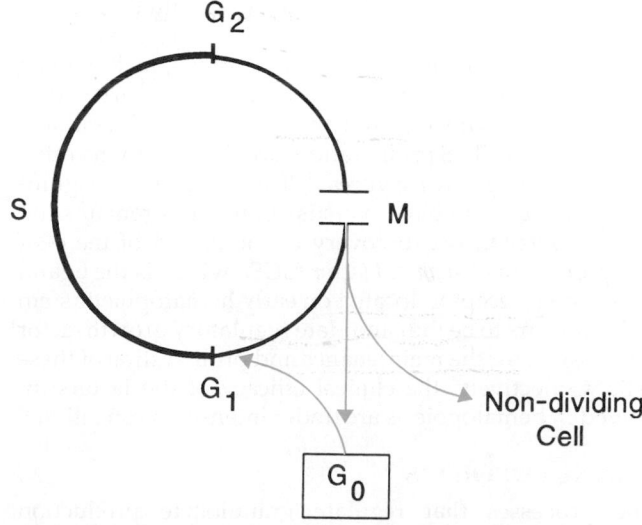

FIGURE 5-6. The cell cycle. G_0 = limbo or resting stage; G_1 = postmitotic, presynthetic stage; S = DNS synthesis stage; G_2 = postsynthetic, premitotic stage; M = mitosis.

(G)—monocyte/macrophage (M) lineage are termed CFU-GM and have limited proliferative capacity.[4,27,28] Erythroid progenitors, termed burst-forming units–erythroid (BFU-E), are the erythroid equivalent of the CFU-GM. The other erythroid progenitor, colony-forming unit–erythroid (CFU-E) is found later in the erythroid maturation sequence (Chap 6).[1]

Less well defined but also considered to be committed stem cells are the megakaryocyte colony-forming unit (CFU-Meg) and eosinophil (and possibly basophil) colony-forming unit (CFU-Eo).[11] Likewise, the lymphoid stem cell is committed to lymphocyte production (Chap. 24).

REGULATION OF STEM CELL DEVELOPMENT—GROWTH FACTORS AND CYTOKINES

The bone marrow microenvironment (surrounding structures and stromal cells) contributes significantly to hematopoiesis through the presentation of an extracellular matrix consisting of collagens, proteoglycans, and various cytokines known as growth factors.[21] Both normal and leukemic progenitor cells require growth factors for their survival, proliferation, maturation, differentiation, and function.[31] These growth factors interact with specific cell surface receptors, causing activation of intracellular pathways and resulting in changes in cell proliferation. Many of the growth factors discussed below have very little lineage specificity in that they act on more than one cell line. For example, interleukin-6 has significant effects on B cells, T cells, neutrophils, and macrophages. Furthermore, growth factors are frequently synergistic in their action. In other words, two or three cytokines produce effects that are far greater than their individual effects combined.

The Myeloid Stem Cell (CFU-S or CFU-GEMM)

Many in vivo studies have demonstrated effects of humoral agents on CFU-S. Phytohemagglutinin (PHA),[8] cyclophosphamide,[17] and concanavalin A[42] all have positive effects on CFU-S. These effects are variable, including an increase in CFU-S number,[8,24] an increase in survival[3] or protection from death,[17] and an increase in proliferation.[17] Inhibitors of CFU-S proliferation have been demonstrated also, including hydroxyurea.[41] The physiologic significance of these inhibitors versus stimulators remains unclear. However, the discovery of the ligand of the c-kit receptor, termed *stem cell factor (SCF)*, which is the ligand for the c-kit receptor, located on early hematopoietic stem cells, appears to be the candidate regulatory growth factor responsible for the maintenance and proliferation of these cells. Collectively, the clinical efficacy of the factors involved in hematopoiesis are under intense investigation.[14]

GRANULOPOIESIS

The processes that regulate granulocyte production (Chap. 22), specifically that of neutrophils, are orderly, originating from the CD34+33− cell to committed stem cell precursors referred to as CFU-GM. These cells have the capability of expanding exponentially in total number and then developing into morphologically recognizable granulocyte-monocyte/macrophage progenitors with the capability for a few more mitotic divisions. Once the cell has made a commitment to the CFU-GM pathway, the process is irreversible.

Maintenance and sustained proliferation of the CFU-GM colony *in vitro* and *in vivo* requires the continual presence of one of a number of molecules, collectively termed *colony-stimulating factors (CSF)*. Macrophages are an important source of CSFs, which are responsible for regulation of granulopoiesis *in vivo*.[27,29] Currently, these molecules are being investigated for their potential clinical use in conditions in which granulocyte production has been faulty or inadequate. Inhibitors of granulopoiesis have also been described,[5,6] although more evidence concerning these proposed inhibitors brings their true physiologic significance into question.[13,40]

Eosinophils, and possibly basophils/mast cells[37], are derived in granulopoiesis from a committed stem cell (CFU-Eo) that appears to be regulated by interleukin-5.

ERYTHROPOIESIS

New information has focused on the dynamics of erythrocyte production (Chap. 6). More primitive red cell precursors, not identifiable by light microscopy, have been detected by assays that measure the precursors' ability to produce new red cells.

Erythropoiesis is regulated by the glycoprotein hormone erythropoietin (EPO), which is present in normal serum in concentrations that vary according to the oxygen-carrying capacity of the blood. EPO is a single-chain acidic glycoprotein with a molecular weight of 30,000 to 34,000 kilodaltons (KD) and a carbohydrate content of approximately 35% to 40%.[32] It augments erythropoiesis by stimulating the production of new erythroblastic cells synthesizing hemoglobin, whether *in vivo* or *in vitro*. These cells are unable to produce hemoglobin without erythropoietin.

Culture systems exist to assay primitive erythropoietic precursor stem cells. *In vitro* studies have demonstrated two types of erythroid progenitor stem cells, burst-forming unit erythrocyte (BFU-E)[1] and colony-forming unit erythrocyte (CFU-E). The BFU-E are more primitive than the CFU-E and have a number of phenotypic differences. Characteristically, BFU-E proliferate in the presence of interleukin-3 (IL-3)[26] and stem cell factor.[25] BFU-E will form large colonies after a long period of incubation with a high concentration of erythropoietin.[8,10] These colonies were described as "bursts" because of their appearance.[1] In contrast, CFU-E form small clusters consisting of 8 to 32 cells. CFU-E are the target cells for erythropoietin.[22]

MEGAKARYOCYTOPOIESIS

Although many of the physiologic mechanisms that control both platelet and megakaryocyte production remain elusive (Chap. 55), it appears that platelet production is regulated by humoral factors such as IL-3[26] and stem cell factor.[43] Plasma harvested from severely thrombocytopenic animals, that is, animals with very low platelet counts, contains factors that significantly increase platelet production in recipient animals. This factor has been termed *thrombopoietin*[34] and, more recently, the *c-mpl ligand*.[12,45] Thrombopoietin, in the presence of early-acting cytokines such as IL-3 and stem cell factor, significantly increases development of committed megakaryocyte progenitors.

A factor that increases CFU-Meg colony formation significantly has been identified in the serum or plasma of patients with hypomegakaryocytic thrombocytopenia.[16,20] It appears that this factor, termed megakaryocyte-colony-stimulating factor (Meg-CSF), responds to the number of bone marrow megakaryocytes rather than the peripheral blood platelet count. Meg-CSF has been purified from the plasma of a patient with selective hypomegakaryocytic thrombocytopenia[31] and proved to be a glycoprotein with a molecular weight of 46,000 kD. Meg-CSF has no effect on other progenitor cells *in vitro* (*e.g.*, BFU-E, CFU-E, or CFU-GM).

The Lymphoid Stem Cell (CFU-L)

There are two distinct classes of lymphocytes, based on their functional characteristics, T lymphocytes and B lymphocytes. Current understanding of the regulatory mechanism of lymphocyte proliferation has resulted from laboratory studies of T and B lymphocytes in culture.[38]

T LYMPHOCYTES

T-cell clonal assays usually require a one-step method in which lymphocytes are incubated in the presence of a mitogen (mitosis-stimulating plant protein), usually phytohemagglutinin (PHA). The ability of lymphocytes to clone in these *in vitro* assays was suggested to differ from that of other hematopoietic cell lines, because it appeared that T cells were able to secrete their own necessary growth factor when plated in the presence of mitogen. Other blood cells (with the exception of macrophages) require the addition of their specific growth hormone by other cells (*e.g.*, erythropoietin produced by renal cells). Therefore, it appears that lymphocytes that have become blast-like because of mitogen exposure can release a lymphocyte growth factor. Production of this factor by T cells can be accelerated by monocytes or macrophages. Studies suggest that the T-cell growth factor is interleukin-2 (IL-2).[39] Proliferation of cytotoxic T cells and natural killer (NK) cells is influenced by IL-12. Interleukin-12 enhances peripheral hematopoiesis *in vivo* by mobilizing stem cells from marrow to peripheral blood.[19]

B LYMPHOCYTES

Understanding of the mechanisms that regulate B-cell proliferation has come from the ability to clone B-cell precursors *in vitro*.[30] These clones require stimulation by a B-cell activator such as a bacterial lipopolysaccharide (LPS). Identification of B-cell progenitors has been made possible by studies using inbred congenitally athymic (nude) mice, which are deficient in functional T cells. Stimulation of their lymphocytes by LPS induces the presence of colonies whose B-cell nature can be confirmed by the presence of cell surface–derived immunoglobulins. A B-cell growth factor is required, which usually can be provided by incubating mononuclear blood cells with mitogen for 72 hours. The requirement for B-cell growth factor is independent of the factor required for T-cell proliferation. IL-2 does not induce B-cell proliferation. See Chapter 23 for additional detail on lymphopoiesis.

ESSENTIALS OF GENETICS

Many genetic terms and definitions are important to understanding the origin of some hematologic disorders. The following discussion serves as a basic genetics reference for this text.

Genetics is the study of heredity, which is the transmission of physical traits from parents to offspring. The differences and resemblances among organisms related by descent are determined by the nuclear information in the gametes or sex cells of an organism. The nucleus houses genes, which are present on structures called chromosomes. Normal human cells contain 46 chromosomes, which may be divided into 22 different pairs of identical chromosomes (autosomes) and one pair of sex chromosomes (female: XX; male: XY). The chromosomes of each pair are referred to as homologous. One of each pair is derived from each of two parents.

Chromosomes make up the chromatin of the nucleus and provide information necessary for production of all substances and structures in the cell. The nucleic acid DNA is the primary constituent of chromosomes and is responsible for the passing on of inherited characteristics from generation to generation.

Mitosis and Meiosis

When the human sperm and egg meet for fertilization, a zygote is formed and begins development. This process requires two types of cell division: mitosis and meiosis.

MITOSIS

Mitosis is the process of cell division that permits the number of cells in an organism to increase or be maintained as necessary. Specifically, mitosis provides for the production of two daughter cells having the same number and type of chromosomes as the parent cell.

Mitosis consists of four stages: (1) *prophase*, in which nuclear chromatin begins to condense into pairs of threadlike structures (chromatids) connected by a centromere. Two pairs of centrioles migrate to opposite poles of the cell with a network of microtubules stretching between them (the spindle); (2) *metaphase*, in which the nuclear envelope disappears and the chromosomes begin to line up at the equator of the cell as they become attached to the microtubules of the spindle; (3) *anaphase*, in which the chromatid pairs separate and the chromatids begin migrating toward the opposite centriole poles; and, (4) *telophase*, in which spindle fibers disappear and a nuclear membrane forms around each set of chromosomes. The chromosomes begin to uncoil, and the cell begins to divide into two cells, each with a nucleus. Between mitoses, a cell is in interphase or the resting phase (Fig. 5-6). Greater detail on the stages of mitoses may be found in standard textbooks on genetics.

MEIOSIS

Meiosis is the cell division process by which the daughter cells receive only half the chromosome number of the parent. This process manufactures the gametes or sex cells, which in humans require only 23 chromosomes (referred to as the haploid number). Fertilization of an egg by a spermatozoan restores the diploid (46 chromosome) number.

Formation of gametes by meiosis requires a two-phase process, meiosis I and II. Meiosis I reduces the number of chromosomes by half by separating homologous pairs of chromosomes *without* prior duplication. Meiosis I is divided into several stages during which the homologous chromosomes align together, gene to gene, in a highly specific manner. They then repel each other and are separated, followed by cell separation. Meiosis II involves the separation of sister chromatids with the ultimate formation of four haploid cells with 23 single chromatids. Details on the stages of meiosis I and II may be found in textbooks on genetics.

The Genetic Code

The basic genetic material is DNA (deoxyribonucleic acid). It contains the code for cellular protein synthesis and is composed of two polynucleotide chains formed in a double helix. The polynucleotide chains consist of a variable sequence of two purines, adenine (A) and guanine (G); and two pyrimidines, thymidine (T) and cytosine (C). Purines and pyrimidines are matched in a sequence that is referred to as base pairing. For example, A binds to T and G with C. This pairing is obligatory and allows the DNA molecule to replicate itself precisely by separation of its strands and the formation of two new complementary strands.

The genetic code in its most basic form consists of sequences of three bases, each referred to as a triplet or codon, which directs the addition of a particular amino acid to a growing peptide or protein. For example, the codon CTC codes for glutamic acid, ATA codes for tyrosine, and AAA codes for phenylalanine. A gene is a sequence of codons that together encode the unique sequence of amino acids that create a particular protein.

The link between the DNA code and the cytoplasm where proteins are manufactured is messenger RNA (mRNA), a single-strand of polynucleotides that is formed from the DNA template by an enzyme, RNA polymerase. mRNA migrates to the cytoplasm, where its message is read by ribosomal RNA (rRNA) and transfer RNA (tRNA), which collects and transfers the proper amino acids to the proper ribosome area.

Alterations or misreading of the DNA code may or may not produce mutations that result in disease. Examples of disorders in hematology include mutations causing amino acid substitutions in the hemoglobin molecule, producing hemoglobinopathies (*e.g.*, sickle cell anemia) and misalignment of homologous chromosomes followed by nonhomologous crossing over of DNA segments between sister chromatids during meiosis (*e.g.*, hemoglobin Lepore).

Genetic Terminology

A basic understanding of genetic terminology will be helpful in studying hematologic abnormalities.

A *hereditary* or inherited condition is always transmitted genetically but may not be detectable at birth. For example, pernicious anemia (Chap. 12) may be hereditary but is usually first detected in adult life.

A *congenital* condition is one that is present at birth although it may not be detectable. It need not be hereditary. For example, a baby born deaf because of *in utero* exposure to rubella virus during the first trimester has a congenital condition that was not caused by genetic transmission and is thus not hereditary. A *familial* condition is present in more than one member of a family and may be hereditary or caused by environmental factors.

Although genes on a homologous chromosome pair code for the same trait, there are often alternate trait forms, such as blue or brown eyes or blood group A or B. Two genes in a homologous pair are referred to as *alleles* and may code for the same or alternate forms of the trait. An individual having two different alleles for a particular genetic trait (*e.g.*, one allele for blue eyes, the other for brown) is said to be *heterozygous*. An individual with identical genes for a given homologous pair from each parent (*e.g.*, both genes code for blue eyes) is *homozygous* for that trait.

Genotype is dependent on the type of alleles present on the chromosome pair. For example, for blood groups the genotype may be AA, AO, or AB. The *phenotype* of an individual is the morphologic, physiologic, or biochemical expression of the genotype. For example, a person will express blood group O only if both alleles coding for the blood group are O. That is, the person must have the homozygous genotype OO to have the phenotype O. On the other hand, a person with the heterozygous genotype AO will have the phenotype A; the blood will type as group A just like the blood of a person with the homozygous genotype AA.

The phenotype concept becomes more clear with an understanding of the terms *dominant* and *recessive*. An allele is dominant (*e.g.*, blood group allele A) when it is expressed regardless of whether the genotype is homozygous or heterozygous. A recessive allele, on the other hand, is expressed phenotypically only when the genotype is homozygous (*e.g.*, blood group allele O).

Probability and Patterns of Gene Transmission

The genetic laws of probability determine the patterns of genetic transmission. Consider a hypothetical crossing of two parents who are each heterozygous for the trait T, making their genotypes Tt. Assume that T is dominant and associated with tall height and that t is recessive and represents short height. Figure 5-7 shows two Punnett squares (developed by R.C. Punnett in the early 1900s), which help to visualize the probable genetic composition. The genetic characteristics of one parent are placed at the top of the square and those of the other parent down the left side. The possible combinations for the zygote are

A

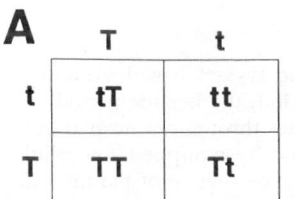

	T	t
t	tT	tt
T	TT	Tt

B

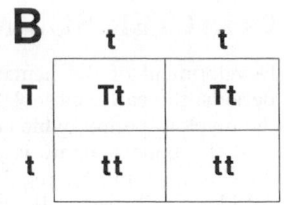

	t	t
T	Tt	Tt
t	tt	tt

FIGURE 5-7. Punnett square showing genetic probabilities. (**A**) Both parents are heterozygous for height (Tt). The resulting probability square indicates that most likely three-fourths of the offspring will be tall (¼ tT, ¼ TT, ¼ Tt) and one-fourth short (tt). (**B**) A heterozygous (Tt) and a homozygous (tt) parent; half of the offspring are expected to be tall and half short.

then figured in the resulting squares. Note that the expected ratios are probabilities, not certainties; offspring of these two hypothetical parents could turn out to be all tall or all short.

There are four basic patterns of gene transmission: (1) Autosomal dominant (*e.g.*, hereditary spherocytosis); (2) Autosomal recessive (*e.g.*, pyruvate kinase deficiency); (3) X-linked or sex-linked dominant (no well-known hematologic disorders in this category); and (4) X-linked or sex-linked recessive (*e.g.*, hemophilia). Autosomal transmission refers to transmission by any of the 22 pairs of chromosomes not involved in the determination of sex. Sex-linked transmission is synonymous with X-linked (the X chromosome); that is, genes associated with the X chromosome are sex-linked. The Y chromosome has few

if any proven loci other than those determining the male sex. Because the Y chromosome is basically inert, any allele present on the male's single X chromosome will be expressed. Thus, X-linked traits are more commonly expressed in men than women.

In the autosomal dominant pattern, the dominant trait generally appears in every generation without skipping and is transmitted by an affected person to at least half of his or her offspring. The trait is expressed whether the genotype is homozygous or heterozygous. In the autosomal recessive pattern the zygote must receive two identical alleles for a trait, one from each parent, for expression of that trait to occur.

In the X-linked dominant pattern, the genetic abnormality is present on the X chromosome and is dominant. Consequently, both males and females will express the abnormality. As with any X-linked abnormality, a father with an abnormal X chromosome will transfer this abnormality to all of his daughters, but it is impossible to transmit the abnormality from father to son because the Y chromosome is normal. Affected heterozygous females are expected to transmit the trait to half of their children. Homozygous females transmit the trait to all of their children.

In the X-linked recessive pattern, expression is far more common in males than females because males are affected by a single X chromosome, whereas females who have two X chromosomes must be homozygous before the abnormality is expressed. Hemophilia is a classic blood

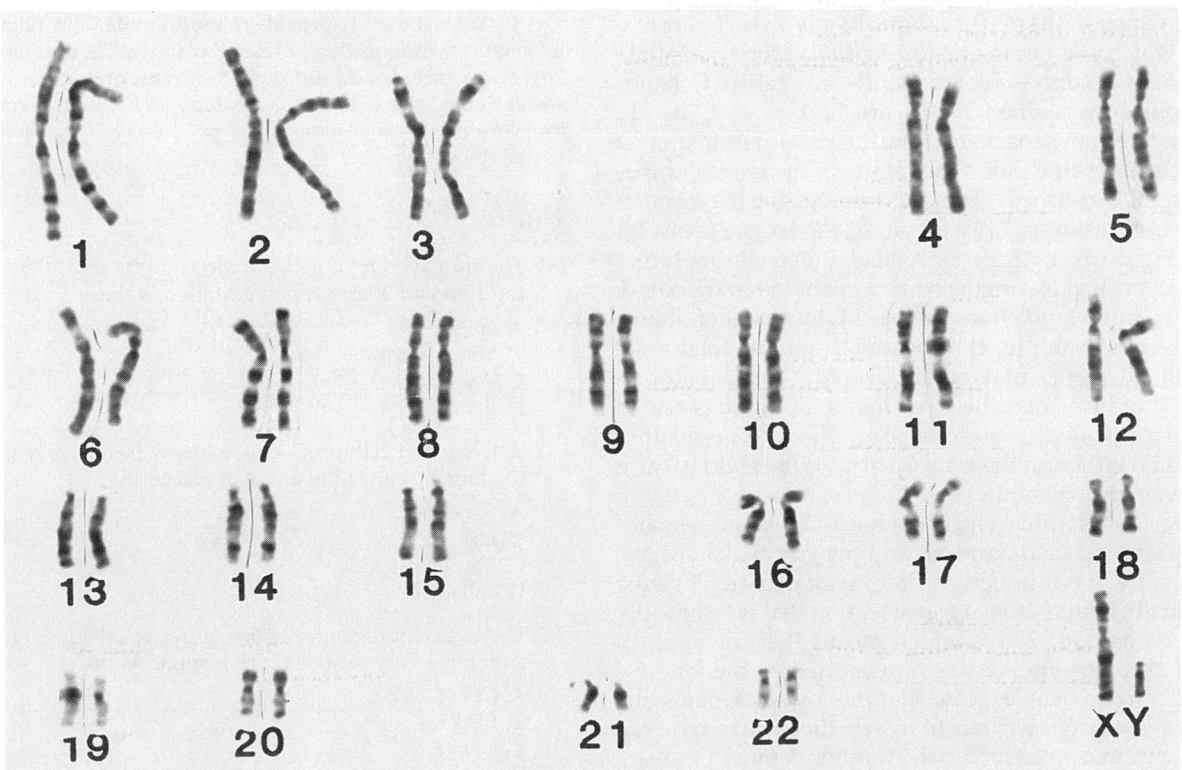

FIGURE 5-8. Normal G-banded male karyotype. (With permission of Ann Cork, Assistant Clinical Cytogeneticist, Section of Cytogenetics, and Dr. JM Trujillo, Head, Division of Laboratory Medicine and Chief, Section of Cytogenetics, The University of Texas System Cancer Center, MD Anderson Hospital and Tumor Institute, Houston, TX.)

disorder in this category. The trait is passed from affected males by way of their single abnormal X chromosome to all daughters, who may transfer the abnormality to half of their offspring, male or female. X-linked recessive traits may never be passed directly from father to son because the Y chromosome is normal. The extent of expression of an X-linked disorder in a female heterozygote (carrier) can vary considerably because of random and fixed inactivation of one of the two X chromosomes during early embryonic life (Lyon hypothesis).

CYTOGENETICS

Cytogenetics is the analysis of chromosomal structure. The examination of chromosomes in blood cells can provide information important to the diagnosis and prognosis of leukemias, lymphomas, and related disorders. Figure 5-8 depicts a normal human male karyotype showing each of the 22 autosomal chromosomal pairs with the sex chromosomes (XY) in the lower-right-hand corner. The chromosomes are matched according to their relative size and centromere location. Each pair has been assigned a unique number for karyotyping purposes.

Development of a karyotype involves culturing hematopoietic cells to obtain dividing cells in the metaphase stage. The mitotic process is then stopped by the addition of colchicine which destroys the mitotic spindle. The cells are fixed and dropped onto a clean microscope slide, where the chromosomes fall in a random pattern. The slides are then stained, usually with Giemsa or quinacrine, both of which stain specific unique bands on each chromosome, which are necessary to identify chromosomal abnormalities. Giemsa-colored bands are called G bands and quinacrine-stained bands are known as Q bands. Whichever stain is used, the banding pattern is unique for every chromosome pair. Once stained, the chromosomes may be photographed. From this photograph the chromosomes are cut out and placed on the karyotype board for study. Figure 5-8 depicts normal G-banded chromosomes that have been placed in the correct positions on the board.

Karyotype study may reveal many types of abnormalities. For example, chromosomes may be totally deleted, or extra ones may be discovered. Parts of chromosomes may be added, deleted, inverted, or translocated (moved from one chromosome to another). Abnormalities are located either on the long (q) arm or the short (p) arm of a given chromosome.

The Philadelphia chromosome is a classic hematologic example of a diagnostic and prognostic karyotypic abnormality. It is found in chronic myelogenous leukemia and usually results from a translocation that is technically described as $t(9q^+.22q^-)$, which means that the long (q) arm of chromosome 22 has translocated to the long (q) arm of chromosome 9. Note that the lower chromosome number is always written first, whether it has received or lost chromosomal material. Another common translocation in leukemias and lymphomas is $t(8q^-;14q^+)$, which refers to translocation from the long arm of chromosome 8 to the long arm of chromosome 14. An abnormality receiving increasing attention in hematology is $5q^-$, which represents deletion of the long arm of chromosome 5.

CHAPTER SUMMARY

Development of the hematopoietic system has three defined periods: the early, mesoblastic period; the hepatic period; and the myeloid period, which continues throughout normal life.

The bone marrow is anatomically equipped for cellular development and for regulation of the release of mature cells. All blood cells except lymphocytes are believed to be derived from a bone marrow cell known as CFU-S or CFU-GEMM. Lymphocytes are produced from the lymphoid stem cell (CFU-L). Both of these stem cells are derived from a more primitive stem cell known as the totipotential stem cell.

Growth factors are necessary for stem cell development, as well as for maturation of these cells into more committed progeny as they develop into granulocytes, lymphocytes, erythrocytes, and megakaryocytes. Stem cell factor, the ligand for c-kit receptor, appears to be the molecule necessary for the proliferation and maintenance of these primitive stem cells. Colony-stimulating factors such as GM- and G-CSF are responsible for regulating granulocyte production. These factors are now being evaluated for their efficacy in clinical medicine. Three classes of lymphocytes exist: B, T, and null cells. The T cell can produce its own growth factor (IL-2), whereas B cells require extrinsic growth factor stimulation. Erythrocyte production is regulated by the hormone erythropoietin (EPO). Regulation of megakaryocyte and platelet production has been linked to thrombopoietin, the ligand for the c-mpl receptor.

Concepts of genetics were reviewed in this chapter to provide a basis for understanding the inheritance of many hematologic abnormalities. The terms defined were genes, chromosomes, alleles, mitosis, meiosis, hereditary, congenital, heterozygous, homozygous, genotype, phenotype, dominant, and recessive. Probability and patterns of gene transmission were defined.

Cytogenetic study provides a useful tool in the diagnosis of leukemias, lymphomas, and related disorders. A normal human karyotype includes 22 autosomal chromosome pairs and the sex chromosomes. Chromosomes may be deleted, inverted, or translocated. Extra chromosomes may also be discovered in a karyotype study.

Review Questions

5-1. The primary site of hematopoiesis in the fetus between the 10th and 30th week of gestation is the

   A. spleen.
   B. bone marrow.
   C. thymus.
   D. liver.

5-2. Active blood cell–producing marrow begins to regress in the fourth year of life and is replaced by

   A. bone.
   B. fat.
   C. fibrous tissue.
   D. collagen.

5-3. The red cell progenitor that requires relatively large amounts of erythropoietin to respond is the

   A. CFU-GEMM.
   B. BFU-E.
   C. CFU-E.
   D. pronormoblast.

5-4. The two cell types that produce their own growth factors are

   A. neutrophils and monocytes.
   B. neutrophils and lymphocytes.

C. neutrophils and eosinophils.

D. lymphocytes and monocytes.

5-5. The metaphase stage of mitosis is characterized by

A. the beginning of chromatin condensation into chromosomes.

B. the lining up of chromosomes along the center of the cell.

C. the separation of chromatids to the two poles of the cell.

D. the initiation of cellular division into two daughter cells.

5-6. The link between the DNA code and the cytoplasm in which proteins are manufactured is

A. RNA polymerase.

B. messenger RNA.

C. transfer RNA.

D. ribosomal RNA.

5-7. An abnormal condition that is present at birth is said to be

A. congenital and may or may not be hereditary.

B. hereditary and may or may not be familial.

C. familial and may or may not be congenital.

D. acquired and may or may not be hereditary.

5-8. A characteristic that is autosomal dominant

A. will appear in every other generation.

B. is manifested in males more than females.

C. requires two alleles to be expressed.

D. appears in every generation.

References

1. Axelrad AA, McLeod DL, Shreeve MM et al: Properties of cells that produce erythrocytic colonies *in vitro*. In Robison WA (ed): Hemopoiesis in Culture, p 226. Washington, DC, US Government Printing Office, 1974

2. Becker AJ, McCulloch EA, Siminovitch L et al: The effect of different demands for blood cell population in DNA synthesis by haematopoietic colony forming cells of mice. Blood 26:296, 1986

3. Blackburn MJ, Patt HM: Increased survival of haematopoietic pluripotent stem cells *in vitro* induced by a marrow fibroblast factor. Br J Haematol 37:337, 1977

4. Bradley TR, Metcalf DD: The growth of mouse bone marrow cells *in vitro*. Aust J Exp Biol Med Sci 44:287, 1966

5. Broxmeyer HE: Inhibition *in vivo* of mouse granulopoiesis by cell-free activity derived from human polymorphonuclear neutrophils. Blood 51:899, 1978

6. Broxmeyer HE, Smithyman A, Egar RR et al: Identification of lactoferrin as the granulocyte-derived inhibitor of colony stimulating activity production. J Exp Med 148:1052, 1978

7. Cairns J: Mutation selection and the natural history of cancer. Nature 225:1197,1975

8. Cerny J: Stimulation of bone marrow haematopoietic stem cells by a factor from activated T-cells. Nature 249:63, 1974

9. Curry JL, Trentin JG: Hemopoietic spleen colony studies. I: Growth and differentiation. Dev Biol 15:395, 1967

10. Dainiak N, Kreczko S, Cohen A et al: Primary human marrow cultures for erythroid bursts in a serum-substituted system. Exp Hematol 13:1073, 1985

11. Denburg JA, Telizyn S, Messner H et al: Heterogeneity of human peripheral blood eosinophil-type colonies: Evidence for a common basophil-eosinophil progenitor. Blood 66:312, 1985

12. deSauvage FJ, Hass PE, Spencer SD et al: Stimulation of megakaryocytopoiesis and thrombopoiesis by the c-mpl ligand. Nature 369:533, 1994

13. Dezza L, Cazzola M, Piacibello W et al: Effect of acidic and basic isoferritins on *in vitro* growth of human granulocyte-monocyte progenitors. Blood 67:789:1986

14. Doukas MA, Gallicchio VS: Cytokine modulation of radiation injury. In Aggarwal BB, Puri R (eds): Human Cytokines: Their Role in Disease and Therapy, p 567. London, Blackwell Scientific, 1995

15. Drinker CK, Drinker KR, Lund CC: The circulation in the mammalian bone marrow. Am J Physiol 62:1, 1922

16. Enomoto K, Kawakita M, Koshimoto S et al: Thrombopoiesis and megakaryocyte colony stimulating factor in the serum of patients with aplastic anemia. Br J Haematol 45:551, 1980

17. Fliedner TM, Cronkite EP, Robertson JS: Granulocytopoiesis. I. Senescence and random loss of neutrophilic granulocytes in human beings. Blood 24:402, 1964

18. Gregory CG: Erythropoietin sensitivity as a differentiation marker in the hemopoietic system: Studies of three erythropoietic colony responses in culture. J Cell Physiol 89:289, 1976

19. Jackson JD, Yan Y, Brunda MJ et al: Interleukin-12 enhances peripheral hematopoiesis *in vivo*. Blood 85:2371, 1995

20. Kawakita M, Miyake T, Kishimoto S et al: Apparent heterogeneity of human megakaryocyte colony- and thrombopoiesis stimulating factors: Studies on urinary extracts from patients with aplastic anaemia and idiopathic thrombocytopenic purpura. Br J Haematol 52:429, 1982

21. Klein G: The extracellular matrix of the hematopoietic microenvironment. Experientia 51:914, 1995

22. Koury MS, Sawyer ST, Bondurant MC: Splenic erythroblasts in anemia-inducing Friend disease: A source of cells for studies of erythropoietin-mediated differentiation. J Cell Physiol 121:526, 1984

23. Lajtha LG: Stem cell concepts. Differentiation 14:23, 1979

24. Lord BI, Mori KJ, Wright EG: A stimulation of stem cell proliferation in regenerating bone marrow. Biomedicine 27:223, 1977

25. Martin FH, Suggs SV, Langley KE et al: Primary structure and functional expression of rat and human stem cell factor DNAs. Cell 63:203, 1990

26. Messner HA, Yanazaki K, Jamal N et al: Growth of human hematopoietic colonies in response to recombinant gibbon interleukin 3. Comparison with human recombinant granulocyte and granulocyte-macrophage colony stimulating factor. Proc Natl Acad Sci USA 84:6765, 1987

27. Metcalf D: The Hemopoietic Colony Stimulating Factors. Amsterdam, Elsevier, 1984

28. Metcalf D: The molecular biology and functions of the granulocyte-macrophage colony stimulating factors. Blood 67:257, 1986

29. Metcalf D, Burgess AW: Analysis of progenitor commitment to granulocyte or macrophage production. J Cell Physiol 111:275, 1982

30. Metcalf D, Warner NL, Nassal GJV et al: Growth of B-lymphocyte colonies *in vitro* from mouse lymphoid organs. Nature 255:630, 1975

31. Minden M: Growth factor requirements for normal and leukemic cells. Semin Hematol 32:162, 1995

32. Miyaki T, Kung CKH, Goldwasser E: Purification of human erythropoietin. J Biol Chem 252:5558, 1977

33. Moffatt DJ, Rose C, Yoffey JM Jr: Identity of the hematopoietic stem cell. Lancet 2:547, 1967

34. Nagahisa H, Cuda Y, Okutomi K et al: Thrombopoietin induces megakaryocyte differentiation in hematopoietic progenitor FDC-P2 cells. J Biol Chem 270:19673, 1995

35. Nakahata T, Gross AJ, Ogawa M: A stochastic model of self renewal and commitment to differentiation of the primary hemopoietic stem cells in culture. J Cell Physiol 113:455, 1982

36. Nakahata T, Ogawa M: Identification in culture of a new

class of hematopoietic colony-forming units with extensive capability to self-renew and generate multipotential colonies. Proc Natl Acad Sci USA 29:3843, 1982

37. Pluznik DH, Sachs L: The cloning of normal mast cells in tissue culture. J Cell Comp Physiol 66:319, 1965

38. Rozenszajn LA, Zeevi A, Gopas J et al: Lymphocyte colony growth *in vitro*. ICN-UCLA Symp Mol Cell Biol 10:261, 1978

39. Ruscetti FW, Gallo RC: Human T lymphocyte growth factor. Regulation of growth and function of T lymphocytes [review]. Blood 57:379, 1981

40. Sala G, Worwood M, Jacobs A: The effect of isoferritins on granulopoiesis. Blood 67:436, 1986

41. Schofield R: The relationship between the spleen colony-forming cell and the haematopoietic cell. Blood Cells 4:7, 1978

42. Schrader JW, Clark-Lewis I: A T cell derived factor stimulating multipotential hemopoietic stem cells: Molecular weight and distinction from T cell derived granulocyte-macrophage colony stimulating factor. J Immunol 139:30, 1982

43. Tanaka R, Katayama N, Ohishi K et al: Accelerated cell-cycling of hematopoietic progenitor cells by growth factors. Blood 86:73, 1995

44. Till JE, McCulloch EA, Siminovitch L: A stochastic model of stem cell proliferation, based on the growth of spleen colony forming cells. Proc Natl Acad Sci USA 78:29, 1964

45. Wang JF, Deng B, Groopman JE et al: Modulation of megakaryocytopoiesis by thrombopoietin: the c-mpl ligand. Blood 86:1331, 1995

46. Weiss L: This histology of the bone marrow. In Gordon AS (ed): Regulation of Hematopoiesis, vol 1, p 79. New York, Appleton-Century-Crofts, 1970

PART II

The Erythrocytes

CHAPTER 6

Normal Erythrocyte Production, Physiology, and Destruction

Marian Schwabbauer

Objectives

1. List the principal sites of erythrocyte production and destruction.
2. Draw a flow diagram of the major erythrocyte morphologic maturation process from pluripotent stem cell to mature erythrocyte.
3. Describe classic morphologic features of each erythrocyte maturation stage.
4. List each major erythrocyte component and its primary function(s).
5. Describe the glycolytic processes that provide the erythrocyte with energy and protection from oxidative stresses.
6. Compare and contrast the destruction of normal and severely damaged red cells.
7. Explain erythrokinetics and how balance between erythrocyte production and destruction is maintained.

Erythrocytes play a vital role in human physiology. To appreciate this role and how it relates to disease states, a basic understanding of erythrocyte development is necessary. In this chapter, normal erythrocyte development and the factors that influence erythrocyte survival, function, physiology, and destruction will be presented.

van Leeuwenhoek first viewed erythrocytes through his primitive microscope in 1673, describing them as "small round globules." At that time erythrocytes were thought to be insignificant. Today he would be amazed to learn of the intricacies of the erythrocyte's internal dynamics, the simple and yet complicated molecular membrane structure, and the numerous internal and morphologic changes that occur as the erythrocyte matures from a primitive cell. Even slight alterations in these complicated features can be associated with numerous disorders, some of which can be life threatening.

Erythrocytes and their precursors can be thought of as a functioning organ called the *erythron*.[9] The primary function of the erythron is to deliver adequate oxygen (O_2) to the tissues. Oxygen, which is used for aerobic metabolism, is bound to hemoglobin (Hb; Chap. 7) within the erythrocyte and carried from the lungs to cells throughout the body. Transport of the waste product carbon dioxide (CO_2) is also a vital erythron function.

To function effectively, the body must maintain approximately 309×10^9 circulating erythrocytes per kilogram of body weight.[17] Remarkable regulatory mechanisms keep the production and destruction of erythrocytes in balance. Normally, whenever there is blood loss or when erythrocytes are destroyed after their normal 120-day life span,[4] they are quickly replaced from various production sites (Fig. 6-1). Erythrocyte production (erythropoiesis) and destruction are a constant process.

ERYTHROCYTE PRODUCTION

Origin

Erythrocytes originate from a pluripotent stem cell called the colony-forming unit–stem (CFU-S; Chap. 5). During

a progressive process, the cell becomes specialized and able to synthesize proteins that are needed for function and survival. As these proteins accumulate and various other changes occur, the morphology of the cell changes. These changes in the maturation process have been divided into stages (Fig. 6-2). The rubriblast, the earliest stage, and the stages that follow will be discussed later. These stages are found in the bone marrow and may be separated morphologically by light microscopy. The precursor cells after the pluripotent stem cell and before the rubriblast are found in small numbers; their presence has been postulated on the basis of the results of *in vitro* studies in the 1970s.

The burst-forming unit—erythroid (BFU-E) is the earliest erythroid-committed cell thus far identified and is thought to be closely related to the CFU-S. The BFU-E is thought to mature gradually through several steps into the colony-forming unit–erythroid (CFU-E),[19,55] which is closely related to the rubriblast.

The terms BFU-E and CFU-E describe the cells' growth patterns in laboratory culture media. The CFU-E was first to be identified. In 1971 Stephenson and associates[76] added erythropoietin (EPO) to a bone marrow cell culture.[36,64] EPO is a glycoprotein long known to be a stimulator of erythropoiesis. After 1 to 2 days, pure colonies of maturing erythroid cells were detected. These investigators postulated that primitive erythroid precursors in the bone marrow culture were stimulated by the EPO and that each precursor formed one colony of maturing erythroid precursors (designated CFU-E).

Axelrad and coworkers[4] did a similar study in which a large amount of EPO was added to a bone marrow culture. The expected CFU-E colonies grew and then diminished. After 7 days, another type of colony appeared[21] whose growth was in clusters or "bursts." This progenitor was designated burst-forming unit—erythroid or BFU-E. Later work confirmed that the BFU-E is actually a precursor of the CFU-E.

Only a few BFU-E normally are present in the bone marrow; therefore, BFU-E are difficult to identify morphologically. They are thought to be different from, although similar to, small to medium-sized lymphocytes. Circulating BFU-E have been grown from the peripheral blood[12] and are thought to reside in the natural killer (NK) cell fraction of lymphocytes (*i.e.*, non-B, non-T, or null lymphocytes) (Chaps. 5 and 23). Recent evidence suggests that they reside specifically in a subpopulation of NK cells that lack the receptor for the Fc fragment of immunoglobulin G.[67] Increased numbers of circulating BFU-E have been demonstrated in some anemias.[58] The CFU-E (which may also be found in peripheral blood) may resemble early erythroid precursors by light microscopy but show much larger nucleoli and many more mitochondria by electron microscopy.[57]

Production Sites

The main sites of adult hematopoiesis or blood cell production include the vertebrae, pelvis, ribs, sternum, and skull and the proximal ends of the femur and humerus.[15] Figure 6-1A demonstrates these production sites as revealed by radioisotopes.

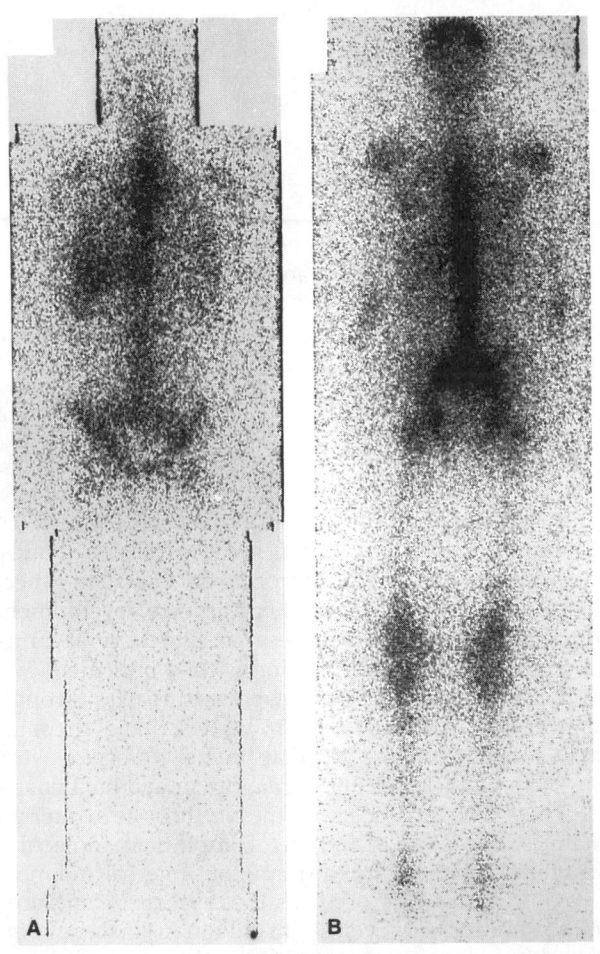

FIGURE 6-1. Radionuclide images that demonstrate erythrocyte production sites. (**A**) ^{52}Fe scan in normal man. (**B**) ^{52}Fe scan in adult with sickle cell disease. Note expansion of active marrow into the long bones and skull. (Courtesy of Dr. EW Fordham.)

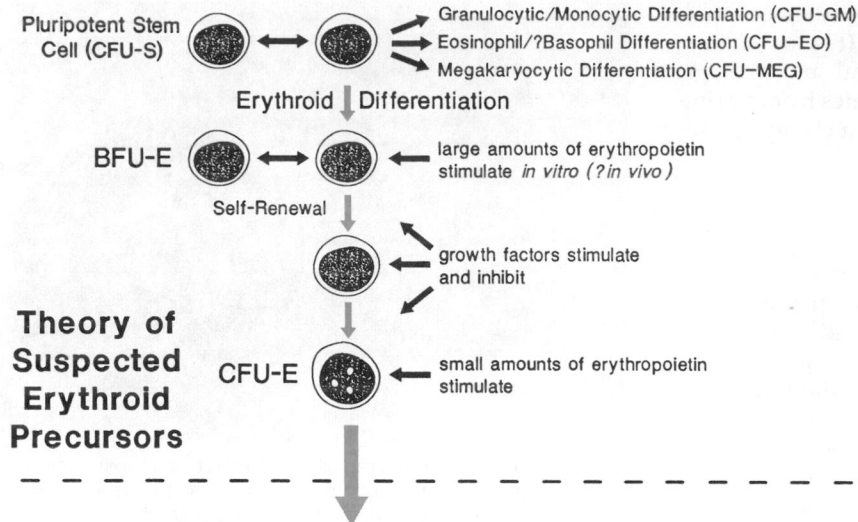

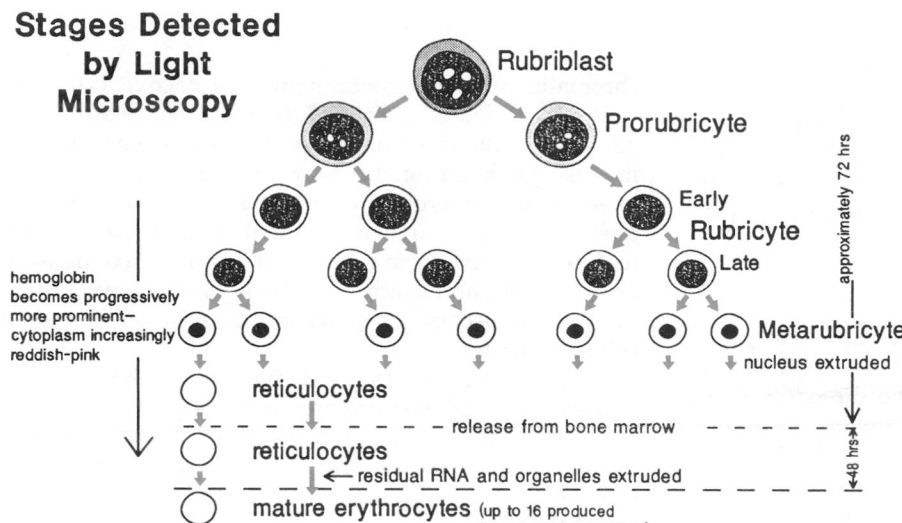

FIGURE 6-2. Steps in erythrocyte maturation.

RADIOISOTOPIC EVALUATION OF PRODUCTION SITES

Historically, radioisotopes of iron (^{59}Fe and ^{52}Fe) have been used in a nuclear medicine technique called radioactive imaging to study sites of erythropoiesis (Fig. 6-1A).[7] The technique involves the intravenous injection of a radioisotope or radioactive tracer element, which is carried by the circulation to the organs that normally metabolize or store that element. After radioisotope injection, total body surface counts are done with an external probe, which shows the locations of radioactivity in the body. Studies of specific organs are performed by selecting the appropriate radioisotope.

Iron was the radioisotope of choice because it mimics ingested iron, which is normally bound to transferrin in the blood, carried to sites of erythropoiesis, incorporated into the erythrocyte, and used for Hb formation. Thus, radioisotopic iron was used to demonstrate both normal erythrocyte production sites and abnormal marrow space expansion into the long bones and extramedullary eryth-

ropoiesis in the spleen and liver as seen in some disease states (Fig. 6-1B).

Many studies have been performed using radioiron to evaluate production sites in anemias and myeloproliferative disorders and after radiation treatment. Since the information gained from these studies has now been correlated with other clinical and laboratory data and since newer imaging techniques such as magnetic resonance imaging (MRI) and computerized axial tomographic (CAT) scans give much more information about the activity of the bone marrow and related organs, it is rarely necessary to use radioiron or other radioisotopes such as technetium-99m (^{99m}Tc) for such studies today.

ERYTHROCYTE MATURATION

Erythropoietin and other growth factors stimulate early erythroid precursors (BFU-E and CFU-E) to differentiate to the rubriblast (pronormoblast) stage of development. The rubriblast is the first precursor that can be recognized by light microscopy. The rubriblast gives rise to 16 mature erythrocytes through four cell divisions (Fig. 6-2) taking approximately 72 hours. Ultrastructural morphologic changes occur as the rubriblast differentiates from a primitive, nucleated cell to a mature, non-nucleated erythrocyte.

Ultrastructure

The organelles in early erythrocyte precursors are necessary for metabolism and synthesis of Hb, enzymes, and other proteins (Fig. 6-3). The function and structure of these organelles are complex and not completely understood. However, as proteins accumulate, the number of organelles gradually diminishes. As erythrocytes differentiate, there are alterations in morphology and membrane properties that result, in large part, from reorganization of the membrane skeletal protein network. An important component of this network is protein 4.1. Protein 4.1 is a phosphoprotein that binds to spectrin-actin complexes which compose the erythrocyte cytoskeleton (Figs. 6-6 and 17-1). Protein 4.1 also binds to the major transmembrane glycoprotein called glycophorin, which is in the lipid bilayer. Thus, protein 4.1 serves as a critical link between the cytoskeleton and the lipid bilayer. The ultrastructural changes that occur as erythrocytes mature correlate with the morphologic changes seen by light microscopy.[11,69]

NUCLEUS

The nucleus is most important in the earliest stages of development, serving as the site for DNA and RNA synthesis and, as such, the center for the direction of cell development and maturation. Chromatin, the major component of the nucleus, contains genetic material. It is composed of DNA, histones, and other proteins. It is finely dispersed and appears either condensed or granular by electron microscopy (EM). The more condensed areas of

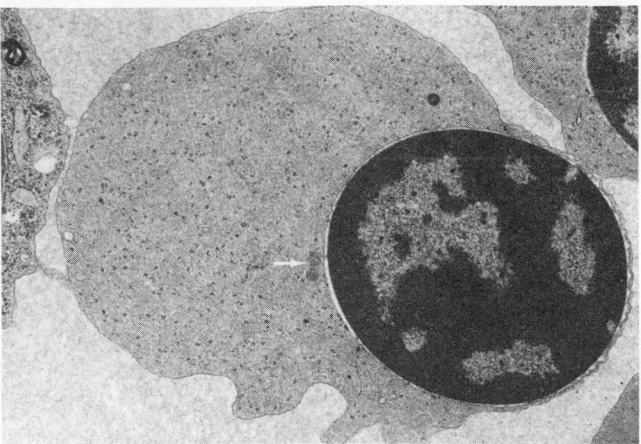

FIGURE 6-4. Electron micrograph of metarubricyte extruding its nucleus. Note residual mitochondria (**arrow**) and ribosomes (**dark granules**) in the cytoplasm and the irregular cytoplasmic borders. Most of the chromatin is condensed, inactive heterochromatin.

chromatin, called heterochromatin, are inactive. When the cells are stained with basic dyes, heterochromatin takes on a basophilic color (dark blue) when viewed by light microscopy. Euchromatin, which is active, appears more open by light microscopy and does not stain with basic dyes. It is not well demonstrated by EM. As the cell matures the chromatin becomes increasingly condensed, and metabolic and synthetic activities decline until finally the nucleus becomes inactive and is extruded from the cell (see Fig. 6-4).

Multiple nucleoli that stain intensely with basic dyes and are electron dense are present in the rubriblast. They contain RNA, proteins, and small amounts of DNA.[29] Nucleoli are involved in the production and distribution of RNA.

CYTOPLASM

Many free ribosomes and clusters of ribosomes called polyribosomes are present in the cytoplasm of the early erythrocyte precursors. They are the site of synthesis of globin (a Hb component) and other proteins. Polyribosomes may also be attached to the endoplasmic reticulum and are thought to form different proteins from those synthesized by free ribosomes. Ribosomes give stained early precursors a deep, dark blue cytoplasm by light microscopy (see Color Plate 6-1). As Hb is formed, the number of ribosomes gradually diminishes, and the dark blue color is gradually replaced with reddish pink.

The Golgi apparatus is located near the nucleus and appears by light microscopy as a pale or lightened area. By EM the Golgi apparatus appears as a cluster of vesicles and plates of different shapes. Glycoproteins enter the organelle to be modified, sorted, and sent to their appropriate destination within the cell. That is, the Golgi acts as "traffic director" for the thousands of protein molecules synthesized.[68]

Mitochondria, as seen by EM, are rod- or oval-shaped organelles in the cytoplasm that serve several functions in erythroid precursors. The most important are aerobic generation of energy for the maturing cell and insertion

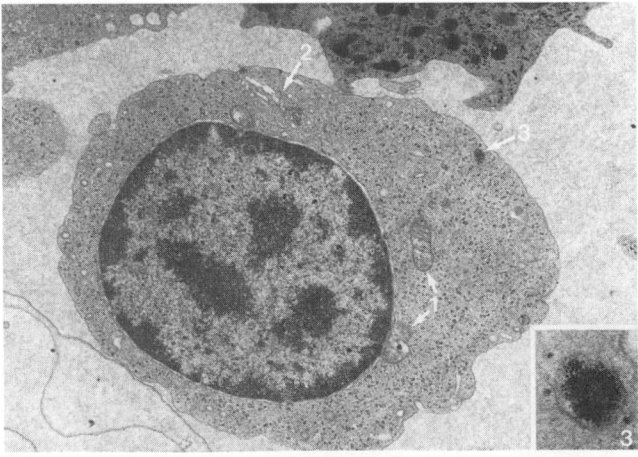

FIGURE 6-3. Electron micrograph of early erythroid precursor (approximately at prorubricyte stage). (1) Mitochondria. (2) Golgi apparatus. Note many ribosomes in cytoplasm, which appear as dark granules. The lighter areas of the nucleus are active (euchromatin); the darker areas are inactive (heterochromatin). **Inset:** (3) Magnified view of a vesicle containing ferritin. (Original magnification ×108,850.)

of ferrous (Fe^{2+}) iron into protoporphyrin IX during heme synthesis (Chap. 7). Mitochondria are not visible by light microscopy.

Iron is also present in the cytoplasm as ferritin and hemosiderin, two storage forms of iron, which can be found freely dispersed or membrane-bound in vesicles. Using light microscopy and an iron stain such as Prussian blue, iron can be demonstrated in small aggregates called siderotic granules (see Fig. 8-24).

Maturation Stages as Seen by Light Microscopy

Staining a bone marrow sample with a modified Romanowsky stain such as Wright stain and observing by light microscopy allow the identification of six morphologic stages of erythrocyte maturation. Because maturation is a continuous process, there is overlap between stages. However, the designation of stages is a helpful diagnostic tool, and these stages can be identified easily by the trained eye.

Normal morphology is dependent on adequate intake and metabolism of many nutrients necessary for maturation. Vitamin B_{12}, folate, and iron are particularly important. The abnormal morphology associated with these nutrient deficiencies is discussed in Chapters 12 and 13.

NOMENCLATURE

There are three nomenclatures used today to describe the six stages of erythrocyte maturation: rubri, normoblast, and erythroblast (Table 6-1). In the late 1800s Paul Ehrlich used the term erythroblast to describe nucleated erythrocyte precursors and divided them into two categories. Normal precursors he called normoblasts. Large abnormal precursors, now known to be caused by impairment of DNA synthesis, he called megaloblasts (Chap. 12).

Through the years, the terms normoblast and erythroblast have been used with descriptive prefixes to describe the first four stages of normal erythrocyte maturation. Use of the word *blast* when referring to a cell beyond the blast stage of development has been confusing. To solve this problem and to develop uniformity in classification, a new nomenclature was proposed by the American Society of Clinical Pathologists (ASCP).[13] *Rubri,* meaning red,

was incorporated into the name of the first four maturation stages (Table 6-1). The rubri nomenclature has not been universally accepted, however, so it is necessary to be familiar with the older terms as well. The rubri and normoblast nomenclatures are most commonly used.

GENERAL GUIDELINES

The College of American Pathologists[10] has published a glossary developed by hematologist Dr. L. W. Diggs to promote uniformity in cell identification, which will be used, in part, in the following descriptions of erythrocyte precursors. The following are some general guidelines for the identification of erythroid precursors:

Progressive decrease in size and the degree of cytoplasmic basophilia (blue color) as the cell matures

Nuclei are round or oval in the blast stage, becoming very round thereafter

Gradual increase in the coarseness and condensation of the chromatin, ranging from fine in the early stages to pyknotic (dense nuclear mass) in the stage just before nuclear extrusion

RUBRIBLAST (PRONORMOBLAST)

The rubriblast is the earliest erythrocyte precursor identifiable by light microscopy in the Romanowsky-stained bone marrow sample (see Color Plates 6-1 through 6-4). Cell size is variable, ranging from 12 to 25 μm. The nuclear:cytoplasmic ratio is high, with the nucleus usually occupying more than 80% of the cell. The cytoplasm is basophilic (intense dark blue) because of the high RNA content, which attracts the basic part of the stain, such as methylene blue. The Golgi apparatus may be visible as a pale area next to the nucleus. The nucleus is usually round to slightly oval, has dispersed fine clumps of chromatin, and contains nucleoli.

At times it is difficult to differentiate the rubriblast from a myeloblast (the earliest identifiable stage of granulopoiesis). However, a myeloblast usually has less cytoplasmic basophilia and a fine, lacy chromatin that stains less intensely than the rubriblast (see Color Plate 6-4). At this stage of maturation the degree of basophilia probably is more helpful than nuclear characteristics in distinguish-

---

TABLE 6-1
Nomenclatures of Erythrocytic Stages of Maturation

Rubri	Normoblast	Erythroblast
Rubriblast	Pronormoblast	Proerythroblast
Prorubricyte	Basophilic normoblast	Basophilic erythroblast
Rubricyte	Polychromatophilic normoblast	Polychromatophilic erythroblast
Metarubricyte	Orthochromic or orthochromatophilic normoblast	Orthochromic erythroblast
Reticulocyte*	Reticulocyte*	Reticulocyte*
Erythrocyte	Erythrocyte	Erythrocyte

* *"Diffusely basophilic erythrocyte" and "polychromatophilic erythrocyte" are terms sometimes applied to the reticulocyte, particularly when seen on the peripheral blood film.*

ing between the two. The rubriblast gives rise to two prorubricytes (Fig. 6-2).

PRORUBRICYTE (BASOPHILIC NORMOBLAST)

The prorubricyte is slightly smaller (12–17 μm) than the rubriblast, with the nucleus usually occupying 75% of the cell (see Color Plates 6-1 and 6-2). The cytoplasm is basophilic, with the Golgi apparatus usually visible as a light area near the nucleus. The nucleus is round; its chromatin is dark violet and definitely coarser and more clumped than that of the rubriblast. Parachromatin, the nonstaining or clear area of the nucleus, is slightly visible between the clumps of chromatin. Usually nucleoli are no longer visible. The coarser chromatin and the absence of nucleoli are the most helpful criteria in distinguishing the prorubricyte from the rubriblast (see Color Plate 6-5). The prorubricyte usually divides two times, giving rise to four rubricytes.

RUBRICYTE (POLYCHROMATOPHILIC NORMOBLAST)

The rubricyte is usually smaller (12–15 μm) than the prorubricyte (see Color Plates 6-1, 6-2, and 6-6). It has a round nucleus that may be eccentric. Throughout this stage of maturation, more cytoplasm becomes apparent as the nucleus becomes smaller. The cytoplasm shows a varied spectrum of blue color as Hb is synthesized. Blue RNA mixed with red Hb gives the cytoplasm an opaque, blue-gray-violet color called polychromasia or polychromatophilia. Early rubricyte cytoplasm is moderately polychromatophilic, differing from the intensely dark blue cytoplasm of the prorubricyte. Late rubricytes have a paler violet-blue-gray to slightly pinkish color. The nuclear chromatin is coarse and condensed. Distinct areas of parachromatin are visible amid clumps of chromatin. This cell can be confused with a lymphocyte (see Color Plate 6-7). Each rubricyte usually gives rise to two metarubricytes. This is the last cell division during maturation.

METARUBRICYTE (ORTHOCHROMIC NORMOBLAST)

The metarubricyte is the last nucleated erythrocyte stage (see Color Plates 6-1, 6-2, and 6-8). It is the same size as or slightly smaller than the rubricyte (8–12 μm). One distinguishing feature of this cell is its paler, violet-blue-gray (polychromatophilic) cytoplasm, which is more pinkish than that of the rubricyte since Hb is the main cytoplasmic constituent. Another feature is the very dense, coarse, and clumped nuclear chromatin pattern. The nucleus is degenerated or pyknotic.

The nucleus is extruded at this stage (Fig. 6-4) and the cell becomes a reticulocyte. Sometimes the nucleus is not completely extruded. The nuclear remnant is called a Howell-Jolly body (see Fig. 8-21). Normally Howell-Jolly bodies are removed (pitted) by the spleen and not seen in circulating red cells; however, they may be seen in certain disease states (Chap. 8).

Not all immature erythrocytes develop normally. Abnormal early cells are removed by macrophages in the bone marrow; these cells never reach maturity and the

circulation. When an abnormally increased number of developing cells do not become normal circulating erythrocytes, the term *ineffective erythropoiesis* is used.

RETICULOCYTE (DIFFUSELY BASOPHILIC ERYTHROCYTE, POLYCHROMATOPHILIC ERYTHROCYTE)

The reticulocyte is slightly larger than the mature erythrocyte. It may have irregular cytoplasmic borders (see Color Plate 6-2). The cytoplasm still contains small amounts of RNA, producing varying amounts of polychromasia.

After nuclear expulsion, reticulocytes are retained in the marrow for 2 to 3 days[24] before release into the marrow sinusoids to appear in the peripheral blood. The mechanism for their release is unknown; many factors probably are involved. Perhaps as the erythrocyte matures, it loses its ability to adhere to fibronectin, a glycoprotein in the bone marrow matrix.[60]

The reticulocyte contains Golgi apparatus remnants and residual mitochondria that permit continued aerobic metabolism and Hb production, which decrease as the cell matures. Reticulocytes also contain residual RNA, which may be stained supravitally (in the living state) using stains such as new methylene blue or brilliant cresyl blue (see Fig. 9-6). Such staining causes the RNA to precipitate and aggregate into a network of strands or clumps visible by light microscopy. Reticulocytes can then be counted and the reticulocyte production index (RPI; Chap. 9) calculated for evaluation of the effectiveness of erythropoiesis in anemic states.

Within 24 to 48 hours of release from the bone marrow, the reticulocyte loses its organelles and assumes a biconcave shape. It is then considered a mature erythrocyte.

MATURE ERYTHROCYTE

The mature erythrocyte is approximately 7.2 μm in diameter (see Color Plate 6-1). In the resting state it is a biconcave disc, thus the name discocyte (see Fig. 6-5). A Wright stain reveals a central pale area that fades gradually into reddish-pink cytoplasm (see Color Plate 6-9). The central pallor corresponds to the indentation in the erythrocyte disc. The mature erythrocyte contains no mitochondria; therefore, neither protein nor Hb is synthesized.

Problems in Erythroid Cell Identification

Problems in bone marrow erythroid cell identification may be encountered unless several precautions are taken. Proper identification requires selection of an area of the slide containing a thin film of bone marrow in which the cells are separated (Chap. 27). The stain should be bright with good contrast between purple, blue, and pink. Granulocyte granules should be distinct. Even with a good stain, however, it can be difficult to distinguish erythroid precursors from other cells such as plasma cells and lymphocytes.

Besides early erythroid precursors, the only other normal cells in the bone marrow that usually display intense, dark blue cytoplasm are plasma cells (see Color

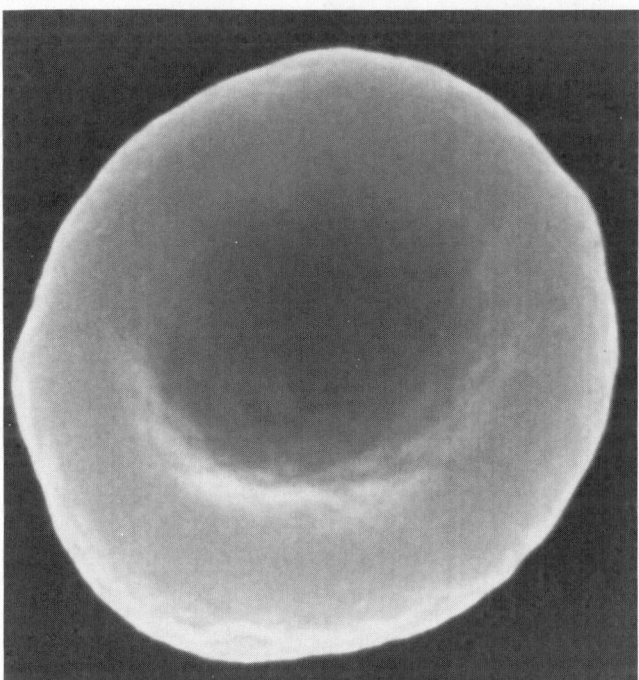

FIGURE 6-5. Scanning electron micrograph of a mature erythrocyte shows the normal discoid shape.

Plates 6-3 and 6-10). Plasma cells tend to have a low nuclear:cytoplasmic ratio and a dense clumped chromatin pattern. Both the rubriblast and prorubricyte have a high nuclear:cytoplasmic ratio. Although the chromatin is fine to coarse at these stages, it is not as coarse or condensed as in a mature plasma cell. The eccentric nucleus and perinuclear halo of the plasma cell also help in its identification.

Rubricytes and metarubricytes are often confused with lymphocytes (see Color Plates 6-2 and 6-7). The nucleus of the lymphocyte tends to be less round (slightly oval), with a dense homogeneous chromatin pattern. The chromatin pattern of the rubricyte and metarubricyte is more clumped with lightened areas (parachromatin). Small lymphocytes usually have scant cytoplasm in contrast to the more abundant cytoplasm of erythroid cells. The polychromatophilic to pinkish appearance of the cytoplasm of rubricytes, particularly metarubricytes, is also a distinguishing feature; lymphocyte cytoplasm should be a distinct light blue.

STRUCTURE AND PHYSIOLOGY OF THE MATURE ERYTHROCYTE

The mature erythrocyte is unique in that it lacks a nucleus and organelles, and yet all components necessary for survival and function are present. The main cell component is hemoglobin. The erythrocyte is surrounded by a specialized membrane that allows it to transport O_2 and CO_2 and to survive in the circulation for approximately 120 days.[3]

Many factors are involved in erythrocyte membrane and Hb maintenance. A source of energy is vital. Membrane shape and deformability are also important; they are influenced by cell composition and structure, internal Hb viscosity, and energy status.[34,52,70]

Shape and Deformability

The biconcave disc shape of the resting mature erythrocyte can be seen by scanning electron microscopy (SEM) (Fig. 6-5). This shape facilitates O_2–CO_2 transport by maximizing the ratio of the surface area to the volume. To a degree it also allows the cell to be flexible. Flexibility, or deformability, allows the cell to adjust to small vessels in the microvasculature (some of which have a smaller diameter than the erythrocyte) and still maintain a constant surface area to volume ratio. Significant alteration in this ratio causes the cell to be less deformable and subject to fragmentation and lysis. For example, a spheroid shape can be caused by membrane loss secondary to fragmentation (decreased surface area) or by increased uptake of cations and water (increased volume).

Membrane Composition and Structure

The composition and structure of its membrane allow the erythrocyte to (1) separate the intracellular fluid environment of the cytoplasm from the extracellular fluid environment of the plasma; (2) selectively pass nutrients and ions into and out of the cell; and (3) deform when required. The membrane is composed of lipids and proteins in approximately equal proportions by weight. Lipids and proteins located on the cytoplasmic side of the membrane are different from those in the membrane interior or from those on the plasma side of the membrane (Fig. 6-6). This asymmetric arrangement allows selective passage of molecules into and out of the cell.

LIPIDS

Phospholipids and unesterified cholesterol predominate in the lipid fraction and are present in approximately equal proportions. Phospholipid molecules are arranged in a double layer called the lipid bilayer leaflet (Fig. 6-6). As in other cell membranes, the hydrophilic phospholipid polar (head) groups are oriented toward the aqueous environment (cytoplasm and plasma), whereas the hydrophobic nonpolar fatty acid chains (tails) face the leaflet interior. This arrangement allows the membrane to act as a liquid sealer. Phospholipids are fluid because the fatty acid tails are free to move laterally within the membrane,[72,73] which allows lipids to interact with one another and with membrane proteins. Significant interactions between lipids and the structural or skeletal proteins spectrin and actin in the membrane (see Proteins, below) are thought to take place.[70]

Cholesterol plays an important role in maintaining the surface area to volume ratio by regulating membrane fluidity and permeability to electrolytes and nonelectrolytes. Lipid exchange, most notably of cholesterol, occurs between the membrane and the plasma. Approximately 98% of membrane cholesterol is unesterified, whereas 70% of plasma cholesterol is esterified. Esterified cholesterol consists of cholesterol with long-chain fatty acids attached.

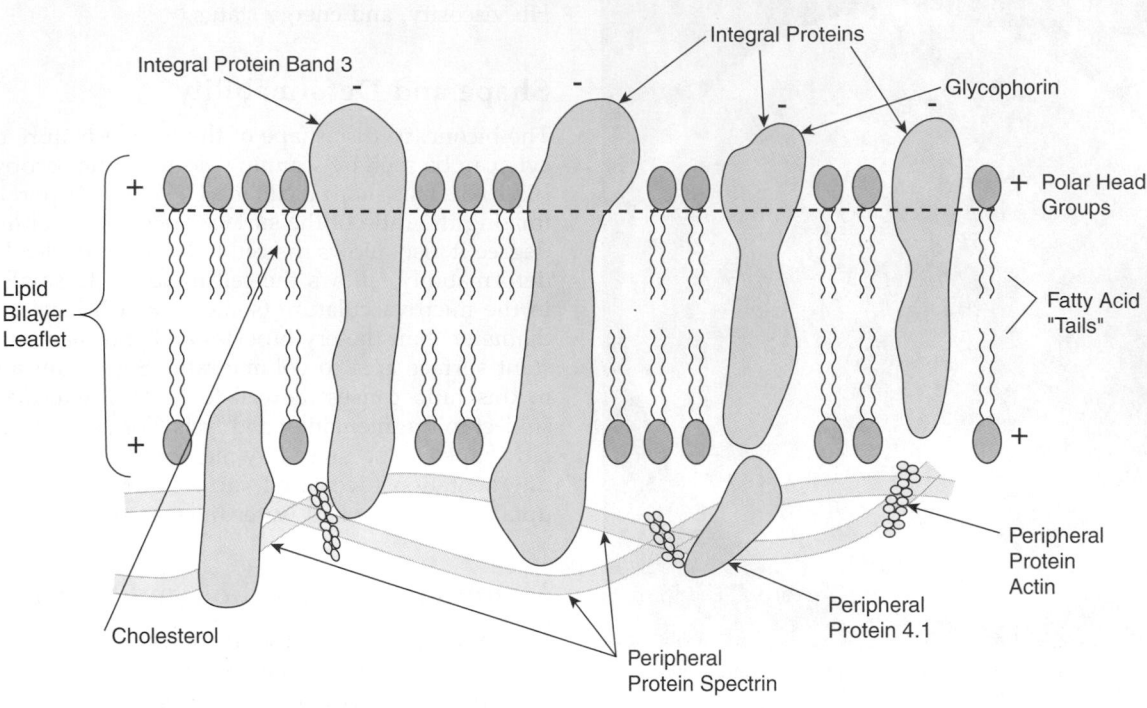

FIGURE 6-6. Simplified diagram of erythrocyte membrane structure.

PROTEINS

Proteins are bound to lipids throughout the membrane. Many membrane proteins have been characterized by the way they separate and form bands on polyacrylamide gel. They have been classified as peripheral or integral, depending on the extraction method and their location in the lipid bilayer (Fig. 6-6). The peripheral proteins are present on the inner portion of the membrane nearest to the cytoplasm. The integral proteins are in contact with both the inner and outer surfaces of the membrane, and thus act as receptors for ions and molecules needed in the cell such as transferrin and EPO.

The peripheral proteins include three important skeletal proteins, α and β spectrin (also called bands 1 and 2) and actin (also called band 5). Spectrin proteins are long, rod-shaped molecules, whereas actin proteins tend to form only short filaments. These two proteins are thought to underlie the lipid bilayer on the cytoplasmic side and to regulate membrane shape and deformability.[52] Their linkage is mediated by a fourth peripheral protein, protein 4.1. These proteins give the membrane appropriate viscoelastic properties. Abnormalities in spectrin have been found in some anemias caused by abnormal erythrocyte shape, such as hereditary spherocytosis[70] and hereditary elliptocytosis[49] (see Fig. 17-1).

The principal integral proteins are the glycoproteins designated glycophorin A and band 3 that span the lipid bilayer. Band 3 is an inorganic anion (Cl^-–HCO_3^-) transport channel. Glycophorin A bears the ABO blood group antigens. Rh proteins are also integral proteins. Integral proteins contain sialic acid, which gives erythrocytes a negative charge. This negativity between the cells, called the *zeta potential*, causes cells to repel one another as they move through the circulation. One cause of a decreased zeta potential is altered plasma proteins. This is reflected by an increase in red cell rouleaux and an increase in the erythrocyte sedimentation rate (ESR; Chaps. 9 and 39).

Membrane proteins are vital to erythrocyte function. In addition to making up the skeletal structure, many enzymes facilitate the movement of substrates and co-factors into and out of the cell. Two very important membrane enzyme systems are Na^+,K^+-ATPase and Ca^{2+},Mg^{2+}-ATPase. The former controls active transport of sodium and potassium. Increased sodium without loss of potassium causes the cell to gain water (increased volume) and subjects it to lysis, whereas increased potassium causes cell shrinkage. The second enzyme system, called the *calcium pump*, moves calcium out of the cell to the plasma against a high concentration gradient. Calcium is thought to be involved in the regulation and stabilization of membrane phospholipid structure.[70] High intracellular calcium concentrations cause the cell to become less deformable and therefore abnormal in shape.

Hemoglobin Viscosity

Normal erythrocyte Hb concentration has a low viscosity and is fluid. Cellular water loss and Hb that is precipitated, polymerized, or crystallized can all cause the cell to be less deformable and subject to lysis. Precipitated Hb, called *Heinz bodies*, forms rigid cellular inclusions that are visible by light microscopy after special staining and are associated with various hematologic disorders (see Fig. 8-26). Some hereditary Hb variants cause Hb to polymerize, such as Hb S in sickle cell anemia, or crystallize, such as Hb C disease (Chap. 14).

Energy Metabolism

ENERGY REQUIREMENTS

Energy is needed to maintain various components of the erythrocyte: preservation of the membrane and its shape, enzymatic reactions, and the movement of calcium, sodium, and potassium. Energy is also required to reduce oxidized proteins. Hemoglobin must be maintained in its reduced state for proper function.

Two sites on the Hb molecule are particularly prone to oxidation: the iron atom in the heme ring and the sulfhydryl (–SH) groups located at certain points on the globin chains.[41] Oxidation of the normal ferrous (Fe^{2+}) state to the ferric (Fe^{3+}) state results in the formation of methemoglobin, which has no O_2 delivery capacity. Normally, 1% to 3% of hemoglobin is oxidized to methemoglobin each day. This occurs by the loss of an electron from Fe^{2+} to O_2 during deoxygenation when water is present in the heme pocket. Hereditary unstable hemoglobins (Chap. 14), methemoglobin reductase deficiency (Fig. 6-7B), or exposure to oxidant drugs may cause large accumulations of methemoglobin. Oxidation of sulfhydryl groups causes Hb precipitation (Heinz body formation).

SOURCES OF ENERGY

Although the erythrocyte can utilize other sugars such as galactose, fructose, and mannose, glucose is the principal energy source. Pentoses and disaccharides are not metabolized. Glycogen is not normally metabolized as an energy source, but the cell does possess enzymes for its degradation if it accumulates. Membrane permeability differs for various sugars. Glucose can diffuse quickly without expense of energy, whereas the membrane is essentially impermeable to sucrose, lactose, and maltose.

Lacking mitochondria, mature erythrocytes depend on two relatively inefficient pathways for energy metabolism. They are the anaerobic Embden–Meyerhof pathway (EMP) and the aerobic hexose monophosphate shunt (HMS; also known as the pentose phosphate pathway). Both are shown in Figure 6-7 and discussed in detail below.

Embden–Meyerhof Pathway (EMP). The EMP is an anaerobic method for energy generation that catabolizes glucose to lactate in order to form adenosine triphosphate (ATP). Approximately 90% to 95% of the glucose used by the cell is normally metabolized by the EMP.

ATP, a high-energy phosphate, is used by the erythrocyte to: (1) maintain membrane shape and deformability, probably by phosphorylation of spectrin and perhaps by chelation of calcium[52]; (2) provide energy for active transport of cations; and (3) help modulate the amount of 2,3-DPG generated. Two molecules of ATP per molecule of glucose are utilized during the first three steps of the EMP, whereas four molecules may be generated–two from the 1,3-DPG to 3-PG step if the Rapoport–Luebering shunt

is not taken, and two at the phosphoenol pyruvate to pyruvate step, which requires the enzyme pyruvate kinase (Fig. 6-7C). Thus, there is a net yield of two ATP molecules for each molecule of glucose catabolized in the EMP.

The rate of glycolysis is pH dependent. Hexokinase and phosphofructokinase, enzymes at the beginning of the EMP, both react optimally at a pH above 7.0. Glycolysis thus increases during hypoxia because of the increased intracellular pH. In addition, ATP affects the glycolysis rate. As the ATP level rises, glycolysis diminishes. As it decreases, glycolysis increases. Through these and other mechanisms, the cell can adjust its energy state as long as glucose is available and normal enzyme levels are present.

Nicotinamide adenine dinucleotides (NAD^+ and NADH) are important cofactors in the EMP. Oxidized NAD^+ and its reduced form NADH are involved in multiple steps along the EMP. NAD^+ is used as a coenzyme with glyceraldehyde-3-phosphate dehydrogenase in the formation of 1,3-DPG. In that same reaction, the NADH formed acts as a coenzyme with methemoglobin reductase to reduce methemoglobin (Hb Fe^{3+}) to Hb (Fe^{2+}). This short pathway is known as the *methemoglobin reduction pathway* (Fig. 6-7B). NADH also acts as a coenzyme with lactate dehydrogenase (LD) to reduce pyruvate to lactate. Lactate is the end product of the EMP.[41]

A number of hereditary enzyme deficiencies or mutants are known to occur in man. Since the EMP is the main energy-generating force in the cell, enzyme deficiencies in the EMP are extremely rare. Of those that do occur, pyruvate kinase deficiency is the most common (Chap. 17).

Rapoport–Luebering Shunt. The erythrocyte EMP is similar to the EMP of other cells except for the formation of 2,3-diphosphoglycerate (2,3-DPG) in the Rapoport–Luebering shunt, a bypass pathway in the EMP (Fig. 6-7C), which helps modulate O_2 transport in the cell. At low tissue O_2 tension, 2,3-DPG binds to the deoxyhemoglobin form. This causes Hb to resist oxygenation by decreasing its O_2 affinity, thus increasing tissue O_2 delivery (Chap. 7).

2,3-DPG is generated from 1,3-DPG in the EMP. 1,3-DPG can be catabolized to 3-phosphogluconate (3-PG) in two ways: (1) by using the shunt, in which 2,3-DPG is an intermediate, or (2) directly by a path in which two molecules of high-energy ATP are generated. Because the erythrocyte needs both 2,3-DPG and ATP to function, intricate regulatory mechanisms direct the way 1,3-DPG will be catabolized. These mechanisms are not completely understood. One important factor is that hypoxia causes catabolism to go through the shunt, probably by increasing intracellular pH. On the other hand, decreased cellular ATP levels will cause direct metabolism of 1,3-DPG to increase ATP generation.

Hexose Monophosphate Shunt (HMS) and Glutathione Reduction Pathway. The HMS (also called the pentose phosphate pathway) is an aerobic method of erythrocyte glycolysis, which processes about 10% of erythrocyte glucose. The primary purpose of the HMS is to provide reducing potential for the cell by generating reduced nicotinamide adenine dinucleotide phosphate (NADPH). The

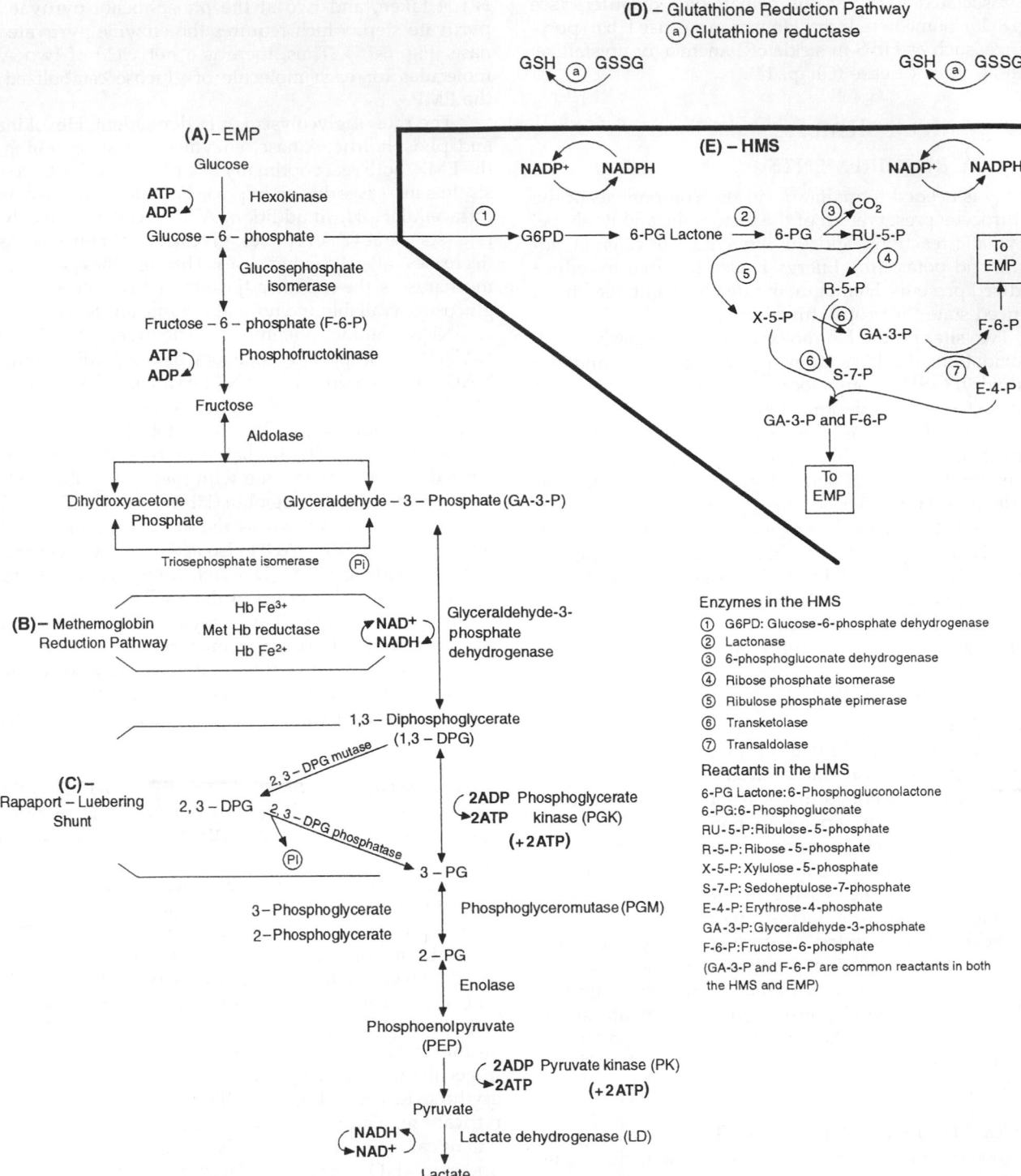

FIGURE 6-7. Diagram of the erythrocyte metabolisms showing the Embden–Meyerhof pathway (EMP) and the hexose monophosphate shunt (HMS).

HMS is an oxidative pathway in that substances are oxidized in order to reduce NADP+ to NADPH. In the HMS, glucose-6-phosphate, generated in the first step of the EMP, is catabolized to 6-phosphogluconate (6-PG) rather than passing though the EMP (Fig. 6-7E). This reaction is driven by an important enzyme in the HMS, glucose-6-phosphate dehydrogenase (G6PD). Two HMS reactions involve reduction of NADP+ to yield NADPH, which is important in the generation of reduced glutathione (Fig. 6-7D).

Reduced glutathione (GSH) is the principal reducing agent in the cell. It is used to reduce oxidized sulfhydryl groups in Hb and other proteins in the red cell membrane and thus keep them intact. The reducing reaction yields reduced sulfhydryl groups and oxidized glutathione (GSSG). Glutathione reductase and NADPH from the HMS then reduce GSSG back to GSH, making it available for further reductions of sulfhydryl groups (Fig. 6-7D). GSH is also required to decompose red cell hydrogen peroxide (H_2O_2) to water. If hydrogen peroxide accumulates, it causes the formation of excess methemoglobin.

The HMS also generates ribose-5-phosphate (R-5-P), which is used by nucleated cells during nucleic acid (*e.g.*, DNA) metabolism. Mature erythrocytes are capable of limited purine metabolism, and the R-5-P produced is usually recycled back into the EMP. The intermediates glyceraldehyde-3-phosphate and fructose-6-phosphate are common reactants in both pathways and are likewise fed back into the EMP (Fig. 6-7E).

The HMS is regulated largely by the $NADP^+$:NADPH ratio. As NADPH is utilized to reduce GSSG, $NADP^+$ is formed, which causes more glucose to be metabolized by the HMS. Upon exposure to an oxidant drug, this mechanism provides the cell with more reducing potential. NADPH also plays a minor role in methemoglobin reduction.[34]

ERYTHROCYTE DESTRUCTION

A red cell that has lived its life span is termed senescent. As the erythrocyte ages, a variety of gradual changes occur that make it susceptible to destruction. Alterations in the membrane such as loss of sialic acid[2] and lipids,[79] decreased ATP levels, and increased calcium,[8] all have been implicated in the aging process. Possibly a senescent antigen that makes the cell a target for removal appears as it ages.[39] Whatever the reason, at approximately day 120, erythrocytes are recognized as abnormal and removed from the circulation by phagocytic cells in the reticuloendothelial system (RES).

The term reticuloendothelial system refers to the total mass of cells, both in the circulation and in the tissues, that comprise the cellular and immunologic defense system in the body. Common use of the term usually refers to phagocytic cells, namely, the histiocytes, monocytes, and macrophages found primarily in the spleen, liver, lymph nodes, bone marrow, and to a lesser extent the lungs and other tissues.[5] The endothelial cells lining the sinuses of those organs are also considered part of the RES, as are circulating monocytes. Most RES cells are either fixed or free macrophages. The liver's RE cells are called Kupffer cells; scavenger cells in the lungs are called alveolar macrophages.

Sites of Erythrocyte Hemolysis

Most destruction of both normal and abnormal erythrocytes occurs in RES organs. The term *extravascular hemolysis* is used to describe red cell destruction that occurs by phagocytosis of intact or fragmented red cells in the RES with release of hemoglobin into the macrophages.

The spleen is the principal site of erythrocyte phagocytosis by tissue macrophages after erythrocyte damage by normal aging or only mild alterations in their discoid shape.[14,35,74] The liver, which has a greater blood flow, plays a more active role in the removal of cells with severe damage or shape alterations.[14,35]

Extremely damaged cells may lyse within the circulation before they reach the liver or spleen. This process is referred to as intravascular hemolysis (Chap. 16).

Role of the Spleen

The spleen consists of two functional parts called the red and the white pulp (Fig. 6-8). The white pulp (lymphatic tissue) consists of a germinal center, where lymphocytes are produced, and the periarterial lymphatic sheath, which contains lymphocytes. Most phagocytic activity occurs in the red pulp. It contains a system of vascular channels called sinuses. The areas separating the sinuses, called splenic cords, contain a high concentration of macrophages. The marginal zone is a spongy network filled with blood cells that separates the red and white pulp.

Blood flows into the spleen through the splenic artery, which branches into multiple central arteries. Right angle vascular branches from the central arteries skim off a portion of the plasma, causing hemoconcentration in the central arteries. A portion of the blood in a central artery empties directly into the sinuses, or very near them, where the venous system collects the blood. The other portion empties into the marginal zone separating the red and white pulp or into the splenic cords of the red pulp. Red cells that arrive in this cordal area must slowly make their way into the venous sinuses, passing through openings in the cordal wall (only 3 μm in diameter) that separates the cords from the sinuses.[6,23,45] Since the average red cell is 7 μm in diameter, this slow, tortuous passage requires that red cells be easily deformable. It also brings them into prolonged contact with macrophages in the splenic cords and exposes them to conditions of low glucose concentration[37] and low pH[53] that may lead to membrane damage. Blood leaves the spleen by way of the venous drainage system in the red pulp. Blood flows out through the trabecular vein into the portal circulation on its way to the liver.

As the erythrocyte ages, its ability to generate energy declines. Repeated passes through the spleen deplete the cells of glucose and decrease their surface area.[23] The spleen apparently recognizes subtle abnormalities in senescent cells, and then sequesters and destroys them. It also removes abnormal red cells, such as those that contain inclusion bodies, that are not yet senescent. This process of removing senescent and abnormal red cells is termed *culling*.

REGULATION OF ERYTHROPOIESIS (ERYTHROKINETICS)

Erythropoiesis and erythrokinetics are best understood in the context of the erythron model.[9] The *erythron* is defined as the entire mass of mature and immature erythrocytes in both intravascular and extravascular locations. Included in the extravascular portion are all immature nucleated erythrocytes and reticulocytes in the bone mar-

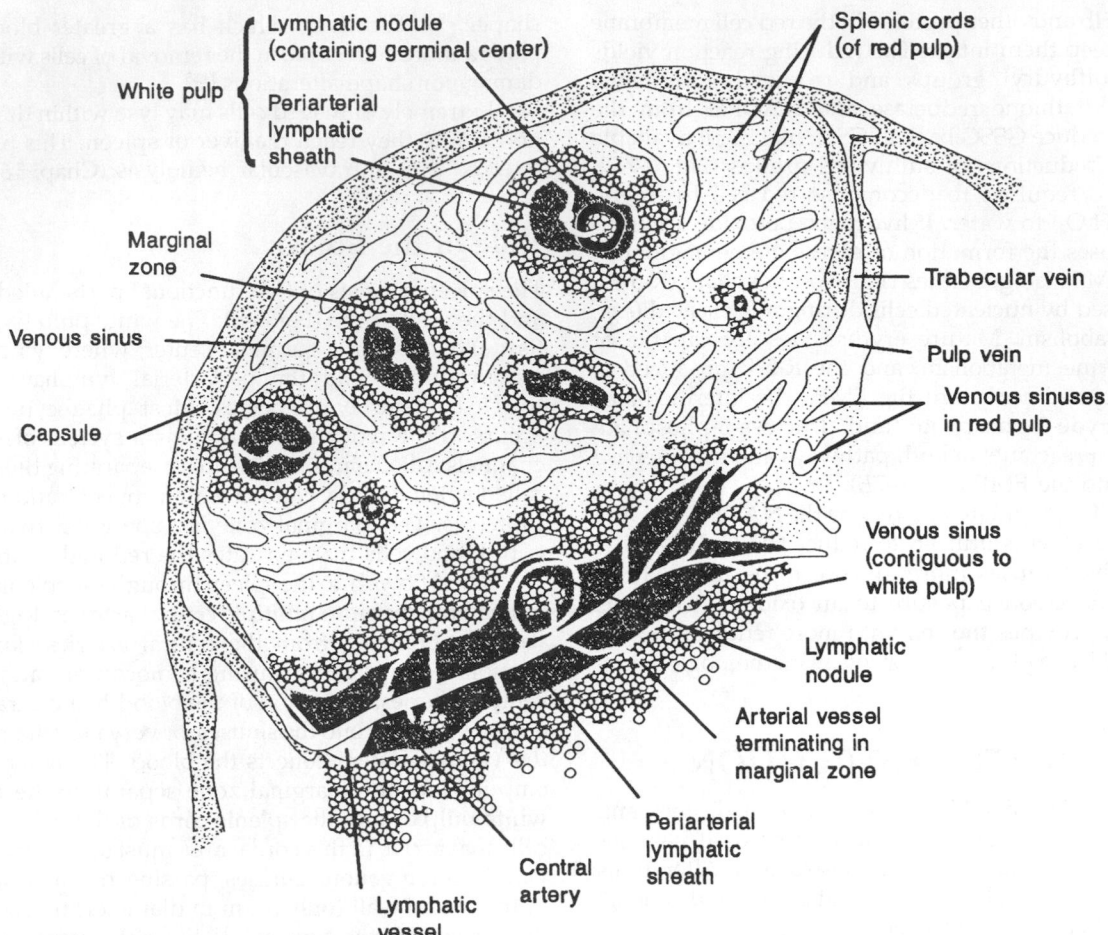

FIGURE 6-8. Structure of the spleen; see text for details. (From Weiss L, Greep RO: Histology. New York, Elsevier Science Publishing Co, Inc, 1977. Reprinted with permission of the publisher.)

row. The intravascular portion includes circulating erythrocytes and the few reticulocytes normally found in the peripheral blood.

The erythron model comprises the three phases of erythrocyte life: erythropoiesis or erythrocyte production, release from the marrow and circulation in the bloodstream, and destruction. A fine balance between production and destruction normally keeps the erythrocyte numbers fairly constant provided each of these phases is functioning normally. Production and maintenance of the erythron require a normally functioning, competent bone marrow as well as adequate levels of EPO, growth factors, and nutrients such as iron, folate, and vitamin B_{12}.

Somewhere between 3×10^9 and 8.5×10^9 erythrocytes per kilogram of body weight are produced every day. The process is controlled by an interacting network of biomolecules called cytokines or growth factors, the most important of which is EPO. The BFU-E and CFU-E are the primitive erythroid-committed stem cells that respond as needed to both humoral and cellular growth factors to replenish the circulating erythrocyte pool.

The two principal disturbances of the erythron are erythrocytosis and anemia (Chap. 10). Erythrocytosis is a condition characterized by an *increase* in circulating erythrocytes (production exceeds destruction or loss).

Anemia is a condition usually characterized by a *decrease* in circulating erythrocytes (destruction or loss exceeds production). However, note that in some conditions, such as thalassemia (Chap. 15), the erythrocyte count is usually normal to increased, whereas the hemoglobin is normal to severely decreased. In such cases, anemia is best defined as a decrease in hemoglobin.

Erythropoietin Production and Regulation

EPO has a well established role in the regulation of erythropoiesis. It is a hormone composed of glycoprotein with a molecular weight of 34,000.[32,80] In contrast to other hematopoietic cytokines, EPO is an erythroid growth factor that has remarkable specificity, triggering only erythrocyte progenitor (mainly CFU-E) cell division and maturation (Fig. 6-2).[65] Stromal and other cells within the marrow microenvironment also affect the fertility and survival of erythrocyte progenitors.[22]

PRODUCTION SITES

EPO is produced primarily in the kidney. EPO levels fall after kidney removal and at times rise above normal after transplantation.[78] Since some EPO remains after kidney removal, there are other production sites, presumably the liver.[27,56,61] However, less than 15% is normally produced outside of the kidney.[21] It has been difficult to actually demonstrate EPO in the kidney. However, development of a technique to synthesize EPO by recombinant DNA has led to the use of a commercial product to relieve anemia in certain patients, particularly those with chronic renal disease.[42,43]

REGULATION OF PRODUCTION

Erythropoiesis is predominantly regulated by renal O_2 tension, which, when decreased, induces expression of the erythropoietin gene and the release of EPO.[65] Tissue O_2 tension is affected by such factors as Hb O_2 saturation, plasma 2,3-DPG levels, pO_2 of the plasma, Hb concentration, erythrocyte mass, basal metabolic rate, and rate of blood flow. When tissue and renal O_2 tension return to normal, EPO levels fall.

Prostaglandins are thought to help regulate EPO production and also to enhance its effect on CFU-E.[25,62] On the other hand, estrogen may inhibit EPO production.[51] The action of estrogen probably explains why young women have lower erythrocyte reference ranges than men.

Erythropoietin Action in Normal and Anemic States

Primitive BFU-E appear to be relatively insensitive to EPO and require other growth factors to differentiate.[19] However, CFU-E are particularly sensitive to EPO; only minute amounts are needed to stimulate growth. From the CFU-E stage of maturation onward, EPO is necessary for cell maturation. EPO enters the cell through a specific membrane receptor. Once in the cell, it stimulates scription of globin mRNA and may also be necessary heme synthesis.[32]

If anemia is present, the increased EPO level produced in response to hypoxia stimulates more progenitors to differentiate. It also shortens the maturation time in the marrow. It was previously thought that this shortened maturation time was caused by cells skipping cell divisions. However, it is more likely that increased EPO simply causes an increased rate of Hb synthesis and earlier reticulocyte release.[59] These early reticulocytes are larger than normal, contain more RNA (and are therefore more polychromatophilic), and retain Hb synthetic capability longer in the peripheral blood. Adequate iron stores are necessary for increased cell proliferation and a shortened cell maturation time.[1] Anemia attributable to blood loss is not associated with as great an erythroid response as that seen with hemolytic anemia, presumably because of the lower iron levels usually associated with chronic blood loss (*i.e.*, Hb iron is lost rather than recycled to the bone marrow).

Normal maturation takes approximately 5 days. During accelerated erythropoiesis, this time can be shortened to 3 to 4 days. Because this response to hypoxia is relatively slow, increased 2,3-DPG levels help reduce hypoxia by causing more O_2 to be released to the tissues until erythrocyte numbers are back in balance. As erythrocyte numbers increase, hypoxia is reduced, and EPO levels and the maturation cycle return to normal (Fig. 6-9).

Growth Factors

In addition to EPO, many other growth factors, including hormones and cytokines secreted by various cells, have now been shown to stimulate erythropoiesis (Table 6-2).

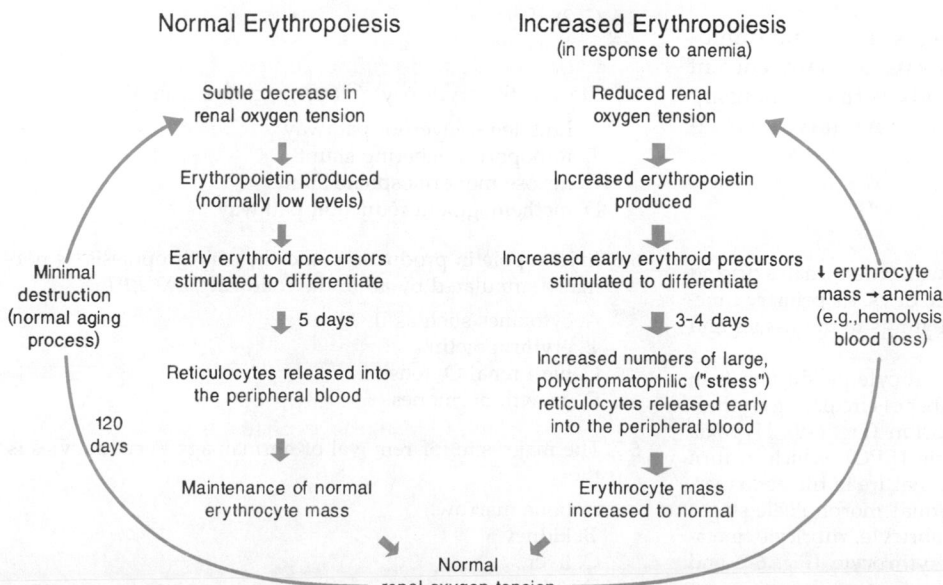

Erythropoiesis Regulation (Erythrokinetics) Normal vs response to anemia

FIGURE 6-9. Erythropoiesis regulation (erythrokinetics): Normal vs response to anemia.

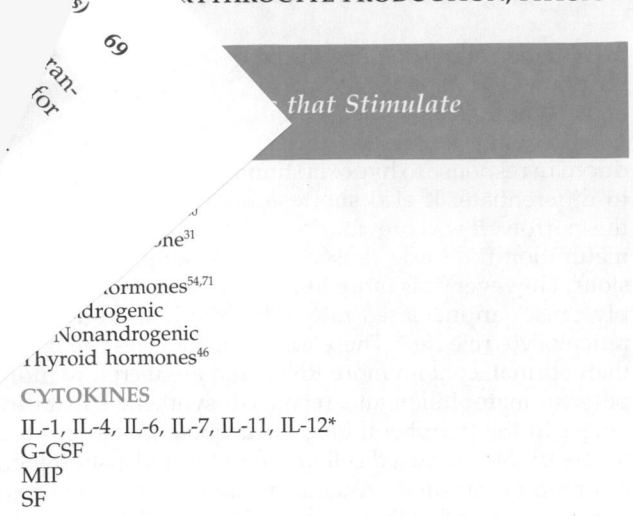

... that Stimulate

...one[31]

...ormones[54,71]
...drogenic
...Nonandrogenic
...hyroid hormones[46]

CYTOKINES

IL-1, IL-4, IL-6, IL-7, IL-11, IL-12*
G-CSF
MIP
SF

IL, interleukin; G-CSF, granulocyte colony-stimulating factor; MIP, macro-phage inflammatory proteins; SF, steel factor.

These cytokines are molecules that have been identified in cell culture supernatants with the help of modern recombinant DNA technology. Many of them are now known collectively as the interleukins (IL). They can be secreted by many types of cells (*e.g.*, T lymphocytes and endothelial cells) and may have different effects on many other types of cells.

Growth factors are involved in both the proliferation and differentiation of maturing erythrocytes.[69] Some growth factors can act in combination with other factors to stimulate erythropoiesis even though they may individually have little stimulatory effect.[16,20,77] On the other hand, monocytes or macrophages alone can be strong enhancers of erythropoiesis,[33,81,82] but in combination with other cells, they have been reported as inhibitors.[18,66] Likewise, different subsets of T lymphocytes can stimulate[28,63] or inhibit[48] erythropoiesis.

Other inhibitors of erythropoiesis include viruses,[75] interferon,[47] uremic toxins produced in renal disease,[26,50] IL-1 alpha, tumor necrosis factor (TNF)–alpha,[38] and alcohol.[30]

Identification of proliferation-enhancing and -inhibiting factors continues to be the focus of many current studies. Another area of current study is the relationship of cell differentiation to the bone marrow microenvironment and adhesion to fibronectin.[44]

CHAPTER SUMMARY

The mature erythrocyte is a blood cell with a deformable discoid shape that has a normal life span of 120 days. Its primary functions are transportation of O_2 from the lungs to the tissues and removal of the waste product CO_2.

Under normal circumstances erythrocyte production is in equilibrium with destruction. The number of circulating erythrocytes is primarily regulated by O_2 tension (Fig. 6-9). Hypoxia stimulates production of erythropoietin (EPO), which in turn stimulates immature erythroid cells to mature in the bone marrow more rapidly through the six normal morphologic stages of development—the rubriblast, prorubricyte, rubricyte, metarubricyte, reticulocyte, and mature erythrocyte (Fig. 6-2 and Table 6-1).

Normal structure and composition of the erythrocyte membrane (Fig. 6-6) and of Hb are necessary for the erythrocyte to function and survive. In addition, there are five important pathways that must be operative to keep erythrocytes functioning normally (Fig. 6-7). They include (1) the anaerobic Embden–Meyerhof pathway (EMP), from which erythrocytes gain ATP for energy; (2) the methemoglobin reduction pathway (part of the EMP), where methemoglobin (Hb^{3+}) is reduced to Hb^{2+} to prevent its denaturation and precipitation; (3) the Rapoport–Luebering shunt, where 2,3-DPG is produced, which controls Hb oxygen affinity; (4) the aerobic hexose monophosphate shunt (HMS), in which NADPH is produced to reduce oxidized glutathione (GSSG) normally produced in red cells; and (5) the glutathione reduction pathway, in which GSSG is reduced to glutathione (GSH). GSH is required to prevent Hb denaturation and oxidation. Normal removal of aging erythrocytes occurs within the reticuloendothelial system (RES), primarily in the spleen (Fig. 6-8).

Review Questions

6-1. The major erythrocyte production site is the

A. bone marrow.
B. kidney.
C. liver.
D. spleen.

6-2. The correct maturation order of erythrocyte morphologic stages is

A. prorubricyte, rubricyte, rubriblast, metarubricyte.
B. rubriblast, prorubricyte, rubricyte, metarubricyte.
C. rubriblast, metarubricyte, rubricyte, prorubricyte.
D. rubriblast, rubricyte, prorubricyte, metarubricyte.

6-3. Compared to a rubricyte, a metarubricyte looks different because of its

A. dark blue cytoplasm.
B. pyknotic nucleus.
C. larger size.
D. nucleoli.

6-4. A normal mature erythrocyte has a life span of

A. 8.2 hours.
B. 5 days.
C. 28 days.
D. 120 days.

6-5. Most of the erythrocyte's energy comes from the

A. Embden–Meyerhof pathway.
B. Rapoport–Luebering shunt.
C. hexose monophosphate shunt.
D. methemoglobin reduction pathway.

6-6. Erythropoietin production (and thus erythropoiesis) is normally stimulated by all of the following *EXCEPT*

A. cytokines such as IL-1.
B. erythropoietin.
C. high renal O_2 tension.
D. growth hormones.

6-7. The major site for removal of normal, aged erythrocytes is the

A. bone marrow.
B. kidney.
C. liver.
D. spleen.

References

1. Adamson JW: The relationship of erythropoietin and iron metabolism to red blood cell production in humans. Semin Oncol 21:9, 1994

2. Aminoff D: Senescence and sequestration of RBC from circulation. Prog Clin Biol Res 195:279, 1985

3. Ashby W: The span of life of the red blood cell: A resume. Blood 3:486, 1948

4. Axelrad AA, McLeod DL, Shreeve MM et al: Properties of cells that produce erythrocytic colonies *in vitro*. In Robinson W (ed): Hemopoiesis in Culture, p 226. Washington, DHEW Publication No. (NIH) 74-205, 1973

5. Beck WS: Reticuloendothelial (mononuclear phagocyte) system, lymphatic system, and spleen. In Beck WS (ed): Hematology, 4th ed. Cambridge, MA, The MIT Press, 1985

6. Bennington JL: Saunders Dictionary & Encyclopedia of Laboratory Medicine and Technology. Philadelphia, WB Saunders, 1984

7. Bernier DR, Christian PE, Langan JK: Nuclear Medicine Technology and Techniques. St. Louis, Mosby, 1994

8. Bookchin RM, Lew VL, Roth Jr EF: Elevated red cell calcium: Innocent bystander or kiss of death? Prog Clin Biol Res 195:369, 1985

9. Boycott AE: The blood as a tissue: Hypertrophy and atrophy of the red corpuscles. Proc R Soc Med 23:15, 1929

10. CAP Survey Manual, Section II, p 24. Skokie, IL, College of American Pathologists, 1986

11. Chasis JA, Coulombel L, Conboy J et al: Differentiation-associated switches in protein 4.1 expression. Synthesis of multiple structural isoforms during normal human erythropoiesis. J Clin Invest 91:329, 1993

12. Clarke BJ, Housman D: Characterization of an erythroid precursor cell of high proliferative capacity in normal human peripheral blood. Proc Natl Acad Sci USA 74:1105, 1977

13. Committee for Clarification of the Nomenclature of Cells and Diseases of the Blood and Blood Forming Organs: Second report. Am J Clin Pathol 19:56, 1949

14. Cosgrove P, Sheetz M: Effect of cell shape on extravascular hemolysis. Blood 59:421, 1982

15. Custer RP: Studies on the structure and function of the bone marrow. J Lab Clin Med 17:952, 1932

16. Dexter TM, Garland JM, Testa NG (eds): Colony Stimulating Factors. New York, Dekker, 1990

17. Donahue DM, Reiff RH, Hanson ML et al: Quantitative measurement of the erythrocytic and granulocytic cells of the marrow and blood. J Clin Invest 37:1571, 1958

18. Eastman CE, Ruscetti FW: Regulation of erythropoiesis in long-term hamster marrow cultures: Role of bone marrow adherent cells. Blood 65:736, 1985

19. Eaves AC, Eaves CJ: Erythropoiesis in culture. Clin Haematol 13:373, 1984

20. Erickson N, Quesenberry PJ: Regulation of erythropoiesis. The role of growth factors. Med Clin North Am 76:745, 1992

21. Erslev AJ, Adamson JW, Eschbach JW et al: Erythropoietin. Molecular, Cellular, and Clinical Biology. Baltimore, The Johns Hopkins University Press, 1991

22. Erslev AJ, Beutler E: Production and destruction of erythrocytes. In Beutler E, Lichtman MA, Coller BS et al (eds): Williams Hematology, 5th ed, p 425. New York, McGraw-Hill, 1995

23. Erslev AJ, Gabuzda TG: Pathophysiology of Blood, 2nd ed. Philadelphia, WB Saunders, 1979

24. Finch CA: Some qualitative aspects of erythropoiesis. Ann NY Acad Sci 77:410, 1959

25. Fisher JW, Hagiwara M: Effects of prostaglandins on erythropoiesis. Blood Cells 10:241, 1985

26. Freedman MH, Cattran DC, Saunders EF: Anemia of ch[ ] renal failure: Inhibition by uremic serum. Nephron 3[ ] 1983

27. Fried W: The liver as a source of extrarenal erythropoieti[ ] production. Blood 40:671, 1972

28. Froom P, Ramot B, Beniaminov M et al: Production of burst-promoting activity by monoclonal antibody defined malignant T lymphocytes from patients with lymphocytic leukemia and lymphoma. Blood 65:997, 1985

29. Ghadially FN: Ultrastructural Pathology of the Cell and Matrix, 2nd ed. London, Butterworths, 1982

30. Giglio MJ, Santoro RC, Bozzini CE: Effect of chronic ethanol administration on production of and response to erythropoietin in the mouse. Alcoholism 8:323, 1984

31. Golde DW, Bersch N, Li CH: Growth hormone: Species-specific stimulation of erythropoiesis *in vitro*. Science 196:1112, 1977

32. Goldwasser E: Erythropoietin and its mode of action. Blood Cells 10:147, 1984

33. Gordon LJ, Wesley JM, Branda RF et al: Regulation of erythroid colony formation by bone marrow macrophages. Blood 55:1047, 1980

34. Grimes AJ: Human Red Cell Metabolism. Oxford, Blackwell Scientific, 1980

35. Jacob HS, Jandl JH: Effects of sulfhydryl inhibition on red blood cells II. Studies *in vivo*. J Clin Invest 41:1514, 1962

36. Jacobson LO, Goldwasser E, Plzak LF et al: Studies on erythropoiesis IV. Reticulocyte response of hypophysectomized and polycythemic rodents to erythropoietin. Proc Soc Exp Biol Med 94:243, 1957

37. Jandl JH, Aster RH: Increased splenic pooling and the pathogenesis of hypersplenism. Am J Med Sci 253:383, 1967

38. Johnson CS, Pourbohloul SC, Furmanski P: Negative regulators of *in vivo* erythropoiesis: Interaction of IL-1 alpha and TNF-alpha and the lack of a strict requirement for T or NK cells for their activity. Exp Hematol 19:101, 1991

39. Kay MMB: Senescent cell differentiation antigen. Prog Clin Biol Res 195:251, 1985

40. Kurtz A, Jelkmann W, Bauer C: Insulin stimulates erythroid colony formation independently of erythropoietin. Br J Haematol 53:311, 1983

41. Lee GR, Bithell TC, Foerster J et al (eds): Wintrobe's Clinical Hematology, 9th ed. Philadelphia, Lea & Febiger, 1993

42. Lee-Huang S: Cloning and expression of human erythropoietin cDNA in *Escherichia coli*. Proc Natl Acad Sci USA 81:2708, 1984

43. Lin FK, Suggs S, Lin CH et al: Cloning and expression of the human erythropoietin gene. Proc Natl Acad Sci USA 82:7580, 1985

44. Long MW, Wicha MS (eds): The Hematopoietic Microenvironment. Baltimore, The Johns Hopkins Press, 1993

45. Macpherson AIS, Richmond J, Stuart AE: The Spleen. Springfield, Charles C Thomas, 1973

46. Malgor LA, Blanc CC, Klainer E et al: Direct effects of thyroid hormones on bone marrow erythroid cells of rats. Blood 45:671, 1975

47. Mamus SW, Beck-Schroeder S, Zanjani ED: Suppression of normal erythropoiesis by gamma interferon *in vitro*: Role of monocytes and T lymphocytes. J Clin Invest 75:1496, 1985

48. Mangan KF, Hartnett ME, Matis SA et al: Natural killer cells suppress human erythroid stem cell proliferation *in vitro*. Blood 63:260, 1984

49. Marchesi SL, Knowles WJ, Morrow JS et al: Abnormal spectrin in hereditary elliptocytosis. Blood 67:141, 1986

50. McGonigle RJ, Wallin JD, Shadduck RK et al: Erythropoietin deficiency and inhibition of erythropoiesis in renal insufficiency. Kidney Int 25:437, 1984

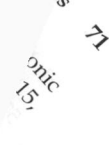

AS: Mechanism of estrogen action in
...nology 78:325, 1966

Control of red cell deformability
..., Yachnin S (eds): Current Topics in
...71. New York, Alan R Liss, 1978

...fluence of pH and temperature on some
...ties of normal erythrocytes and erythrocytes
...s with hereditary spherocytosis. J Lab Clin Med
...67

...y MJ Jr: In Vitro Aspects of Erythropoiesis. New York,
...inger-Verlag, 1978

...Nathan DG, Sytkowski A: Editorial retrospective: Erythropoietin and regulation of erythropoiesis. N Engl J Med 308:520, 1983

56. Naughton GK, Naughton BA, Gordon AS: Erythropoietin production by macrophages in the regenerating liver. J Surg Oncol 30:184, 1985

57. Nijhof W, Wierenga PK: Isolation and characterization of the erythroid progenitor cell: CFU-E. J Cell Biol 96:386, 1983

58. Ogawa M, Grush OC, O'Dell RF et al: Circulating erythropoietic precursors in culture: Characterization in normal men and patients with hemoglobinopathies. Blood 50:1081, 1977

59. Papayannopoulou T, Finch CA: Radioiron measurements of red cell maturation. Blood Cells 1:535, 1975

60. Patel VP, Ciechanover A, Platt O et al: Loss of adhesion of erythrocyte precursors to fibronectin during erythroid differentiation. Prog Clin Biol Res 184:355, 1985

61. Paul P, Rothman SA, McMahon JT et al: Erythropoietin secretion by isolated rat Kupffer cells. Exp Hematol 12:825, 1984

62. Pavlovik-Kentera V, Susic D, Biljanovic-Paunovic et al: Prostaglandin synthesis inhibitors in erythropoiesis. Haematologia (Budap) 17:161, 1984

63. Pistoia V, Ghio R, Nocera A et al: Large granular lymphocytes have a promoting activity on human peripheral blood erythroid burst-forming units. Blood 65:464, 1985

64. Reissmann KR: Studies on the mechanism of erythropoietin stimulation in parabiotic rats during hypoxia. Blood 5:372, 1950

65. Rich IN, Lappin TRJ: Molecular, cellular, and developmental biology of erythropoietin and erythropoiesis. Ann N Y Acad Sci 718:123-124, 1994

66. Roodman GD, Horadam VW, Wright TL: Inhibition of erythroid colony formation by autologous bone marrow adherent cells from patients with the anemia of chronic disease. Blood 62:406, 1983

67. Rosenthal CJ, Hassan M, Rieder RF et al: Identification of erythroid colony progenitors in a subset of human peripheral

lymphocytes devoid of Fc receptors. Am J Hematol 19:109, 1985

68. Rothman JE: The compartmental organization of the Golgi apparatus. Sci Am 253:74, 1985

69. Sachs L, Abraham NG, Weedermann CJ et al: Molecular Biology of Haematopoiesis. Andover Hampshire, Intercept, 1989

70. Schwartz RS, Chiu DTS, Lubin B: Plasma membrane phospholipid organization in human erythrocytes. In Piomelli S, Yachnin S (eds): Current Topics in Hematology, vol 5, p 63. New York, Alan R Liss, 1985

71. Singer JW, Samuels AI, Adamson JW: Steroids and hematopoiesis I. The effect of steroids on in vitro erythroid colony growth: Structure/activity relationships. J Cell Physiol 88:127, 1976

72. Singer SJ, Nicholson GL: The fluid mosaic model of the structure of cell membranes. Science 175:720, 1972

73. Singer SJ: The molecular organization of membranes. Annu Rev Biochem 43:805, 1974

74. Smedsrød B, Aminoff D: Use of ^{75}Se-labeled methione to study the sequestration of senescent red blood cells. Am J Hematol 18:31, 1985

75. Socinski MA, Ersler WB, Tosato G et al: Pure red cell aplasia associated with Epstein Barr virus infection: Evidence for T cell-mediated suppression of erythroid colony forming units. J Lab Clin Med 104:995, 1984

76. Stephenson JR, Axelrad AA, McLeod DL et al: Induction of colonies of hemoglobin-synthesizing cells by erythropoietin in vitro. Proc Natl Acad Sci USA 68:1542, 1971

77. Tanaka R, Katayama N, Ohishi K et al: Accelerated cell-cycling of hematopoietic progenitor cells by growth factors. Blood 86:73, 1995

78. Thevenod F, Radtke HW, Grutzmacher P et al: Deficient feedback regulation of erythropoiesis in kidney transplant patients with polycythemia. Kidney Int 24:227, 1983

79. Wagner G, Chiu DTY, Schwartz RS et al: Membrane phospholipid abnormalities in pathologic erythrocytes: A model for cell aging. Prog Clin Biol Res 195:237, 1985

80. Wang FF, Kung CKH, Goldwasser E: Some chemical properties of human erythropoietin (abstract). Fed Proc 42:1872, 1983

81. Zuckerman KS, Bagby GC Jr, McCall E et al: A monokine stimulates production of human erythroid burst-promoting activity by endothelial cells in vitro. J Clin Invest 75:722, 1985

82. Zuckerman KS: Human erythroid burst-forming units: Growth in vitro is dependent on monocytes, but not T lymphocytes. J Clin Invest 67:702, 1981

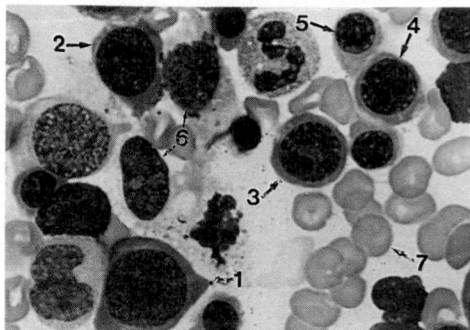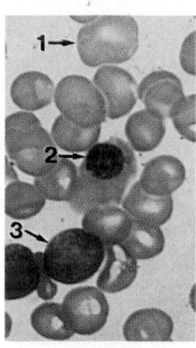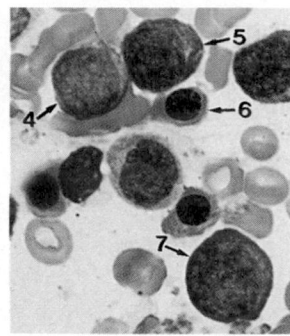

PLATE 6-1. Bone marrow erythrocyte precursors surrounding two histiocytes. (*1*) Rubriblast. (*2, 3*) Prorubricytes. (*4*) Early rubricyte. (*5*) Early metarubricyte. (*6*) Two histiocytes. (*7*) Mature erythrocyte (background). Erythroid precursors often are in contact with iron-containing histiocytes.

PLATE 6-2. Contrasting morphology between bone marrow erythrocyte precursors, lymphocytes, and a myeloblast. (*1*) Reticulocyte (polychromatophilic erythrocyte). (*2*) Metarubricyte. (*3*) Lymphocyte. (*4*) Myeloblast. (*5*) Prorubricyte. (*6*) Metarubricyte. (*7*) Rubriblast.

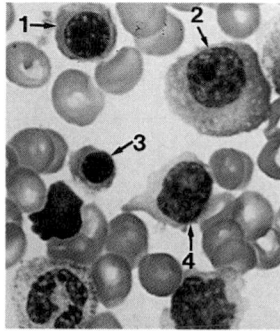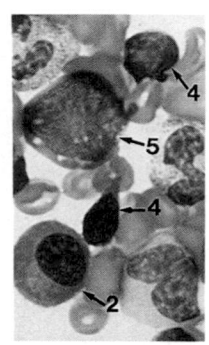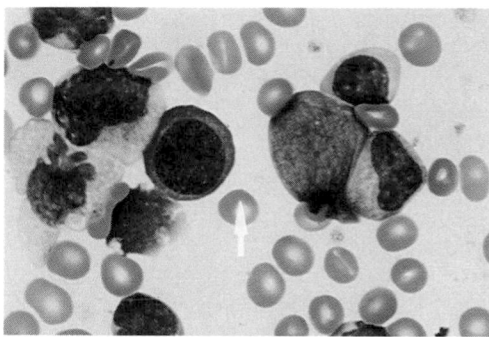

PLATE 6-3. Contrasting morphology between bone marrow erythroid precursors, plasma cells, and lymphocytes. (*1*) Rubricyte. (*2*) Plasma cell. (*3*) Metarubricytes. (*4*) Lymphocytes. (*5*) Rubriblast. Note that the three lymphocytes display slightly different morphologic characteristics.

PLATE 6-4. Rubriblast vs myeloblast. The *arrow* is pointing between two blue cells. To the left—the bluer cell—is a rubriblast (pronormoblast). To the right is a large myeloblast with a medium lymphocyte (upper) and a neutrophil metamyelocyte (lower) touching it. (1000×)

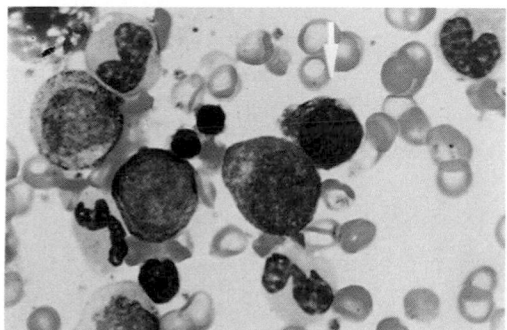

PLATE 6-5. Prorubricyte (basophilic normoblast) vs rubriblast (pronormoblast). The *arrow* is pointing to a prorubricyte. The cell immediately below and touching it is a rubriblast. Note the difference in size and in chromatin pattern. (1000×)

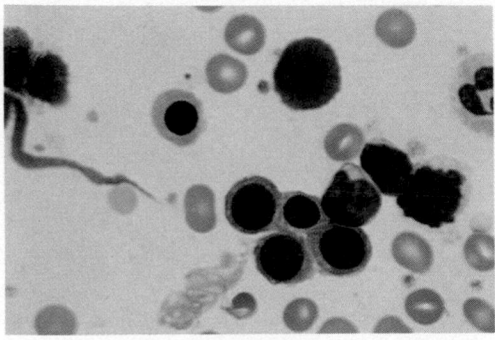

PLATE 6-6. Metarubricyte vs rubricyte. The single nucleated red cell precursor (upper left) is a metarubricyte (orthochromic normoblast). Note the dense, pyknotic chromatin. To the lower right is a group of six cells: four rubricytes and two lymphocytes. Can you tell which are the lymphocytes? (1000×)

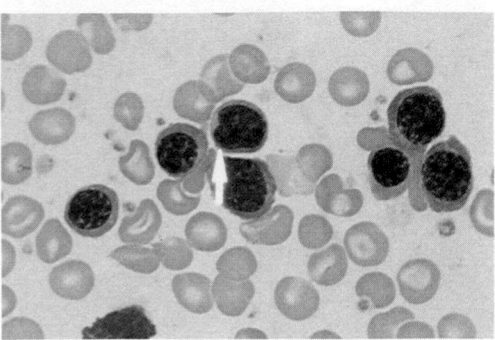

PLATE 6-7. Rubricyte vs lymphocyte. The *arrow* is pointing to a lymphocyte. All the other cells in the field are rubricytes (polychromatic normoblasts). (1000×)

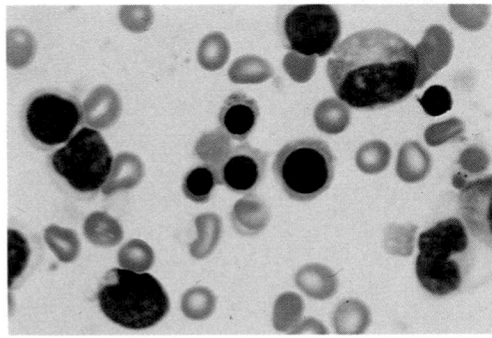

PLATE 6-8. Metarubricytes (orthochromic normoblasts). In the center of the field are four metarubricytes with their very dense nuclear chromatain. (1000×)

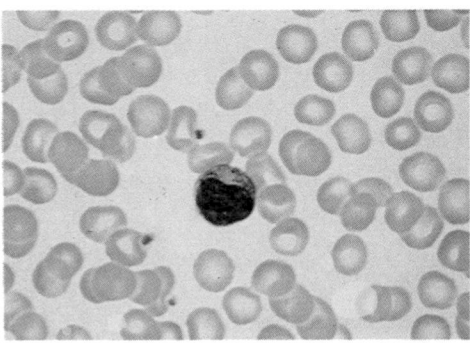

PLATE 6-9. Normal erythrocytes in peripheral blood with a small lymphocyte in the center of the field. Note that the size of the individual red cells is just slightly smaller than the nucleus of the small lymphocyte. Also note that the diameter of the central pallor in the erythrocytes is roughly 30% to 40% of the erythrocyte. (1000×)

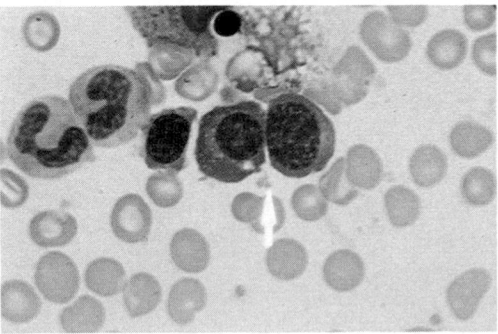

PLATE 6-10. Plasma cell vs prorubricyte. The *arrow* is pointing between two blue cells, both of which are busy making proteins. To the left is a plasma cell synthesizing immunoglobin, whereas the prorubricyte, which is synthesizing hemoglobin, is on the right. Note the difference in nuclear:cytoplasmic ratio. The plasma cell has much more cytoplasm to nucleus than does the red cell precursor. (1000×)

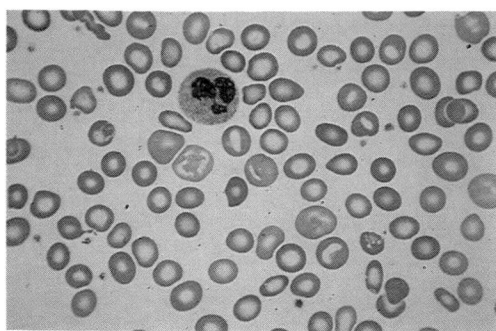

PLATE 9-1. Shift reticulocytes. This term refers to young non-nucleated red cells that have left the bone marrow prematurely. They are large, lumpy and have a distinct bluish cast. This blood sample is from an iron-deficient individual who had recently been treated with iron. In response, the bone marrow increased erythropoiesis, which is reflected by the large polychromatophilic red cells (shift reticulocytes). At least three are in the center of the field. (1000×)

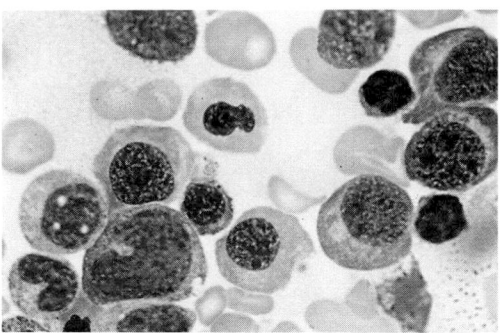

PLATE 12-1. Megaloblastic marrow. Several megaloblastic red cell precursors at various stages of maturation are present in this field. Metarubricytes, such as the one with the peanut-shaped nucleus, best reflect the asynchronism between cytoplasm and nucleus (the nucleus appears younger than the cytoplasm due to the difficulty these cells have in synthesizing DNA). Compare this metarubricyte with those in Color Plate 6-8. The nucleus in the megaloblastic metarubricyte is more open (less dense). (1000×)

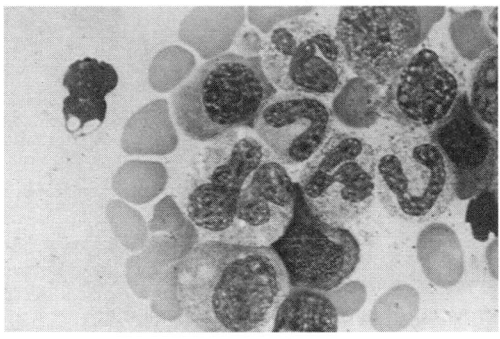

PLATE 12-2. Megaloblastic marrow. In the center of the field is a giant, band form neutrophil with a highly contorted nucleus. This cell will develop into a large hypersegmented neutrophil. Immediately above is a megaloblastic rubricyte. (1000×)

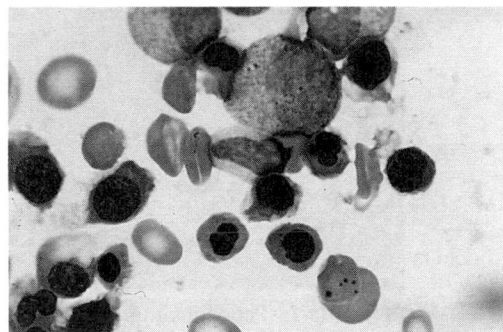

PLATE 12-3. Megaloblastic marrow. This field represents the reversed myeloid:erythroid ratio characteristic of numerous types of anemias, including megaloblastic anemia (sometimes referred to as the granulocyte:erythrocyte ratio). Normally, there should be three granulocyte precursors (myeloid cells) for every erythrocyte precursor. In this field, however, there are at least 11 red cell precursors to only four granulocyte precursors (two of which are half out of the field at the upper edge). (1000×)

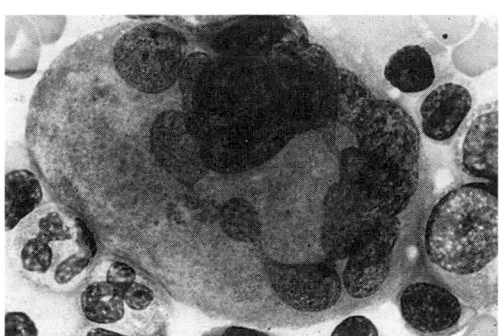

PLATE 12-4. Megaloblastic marrow. This field is dominated by a megakaryocyte. Compare it with the normal megakaryocytes in Color Plate 55-4. The megaloblastic process affects megakaryocytes in that they are larger and their nucleus is hypersegmented (for the same reasons that neutrophils tend to be large and hypersegmented, *i.e.*, difficulty in synthesizing DNA). (1000×)

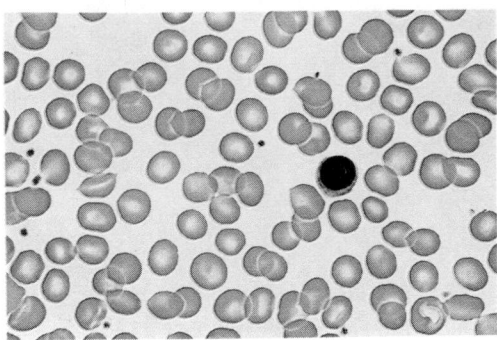

PLATE 22-7. Small resting lymphocyte. Note that the size of the nucleus is only slightly larger than the surrounding erythrocytes. This blood film was stained manually at a pH of 6.4. (500×)

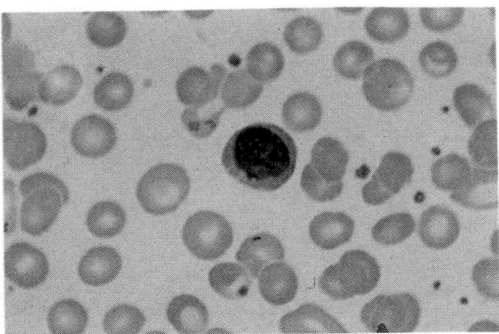

PLATE 22-8. Small-to-medium-sized lymphocyte in peripheral blood. This blood film was stained using an automated dip-type method at a pH of 6.8. (1000×)

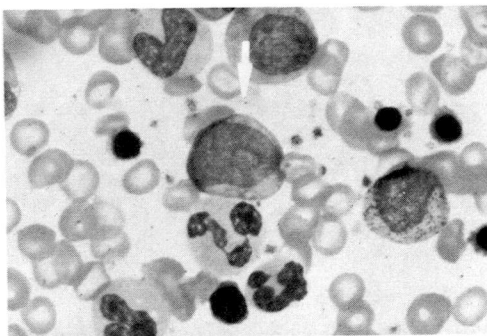

PLATE 22-9. Agranular myeloblast (type I) as seen in bone marrow. Note the large oval nucleolus and the delicate, pale-staining chromatin. (1000×)

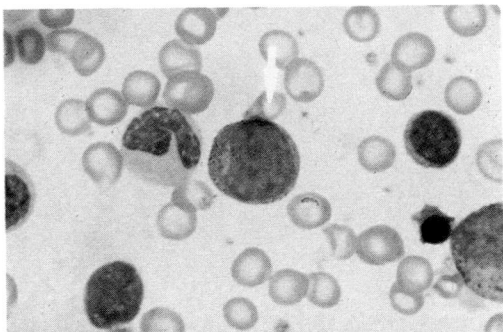

PLATE 22-10. A type II myeloblast containing a few primary granules in its cytoplasm (best seen to the left of the nucleus).

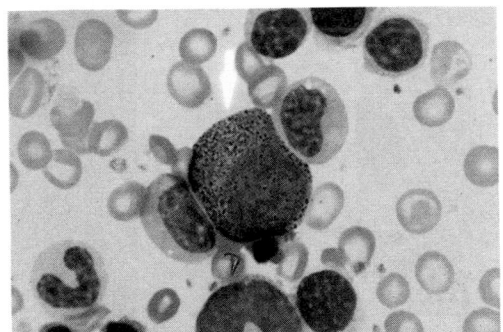

PLATE 22-11. In this promyelocyte (progranulocyte), note the eccentric nucleus and the large number of primary (purple) granules in the cytoplasm. (1000×)

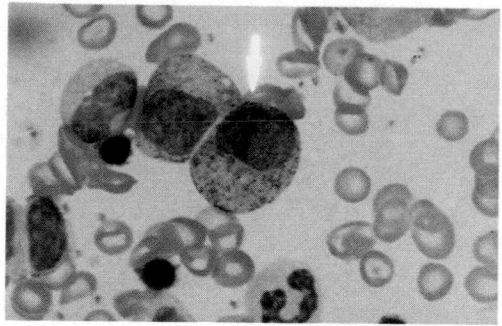 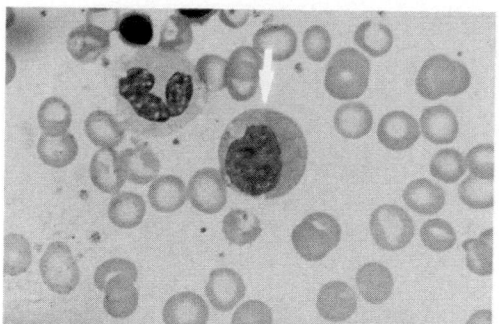

PLATE 22-12. Neutrophilic myelocytes. **(A)** The *arrow* points to an early form; **(B)** a later form. (1000×)

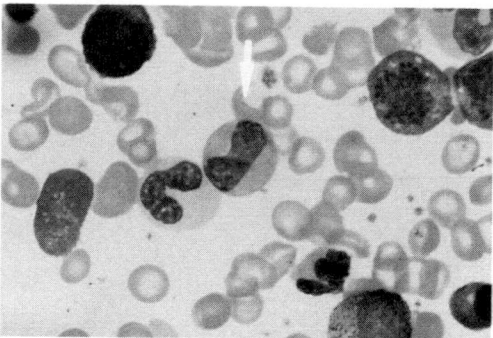

PLATE 22-13. Neutrophil metamyelocyte (*arrow*). The cell immediately adjacent to it is a neutrophil band form. (1000×)

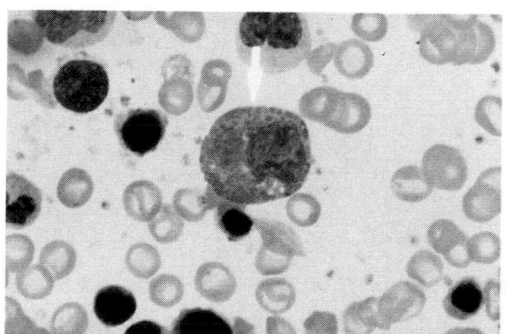 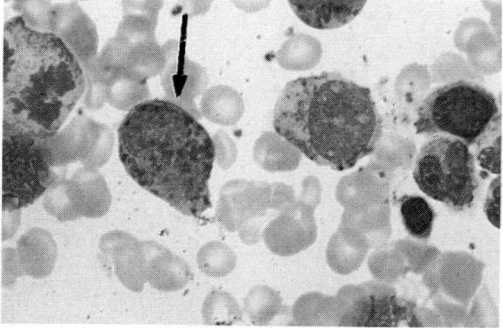

PLATE 22-14. Two examples of eosinophil myelocytes from bone marrow. **(A)** is slightly older than **(B)** in that cytoplasmic RNA (blue color) is almost gone. Its rounded nucleus requires that it be staged as a myelocyte. Note the blue background cytoplasm in cell **(B)** and the presence of large granules—some of which stain purple, indicating granule immaturity. Pale, light orange granules can be seen in the lower part of the cell. Note that these latter granules have not yet acquired the refractile characteristics of the more mature eosinophil granules. (1000×)

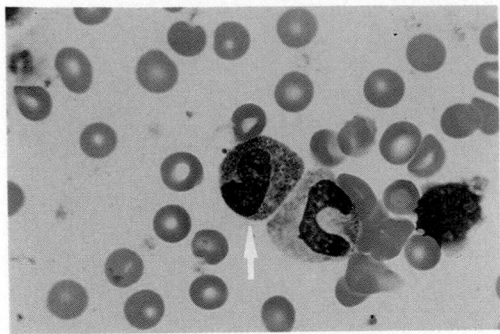

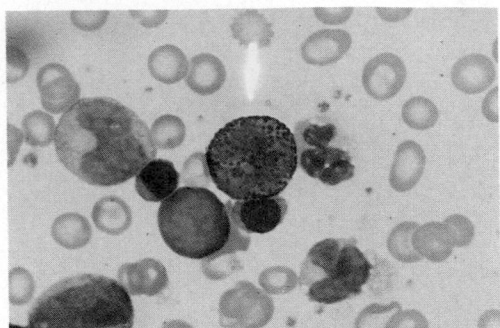

PLATE 22-15. Eosinophil metamyelocyte (*arrow*). Compare this with Color Plate 22-14 (**B**). The granules in the metamyelocyte are more mature and have acquired refractile properties. Bluish-purple granules are no longer apparent. Also, note the difference in granule characteristics between the eosinophil and the neutrophil band form to its right. (1000×)

PLATE 22-16. An immature basophil found in bone marrow. The nucleus occupies most of the cell, and the background cytoplasm still contains RNA (bluish color). (1000×)

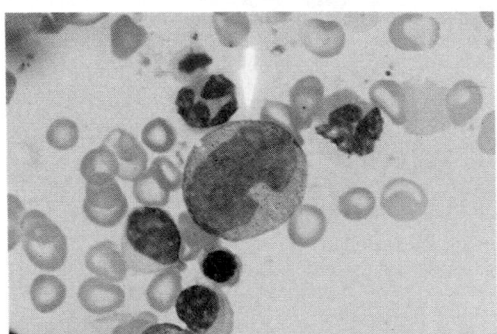

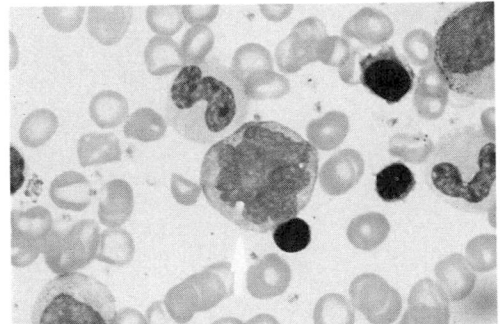

PLATE 22-17. (**A and B**). Two examples of promonocytes found in non-neoplastic marrow.

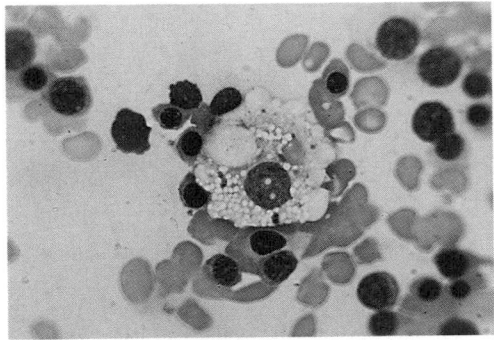

PLATE 22-18. Macrophage. Note the small, eccentric nucleus, abundant foamy cytoplasm, and evidence of ingested cells (debris).

CHAPTER 7

Hemoglobin Synthesis and Function

F. Bernhard Ludvigsen

Objectives

1. Describe the composition and structure of hemoglobin.
2. List and describe normally occurring variants of the hemoglobin molecule.
3. Explain the behavior of hemoglobin at different levels of oxygen tension, and list and discuss several factors that affect this behavior.
4. Name three hemoglobin derivatives that affect the efficiency of oxygen transport, and briefly describe causes for their formation.
5. Name and define the group of diseases resulting from faulty heme synthesis.

The single most common complex organic molecule in vertebrates is hemoglobin (Hb). In humans the weight of Hb represents a little more than 1% of total body weight. Nearly all of this metalloprotein is found in the erythrocytes. Hemoglobin is synthesized within maturing nucleated erythrocytes in the bone marrow. Upon release of erythrocytes into the vascular system, Hb normally remains in the intracellular space of erythrocytes as they travel through the vascular system. Hemoglobin has several functions, most of which affect the extracellular fluid portion of the blood called plasma in which erythrocytes circulate (*e.g.*, maintaining blood pH).

Body tissues and organs require oxygen (O_2) to function and survive. The primary functions of Hb are to deliver O_2 to these tissues and organs and to transport the waste product carbon dioxide (CO_2) away to the lungs, where it is exhaled from the body.

Hemoglobin is the primary biologic substance that permits adequate oxygenation of the body mass of man and other vertebrates. Oxygenation of plasma on its own is not at all adequate to support the O_2 requirements of the large body mass of any vertebrate.

COMPONENTS OF HEMOGLOBIN

The complete adult Hb molecule consists of four significantly different constituents:

1. A protein component called *globin* composed of two sets (dimers) of two different polypeptide chains
2. Four molecules of the nitrogenous substance protoporphyrin IX
3. Four iron atoms in the ferrous (Fe^{2+}) state that combine with protoporphyrin IX to form four heme molecules
4. One 2,3-diphosphoglycerate (2,3-DPG) molecule as a sometime resident in the center of the Hb unit

Globin Chains

Globin chains consist of varied sequences of amino acids; thus they are polypeptide chains. The chains are designated by the Greek letters $\alpha, \beta, \gamma, \delta, \varepsilon$, and ζ. The difference in the globin chain designations relates both to the sequence and to the number of amino acids in the chain. Table 7-1 lists some characteristics of each of the chain types.

The amino acid sequences forming globin polypeptide chains and the proportions of these chains undergo

TABLE 7-1
Globin Chains in Hemoglobin

Greek Designation	Greek Name	No. of Amino Acids	Comments
α	Alpha	141	
β	Beta	146	
γ	Gamma	146	Differs from beta chain by 39 amino acids
δ	Delta	146	Differs from beta chain by 10 amino acids
ε	Epsilon	146	Embryonic only*
ζ	Zeta	146	Embryonic only*

Found only in the first 3 months of embryonic life.

a series of changes during fetal and early infant life. Soon after birth, however, the chains take on the proportions they will retain throughout life.

Protoporphyrin IX and Iron

Protoporphyrin IX is a nitrogenous substance synthesized partly inside the mitochondria and partly in the cytoplasm of the nucleated erythrocyte during maturation. When Fe^{2+} is added to the center of protoporphyrin IX, a substance called ferroprotoporphyrin IX, otherwise known as heme, is formed (Fig. 13-1). The connection of heme and globin through chemical bonds forms the basis of the Hb molecule.

2,3-Diphosphoglycerate

2,3-DPG is a substance produced in the anaerobic glycolytic (Embden–Meyerhof) pathway. This pathway generates energy for the erythrocyte (Fig. 6-7). Specifically, 2,3-DPG is produced in the Rapoport–Luebering shunt. When Hb binds 2,3-DPG, O_2 affinity decreases. Conversely, when the plasma level of 2,3-DPG decreases, Hb 2,3-DPG is released, and the Hb affinity for O_2 increases. Thus, there is an inverse relation between the amount of

2,3-DPG available for binding by Hb and the affinity of hemoglobin for O_2. Adequate tissue oxygenation requires, among other factors, adequate supplies of 2,3-DPG to encourage Hb to release O_2 to the tissues.

NORMAL HEMOGLOBIN VARIANTS

During the first 3 months after conception, the fetus produces three embryonic types of Hb called Portland, Gower I, and Gower II, composed of different types of globin chains as well as heme and iron (Table 7-2). In the fourth month of embryonic development, α and γ globin chains are produced, which together form fetal hemoglobin, designated Hb F. This becomes the predominant variant at this point in fetal life, whereas the concentrations of the embryonic Hb decrease so that none is detectable at birth. The molecular structure of Hb F is $\alpha_2\gamma_2$. In other words, Hb F consists of two alpha globin chains and two gamma globin chains. At birth Hb F comprises about 80% of the total Hb, the remainder being Hb A_1 and Hb A_2 (Table 7-2). By 1 year of age essentially all the child's Hb is in the adult forms: Hb A_1 ($\alpha_2\beta_2$), also called Hb A, accounts for approximately 97% of the Hb by this age and throughout life; Hb A_2 ($\alpha_2\delta_2$) accounts for approximately 2%; and the remainder, usually less than 1%, is Hb F.

Hemoglobin variants, normal and abnormal, may be identified by electrophoresis (Chap. 14). Special quantitative analyses of Hb A_2 and Hb F are useful in the diagnosis of some hematologic disorders (Chap. 15).

HEMOGLOBIN STRUCTURE AND SYNTHESIS

Because so many factors are involved in the synthesis and final structure of Hb, it is not surprising that a multitude of hematologic disorders are associated with both structural and synthetic defects in Hb. Structural defects (most commonly one or more incorrect amino acid[s] substituted into a globin chain's amino acid sequence) lead to abnormal variants that cause disorders called hemoglobinopathies (Chap. 14). Synthetic defects (most commonly de-

TABLE 7-2
Normal Human Hemoglobin Variants

Hemoglobin	Molecular Structure	Stage of Life	Proportion (%)	
			Newborns	*Adults**
Portland	$\zeta_2\gamma_2$	Embryonic†	0	0
Gower I	$\zeta_2\varepsilon_2$	Embryonic†	0	0
Gower II	$\alpha_2\varepsilon_2$	Embryonic†	0	0
Fetal (F)	$\alpha_2\gamma_2$	Newborn and adult	80	<1
A_1	$\alpha_2\beta_2$	Newborn and adult	20	97
A_2	$\alpha_2\delta_2$	Newborn and adult	<0.5	2.5

*Older than 1 yr.
†The Portland, Gower I, and Gower II Hbs are found only during embryonic life.

creased or nonexistent production of one or more globin chain types) cause thalassemic disorders (Chap. 15). It is therefore important to have knowledge of the intricate structure and complex synthetic process of Hb.

Three-Dimensional Structure

As the name hemoglobin implies, the molecule has a globular shape. However, the locations and characteristic behaviors of the individual components of the molecule can easily be depicted in a two-dimensional simplification (Fig. 7-1).

STRUCTURAL RELATIONS OF GLOBIN, 2,3-DPG, AND HEME

Figure 7-1 shows two Hb A molecules, each with four globin chains, two α and two β chains. There is a central cavity in which one molecule of 2,3-DPG is bonded to the β chains when the Hb molecule is in its nonoxygenated state (note that the terms "reduced" and "deoxygenated" are frequently used but may not be as appropriate as "nonoxygenated"). The 2,3-DPG is expelled when Hb A is in its oxygenated state. On each outside corner, one heme group is contained in a pocket formed by a globin chain.

HEMOGLOBIN $\alpha\beta$ DIMERS

The α and β globin units on the left and right sides of Figure 7-1 each form a structure called a *dimer*. Thus, each Hb molecule contains two dimers. The bonds between the α and β units, indicated by an "a" for each dimer, are very strong, whereas the bonds between the two $\alpha\beta$ dimers, indicated by a "b," are of lesser strength. The two dimers can therefore move relative to each other, approaching and separating as well as twisting, thus allowing for the change between the tense and relaxed forms of Hb (Fig. 7-1) as required by the body's tissue O_2 needs.

NONOXYGENATED HEMOGLOBIN STRUCTURE: TENSE (T) FORM

In its nonoxygenated state, Hb takes on its tense or T form. The beta chains of the molecule move farther apart, and the molecule binds 2,3-DPG, with the formation of anionic salt bridges between the β chains. The presence of 2,3-DPG in Hb encourages improved O_2 delivery to the tissues.

OXYGENATED HEMOGLOBIN STRUCTURE: RELAXED (R) FORM

On partial oxygenation of Hb, 2,3-DPG is expelled, and Hb takes on its relaxed or R form. This permits further O_2 binding. The salt bridges are broken, and the β chains move closer together. This form of Hb has an increased affinity for O_2 binding.[22]

Genetic Coding for Globin Chains

The human chromosomes 11 and 16 contain all the genetic information necessary to direct the synthesis of the various globin chains required for normal Hb production. An illustration of these chromosomes is provided in Figure 15-2. Chapter 15 also provides details on the genetics of globin chain production in relation to thalassemia, which is caused by genetic defects leading to reduced globin chain production. The chromosome ends are designated as 3' and 5' to serve as points of reference. Note that chromosome 16 codes for α and ζ chains, whereas chromosome 11 codes for β, γ, δ, and ε chains.

Globin Chain Production

Globin chains are simple (nonconjugated) proteins consisting only of amino acids (NH_2–CH(R)–COOH). The amino acids are connected by peptide bonds (–CO·NH–) in a specific sequence to form a given globin chain type. Genes along chromosomes 11 and 16 provide the unique

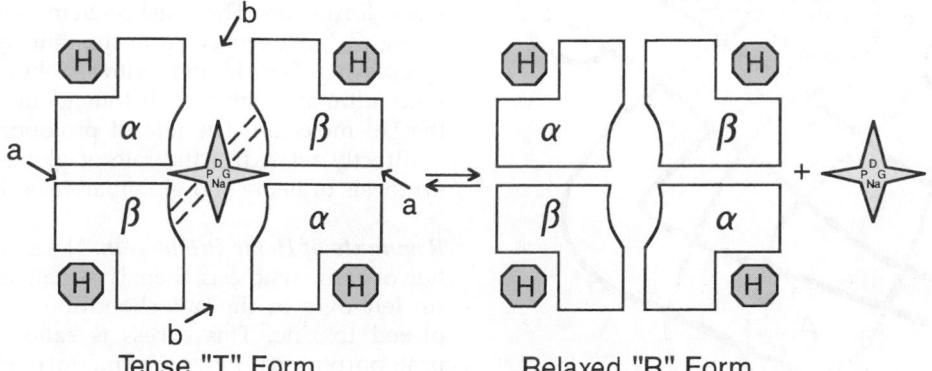

Tense "T" Form   Relaxed "R" Form

FIGURE 7-1. Structure of the Hb A hemoglobin molecule. α and β indicate globin chains, H represents a heme molecule, DPG is 2,3-diphosphoglycerate, and a $\rightarrow$ represents the strong bonds inside each set of α and β chains. Each set forms a dimer; b $\rightarrow$ represents the weak bond between the two dimers. The dashed lines indicate anionic salt bridges between the β chains. (**Left**) The nonoxygenated state, also called the "tense," or "T" form. (**Right**) The "relaxed" or "R" form. It is formed after partial oxygenation of hemoglobin, in which the central cavity of the molecule shrinks to expel the 2,3-DPG molecule, and the β chain salt bridges are broken. See text for details.

DNA code for each type of globin chain. For details on protein synthesis, the reader is referred to a standard biology text.

Globin Chain Structure

Globin chains are best described by their primary and secondary structures. The primary globin structure is defined as a specific sequence of amino acid residues that together form a certain type of globin chain. Those of the α chain are numbered beginning with 1 at the beginning (N-terminal) of the chain to 141 at the end (C-terminal) of the chain. Amino acid residues of the β, γ, and δ chains are similarly numbered from 1 through 146.

The secondary globin structure is defined by dividing the chain into eight separate helical segments. These segments are designated by the letters A through H (Fig. 7-2) and are structurally rigid. There are also seven nonhelical segments (NA, AB, CD, EF, FG, GH, and HC) that lie between the eight helical segments and provide the flexibility that allows physical bending of the globin chain to form the tertiary structure.[12] Figure 7-2 shows where such bending occurs.

Heme Production and Structure

Heme production requires the formation of protoporphyrin IX and the availability of iron. Like all porphyrins, protoporphyrin is a derivative of porphin. This substance, also called tetramethenetetrapyrrole, is a cyclic compound consisting of four pyrrole rings (designated A, B, C, and

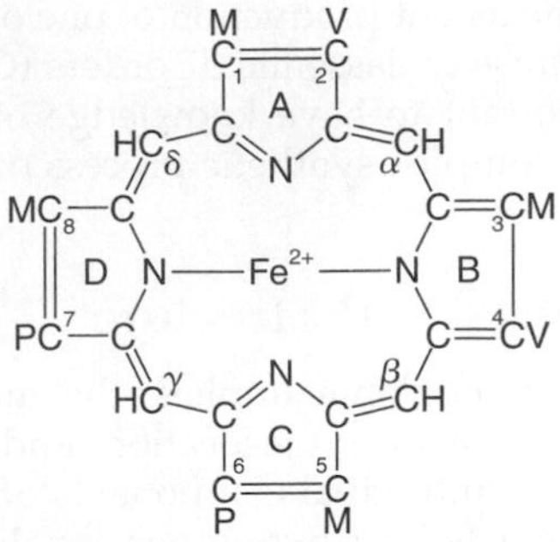

FIGURE 7-3. The heme or protoheme molecule. A, B, C, D = pyrrole rings; α, β, γ, δ = methene bridges connecting pyrrole rings; M = methyl ($-CH_3$); V = vinyl ($-CH=CH_2$); P = propionic acid ($-CH_2-CH_2-COOH$); C = carbon; N = nitrogen; H = hydrogen.

D) connected with four methene (=CH–) bridges (designated α, β, γ, and δ). Figure 7-3 depicts the heme molecule, a protoporphyrin IX molecule into which a Fe^{2+} atom has been inserted. Heme protoporphyrin is named IX because it was the ninth of 15 possible isomers synthesized by Hans Fischer, who was the first to study and describe porphyrins.

FORMATION OF PROTOPORPHYRIN IX AND HEME

Protoporphyrin IX is the last compound produced in a series of reactions leading to the formation of heme. These reactions are all enzymatically directed and take place in nucleated red blood cells (NRBCs). The initial and final steps take place in the mitochondria of NRBCs, whereas the intermediate steps take place in the cell cytoplasm. See Figure 13-1 for details of these steps, the enzymes involved, and the locations of the reactions.

In the final reaction, the insertion of Fe^{2+} into the protoporphyrin IX molecule is catalyzed by the enzyme ferrochelatase to form heme. Iron is provided to NRBCs in the ferric (Fe^{3+}) state by a transport protein named transferrin (see Iron Transport section below). Once inside the mitochondrion, Fe^{3+} is reduced to Fe^{2+} needed for heme formation. The finished heme molecule, depicted in Fig. 7-3, is expelled from the mitochondrion into the cytoplasm, where it binds with a globin chain. Four heme units ultimately bind with four globin chains to create the Hb molecule. The rate of protoporphyrin synthesis is directly related to the rate of globin synthesis. Thus synthesis of heme and globin are closely synchronized.[1]

Remnants of Heme Production. Normally at the completion of heme synthesis, there is a small amount of porphyrin left over in the mitochondrion that becomes complexed to zinc. This excess is called free erythrocyte protoporphyrin (FEP).[32] The amount of FEP in the erythrocyte is elevated when the iron supply is diminished. Free erythrocyte protoporphyrin can be measured in the laboratory and is a useful test in the diagnosis of certain disorders (Chap. 13). The iron not used in heme production is found normally in the cytoplasm as ferritin aggregates (see Iron Transport below).[13]

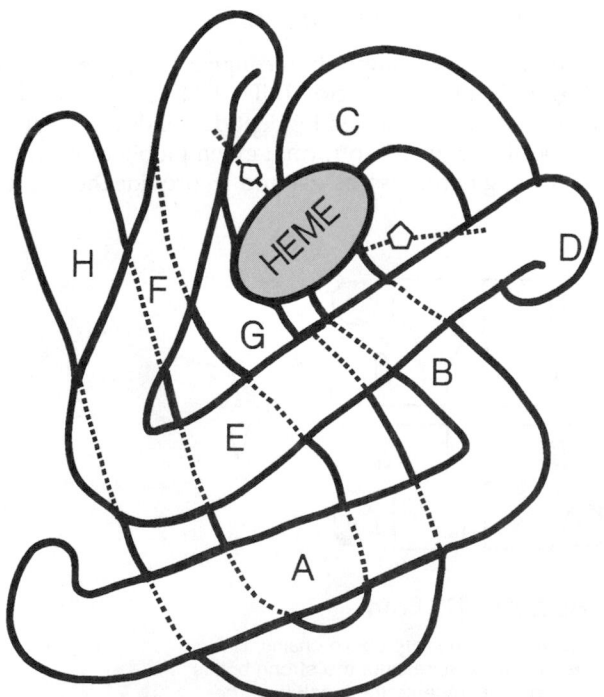

FIGURE 7-2. The tertiary structure of a β globin chain. Heme is contained in a pocket between the E and F helices. (Courtesy of C A Finch, MD.)

Iron Metabolism for Heme Synthesis

Iron in the ferrous (Fe^{2+}) state is required to convert protoporphyrin to heme. Knowledge of the process by which iron is made available to the erythrocytes is necessary to understand some of the disorders of iron metabolism (Chap. 13).

PHYSIOLOGIC LOCATIONS OF IRON

Iron is present throughout the body. Most of it is physiologically active, but some is stored for future use. Most of the stored iron is found in the intracellular space of the liver and bone marrow. Iron is stored for the most part in the form of ferritin, which is composed of iron and a protein called apoferritin. When apoferritin is unavailable, iron is stored as hemosiderin.

SOURCES, RECYCLING, AND LOSS OF IRON

Proper nutrition provides the body with adequate iron. Dietary iron is ingested in both the ferric (Fe^{3+}) and ferrous (Fe^{2+}) states; however, only the ferrous (reduced) form is absorbed. Reduction is accomplished by the acid pH of the stomach and certain reducing substances. A small amount of iron is absorbed in the stomach, but most absorption occurs in the duodenum and jejunum. Only about 10% of the daily dietary iron intake is absorbed, because the body conserves iron so well by recycling it. Once the iron is absorbed, intestinal mucosal cells oxidize it to its ferric state, and the iron is stored temporarily in these cells as ferritin. When saturated, the mucosal cells will no longer absorb iron. Unabsorbed iron is then retained in the bowel and subsequently excreted in the feces.

An overwhelming amount of stored iron is derived from the natural turnover of erythrocytes. On their natural destruction at approximately 120 days of age, erythrocyte iron is released for recycling. However, significant amounts of iron may be lost in episodes of chronic or acute blood loss.

IRON TRANSPORT

When iron is needed, Fe^{3+} is released from the intestinal mucosal cells. It then attaches to transferrin, the plasma iron transport protein, for circulation in the blood as ferric–transferrin. Transferrin can transport two atoms of iron simultaneously. It delivers iron for Hb, myoglobin, cytochrome, and other protein synthesis to the iron storage sites and to most body tissues.

Developing erythrocyte precursors have ferric–transferrin membrane receptors. When a ferric–transferrin complex binds to a receptor, the membrane invaginates, and a vacuole is formed that contains the ferric–transferrin–receptor complex. Most iron is then delivered to the mitochondria for synthesis of heme, and the remainder is stored as crystalline aggregates of ferritin in the cytoplasm. Special studies (*e.g.,* electron microscopy) can reveal ferritin stores in nucleated and mature erythrocytes. Nucleated erythrocytes with stored ferritin are referred to as *sideroblasts,* and mature erythrocytes with ferritin are called *siderocytes.* Aggregated ferritin in sideroblasts or siderocytes can be seen microscopically in a bone marrow or peripheral blood sample after staining with Prussian blue (Fig. 8-24). After releasing iron, the transferrin–receptor complex moves back to the cell membrane, and the transferrin is returned to the plasma for transport of more iron.

Assembly of the Hemoglobin Molecule

Formation of Hb requires iron (ferritin), globin chains, protoporphyrin IX, and the sometimes-resident 2,3-DPG. The source and synthesis of each of these components were described above.

To assemble the molecule, a Fe^{3+} atom must be obtained from ferritin; it must be chemically reduced and then inserted as Fe^{2+} into the center of the protoporphyrin IX molecule. This process is aided by the enzyme ferrochelatase.

When a globin chain is completed on the ribosome, it is released to the cytoplasm. Individual α and β chains spontaneously and quickly form $\alpha\beta$ dimers, to which two heme molecules bind in the crevice between the E and F helices (Fig. 7-2). Two of these dimers quickly form $\alpha_2\beta_2$ Hb tetramers and assume the final three-dimensional (quaternary) structure (Fig. 7-4). Finally, one 2,3-DPG molecule is inserted in the central cavity of the Hb structure.

Assembly of Myoglobin

Myoglobin is discussed here because it is a molecule with many similarities to Hb, although there are also many differences. Myoglobin is a heme pigment found in striated muscle. It has a small molecular weight (17,000). Myoglobin production, like Hb production, requires amino acids, iron, and protoporphyrin IX as raw materi-

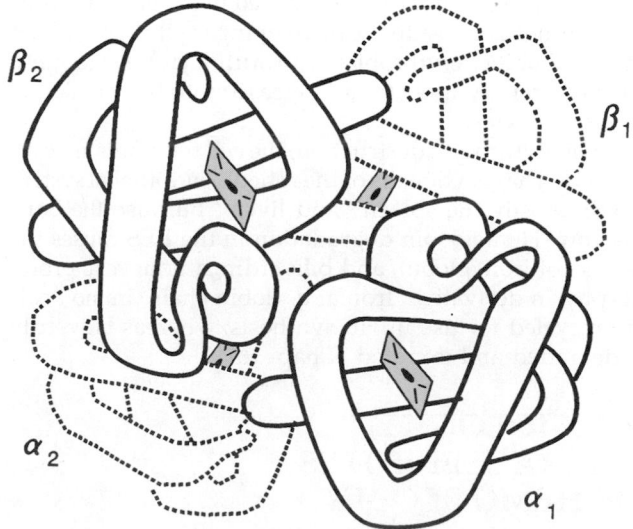

FIGURE 7-4. The three-dimensional Hb A (adult hemoglobin) molecule. It comprises two α and two β chains, each forming its own pocket containing a heme group (indicated by the four small rectangles). (Courtesy of Anne Stiene-Martin.)

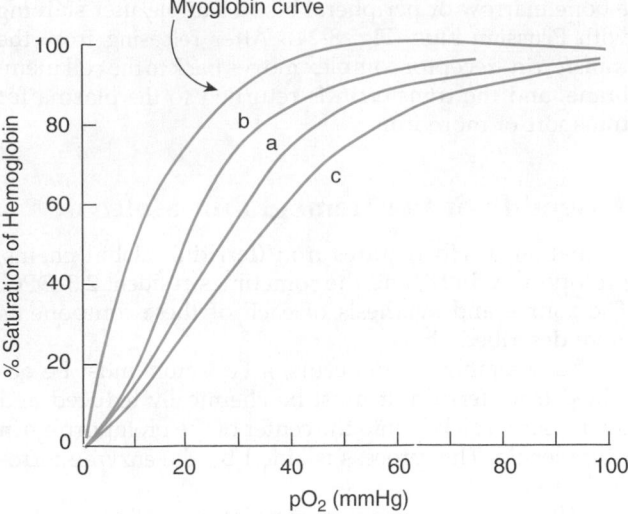

FIGURE 7-5. Oxyhemoglobin dissociation curves under various influences. a = normal dissociation curve; b = "shift to the left" indicating increased Hb affinity for O_2; c = "shift to the right" indicating decreased Hb affinity for O_2. Compare these sigmoidal (S) shaped curves to the parabolic myoglobin dissociation curve. See text for details.

als. Myoglobin has a single polypeptide chain very similar to a globin chain in hemoglobin. It has one heme molecule attached to the polypeptide chain, and the heme can bind O_2. A significant difference between myoglobin and Hb is that the O_2 dissociation curve for myoglobin is hyperbolic, whereas that for Hb is sigmoid (S-shaped; Fig. 7-5).[2] Thus, unlike Hb, myoglobin binds O_2 very tightly and will release it only at very low values of tissue pO_2.

LOCATIONS OF HEMOGLOBIN DURING FUNCTION AND DEGRADATION

Except during fetal life, Hb is formed in the bone marrow. It is synthesized inside the developing erythrocytes, from the basophilic erythroblast (prorubricyte) stage until shortly after erythrocytes are released into the circulation as reticulocytes.

On erythrocyte destruction, the cell remnants are captured by phagocytic cells of the reticuloendothelial system (RES), mostly the spleen[10] and liver,[28] but also the bone marrow. Hemoglobin degradation in the RES causes the release of iron, globin, and biliverdin, a noncyclic protoporphyrin derivative. Iron and globin chain amino acids are recycled for use in Hb synthesis, whereas biliverdin is degraded and excreted (Chap. 16).

PHYSIOLOGIC CHARACTERISTICS OF HEMOGLOBIN

Functions of Hemoglobin

Hemoglobin performs three functions, each of which is essential for life: (1) transport of molecular O_2 from the lungs to the tissues; (2) transport of CO_2 from the tissues

to the lungs; and (3) buffering of the blood to prevent changes in pH that may be incompatible with life. The structure and composition of Hb make it eminently suited for such purposes.

Oxygen Transport

HEME–HEME INTERACTION

Oxygen affinity is affected by the phenomenon of heme–heme interaction. At any time the Hb molecule may be carrying one, two, three, or four O_2 molecules. Because of the nature of heme–heme interaction, the binding of one molecule causes an increased affinity of the other heme groups for O_2. In other words, the more O_2 bound by a Hb molecule, the greater its affinity for O_2. This increase in affinity coincides with the expulsion of 2,3-DPG and conversion of Hb to the R form (Fig. 7-1).

OXYGEN TRANSPORT MECHANISM

Each heme–globin unit of the Hb molecule has the ability to bind one O_2 molecule, so that a fully oxygenated Hb molecule should be represented by the symbol $Hb(O_2)_4$ rather than by the common form HbO_2. Hemoglobin acquisition of O_2 takes place in the alveolar capillaries of the lungs. The atmospheric air entering the lungs contains approximately 21% O_2 at all altitudes on earth. At sea level the partial pressure of inspired O_2 (pressure of air caused only by O_2) is approximately 149 mm Hg. However the final tension (pO_2) in the alveoli of the lungs is approximately 100 mm Hg, because inspired air is mixed with "used" air on its way out. The difference in pO_2 between the venous blood in the lungs (approximately 40 mm Hg) and alveoli (100 mm Hg) favors the movement of O_2 into the blood. Also the minute distance between the O_2 in the alveoli and the blood in the capillary network of the lungs makes the diffusion of O_2 into the blood very rapid. In the lungs, Hb becomes about 95% saturated with O_2 as a result of diffusion from alveolar O_2.

Hemoglobin is essential to the adequate oxygenation of body tissues because O_2 is only slightly soluble in water, the solvent for blood. At rest a human adult of 70 kg requires about 250 mL of O_2 per minute. Therefore, without the O_2 transport capability of Hb, an adult's activities would be restricted to about one-fiftieth of that possible with Hb. Thus, a person with a normal Hb level of 15.0 g/dL can carry out normal daily activities, whereas an anemic person with, for example, 8.0 g/dL of Hb obviously cannot place nearly the same demand on the reduced oxygen reserve.

Breathing pure O_2 or hyperbaric (high pressure) O_2 is sometimes required to treat conditions such as carbon monoxide (CO) poisoning and infant respiratory distress syndrome. Hyperbaric therapy requires that the patient be put into a special chamber that provides O_2 at two and one-half to three times atmospheric pressure.

Since CO has an affinity for hemoglobin of more than 200 times that of oxygen, the goal of O_2 therapy is to increase the pO_2 without dependence on the Hb molecule. As pO_2 is increased, there is a significant increase in the plasma O_2 concentration without any significant change in the amount of O_2 bound to Hb. Breathing pure O_2 raises the pO_2 to more than 600 mm Hg in the alveoli of the lungs and significantly elevates the available plasma O_2 content from 0.08 to 0.78 mmol/L.

OXYHEMOGLOBIN DISSOCIATION CURVE

Hemoglobin has the ability to bind large quantities of O_2; however, Hb must also be willing to release O_2 when needed. The Hb molecule can perform this feat because of its configuration (quaternary structure), which is altered with changes in the circulatory environment. These changes cause alterations in the chemical and physical characteristics of the molecule, particularly movement between the T and the R forms, both of which are related to O_2 affinity as previously discussed. Factors that affect Hb affinity for O_2 are listed in Table 7-3 and discussed in more detail later in this chapter.

It is common to represent the affinity of Hb for O_2 in a graph called the oxyhemoglobin dissociation curve. Figure 7-5 presents the normal curve (curve a) and the influences of environmental factors on Hb O_2 affinity (curves b and c). The curve for the O_2 affinity of myoglobin (discussed previously) is also shown. The y axis reflects the percentage of Hb saturated with oxygen, sO_2, for a Hb solution at pH 7.4. This is plotted against the partial pressure of oxygen at equilibrium, pO_2, on the x axis. Curve b represents a "shift to the left" from normal, and curve c, a "shift to the right." Note the physiologically important sigmoidal (S) shape of the curves.

Normal Curve. The S shape reflects the following important points under normal conditions:

When the pO_2 is less than 20 mm Hg, Hb has a very low affinity for O_2.

When the pO_2 is between 20 and 60 mm Hg, the levels generally found in the tissues, O_2 affinity of Hb increases substantially. Note that the curve in this range is steep, indicating that Hb can release O_2 rapidly. This steep slope also shows that, if necessary, the quantity of O_2 released may be large for a relatively small change in pO_2, thus permitting maximum O_2 delivery to the tissues when needed.

When the pO_2 is above 60 mm Hg, the curve begins to flatten rapidly toward the area of 100% Hb saturation, indicating an almost complete saturation of Hb with O_2. This situation is found in the alveoli of the lungs.

Shift to the Left. When the curve is shifted to the left, Hb has an increased affinity for O_2 and does not readily release it to the tissues. Certain environmental conditions can cause this left shift (Table 7-3), including a decrease in body temperature, a decrease in 2,3-DPG or carbon dioxide (CO_2) concentration, and an increase in blood pH, all of which increase the affinity of Hb for O_2.

One example of such a condition is hyperventilation, in which larger than normal amounts of CO_2 are lost as the individual breathes excessively, often because of severe anxiety. This CO_2 loss causes an increase in blood pH (*i.e.,* an excessively alkaline environment). Hemoglobin binding of O_2 causes Hb to release free hydrogen ions (H^+), which eventually reduces the pH to normal and is reflected by a shift of the curve back to its normal position. Oxygenation of Hb also causes it to release 2,3-DPG, resulting in decreased levels of erythrocyte 2,3-DPG and allowing for further O_2 binding.

Shift to the Right. A shift to the right in the oxyhemoglobin dissociation curve represents a decreased affinity of Hb for O_2. This may result from increased body temperature, increased concentrations of 2,3-DPG or CO_2, or decreased blood pH (acidic state), all of which necessitate increased delivery of O_2 to the tissues (Table 7-3). Examples of such conditions are the physiologic state during exercise, in which the muscle tissue temperature rises, and the abnormal buildup of H^+ ions in renal failure. An acidic state results from excess H^+ ions that are released into the blood.

Nonoxygenated Hb binds more excess H^+ ions than oxygenated Hb. Increased amounts of nonoxygenated Hb are made available by the decrease in the O_2 affinity of hemoglobin caused by the decrease in pH (see Blood pH [The Bohr Effect] below). By binding with H^+, the Hb plays its role as a buffer, and eventually, the pH is brought back to normal, thus shifting the dissociation curve in the direction of normal. In the deep tissues, the high concentrations of CO_2 encourage Hb to release O_2 as well.

Factors Affecting Hemoglobin Affinity for Oxygen

BLOOD (BODY) TEMPERATURE

The solubility of a gas in an aqueous liquid is inversely related to the temperature of the liquid, at constant pressure. When the temperature of the body, and therefore of the blood, increases, the equilibrium in plasma shown in this reaction

$$Hb + O_2 \leftrightarrows HbO_2$$

shifts to the left because the O_2 concentration diminishes. This is equivalent to a decrease in Hb affinity for O_2, which is symbolized in a shift to the right of the O_2 dissociation curve. Conversely, a lowering of the body temperature causes the equilibrium to move to the right,

---

TABLE 7-3
Effects of Various Factors on Oxyhemoglobin Dissociation Curve

Factor	Shift Caused by*	
	Factor Increase	*Factor Decrease*
Blood temperature	R	L
pH	L	R
Erythrocyte 2,3-DPG	R	L
CO_2	R	L
Hb F admixture	L	NA†

*A shift to the left (L) is associated with an increased affinity for O_2. A shift to the right (R) is associated with a decreased affinity for O_2.
†Not applicable.

increasing the Hb affinity for O_2, and causing a left shift in the curve. Put simply, increased blood temperature causes Hb to release O_2 more readily. The opposite is true for decreased blood temperature.

ERYTHROCYTE 2,3-DIPHOSPHOGLYCERATE (2,3-DPG)

A similar shifting of the oxyhemoglobin dissociation curve is seen as a result of variation in the erythrocytic 2,3-DPG concentration.[4] With increasing 2,3-DPG concentration, 2,3-DPG is bound by the salt bridges between the β chains, the curve shifts to the right, the Hb affinity for O_2 is diminished, and bound O_2 is released. This is of specific importance in blood storage, in that some anticoagulants cause whole blood or packed cells to lose most of their native 2,3-DPG during storage. If blood with decreased 2,3-DPG levels is transfused to a patient, its Hb may not release O_2 when and where needed until adequate concentrations of 2,3-DPG have been built up from metabolic activities in the erythrocytes after transfusion.

FETAL HEMOGLOBIN (Hb F)

Hemoglobin F, the normal Hb variant present in high concentrations at birth, has an increased affinity for O_2 and therefore shows an oxyhemoglobin dissociation curve slightly to the left of normal. This is due to the fact that 2,3-DPG is not as strongly attached to γ chains in the nonoxygenated state of Hb F as it is to β chains in Hb A_1. Therefore 2,3-DPG slips out of Hb F more easily, thus increasing its O_2 affinity.

Since a fetus exists in an environment with generally lower O_2 tension, it is important that Hb F has a higher than normal affinity for O_2; however, release of the O_2 to the tissues becomes more difficult. Nature has overcome this problem by providing a high erythrocyte count during fetal life.

BLOOD pH (THE BOHR EFFECT)

The change in Hb O_2 affinity caused by changes in blood pH is referred to as the Bohr effect.[25] An increase in pH (decrease in acidity) increases Hb O_2 affinity and shifts the dissociation curve to the left. Thus, the conditions in the lungs, where pH is at its highest, favor uptake of O_2 by Hb. Conversely, in the peripheral tissues where acidic metabolites are produced, the pH is lower, Hb O_2 affinity is decreased, the curve shifts to the right, and O_2 is released readily.

Usually the arteriovenous pH difference is small (0.04). Nevertheless, when local acidic conditions occur, the characteristics of the dissociation curve and the Bohr effect provide for a rapid increase in O_2 delivery and Hb uptake of H^+.

ABNORMAL HEMOGLOBIN VARIANTS

A number of abnormal Hb variants show dissociation curve shifts, either right or left, compared with Hb A under identical environmental circumstances. This results from their structural abnormalities, often caused by globin chain amino acid substitutions (Chap. 14).

Hemoglobin Transport of Carbon Dioxide

Hemoglobin not only provides oxygen for the tissues but also participates in the removal and transport of CO_2 from tissues to the lungs for subsequent expiration. Although about 70% of CO_2 is carried in the plasma, mostly in the form of bicarbonate (HCO_3^-), 30% is carried by the erythrocytes. Of this 30%, 25% is in the form of bicarbonate and 2% is nonionized CO_2, both dissolved in the water of erythrocytes; the remainder (about 3%) is in the form of carbamino-hemoglobin ($Hb\text{-}NH\text{-}COO^-$). The reactions in this transport method not only remove CO_2 from the body but also buffer the blood.[23]

Carbon dioxide (CO_2) exerts an effect on Hb O_2 uptake and delivery similar to the Bohr effect. In the tissues, increased blood CO_2 levels cause a shift to the right in the oxyhemoglobin dissociation curve, with a decreased Hb affinity for O_2. This encourages release of O_2 and increased binding of CO_2, thus removing it from the tissues. In the lungs, decreased CO_2 levels cause the opposite effect. There, CO_2 is excreted by means of expired air.

Blood containing nonoxygenated Hb has a greater affinity for CO_2 than does oxygenated blood because of the Bohr effect. Further, a CO_2 dissociation curve (Fig. 7-6) reflects the relation between blood CO_2 content and the pCO_2 for 0% HbO_2, nonoxygenated blood, and 97.5% HbO_2, oxygenated blood. The difference in these curves demonstrates the Haldane effect. This mechanism allows Hb to play its role as a buffer, decreasing the acidity caused by dissolved CO_2 in the blood (see Hemoglobin's Role in Acid–Base Balance below).

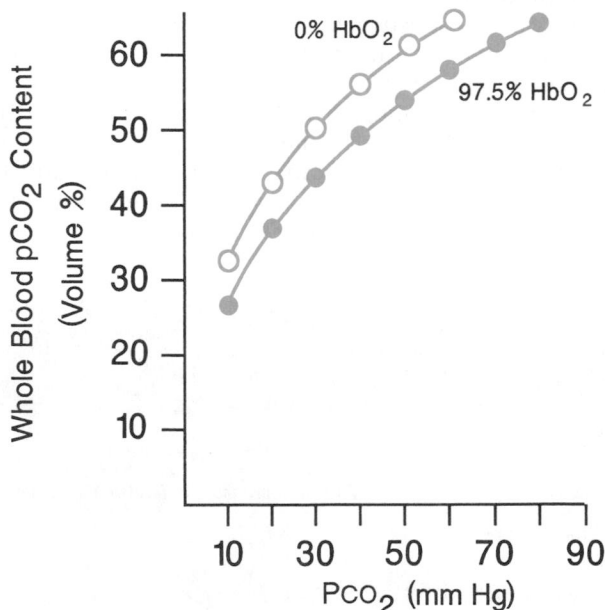

FIGURE 7-6. The carbon dioxide dissociation curve of whole blood. The curve is relatively linear between pCO_2 40 and 60 torr (torr = 1/760 of normal atmospheric pressure). The Haldane effect is represented by the difference between the two curves, which reflect a comparison of oxygenated (97.5% HbO_2) and deoxygenated (0% HbO_2) blood.

Hemoglobin's Role in Acid–Base Balance

Nonoxygenated hemoglobin (Hb^-) is a stronger base than oxyhemoglobin ($Hb[O_2]_4$ or HbO_2); therefore, it can more easily accept and neutralize H^+ ions (protons) formed as a result of increased blood CO_2 levels. However, both Hb^- and $Hb(O_2)_4$ are capable of accepting H^+ ions. The following two reactions are responsible for physiologic acid–base balance involving Hb:

$$Hb(O_2)_4 + H_2O + CO_2 \xrightarrow{CA} Hb^- + H_2CO_3 + 4O_2 \quad (1)$$

$$Hb^- + H^+ + HCO_3^- \longleftrightarrow HHb + HCO_3^- \quad (2)$$

The net result of these two reactions is that there is a very small difference in the arterial and venous pH.

In reaction 1, $Hb(O_2)_4$ releases O_2 to the tissues while CO_2 diffuses into the erythrocyte and combines with H_2O to form carbonic acid (H_2CO_3). This reaction is catalyzed by the enzyme carbonic anhydrase (CA). In reaction 2, Hb^- acts as a base and accepts and neutralizes the H^+ ion to form HHb, reduces carbonic acid content, and increases bicarbonate (HCO_3^-) ions.

The reaction in which oxygenated Hb (HbO_2) accepts and neutralizes the H^+ ion is illustrated in Figure 7-7. The binding of the H^+ ion encourages Hb to release its oxygen to the tissues. The buildup of bicarbonate ions in the erythrocyte eventually causes a concentration gradient between the cell and plasma, and bicarbonate begins to diffuse into the plasma. This loss of negative ions causes chloride ions (Cl^-) to diffuse into the cell to maintain electroneutrality. This is called the *chloride shift* (Fig. 7-7).

The erythrocyte then travels back to the lungs, where the reactions go in the opposite direction. Hemoglobin again becomes oxygenated, making it a stronger acid and causing carbonic acid to convert back to water and CO_2, which is expelled.

In addition, as with any other protein, acidic groups (primarily carboxyl groups [—COOH]) and basic groups (primarily amino groups [—NH$_2$]) on the surface of Hb cause it to act as an amphoteric substance; that is, one that may act both as an acid (proton donor) and as a base (proton acceptor). Although most carboxyl and amino groups are tied up in peptide bonds, a sufficient number are available to play a significant role in acid–base balance in the blood. Because Hb is present in the bloodstream in such a high concentration, it is an effective buffer.

HEMOGLOBIN DERIVATIVES AND THEIR ASSOCIATED DISORDERS

Hemoglobin derivatives are abnormal forms in which the heme is altered in some way but the globin chains are unaffected. These derivatives are nonfunctional and may or may not be reversible to a normal variant.

Hemoglobin is a very stable protein and functions during the full 120-day life span of the erythrocyte. It might function even longer if it were not dependent on the erythrocyte for its transportation. During the 120-day period, Hb passes through an incomprehensible number of metabolic cycles, each time without showing signs of aging. Nevertheless, the substance is not immune to reversible and irreversible conversions to the nonfunctional derivative states, which include methemoglobin, sulfhemoglobin, and carboxyhemoglobin. Each of these can cause an abnormal clinical state of varying severity.

Methemoglobin and Methemoglobinemia

Methemoglobin (also referred to as hemiglobin or Hi) is well known in the laboratory for its use as an intermediary in the cyanmethemoglobin method for quantitation of whole blood Hb. It is formed by gentle oxidation in which the iron in the heme groups is oxidized to its ferric (Fe^{3+}) state. In this form, heme cannot bind O_2.[16]

Normal endogenous production is a continuing event. Approximately 0.5% to 3% of the total body Hb is spontaneously converted to methemoglobin daily.[16] However, this seldom causes any problems because of an enzyme, NADH-methemoglobin reductase (diaphorase), which is present in erythrocytes at a level sufficient to counter methemoglobin produced at rates many times those normally encountered. Methemoglobin reduction, or rather reduction of its associated heme–Fe^{3+}, also requires a properly functioning Embden–Meyerhof pathway to produce NADH (Chap. 6), which is the main source for electron donation in the reduction process. Specifically, the reduction takes place in the methemoglobin reduction pathway (see Fig. 6-7). In this pathway, heme is reduced to its functional ferrous (Fe^{2+}) form. With this protection system in place, methemoglobin levels are rarely above 1% of the total hemoglobin.[27]

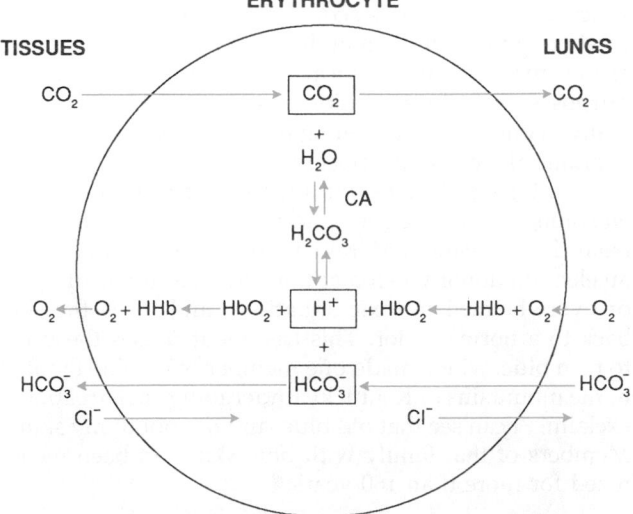

Hemoglobin and Erythrocyte Function

ERYTHROCYTE

FIGURE 7-7. The interrelations of oxygen and carbon dioxide transport in the erythrocyte that affect the whole blood acid–base balance. Arrows to the left indicate the direction of reactions taking place in the tissues; those to the right, in the lungs. (From Telen MJ: The mature erythrocyte. In Lee GR, Bithell TC, Foerster J et al [eds]: Wintrobe's Clinical Hematology, 9th ed, p 122. Philadelphia, Lea & Febiger, 1993, with permission).

Methemoglobinemia is characterized by elevated erythrocyte methemoglobin concentrations. The clinical manifestations are few and generally mild. Rarely, the disorder is inherited; more often, it is acquired. Five inherited Hb variants, each a form of Hb M (M for methemoglobin; Chap. 14), also cause methemoglobinemia.

PATHOPHYSIOLOGY

Whether acquired or inherited, methemoglobinemia stems from the inability to adequately reduce methemoglobin that builds up in the circulation, thus causing cyanosis. Characteristically, the patient responds to therapeutic doses of methylene blue (except patients with a Hb M disorder), as evidenced by the return of normal skin color shortly after therapy is initiated.

Inherited Methemoglobinemia. When inherited, methemoglobinemia is most commonly attributed to inheritance of an NADH-methemoglobin reductase enzyme deficiency. This is also called diaphorase deficiency. Without this enzyme, even with sufficient NADH produced in the Embden–Meyerhof pathway, methemoglobin is not adequately reduced, causing increased circulating levels of methemoglobin. These patients respond to methylene blue treatment.[8]

Acquired Methemoglobinemia. Abnormal and toxic methemoglobin production may be caused by a variety of substances, either ingested or absorbed. These include oxidants from a plethora of sources, including antimalarial drugs, therapeutic drugs such as sulfonamides (among others), drugs of abuse, aniline dyes (*e.g.*, fresh dye on shoes), nitrate-rich water and foodstuffs, and many common aromatic chemicals. These patients also respond to methylene blue treatment.

Inherited Hemoglobin M Methemoglobinemia. The five Hb M variants are the result of various amino acid substitutions in the globin chains that directly affect the heme group, causing it to enter the ferric or oxidized state, which leads to a methemoglobin buildup in the blood. Patients with these disorders characteristically *do not* respond to methylene blue treatment. Treatment is actually not possible, nor is it necessary, because the patients show no clinical abnormalities other than their cyanotic appearance (Chap. 14).

DEMOGRAPHICS AND GENETICS

Diaphorase deficiency is rare and inherited as an autosomal recessive trait. It was first described in Europe[8]; however, it is now found practically worldwide. Most cases involve inbreeding among siblings or other close relatives.

SYMPTOMS AND PHYSICAL FINDINGS

Cyanosis (a bluish skin discoloration) appears when the methemoglobin level exceeds 10% of the total Hb. This is mainly a cosmetic problem, and affected patients do not report any specific symptoms. Although the cyanosis affects the skin color of the entire body, it is particularly evident on the lips, mucous membranes of the mouth, ears, cheeks, and nail beds. If the methemoglobin level exceeds 35%, symptoms of hypoxia such as shortness of breath, dizziness, headaches, or tachycardia may occur. Levels of 60% to 70% or even greater are rare and are usually fatal.[17]

LABORATORY FINDINGS AND CORRELATIONS WITH DISEASE

Peripheral Blood Film. Heinz bodies (See Fig. 8-29), which reflect denatured Hb, may be demonstrated in the erythrocytes of cells affected by ingested toxins. This requires the use of special stains (Chap. 14).

Diaphorase Enzyme Screening Tests. Diaphorase screening tests are rapid.[18,26] Specific enzyme assays for use with prepared hemolysates are also available.[15]

Methemoglobin Quantitation. This test is based on the small but characteristic absorbance peak of methemoglobin at 630 to 635 nm. After measuring absorbance of a hemolysate at 632 nm, KCN is added, which causes conversion of methemoglobin to cyanmethemoglobin, which does not absorb at 632 nm.[5] The difference in the absorbance of the specimen at 632 nm before and after addition of KCN is proportional to the methemoglobin concentration.

Any methemoglobin level above 1.5% of the total Hb concentration is considered abnormal. Levels in individuals with acquired methemoglobinemia secondary to toxic substances may range from 10% to greater than 70%, depending on the circumstances. Levels in untreated individuals with diaphorase deficiency usually stay between 15% and 30%.[19]

Laboratory investigation of the Hb M disorders is discussed in Chapter 14.

EFFECTS OF TREATMENT ON LABORATORY RESULTS

Whether the disorder is acquired or inherited, therapy is rarely required. Other than the bluish skin color, patients are normal and live a normal life span.[17] For cosmetic purposes, oral administration of methylene blue will generally maintain the methemoglobin level below 10%, thus avoiding the cyanotic appearance.

For toxic situations, intravenous infusion of methylene blue is suggested for rapid methemoglobin clearance from the circulation. Methylene blue is very effective as an electron donor when diaphorase levels are insufficient or overwhelmed in toxic situations, and turns the skin back to a normal color. This treatment causes the urine to turn blue, which made one member of a "blue family" in the mountains of Kentucky undergoing such treatment exclaim, "I can see that old blue running out of my skin." Members of that family with blue skin had been recognized for more than 160 years.[30]

Sulfhemoglobin and Sulfhemoglobinemia

Sulfhemoglobin is another derivative formed during the oxidative denaturation of Hb by the addition of a sulfur (S) atom to each heme molecule. Sulfhemoglobin retains iron in the ferrous form, but its affinity for O_2 is only one hundredth of normal Hb. It does not form as a result of normal metabolic activities, and it is probably always an acquired condition. Patients may have a significantly cyanotic appearance.

In vitro, sulfhemoglobin forms when hydrogen sulfide (H_2S) is added to Hb; thus the name sulfhemoglobin. *In vivo,* sulfhemoglobin forms in the occasional patient as a result of exposure to certain drugs and chemicals (*e.g.,* acetanilid, phenacetin, and sulfonamides).[7,21,24] It is unclear why some patients, on the same drug exposure, form sulfhemoglobin whereas others form methemoglobin, and still others develop erythrocyte globin precipitates.

Sulfhemoglobinemia results from excessive sulfhemoglobin concentrations in the blood, although they hardly ever exceed 20% of the total Hb. Such levels are not life threatening, and the only significant effect is cyanosis. The condition generally is benign. Once formed, sulfhemoglobin stays in the erythrocyte during the remainder of its 120-day life span. Sulfhemoglobin cannot be converted back to normal, functional Hb.

Sulfhemoglobin quantitation may be performed by examination of a prepared hemolysate for a distinct, broad increase in the absorption curve in the range of 600 to 620 nm.[14] Treatment of the patient consists of removal of the offending agent.

Carboxyhemoglobin and Carboxyhemoglobinemia

Carboxyhemoglobin is a carbon monoxide (CO) derivative of Hb normally found in blood at levels of less than 1% of the total hemoglobin.

PATHOPHYSIOLOGY

Hemoglobin has more than 200 times the affinity for CO than it has for O_2. Exposure to even small percentages of CO in the inspired air therefore prevents a substantial amount of Hb from carrying out its function in O_2 transport. This can lead to asphyxiation. Automobile exhaust is a well-known source of toxicity,[3] and exposure to this exhaust is a common method in attempted suicides. Industrial wastes such as coal gas (*e.g.,* gas from burning charcoal) are also recognized sources of toxicity.[20]

SYMPTOMS AND PHYSICAL FINDINGS

Carbon monoxide poisoning may be insidious, with the effects of hypoxia suddenly overwhelming an individual, particularly because the gas is colorless and odorless. The skin turns a bright cherry red with increasing levels of carboxyhemoglobin. With lower levels of exposure, symptoms such as dizziness, nausea, headache, vomiting, and confusion may occur. At high levels (approximately 50% to 70% of total Hb), an individual can be asphyxiated.

LABORATORY FINDINGS AND CORRELATIONS WITH DISEASE

A level of 0.5% carboxyhemoglobin is typical in nonsmokers, whereas 5% is common among smokers. With only 0.04% (v/v) CO in air, the carboxyhemoglobin level can increase to 10%, which is associated with shortness of breath on exertion. Long exposure at this level impairs judgment. With exposure to a CO level of 0.1% (v/v), the carboxyhemoglobin level can reach 50% to 70%, resulting in unconsciousness, respiratory failure, and death. A level of 0.4% (v/v) causes the blood carboxyhemoglobin level to rise quickly to 80%, which is immediately fatal.[31]

Laboratory screening tests for carboxyhemoglobin are available. One spot test calls for hemolyzing 0.5 mL of whole blood with 20 mL of distilled water, then adding 1 mL of NaOH, 1.0 mol/L. Blood containing more than 20% carboxyhemoglobin will cause the appearance of a light cherry-red color; with normal blood the mixture will turn brown.[11]

Quantitation of CO can be performed by gas chromatography,[9] spectrophotometry,[29] and other techniques.[6] Dedicated spectrophotometric instruments now yield instantaneous highly accurate readings of Hb, carboxyhemoglobin, and oxygen saturation of Hb.

EFFECTS OF TREATMENT ON LABORATORY RESULTS

Therapeutic measures in CO poisoning consist of removing the source of toxicity and administration of high levels of O_2, including, in some cases, hyperbaric O_2 therapy; proper ventilation must be maintained. The carboxyhemoglobin level should then return to normal. Unless brain damage occurs, there are no long-term effects from such a toxic exposure as long as the patient receives proper and prompt treatment. Neither chemical nor hematologic data are affected.

ABNORMAL HEME SYNTHESIS: THE PORPHYRIAS

Disorders of heme synthesis known as porphyrias will be addressed here. Addressed elsewhere are disorders of globin synthesis, both qualitative (Chap. 14) and quantitative (Chap. 15).

The laboratory analysis of abnormalities in heme synthesis is necessary to detect the deficiency of, or a defect in, one or more of the hematopoietic enzymes involved in heme production (see Fig. 13-1). Such deficiencies or defects constitute a group of disorders, commonly known as porphyrias, which may be inherited or acquired.

Pathophysiology

The porphyrias lead to the accumulation of porphyrin precursors or one or more of the porphyrin(ogen)s in the bone marrow (erythropoietic porphyrias) or in the liver (hepatic porphyrias). Decreased Hb production is the result. With the exception of ALA synthase, deficiencies of all other enzymes have been described.

Primary porphyrias are inherited disorders. Table 7-4 lists characteristics of the enzymatic defects of primary porphyrias that are associated with erythropoietic abnormalities. All other enzyme abnormalities of the heme syn-

TABLE 7-4
The Primary Erythropoietic Porphyrias

Porphyria	Enzyme Defect	Inheritance	Clinical Presentation	Laboratory Findings and Comments
Hereditary PBG synthase deficiency	Porphobilinogen synthase*	Autosomal dominant	Not well known; possible neurologic abnormalities	Only decreased enzyme activity
Congenital erythro-poietic porphyria (CEP)	Uroporphyrinogen III cosynthase	Autosomal recessive	Severe photocutaneous lesions; teeth fluoresce red under UV light, patients rarely survive past middle age	Rarest porphyria; hemolytic anemia; marked increase in RBC coproporphyrin; marked increase in urine uroporphyrin, causing red urine; marrow morphology shows erythroblastic hyperplasia; possible anisocytosis, poikilocytosis, polychromasia
Protoporphyria (PP)	Ferrochelatase	Autosomal dominant	Photocutaneous lesions; mild to severe hepatobiliary disease	Possibly second most common porphyria; marked increase in FEP†; marrow morphology normal

*Porphobilinogen synthase = ALA dehydrase.
†Free erythrocyte protoporphyrin.

thesis pathway are associated with hepatic porphyrias that show no hematologic abnormalities.

Secondary porphyrias are acquired disorders stimulated by certain drugs or chemicals through various mechanisms. The secondary porphyrias mainly affect the liver and seldom affect the bone marrow. The most important exception to this is the secondary porphyria caused by lead poisoning, which causes abnormalities in both the peripheral blood and bone marrow (Chap. 13).

Symptoms and Physical Findings

Patients with primary porphyrias are generally either (1) asymptomatic; (2) suffering from characteristic skin lesions easily recognized by a physician; or (3) suffering from neurologic disturbances (Table 7-4). The skin lesions, referred to as photocutaneous lesions, are formed on exposure of the skin to sunlight, indoors or outdoors, because of the patient's increased porphyrin level. Porphyrins absorb sunlight very strongly. Symptoms of anemia may be reported in cases of congenital erythropoietic porphyria (CEP), in which case hemolytic anemia may be observed.

Laboratory Findings and Correlations with Disease

Laboratory findings for the inherited erythropoietic porphyrias are summarized in Table 7-4. Note the characteristic increase in FEP in protoporphyria. This increase is caused by the lack of iron chelation to protoporphyrin IX secondary to the ferrochelatase enzyme deficiency. The FEP cannot be used in Hb synthesis and thus does not bind to globin. Elevated FEP levels are also found in iron deficiency anemia and anemia of chronic disease because of insufficiency of iron available to the erythron for Hb synthesis (Chap. 13).

Effects of Treatment on Laboratory Results

A variety of therapeutic measures have been used to alleviate the skin lesions, some of which have no effect on laboratory results, whereas others are said to reduce porphyrin levels. Hemolysis in CEP, as well as porphyrin levels, can sometimes be reduced by transfusions, splenectomy, or steroids, although these measures do not prevent the recurrence of hemolysis. The reader is referred to a textbook of clinical chemistry for more details on the porphyrias.

LABORATORY EVALUATION OF HEMOGLOBIN AND IRON AVAILABILITY

Hemoglobin analysis has played an important role in clinical diagnosis since early times. Of the many techniques proposed or used in the past to quantitate Hb, essentially only two analytical principles remain in use: the cyanmethemoglobin method for measurement of total Hb in whole blood (Chap. 9) and analysis of oxyhemoglobin to measure plasma Hb (Chap. 16).

Because Hb synthesis requires iron, the laboratory measurement of iron availability has long been a useful tool in the evaluation of anemias secondary to disorders of iron metabolism (Chap. 13). There are a number of chemical analyses for the evaluation of iron availability to the erythron. Most of these tests are performed in the chemistry laboratory, and a brief description of each may be found in Chapter 13.

CHAPTER SUMMARY

Hemoglobin (Hb) is necessary for adequate tissue oxygenation in vertebrates because O_2 is minimally soluble in plasma. Hemoglobin also plays a role in the removal of CO_2 from the tissues. Hemoglobin is synthesized in maturing nucleated red cells in the bone marrow and consists of globin, heme, and sometimes 2,3-DPG (Fig. 7-1). Globin chain composition (*i.e.,* amino acid sequence and number; Table 7-1) determines the Hb variant. For example, the variant Hb A_1, which constitutes most adult Hb, consists of two α and two β chains ($\alpha_2\beta_2$; Table 7-2). Heme consists of ferrous iron and protoporphyrin IX (Fig. 7-3). Excess protoporphyrin produced during heme synthesis is called free erythrocyte protoporphyrin (FEP), which can be measured in the laboratory. Elevated FEP often indicates some form of iron metabolism disorder.

2,3-DPG is synthesized in the Embden–Meyerhof pathway. When Hb binds 2,3-DPG, its affinity for O_2 decreases; on release of 2,3-DPG, the affinity increases. Heme–heme interaction increases affinity for O_2 of hemoglobin; Hb can bind four O_2 molecules.

The oxyhemoglobin dissociation curve (Fig. 7-5) is sigmoidal (S) shaped. Normally when pO_2 is below 20 mm Hg, Hb has a low O_2 affinity; when pO_2 is between 20 and 60 mm Hg (normal tissue levels), Hb can readily bind or release O_2 to respond quickly to small changes in the pO_2 of its environment. When Hb O_2 affinity is increased, the dissociation curve shifts to the left. When decreased, the shift is to the right (Table 7-3). In general, body temperature, blood pH (Bohr effect), 2,3-DPG levels, blood CO_2 levels, amount of fetal Hb, and abnormal variants of Hb all affect the O_2 affinity of hemoglobin.

Hemoglobin derivatives contain an abnormal heme component (but normal globin chains), making them unable to carry O_2. They include methemoglobin, in which heme contains Fe^{3+} instead of Fe^{2+}; sulfhemoglobin, in which sulfur is permanently bound to heme during oxidative Hb denaturation; and carboxyhemoglobin, in which carbon monoxide (CO) is bound reversibly to heme. Certain hereditary and acquired clinical disorders are caused by these derivatives, and a number of laboratory tests exist for their diagnosis.

The porphyrias are inherited or acquired disorders of heme synthesis that lead to accumulation in the liver or bone marrow of porphyrins or their precursors. Laboratory features are presented in Table 7-4.

Review Questions

7-1. The hemoglobin (Hb) structure includes all of the following *EXCEPT*

A. protoporphyrin IX.
B. polypeptide chains.
C. transferrin.
D. iron.

7-2. The molecular structure of Hb A_1 is

A. $\alpha_2\beta_2$.
B. $\alpha_2\delta_2$.
C. $\alpha_2\varepsilon_2$.
D. $\alpha_2\gamma_2$.

7-3. One oxygenated Hb A_2 molecule consists of

A. 2 α and 2 γ chains; 4 heme molecules; and 4 O_2 molecules.
B. 2 α and 2 δ chains; 4 heme molecules; and 8 O_2 molecules.
C. 2 α and 2 δ chains; 4 heme molecules; and 4 O_2 molecules.
D. 2 α and 2 δ chains; 8 heme molecules; and 4 O_2 molecules.

7-4. The addition of iron to the protoporphyrin IX molecule to form heme occurs

A. spontaneously.
B. with the aid of ferrochelatase.
C. with the aid of 2,3-DPG.
D. through the delivery of iron by ferritin.

7-5. Hemoglobin affinity for O_2 is regulated by

A. heme.
B. globin.
C. iron.
D. 2,3-DPG.

7-6. Hemoglobin will release O_2 more easily if

A. body temperature decreases.
B. erythrocyte 2,3-DPG increases.
C. plasma CO_2 decreases.
D. blood pH increases.

7-7. Methemoglobin in the bloodstream

A. is disastrous.
B. causes the skin to turn cherry red.
C. replaces carboxyhemoglobin after exposure to carbon monoxide.
D. is usually convertible to normal Hb.

7-8. Carboxyhemoglobin is characterized by all of the following *EXCEPT*

A. it is rapidly fatal at levels of more than 80% of the total blood Hb.
B. it is found in higher blood levels in smokers than nonsmokers.
C. it cannot be removed from Hb after binding.
D. it is detectable in blood by a spot screening test.

7-9. Porphyrias are a group of diseases that are caused by

A. excessive heme precursor accumulation.
B. excessive heme accumulation.
C. insufficient iron supply.
D. insufficient globin production.

References

1. Adamson SD, Herbert E, Godchaux W: Factors affecting the rate of protein synthesis in lysate systems from reticulocytes. Arch Biochem 125:671, 1968
2. Bauer JD: Hemoglobin. In Kaplan LA, Pesce AJ (eds): Clinical Chemistry: Theory, Analysis and Correlation, 2nd ed, p 514. St Louis, CV Mosby, 1989
3. Beck HG, Schulze WH, Suter GM: Carbon monoxide—A domestic hazard. JAMA 115:1, 1940
4. Benesch R, Benesch RE: Effect of organic phosphate from human erythrocytes on allosteric properties of hemoglobin. Biochem Biophys Res Commun 26:162, 1967
5. Betke K, Steim H, Tonz O: A family with congenital methaemoglobinaemia due to reductase deficiency. Germ Med Month 7:217, 1962
6. Blanke RV, Decker WJ: Analysis of toxic substances. In Tietz NW (ed): Fundamentals of Clinical Chemistry, p 885. Philadelphia, WB Saunders, 1987
7. Brandenburg RO, Smith HL: Sulfhemoglobinemia: Study of 62 clinical cases. Am Heart J 42:582, 1951
8. Codounis A: Hereditary methaemoglobinaemic cyanosis. Acta Genet Statist Med 7:131, 1957

9. Collison HA, Rodkey FL, O'Neal JD: Determination of carbon monoxide in blood by gas chromatography. Clin Chem 14:162, 1968

10. Cooper RA, Shattil SJ: Mechanisms of hemolysis: The minimal red cell defect. N Engl J Med 285:1514, 1971

11. Decker WJ, Treuting JJ: Spot tests for rapid diagnosis of poisoning. Clin Toxicol 4:89, 1971

12. Dickerson RE: X-ray analysis and protein structure. In Neurath H (ed): The Proteins: Composition, Structure and Function, vol 2, p 603ff. New York, Academic Press, 1964

13. Douglas AS, Dacie JV: The incidence and significance of iron containing granules in human erythrocytes and their precursors. J Clin Pathol 6:307, 1953

14. Fairbanks VF, Klee GG: Biochemical aspects of hematology. In Tietz NW (ed): Fundamentals of Clinical Chemistry, 3rd ed, pp 805–806. Philadelphia, WB Saunders, 1987

15. Hegesh E, Calmanovici N, Avron M: New method for determining ferrihemoglobin reductase (NADH-methemoglobin reductase) in erythrocytes. J Lab Clin Med 72:339, 1968

16. Hsieh H-S, Jaffe ER: The metabolism of methemoglobin in human erythrocytes. In Surgenor DM (ed): The Red Blood Cell, 2nd ed, p 799. New York, Academic Press, 1975

17. Jaffe ER, Heller P: Methemoglobinemia in man. In Moore CV, Brown EB (eds): Progress in Hematology, vol 4, p 48. New York, Grune & Stratton, 1964

18. Kaplan JC, Nicolas AM, Hanzlickova-Leroux A et al: A simple spot screening test for fast detection of red cell NADH-diaphorase deficiency. Blood 36:330, 1970

19. Lukens JN: Methemoglobinemia and other disorders accompanied by cyanosis. In Lee GR, Bithell TC, Foerster J et al (eds): Wintrobe's Clinical Hematology, 9th ed, p 1266. Philadelphia, Lea & Febiger, 1993

20. Mayers MR: Carbon monoxide poisoning in industry and its prevention. Albany, NY State Dept of Labor, Special Bull 194, 1938

21. McCutcheon AD: Sulphaemoglobinaemia and glutathione. Lancet 2:240, 1960

22. Perutz MF: Hemoglobin structure and respiratory transport. Sci Am 239:92, 1978

23. Pruden EL, Siggaard–Andersen O, Tietz NW: Blood gases and pH. In Burtis CA, Ashwood ER (eds): Tietz Textbook of Clinical Chemistry, p 1379. Philadelphia, WB Saunders, 1994

24. Reynolds TB, Ware AGL: Sulfhemoglobinemia following habitual use of acetanilid. JAMA 149:1538, 1952

25. Riggs A: Functional properties of hemoglobins. Physiol Rev 45:619, 1965

26. Rogers LE: Rapid method for detection of erythrocyte NADH-methemoglobin reductase deficiency. Am J Clin Pathol 57:186, 1972

27. Scott EM: Congenital methemoglobinemia due to DPNH-diaphorase deficiency. In Beutler E (ed): Hereditary Disorders of Erythrocyte Metabolism, p 102. New York, Grune & Stratton, 1968

28. Singer K, Weisz L: The life cycle of the erythrocyte after splenectomy and the problems of splenic hemolysis and target cell formation. Am J Med Sci 210:301, 1945

29. Tietz NW, Fiereck EA: The spectrophotometric measurement of carboxyhemoglobin. Ann Clin Lab Sci 3:36, 1973

30. Trost C: The blue people of Troublesome Creek. Science 82, 3(9):24, 1982

31. Winter PM, Miller JN: Carbon monoxide poisoning. JAMA 236:1502, 1976

32. Wranne L: Free erythrocyte copro- and protoporphyrin. Acta Paediatr Scand 49:1, 1960

CHAPTER 8

Morphologic Evaluation of Erythrocytes

Ann Bell

Objectives

1. Recognize the difference between rouleaux and ag-glutination.
2. Define and describe microcytic, hypochromic red cells and macrocytic red cells.
3. Describe and differentiate spherocytes, stomato-cytes, codocytes, and dacryocytes.
4. Define and describe differences among schistocytes, burr cells, acanthocytes, and pyropoikilocytes.
5. Differentiate sickle cells, Hb CC crystals, and Hb SC crystals.
6. Define and differentiate Howell-Jolly bodies, Heinz bodies, Pappenheimer bodies, siderotic granules, and basophilic stippling.
7. Define and describe polychromatophilic red cells and explain their significance.
8. List five major categories that must be evaluated when reviewing erythrocyte morphology on a blood film.

A careful and thorough examination of erythrocytes by light microscopy in the optimal area on a well-made, well-stained peripheral blood film provides an experienced observer with valuable information about morphology, normal or abnormal. Erythrocytes should be examined for deviation in size, shape, distribution, concentration of hemoglobin (Hb), and inclusions. A systematic manner of reporting abnormal findings should be established in each laboratory. The morphologist should also be aware of artifacts that hinder proper evaluation of erythrocytes.

Some features of erythrocytes will be diagnostic, whereas others may provide clues to suggest a particular disease state. Certain characteristics may indicate the ne-cessity for additional procedures to confirm a diagnosis. A thorough examination of red cell morphology serves as a check on red cell indices and other hematologic proce-dures.

DISTRIBUTION

Normal Distribution

An ideal normal blood film has an even distribution of erythrocytes in the thin portion adjacent to the feather end of the film. In this thin area red cells should be slightly separated from one another or barely touching without overlapping. The thin area should represent at least one-third of the entire film. Normal red cells should be circular with a smooth edge and a central pale area that gradually fades into reddish-pink cytoplasm (Fig. 8-1).

At the feather end of the film and often at the edges, the red cell distribution is irregular with artifactual shapes and colors and size distortions. In the thicker portions of the film, red cells may overlap or lie on top of one another, making them unsuitable for evaluation.

Abnormal Distribution

ROULEAUX

Formation of rouleaux is reflected in the usual observation area by erythrocytes that are not separated from one an-other; rather, they appear in short or long stacks *(rouleaux)* resembling coins or flat plates. The entire outline of each cell is not visible. Rouleaux is the arrangement of red cells with their biconcave surfaces in apposition (Fig. 8-2).

Rouleaux is characteristic of hyperproteinemia and multiple myeloma (Chap. 39) because of an increased amount of plasma globulin. In macroglobulinemia, rou-leaux formation is often pronounced and creates lengthy chains. The first clue to the presence of a paraprotein or protein abnormality is rouleaux along with an increased erythrocyte sedimentation rate. Making satisfactory blood films in protein dyscrasias may be difficult or even impos-

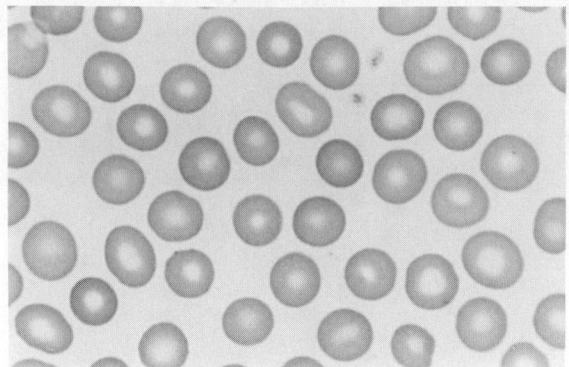

FIGURE 8-1. Normal adult peripheral blood film showing normocytic, normochromic cells. ×1000.

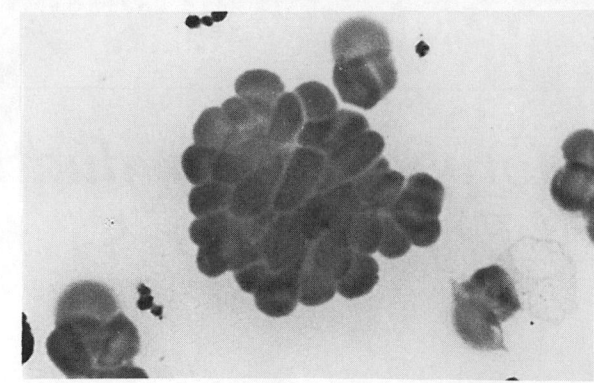

FIGURE 8-3. Autoagglutination. ×1000.

sible. Cell size and shape cannot always be evaluated in the presence of rouleaux formation.

When fibrinogen is significantly increased (*e.g.*, in infections, tissue necrosis, or pregnancy), rouleaux forms long stacks. Even normal red cells may form rouleaux in a thick moist preparation of blood under a coverslip. Spherocytes (see section on Spherocytes later in this chapter), on the other hand, cannot form rouleaux.

AGGLUTINATION

Erythrocyte agglutination occurs as cells aggregate into random clusters or masses (Fig. 8-3) when exposed to various red cell antibodies. Thus, the outline of each individual cell is not seen. Rouleaux does *not* form in the presence of red cell antibodies.

Autoagglutination occurs when an individual's red cells agglutinate in his or her own plasma or serum that contains no known specific agglutinins. Sometimes, autoagglutination is seen in the blood of apparently normal individuals but is more likely to be observed in connection with certain hemolytic anemias, atypical pneumonia, staphylococcal infections, and trypanosomiasis.[7,39,70] Autoagglutination may cause anticoagulated blood to appear somewhat "grainy" or granular as the tube is being rotated at room temperature.[21]

A common form of autoagglutination is seen in cold agglutinin disease. Here clumps of red cells may be noted

on a blood film when the temperature is below 31°C and particularly below 25°C, which enhances autoantibody activity.[54] Blood film preparation and red cell description are almost impossible without warming of the blood and the glass slide prior to preparation. The clumps of agglutinated cells disintegrate on warming of the tube. Evaluation of red cells on films made from warmed samples does not correlate with red cell indices measured on electronic counters, because cell clumping interferes with accurate automated red cell evaluation. The mean corpuscular volume (Chaps. 9 and 42) is artifactually elevated by clumps of red cells being counted as single large cells.

NORMAL MORPHOLOGY

A normal red cell *in vivo* is a biconcave disc and thus has been named a discocyte. This shape is well suited for the erythrocyte's task of gas transport and its survival in the circulation.[51] On the slide the cell has been flattened and thus has a round appearance with an area of central pallor representing the indented region of the disc. Normal red cells are almost uniform in size, shape, and Hb concentration. They stain a light red to pink with Wright stain and have a relatively clear central area that gradually leads to a more deeply stained periphery. The diameter of the central clear area should not be more than one-third of the cell diameter. The gradual transition to deeper stain is an important morphologic feature because it distinguishes normal cells from those with artifactual morphologic changes (see Artifacts section). There are no inclusions in normal red cells (Fig. 8-1).

The diameter of a normal red cell varies slightly, with a mean of 7 to 8 μm,[6,52] and is approximately the same size as or slightly smaller than the nucleus of a small lymphocyte (see Color Plate 6-9). Other characteristics include an average thickness of 2.5 μm,[7] an average volume of 90 fL[27] (1 fL = 10^{-15}/L), and an average surface area of 160 μm.[11]

The relationship between the limited metabolic factors in the non-nucleated erythrocyte and certain proteins within the cell membrane, as well as the external environment, help to maintain the disc shape throughout the life of the cell. If any of these factors is altered, the cell usually becomes spherical.

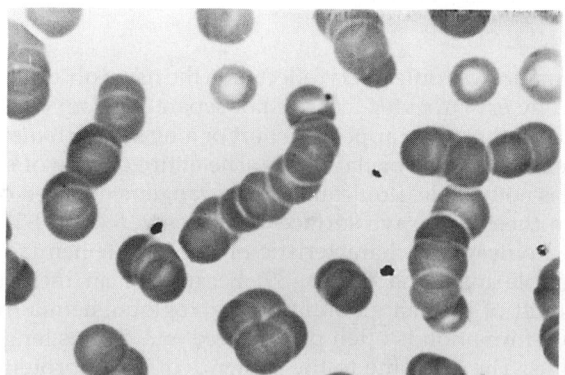

FIGURE 8-2. Rouleaux formation by erythrocytes. ×1000. (From Bell A, Lofsness KG: A photo essay on red cell morphology. J Med Technol 3:85, 1986, with permission.)

SIZE
Average Size Correlated with Mean Corpuscular Volume

NORMOCYTIC

Automated complete blood counts usually include measurement of the mean corpuscular volume (MCV), which is important because this value indicates the average size of erythrocytes. Observation of red cell morphology on the blood film provides a quality control check on the electronic MCV, as well as the other two red cell indices, mean corpuscular hemoglobin (MCH) and mean corpuscular hemoblobin concentration (MCHC; Chap. 9). An MCV in the reference range (80 to 100 fL for adults) suggests that the red cells are generally of normal size (normocytic); however, the film may demonstrate a minor population of smaller or larger cells, which may not significantly alter the MCV. There may be a mixture of different populations of erythrocytes on the film, in which case the MCV should be in the normal range because of the averaging of large and small cell sizes.

MACROCYTIC

Erythrocytes are generally described as macrocytic if the diameter exceeds 8.5 to 9.0 μm and the MCV exceeds 100 fL.[7] Automated blood counts have led to increasing awareness of macrocytosis with or without anemia.[26] A slight macrocytosis is observed frequently in hospital patients and probably does not warrant investigation. Low vitamin B_{12} or folate levels are common causes of macrocytosis (Chap. 12).

Common causes of a slight to moderate increase in MCV and of round macrocytes are alcoholism (see Fig. 8-4*A*) with or without hepatic disease; cancer chemotherapy because it interferes with DNA synthesis; chronic hemolytic anemia with reticulocytosis; myeloma; leukemia; lymphoma; metastatic carcinoma; hypothyroidism; and hemolytic disease of the newborn.[7,26] Large red cells are seen occasionally in stem cell disorders, particularly aplastic anemia, refractory anemia, pure red cell aplasia, myelofibrosis, and sideroblastic anemia.[26] Occasionally, macrocytes are found in chronic obstructive pulmonary disease. However, a cause for macrocytosis often is not apparent.

Patients with liver disease may have macrocytosis; however, whether the macrocytosis is real is debated.[26] Excess plasma cholesterol may be taken up by the red cell membrane, increasing the surface area of the cell. When the erythrocyte is spread on the slide, a thin macrocyte is formed. True macrocytes with MCV exceeding 100 fL probably are rare in liver disease without folate deficiency.[26]

The presence of oval macrocytes (usually also lacking central pallor), increased MCV, and low levels of vitamin B_{12} or folate suggest a nuclear maturation defect, which may be observed in megaloblastic red cells in the bone marrow (Chap. 12). The developmental abnormality of oval macrocytic cells (Fig. 8-4*B*) is discussed later in this chapter.

Normal non-nucleated erythrocytes that have just left the bone marrow sinusoids are slightly macrocytic and appear in stained peripheral blood films as diffusely basophilic (polychromatophilic) cells. Prematurely released red cells, called "shift" cells, occur as a result of stimulated erythropoiesis in acute hemolytic anemia. These polychromatophilic cells have an increased MCV, suggesting a macrocytosis.[14]

When the blood glucose is above 600 mg/dL, the high intracellular osmolarity causes fluid to be taken into the cell when it is placed in isotonic diluent. The result is a spurious macrocytosis if the count is performed before equilibration.[41]

With *Mycoplasma pneumoniae* infection or high titers of cold agglutinins, the MCV may be artifactually high because red cells in doublets or triplets (autoagglutination) may pass the aperture of an electronic counter.[44]

MICROCYTIC

Small erythrocytes with reduced volume are termed *microcytes.* Microcytes have normal or decreased Hb content and reduced, normal, or increased diameters. These electronic and visual changes in morphology are not apparent until iron stores have been completely exhausted and additional iron depletion restricts iron to the erythron.

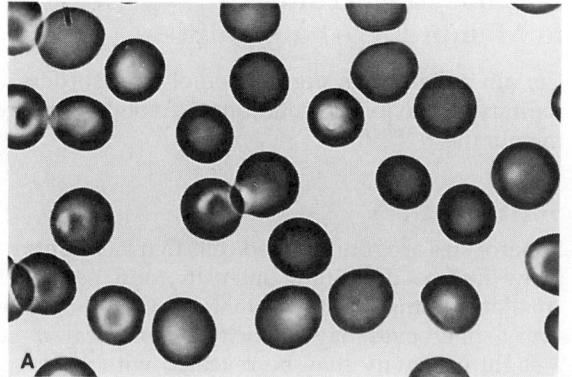
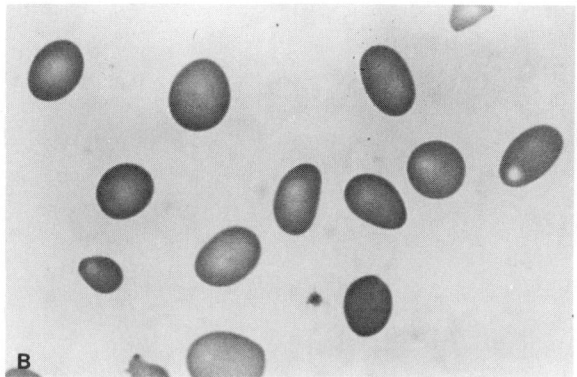

FIGURE 8-4. Types of macrocytosis. (**A**) Macrocytes in film of patient with alcoholism and liver disease. (From Bell A, Lofsness KG: A photo essay on red cell morphology. J Med Technol 3:85, 1986, with permission.) (**B**) Oval macrocytes in film of patient with vitamin B_{12} deficiency. Both ×1000.

Iron deficiency is first apparent in biochemical iron studies (Chap. 13). As anemia develops, Hb concentration is depressed, and red cells become more microcytic and hypochromic.

Microcytes occur on the blood film when the MCV is below 80 fL. However, only a few microcytic cells may not cause a decreased MCV. Significant numbers of microcytes are not produced until storage iron has been depleted for many weeks.

Microcytes with a diameter of 6 μm or less are characteristic of iron deficiency anemia (Fig. 8-5). Inflammation may also cause a slight microcytosis.

Decreased globin synthesis in β-thalassemia (Chap. 15) results in a variable number of microcytic, hypochromic red cells along with target cells. Because blood films in iron deficiency and thalassemia may be similar, special Hb determinations and family studies are needed for the differential diagnosis.

Erythrocytes that are small, lack central pallor, and appear to have an increased Hb concentration are seen in some hemolytic anemias. Such cells are called *spherocytes*.

Erythrocytes that are thinner than normal and have a colorless center are designated by the term *leptocyte* (from the Greek word lepto, "thin"). A leptocyte has an increased surface area that is out of proportion to the volume. Leptocytes may be normocytic or microcytic. Microcytic leptocytes are formed because of a lack of Hb, as seen in severe iron deficiency. Small leptocytes may be seen in thalassemia and hemoglobinopathies such as Hb C, occasionally in sideroblastic anemia and obstruction of the bile ducts, and sometimes in cirrhosis and steatorrhea (fatty feces).[7]

Variation in Size (Anisocytosis) Correlated with Red Cell Distribution Width (RDW)

Variation in red cell population size or diameter is termed *anisocytosis*. To report anisocytosis the examiner should see a mixture of normal cells with small or large cells, or both. Anisocytosis should be estimated in a semiquantitative manner: slight, moderate, or marked. If the variation is primarily microcytes or macrocytes, or both, this should be reported also.

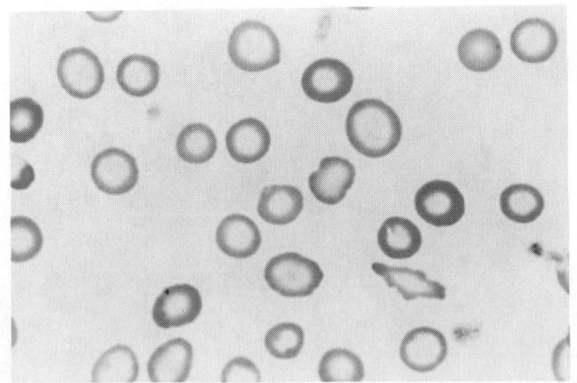

FIGURE 8-5. Microcytic, hypochromic red cells in a patient with iron deficiency anemia. ×1000.

Some automated cell counters generate the red cell distribution width (RDW), which is reported to quantitate anisocytosis. The RDW is said to identify minor populations of microcytic or macrocytic cells[10] that are not apparent from the MCV, although the clinical significance of the RDW requires further study (Chap. 10).[27]

SHAPE VARIATION— POIKILOCYTOSIS

Normal erythrocytes show little or no shape variation. Variation only on the edges of films primarily is an artifact of preparation.

The term used for variation in red cell shape is *poikilocytosis*. Recognition of various shapes or poikilocytes on the film is helpful in the differentiation of anemias. Examples of poikilocytes characteristic of certain anemias include elliptical, sickled, fragmented, and spherical forms. Generally a descriptive term of Greek origin is used to identify the poikilocyte. Poikilocyte shapes can sometimes be explained by structural and biochemical changes in the membrane, an abnormal metabolic state in the cell, Hb molecule abnormalities, an abnormal microenvironment, changes in the red cell's ability to deform, or red cell age. Electron microscopy has greatly advanced our understanding of the mechanism of poikilocyte production.

Poikilocytes Secondary to Developmental Macrocytosis (Oval Macrocytes)

A markedly increased MCV (more than 125 fL) strongly implicates megaloblastic erythropoiesis caused by vitamin B_{12} or folate deficiency (Chap. 12). A nuclear maturation defect in the early nucleated red cells of the bone marrow leads to development of macrocytes, which are mostly oval (oval macrocytes or macroovalocytes) (Fig. 8-4B). Even a few oval macrocytes are significant and suggest megaloblastic anemia. The cells appear well filled with Hb because of their increased thickness. Hb content increases as the cell increases in size, thereby forming a macrocyte that no longer has a central pale area.

Poikilocytes Secondary to Membrane Abnormalities

Certain poikilocytes suggest hemolytic disorders and hereditary or acquired conditions involving the red cell membrane.[11,38,40,65,66]

SPHEROCYTES

Spherocytes are rounded red cells that lack central pallor, show increased staining intensity, and usually have a smaller volume than a normal cell (Fig. 8-6). However, every spherocyte may not be truly spherical *in vivo*, and a slight concavity may be revealed with stereoscan microscopy. Spherocyte diameter is approximately 6.2 to 7.0 μm, and the thickness ranges from greater than 2.2 up to 3.4 μm.[31,62]

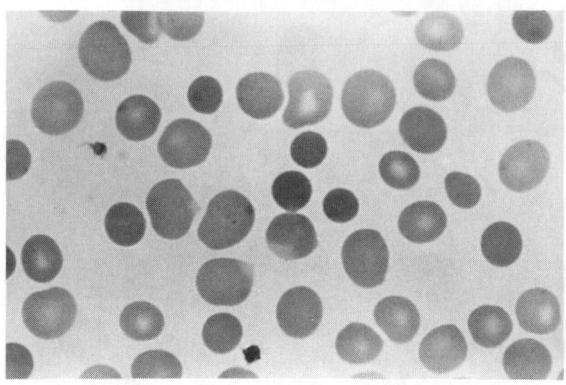

FIGURE 8-6. Spherocytes in film of patient with hereditary spherocytosis. ×1000.

Spherocytes may be caused by a hereditary or an acquired condition. Several molecular defects in membrane proteins have been identified in hereditary spherocytosis (Chap. 17); spectrin deficiency has been found in many patients.[11,35,43] Spherocytes are not easily deformed and therefore may lose their membrane by fragmentation during passage through the circulation. These cells become smaller and denser with increased Hb content and become less deformable with age. When the cell is deprived of membrane as it ages, it assumes the spherical shape. Spherocytes have a shortened survival time because they are sequestered in the spleen and hemolyzed.[67]

The presence of spherocytes indicates a hemolytic process because hemolysis results from a membrane abnormality. The hallmark of hereditary spherocytosis is a spherocyte that is fairly uniform in size and density with a decreased membrane surface:volume ratio. The MCV may be normal or slightly decreased; the MCHC is often increased. Spherocytes show increased fragility when placed in increasing dilutions of hypotonic saline in the osmotic fragility test (Chap. 17). After splenectomy in patients with hereditary spherocytosis, hemolysis decreases but spherocytes persist,[17] indicating that the abnormality involves the red cell membrane itself rather than splenic damage to the cells.

Frequent causes of acquired spherocytosis are immunohemolytic anemia secondary to autoimmune or isoimmune antibodies, Heinz body hemolytic anemia, microangiopathic hemolytic anemia, and hemolysis secondary to water dilution.[11] Banked blood stored for long periods of time develops spherocytes. Transfused cells are often spherical when viewed on a blood film and can be differentiated from the patient's cells.

ELLIPTOCYTES AND OVALOCYTES

Elliptocytes or ovalocytes are erythrocytes that have an elliptical or oval shape (Fig. 8-7). These cells result from hereditary or acquired conditions and range from egg-shaped or slightly oval to sausage, rod, or pencil forms.[25] With electron microscopy, Hb appears to be concentrated at the two ends of the cell, leaving a normal central area of pallor.[21,45]

Late nucleated red cells in the bone marrow of patients with elliptocytosis are not elliptical except in rare cases of hereditary elliptocytosis.[21,45]

Usually no more than 1% of the red cells in normal individuals are slightly elliptical.[29] Ovalocytes or elliptocytes may be acquired in iron deficiency anemia, megaloblastic anemia, and myelophthisic anemia, in which as many as 10% of the cells may be oval. Megaloblastic anemia is characterized by oval macrocytes (Fig. 8-4B), which may be 9 μm or more in diameter and lack central pallor. Elliptocytes are also observed in thalassemia and sickle cell anemia.

Hereditary elliptocytosis (Chap. 17) is characterized on the blood film by 25% to 90% elliptocytes, but it is not typically associated with hemolysis.[21] The principal defect is considered to be in the cytoskeleton, with a decrease in the skeletal membrane protein band 4.1.[1] An increased heat sensitivity of spectrin in some families with hereditary elliptocytosis has been reported.[59] The life span of elliptocytes may be somewhat shortened in a few individuals; however, elliptocytes usually function normally. The osmotic fragility is normal.

ECHINOCYTES AND BURR CELLS

Echinocytes (from the Greek *echinos*, ''sea urchin'') have evenly distributed, uniform-size blunt spicules or bumps on their surfaces (Figs. 8-8A, 8-13). Echinocytes or crenated red cells may be seen on films made from anticoagulated blood that is several hours old, but such cells are artifacts not normally present *in vivo*. Bessis[7] states that crenation is caused by release of basic substances from glass slides that change the pH and transform the cells into echinocytes. In stored blood echinocytes may be numerous because of depletion of ATP and biochemical abnormalities in plasma. Echinocytes formed *in vitro* can be reversed to normal shape, whereas those formed *in vivo* cannot.[7] Transformation of discocytes to echinocytes can be observed on a glass slide using a moist saline preparation of red cells in the presence of an elevated (basic) pH.[7]

In anemia associated with renal insufficiency (Chap. 18), some red cells acquire a membrane abnormality with irregularly sized and unevenly spaced spicules.[55] Such red cells are called *burr cells* (Figs. 8-8B, 8-13). The number of burr cells often increases as blood urea nitrogen (BUN) increases. This membrane alteration is probably related to plasma chemical abnormalities. The spicules of burr

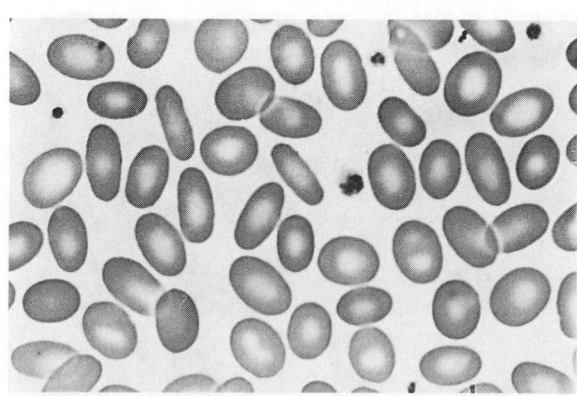

FIGURE 8-7. Elliptocytes in film of patient with hereditary elliptocytosis. ×1000.

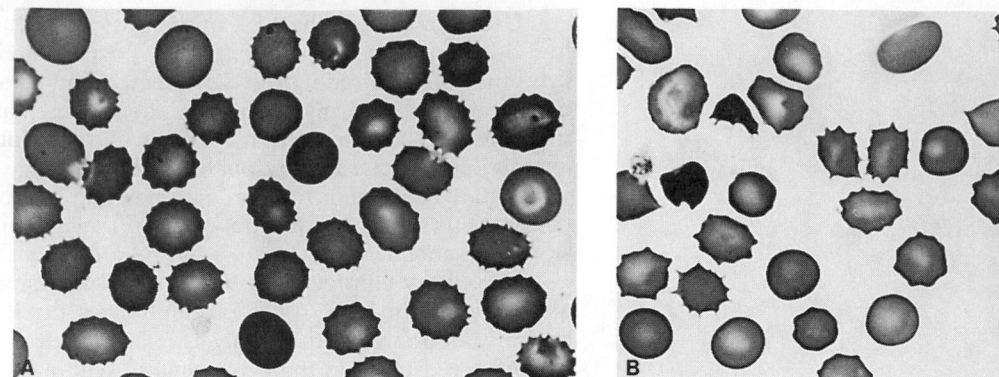

FIGURE 8-8. (**A**) Echinocytes or crenated cells in film of normal peripheral blood. (**B**) Burr cells in film of patient with uremia. Note resemblance to echinocytes. Both ×1000.

cells are usually reversible, as the cells can be induced to revert to normal shape.

The differences between crenated cells (echinocytes) and burr cells may be minimal and not always recognizable. Crenated cells with uniform blunt spicules represent an artifact that is evident in practically every cell in the thin portion of the film and should *not* be reported. In contrast, burr cells may be distinguished by their irregularly sized spicules and variable number in different microscopic fields and should be reported. A burr cell has also been called an echinocyte by several hematologists because of its membrane irregularities.

ACANTHOCYTES

Acanthocytes (from the Greek word *acantho,* ''thorn'' or ''spike'') are small, densely stained red cells that are no longer disc shaped and have a few irregularly spaced, pointed spicules or thornlike projections of various lengths and widths over their surfaces (Fig. 8-9). The spicules may appear clublike. Acanthocytes may be acquired or inherited and are smaller than normal red cells because they are becoming spheroidal. Generally acanthocytes have fewer, more irregular, and more blunted points than burr cells. Also, unlike burr cells, acanthocytes cannot be induced to regain a normal shape. Acanthocytes may be caused by changes in the ratio of plasma lipids (lecithins and sphingomyelins).[64]

Acanthocytes have been observed in alcoholic cirrhosis with hemolytic anemia, malabsorption states, postsplenectomy states, hepatitis of newborns, pyruvate kinase deficiency, and disorders of lipid metabolism.[7] Cells similar to acanthocytes have been named *spur cells* in severe hemolytic anemia associated with cirrhosis and in metastatic liver disease because of their sharp points.[21,45]

Increased numbers of acanthocytes have been reported in a rare congenital syndrome called abetalipoproteinemia (Chap. 17), which is characterized by mild hemolytic anemia, retinal degeneration, and steatorrhea.[3,33]

STOMATOCYTES

Stomatocytes on a fixed and stained film have an elongated or slitlike area of central pallor (Fig. 8-10) instead of the usual circular form. These cells may be hereditary or acquired. The Greek word *stoma* means mouth. Stomatocytes are so named for their mouth-shaped central pallor. These cells appear bowl shaped in a moist preparation and by stereoscan microscope.[6]

Blood films from normal individuals may demonstrate a few stomatocytes, but stomatocytes are usually observed in patients with alcoholism, cirrhosis, obstructive liver disease,[11] and Rh null disease.[58] These cells also may occur as artifacts of blood film preparation.

Hereditary stomatocytosis is characterized by numerous stomatocytes, but anemia is usually mild.[42] One of

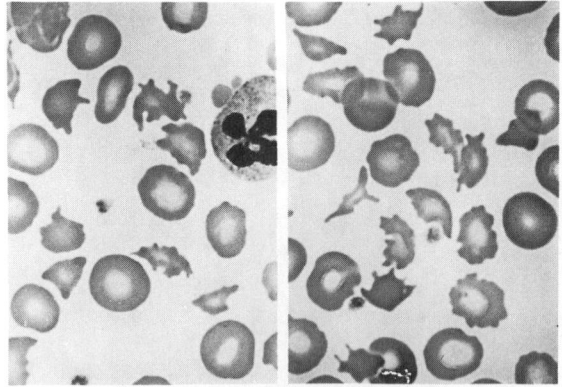

FIGURE 8-9. Acanthocytes. As seen in film of patient with microangiopathic hemolytic anemia. ×1000.

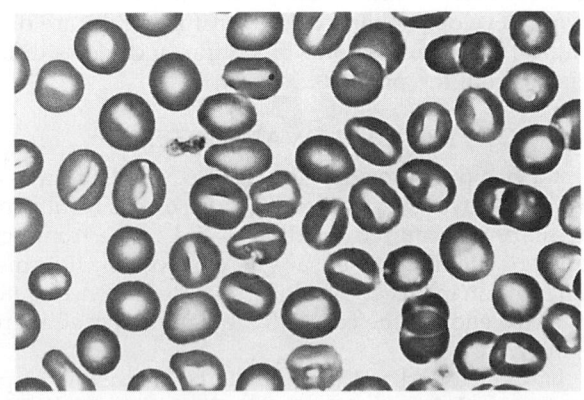

FIGURE 8-10. Stomatocytes in film of patient with hereditary stomatocytosis. ×1000.

the suggested consequences involves a membrane defect that results in high cellular sodium and low potassium content (Chap. 17). The heterogeneous clinical picture results from an abnormal sodium to potassium transport ratio and a greatly increased rate of active cation transport.[42] Because of the shape of the red cell and the somewhat impaired deformability, stomatocytes may be retained in the spleen.

CODOCYTES (TARGET CELLS)

Codocytes or target cells have a central area of Hb surrounded by a relatively colorless ring and a peripheral ring of Hb (Fig. 8-11). By scanning electron microscopy the codocyte has a bell or tall hat shape and appears to be thin walled and concave. A codocyte (Greek *kodon*, "bell") is also called a Mexican hat cell. This shape is always acquired. Codocytes appear when the membrane surface is increased after loading of the membrane with cholesterol and phospholipids.[19] In other words, a target cell is similar to a bag too large for its contents. Its greater osmotic resistance (or decrease in osmotic fragility) is explained by the increase in surface to volume ratio.

Finding target cells in only one portion of the film suggests an artifact of film preparation. Fixing blood films in methanol before staining may help avoid this problem. In pathologic states, target cells are observed throughout the usual examination area. Target cells do not appear at the ends of a film where cells are flattened nor in thick portions of the film.

Codocytes are characteristic of thalassemia; hemoglobinopathies SS, CC, DD, EE, and S-thalassemia; obstructive liver disease; postsplenectomy state; and iron deficiency anemia (Chaps. 13, 14, 15).[11,19,21]

Poikilocytes Secondary to Trauma

Erythrocytes may fragment and lyse when subjected to excessive physical trauma in the cardiovascular system. Intravascular hemolysis and shortened red cell survival may result from severe trauma. The hallmark of hemolytic anemia secondary to red cell fragmentation is the schistocyte, which takes several forms. Other cells caused by trauma are included in this section.

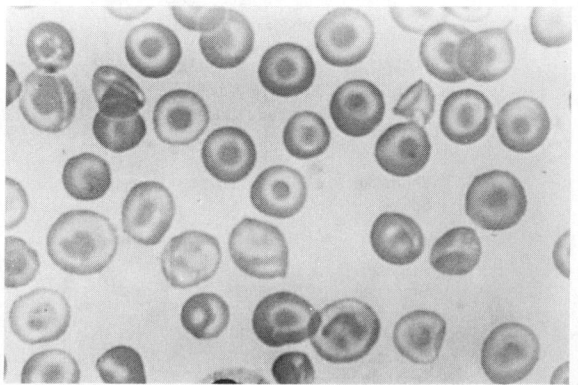

FIGURE 8-11. Codocytes (target cells) in film of patient with liver disease. ×1000.

SCHISTOCYTES

When a red cell attempts to pass between fibrin strands,[15] altered vessels, or damaged heart valve prostheses,[53,56] it may be cleaved and fragmented and become a schistocyte (Figs. 8-12*A* and *B*, 8-13). The erythrocyte trying to squeeze through an opening half its diameter becomes stretched and develops a blister (Fig. 8-12*C*) because of the shear stress of the flowing blood. When this cell passes through the spleen, it is fragmented into two pieces, and the membrane is less deformable. Fragmented red cells do not survive long in the circulation.[67]

Schistocytes (Greek word *schistos*, "cloven") or *schizocytes* (Greek *schizo*, "split") result from membrane damage; they are not hereditary. Schistocytes include helmet, triangular, and a variety of small, irregular shapes with a few pointed extremities. The finding of helmet and fragmented cells is strongly suggestive of a microangiopathic hemolytic anemia or traumatic hemolytic anemia (Chap. 18).[13] Schistocytes occur in patients with severe burns, renal graft rejection, glomerulonephritis, vasculitis, thrombotic thrombocytopenic purpura, and diffuse intravascular coagulation.[7,11] Schistocytes accompanying march hemoglobinuria most likely are attributable to mechanical damage to the cells in the feet of individuals on long walking expeditions.

SCHISTOCYTES AND KERATOCYTES

A schistocyte with one or more hornlike projections has been identified as a *keratocyte* (Greek *keras*, "horn") (Fig. 8-12*D*). These cells may or may not have a normal volume and usually no area of central pallor. A keratocyte is the result of an erythrocyte being caught on a fibrin strand, which could cut the cell in two. As the sides of the erythrocyte are pushed against the fibrin strand, they tend to fuse together. When this cell escapes from the fibrin strand, it may have a vacuole-like area in the fused portion (this is known as a *blister cell*; Fig. 8-12*C*). This vacuole ruptures to form the keratocyte—a damaged red cell with horns. Keratocytes do not remain in circulation for more than a few hours, as they are fragile.[7] A keratocyte is a rare and interesting phenomenon. Some morphologists report helmet cells, which actually look like a helmet, as keratocytes.

DACRYOCYTES (TEARDROPS)

Dacryocytes (teardrops) have been so labeled because of their shape (Greek *dakry*, "tear") (Fig. 8-14). They may also be pear shaped with a blunt pointed projection and may be normal size, small, or large.[6,60] If a red cell contains a rigid inclusion, such as a Heinz body, the portion with the inclusion cannot pass through small openings of splenic sinuses and thus remains behind. As the red cell squeezes through the small opening, it is stretched beyond its ability to regain its original shape. Thus, a teardrop or pear shape is created.[6]

Teardrop cells typically are observed in myelofibrosis with myeloid metaplasia (Chap. 35) because of the large size of the spleen. Other conditions with dacryocytes include myelophthisic anemia, pernicious anemia, β-thalassemia, drug-induced Heinz body formation, tuberculosis, and tumor metastasized to the marrow.[7,60,69]

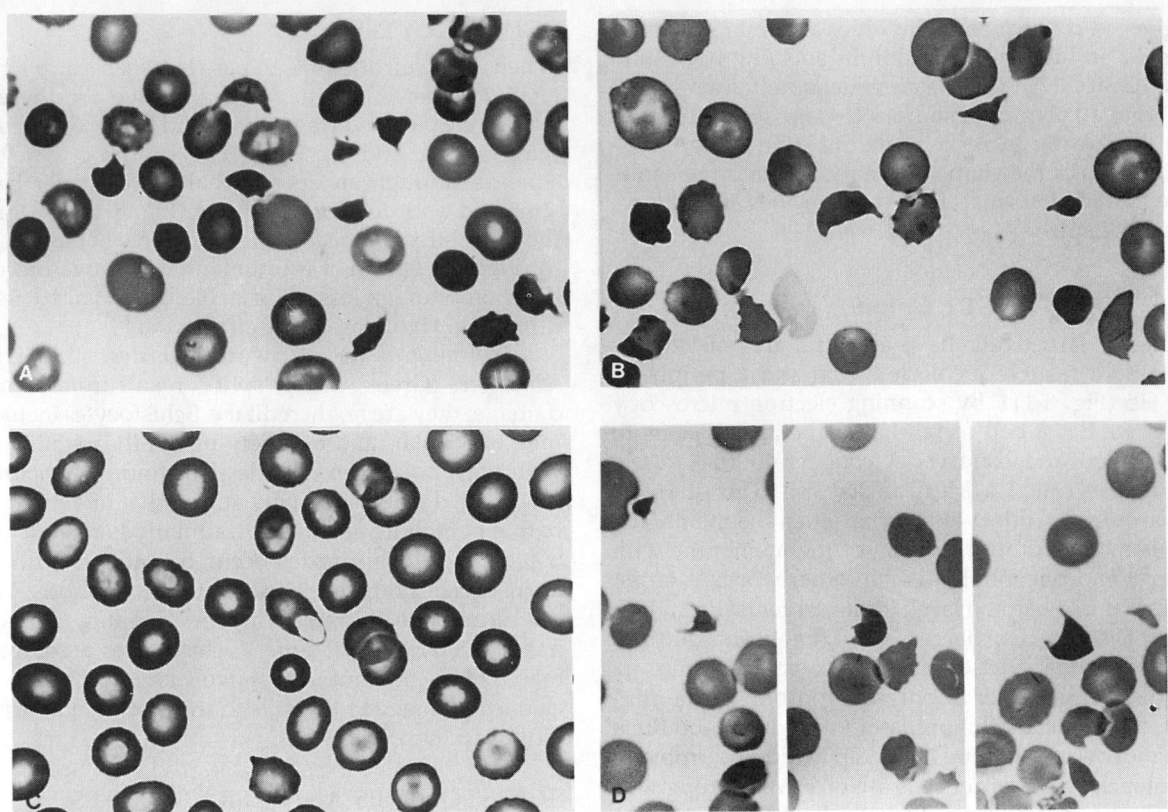

FIGURE 8-12. Schistocytes. (**A, B**) In film of patient with thrombotic thrombocytopenic purpura. Note helmet, triangular, fragmented, and bizarre shapes. (**C**) Blister cell in film of patient with probable microangiopathic hemolytic anemia. (**D**) Keratocytes (horn cells) in film of patient with microangiopathic hemolytic anemia. All ×1000.

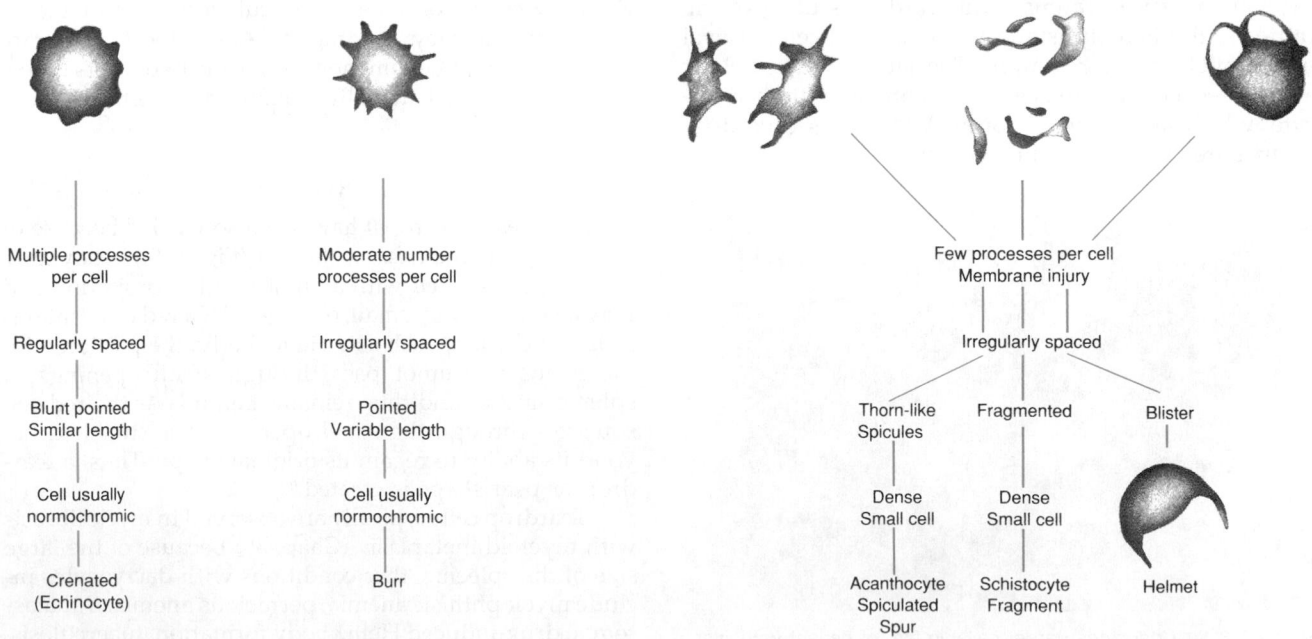

FIGURE 8-13. Analysis of membrane irregularities in red blood cells.

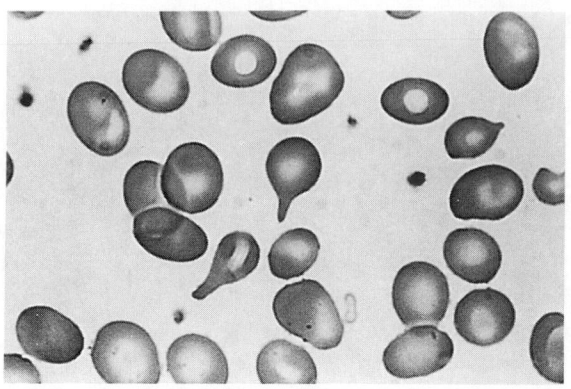

FIGURE 8-14. Dacryocytes (teardrop cells) in film of patient with vitamin B$_{12}$ deficiency. ×1000.

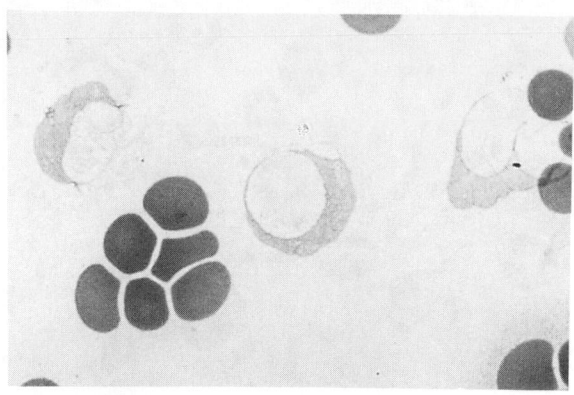

FIGURE 8-16. Semilunar bodies (red cell ghosts) in film of patient with malaria. ×1000.

MICROSPHEROCYTES AND PYROPOIKILOCYTES

Microspherocytes (Fig. 8-15A) occur in severe burns as small, round cells that may be smaller than platelets. They are the result of thermal damage to the cell membrane.[57] Another name for these round fragments is microspherules.

A rare hereditary hemolytic anemia designated pyropoikilocytosis (Chap. 17) presents a striking picture of fragments and microspherocytes (Fig. 8-15B) associated with heat sensitivity. The red cell abnormality probably is in the membrane protein spectrin (Chap. 17). These tiny, round, fragmented cells are greatly increased when blood cells are heated *in vitro* to 45°C, in contrast to normal red cells, which fragment around 49°C.[71] The mean diameter of the spherical fragments is approximately 2 to 3 μm, and the MCV is extremely low (less than 60 fL).[16,68]

SEMILUNAR BODIES

A semilunar body (half-moon cell; crescent cell) is a large, pale-pink staining ghost of a red cell—the membrane remaining after the contents have been released (Fig. 8-16). Semilunar bodies are as large as leukocytes and are always acquired.[24] They are frequently seen in malaria

(see Protozoan Inclusions later in this chapter) and in other conditions causing overt hemolysis.

Poikilocytes Secondary to Abnormal Hemoglobin Content

Poikilocytes can be diagnostic of a chronic hereditary hemolytic anemia. Three types of poikilocytes are characteristic of three abnormal hemoglobins: drepanocytes (from Hb S), Hb CC crystals, and Hb SC crystals (Chap. 14).

DREPANOCYTES (SICKLE CELLS)

Drepanocytes (sickle cells) (Greek *drepane*, "sickle") have been changed from the normal disc shape by the long rod-shaped polymers of the inherited abnormal Hb S. A red cell does not appear sickled until it has lost its nucleus and has been fully hemoglobinized. Sickle cells are thin and elongated with pointed ends and are well filled with Hb (Fig. 8-17). They may be curved or straight or have S, V, or L shapes.[24] This change is striking and irreversible secondary to permanent membrane damage by the polymerization of Hb S.[5,48]

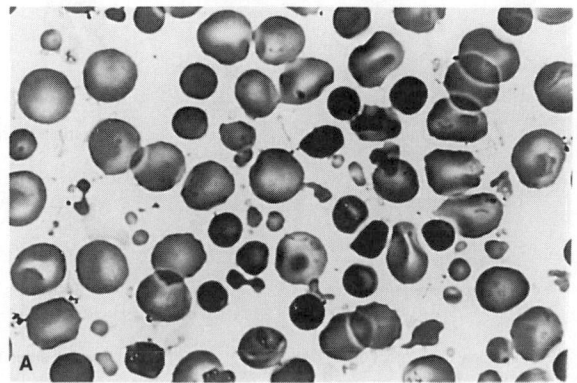

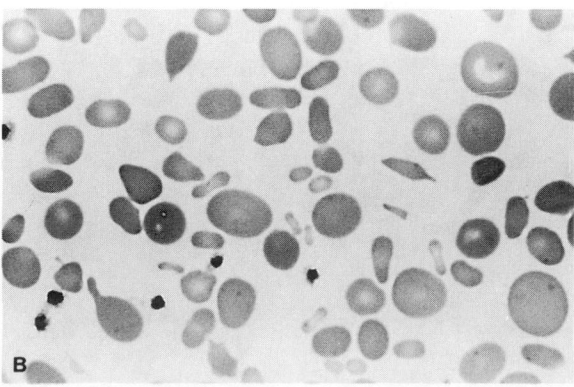

FIGURE 8-15. Microspherocytes. (**A**) As a result of thermal damage in film of patient with severe burns. (**B**) As a result of heat sensitivity in film from patient with hereditary pyropoikilocytosis. (From Bell A, Lofsness KG: A photo essay on red cell morphology. J Med Technol 3:85, 1986, with permission.)

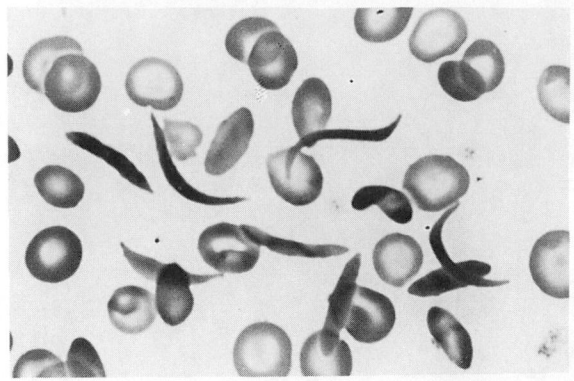

FIGURE 8-17. Drepanocytes (sickled red cells) in film of patient homozygous for Hb S (sickle cell anemia). ×1000. (From Bell A, Lofsness KG: A photo essay on red cell morphology. J Med Technol 3:85, 1986, with permission.)

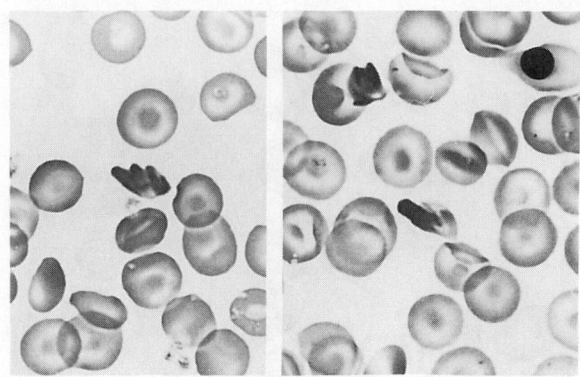

FIGURE 8-19. Hemoglobin SC crystals in film of patient with Hb SC disease. ×1000. (From Bell A, Lofsness KG. A photo essay on red cell morphology. J Med Technol 3:85, 1986 with permission.)

Typical sickle cells are observed in films from patients with homozygous Hb S disease (Hb SS) but are not often seen in heterozygous Hb S (Hb AS; sickle trait) except under unusual situations when there is low *in vivo* oxygen tension. Therefore, morphology is not very helpful in the diagnosis of Hb AS. A few sickled cells may be seen in the abnormal Hb SC, Hb S-β-thalassemia, Hb C-Harlem, and Hb S-Memphis disorders.

HEMOGLOBIN CC CRYSTALS

Intraerythrocytic Hb CC crystals in homozygous C (Hb CC) disease tend to be hexagonal with blunt ends and darkly stained (Fig. 8-18). These angular crystals form within the cell membrane when Hb C crystallizes, often leaving the remainder of the cell relatively Hb free and colorless (Fig. 8-20). Frequently, the cell membrane is not visible, and the crystal appears to be free. At times, several smaller CC crystals form within the red cell.[23]

Crystals of Hb CC are not observed in every patient with electrophoretically proven Hb CC and in most instances are seen only after searching. Actually, the crystals are more frequent after splenectomy. Crystals are not seen in Hb C trait (Hb AC).

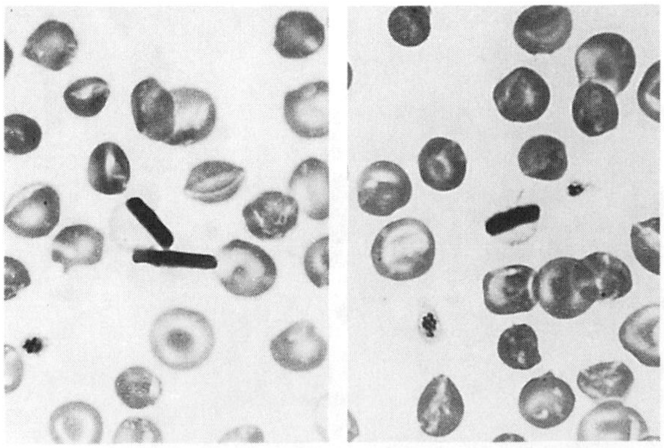

HEMOGLOBIN SC CRYSTALS

Hb SC crystals within erythrocytes in Hb SC disease can be seen on searching. These dark-hued crystals of condensed Hb distort the red cell membrane (Fig. 8-19). The characteristic type of crystalline projection is often straight with parallel sides and one blunt, pointed, protruding end ("Washington monument" shape).[22] Another erythrocyte typical in Hb SC disease contains multiple crystals that protrude in different directions as finger-like projections from a common crystalline center (Fig. 8-20).

Hb condensed in one portion of the cell often is accompanied by relative pallor in the opposite portion. In occasional elongated cells, crystals form at opposite poles, leaving a hypochromic area in the center. Another feature is the bent or curved cellular shape caused by polymers of soluble Hb consisting of Hb S tactoids mixed with Hb C crystals.

Diggs and Bell[22] reported intraerythrocytic crystals in 70% of the blood films from 60 cases of electrophoretically proven Hb SC disease. The incidence of intracellular Hb SC crystals was found to be 0 to 23 per 1000 red cells,

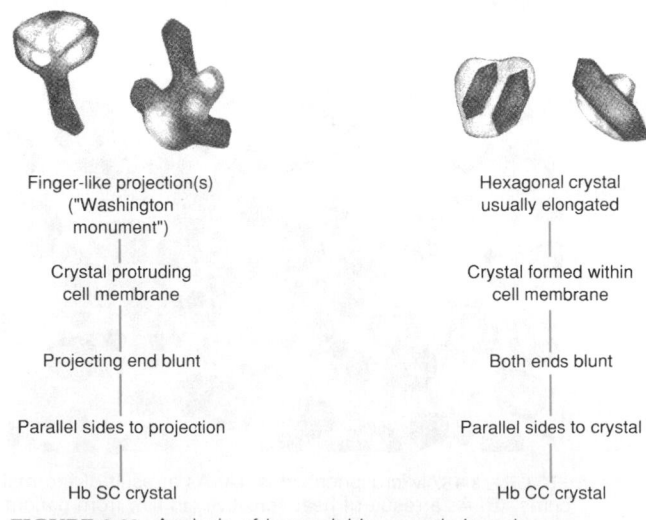

Finger-like projection(s) ("Washington monument")	Hexagonal crystal usually elongated
Crystal protruding cell membrane	Crystal formed within cell membrane
Projecting end blunt	Both ends blunt
Parallel sides to projection	Parallel sides to crystal
Hb SC crystal	Hb CC crystal

FIGURE 8-20. Analysis of hemoglobin crystals in red blood cells.

FIGURE 8-18. Hemoglobin CC crystals in film of patient with homozygous Hb C disease. ×1000. (From Bell A, Lofsness KG: A photo essay on red cell morphology. J Med Technol 3:85, 1986, with permission.)

with an average of 3.2 per 1000. No correlation between the number of crystals and the clinical findings was apparent. The Hb SC erythrocytic abnormalities have not been observed with other abnormal hemoglobins.

Crystals of Hb SC are distinguished by the one or more fingerlike, blunt-pointed projections that protrude from the cell membrane in Hb SC disease, leaving a pale area at the opposite end, and by the fact that the SC crystal is not hexagonal (Fig. 8-20). On the other hand, Hb CC crystals are hexagonal, form within the membrane, and have blunt ends. Suspected Hb SC or CC crystals on the blood film should always be confirmed by Hb electrophoresis (Chap. 14).

HEMOGLOBIN CONTENT

Erythrocytes with a normal Hb content have a clear central pallor that occupies about one-third of the cell diameter. Such cells are described as *normochromic*. There may be slight variations in the amount of central pallor in different areas of the normal blood film.

With decreasing Hb concentration, there is increased central pallor, and the cells are then described as *hypochromic*. Hypochromia is caused by impaired Hb synthesis and ranges from slight pallor to marked pallor, in which there may be only a thin rim of Hb. The changes in Hb content in severe iron deficiency anemia (Chap. 13) are evident in the MCH and MCHC (Chap. 9). Hypochromia is associated most often with microcytosis. Examples of hypochromic, microcytic anemias include iron deficiency anemia, thalassemia, and sideroblastic anemia. Hypochromia is sometimes associated with normocytic (normal-size) red cells in disorders such as rheumatoid arthritis, chronic infection, or inflammation. These conditions result from defective macrophage iron release, which prevents iron from reaching the normoblasts for proper red cell maturation.

Anisochromia is the term used to describe the variation in Hb content when both hypochromic and normochromic cells are present. In sideroblastic anemia, hypochromic and normochromic cells are seen, indicating the marrow production of two populations of red cells. After transfusions for hypochromic anemia, anisochromia is often present because the patient's hypochromic cells are visible along with the transfused normal cells.

Macrocytic cells usually do not have an area of central pallor because of their increased thickness. Spherocytes have reduced central concavity and no central pallor because of their increased thickness.[7] Sickled red cells do not show normal central pallor. Hb is concentrated within a crystal in the abnormal Hb genotypes CC and SC. Technically, these erythrocytes are *hyperchromic* because of their lack of central pallor even though they lie in a desirable area for morphologic observation. Erythrocytes along the extreme feather edge often appear hyperchromic; however, this is an artifact. True hyperchromia exists when the MCHC is elevated. Hyperchromia is common on films from patients with hemolytic anemias, including hemolysis caused by burns, resulting in microspherocytes with a reduced surface to volume ratio, causing an increased MCHC. Although cells may be hyperchromic, hyperchromia is almost never reported by the laboratory.

By convention, reporting the type of hyperchromic cell present is, *de facto*, an indication of hyperchromia.

INCLUSIONS

Normally erythrocytes do not contain inclusions. However, many different inclusions may be seen in various hematologic disorders.

Developmental Organelles

Inclusions that have developed in erythrocytes due to certain types of anemia not only are visible in Wright stain but also are identifiable as cell organelles on ultrastructural analysis. These inclusions are Howell-Jolly bodies, basophilic stippling, Pappenheimer bodies, polychromatophilic red cells, and Cabot rings.

HOWELL-JOLLY BODIES

Howell-Jolly bodies are small, round fragments of the nucleus (resulting from karyorrhexis or nuclear disintegration) of a late nucleated red cell or metarubricyte; they stain reddish-blue to blue-black with Wright stain (see Figs. 8-21 and 8-28). These inclusions may also result from incomplete extrusion of the nucleus or from chromosomes that were separated from the spindle during abnormal mitotic division. Howell-Jolly bodies give a positive Feulgen reaction (a test for DNA in nuclear chromatin) and thus are presumed to contain DNA. A Howell-Jolly body usually appears singly in a cell and is ordinarily less than 1 μm in diameter; however, two or more may be noted in a cell in severe anemias and alcoholism.[37]

Normally as the immature erythrocyte passes through the endothelial slits in the splenic sinuses, the Howell-Jolly body is pitted from the cell. Thus, after splenectomy, increased numbers of these inclusions are noted on the blood film. Howell-Jolly bodies are seen in sickle cell anemia (secondary to splenic fibrosis), other hemolytic anemias, megaloblastic anemia, congenital absence of the spleen, or splenic atrophy after multiple infarctions.[37]

BASOPHILIC STIPPLING

Basophilic stippling is the fine or coarse, deep blue to purple staining inclusion that appears in erythrocytes on

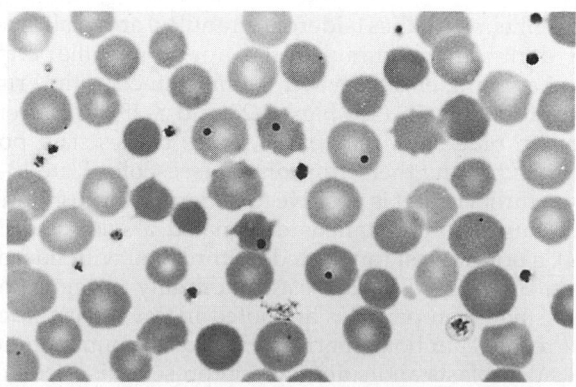

FIGURE 8-21. Howell-Jolly bodies in film of patient after splenectomy. ×1000.

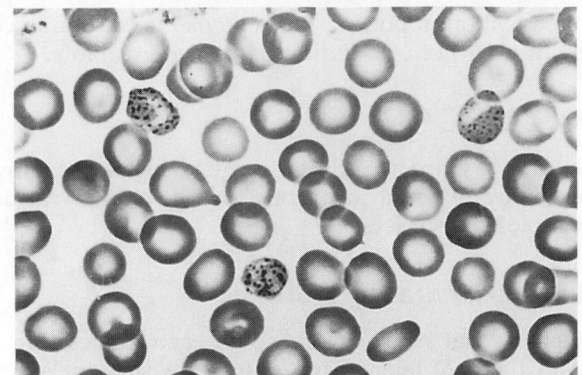

FIGURE 8-22. Stippled red blood cells in film of patient with lead poisoning. ×1000.

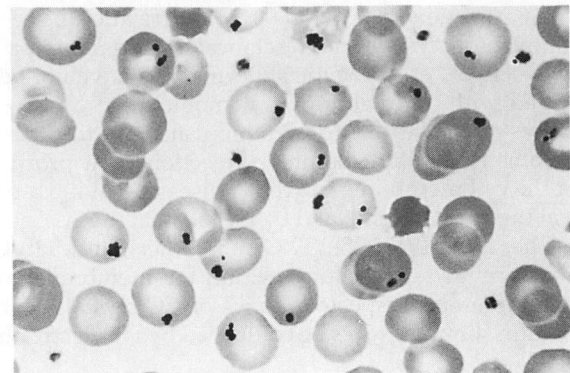

FIGURE 8-23. Pappenheimer bodies in film of patient with sideroblastic anemia. ×1000.

a dried Wright-stained film (see Figs. 8-22 and 8-28). They are much smaller than Howell-Jolly bodies, are usually irregularly shaped, and appear homogeneously throughout the Hb portion of the erythrocyte. Bessis[6] states that these inclusions do not exist in the living cell, but they can be observed in well-made preparations for electron microscopic study.[36] Stippling represents aggregates of ribosomes that appear during the drying and staining of films.[6,36] Punctate basophilia may be found in nucleated red cells or diffusely basophilic cells.

Whenever there is alteration in the biosynthesis of Hb, such as in thalassemia, stippling in erythrocytes may be seen frequently. Stippling also is found in megaloblastic anemias (Chap. 12) and alcoholism. Marked basophilic stippling occurs in a deficiency of erythrocyte pyrimidine-5'-nucleotidase.[4] Stippling is likewise prominent in lead (Chap. 13) and arsenic intoxication, but it may not always be observed, because formation is dependent on the manner in which the film is dried.

Basophilic stippling is an inclusion that may be confused, even by experienced observers, with Pappenheimer bodies (see next section). The main differentiating factors are that stippling appears homogeneously over the cell, whereas Pappenheimer bodies tend to appear in groups at the cell periphery; also, Pappenheimer bodies stain positively with an iron stain (Prussian blue), whereas stippling does not (see Fig. 8-28).

PAPPENHEIMER BODIES

Pappenheimer bodies (siderotic granules) are small, irregular, dark-staining granules[49] that appear near the periphery of a young erythrocyte in a film stained with Wright or supravital stain (see Figs. 8-23 and 8-28). With Perls' Prussian blue stain (Chap. 29), these bodies stain positively, indicating their iron content (see Color Plate 13-1). An erythrocyte that is positive for siderotic (iron) granules in a Prussian blue stain is designated a *siderocyte* (Fig. 8-24); a normoblast (nucleated erythrocyte) with siderotic granules is called a *sideroblast*. Normally no more than three small iron particles are noted in developing nucleated red cells in bone marrow. Siderotic granules in normal sideroblasts and siderocytes represent dispersed ferritin (a storage form of iron) molecules. They may exist as one granule or as aggregates of seven or eight particles

of ferritin. Tiny particles are readily revealed in electron micrographs, but only aggregates may be seen by light microscopy.[8]

The spleen normally removes these inclusions without destroying the cell. The term *pitting* was introduced by Crosby[20] to describe this action by the spleen. However, after splenectomy Pappenheimer bodies are visible on the blood film. The spleen is thus responsible for removing excess iron-containing granules from young red cells in which Hb synthesis is complete. These granules are also found in hyposplenism, in which the spleen does not function normally.

With severe disturbances of Hb synthesis, pathologic sideroblasts and siderocytes are present in the bone marrow and peripheral blood. Siderotic granules may be present in sideroblastic anemia, thalassemia, refractory anemias, and dyserythropoietic anemias (Chaps. 13 and 15).

In sideroblastic anemia (a myelodysplastic disorder; Chaps. 13 and 33), numerous siderotic granules are found within the mitochondria and form a ring around at least one-third of the nucleus. Such cells are called *pathologic ringed sideroblasts* (Fig. 8-24; see Color Plate 13-2).[9,12,42,46]

Iron overload in hemosiderosis and hemochromatosis (Chap. 13) is associated with an increase in the number of siderotic granules (approximately 20 per cell) and an increase in the size of the siderotic granules.

On a Wright-stained film it is possible to misidentify Pappenheimer bodies as basophilic stippling when the iron overload is severe (Fig. 8-28). Therefore, when disorders of Hb synthesis or iron overload are suspected and there is doubt concerning the red cell inclusions observed, a Prussian blue stain for iron should be performed for confirmation.

POLYCHROMATOPHILIC RED CELLS

Diffusely basophilic red cells or polychromatophilic cells[50] are young red cells that no longer have a nucleus but still contain some RNA (Fig. 8-28). As the name implies, this RNA stains diffusely blue with Wright stain (see Color Plate 9-1). Such cells are slightly larger than mature red cells and contain ribosomes, mitochondria, and other organelles.

When polychromatophilic cells are stained supravitally with new methylene blue, they are identified as

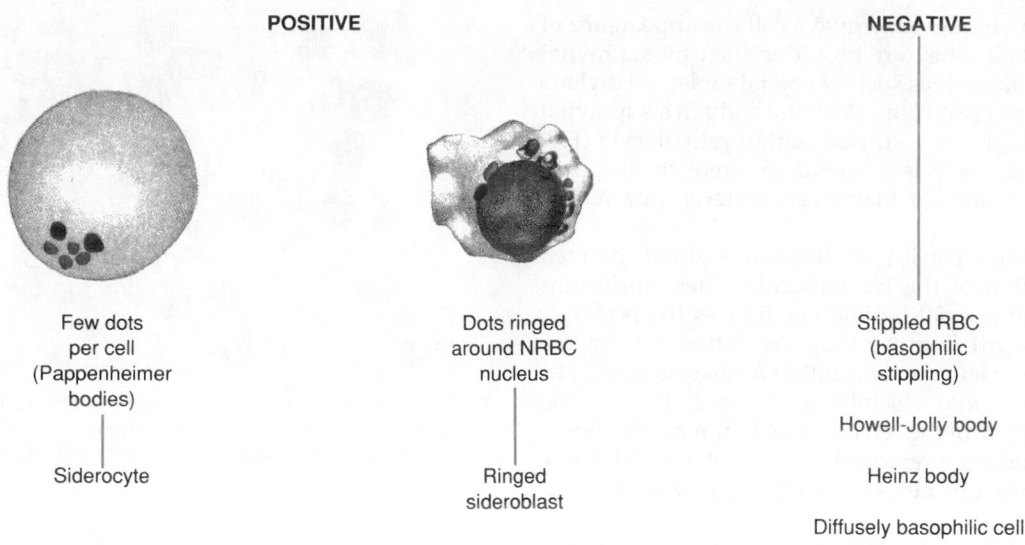

POSITIVE

Few dots
per cell
(Pappenheimer
bodies)

|
Siderocyte

Dots ringed
around NRBC
nucleus

|
Ringed
sideroblast

NEGATIVE

Stippled RBC
(basophilic
stippling)

Howell-Jolly body

Heinz body

Diffusely basophilic cell

FIGURE 8-24. Analysis of findings with Prussian blue stain for iron.

reticulocytes because of their granulofilamentous pattern (see Figs. 8-29 and 9-6). The supravital dye precipitates the ribosomes and other organelles in the living state to give this reticulated appearance. Thus, a diffusely basophilic cell is called a reticulocyte when a supravital dye is used.[32]

Normally these cells are seen in only an occasional oil immersion (1000 × magnification) field. If more are seen, increased erythrocyte production is indicated secondary to increased erythropoietin stimulation of the marrow. Depending on the pH of the Romanowsky stain or buffer, basophilia may be more or less prominent. More acidic solutions tend to obscure basophilia.

Very large diffusely basophilic cells are known as *shift cells* and indicate premature release from the marrow during intense erythrocyte production.

CABOT RINGS

A thin ringlike structure called a *Cabot ring* (Figs. 8-25, 8-28) may appear in erythrocytes in megaloblastic anemia or other severe anemias, in lead poisoning, and in dyserythropoiesis, in which erythrocytes are destroyed be-

fore being released from the marrow. A Cabot ring stains reddish-blue to violet in Wright stain. It may be circular and appear at the cell periphery, or it may form a figure eight, incomplete rings, or other configurations.[24] More than one ring may be present in a single cell.

A Cabot ring may be observed in a nucleated red cell or be associated with stippling or a Howell-Jolly body in the same erythrocyte. This threadlike structure may represent a part of the mitotic spindle, remnants of microtubules, or a fragment of the nuclear membrane. However, its origin is still unclear.[61]

Abnormal Hemoglobin Precipitation

HEINZ BODIES

Heinz bodies are round, refractile inclusions not visible on a Wright-stained film. They range in size from about 1 to 3 μm and are attached to the erythrocyte membrane (Fig. 8-26). When appearing singly, a Heinz body is large, but when several are present in one cell, they are small.

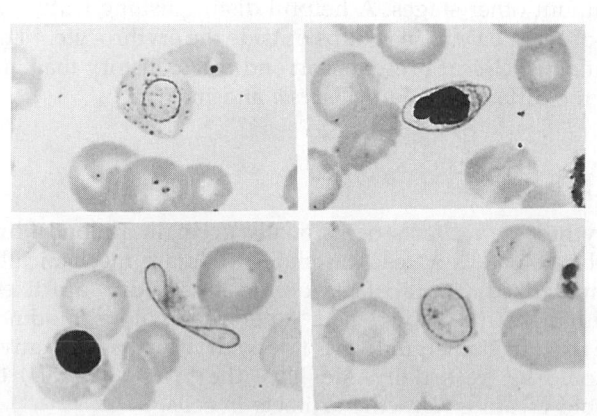

FIGURE 8-25. Cabot rings in film of patient with vitamin B$_{12}$ deficiency. ×1000.

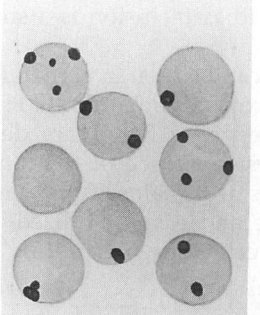 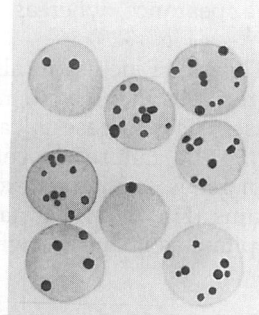

FIGURE 8-26. Heinz bodies in erythrocytes after 4-hour incubation with acetylphenylhydrazine followed by staining with crystal violet. (**Left**) Normal blood with one to four Heinz bodies in most cells. (**Right**) Five or more Heinz bodies per cell from a patient with G6PD deficiency. (From Diggs LW, Sturm D, Bell A: Morphology of Human Blood Cells, 5th ed. N Chicago, IL: Abbott Laboratories, 1985, with permission.)

Multiple Heinz bodies may give a cell the appearance of a pitted golf ball. They are best identified by supravital staining with basic dyes such as crystal violet, methylene blue, or brilliant cresyl blue. A Heinz body in a supravital preparation might be confused with a reticulocyte (Fig. 8-29). A Heinz body is a round, discrete inclusion in contrast to the reticular filamented material in a reticulocyte.

Heinz bodies consist of denatured globin derived from destruction of the Hb molecule. These inclusions are not seen in normal individuals (unless the person is acutely poisoned) because they are pitted out by the spleen. When a Heinz body is pitted from an erythrocyte, the resulting cell may resemble a "bite cell" (keratocyte) in which a portion of the cell has been removed. However, if the spleen has been removed or is atrophic or infarcted, these inclusions can be noted frequently with supravital stains.[34]

Heinz bodies are produced in the blood of normal persons who have been poisoned by aromatic nitro-compounds, amino-compounds, and inorganic oxidizing agents used in treatment protocols. With large doses of the drugs that cause Heinz bodies, hemolysis is present. Heinz bodies also occur in individuals with a hereditary deficiency of the enzymes glucose-6-phosphate dehydrogenase (G6PD) or glutathione as a result of exposure to drugs or agents containing the above compounds (Chaps. 6 and 17). In rare hereditary hemolytic anemias secondary to instability of the Hb molecule (*e.g.*, Hb Zurich and Hb Köln; Chap. 14), such bodies are formed spontaneously in young and mature erythrocytes and also after exposure to sulfonamides or similar drugs. The blood film from a patient with an unstable Hb reveals at least one large Heinz body in almost every red cell after splenectomy.[34]

HEMOGLOBIN H INCLUSIONS

In patients with Hb H disease, an α-thalassemia with a moderate hemolytic anemia (Chap. 15), small greenish-blue inclusion bodies appear in many erythrocytes after four drops of blood are incubated with 0.5 mL of 1% brilliant cresyl blue for 20 minutes at 37°C. These inclusions represent precipitated Hb H (Fig. 8-27). They must be differentiated from reticulocytes, which also stain with brilliant cresyl blue. A reticulocyte has a granulofilamentous appearance, whereas a Hb H inclusion is a single body (see Fig. 8-29).

The Hb H inclusions also can be seen in early nucleated red cells in the bone marrow of patients with Hb H disease.[28] The disease is caused by a hereditary defect leading to a failure of synthesis of three of the four α globin genes, leaving an excess of β chains. Tetramers of β chains (Hb H) are unstable and easily oxidized and precipitate as inclusions with cell aging (Chap. 15).

Protozoan Inclusions

MALARIA

There are four species of human malarial parasites that invade erythrocytes. They are transmitted to man by the bite of the *Anopheles* mosquito and include *Plasmodium vivax* (Fig. 8-30), *Plasmodium malariae, Plasmodium falci-*

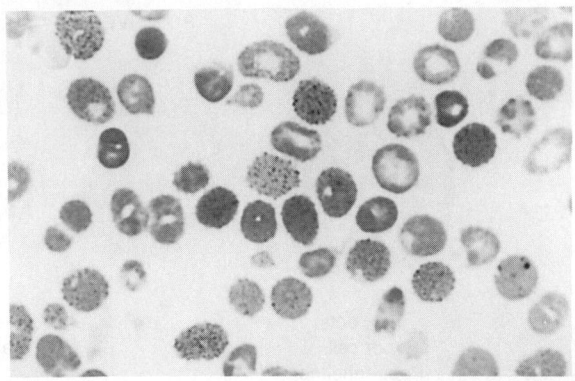

FIGURE 8-27. Hemoglobin H inclusions in film stained with brilliant cresyl blue from patient with hemoglobin H. ×1000. (Courtesy of the Hemoglobinopathy Laboratory, US Centers for Disease Control, Atlanta.)

parum, and *Plasmodium ovale*. Refer to standard parasitology textbooks for details on these protozoa and their effects on erythrocytes. An atlas by Diggs, Sturm, and Bell[24] contains color drawings of these effects.

A malarial organism may be mistakenly identified as a platelet. The observer should note that a malarial ring has a central area that lacks color, whereas the platelet stains completely and has a surrounding halo under light microscopy.

BABESIA

Babesia organisms are transmitted to humans by a tick bite. *Babesia* in a red cell forms ringlike structures resembling the ring stages of malarial parasites.[2] *Babesia* rings may be round, oval, elongated, amoeboid, or pear-shaped and are often tiny, ranging in size from 1 to 5 μm (Figs. 8-28, 8-31). *Babesia microti* appears as tiny rings (usually less than 2 μm) with minimal blue tufts of cytoplasm and a little dot of chromatin. Reproduction occurs asexually by a division that results in a tetrad of organisms that somewhat resembles a cross. One or two chromatin dots with little evidence of cytoplasm is sometimes seen.

Red cells infected with *Babesia* are not enlarged, and pigment is not present. Schüffner's stippling is not observed. Babesiosis, rather than malaria, may be suspected when there are small (or tiny) rings and the tetrad form without other stages. A helpful distinguishing feature is to observe *Babesia* in groups outside the erythrocyte.[24] The patient's clinical presentation and travel history may aid in the differentiation of *Babesia* and malaria.

ARTIFACTS

Erythrocyte artifacts occasionally occur in a blood film. When blood is spread on slides, cells are mechanically traumatized, and artifacts occur as cells dry, are fixed with methanol, and stained. A peripheral film should not be fixed or stained until it is totally dry. Methanol fixative should be fresh daily and have the proper *p*H (8.4) to avoid creating refractile artifacts in cells.

Allowing Wright stain to remain longer than usual on the film leads to evaporation of the methanol in the

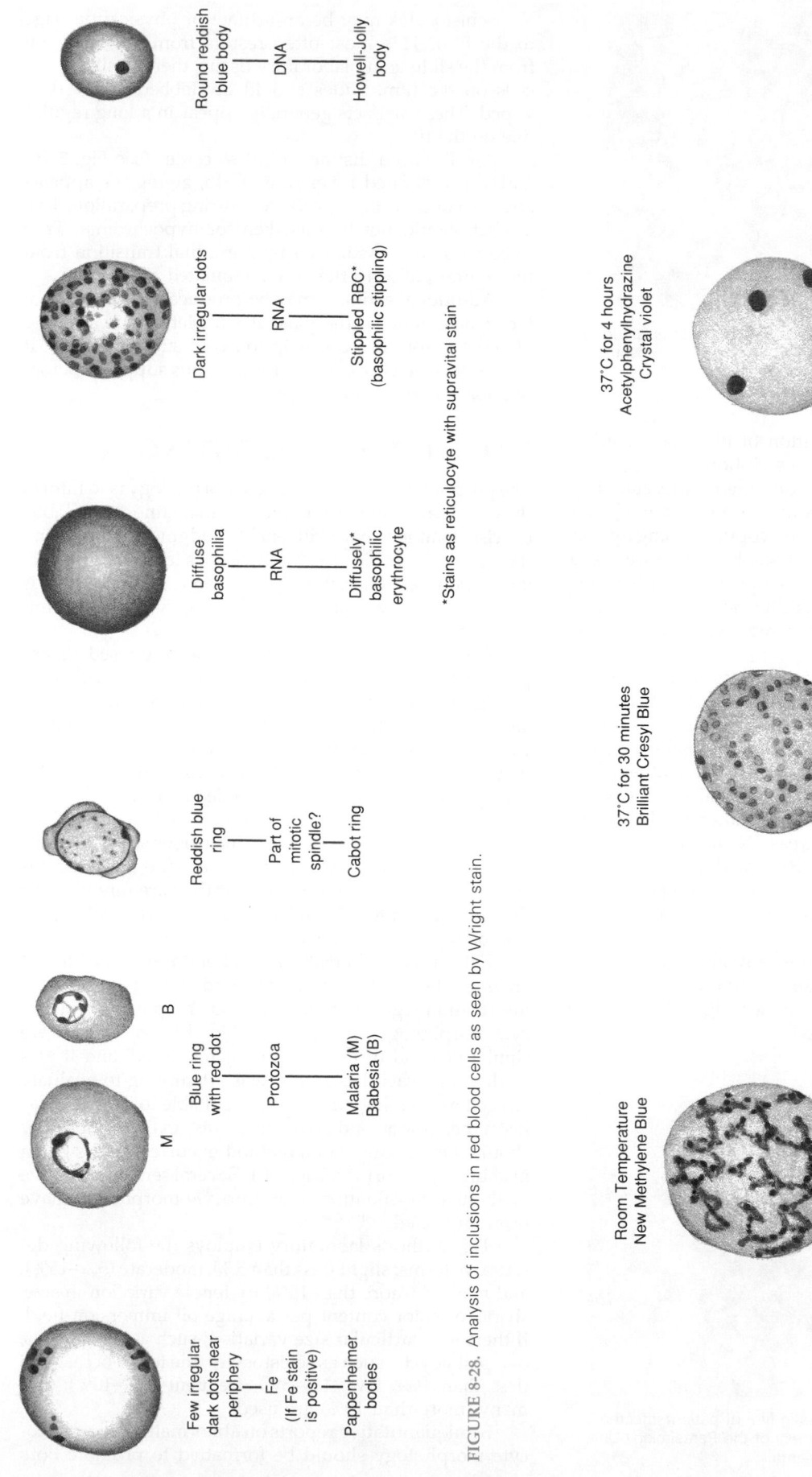

Round reddish
blue body ─── DNA ─── Howell-Jolly
body

Dark irregular dots ─── RNA ─── Stippled RBC*
(basophilic stippling)

Diffuse
basophilia ─── RNA ─── Diffusely*
basophilic
erythrocyte

*Stains as reticulocyte with supravital stain

Reddish blue
ring ─── Part of
mitotic
spindle? ─── Cabot ring

M   B

Blue ring
with red dot ─── Protozoa ─── Malaria (M)
Babesia (B)

Few irregular
dark dots near
periphery ─── Fe
(If Fe stain
is positive) ─── Pappenheimer
bodies

FIGURE 8-28. Analysis of inclusions in red blood cells as seen by Wright stain.

37°C for 4 hours
Acetylphenylhydrazine
Crystal violet

Round bodies
Normal: <5 per cell in ≥70% of cells ─── Denatured hemoglobin ─── Heinz bodies

37°C for 30 minutes
Brilliant Cresyl Blue

Multiple small dots in
nearly every cell ─── Precipitates of Hb H ─── Hemoglobin H

Room Temperature
New Methylene Blue

Granulofilamentous pattern
in some cells ─── RNA ─── Reticulocyte

FIGURE 8-29. Analysis of inclusions in red blood cells as seen by supravital stains.

101

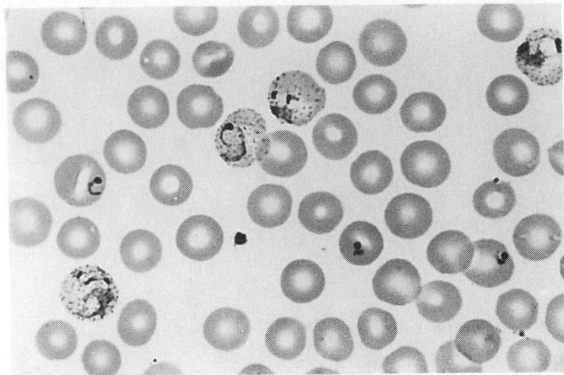

FIGURE 8-30. Malarial ring and trophozoite stages in enlarged erythrocytes in film from patient with *Plasmodium vivax*. Note Schüffner's granules. ×1000.

stain and may cause precipitation of the dye granules, which interferes with red cell description.

Refractile artifacts must be identified if present. They may be caused by water contamination of the methanol or Wright stain. Under light microscopy, focusing up and down with the fine adjustment knob will cause these artifacts to refract rather than disappear, and use of this technique will help in their identification. Refractile artifacts must not be confused with red cell inclusions and should not be reported.

When examining a film several areas should be studied. For example, codocytes may be observed in some areas but not others. Therefore, codocytes should not be reported unless they appear in every acceptable area examined. On the sides and at the pushed-out (feather edge) end of the film, erythrocytes lack normal central pallor and appear solid (see Fig. 3-5A). Evaluation of Hb content should be avoided in such areas. Near the sides of a film, there may be shape distortion with elongated cells arranged in the same direction, much like a school of fish swimming in the same direction; this formation is an artifact of spreading.

Echinocytes or crenated cells may also be artifacts if practically every cell in the thin portion of the film has a uniformly spiculed membrane (see Fig. 3-13A). These features should not be reported.

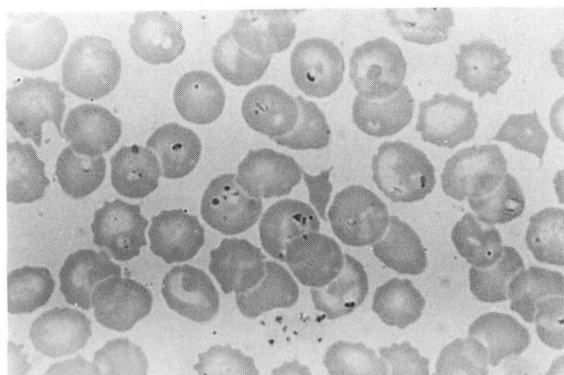

FIGURE 8-31. Rings in erythrocytes in film of patient infected with *Babesia microti*. ×1000. (Courtesy of the Parasitology Unit, US Centers for Disease Control, Atlanta.)

Schistocytes may be an artifact of physical damage to the film. This most often results from removing oil from the slide using laboratory tissue, thereby slicing the cells on the film. Slides should be dabbed rather than wiped. These artifacts generally appear in a long regular line on the film.

A cell with a distinct colorless center (see Fig. 3-16) and a well-defined inner ring of Hb, giving the appearance of a doughnut, is produced during preparation. This artifact should not be mistaken for hypochromia. True hypochromia is evidenced by a gradual transition from the central pallor to the hemoglobinated cytoplasm.

Additional artifacts may be produced by particles of fat or detergent on the glass itself. Meticulous cleaning of slides before use can help to avoid such problems. It may be wise to check slides from various suppliers before purchasing larger quantities.

MORPHOLOGY REPORTING

The purpose of reporting red cell morphology is to inform the physician of abnormal findings in an understandable, concise manner that will enable judgment concerning their clinical significance.[38] To achieve a level of reproducibility between observers in the same laboratory, it is necessary to have set criteria that everyone must uniformly follow.[63]

Appropriate oil immersion fields composed of approximately 200 red cells should be examined with 1000 x magnification. The overall impression of size, shape, and Hb content should be expressed in a semiquantitative way. Emphasis should be placed on the abnormalities that seem significant. Specific size variation and shape changes should be reported. If rouleaux formation or agglutination are truly present, a statement to this effect should be made. The presence of inclusions should always be reported. Likewise, schistocytes and spherocytes should always be reported, even if they are rare because they may indicate a hemolytic process. Sickle cells must also be reported whenever seen.

Fifteen large hematology laboratories in different areas of the United States responded to a request for information regarding their method of reporting erythrocyte morphology on peripheral blood films. There were similarities and differences for each method, and it was evident that each laboratory was attempting to evaluate red cell morphology in a manner suitable to its particular instrumentation and personnel, as every laboratory should. One example of a method in current use is given in abbreviated form in Table 8-1. Several semiquantitative methods for evaluation of erythrocyte morphology have been published.[18,30,38,47,63]

This author's laboratory employs the following descriptive terms: slight (less than 5%), moderate (5%–15%), and marked (more than 15%) to denote variation in size, shape, or color content per average oil immersion field. If there is a particular size variation, such as macrocytes, or a poikiloycte, such as schistocytes, the terms occasional (less than 1%), few (1%–5%), frequent (5%–10%), and many (more than 10%) are used.

Semiquantitative reports on abnormalities in erythrocyte morphology should be formatted to promote both

TABLE 8-1
Sample Criteria for Erythrocyte Morphology Evaluation*

Morphologic Characteristic	WNL†	1⁺	2⁺	3⁺	4⁺
Macrocytes > 9 μm diameter	0–5	5–10	10–20	20–50	>50
Microcytes <6 μm diameter	0–5	5–10	10–20	20–50	>50
Hypochromia	0–2	3–10	10–50	50–75	>75
Poikilocytosis (generalized variations in shape)	0–2	3–10	10–20	20–50	>50
Burr cells	0–2	3–10	10–20	20–50	>50
Acanthocytes	<1	2–5	5–10	10–20	>20
Schistocytes	<1	2–5	5–10	10–20	>20
Teardrop poikilocytes (dacryocytes)	0–2	2–5	5–10	10–20	>20
Target cells (codocytes)	0–2	2–10	10–20	20–50	>50
Spherocytes	0–2	2–10	10–20	20–50	>50
Ovalocytes	0–2	2–10	10–20	20–50	>50
Stomatocytes	0–2	2–10	10–20	20–50	>50
Sickle cells (drepanocytes)	Absent	Report as 1⁺ to indicate presence; do not quantitate			
Polychromatophilia					
Adult	<1	2–5	5–10	10–20	>20
Newborn	1–6	7–15	15–20	20–50	>50
Basophilic stippling	0–1	1–5	5–10	10–20	>20
Howell-Jolly bodies	Absent	1–2	3–5	5–10	>10
Siderocytes (Pappenheimer bodies)	Absent	1–2	3–5	5–10	>10

*Guidelines for semiquantitation are expressed in numbers of occurrences per oil immersion field (applies to fields of approximately 200 to 250 cells per 100× oil objective).
†Within normal limits.
From University of California Medical Center, San Diego, Hematology Laboratory, with permission.

effective communication with the physician and laboratory reproducibility.

APPROACHING ERYTHROCYTE ABNORMALITIES ON THE UNKNOWN FILM

To aid in comparing particular erythrocyte abnormalities on an unknown film, several decision trees have been presented. These trees should help the observer differentiate red cell inclusions by Wright stain (Fig. 8-28), supravital stain (Fig. 8-29), and Prussian blue stain for iron (Fig. 8-24). They should also help to differentiate cells with membrane irregularities (Fig. 8-13) and red cells containing Hb crystals (Fig. 8-20).

CHAPTER SUMMARY

Careful evaluation of red cell morphology on blood films can provide useful diagnostic information. The examiner should describe any variation in red cell size, shape, and Hb content. Red cells may be normocytic, microcytic, or macrocytic in size. Red cells may be normochromic, hypochromic, or hyperchromic, indicating their Hb content.

The morphologist should observe any abnormal shapes that suggest acquired or hereditary hemolytic disorders involving the red cell membrane: spherocytes, elliptocytes, echinocytes, burr cells, acanthocytes, stomatocytes, and codocytes. Schistocytes, keratocytes, dacryocytes, and microspherocytes may ap-

pear secondary to trauma. Poikilocytes that may appear secondary to abnormal Hb content include drepanocytes (sickle cells) and Hb CC and SC crystals.

Inclusions that should be looked for are Howell-Jolly bodies, Pappenheimer bodies, polychromatophilic red cells, and Cabot rings. The protozoan infections of malaria and *Babesia* should not be overlooked.

Artifacts may occur on blood films due to poor staining quality, slow drying, poor preparation, cell damage, and fat particles.

Erythrocyte abnormalities must be recognized microscopically by the examiner to ensure accurate morphologic reports and high quality patient care.

Review Questions

8-1. A Wright-stained erythrocyte that is 9μ, bluish in color and with one small, round nuclear fragmented body is a

A. macrocyte with a siderotic granule.
B. polychromatophilic normocyte with stippling.
C. normocyte containing a malarial ring.
D. polychromatophilic macrocyte with a Howell-Jolly body.

8-2. A Wright-stained erythrocyte which is thin and elongated and has a point at each end is a(n)

A. elliptocyte.
B. Hb CC crystal.
C. helmet cell.
D. drepanocyte.

8-3. An erythrocyte inclusion that appears as a few small irregularly shaped granules and stains positively with Prussian blue is

A. a Heinz body.
B. Schüffner's granules.
C. siderotic granules.
D. basophilic stippling.

8-4. Finding target cells in only one portion of the acceptable area of a blood film suggests

A. an artifact that should not be reported.
B. an artifact that should be reported.
C. a significant morphologic finding that should be reported.
D. the blood film was fixed in methanol prior to staining.

8-5. Which of the following statements is FALSE concerning spherocytes?

A. Spherocytes lack central pallor.
B. Spherocytes commonly indicate hemolysis.
C. Spherocytes have an increased mean corpuscular volume.
D. Spherocytes should always be reported, even if they are rare.

Matching

8-6. drepanocyte
8-7. dacryocyte
8-8. codocyte
8-9. microcytic and macrocytic cells on the blood film together
8-10. red cell with increased central pallor
8-11. red cell with abnormal shape
8-12. schistocyte
8-13. red cell with decreased MCV

a. teardrop
b. poikilocyte
c. red cell fragment
d. hypochromic
e. microcytic
f. anisocytosis
g. target cell
h. sickle cell

References

1. Alloisio N, Dorleac E, Girot R et al: Analysis of the red cell membrane in a family with hereditary elliptocytosis: Total or partial absence of protein 4.1. Hum Genet 59:68, 1981
2. Ash LR, Orihel TC: Atlas of Human Parasitology, 2nd ed. Chicago, American Society of Clinical Pathology Press, 1984
3. Bassen FA, Kornzweig AL: Malformation of the erythrocytes in a case of atypical retinitis pigmentosa. Blood 5:381, 1950
4. Ben-Bassat I, Brok-Simoni F, Kende G et al: A family with red cell pyrimidine-5'-nucleotidase deficiency. Blood 47:919, 1976
5. Bertles JF, Milner PFA: Irreversibly sickled erythrocytes: A consequence of heterogenous distribution of hemoglobin types in sickle cell anemia. J Clin Invest 47:1731, 1968
6. Bessis M: Living Blood Cells and Their Ultrastructure. New York, Springer-Verlag, 1973
7. Bessis M: Blood Smears Reinterpreted. G Brecher (trans). New York, Springer International, 1977
8. Bessis M, Breton-Gorious J: Ferritin and ferruginous micelles in normal erythroblasts and hypochromic hypersideremic anemias. Blood 14:423, 1959
9. Bessis M, Jensen WN: Sideroblastic anaemia, mitochondria and erythroblastic iron. Br J Haematol 11:49, 1965
10. Bessman JD: Automated Blood Counts and Differentials: A Practical Guide. Baltimore, Johns Hopkins University Press, 1986
11. Beutler E, Erslev AJ, Coller BS et al (eds): Williams' Hematology, 5th ed. New York, McGraw-Hill, 1995
12. Bowman WD Jr: Abnormal (ringed) sideroblasts in various hematologic and nonhematologic disorders. Blood 18:662, 1961
13. Brain MC, Dacie JV, Hourihane D: Microangiopathic haemolytic anaemia: The possible role of vascular lesions in pathogenesis. Br J Haematol 8:358, 1962
14. Brecher G, Haley JE, Prenant M et al: Macronormoblasts, macroreticulocytes and macrocytes. Blood Cells 1:547, 1975
15. Bull BS, Kuhn IN: The production of schistocytes by fibrin strands (a scanning electron microscope study). Blood 35:104, 1970
16. Chang K, Williamson JR, Zarkhowsky HS: Effect of heat on the circular dichroism of spectrin in hereditary pyropoikilocytosis. J Clin Invest 64:326, 1979
17. Chapman RG: Red cell life span after splenectomy in hereditary spherocytosis. J Clin Invest 47:2263, 1968
18. Connors DM, Wilson MK: A new approach to the reporting of red cell morphology. J Med Technol 3:94, 1986
19. Cooper RA, Jandl JH: Bile salts and cholesterol in the pathogenesis of target cells in obstructive jaundice. J Clin Invest 47:809, 1968
20. Crosby WH: Siderocytes and the spleen. Blood 12:165, 1956
21. Dacie JV: The Haemolytic Anaemias, 3rd ed, vol 1. Edinburgh, Churchill Livingstone, 1985
22. Diggs LW, Bell A: Intraerythrocytic hemoglobin crystals in sickle cell–hemoglobin C disease. Blood 25:218, 1965
23. Diggs LW, Kraus AP, Morrison DB et al: Intraerythrocytic crystals in a white patient with hemoglobin C in the absence of other types of hemoglobin. Blood 9:1172, 1954
24. Diggs LW, Sturm D, Bell A: Morphology of Human Blood Cells, 5th ed. Abbott Park, IL, Abbott Laboratories, 1985
25. Dresbach M: Elliptical human red corpuscles. Science 19:469, 1904
26. Eichner ER: Macrocytic anemia. In Spivak JL (ed): Fundamentals of Clinical Hematology, 2nd ed. Philadelphia, Harper & Row, 1985
27. England JM, Down MC: Red cell volume distribution curves and the measurement of anisocytosis. Lancet 1:701, 1974
28. Fessas P, Yataghanas X: Intraerythroblastic instability of hemoglobin $\beta 4$ (Hgb H). Blood 31:323, 1968
29. Florman AL, Wintrobe MM: Human elliptical red corpuscles. Bull Johns Hopkins Hosp 63:209, 1938
30. Glasser L: Grading red cell morphology. Diag Med 3:15, 1980
31. Haden RL: The mechanism of the increased fragility of the erythrocytes in congenital hemolytic jaundice. Am J Med Sci 188:441, 1934
32. Hillman RS: Characteristics of marrow production and reticulocyte maturation in normal man in response to anemia. J Clin Invest 48:443, 1969
33. Isselbacher KJ, Scheif R, Plotkin GR et al: Congenital β-lipoprotein deficiency: A hereditary disorder involving a defect in the absorption and transport of lipids. Medicine 43:347, 1964
34. Jacob HS: Mechanism of Heinz body formation and attachment to red cell membrane. Semin Hematol 7:341, 1970
35. Jacob HS, Ruby A, Overland ES et al: Abnormal membrane protein of red blood cells in hereditary spherocytosis. J Clin Invest 50:1800, 1971
36. Jensen WN, Moreno GD, Bessis M: An electron microscopic description of basophilic stippling in red cells. Blood 25:933, 1965

37. Koyama S: Studies on Howell-Jolly body. Acta Haematol Jpn 23:20, 1960
38. Krause JR: Red cell abnormalities in the blood smear: Disease correlations. Lab Management 23:29, 1985
39. Lee GR: The hemolytic anemias: General conderations. In Lee GR, Bithell TC, Foerster J et al (eds): Wintrobe's Clinical Hematology, 9th ed. Lea & Febiger, Philadelphia, 1993
40. Lessin L, Klug P, Jensen W: Clinical implications of red cell shape. Adv Intern Med 21:451, 1976
41. Lindenbaum J: Brief review: Status of laboratory testing in the diagnosis of megaloblastic anaemia. Blood 61:684, 1983
42. Lock SP, Smith RS, Hardisty RM: Stomatocytosis: A hereditary red cell anomaly associated with haemolytic anaemia. Br J Haematol 7:303, 1961
43. Lux SE: Spectrin–actin membrane skeleton of normal and abnormal red cells. Semin Hematol 16:21, 1979
44. McPhedran P, Barnes MG, Weinstein JS et al: Interpretation of electronically determined macrocytosis. Ann Intern Med 78:677, 1973
45. Miale JB: Laboratory Medicine: Hematology, 6th ed. St Louis, CV Mosby, 1982
46. Mollin DL: Sideroblasts and sideroblastic anaemia. Br J Haematol 11:41, 1965
47. Napoli VM, Nichols CW, Cleck S: A semiquantitative estimate method for reporting abnormal RBC morphology. Lab Med 11:111, 1980
48. Padilla F, Bromberg PA, Jensen WN: The sickle–unsickle cycle: A cause of cell fragmentation leading to permanently deformed cells. Blood 41:653, 1973
49. Pappenheimer AM, Thompson WP, Parker DD et al: Anaemia associated with unidentified erythrocytic inclusions. Q J Med Sci 14:75, 1945
50. Perrotta AL, Finch CA: The polychromatophilic erythrocyte. Am J Clin Pathol 57:471, 1972
51. Ponder E: Hemolysis and Related Phenomena. New York, Grune & Stratton, 1948
52. Price-Jones C: Red Blood Cell Diameters. London, Oxford Medical Publications, 1933
53. Sayed HN, Dacie JV, Handley DA et al: Haemolytic anaemia of mechanical origin after open heart surgery. Thorax 16:356, 1961
54. Schubothe H: The cold hemagglutinin disease. Semin Hematol 3:27, 1966
55. Schwartz SO, Motto SA: The diagnostic significance of "burr" red blood cells. Am J Med Sci 218:563, 1949
56. Sears DA, Crosby WH: Intravascular hemolysis due to intracardiac prosthetic devices. Am J Med 39:341, 1965
57. Shen SC, Ham TH, Fleming EM: Studies on the destruction of red blood cells III. Mechanism and complications of hemoglobinuria in patients with thermal burns: Spherocytosis and increased osmotic fragility of red blood cells. N Engl J Med 229:701, 1943
58. Sturgeon P: Hematological observations on the anemia associated with blood type Rh null. Blood 36:310, 1970
59. Tomaselli MB, John KM, Lux SE: Elliptical erythrocyte membrane skeletons and heat-sensitive spectrin in hereditary elliptocytosis. Proc Natl Acad Sci USA 78:1911, 1981
60. van Assendelft OW: Interpretation of the quantitative blood cell count. In Koepke JA (ed): Practical Laboratory Hematology. New York, Churchill Livingstone, 1991
61. Van Oye E: L'origine des anneaux de Cabot. Rev Hematol 9:173, 1954
62. Vaughan JM: Red cell characteristics in acholuric jaundice. J Pathol Bacteriol 45:461, 1937
63. Walton JR: Uniform grading of hematologic abnormalities. Am J Med Technol 39:517, 1973
64. Ways P, Reed CF, Hanahan DJ: Red-cell and plasma lipids in acanthocytosis. J Clin Invest 42:1248, 1963
65. Weed RI: The importance of erythrocyte deformability. Am J Med 49:147, 1970
66. Weed RI, Reed C: Membrane alterations and red cell destruction. Am J Med 41:681, 1966
67. Weiss L, Tavassoli M: Anatomical hazards to the passage of erythrocytes through the spleen. Semin Hematol 7:372, 1970
68. Wiley JS, Gill FM: Red cell calcium leak in congenital hemolytic anemia with extreme microcytosis. Blood 47:197, 1976
69. Wintrobe MM, Lukens JN, Lee GR: The approach to the patient with anemia. In Lee GR, Bithell TC, Foerster J et al (eds): Wintrobe's Clinical Hematology, 9th ed, p 715. Lea & Febiger, Philadelphia, 1993
70. Woodruff AW, Topley E, Knight R et al: The anaemia of kala azar. Br J Haematol 22:319, 1972
71. Zarkowsky HS, Mohandas N, Speaker CB et al: A congenital haemolytic anaemia with thermal sensitivity of the erythrocyte membrane. Br J Haematol 29:537, 1975

CHAPTER 9

Quantitative Laboratory Evaluation of Erythrocytes

Tina M. Riedinger
Bernadette F. Rodak

Objectives

1. State the principle, sources of error, and the adult reference ranges for the cyanmethemoglobin method for hemoglobin determination and the centrifuged microhematocrit determination.
2. Using the results of a standard curve for manual hemoglobin determinations, find the hemoglobin concentration of an unknown specimen given its absorbance or percent transmittance at 540 nm.
3. Apply the "rule of three" to quickly check the accuracy of an erythrocyte count and hemoglobin and hematocrit values to determine if a discrepancy exists and further investigation is required.
4. Define, calculate, and state the adult reference range for the mean corpuscular volume (MCV), mean corpuscular hemoglobin (MCH), and mean corpuscular hemoglobin concentration (MCHC).
5. Identify four major reasons for discrepancies in reticulocyte counts and list other interfering, supravitally staining substances.
6. Calculate reticulocyte percentage and state the adult reference range.
7. Calculate and interpret the absolute reticulocyte count (ARC), the corrected reticulocyte count (CRC), and the reticulocyte production index (RPI).
8. State the principle, common sources of error, and adult reference ranges for the erythrocyte sedimentation rate (ESR), and describe the different ESR methods available.
9. Recognize physiologic conditions that may affect ESR results.
10. Convert hematologic units of measurement from conventional units to the International System of Units (SI).

The evaluation of erythrocytes is an important part of the complete blood count (CBC), which is performed routinely in most clinical laboratories. This chapter discusses basic laboratory procedures relating to the qualitative and quantitative evaluation of erythrocytes and their composition. Although many of these tests are now performed by automated methods, every laboratory maintains procedures and equipment for their manual performance, because some specimens have abnormalities that interfere with accurate automated hematologic testing.

An exception is the manual erythrocyte count using Thoma pipettes and a hemocytometer, which is no longer performed because of its lack of accuracy and reliability. Now this task is reserved for multiparameter instruments (Chap. 42).

Other erythrocyte evaluation procedures are routinely performed manually, including the reticulocyte count and the erythrocyte sedimentation rate (ESR). Skill in performing these tests, as well as other tests that are infrequently performed manually, is essential for hematology laboratory personnel.

For all procedures in this chapter a whole blood specimen, anticoagulated with EDTA and less than 24 hours old, is required unless otherwise noted. Table 9-1 presents a sample reference range for the peripheral blood erythrocyte count and other related erythrocyte measurements presented in this chapter. Note that these ranges are meant to give only general guidelines: every laboratory should determine the reference range for each of these measurements based on its own patient population.

SPECTROPHOTOMETRIC DETERMINATION OF HEMOGLOBIN CONCENTRATION (HEMOGLOBINOMETRY)

Review of Spectrophotometry

The manual procedure for determining hemoglobin (Hb) concentration in whole blood requires the use of a spectrophotometer. This instrument measures monochromatic

TABLE 9-1
Hematology References Ranges (Mean ± 2 SD)*

Age (Years)	Erythrocyte Count (× 10^{12}/L)†	HB (g/dL)†‡	Hematocrit (L/L)†	MCV (fL)	MCH (pg)	MCHC (g/dL)
Birth (cord blood)	3.9–5.5	13.5–19.5	0.42–0.60	98–118	31–37	30–36
1 to 3 days (capillary blood)	4.0–6.6	14.5–22.5	0.45–0.67	95–121	31–37	29–37
0.5 to 2	3.7–5.3	10.5–13.5	0.33–0.39	70–86	23–31	30–36
2 to 6	3.9–5.3	11.5–13.5	0.34–0.40	75–87	24–30	31–37
6 to 12	4.0–5.2	11.5–15.5	0.35–0.45	77–95	25–33	31–37
12 to 18 (male)	4.5–5.3	13.0–16.0	0.37–0.49	78–98	25–35	31–37
12 to 18 (female)	4.1–5.1	12.0–16.0	0.36–0.46	78–102	25–35	31–37
18 to 49 (male)	4.5–5.9	13.5–17.5	0.41–0.53	80–100	26–34	31–37
18 to 49 (female	4.0–5.2	12.0–16.0	0.36–0.46	80–100	26–34	31–37

Data from Dallman PR: Blood and blood forming tissues. In Rudolph A (ed): Pediatrics, 16th ed, p 1111. New York, Appleton-Century-Crofts, 1977; with permission. Compiled from the following sources: Dutcher: Lab Med 2:32, 1971; Koerper et al: J Paediatr 89:580, 1976; Marner: Acta Paediatr Scand 58:363, 1969; Matoth et al: Acta Paediatr Scand 60:317, 1971; Moe: Acta Paediatr Scand 54:69, 1965; Okuno: J Clin Pathol 25:599, 1972; Oski and Naiman: Hematological Problems in the Newborn. Philadelphia, WB Saunders, 1972, p 11; Penttila et al: Suomen Laakarilehti 26:2173, 1973; and Viteria et al: Br J Haematol 23:189, 1972.

* Emphasis was given to studies employing electronic counters and to the selection of populations that are likely to exclude individuals with iron deficiency. The mean ± 2 SD can be expected to include 95% of the observations in a normal population.

† Erythrocyte count, Hb, and hematocrit are slightly lower in three significant situations: (1) after age 50; (2) in recumbency (i.e., a blood sample is taken when the patient is lying down); and (3) after meals (as much as 10% lower). Values may be significantly lower in runners than in nonrunners but seldom reflect true anemia.[8]

‡ Hemoglobin may be elevated in heavy smokers because of the increase in carboxyhemoglobin, which is not capable of carrying oxygen to tissues.

light transmitted through a solution to determine the concentration of the light-absorbing substance in that solution.

SPECTROPHOTOMETER COMPONENTS

A basic spectrophotometer has five components: (1) a stable source of radiant energy (lamp); (2) a wavelength selector or monochromator (prism, diffraction grating); (3) a container to hold the substance to be measured (cuvette); (4) a radiant energy detector (photomultiplier tube); and (5) a device to provide a readout of the electronic signal generated by the detector (*e.g.*, galvanometer). Light from the lamp passes through the diffraction grating or prism, which allows light of only a chosen wavelength to pass through the cuvette. This transmitted light strikes a detector, where it is converted into electrical energy and presented to the readout device.

BEER'S LAW

The principle of spectrophotometry follows Beer's law, which states that absorbance of light is directly proportional to the concentration of the absorbing substance and to the length of the light path through the substance:

$$A = \varepsilon \times b \times c$$

where A = absorbance; amount of light absorbed by a substance

ε = molar absorptivity; the fraction of a specific wavelength of light absorbed by a given type of molecule

b = length of light path through substance

c = concentration of substance.

Since the path length and molar absorptivity are constant for a given cuvette and wavelength, respectively, absorbance (A) is directly proportional to concentration (c). For example, plotting concentration versus absorbance of a 1% solution with an absorbance of 0.1, a 2% solution with an absorbance of 0.2, and a 3% solution with an absorbance of 0.3 would yield a straight line, thus demonstrating Beer's law, as each solution has a concentration directly proportional to its absorbance. Absorbance is also known as optical density (O.D.), a term now obsolete.

Beer's law also shows that the concentration of a substance is inversely proportional to the logarithm of transmitted light. *Percent transmittance (%T)* is the term used for the amount of light transmitted by a substance. Many spectrophotometers have both an A and a %T scale. If absorbance cannot be measured directly by a spectrophotometer, it is derived mathematically from %T: A = 2 − log %T (refer to Appendix C for %T to A conversion chart).

Because absorbance is directly proportional to concentration, it is easier to use than the absorbance and %T relation. The concentration (c) of an unknown may be determined by the following ratio:

$$\frac{c_{unknown}}{A_{unknown}} = \frac{c_{standard}}{A_{standard}} \quad \text{or} \quad c_{unknown} = \frac{c_{standard} \times A_{unknown}}{A_{standard}}$$

This formula may be applied to calculation of a specimen's Hb concentration based on a cyanmethemoglobin standard (discussed below).

QUALITY CONTROL

To ensure accuracy, function verification should include checks on wavelength accuracy, stray light, and linearity of the detector response for any spectrophotometer used in the laboratory.[32] Details on such function verification may be found in standard textbooks of clinical chemistry.

Hemoglobin Concentration Determination

Hemoglobin concentration provides an estimate of the oxygen-carrying capacity of blood. The International Committee for Standardization in Haematology[19,21] and the National Committee for Clinical Laboratory Standards (NCCLS)[29] recommend the cyanmethemoglobin (hemiglobincyanide) method for Hb determination. This method was selected as the international preferred method because it has a very broad absorption peak (Fig. 9-1). If the wavelength is set between 535 and 545 nm, the readings will still be similar, since the spectral peak is broad. A formerly popular method for Hb determination is the oxyhemoglobin procedure, which is faster and uses a much less complex reagent than the cyanmethemoglobin method. However, the oxyhemoglobin method was not chosen as the international preferred method because it must be standardized against an oxygen capacity method, which is quite difficult to perform accurately. Additionally the absorption peak is very narrow at 540 nm, and thus the method requires more sophisticated and expensive spectrophotometers.

HEMOGLOBIN STANDARD CURVE

A standard curve must be set up using the cyanmethemoglobin standard before testing patient specimens. Cyanmethemoglobin, a secondary standard, is available commercially. It is the only commercially available *stan-dard* used in routine hematology; all other products for quality control maintenance are known as *controls* (Chap. 45). The curve is set up by diluting Cyanmethemoglobin Certified Standard with cyanmethemoglobin reagent and measuring the absorbance of each dilution at 540 nm.[2,3]

Standard Curve Preparation

PROCEDURE
1. For instruments that require cuvette volumes of 5.0 mL or less, make dilutions to achieve certain concentrations (Table 9-2; see Comments below for an explanation of how these concentrations are calculated). The amount of dilution will depend on the concentration of the standard and the total volume required by the cuvette. For further information on setting up standard curve dilutions, see the standard package insert.[2]
2. Transfer these solutions to matched cuvettes and read absorbance of each dilution against a reagent blank on a spectrophotometer at 540 nm. Use the same instrument and wavelength for standards and unknowns.
3. Plot absorbance of each standard against its concentration on linear graph paper. Alternatively, on semilogarithmic paper, plot %T against concentration (Fig. 9-2). This curve may be used to read Hb concentration of controls and unknowns.

COMMENTS
1. Set up a new standard curve with each new lot of reagent prepared. Note that the "curve" should be a straight line (Fig. 9-2).
2. It is recommended that the standard curve be checked whenever repairs, relocations, or other alterations are made in the instrument (*e.g.*, whenever a bulb is changed).[2]
3. To understand how the Hb concentrations are calculated in Table 9-2, consider the following. The stock undiluted cyanmethemoglobin standard contains 80 mg/dL or 80 mg/100 mL of cyanmethemoglobin. This is equal to a whole blood Hb value of 20 g/dL if 0.02 mL of a blood sample is diluted to 5.0 mL with cyanmethemoglobin reagent. Why are these equal? Because 80 mg of cyanmethemoglobin in 100 mL is equal to 4 mg of cyanmethemoglobin in 5 mL (which formed from 4 mg of Hb). Therefore, if a 0.02-mL blood sample contains 4 mg of Hb, then a 100-mL (1 dL) blood sample contains

$$\frac{4\,mg}{0.02\,mL} \times 100\,mL \times \frac{1\,g}{1000\,mg}$$
$$= 20\,g\text{ of Hb (i.e., the standard equivalent of 20 g/dL)}$$

Cyanmethemoglobin Method for Hemoglobin Determination

PRINCIPLE AND SPECIMEN REQUIREMENTS. In the cyanmethemoglobin method, whole blood is mixed with a solution of potassium ferricyanide (K_3FeCN_6) to convert Hb in the ferrous (Fe^{2+}) state, to methemoglobin (Hi; also called hemiglobin) in the ferric (Fe^{3+}) state, which then reacts with potassium cyanide (KCN) to form cyanmethemoglobin, also called hemiglobincyanide (HiCN). HiCN is very stable and has a broad absorption maximum around 540 nm. The reaction is

$$Hb(Fe^{2+}) \xrightarrow{K_3Fe(CN)_6} \underset{\text{methemoglobin}}{Hi\,(Fe^{3+})} \xrightarrow{KCN} \underset{\text{cyanmethemoglobin}}{HiCN}$$

The absorbance of the solution at 540 nm is directly proportional to the amount of Hb present. All forms of Hb except sulfhemoglobin are measured. Either venous blood collected in EDTA or capillary blood may be used.

REAGENTS. The recommended cyanmethemoglobin reagent contains KCN, 0.050 g; K_3FeCN_6, 0.200 g; KH_2PO_4 (anhydrous), 0.140 g; and nonionic detergent, 0.5 to 1.0 mL in 1 liter of distilled

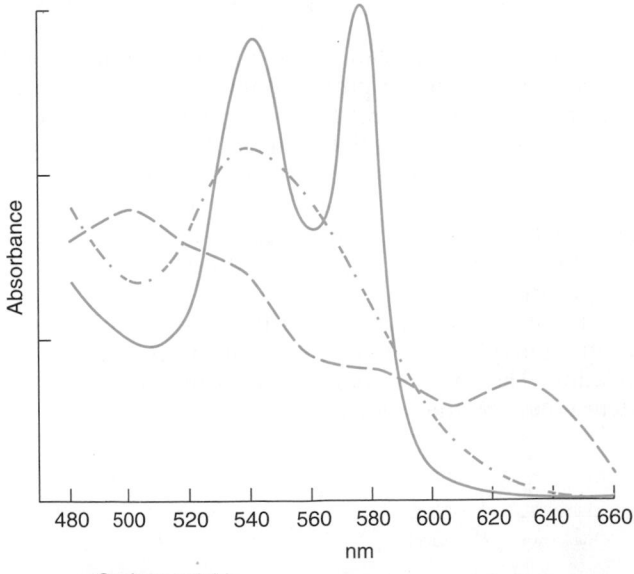

FIGURE 9-1. Absorption spectra of hemoglobin derivatives. At 540 nm, note the broad absorption peak for cyanmethemoglobin compared to the narrow peak for oxyhemoglobin.

——— Oxyhemoglobin
— · — Cyanmethemoglobin
— — Methemoglobin

TABLE 9-2
Dilutions and Resulting Concentrations for Cyanmethemoglobin Standard Curve*

Hemoglobin concentration (g/dL)	Blank	5	10	15	20
Cyanmethemoglobin standard (mL)	0.0	1.5	3.0	4.5	6.0
Cyanmethemoglobin reagent (mL)	6.0	4.5	3.0	1.5	0.0

* This is an example using a standard containing 80 mg/dL cyanmethemoglobin.

water (available commercially).[29] The original and modified Drabkin's reagents formerly used widely in Hb determinations are no longer recommended for use in the cyanmethemoglobin procedure because of their long reaction times and problems with turbidity in the reaction solutions.[29]

QUALITY CONTROL. Commercial controls are available to determine accuracy of equipment and procedure. Proficiency testing also serves as a check (Chap. 45). A control should be run with each batch of specimens.

PROCEDURE

1. Using Sahli or disposable "to contain" pipettes, make a 1:251 dilution by adding 0.02 mL (20 μL) of venous or capillary blood to 5.0 mL of cyanmethemoglobin reagent and rinsing the pipette in the specimen mixture several times to ensure accurate dilution. Cover and invert the tube to mix. Depending on reagent manufacturer, conversion of hemoglobin to cyanmethemoglobin takes from 3 minutes[11] (DMA, Data Medical Associates, Arlington, TX) to 10 minutes[3] (Boehringer-Mannheim, Indianapolis, IN). DMA has added a buffer to the reagent that has shortened the reaction time.[11]
2. Set spectrophotometer wavelength to 540 nm. Blank spectrophotometer with cyanmethemoglobin reagent in one of two matched cuvettes.
3. Read absorbance (A_u) of specimen on spectrophotometer using other matched cuvette. Alternatively, %T may be read using a colorimeter and a green filter (540 nm).
4. Convert reading into grams of Hb per dL (g/dL) using a standard curve set up with the same equipment and reagents used for the specimen or calculate specimen concentration (C_u) based on Beer's law as follows[13]:

$$C_u(g/dL) = 0.251 \frac{A_u \times C_s}{A_s}$$

where A_u is the absorbance of the unknown, C_s is the concentration of the standard (usually 80 mg/dL), and A_s is the absorbance of the standard run most recently under the same conditions as the patient specimen. For example, given $A_u = 0.480$, $C_s = 80$ mg/dL, and $A_s = 0.800$, then

$$C_u = \frac{0.251 \,(0.480 \times 80)}{0.800} = 12.0 \,g/dL$$

Semiautomated Measurement of Hemoglobin Concentration

PRINCIPLE. The cyanmethemoglobin method is also employed when using semiautomated instruments such as the hemoglobinometer (Coulter Diagnostics, Hialeah, FL).

PROCEDURE

1. Make a 1:501 dilution by adding 20 μL of blood to a 10-mL volumetric flask. Dilute to volume with isotonic saline.
2. Add three drops of lysing and hemoglobin reagent. This reagent contains a cationic surfactant (that lyses erythrocytes) and potassium ferricyanide, which converts Hb to cyanmethemoglobin. Invert tube to mix. Let stand for 2 minutes for complete chemical reaction. If sample is turbid, it must be

centrifuged to clear before reading (see Comments and Sources of Physiologic Error below).
3. Introduce dilution into instrument (instrument blanks itself). Instrument provides a direct readout of Hb in g/dL. Readings of duplicate dilutions should agree within 0.2 g/dL.
4. Waste should be treated as any blood-contaminated product.

HEMOGLOBIN REFERENCE RANGES. Refer to Table 9-1 for reference ranges at various ages.

COMMENTS AND SOURCES OF TECHNICAL ERROR IN HEMOGLOBIN MEASUREMENT. Sources of technical error include pipetting error; use of dirty, scratched, or unmatched cuvettes; and use of deteriorated reagents. All instruments and pipettes must be properly standardized. Cyanmethemoglobin reagent is unstable if exposed to light and must therefore be kept in a dark cabinet, a container covered with foil, or a dark glass bottle. The reagent should be tightly capped.

Cyanmethemoglobin reagent contains cyanide and is considered dangerous; it must be used with caution. However, a lethal dose would require ingestion of 4 to 16 L of reagent. Because hydrogen cyanide gas is liberated on acidification of the reagent, samples and spent reagents should be discarded into running water in a sink (free of acids) followed by copious flushing with water or into a hazardous waste container, depending on local laws.[12]

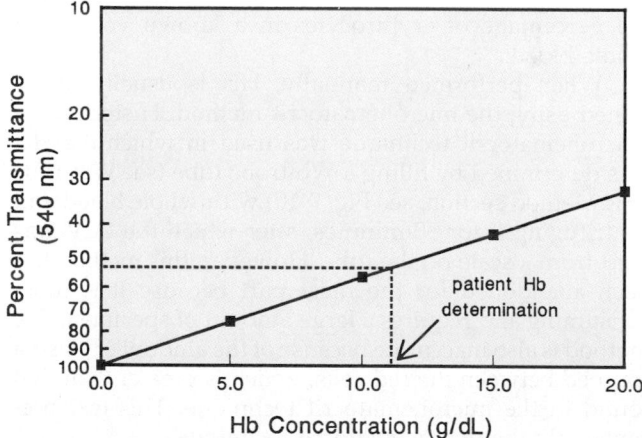

FIGURE 9-2. Cyanmethemoglobin standard curve developed on the basis of the following percent transmittance (T) readings obtained after preparing the hemoglobin concentrations as illustrated in Table 9-2: 0 g/dL = 100% T, 5 g/dL = 75% T, 10 g/dL = 56% T, 15 g/dL = 42.5% T, 20 g/dL = 32% T. This curve is presented for illustrative purposes only; every laboratory should develop its own standard curve using its own reagents and equipment. With the aid of the curve developed specifically for any given laboratory, any patient's hemoglobin concentration can be determined manually by finding the sample percent T on the y axis and then point of intersection with the x axis along the standard curve. For example, using this graph, if a patient's sample gave a T of 52%, the hemoglobin concentration (using these reagents and equipment) would be approximately 11 g/dL.

COMMENTS AND SOURCES OF PHYSIOLOGIC ERROR IN HEMOGLOBIN MEASUREMENT. Several patient conditions can cause erroneous Hb values. Turbidity in the mixture will cause falsely elevated values. Turbidity may be the result of the following:

1. Lipemia. Correct by adding 0.02 mL (20 μL) of patient's plasma to 5.0 mL of cyanmethemoglobin reagent and use this mixture as a patient blank.
2. Extremely high leukocyte counts (greater than 30.0×10^9/L). Correct by centrifuging test mixture and determining the Hb in supernatant fluid.
3. Hb S and Hb C. Cells containing these variants (Chap. 14) have a relative resistance to hemolysis, which causes test mixture turbidity. It is corrected by diluting hemoglobin mixture 1:2 by taking one part of mixture and adding one part distilled water. The absorbance result must be multiplied by the dilution factor, which is 2.
4. Easily precipitated globulins (*e.g.*, those found in Waldenström's macroglobulinemia or multiple myeloma; Chap. 39). This was a problem in the past; however, because the cyanmethemoglobin reagent contains KH_2PO_4 salt, this problem is not likely to occur. Using the original Drabkin's reagent, this problem was corrected by adding 0.1 g of potassium carbonate to 1 L of Drabkin's before use. This increased the alkalinity of the reagent, causing globulins to remain in solution and thus prevented interference with absorbance readings.

In heavy smokers carboxyhemoglobin may represent as much as 10% of the total Hb. Carboxyhemoglobin takes up to 1 hour to convert completely to cyanmethemoglobin. Readings taken at the usual development time may be erroneous; however, the degree of error probably is not clinically significant.

CENTRIFUGED MICROHEMATOCRIT

The term *hematocrit* (Hct) actually refers to the instrument used to determine packed cell volume (PCV). However, Hct is commonly used synonymously with PCV to denote the percentage of erythrocytes in a known volume of whole blood.

When performed manually, Hct is usually determined using the microhematocrit method. Historically a macrohematocrit technique was used in which the Hct was determined by filling a Wintrobe tube (see Wintrobe ESR Method section; see Fig. 9-10) with whole blood and centrifuging it for 30 minutes, after which the PCV was read from a scale on the tube. However, this method has been abandoned for the most part because it is time-consuming and requires a large amount of specimen. The method is also inaccurate because of the amount of plasma trapped between the red cells, which is greater than that found in the microhematocrit technique. This text presents only the microhematocrit technique.

Microhematocrit Technique

PRINCIPLE AND SPECIMEN REQUIREMENTS. A small amount of whole blood is centrifuged to determine maximum packing of erythrocytes, expressed as PCV or Hct. Whole blood anticoagulated with EDTA (1.5–1.8 mg/mL of blood) is recommended.[28] Capillary blood collected in heparinized capillary tubes may also be used. Note that if blood from a vacuum tube containing EDTA requires a manual Hct, non-anticoagulated capillary tubes must be used to avoid overanticoagulation of specimen. Specimens should be stored at 22 ± 4°C. Manual Hcts should be performed within 6 hours after blood collection.

REAGENTS AND EQUIPMENT

Capillary hematocrit tubes containing heparin (for skin puncture collection; color coded with a red band) or plain (for blood already anticoagulated; may be color coded with a blue band). Capillary tubes should meet specifications described elsewhere.[28]

Nonabsorbent sealing clay

Microhematocrit reader device (Figs. 9-3 and 9-4)

Microhematocrit centrifuge capable of sustaining a relative centrifugal force (RCF) of 10,000 to 15,000 g (number of times greater than gravity) without the rotor exceeding a temperature of 45°C.

Calculation of RCF is explained in Appendix D. The calculation requires measurement of centrifuge rotating speed in revolutions per minute (rpm), which may be obtained using a tachometer. RCF calculation also requires the centrifuge rotating radius, which should be listed in the manufacturer's instrument operation manual. Most standard American microhematocrit centrifuges develop the required force when rotating at 10,000 to 12,000 rpm.

QUALITY CONTROL

1. Accuracy and reproducibility of centrifuge timer should be checked periodically with a stopwatch.
2. RCF or rpm must be verified periodically using a calibrated tachometer.
3. Minimum time to achieve maximum cell packing should be determined for each instrument, both when it is new and on a periodic basis. This is determined as follows:
   a. Fill 10 to 14 microhematocrit tubes with EDTA-anticoagulated blood. Repeat this procedure for a second specimen. One of the two specimens should have a Hct greater than

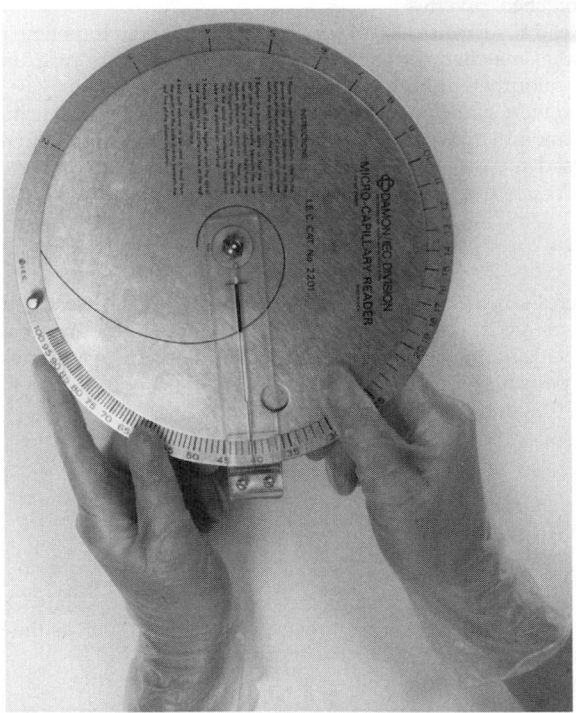

FIGURE 9-3. Hematocrit sample prepared for reading on Micro-Capillary Reader (Damon/IEC Division, Needham Hgts, MA). Hematocrit for this sample is 40.5% or 0.405 L/L. Caution: hematocrits may be misread by the untrained eye. Note that this value would mistakenly be read as 49.5% or 0.495 L/L if the scale were read in the wrong direction. The hematocrit numbers ascend from right to left. (Photograph by Steve Kasper, MT [ASCP].)

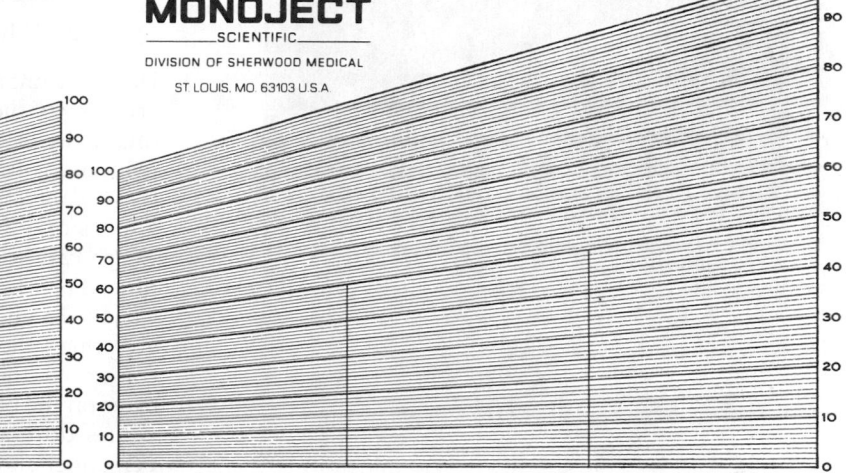

HRI

8889-111004   LOT NO. 33651

CRITOCAPS™

Micro-Hematocrit Capillary Tube Reader

Permits Reading of Packed Cell
Volume Directly in Percentage

For In Vitro Diagnostic Use

DIRECTIONS FOR USE:
Place the centrifuged Micro-Hematocrit Tube vertically on the chart with the bottom edge of the CRITOCAP just touching the red line below the "0" percent line. The bottom of the column of blood should then be at the "0" percent line. Slide the tube along the chart until the meniscus of the plasma intersects the "100" percent line. The height of the packed red cell column is then read directly as percent cell volume.

MANUFACTURED FOR

MONOJECT
____SCIENTIFIC____
DIVISION OF SHERWOOD MEDICAL
ST. LOUIS, MO. 63103 U.S.A.

M-29-3

FIGURE 9-4. The CRITOCAPS Micro-Hematocrit Capillary Tube Reader (Monoject Scientific, St. Louis) provides an alternative to the Micro-Capillary Reader wheel. The lower RBC column in the tube is matched up with the 0 mark, and the plasma meniscus is lined up with 100%. The hematocrit is then read at the top of the RBC column from the scale on either side.

0.50 L/L. Such a specimen can be prepared by removing plasma from a specimen with a lower Hct.

b. Using two capillary tubes for each specimen, perform microhematocrits with a spin time of 2 minutes. Record results of all four tubes. Repeat this procedure a number of times, each time increasing spin time by 30 seconds. When Hct has remained at the same value for two consecutive spins, minimum time for maximum packing has been determined.

c. The second (longer) time interval in which the Hct value has remained the same is the spin time used for all future specimens to ensure that enough time is allowed for optimal packing of RBCs. Specimens with Hcts greater than 0.50 L/L may take longer to pack; using the second time interval allows for this possibility without spinning any longer than necessary to obtain an accurate result on all specimens. Packing times longer than 5 minutes are unacceptable, and the centrifuge rotation speed should be rechecked if such a time is obtained.[28]

4. Controls must be run periodically at intervals specified by each laboratory. For example, a control sample may be run after every 20 specimens, but this may vary depending on workload, instrument stability, and regulatory requirements.

5. Centrifuge brushes should be checked and replaced whenever they are less than half their original size.

6. Centrifuges should be cleaned immediately if blood is spilled using an effective germicidal agent such as 10% bleach.

PROCEDURE

1. Fill at least two capillary tubes approximately two-thirds full. If using tubes with a colored band at one end, fill from opposite end.

2. Seal unfilled end (end with color-coded band) with nonabsorbent material (*e.g.*, clay).

3. Place capillary tubes in opposite slots of microhematocrit centrifuge with their clay-filled ends against gasket. Be sure to note position number if spinning specimens from more than one patient.

4. Place head cover on centrifuge; tighten securely and close top. Centrifuge for the minimum time determined for maximum cell packing on that centrifuge. Open lid, remove cover, and remove capillary tubes one at a time for reading Hct.

5. Using a microhematocrit reading device (Figs. 9-3 and 9-4), determine Hct. Buffy coat (leukocytes and platelets) should *not* be included in the reading, which should be taken below the buffy coat.

6. Note presence of a buffy coat (Fig. 9-5) and plasma color (normal, icteric, lipemic, or hemolyzed) on patient requisition.

7. Results should agree within 0.02 L/L for the duplicate patient samples.

MICROHEMATOCRIT REFERENCE RANGES. Refer to Table 9-1 for ranges at various ages.[9]

COMMENTS AND SOURCES OF TECHNICAL ERROR. The Hct may be falsely increased or decreased for many reasons relating to technical laboratory errors as outlined below.

1. Excess anticoagulant decreases Hct value because of shrinkage of erythrocytes.

2. Insufficient mixing of blood prior to obtaining Hct sample may decrease or increase Hct, depending on which part of specimen (plasma or cells) is principally drawn into microhematocrit tube.

3. Improper sealing of capillary tube decreases Hct because of leakage of specimen; erythrocyte loss is greater than plasma loss.

4. Inadequate centrifugation or allowing tubes to stand too long

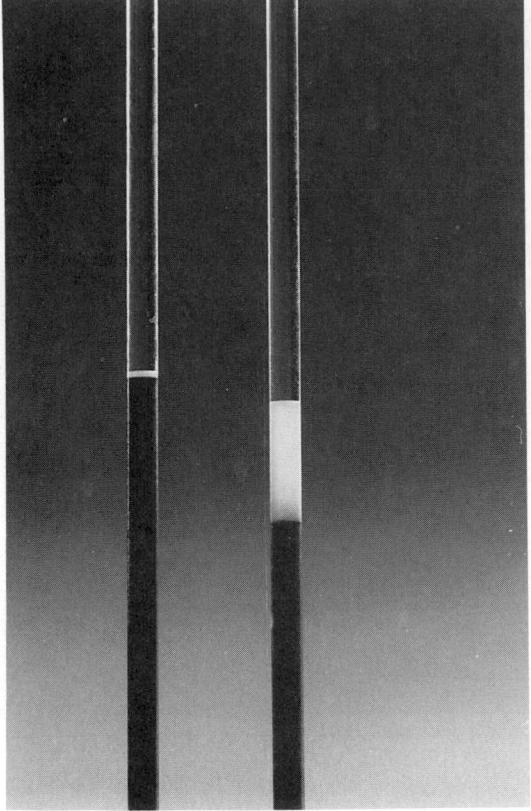

FIGURE 9-5. Comparison of a small (**left**) and large (**right**) buffy coat in hematocrit samples from two patients. A large buffy coat results from increased WBC and platelet counts.

after centrifugation increases Hct. Results should be read within 10 minutes of centrifugation.

5. Including a large buffy coat in the reading increases Hct.
6. Improper use of Hct reader may increase or decrease Hct.
7. Heat sealing of capillary tubes may damage the blood sample and is therefore not recommended.

COMMENTS AND SOURCES OF PHYSIOLOGIC ERROR

1. Trapped plasma may cause the Hct to be falsely increased by as much as 0.02 L/L. (Trapped plasma is the small amount of plasma that remains in the erythrocyte portion of the spun Hct even when proper centrifugal force is obtained.) More plasma is trapped in sickle cell anemia, hypochromic anemia, spherocytosis, macrocytosis, and thalassemia. The amount of plasma trapped increases with the Hct. When determined by fully automated methods, the Hct may be 0.01 to 0.03 L/L lower than the microhematocrit method because it is electronically calculated and therefore is unaffected by trapped plasma.
2. Certain abnormal erythrocyte shapes (*e.g.*, spherocytes and sickle cells) interfere with complete packing.
3. During the first few hours after acute blood loss, both the Hct and Hb appear normal. Therefore, neither is a reliable estimate of the degree of anemia immediately following acute blood loss because the plasma volume has not yet been replaced (Chap. 20). Actually, the Hct and Hb do not reach their minimum levels for several days following acute blood loss.
4. Dehydration can increase the Hct because of fluid loss, which causes a decrease in plasma volume.
5. Specimen collection errors may alter the Hct. Leaving the tourniquet on the arm too long causes hemoconcentration, which falsely increases Hct. Difficult venipuncture or skin puncture may introduce interstitial fluid into the sample, caus-

ing a falsely decreased Hct. Hemolysis also causes a falsely decreased Hct.

6. Refer to Chapter 42 for details on automated methods for hemoglobin and hematocrit.

CORRELATIONS AND CALCULATIONS BASED ON ERYTHROCYTE MEASUREMENTS

Rule of Three

Under ordinary circumstances, it is possible to check the accuracy of the erythrocyte count and Hb and Hct values (manually or by automated instruments) by quick visual inspection of the values. This is accomplished by applying the *"rule of three,"* as shown in Table 9-3. The rule of three applies only to normocytic, normochromic erythrocytes, which can be verified by visual inspection of the blood film. (For erythrocytes that do not fit these criteria, see Chaps. 12 and 13.) If the erythrocytes are found to be abnormal, the automated values cannot be expected to conform to these rules. On the other hand, if the erythrocytes on the blood film appear normal but the automated values do not conform to the rule of three, laboratory personnel should check to ensure that a random error has not occurred (Chap. 46). *Random error* is an error that occurs by chance. An example is sample or blood film misidentification. The possibility of a systematic error should also be considered. Such errors affect all samples equally in a proportionate or constant manner and often involve an instrument malfunction (Chap. 45).

Table 9-3 provides an example of two blood counts. In case A the assay conforms to the rule of three. In case B there appears to be a problem with the Hb: it is unrealistically low because it does not conform to the rules of matching with the erythrocyte count or Hct. In this case, because the problem seems to be isolated to the Hb and the error seems so great, a systematic error should be considered. Reports from specimens run before and after this one should also be checked to see if the Hb was unrealistically low compared with the erythrocyte count and Hct. Problems such as a malfunctioning Hb reading device should be investigated. A control blood sample could also be run at this time if no instrument malfunction can be detected to ensure that the Hb procedure is in control.

Consider an automated report in which the Hb appears to be too high when compared with the erythrocyte count and Hct. If erythrocyte morphology appears normal and the Hb was valid on the samples run before and after this specimen, a common problem to consider is a markedly elevated leukocyte count. In such cases the Hb concentration must be obtained manually (see method described earlier), the solution centrifuged to clear turbidity, and the Hb determined on the supernatant in order to avoid leukocyte interference with the spectrophotometric reading of Hb concentration. Alternatively the Hb can be determined using an instrument such as the HemoCue (see Point of Care Testing section below), which compensates for interference from turbidity.[37]

Whenever the rule of three indicates a problem with any specimen, a systematic approach to investigation of

TABLE 9-3
The Rule of Three

BASIC EQUATIONS

$$3 \times RBC = Hb$$
$$3 \times Hb = HCT \pm 3\ (\%)$$

CASE A: ACCURATE SPECIMEN/NORMOCYTIC, NORMOCHROMIC

Patient Results	Accuracy Check	Confirmation
RBC = 3.0×10^{12}/L	$3 \times 3.0 = 9.0$	RBC checks with Hb
Hb = 9.2 g/dL	$3 \times 9.2 = 27.6$	Hb checks with HCT (26 $\pm$ 3)
HCT = 26% (0.26 L/L)		

CASE B: INACCURATE SPECIMEN OR NOT NORMOCYTIC, NORMOCHROMIC

Patient Results	Accuracy Check	Confirmation
RBC = 4.0×10^{12}/L	$3 \times 4.0 = 12.0$	RBC does not check with Hb
Hb = 3.5 g/dL	$3 \times 3.5 = 10.5$	Hb does not check with HCT (37 $\pm$ 3)
HCT = 37% (0.37 L/L)		

the discrepancy must be undertaken until the nature of the problem is determined. If necessary, corrective action should be taken, whether it involves the specimen or the instrument.

Erythrocyte Indices

In addition to serving as quality control checks on one another, the erythrocyte count, Hb, and Hct can be utilized in calculations to determine the erythrocyte indices: mean corpuscular volume (MCV), mean corpuscular Hb (MCH), and mean corpuscular Hb concentration (MCHC). The indices are used both in quality control (Chap. 45) and in classifying and differentiating anemias (Chap. 10). The diagnostic interpretation of the indices should always be combined with a careful examination of the blood film, because indices are *average* values for many cells examined either manually or electronically.

Mean Corpuscular Volume

PRINCIPLE. MCV indicates the average volume of a single erythrocyte in a given blood sample. It is expressed in SI units (see below) as femtoliters (fL; 1 fL = 10^{-15} L). Formerly, MCV was expressed in μ^3 (see Table 9-6).

CALCULATION AND REFERENCE RANGES

$$MCV = \frac{Hct(\%) \times 10}{RBC\ (10^2/L)}$$

For example, if Hct equals 0.36 L/L (36%) and RBC equals 4.0 $\times 10^{12}$/L, then

$$MCV = \frac{36 \times 10}{4.0} = 90\ fL$$

Refer to Table 9-1 for reference ranges at various ages.[9]

TERMINOLOGY AND INTERPRETATION. Values of 80 to 100 fL are described as normocytic, those less than 80 as microcytic, and those more than 100 as macrocytic.

MCV will be discussed in relation to all anemias and hematologic disorders in appropriate chapters in this text. In general MCV is increased in megaloblastic anemias such as folate or vitamin B_{12} deficiencies. It may also be elevated in nonmegaloblastic macrocytic anemias, which are sometimes caused by chronic hemolytic anemias, liver disease, and hypothyroidism. A decreased MCV is associated with such conditions as iron deficiency, defective iron utilization (anemia of chronic disease), and thalassemia.

COMMENTS AND SOURCES OF ERROR. Because the MCV is, as it says, a mean or average value for many cells examined, a dimorphic population of microcytes and macrocytes, which may be observed on a peripheral blood film, yields an average normal calculated MCV value. This baseline MCV is misleading without the blood film comments. An increased number of reticulocytes, which are larger in volume, may elevate the MCV. However, if the patient's baseline MCV is at the low end of the reference range, the elevation may not be significant enough to put the MCV above the reference range.

Mean Corpuscular Hemoglobin

PRINCIPLE. MCH indicates the mean weight of Hb per erythrocyte, expressed in SI units as picograms (pg; 1 pg = 10^{-12} g). Formerly, MCH was expressed in $\mu\mu g$ (see Table 9-6).

CALCULATION AND REFERENCE RANGES

$$MCH = \frac{Hb\ (g/dL) \times 10}{RBC\ (10^{12}/L)}$$

As an example, if Hb equals 12.0 g/dL and RBC equals 4.0 $\times 10^{12}$/L, then

$$MCH = \frac{12.0 \times 10}{4.0} = 30\ pg$$

Refer to Table 9-1 for reference ranges at various ages.[9]

TERMINOLOGY AND INTERPRETATION. Values of 26 to 34 pg are considered normal, those less than 26 decreased, and those more than 34 increased.

MCH should correlate with the MCV and MCHC. There is a higher MCH in macrocytic anemias because the erythrocytes are larger and carry more Hb. A lower MCH is found in hypochromic anemias and in microcytic anemias unless the erythrocytes are also spherocytic. However, when describing anemias, MCH is rarely used; the MCV and MCHC are more commonly used.

Mean Corpuscular Hemoglobin Concentration

PRINCIPLE. MCHC indicates the average concentration of Hb in the erythrocytes in a specimen. It is expressed in SI units as g/dL. Formerly, MCHC was expressed in percent (see Table 9-6).

CALCULATION AND REFERENCE RANGES

$$MCHC = \frac{Hb\ (g/dL) \times 100}{Hct\ (\%)}$$

As an example, if Hb equals 12.0 g/dL and Hct equals 0.36 L/L (36%), then

$$MCHC = \frac{12.0 \times 100}{36} = 33.3 \text{ g/dL}$$

Refer to Table 9-1 for reference ranges at various ages.[9]

TERMINOLOGY AND INTERPRETATION. Values of 31 to 37 g/dL are considered normochromic, those less than 31 are hypochromic and those more than 37 are hyperchromic.

Hypochromic erythrocytes occur commonly in iron deficiency, thalassemias, and defective iron utilization. Hyperchromic erythrocytes are actually caused by a shape change such as that found in spherocytes. "Hyperchromia" is not used in actual descriptions of erythrocyte morphology in the laboratory (Chap. 8). Erythrocytes cannot accommodate more than 37 g/dL of Hb; therefore, a result above 37 g/dL should be recalculated to ensure that all values were correctly measured and no interfering substances are present (see Sources of Error sections for both Hb and Hct determinations earlier in this chapter).

Problem Solving for Erythrocyte Indices. To obtain accurate erythrocyte indices, the values used in the calculations must be accurate. All of the fully automated cell counters either calculate indices automatically or measure the MCV directly and calculate the Hct and other indices. The erythrocyte count may be falsely decreased in the presence of strong cold agglutinins (Chap. 19), thus falsely elevating the MCV and also causing an abnormal MCH and MCHC. This problem may be eliminated by warming the specimen just before running it on an automated counter.

RETICULOCYTE COUNTS

A reticulocyte is an immature erythrocyte that has lost its nucleus but retains aggregates of ribonucleic acid (RNA) within its ribosomes (Chap. 6). The amount of RNA decreases as the erythrocyte matures. After the normoblast loses its nucleus, the reticulocyte usually remains 2 days in the bone marrow and 1 day in the peripheral blood before becoming a mature erythrocyte. The reticulocyte count, with its associated corrections, can be used to assess bone marrow erythropoietic activity.

Routine Reticulocyte Count

PRINCIPLE AND SPECIMEN REQUIREMENTS. The ribosomal RNA of reticulocytes must be stained supravitally; that is, with the erythrocytes in the living state. A *reticulocyte* (Fig. 9-6) is defined as any non-nucleated erythrocyte that contains two or more particles of blue-stained, granulofilamentous material after new methylene blue (supravital) staining.[23] Whole blood anticoagulated with EDTA is recommended. Capillary blood is also acceptable.

REAGENTS AND EQUIPMENT. No special equipment is required, but enumeration may be facilitated by use of a calibrated disk placed in the ocular of the microscope (see procedure below). See Chapter 43 for a discussion on reticulocyte analysis by flow cytometry, which is more rapid, accurate, and precise.

Supravital stains in common use include new methylene blue and brilliant cresyl blue. New methylene blue is recommended by the NCCLS.[27] The stain should be filtered before use.

QUALITY CONTROL. A tri-level whole blood control for reticulocytes called ReticChex is available from Streck Laboratories (Omaha, NE). There are four important reasons for discrepancies

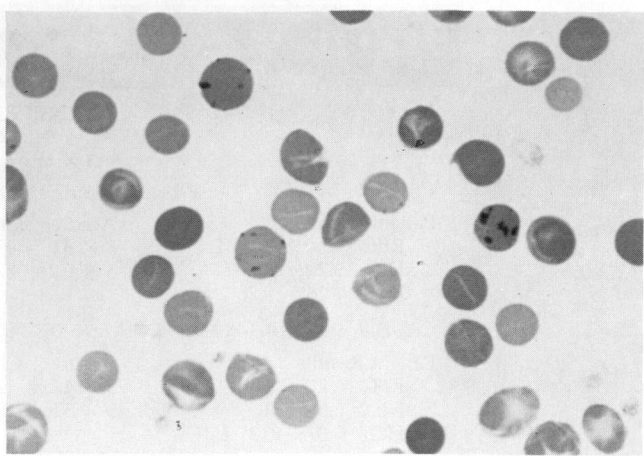

FIGURE 9-6. Reticulocytes are non-nucleated erythrocytes that contain two or more particles of blue-stained, granulofilamentous material after new methylene blue (supravital) staining.

in reticulocyte counting: (1) Interobserver variation in the definition of a reticulocyte (at least two ribosomal remnants should be seen in an erythrocyte); (2) Size of sample evaluated (at least 1000 erythrocytes should be examined); (3) Type of film examined (wedge *versus* spun); and (4) Lack of standardized area if a calibrated disk is not used (see below).

Until uniformity of these variables can be achieved, there are several ways to increase the accuracy of reticulocyte counts. One technologist can count 500 cells on each of two slides, or two technologists can each count 500 or 1000 cells independently. Precision limits between slides should be established. It has been suggested that results obtained by two technologists should agree within 20%.[7]

On high reticulocyte counts the percentage of reticulocytes should correlate roughly with the number of polychromatophilic erythrocytes seen on the peripheral blood film. The higher the reticulocyte count, the more precise the measurement.

SPECIMEN PREPARATION
1. Mix equal amounts of whole blood and stain in a small tube. The amounts do not have to be exactly equal. A slightly higher proportion of blood should be used for specimens with low hematocrits and a slightly lower proportion of blood for specimens with very high hematocrits.[7]
2. Incubate mixture at room temperature. *Note:* Although many references state that the mixture should incubate for no less than 10 minutes[7] to as much as 15 minutes,[6] one report notes that staining is rapid and need not be done for more than 2 minutes.[23] In flow cytometric methods (*e.g.*, the Sysmex R-1000 [Sysmex Corp, Long Grove, IL]), staining is almost instantaneous.
3. After incubation, thoroughly mix the blood and stain solution and immediately prepare two or three films. Allow films to air dry.

There are several methods for counting reticulocytes. The methods presented here are the routine light microscope method and the calibrated Miller disk method.

PROCEDURE—ROUTINE LIGHT MICROSCOPE METHOD
1. Switch to 100× oil immersion objective (oculars should be standard 10×).
2. Select an area where erythrocytes are close but not overlapping, and reticulocytes appear to be well stained.
3. Count the reticulocytes and erythrocytes in each field using the same pattern normally used for performing a leukocyte

differential count (Chap. 24). Reticulocytes should also be counted as erythrocytes.

4. Continue counting until 1000 erythrocytes have been observed.

5. Calculate reticulocytes using this formula:

$$\text{Reticulocyte (\%)} = \frac{\text{No. of Reticulocytes}}{1000 \text{ RBC observed}} \times 100$$

For example, if 10 reticulocytes were seen among 1000 RBCs, the reticulocyte percentage would be calculated as:

$$\text{Reticulocyte (\%)} = \frac{10}{1000} \times 100 = 1.0\%$$

PROCEDURE—CALIBRATED MILLER DISK METHOD

1. A calibrated Miller disk is placed in one microscope ocular to aid in the counting process. The Miller disk appears in the field of view with two squares, one inside the other (Fig. 9-7), the smaller square (B) being one-ninth the size of the larger square (A). Locate an acceptable area to begin count, as in standard reticulocyte count method.

2. Count the erythrocytes in the small square B and the reticulocytes in the large square A in 20 fields where cells are close but not touching or overlapping. A reticulocyte in square B is counted as an erythrocyte and is included in the reticulocyte count, since square B is a part of the large square A. Cells that touch the top or left lines in both squares A and B are counted; those that touch the bottom or right lines are not counted (as in manual cell counts, see Figure 24-4). At this point, theoretically, the number of reticulocytes in 4500 erythrocytes has been counted. If larger numbers of red cells (and reticulocytes) are counted, the precision of the reticuloycte count will, of course, improve.

3. Compute reticulocyte count as

$$\text{Reticulocyte (\%)} = \frac{\text{Total reticulocytes in square A} \times 100}{\text{Total RBCs in square B} \times 9}$$

For example, if a total of 150 reticulocytes were seen in square A (including those in square B) after counting 500 RBCs in 20 fields of square B, the reticulocyte (%) would be calculated as:

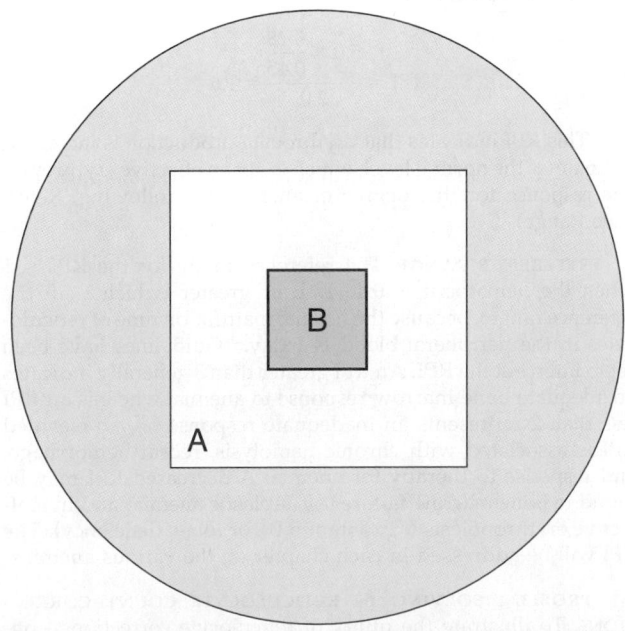

FIGURE 9-7. Miller disk for microscopic reticulocyte counting.

$$\text{Reticulocyte (\%)} = \frac{150}{500 \times 9} \times 100 = 3.3\%$$

Any calibrated disk may be used in the same manner. Refer to manufacturer's instructions.

RETICULOCYTE REFERENCE RANGES. Reticulocyte counts are expressed as a percentage, as shown in the calculations above, or in absolute numbers per liter. The reference range for adults in some laboratories is 0.5% to 1.5%, whereas in others, a broader range of 0.5% to 2.0% is used. The range may be slightly higher in women[10] and persons living at an altitude higher than 6000 feet above sea level.[27] It is higher in newborns (2.0%–6.0%) but drops to adult levels within 1 to 2 weeks.[25] In absolute numbers the adult reference range is approximately 10 to 110 $\times 10^9/\text{L}$.[27]

COMMENTS AND SOURCES OF TECHNICAL ERROR

1. When using the Miller disk, failure to follow the "edge" rule may yield erroneous results; that is, counting reticulocytes touching all four lines of either of the two squares. Only reticulocytes touching the top or left lines should be counted.

2. The use of a Romanowsky counterstain is no longer advised because it may obscure the supravitally stained granulofilamentous material of the reticulocyte.[27]

3. Refractive artifacts in erythrocytes caused by moisture in the air and poor drying of the blood film must not be confused with RNA filaments, which do not appear refractory when adjusting the fine focus on the microscope. The RNA filaments simply disappear when out of focus.

4. Blood and stain must be well mixed before making films, because reticulocytes have a lower specific gravity than mature erythrocytes and thus go to the top of the mixture during incubation.

5. Increased levels of glucose in the blood may inhibit staining of reticulocytes.[7]

6. Pappenheimer, Howell-Jolly, and Heinz bodies will also stain supravitally. (See Figs. 8-28 and 8-29 for a summary of the differentiating factors among and between these inclusions and those of the reticulocyte.) Howell-Jolly bodies stain supravitally as a deep purple and appear either singly or in pairs. If Pappenheimer or Howell-Jolly bodies are suspected, examination of the Romanowsky-stained peripheral blood film will confirm their presence, because these inclusions will stain, whereas reticulocyte granulofilamentous material will not. Pappenheimer bodies must also be confirmed by an iron stain; they are the most difficult to distinguish from reticulocytes. Heinz bodies do not stain with Romanowsky stain. However, on supravitally stained films, they stain a light blue-green and may be differentiated from reticulocytes because they usually are found on the periphery of the erythrocyte and are usually larger than ribosomal RNA. Heinz bodies often make the cell look like a pitted golf ball (see Figs. 8-29 and 17-7).

COMMENTS AND SOURCES OF PHYSIOLOGIC ERROR. The reticulocyte percentage may be misleading if one does not consider the degree of anemia or of intense erythropoietic stimulation. The reticulocyte count may be truly elevated, indicating increased effective erythropoiesis, or it may only appear elevated because the total number of erythrocytes is decreased. Therefore, reticulocyte counts should be corrected for anemia. Several corrections may be made to this percentage taking into consideration total erythrocyte count, Hct, and early release of reticulocytes from the bone marrow. These corrections are considered next.

Absolute Reticulocyte Count

PRINCIPLE. The *absolute reticulocyte count (ARC)* reflects the actual number of reticulocytes in one liter of whole blood.[23] This measurement is beneficial in monitoring bone marrow transplant patients and patients on chemotherapy. It is not yet routinely reported; however, some flow cytometric methods automatically measure the red cell count and report reticulocytes in absolute numbers.

CALCULATION AND REFERENCE RANGE

$$ARC = \frac{Reticulocyte\ (\%)}{100} \times RBC(10^{12}/L)$$

For example, if a patient's reticulocyte count is 4% and the RBC count is $3.30 \times 10^{12}/L$, the ARC would be

$$ARC = \frac{(4) \times (3.30 \times 10^{12}/L)}{100} = 132 \times 10^9/L$$

Values between 10 and $110 \times 10^9/L$ are considered to fall within the reference range.[27]

Corrected Reticulocyte Count

PRINCIPLE. The *corrected reticulocyte count (CRC)* is sometimes referred to as a reticulocyte index (RI) or hematocrit correction. The percentage of reticulocytes may appear increased because of early reticulocyte release into the circulation or because of a decrease in the number of mature red cells in circulation. The CRC corrects the observed reticulocyte count to a "normal" Hct of 0.45 L/L to correct for the degree of anemia.

CALCULATION

$$CRC = Reticulocytes\ (\%) \times \frac{Hct\ (L/L)}{0.45\ L/L}$$

For example, if a patient's reticulocyte count is 4.5% and the Hct is 0.30 L/L, the CRC would be

$$CRC = 4.5 \times \frac{0.30}{0.45} = 3.0\%$$

REFERENCE RANGE. The expected value of CRC depends on the degree of anemia. Normally, CRC should be approximately 1%. Patients with a Hct of 0.35 L/L are expected to have a CRC of 2 to 3%; those at or below 0.25 L/L should have a CRC greater than 3%.

COMMENTS. CRC is most often used as part of the reticulocyte production index (RPI) calculation (discussed below). RPI is clinically more useful than CRC.

Reticulocyte Production Index

PRINCIPLE. RPI (also known as shift correction) provides a further refinement of the CRC. It is a general indicator of the rate of effective erythrocyte production in anemias. During intense erythropoietic stress the maturation time in the bone marrow may be shortened from the usual 3.5 days to as little as 1 day, allowing the reticulocytes to circulate longer than usual in the peripheral blood (Fig. 9-8). Cells released early to the peripheral blood are referred to as shift cells and have a polychromatophilic appearance (see Color Plate 9-1).

Under such intense erythropoietic stress, the number of reticulocytes in the peripheral blood may be markedly increased without a corresponding increase in the bone marrow. Because the life span of the reticulocyte in the peripheral blood corresponds to the degree of anemia, the RPI is corrected for both the Hct and maturation time in the peripheral blood.

CALCULATION

$$RPI = \frac{Reticulocytes\ (\%) \times \frac{Hct\ (L/L)}{0.45\ L/L}}{Maturation\ time\ in\ peripheral\ blood}$$

or

$$RPI = \frac{CRC}{Maturation\ time\ in\ peripheral\ blood}$$

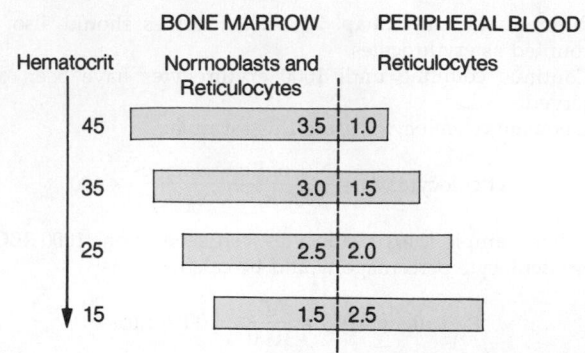

FIGURE 9-8. Correlation of hematocrit with marrow and blood reticulocyte maturation times. Ordinarily, erythropoietin increases in proportion to the degree of anemia present. With increasing erythropoietin stimulation, the maturation time of the marrow erythroblasts and marrow reticulocytes shortens progressively from a normal of 3.5 days to as little as 1.5 to 1.0 day. Much of this shortening is secondary to a shift of marrow reticulocytes into the circulation. This results in a prolongation of the maturation time of circulating blood reticulocytes from a normal of 1 day to as much as 2.5 to 3.0 days with severe anemia. This needs to be taken into account when calculating the reticulocyte production index. The maturation time values shown for the blood retinculocytes can be used as a correction factor in this calculation (see text). (From Hillman RS, Finch CA: Red Cell Manual. Philadelphia, FA Davis, 1985, with permission.)

The approximate maturation time varies with Hct as follows (Fig. 9-8), and these figures are to be used in RPI calculation[18,22]:

Hct (L/L)	Maturation Time (Days)
0.40–0.45	1.0
0.35–0.39	1.5
0.25–0.34	2.0
0.15–0.24	2.5
<0.15	3.0

For example, if a patient has a reticulocyte count of 5.0% and a Hct of 0.28 L/L, the maturation time correction factor is 2.0. The RPI calculation is

$$RPI = \frac{5.0 \times \frac{0.28}{0.45}}{2.0} = 1.6$$

This RPI indicates that erythrocyte production is increased to 1.6 times the normal level, which is not an effective erythropoietic response for this degree of anemia (see following, Reference Range).

REFERENCE RANGE. The reference range for the RPI is 1 when the hematocrit is 0.40 L/L or greater (which is in the reference range), because the normal maturation time of reticulocytes in the peripheral blood is 1 day.[23] Guidelines have been set to interpret the RPI. An RPI greater than 3 generally indicates an adequate bone marrow response to anemia, whereas an RPI less than 2 represents an inadequate response.[17,23] An elevated RPI is associated with chronic hemolysis, recent hemorrhage, and response to therapy for anemia. A decreased RPI may be found in bone marrow failure (*e.g.*, aplastic anemia) and in ineffective erythropoiesis (*e.g.*, vitamin B_{12} or folate deficiency). The RPI will be addressed in each chapter on the various anemias.

PROBLEM SOLVING IN RETICULOCYTE COUNT CORRECTIONS. To illustrate the utility of reticulocyte corrections, consider the example in Table 9-4. At first glance the 4.0% uncor-

TABLE 9-4
Sample Calculations of Absolute Reticulocyte Count (ARC), Corrected Reticulocyte Count (CRC), and Reticulocyte Production Index (RPI) from Sample Patient Results

	Calculation/Result	Comments
Patient RBC	$2.1 \times 10^{12}/L$	Anemic
Hct	0.18 L/L	Anemic
Reticulocyte	4.0%	Increased
ARC	$\dfrac{(4.0 \times 2.1 \times 10^{12}/L)}{100} = 84.0 \times 10^{9}/L$	Inadequate for 0.18 L/L Hct
CRC	$\dfrac{4.0 \times 0.18}{0.45} = 1.6\%$	Inadequate for 0.18 L/L Hct
RPI	$\dfrac{4.0 \times \left(\dfrac{0.18}{0.45}\right)}{2.5} = 0.64$	Inadequate for 0.18 L/L Hct

rected reticulocyte count seems to indicate an adequate marrow response, but after appropriate corrections, the RPI of 0.64 indicates that there is an inadequate response for the degree of anemia.

COMMENTS. There are several other methods of reticulocyte counting, some of which involve automated instruments that identify reticulocytes utilizing pattern recognition.[15,33] Pattern recognition instruments are not available for purchase at this time; however, many of these instruments are still in use in the United States. Flow cytometry (Chap. 43), combined with fluorescent staining techniques, increases the possibility of a more accurate and precise assessment of effective erythrocyte production.[34-36] These methods count large numbers of cells, reducing statistical error, and are capable of assessing the degree of maturation of the reticulocyte population. Both pattern recognition and flow cytometry have been found to be acceptable alternatives to manual reticulocyte counts.[15] The reader is referred to Chapter 10 for further discussion of reticulocytes and RPI in anemia.

ERYTHROCYTE SEDIMENTATION RATE

PRINCIPLE. The ESR is a measure of the degree of settling of erythrocytes in plasma in an anticoagulated whole-blood specimen during a specified period of time. Erythrocyte rouleaux formation is enhanced by increased concentrations of fibrinogen or of alpha or beta globulins, all of which increase the ESR. In general, the ESR is directly proportional to the size or mass of the falling red cells (*e.g.*, red cells that form rouleaux in certain diseases are heavier and therefore have an increased ESR) and inversely proportional to plasma viscosity (*i.e.*, the higher the viscosity, the lower the ESR). Normally erythrocytes settle slowly because normal red cells do not form rouleaux, and therefore their mass is not increased.

SPECIMEN REQUIREMENTS. Whole blood anticoagulated with EDTA drawn atraumatically within no more than 30 seconds is the recommended specimen for performance of the modified Westergren method,[31] since EDTA blood is readily available in most laboratories. Some laboratories prefer the original Westergren method, which calls for drawing blood into 3.8% sodium citrate as the anticoagulant. A special vacuum collection tube is available that allows for the automatic collection of four parts blood into one part 3.8% sodium citrate. No matter which anticoagulant is used, the specimen must be well mixed immediately after drawing.

Blood kept at room temperature must be set up within 4 hours; at 4°C specimens have been reported to be stable for up to 12 hours.[13] In any case, a specimen should be brought to room temperature and well mixed before testing.[31]

Two principal methods have been used for the ESR: the Westergren and the Wintrobe methods. The Westergren method is recommended by both the NCCLS[31] and the International Committee for Standardization in Haematology (ICSH).[20] Both methods will be discussed below, as well as a disposable Westergren ESR method that has gained popularity but may be slightly more expensive. The Ves-Matic automated ESR system will also be discussed.

Westergren ESR Method

EQUIPMENT. The Westergren pipette, as specified by the NCCLS,[31] should be made of disposable glass or plastic with a sufficient length to allow for 200 mm of red cell sedimentation. The plastic must not show adhesive properties toward blood cells. The tube bore (internal diameter) should be not less than 2.55 mm, and tube bore uniformity should be constant (within 5%) throughout the tube length. Markings on the tube should extend from 200 mm at the bottom up to 0 at the top of the scale in divisions of 1 mm.

The rack to hold the Westergren tubes must not allow leakage from the pipettes and must be held motionless in a vertical position. Racks equipped with a leveling bubble or plumb box ensure this vertical position to within ±2°.

QUALITY CONTROL. The NCCLS has published a reference ESR method whose procedure can be found in the NCCLS document on ESR methods.[31] The reference method requires an undiluted specimen anticoagulated with EDTA with a Hct of ≤0.35 L/L. It is recommended that whenever pipettes, personnel, or other variables related to the ESR procedure are changed, and at periodic intervals, the reference ESR method should be performed. In brief, the NCCLS reference ESR method and the laboratory's working ESR procedure (*e.g.*, the Wintrobe method) are performed on the same specimen simultaneously. The NCCLS ESR reference procedure[31] calls for testing of an undiluted EDTA sample in a disposable Westergren pipette. The NCCLS document contains a table showing how to convert the reference ESR reading to an expected result for the laboratory's working procedure. This expected result is then compared with the actual results obtained using the laboratory's working procedure to ensure accurate results.

PROCEDURE. The original and modified Westergren methods differ only in the anticoagulant used and the time at which the blood is diluted; both methods will be discussed in this section.

1. Specimen Preparation
   A. Original Westergren Method. Whole blood is drawn into 3.8% sodium citrate (one volume of sodium citrate to four volumes of blood) using a specially prepared vacuum collection tube (available commercially). No further dilution is performed when using this type of specimen.
   B. Modified Westergren Method. This is the specimen recommended by the NCCLS and ICSH. Mix EDTA-anticoagulated whole blood very thoroughly. Standard 10 to 12 × 75-mm tubes containing 5 mL of blood should be inverted a minimum of eight times; nonstandard tubes may need more inversions. Combine 2.0 mL of well-mixed EDTA-anticoagulated whole blood with 0.5 mL of 0.85% NaCl. This method is much more convenient in most laboratories because EDTA-anticoagulated blood is readily available.
2. Place blood container in pipette rack directly under a hole. Insert a Westergren pipette through the hole into the blood mixture.
3. Firmly press a safety bulb or hand pump on top of the Westergren pipette and aspirate the blood to the 0 mark. If using a plugged pipette (Ulster Scientific, Highland, NY), the plug should be well soaked with blood. Repeat for all specimens to be tested.
4. After exactly 60 minutes, record the distance, in millimeters, from the bottom of the plasma meniscus (at 0 mark) to the top of the column of sedimented erythrocytes. Do not include the buffy coat (leukocytes and platelets) in the reading.
5. Report results as "ESR (Westergren, 1 hour) = ___ mm." Note that this test does not measure a rate (*i.e.*, distance per time interval [mm/h]). Rather, it measures distance after a specified time.[31]
6. Dispose of all Westergren tubes containing blood carefully in biohazardous puncture-proof waste containers.

DISPOSABLE WESTERGREN ESR SYSTEM. Several completely disposable systems are available for performing ESRs. One such system is the Dispette (Ulster Scientific, Highland, New York) (Fig. 9-9). This system automatically dilutes the EDTA blood specimen. The tube has a safety plug made of nonwettable, and therefore nonabsorbent, material that provides automatic zeroing (at the 0-mm mark) of the specimen; any excess blood adheres to the plug, which also holds the column of blood in place. The procedure for this system is shown in Figure 9-9.

WESTERGREN ESR REFERENCE RANGES. Each laboratory should establish its own Westergren ESR reference ranges. Approximate values are as follows (1 h = 1 hour):

Males[4]	<50 years	1 h = 0–15 mm
	>50 years	1 h = 0–20 mm
Females[4]	<50 years	1 h = 0–20 mm
	>50 years	1 h = 0–30 mm
Children[38]		1 h = 0–10 mm

Among people older than 65 years, the reference range may be even higher; the reason is not apparent.[5,14]

Wintrobe ESR Method

SPECIMEN REQUIREMENTS. Whole blood anticoagulated with EDTA or ammonium-potassium oxalate is used.

EQUIPMENT. The Wintrobe tube (Fig. 9-10) is 115 mm long with an internal bore of 3 mm. It has two series of graduations from 0 to 10, one ascending and one descending. For the sedimentation rate, the scale on the left side of the tube is used (0 is at the top). The scale on the right (10 at the top) was historically used to read a macrohematocrit, which is no longer considered an acceptable procedure.

GENERAL PROCEDURE
1. Fill a Wintrobe tube to 0 mark using a disposable Pasteur pipette. The column of blood must be bubble free.
2. Place tube in the rack and set timer for 60 minutes.
3. After 60 minutes read the level of sedimented erythrocytes from the scale on the left side of tube and record as ESR (Wintrobe, 1 hour) = ___ mm. Each cm = 10 mm.

REFERENCE RANGE. The range for males is 1 hour = 0 to 9 mm; that for females is 1 hour = 0 to 20 mm. The range for children is 1 hour = 0 to 13 mm.[39]

COMMENTS AND SOURCES OF ERROR
1. ESR is considered a nonspecific indicator of tissue damage, and it is increased in a number of disorders. Some of the more significant conditions are listed in Table 9-5.
2. Because the ESR depends on the ability of erythrocytes to form rouleaux, conditions in which rouleaux formation is inhibited, such as sickle cell anemia, Hb CC, and spherocytosis, may be accompanied by normal sedimentation rates (*i.e.*, the ESR may not be as elevated as expected for the degree of anemia in these specimens).
3. The ESR should be performed within 4 hours of blood collection. Leaving the specimen for more than 4 hours at room temperature may cause erythrocytes to become spherical and inhibit rouleaux formation. Specimens containing EDTA anticoagulant that are refrigerated may be used for ESR testing up to 12 hours after collection but must be brought to room temperature before testing.
4. Overanticoagulation causes lower values.
5. The rack that holds the tubes must be level. Even slight tilting of the tube increases the ESR. The table on which the rack sits must be free from vibrations.
6. If the area of RBC–plasma separation is hazy, read the level where complete RBC packing is apparent.
7. The testing area must be free from direct sunlight or drafts. Marked changes in ambient temperature will increase (in high temperatures) or decrease (in low temperatures) the ESR.
8. The presence of anemia invalidates the ESR as a tool to detect rouleaux (as an indication of some disease process), since anemia itself increases the ESR value. Correction of ESR results for anemia is not recommended.
9. Inadequate mixing of the blood specimen prior to dilution with 0.85% NaCl in the modified Westergren method is a major source of error.

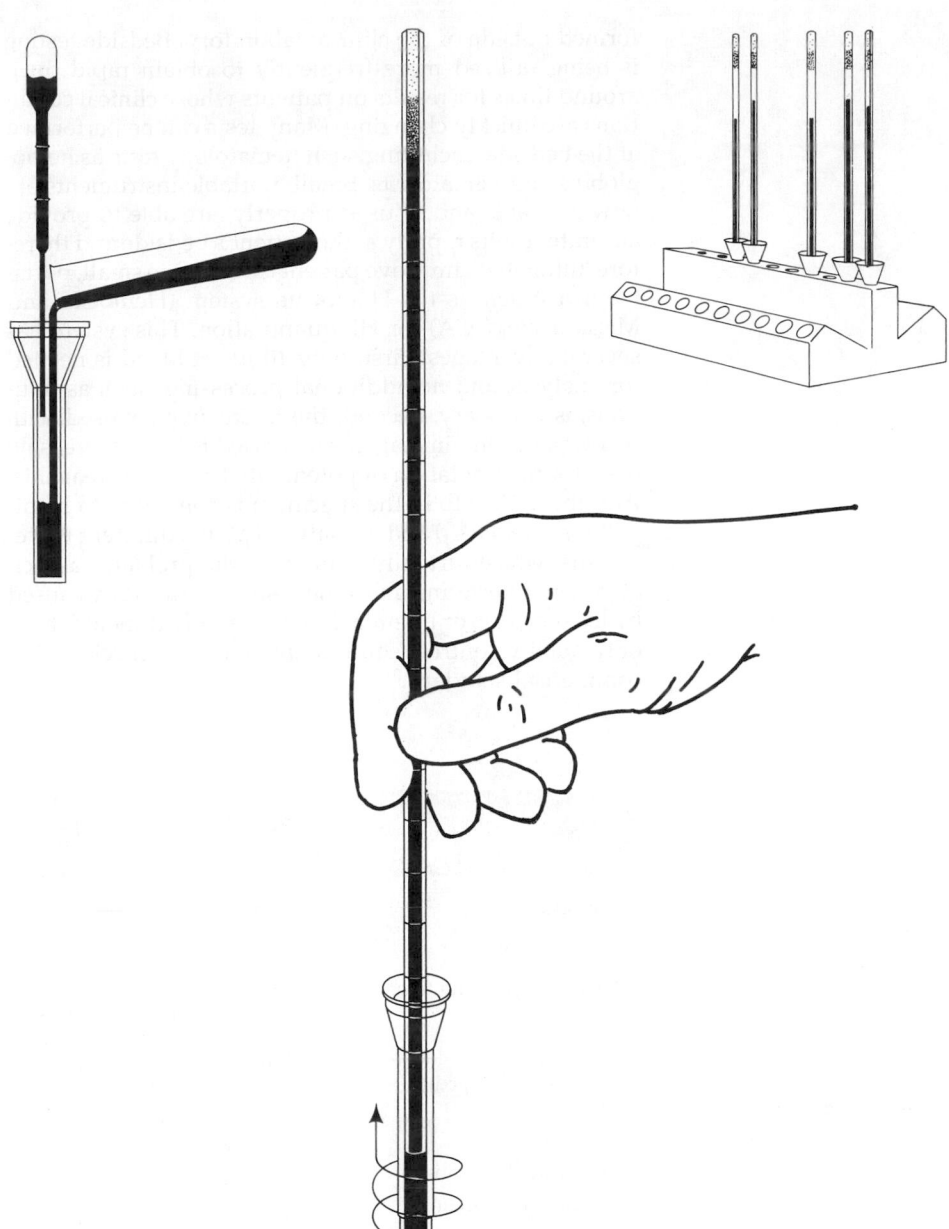

FIGURE 9-9. Westergren Dispette System for erythrocyte sedimentation rate (ESR) determination. (**Left**) After mixing 4 parts EDTA-anticoagulated whole blood with 1 part 0.85% saline, the mixture is poured into vial. (**Center**) Dispette is placed in vial using a twisting motion until blood reaches bottom of safety automatic zeroing plug. (**Right**) Vial and Dispette are placed vertically in a special rack for 60 minutes before reading the ESR. (Courtesy of Ulster Scientific, Highland, NY.)

10. Care must be taken when performing the whole blood dilution with 0.85% NaCl to ensure that the correct dilution is made. Improper dilutions are another major source of error.

Ves-Matic Automated ESR System

EQUIPMENT AND SPECIMEN REQUIREMENTS. The Ves-Matic and Mini-Ves (HiChem Diagnostics, Smithfield, RI) are automated, completely closed systems for erythrocyte sedimentation determination. Specimens are drawn directly into specialized Vacu-Tec tubes, which also serve as the measurement cuvettes. The automated system can give results in 20 minutes. The system is able to produce results rapidly because the sedimentation rate is accelerated by use of an 18° slant. The changes in the opacity of the blood column are measured as the sedimentation occurs, and the results, which are automatically read by an opto-electronic sensor, are comparable to those of a 1-hour Westergren

sedimentation rate. Three models are available, depending on the laboratory's ESR workload and needs, and each of the models offer improved safety for the laboratory worker due to less manipulation of the specimen and the walkaway convenience of an automated system (Fig. 9-11).[26]

Specimens are drawn directly into Vacu-Tec tubes, which draw 1 mL of blood that is anticoagulated with sodium citrate. See manufacturer's instructions for details on operation of the equipment.

Comparison of Erythrocyte Sedimentation Rate Methods

The Westergren method is more sensitive for higher ESRs, but the Wintrobe method is more sensitive for the lower but still abnormal ESRs. The Wintrobe method requires a smaller amount of blood and involves no dilution. In

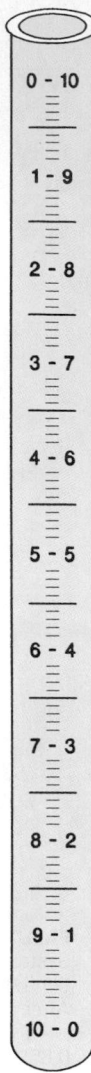

FIGURE 9-10. Wintrobe tube for erythrocyte sedimentation rate determination.

formed outside of the clinical laboratory. Bedside testing is being utilized more frequently to obtain rapid turn-around times for results on patients whose clinical conditions are quickly changing. Many tests can be performed at the bedside, including such hematology tests as hemoglobins and hematocrits. Small, portable instruments are now available and, if used properly, are able to provide accurate results rapidly at the patient's bedside and therefore, ultimately, improve patient care.[1,16] One small, portable instrument is the HemoCue system (HemoCue Inc, Mission Viejo, CA) for Hb quantitation. This system has several advantages. First, only 10 μL of blood is needed for analysis, and no additional processing, such as dilutions, is necessary. Second, the microcuvettes used with this system contain reagents in a dried form so there is no need for manipulation of potentially hazardous reagents. And third, the Hb in the specimen is converted to hemiglobinazide (HiN_3) and is analyzed at two different wavelengths, which virtually eliminates the problems associated with interfering substances such as turbidity caused by leukocytosis or lipemia. It is a small instrument whose only quality control requirement is a daily check with a commercial standard.[37]

addition, once the ESR has been read, the Wintrobe tube can be centrifuged, and blood films can be made from the buffy coat if necessary. However, because of the shorter column of blood, the Wintrobe method is not as sensitive for the higher ESRs as the Westergren method. The disposable ESR methods have the advantage of disposable equipment and ease of setup.

The Ves-Matic system has the advantages of being a closed (less hazardous) system, of providing rapid results in comparison to the other methods, and the convenience of disposable equipment. However, it does require a special analyzer and specialized Vacu-Tec collection tubes.

POINT OF CARE TESTING

Point of care (POC) testing, bedside testing, decentralized testing, ancillary testing, and alternate-site testing are all terms that are currently used to describe testing per-

TABLE 9-5
Expected ESR in Various Conditions

Condition	Comments
ESR INCREASED	
Inflammatory conditions	Associated with elevated plasma proteins, in particular, fibrinogen and α and β globulins
Acute and chronic infections	
Rheumatic fever	
Rheumatoid arthritis	
Myocardial infarction	
Nephrosis	
Tuberculosis	
Multiple myeloma	
Waldenström's macroglobulinemia	
Subacute bacterial endocarditis	
Hepatitis	
Menstruation	
Pregnancy	After the third month
ESR NORMAL	
Polycythemia	
Spherocytes	When large numbers present in peripheral blood
Sickle cells	When large numbers present in peripheral blood
Sickle cell anemia	
Hemoglobin CC disease	
Hereditary spherocytosis	

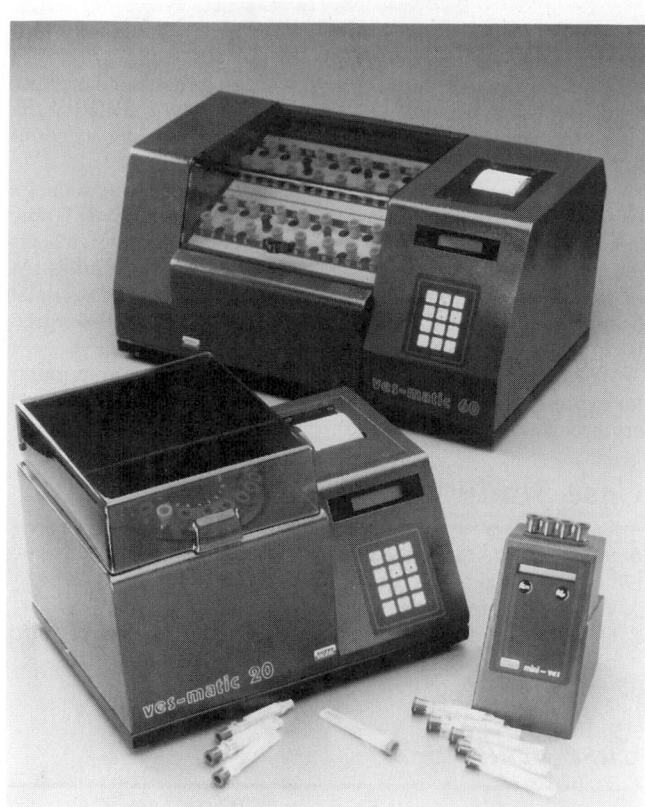

FIGURE 9-11. The Ves-Matic automated ESR system, a completely closed system for erythrocyte sedimentation rate (ESR) determination. Pictured are the three models of the Ves-Matic system that are currently available. The Mini-Ves runs 4 samples concurrently, while the Ves-Matic 20 and Ves-Matic 60 can simultaneously run 20 and 60 samples, respectively. The specialized collection tubes are also pictured (black-stoppered tubes in the foreground) along with the quality control tubes (orange-stoppered tubes). (Courtesy of HiChem Diagnostics, Smithfield, RI.)

TABLE 9-6

Common Prefixes Indicating Multiples and Their Equivalents and Conventional Unit with SI Unit Report Format for Hematologic Measurements

Prefix		Multiple	Equivalents		
deci (d)	=	10^{-1}	1 dL	=	1×10^{-1} L = 0.1 L
milli (m)	=	10^{-3}	1 mL	=	1×10^{-3} L = 0.001 L
micro (μ)	=	10^{-6}	1 μL	=	1×10^{-6} L = 0.000001 L
pico (p)	=	10^{-12}	1 pg	=	1×10^{-12} g = 0.000000000001 g
femto (f)	=	10^{-15}	1 fL	=	1×10^{-15} L = 0.000000000000001 L
			1 mm^3	=	1.00003 μL*

	Conventional Units Report Format	Example (Conventional)	SI Units Report Format	Example (SI)
WBC	$\times 10^3/$mm^3 or $\times 10^3/$uL	$4.5 \times 10^3/\mu$L	$\times 10^9/$L	$4.5 \times 10^9/$L
RBC	$\times 10^6/$mm^3 or $\times 10^6/$uL	$5.21 \times 10^6/\mu$L	$\times 10^{12}/$L	$5.21 \times 10^{12}/$L
Hb†	g/dL	15.4 g/dL	mmol/L	2.39 mmol/L
HCT	%	45.1%	L/L	0.451 L/L
MCV	μ^3 or μm^3	88 μ^3 or μm^3	fL	88 fL
MCH	$\mu\mu$g	29 $\mu\mu$g	pg	29 pg
MCHC	%	33%	g/dL	33 g/dL
PLT	$\times 10^3/$mm^3 or $\times 10^3/$uL	$182 \times 10^3/\mu$L	$\times 10^9/$L	$182 \times 10^9/$L

* The difference between 1 mm^3 and 1 μL is so insignificant that the two volumes are considered equivalent. Therefore, conventionally, cells have been reported using either cells/mm^3 or cells/μL as indicated for WBC, RBC, and PLT.

†Hb will be reported in g/dL in this text because the conversion from conventional to SI units is not easily translated or compared with RBC or HCT values using the rule of three, as can be seen from the SI unit example. The multiplication factor to convert conventional Hb to SI units is 0.155 (in the example above, 15.4 g/dL × 0.155 = 2.39 mmol/L).

UNITS OF HEMATOLOGIC MEASUREMENT

In recent years the hematology community has been steered away from using conventional units for hematologic measurements to using the International System of Units (SI; from the French *Système International d'Unités*) to promote worldwide communication in laboratory measurements.[24,30] Throughout this text SI units are used for measurement of leukocytes, erythrocytes, platelets, and hematocrit, all of which are easy to translate from conventional units. In addition, the SI unit of measurement will be used for erythrocyte indices.

Conventional units of measure used in hematology and their SI equivalents are listed in Table 9-6. Table 9-6 also presents an overview of all common hematologic measurements with examples in their conventional format and their SI unit equivalents. It is easy to see that conversions are simple, requiring no calculation—just a change in unit format (with the exception of Hb, which requires multiplication by 0.155 to obtain the SI unit equivalent). Fortunately, the International Committee for Standardization in Haematology has recommended that the convention g/dL be used instead of SI units for Hb. The NCCLS has published a report summarizing many laboratory measurements according to their conventional units of expression and the proposed SI units.[30]

CHAPTER SUMMARY

Laboratory tests to assess the qualitative and quantitative adequacy of erythrocytes include hemoglobin (Hb), hematocrit (Hct), erythrocyte count, erythrocyte indices, reticulocyte count, and sedimentation rate. The Hb concentration provides an estimate of the oxygen-carrying capacity of the blood. The standard method for manual and automated quantitation is based on the cyanmethemoglobin reaction. When quantitated manually, Hb concentration must be determined on the basis of a standard curve generated by each laboratory using the cyanmethemoglobin standard.

Errors in Hb determination may be caused by poor technique, spectrophotometer malfunction, reagent deterioration, or abnormal specimens. Specimens may be turbid because of lipemia or elevated leukocyte counts. Turbidity may cause false increases in Hb readings; however, these problems may be overcome by using special manual techniques.

Hematocrit refers to the packed cell volume of whole blood. The timer, rpm indicator, brushes, and minimum time to achieve maximum packing must be checked periodically for each microhematocrit centrifuge to ensure accurate results. When reading an Hct, a number of errors may be made. For example, the buffy coat, which contains leukocytes and platelets, must not be included in the Hct value.

The rule of three demonstrates the correlation of Hb, Hct, and the erythrocyte count to check the accuracy of manual or automated methods (Table 9-3). Only normochromic, normocytic erythrocytes can be expected to conform to this rule.

Erythrocyte indices aid in the diagnosis of anemias. They include mean corpuscular volume (MCV), mean corpuscular Hb (MCH), and mean corpuscular Hb concentration (MCHC). The MCV indicates that the average erythrocyte is either normocytic, macrocytic, or microcytic. The MCH indicates the average weight of Hb per erythrocyte. The MCHC determines whether erythrocytes are normochromic, hypochromic, or hyperchromic

(the last condition is not normally reported). Indices are also helpful in quality control (Chap. 45).

The reticulocyte count provides a measure of bone marrow erythrocyte activity. It can be refined further by calculating the absolute reticulocyte count (ARC), corrected reticulocyte count (CRC), or reticulocyte production index (RPI) (Table 9-4).

A nonspecific indicator of inflammation or tissue damage is provided by the erythrocyte sedimentation rate (ESR) (Table 9-5). In this test anticoagulated whole blood is placed in a standardized tube and allowed to settle for exactly 60 minutes. At that time the erythrocyte level is recorded. Test conditions must be carefully controlled. Of the available methods, the Westergren is clinically the most sensitive.

SI units, rather than conventional units, are now popular for expression of the Hct, erythrocyte and leukocyte counts, and erythrocyte indices (Table 9-6).

Case Study 9-1

A technologist obtained a Hb of 15.0 g/dL and a Hct of 0.36 L/L on the same specimen.
1. What is the discrepancy indicated in the results?
2. Other than technical error, what four sources of error could cause this discrepancy?
3. How could each of these problems be resolved?

Case Study 9-2

A woman severely burned in a house fire had blood drawn in the trauma center. Her Hb was 18.0 g/dL, and the Hct was 0.54 L/L.
1. Are these values normal for a woman? Explain why or why not.
2. Are the Hb and the Hct technically and physiologically accurate? Why or why not?

Case Study 9-3

A technologist received a STAT order for a manual Hb and Hct on three specimens. To save time, while centrifuging the Hct specimens, the technologist read the Hbs on the three patients 2 minutes after making the test dilutions. The Hb levels are all lower than expected compared with the Hcts.
1. List two possible explanations for this discrepancy.

Case Study 9-4

Because of lack of space in the laboratory, the rack for sedimentation rate tubes was placed directly on top of a small refrigerator.
1. List three ways in which the results could be adversely affected.

Case Study 9-5

A technologist consistently reads Hcts higher than other coworkers.
1. What could cause a technologist to read such higher Hcts?

Case Study 9-6

A leukemia patient with an elevated leukocyte count (200.0 × 10^9/L) had the following result on erythrocyte measurements performed manually: RBC 2.60 × 10^{12}/L; Hb 12.0 g/dL; and Hct 0.41 L/L.
1. Which result(s) should be questioned?

2. What is the most likely reason for these abnormalities?
3. How could the discrepancies be resolved or verified?

Review Questions

9-1. The following results were obtained on a patient's CBC: WBC 173.0 × 10⁹/L; RBC 3.35 × 10¹²/L; Hb 11.2 g/dL; Hct 0.307 L/L; MCV 91.6 fL; MCH 33.3 pg; MCHC 34.4 g/dL; PLT 18.0 × 10⁹/L. Based on these results, which of the following can be determined?

  A. Results fit the "rule of three"; nothing further needs to be done.
  B. Hb is falsely elevated due to leukocytosis and should be corrected.
  C. Hb is falsely elevated due to lipemia and should be corrected.
  D. Hb is falsely decreased due to hemolysis.

9-2. A technologist performed a manual hematocrit on a specimen on which a manual platelet count had been performed 4 hours earlier that day. The technologist filled two heparinized capillary tubes with the EDTA-anticoagulated blood and proceeded to perform a spun hematocrit. The hematocrit result was

  A. falsely decreased due to the age of the specimen.
  B. falsely elevated due to excess anticoagulant.
  C. falsely decreased due to excess anticoagulant.
  D. accurate if the technologist read the results within 10 minutes of centrifugation.

9-3. Before preparing slides for reticulocyte counting, one must be sure to adequately mix the stained blood specimen because

  A. reticulocytes have a lower specific gravity than mature erythrocytes and will therefore go to the top of the mixture during incubation.
  B. too much stain will completely stain all of the red blood cells and therefore falsely elevate the reticulocyte count.
  C. reticulocytes have a higher specific gravity than mature erythrocytes and will therefore settle at the bottom of the mixture during incubation.
  D. too much stain will create refractive artifacts in the erythrocytes and therefore falsely elevate the reticulocyte count.

9-4. Given the following patient results, calculate the reticulocyte production index (RPI): Reticulocytes 14.3%; RBC 3.2 × 10¹²/L; Hb 9.6 g/dL; and Hct 0.282 L/L. The calculated RPI indicates that there is _____ erythrocyte production and/but an _____ erythropoietic response for this degree of anemia.

  A. increased; effective
  B. increased; inadequate
  C. decreased; inadequate
  D. decreased; adequate

9-5. A false increase in the erythrocyte sedimentation rate (ESR) value can be caused by

  A. cold room temperatures.
  B. slight tilting of the ESR tube rack.
  C. reading the ESR value after exactly 30 minutes.
  D. overanticoagulation of the blood specimen.

For the following questions, choose from these answers:
  A. 1, 3
  B. 2, 4
  C. 1, 2, and 3
  D. 4 only
  E. All are correct

9-6. Which of the following statements concerning reticulocyte counts is/are true?

  1. The adult reference range is approximately 0.5 to 5.0%.
  2. Newborns have a higher reference range than adults.
  3. The material that stains in reticulocytes is DNA.
  4. The Miller disk is a device used to aid in reticulocyte counting.

9-7. Which of the following reference ranges is/are correct for an adult male?

  1. Hb = 13.5 − 17.5 g/dL
  2. Hct = 0.41 − 0.53 L/L
  3. MCV = 80 − 100 fL
  4. MCHC = 31 − 37 g/dL

Exercises

9-1. For the patient results given in review question 9-4, calculate the MCV, MCH, MCHC, RPI, ARC, and CRC.
9-2. If 20 reticulocytes are counted among 1000 erythrocytes, what is the reticulocyte percentage?

References

1. Baer DM: Hematology testing at the bedside. Lab Med 26(1):48, 1995
2. Boehringer Mannheim Corporation: Cyanmethemoglobin certified standard package insert. Indianapolis, IN, 1990
3. Boehringer Mannheim Corporation: Cyanmethemoglobin reagent package insert. Indianapolis, IN, 1990
4. Bottiger LE, Svedberg CA: Normal erythrocyte sedimentation rate and age. Br Med J 2:85, 1967
5. Boyd RD, Hoffbrand BI: Erythrocyte sedimentation rate in elderly hospital in-patients. Br Med J 1:901, 1966
6. Brecher G: New methylene blue as a reticulocyte stain. Am J Pathol 19:895, 1949
7. Brown BA: Routine hematology procedures. In Brown BA: Hematology Principles and Procedures, 6th ed, p 83. Philadelphia, Lea & Febiger, 1993
8. Bunch TW: Blood test abnormalities in runners. Mayo Clin Proc 55:113, 1980
9. Dallman PR: Blood and blood forming tissues. In Rudolph A (ed): Pediatrics, 19th ed, p 1091. Norwalk, CT, Appleton & Lange, 1991
10. Deiss A, Kurth D: Circulating reticulocytes in normal adults as determined by the new methylene blue method. Am J Clin Pathol 53:481, 1970
11. DMA Data Medical Associates, Inc: Cyanmethemoglobin reagent package insert. Arlington, TX 76011
12. Fairbanks VF, Klee GG: Biochemical aspects of hematology. In Tietz NW (ed): Fundamentals of Clinical Chemistry, p 804. Philadelphia, WB Saunders, 1987
13. Gambino SR, DiRe JJ, Monteleone M et al: The Westergren sedimentation rate using K₃EDTA. Am J Clin Pathol 43:173, 1965
14. Gilbertsen VA: Erythrocyte sedimentation rate in older patients: A study of 4,341 cases. Postgrad Med 38:A44, 1965
15. Hackney JR, Cembrowsi GS, Prystowsky MB et al: Automated reticulocyte counting by image analysis and flow cytometry. Lab Med 20:551, 1989
16. Haeberlein L: 'Whole new horizon' awaits MTs who participate in POC testing. Advance 7(12):12, 1995

17. Hillman RS, Finch CA: The detection of anemia. Red Cell Manual, 5th ed, p 49–50. Philadelphia, FA Davis, 1985

18. Hillman RS, Finch CA: Erythropoiesis: Normal and abnormal. Semin Hematol 4:327, 1967

19. International Committee for Standardization in Haematology: Recommendations for reference method for haemoglobinometry in human blood (ICSH Standard 1986) and specifications for international haemiglobincyanide reference preparation, 3rd ed. Clin Lab Haemat 9:73, 1987

20. International Committee for Standardization in Haematology: ICSH recommendations for the measurement of erythrocyte sedimentation rate. J Clin Pathol 46:198, 1993

21. International Committee for Standardization in Haematology: Recommendations for haemoglobinometry in human blood. Br J Haematol 13 (Suppl):71, 1967

22. Kjeldsberg C, Beutler E, Bell C et al: Practical Diagnosis of Hematologic Disorders, revised, p 13. Chicago, ASCP Press, 1991

23. Koepke JF, Koepke JA: Reticulocytes. Clin Lab Haematol 8:169, 1986

24. Lehmann HP: Metrication of clinical laboratory data in SI units. Am J Clin Pathol 65:2, 1976

25. Lowenstein L: The mammalian reticulocyte. Int Rev Cytol 8:135, 1959

26. Mini-Ves Erythrocyte Sedimentation Rate (manual), pp 4–8. Lincoln, RI, Diesse-Vega Biomedical, April 1991

27. National Committee for Clinical Laboratory Standards: Reticulocyte Counting by Flow Cytometry; Approved Guideline, NCCLS document H44-A. Wayne, PA, NCCLS, 1996

28. National Committee for Clinical Laboratory Standards: Procedure for Determining Packed Cell Volume by the Microhematocrit Method, 2nd ed. Approved Standard, NCCLS document H7-A2, vol 13, no 9. Villanova, PA, NCCLS, 1993

29. National Committee for Clinical Laboratory Standards: Reference and Selected Procedures for the Quantitative Determination of Hemoglobin in Blood, 2nd ed. Approved Standard, NCCLS document H15-A2, vol 4, no 3. Villanova, PA, NCCLS, 1994

30. National Committee for Clinical Laboratory Standards: Quantities and Units, SI, NCCLS document C11-CR, vol 3, no 3. Villanova, PA, NCCLS, 1983

31. National Committee for Clinical Laboratory Standards: Methods for the Erythrocyte Sedimentation Rate (ESR) Test, 3rd ed. Approved Standard, NCCLS document H2-A3, vol 13, no 8. Villanova, PA, NCCLS, 1993

32. Onigbinde T, Wu AHB: Analytical techniques and instrumentation. In Bishop ML, Duben-Engelkirk JL, Fody EP (eds): Clinical Chemistry—Principles, Procedures, Correlations, 2nd ed, pp 108–109. Philadelphia, JB Lippincott, 1992

33. Perel I, Hermann N, Watson L: Automated differential leukocyte counting by the Geometric Data Hematrak system: Eighteen months' experience in a private pathology laboratory. Pathology 12:449, 1980

34. Sage B, O'Connell J, Mercolino T: A rapid, vital staining procedure for flow cytometric analysis of human reticulocytes. Cytometry 4:222, 1983

35. Tanke H, Rothbarth P, Vossen J et al: Flow cytometry of reticulocytes applied to clinical hematology. Blood 61:1091, 1983

36. Tanke H, Nieuwenhuis I, Koper G et al: Flow cytometry of human reticulocytes based on RNA fluorescence. Cytometry 1:313, 1980

37. Schenck H, Falkensson M, Lundberg B: Evaluation of "HemoCue," a new device for determining hemoglobin. Clin Chem 32:526, 1986

38. Westergren A: Die Senkungsreaction. Ergeb Inn Med Inderheild 26:577, 1924

39. Wintrobe MM, Landsberg JW: A standardized technique for blood sedimentation test. Am J Med Sci 189:102, 1935

PART III

Erythrocyte Abnormalities

CHAPTER 10

Introduction to Erythrocyte Abnormalities

Dona D. Knapp

Objectives

1. Describe the difference between relative and absolute anemia and relative and absolute erythrocytosis.
2. Identify the six major etiologic classifications of anemia.
3. Identify the three major morphologic classifications of anemia based on mean corpuscular volume (MCV).
4. Define red cell distribution width (RDW) and describe its use together with the MCV in the classification of anemia.
5. Define reticulocyte production index (RPI) and describe its use in the physiologic classification of anemia.
6. Define effective and ineffective erythropoiesis and the two major categories of anemia associated with each.
7. Define and discuss the differentiation of relative and absolute erythrocytosis and further identify and describe the major subcategories of absolute erythrocytosis.
8. List at least four laboratory tests that are useful in the differential diagnosis of erythrocytosis.

This chapter is an introduction to hematologic disorders involving quantitative changes in erythrocytes and how they are classified. Under normal conditions, red cell production and the circulating red cell mass (RCM) remain at a constant level regulated by the erythropoietic mechanism, which functions to meet the body's oxygen requirement. If the RCM is either excessively decreased or increased, significant clinical problems occur. *Anemia* is the term used to denote conditions associated with decreased hemoglobin that are frequently accompanied by decreased numbers of red cells in the circulation (decreased RCM); *erythrocytosis* and *polycythemia* designate conditions involving the presence of too many red cells in the circulation (increased RCM).

Assisting in the diagnosis of red cell disorders is a significant challenge in the hematology laboratory. The goal is prompt detection and recognition of anemic or polycythemic states so that a physician can reach a definitive diagnosis and administer proper treatment. Anemia or erythrocytosis is only a sign that points to the existence of an underlying pathophysiologic process.

ABSOLUTE VERSUS RELATIVE ERYTHROCYTE ABNORMALITIES

Conditions associated with anemia and erythrocytosis can be subdivided into two groups on the basis of whether the change in RCM is absolute or only relative (*i.e.*, secondary to a change in the plasma volume). In absolute anemia or polycythemia there is a true decrease or increase in the RCM, respectively. In relative anemia there is a fluid shift from the extravascular to the intravascular compartment, expanding plasma volume and diluting the RCM. This is most often seen in association with pregnancy and in individuals with diseases associated with hyperproteinemia. Relative erythrocytosis, on the other hand, is the result of a decrease in the plasma volume. The RCM is normal. This most commonly occurs in conditions associated with dehydration. Although neither relative anemia nor relative erythrocytosis is a true hematologic disorder, they must be differentiated from conditions involving an absolute change in RCM (Fig. 10-1).

LABORATORY DEFINITION OF ERYTHROCYTE ABNORMALITIES

Anemic and polycythemic conditions are detected by red cell measurements that are outside the established reference range. Anemia is best defined in relation to a hemoglobin (Hb) level below the reference range, as a patient's physiologic consequences and symptoms are the direct result of the decreased oxygen-carrying capacity of the blood. Polycythemia or erythrocytosis is best defined in relation to a hematocrit (packed red cell volume; Hct) level above the established reference range. The primary clinical consequences include an expanded blood volume and increased blood viscosity.

Reference ranges for red cell measurements (Chap. 9) vary with test methodology, environmental factors, gender, and age. They are based on statistical studies of a representative sample of a healthy population. Each determined range encompasses 95% of the sample results (*i.e.*, 2 standard deviations from the mean); in other words, 5% of healthy individuals are expected to have values above or below the reference range. See Chapter 44 for details on determination of reference ranges.

Even accurately determined reference ranges are of limited value when used to define quantitative erythrocyte abnormalities. Each laboratory value must be interpreted by the physician, taking into account the patient's baseline physiologic state. An occasional patient will have a red cell measurement that is within the population reference range yet physiologically inadequate for him or her as an individual. The converse is also true.

DISORDERS CHARACTERIZED BY DECREASED ERYTHROCYTE CONCENTRATION

The detection of anemia suggests the presence of an underlying disease process. However, establishing a definitive diagnosis is complicated by the fact that there are many possible causative mechanisms. Basically, anemias can be categorized into four groups: (1) hypoproliferative; (2) maturation disorders; (3) hemolytic disorders; and (4) blood loss. The first two groups are characterized by decreased or *ineffective* bone marrow erythrocyte production, whereas the last two are the result of increased red cell destruction or blood loss. The discussion of anemia in this text will follow these categories and is outlined in Table 10-1.

Physiologic Response to Anemia
CHEMICAL AND PHYSICAL RESPONSE

Anemia results in a reduction in the oxygen-carrying capacity of the blood and subsequent tissue hypoxia. The body normally attempts to compensate. The first adjustment involves an increase in erythrocyte 2,3-diphosphoglycerate (2,3-DPG), which increases Hb release of oxygen to the tissues and is represented by a shift to the right in the oxyhemoglobin dissociation curve (see Fig. 7-5). A second response involves the selective redistribution of blood flow to areas of highest oxygen demand. Finally, cardiac output is increased. In mild to moderate anemic

---

TABLE 10-1
The Categories of Anemia

HYPOPROLIFERATIVE ANEMIAS (Chap. 11)

Anemias of bone marrow failure

Anemias of systemic disorders

MATURATION DISORDERS

Anemias of abnormal nuclear development (Chap. 12)

Anemias of abnormal iron metabolism (Chap. 13)

Anemias of abnormal globin development—thalassemias (Chap. 15)

HEMOLYTIC DISORDERS

Hereditary hemolytic anemias
    Hemoglobinopathies (Chap. 14)
    Membrane and enzyme disorders (Chap. 17)

Acquired hemolytic anemias
    Nonimmune (Chap. 18)
    Immune (Chap. 19)

ANEMIAS OF BLOOD LOSS (Chap. 20)

Acute blood loss

Chronic blood loss

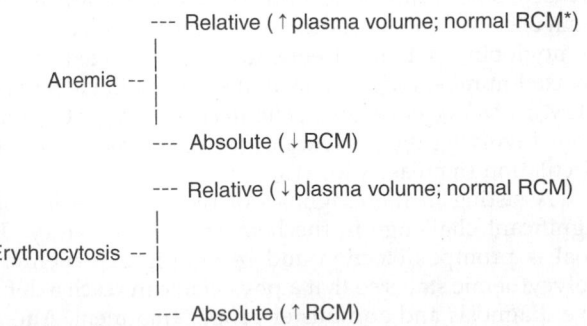

FIGURE 10-1. Absolute and relative erythrocyte disorders. *RCM, red cell mass.

states, these three mechanisms together are effective in maintaining the oxygen pressure at close to normal levels, and the patient remains asymptomatic. More severe anemia leads to increasing cardiac output and greater cardiac stress; at this point, signs such as tachycardia are manifested.

HEMATOLOGIC RESPONSE

A slower but more effective response to anemia involves the triggering of increased erythrocyte production. Tissue hypoxia resulting from anemia normally leads to increased erythropoietic marrow stimulation. Receptors in the kidney are sensitive to decreased oxygen tension and trigger increased production of erythropoietin. Erythropoietin acts on the marrow to increase the number of erythroid precursors, increase their rate of proliferation and maturation, and accelerate their release from the bone marrow (see Fig. 6-9). As a result, "shift reticulocytes" or young polychromatophilic erythrocytes are seen in the peripheral blood, causing an increased reticulocyte count and reticulocyte production index (RPI). The RPI indicates whether or not the bone marrow is responding adequately to anemia (Chap. 9). A normal bone marrow is capable of increasing erythropoiesis approximately six- to eightfold; however, it takes at least 1 week for a full response to be manifested. The marrow may fail to respond because of intrinsic disease, lack of essential hematopoietic factors, or a failure in the erythropoietic mechanism itself.

Clinical Manifestations

Mild anemic states often cause no symptoms because of the body's ability to compensate. Palpitations and dyspnea may be manifested during exercise. With increasing severity, the increased cardiac stress may cause tachycardia, shortness of breath, and headaches. Pallor is the result of vasoconstriction in the vessels of the skin and blood redistribution. Leg cramps, dizziness, fatigue, and insomnia, all of which are common as anemia progresses, are secondary to tissue hypoxia. In its most severe form, anemia may lead to coma and death. The rate of development of anemia also impacts on the severity of the clinical symptoms. In an anemia of acute onset, the symptoms may manifest themselves sooner than in a slowly developing anemic state.

Classification of Anemia

Once anemia has been detected, classifying it is usually beneficial, as it assists in the establishment of a definitive diagnosis. Three basic formats are used: etiologic, morphologic, and physiologic.

ETIOLOGIC CLASSIFICATION

The etiologic classification approach focuses on the principal underlying pathophysiologic mechanisms. Table 10-2 lists six groups of anemias, and each group is expanded to list the types of anemias in each category and their primary causative mechanism.

It is often difficult to classify anemias by etiology because they are often caused by multiple factors. For example, iron deficiency may coexist with folate deficiency. Anemia also frequently involves more than one underlying pathophysiologic mechanism. Megaloblastic anemias may display both disordered maturation and decreased red cell survival.

MORPHOLOGIC CLASSIFICATION

The morphologic classification of anemia can be established using red cell indices and direct examination of their morphology. Red cell morphology is observed and described using a properly prepared and stained blood film (Chap. 8). Anemia can be classified according to erythrocyte size and Hb content. Although widely used and accepted, this approach has been criticized for lack of sensitivity and standardization.[12] In recent years, standardized procedures and reporting formats have been presented in the literature,[5,19,21] and morphology review remains important in the classification of anemias.

The definition of and procedure for determining red cell indices are described in Chapter 9. As early as 1934, Wintrobe presented a scheme for classifying anemias morphologically, based on indices calculated from manually determined red cell measurements.[27] The indices, including the mean corpuscular volume (MCV), mean corpuscular hemoglobin (MCH), and mean corpuscular hemoglobin concentration (MCHC), became the basis for classifying anemias into four categories: (1) normocytic, normochromic; (2) microcytic, hypochromic; (3) microcytic, normochromic; and (4) macrocytic, normochromic. Although this format has been widely used for many years, problems sometimes occur.[1] In prior years, indices derived from manually determined red cell measurements were questioned because of the high level of procedural variability and error, especially in the manual red cell count.[4] Today red cell indices are measured directly or computed automatically by sophisticated electronic cell counters (Chap. 42). Although results are now more reliable, the reported indices are still only as good as the instrumentation and data used to calculate them. Table 10-3 provides a general morphologic classification of anemia, based on the MCV that differentiates microcytic, macrocytic, and normocytic anemias.

Electronic determination of red cell indices has increased the clinical value and usefulness of the MCV and decreased that of the MCH and MCHC. The MCV is now derived directly from red cell size distribution data. Most instruments now calculate the hematocrit (MCV × RBC count) in addition to the MCH and MCHC. The MCH varies in a linear relation to the MCV and provides no additional diagnostic information. Also, it is now recognized that calculated hematocrits may be low in comparison with spun microhematocrits because of plasma trapping in the latter (Chap. 9) or calibration bias. The MCHC derived from a calculated hematocrit that is low is, in turn, artifactually high and loses its sensitivity as an indicator of iron deficiency; it is decreased only in severe microcytic anemias. Although the MCH and MCHC have lost some clinical value, all red cell indices are useful quality control tools and aid in the detection of instrument malfunctions. The use of red cell indices in quality control is discussed in Chapter 45.

TABLE 10-2
Etiologic Classification of Anemias

Type	Causes
RELATIVE ANEMIA	
Pregnancy	Increased plasma volume
Hyperproteinemia	
Intravenous fluids	
ANEMIA ASSOCIATED WITH DEFECTIVE HEMOGLOBIN SYNTHESIS	
Iron deficiency	Excessive loss
	Increased requirements
	Deficient intake
	Defective absorption
Sideroblastic anemia	Enzymatic defect in heme synthesis
Primary	
Secondary	
Anemia of chronic disease	Defective iron utilization
	Infection
	Inflammation
	Neoplasm
Thalassemia syndromes	Imbalanced globin synthesis
ANEMIA ASSOCIATED WITH VITAMIN B_{12} OR FOLATE DEFICIENCY	
Vitamin B_{12} deficiency	Inadequate dietary intake
	Defective absorption
	Increased requirements
	Defective production of intrinsic factor
Folate deficiency	Inadequate dietary intake
	Defective absorption
	Increased requirements
	Impaired utilization—folate antagonists
ANEMIA ASSOCIATED WITH IMPAIRED BONE MARROW OR STEM CELL FUNCTION	
Bone marrow injury	Reduced hematopoietic tissue
Primary aplastic anemia	Idiopathic defect
Secondary aplastic anemia	Injury by drugs, radiation, chemicals, infectious agents
Bone marrow replacement	Infiltration with abnormal tissue
Myelophthisic anemia	Myelofibrosis, leukemia, lymphoma, myeloma, metastatic neoplasm, storage disease
Ineffective hematopoiesis	Hematopoietic stem cell disorder: abnormal proliferation and maturation
Myelodysplastic anemias	Refractory anemia
	Refractory anemia with ringed sideroblasts
	Refractory anemia with excess blasts
	Refractory anemia with excess blasts in transformation
	Chronic myelomonocytic leukemia
Decreased marrow stimulation	Reduced secretion of erythropoietin
Anemia of renal failure	
Anemia of endocrine disorders	
Anemia of chronic disease	
Constitutional anemia	Congenital or genetic predisposition to bone marrow failure
Diamond-Blackfan anemia	
Faconi anemia	
Familial aplastic anemia	
Acquired pure red cell aplasia	Erythroid marrow suppression
Acute self-limited	Associated with viral agents
Thymoma	Immunologic suppression
Paroxysmal nocturnal hemoglobinuria	Acquired stem cell disorder

(continued)

TABLE 10-2
Etiologic Classification of Anemias Continued

Type	Causes
ANEMIAS ASSOCIATED WITH DECREASED RED CELL SURVIVAL AND INCREASED RED CELL DESTRUCTION	
Intrinsic red cell defect	
Membrane defect	Defect in membrane resulting in shortened survival
Hereditary spherocytosis	Structural defect
Hereditary elliptocytosis	Structural defect
Hereditary stomatocytosis	Structural defect
Hereditary pyropoikilocytosis	Structural defect
Hereditary acanthocytosis	Abetalipoproteinemia/abnormal lipid content
Lecithin–cholesterol acyltransferase deficiency	Decreased membrane cholesterol esters
Paroxysmal nocturnal hemoglobinuria	Membrane sensitive to complement lysis
Enzyme defect	Enzyme defect resulting in shortened RBC survival
G6PD deficiency	Oxidative damage
Pyruvate kinase deficiency	Failure to generate normal ATP levels
Others	
Hemoglobinopathies	Defective globin chain synthesis
Qualitative defects	Structural abnormality in globin chain
Sickle cell disease	
Hemoglobin C disease	
Unstable hemoglobins	
Other	
Quantitative defects	Imbalanced globin chain synthesis
β-Thalassemia	β-Chain defect
α-Thalassemia	α-Chain defect
Other	
Qualitative and quantitative defect	Structural abnormality and defective globin chain synthesis combined
Hb S/β-Thalassemia	
Others	
Extrinsic red cell defect	
Immune	Immune destruction
Isoimmune hemolytic anemia	
Hemolytic disease of the newborn	
Hemolytic transfusion reactions	
Autoimmune hemolytic anemia	
Warm antibodies	
Cold antibodies	
Drug-induced immune hemolytic anemia	
Nonimmune	
Microangiopathic hemolytic anemia	Destruction secondary to fibrin deposition
Disseminated intravascular coagulation	
Thrombotic thrombocytopenic purpura	
Hemolytic uremic syndrome	
Hemolytic anemia associated with infection (bacterial, viral, protozoal)	Premature destruction secondary to interaction with infectious agent
Hemolytic anemia associated with toxic agents, chemicals, drugs	Toxic damage
Hemolytic anemia associated with physical agents (vascular prosthesis, march hemoglobinuria, burns)	Physical damage
Hypersplenism	Premature destruction in spleen
ANEMIA SECONDARY TO BLOOD LOSS	
Acute	Decreased blood volume
Chronic	

The MCV also has limitations. It represents the mean (average) size of a given heterogeneous red cell population and does not reflect size variation (anisocytosis) within the population. This shortcoming has been overcome somewhat with the development of a new hematologic parameter that provides a measure of red cell size variation. This parameter, most commonly known as the *red cell distribution width* (RDW), is a size distribution measurement generated from a red cell histogram. It functions as an index of red cell population heterogeneity and can reflect anisocytosis on the peripheral blood film. It is expressed as the ratio of standard deviation (width of histogram) to the MCV or the coefficient of variation of red cell size within a given red cell population.[2] Many automated hematology instruments, both electrical impedance and light scatter systems, now provide RDW-

TABLE 10-3
Morphologic Classification of Anemias

MICROCYTIC (MCV < 80 fL)

Commonly microcytic
Iron deficiency
Thalassemias
Hereditary sideroblastic anemia

Occasionally microcytic
Anemia of chronic disease
Hemoglobinopathies

MACROCYTIC (MCV > 100 fL)

Commonly macrocytic
Folic acid deficiency
Vitamin B_{12} deficiency

Occasionally macrocytic
Hypoproliferative anemia
Refractory anemia
Liver disease
Hemolytic anemia
Blood loss anemia

NORMOCYTIC (MCV 80–100 fL)

Commonly normocytic
Hypoproliferative anemia
Myelophthisic anemia
Refractory dysmyelopoietic anemia
Hemolytic anemia
Hemoglobinopathies
Blood loss anemia
Anemia of chronic disease
Acquired sideroblastic anemia

Occasionally normocytic
Early iron deficiency
Refractory anemia

increased in iron deficiency but normal in heterozygous thalassemias and anemias associated with chronic disease. The RDW has also been reported to be more sensitive than other indicators in detecting early iron deficiency anemia.[7,20]

The use of the RDW in classifying anemias has been criticized.[8,14,23] Many studies have concluded that it is a poor discriminator among microcytic anemias and that it must be used with caution and should not replace other diagnostic tests, such as iron studies and Hb electrophoresis. It is apparent that further studies are needed to clarify the diagnostic value of the RDW.

PHYSIOLOGIC CLASSIFICATION

The physiologic classification system is based on the ability of the bone marrow to respond to anemia with increased erythropoiesis. It involves assessing erythrocyte production using the reticulocyte count (either proportional [%] or absolute) and calculated RPI. When anemia occurs, if the bone marrow is capable of responding, increased numbers of young, nonnucleated red cells enter the circulation. These young polychromatophilic red cells, released prematurely from the marrow because of erythropoietin stimulation, are called *shift reticulocytes*, a term reflecting their premature shift from the bone marrow to the peripheral blood. Thus, reticulocytes may be significantly increased in the circulation without an actual increase in marrow red cell production.

To use the reticulocyte count as an index of marrow red cell production effectiveness, it must be converted to the RPI using two mathematical corrections (Chap. 9). The first correction determines the absolute number of circulating reticulocytes, and the second compensates for the reticulocytes being shifted out of the marrow early and spending a longer time in the circulation.[16]

The accuracy and reliability of the manually determined reticulocyte count (and thus the RPI) have been questioned. Studies suggest unacceptable interlaboratory and intralaboratory variability.[15,22,24] However, greater attention is being given to standardization of the manual procedure, and new flow cytometer methodology has greatly enhanced accuracy (Chaps. 42 and 43). Furthermore, great accuracy is not absolutely necessary for the RPI to be of value. Significantly increased RPIs, whether four or five for example, indicate an increased and effective marrow response to anemia. On the other hand, accuracy does become more critical at the cutoff point between

type measurements. Each instrument derives this parameter differently, and data must be carefully interpreted in light of each laboratory's established reference ranges.

The application of the RDW in classifying anemias has been investigated, and a schematic using the RDW in conjunction with the MCV has been proposed.[3,17] Table 10-4 displays this schematic and divides anemias into six categories on the basis of MCV and RDW. The RDW provides a measure of homogeneity (normal RDW) or heterogeneity (high RDW) within the red cell population. The investigations of this proposed system have focused primarily on its utilization in the differential diagnosis of microcytic anemias. The RDW has been reported to be

TABLE 10-4
Classification of Anemia Using the MCV and RDW

	MCV Low	MCV Normal	MCV High
RDW NORMAL	Microcytic Homogeneous	Normocytic Homogeneous	Macrocytic Homogeneous
RDW HIGH	Microcytic Heterogeneous	Normocytic Heterogeneous	Macrocytic Heterogeneous

TABLE 10-5 *Physiologic Classification of Anemias*			
RPI < 2.0 (Ineffective Erythropoiesis)		**RPI > 3.0 (Effective Erythropoiesis)**	
Hypoproliferative anemias	Maturation disorders	Hemolytic anemias	Blood loss anemias

effective and ineffective marrow production. At that point RPI interpretation is more difficult.

Table 10-5 demonstrates how the RPI can be used to classify anemia into two principal groups, effective and ineffective erythropoiesis, based on the marrow response. An RPI higher than 3.0 indicates an effective bone marrow response, whereas an RPI lower than 2.0 suggests an ineffective bone marrow response.[16] Each group can be subdivided into two categories. An ineffective response is associated with hypoproliferative anemias and anemias resulting from maturation disorders. An effective response is characteristic of hemolytic anemias and anemias secondary to blood loss. See the later discussion on effective and ineffective erythropoiesis.

COMBINED MORPHOLOGIC AND PHYSIOLOGIC CLASSIFICATION

The schematics in Figures 10-2 and 10-3 integrate the physiologic and morphologic classification formats and provide a systematic approach to classifying anemias. Anemias are divided into the four major groups shown in Table 10-5 on the basis of the RPI.

Ineffective Erythropoiesis. Ineffective erythropoiesis (RPI lower than 2.0) is caused by a defective bone marrow, either from intrinsic disease, lack of essential hematopoietic factors, or a failure in the erythropoietic mechanism itself. The two groups demonstrating ineffective erythropoiesis are hypoproliferative anemias and anemias secondary to maturation disorders (Fig. 10-2).

Hypoproliferative anemias tend to be normocytic, normochromic (N/N). This group encompasses a wide variety of anemias, including hypoplastic anemias, myelophthisic anemias, refractory anemia, and a group of moderate anemias associated with diseases that cause decreased hormonal stimulation of the marrow. In hypoplastic anemias, the bone marrow cellularity is severely decreased. Hypoplastic anemias may be idiopathic or associated with exposure to certain chemicals, infectious agents, or drugs that cause maturation arrest. Myelophthisic anemia occurs secondary to marrow infiltration and replacement by abnormal cells (*e.g.,* leukemia). Refractory anemia (a dysmyelopoietic syndrome) is caused by a failure in stem cell maturation and is characterized by dysplasia (abnormal development) of precursor cells in the marrow. Examples of anemias causing decreased marrow stimulation include renal, endocrine, and other chronic diseases. Differentiation of the hypoproliferative anemias often requires a bone marrow examination. Depending on the anemia, the marrow appearance ranges from normal to neoplastic.

Anemias associated with maturation disorders can be further separated into two groups based on the MCV. Microcytic anemias have a decreased MCV; macrocytic anemias, an increased MCV. Macrocytic anemias must be differentiated into those that are megaloblastic anemias associated with vitamin B_{12} or folate deficiency (MCV may exceed 115 fL) and those that are nonmegaloblastic (MCV usually less than 115 fL), including hemolytic anemia with reticulocytosis and liver disease. Red cell morphology also is helpful in differentiating macrocytic anemias (Fig. 10-2). Microcytic anemias include, in order of prevalence, iron deficiency, some anemias of chronic disease, heterozygous thalassemia, and some sideroblastic anemias. Iron studies and Hb electrophoresis are often required in their differential diagnosis. Red cell morphology provides useful clues. The RDW may be helpful in differentation (Fig. 10-2); however, this awaits substantiation.

Effective Erythropoiesis. In the case of effective erythropoiesis (RPI higher than 3.0), the bone marrow is intact, the hematopoietic mechanism is functional, and the components necessary for red cell production are available. The two groups of anemias usually demonstrating effective erythropoiesis are hemolytic anemias and those associated with chronic or acute blood loss. These anemias tend to be normocytic and normochromic with a normal to slightly elevated MCV (Fig. 10-3). In the presence of a significant anemia, an effective bone marrow response will be seen after a sufficient span of time. However, the bone marrow of an occasional individual with hemolytic anemia or blood loss will fail to respond because of an underlying defect in the marrow or the erythropoietic mechanism, a so-called aplastic crisis.

The hemolytic anemias are a diverse group that are caused by hereditary and acquired red cell defects or by an abnormal red cell environment (*e.g.,* abnormal blood vessels; Chap. 18). Red cell morphology is useful in differentiating the hemolytic anemias into four groups (Fig. 10-3). The presence of a predominant red cell morphologic variant is suggestive of a hereditary defect involving the red cell membrane (Chap. 17). Predominant target cells suggest a hemoglobinopathy (Chaps. 14 and 15). Fragmented red cells may suggest a microangiopathic hemolytic process (Chap. 18). Normal morphology or only minor changes, including spherocytes and spiculated red cells, are seen in many types of hemolytic anemia, including immune hemolytic anemias (Chap. 19) and red cell enzyme deficiencies (Chap. 17).

A third, less common group of anemias demonstrating effective erythropoiesis is that associated with hemoglobin variants with decreased oxygen affinity. Decreased oxygen affinity hemoglobins cause increased release of oxygen to the tissues and, therefore, may cause a decrease in the red cell number and anemia. The best known variant in this group is Hb Kansas (Chap. 14).

After initial classification of an anemia, a definitive diagnosis may require additional laboratory studies, as discussed in appropriate chapters. Periodic referral to Figures 10-2 and 10-3 as subsequent chapters are read may be helpful during the initially complex study of this subject.

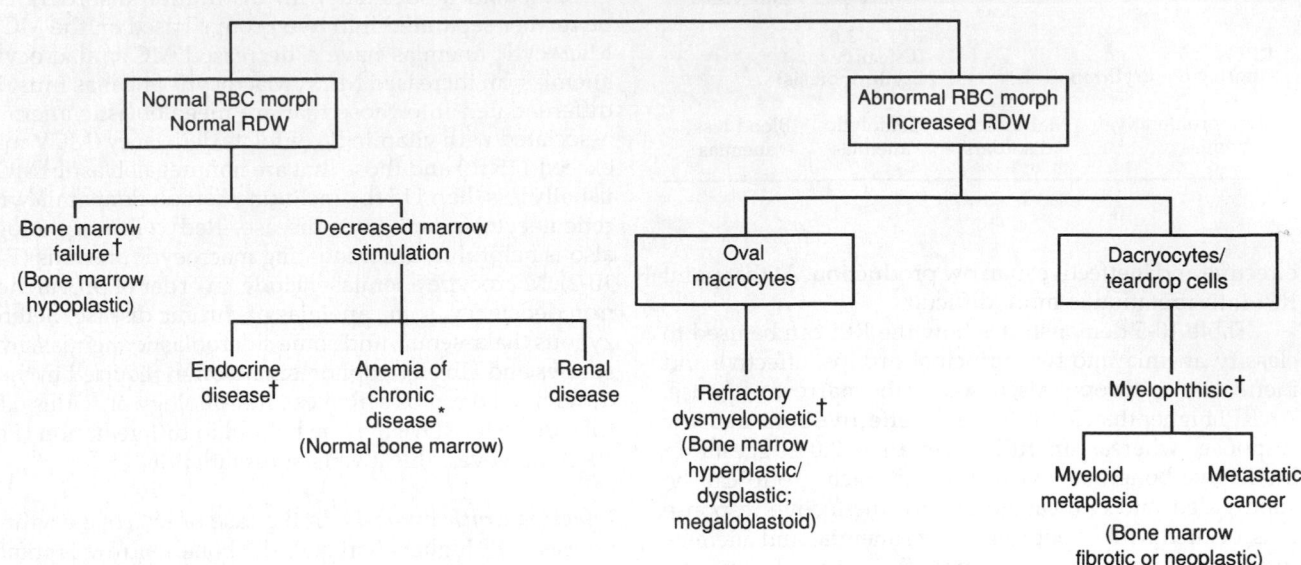

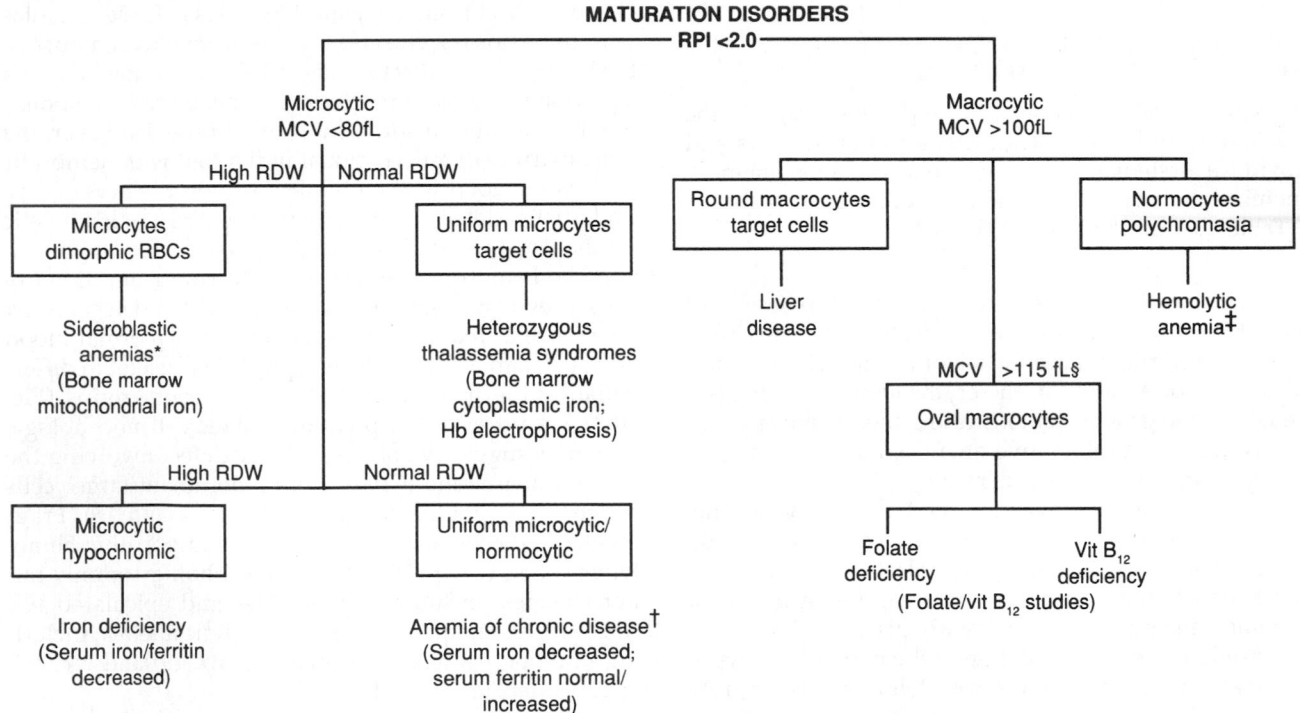

FIGURE 10-2. Systematic approach to the classification of anemias with ineffective erythropoiesis: hypoproliferative anemias (**above**) and disorders of maturation (**below**). Laboratory tests in parentheses are used to differentiate the disorders in that category.

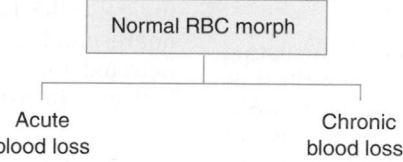

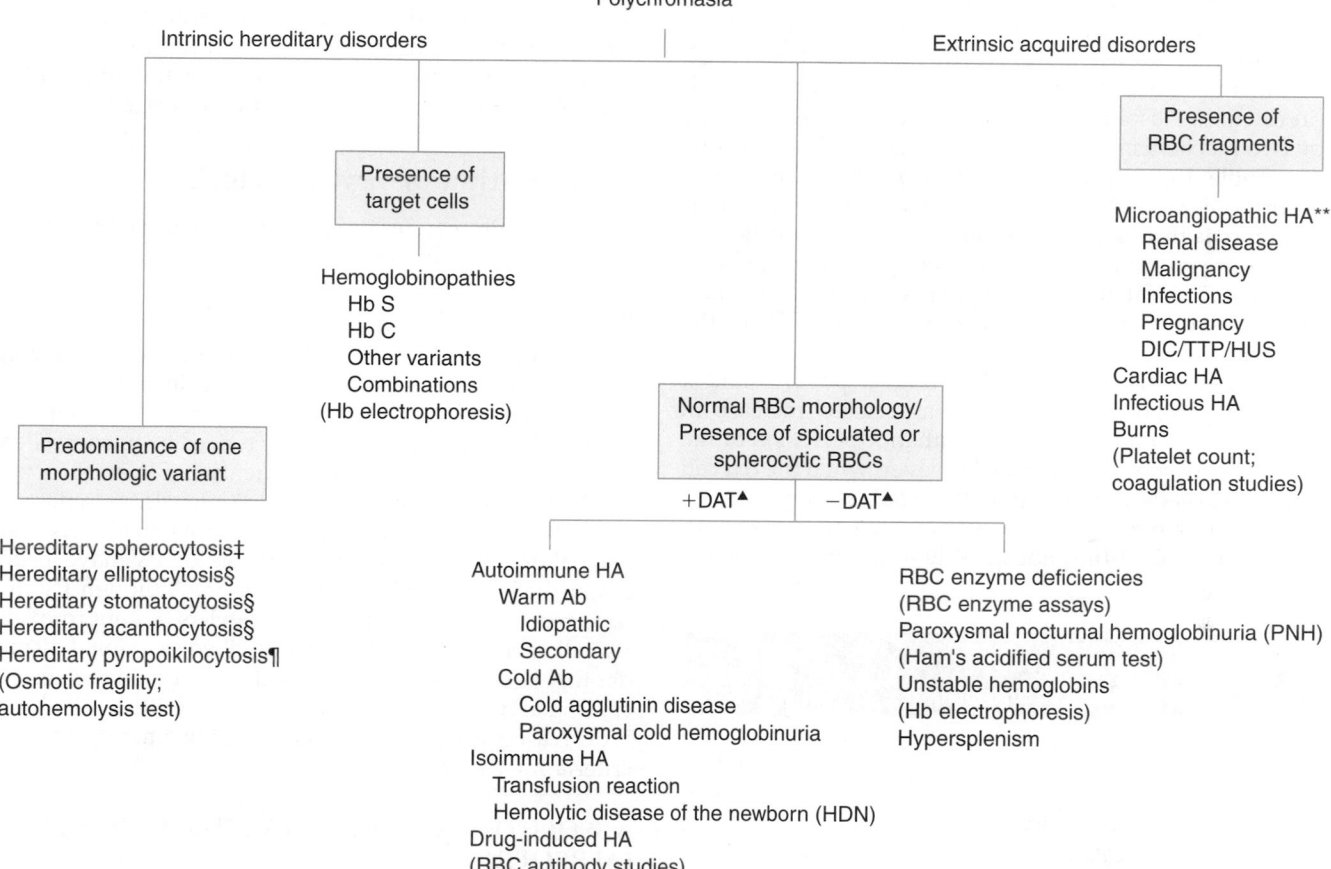

BLOOD LOSS ANEMIAS
RPI > 3.0*
Normocytic, Normochromic Indices

Normal RBC morph

Acute
blood loss

Chronic
blood loss+

*Given adequate response time
+Without treatment, becomes microcytic, hypochromic

HEMOLYTIC ANEMIAS
RPI > 3.0*
Normocytic, Normochromic Indices†
Polychromasia

Intrinsic hereditary disorders

Extrinsic acquired disorders

Presence of
RBC fragments

Microangiopathic HA**
   Renal disease
   Malignancy
   Infections
   Pregnancy
   DIC/TTP/HUS
Cardiac HA
Infectious HA
Burns
(Platelet count;
coagulation studies)

Presence of
target cells

Hemoglobinopathies
   Hb S
   Hb C
   Other variants
   Combinations
(Hb electrophoresis)

Normal RBC morphology/
Presence of spiculated or
spherocytic RBCs

+DAT▲   −DAT▲

Predominance of one
morphologic variant

Hereditary spherocytosis‡
Hereditary elliptocytosis§
Hereditary stomatocytosis§
Hereditary acanthocytosis§
Hereditary pyropoikilocytosis¶
(Osmotic fragility;
autohemolysis test)

Autoimmune HA
   Warm Ab
      Idiopathic
      Secondary
   Cold Ab
      Cold agglutinin disease
      Paroxysmal cold hemoglobinuria
Isoimmune HA
   Transfusion reaction
   Hemolytic disease of the newborn (HDN)
Drug-induced HA
(RBC antibody studies)

RBC enzyme deficiencies
(RBC enzyme assays)
Paroxysmal nocturnal hemoglobinuria (PNH)
(Ham's acidified serum test)
Unstable hemoglobins
(Hb electrophoresis)
Hypersplenism

* In the presence of a significant anemia and after a sufficient response time.
** HA, hemolytic anemia.
▲ DAT, direct antiglobulin test.
† May be macrocytic with extreme polychromasia.
‡ May be microcytic (↓MCV) and hyperchromic (↑MCHC)
§ Anemia often not exhibited because of bone marrow compensation.
¶ Microcytic red cells displaying extreme morphologic variability.

FIGURE 10-3. Systematic approach to the classification of anemias with effective erythropoiesis:
blood loss anemias (**above**) and hemolytic anemias (**below**). Laboratory tests in parentheses are used
to differentiate the disorders in that category.

DISORDERS CHARACTERIZED BY INCREASED ERYTHROCYTE CONCENTRATION

Disorders involving an increased number of circulating red cells, and thus an increased RCM, are described as erythrocytosis or polycythemia. Erythrocytosis is associated with increased red cells, Hb content, hematocrit (Hct), or some combination thereof. A Hct of more than 0.55 L/L (55%) in men and 0.47 L/L (47%) in women is often used as the diagnostic criterion. Erythrocytosis may be classified as absolute or relative (Table 10-6).

Pathophysiology

Absolute erythrocytosis may be primary or secondary (Table 10-6). Primary erythrocytosis refers to a true increase in RCM associated with a chronic myeloproliferative disorder known as polycythemia vera (Chap. 35). The increased RCM is the result of unregulated red cell production. Absolute secondary erythrocytosis is caused by two mechanisms, termed appropriate and inappropriate (Table 10-6). In an appropriate response, increased erythropoietin (EPO) is generated in an attempt to alleviate hypoxia through stimulation of red cell production. In an inappropriate response, increased generation of EPO is the result of localized renal hypoxia or tumor generation of a substance that mimics the action of EPO on the bone marrow.

Absolute erythrocytosis has both a positive and a negative physiologic effect. The associated increase in blood volume and vasodilation enhance perfusion of the blood and tissue oxygenation; however, when the red cell volume exceeds a certain limit, the resulting hyperviscosity decreases blood flow and tissue oxygenation and increases the risk of thrombosis. When this critical point is exceeded, the benefits of enhanced oxygen delivery are outweighed by the potential negative effect of increased blood viscosity and the accompanying cardiac stress. Fortunately, the kidney and erythropoietic mechanism do not respond to hypoxia when excessive blood viscosity is detected, thereby preventing a damaging spiral of further increases in red cell production and blood viscosity.[9]

Clinical Manifestations

The general symptoms of absolute and relative erythrocytosis are vague and depend on the severity and underlying pathologic mechanism. Management of erythrocytosis depends on whether the increase in RCM is an appropriate response to hypoxia or is unrelated to it, the severity of hypoxia, the extent of erythrocytosis, and the individual's clinical state. At times, phlebotomy is used to lower the RCM. It is usually effective in controlling the symptoms associated with erythrocytosis. It lowers the risk of thromboembolic complications while maintaining adequate blood flow to the brain and other organs.

Classification of Erythrocytosis

Table 10-6 summarizes the classification of erythrocytosis defined in the following sections.

ABSOLUTE PRIMARY ERYTHROCYTOSIS

An absolute increase in RCM resulting from a clonal, pluripotent stem cell disorder is seen in polycythemia vera (PV), which is one of a group of chronic myeloproliferative disorders (Chap. 35) characterized by uncontrolled proliferation of bone marrow elements. In PV, erythrocyte production is not controlled by EPO levels, as reflected by the fact that EPO is decreased or normal in PV. Clinical and laboratory criteria for diagnosis of PV have been established,[1] as detailed in Chapter 35. Although PV affects red cells, leukocytes, and platelets, a subgroup of PV called erythremia has been described as a clonal disorder that affects bone marrow production of only red cells, causing an increase in red cell mass.[10] In erythremia, EPO is decreased as in PV; however, all of the other diagnostic criteria for PV are absent.

ABSOLUTE SECONDARY ERYTHROCYTOSIS (APPROPRIATE)

The disorders classified as absolute secondary erythrocytosis with an appropriate response to hypoxia may be caused by high-altitude adjustment, pulmonary disease, cardiovascular disease, alveolar hypoventilation (lack of adequate oxygenation of the lung alveoli), or defective oxygen transport. Secondary erythrocytosis is appropriate for individuals living at high altitudes because of the low pO_2 of the air, which reduces arterial oxygen saturation. Except at very high altitudes, physiologic adjustments are normally made to compensate and satisfy unusual oxygen needs. Such adjustments include increased blood volume, increased oxygen-carrying capacity of blood, increased levels of erythrocyte 2,3-DPG to reduce Hb affinity for oxygen, and increased cardiac output and pulmonary function. Chronic mountain sickness

---

TABLE 10-6
Classifications of Erythrocytosis

ABSOLUTE ERYTHROCYTOSIS

Primary
    Polycythemia vera
    Erythremia

Secondary
    Appropriate
        High altitude
        Pulmonary disease
        Cardiovascular disease
        Alveolar hypoventilation
        Hemoglobinopathy
        Tobacco/carboxyhemoglobin
    Inappropriate
        Essential (idiopathic)
        Renal disease
        Extrarenal tumors

RELATIVE ERYTHROCYTOSIS

Dehydration

Gaisböck's syndrome

Stress/spurious

Tobacco

(Monge's disease) is seen in individuals who become intolerant to living at high altitudes. The causative factor appears to be alveolar hypoventilation secondary to an impaired respiratory response to hypoxia.

Chronic obstructive pulmonary diseases with decreased arterial oxygen tension occasionally cause erythrocytosis; however, the erythropoietic response usually is not as great as necessary. Cardiac diseases, both congenital and acquired, occasionally are recognized as causing erythrocytosis. Alveolar hypoventilation, especially in association with extreme obesity, is associated with erythrocytosis. Hypoventilation with erythrocytosis may also be secondary to mechanical interference with the oxygenation process, such as in poliomyelitis and muscle dystrophies, or to an impaired cerebral respiratory center due to thrombosis, encephalitis, or barbiturate intoxication.

Hemoglobin variants are rare causes of secondary erythrocytosis. Structural changes in the Hb molecule may cause a shift to the left in the oxyhemoglobin dissociation curve (see Fig. 7-5), resulting in increased Hb affinity for oxygen, tissue hypoxia, and increased EPO production, and hence secondary erythrocytosis. Examples of such conditions are Hb Chesapeake and some Hb M disorders (Chap. 14).

It is now recognized that carbon monoxide (CO) exposure from excessive smoking is the most common cause of secondary erythrocytosis. It is estimated that 3% of cigarette smokers have elevated hematocrits.[25] Hb's affinity for CO is 200 times greater than its affinity for oxygen. Hb binding with CO results in the formation of nonfunctional carboxyhemoglobin. As carboxyhemoglobin levels increase, there is a shift to the left in the oxyhemoglobin dissociation curve and a decrease in P_{50} (the partial pressure of oxygen at which Hb is half saturated). This increases Hb oxygen affinity, reduces oxygen delivery to the tissues, and triggers erythrocytosis. In addition, smoking often causes a decrease in the plasma volume. In some persons there is a low plasma volume but a normal RCM. Therefore, changes in the red cell volume and plasma volume among smokers may result in an absolute erythrocytosis in some individuals and a relative erythrocytosis in others.

ABSOLUTE SECONDARY ERYTHROCYTOSIS (INAPPROPRIATE)

When secondary erythrocytosis is not associated with generalized hypoxia, it is considered an inappropriate response. This is seen most often in association with a variety of renal disorders, including tumors, renal artery stenosis, pyelonephritis, urethral obstruction, and renal cystic disease.[13] Renal tumors and disease may interfere with renal blood flow, causing localized hypoxia which, in turn, triggers EPO production. Also it is suggested that some tumors involving the kidneys secrete an EPO-like substance capable of stimulating erythropoiesis. Erythrocytosis is seen in about 10% of kidney transplant recipients.[28] A variety of extrarenal tumors can also inappropriately trigger increased erythropoiesis through secretion of humoral substances with an EPO-like activity. Such tumors include those of the brain, liver, ovary, uterus, prostate, thymus, and adrenal glands.[13]

Rarely an idiopathic overproduction of EPO occurs. It has been suggested that this disorder be designated as a subgroup of secondary erythrocytosis called "essential erythrocytosis."[10]

RELATIVE ERYTHROCYTOSIS

The decreased plasma volume causing relative erythrocytosis may be the result of dehydration secondary to diarrhea, vomiting, excessive sweating, increased vascular permeability (burns or anaphylaxis), or the use of diuretics. Relative erythrocytosis also has been associated with a condition seen in individuals experiencing anxiety and stress. This condition has been called stress syndrome, spurious erythrocytosis, or Gaisböck's syndrome.[26] Affected persons are usually middle-aged, overweight men complaining of headaches, dizziness, and fatigue. It has been suggested that smoking is a critical causative factor and that this syndrome should be recognized as "tobacco polycythemia." In most cases it has been suggested that there probably was an absolute increase in RCM accompanied by a decrease in plasma volume.[25]

Relative erythrocytosis is not a hematologic disorder; however, it must be differentiated from absolute erythrocytosis (see the following differential diagnosis section).

Differential Diagnosis of Erythrocytosis

Figure 10-4 provides a model for the differential diagnosis of erythrocytosis. Relative and absolute erythrocytosis are differentiated on the basis of blood volume studies from which the RCM may be determined. This is accomplished using radioisotopic dilution techniques. Values in excess of 36 mL/kg of body weight for males and 32 mL/kg for females are considered excessive. If the erythrocytosis is absolute, it must be determined whether it is primary (Chap. 35) or secondary (Table 10-6). According to one report,[18] EPO levels measured by radioimmunoassay tend to be decreased in primary conditions, but normal or increased in secondary conditions. However, some investigators have reported conflicting data, suggesting that the EPO level is a poor discriminator of primary versus secondary erythrocytosis.[6]

Arterial blood gas measurements also aid in the differential diagnosis of the absolute erythrocytoses. Arterial blood oxygen saturation (sO_2) is normal (92%) in primary erythrocytosis. Appropriate and inappropriate secondary erythrocytosis usually can be differentiated on the basis of sO_2. Cardiac and pulmonary erythrocytosis demonstrate a decreased sO_2 value. However, most other secondary erythrocytoses demonstrate a normal sO_2 (*e.g.*, abnormal Hbs with high oxygen affinity).

The definitive diagnosis for abnormally high oxygen affinity Hbs usually requires studies of the oxyhemoglobin dissociation curve (see Fig. 7-5) and determination of the partial pressure of oxygen at which Hb is 50% saturated (P_{50}). A decreased P_{50} value confirms a nonfunctional Hb with increased O_2 affinity, which causes a shift to the left in the dissociation curve. Electrophoresis can detect some of these abnormal Hbs (Chap. 14).

Increased carboxyhemoglobin is useful in confirming tobacco-related erythrocytosis. Erythrocytosis associated

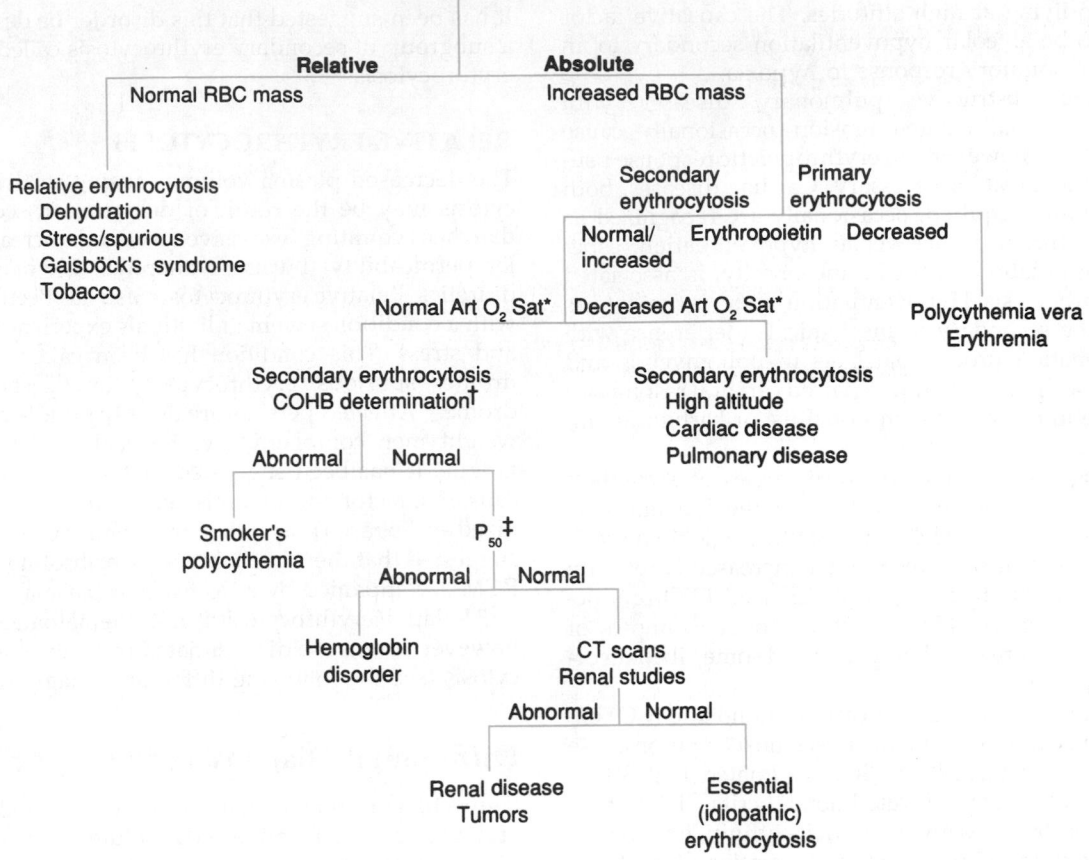

* Art O_2 Sat = arterial O_2 saturation (normal >92%).
† COHB = carboxyhemoglobin.
‡ P_{50} = partial pressure at which hemoglobin is half saturated.

FIGURE 10-4. Differential diagnosis of erythrocytosis.

with carboxyhemoglobin may be accompanied by an abnormal P_{50}. The diagnosis of inappropriate erythrocytosis associated with renal disease or tumors requires computed tomograpy (CT) scanning or magnetic resonance imaging (MRI) and other renal studies.

CHAPTER SUMMARY

The diagnosis of disorders involving red cells provides a challenge to the laboratory. Anemias are disorders characterized by a decreased hemoglobin, which is frequently accompanied by a decreased red cell count, whereas polycythemias or erythrocytoses are characterized by an increased red cell count. Both conditions can be relative, secondary to a change in the plasma volume, or absolute, with a quantitative decrease or increase in the RCM.

Classification of these disorders facilitates diagnostic evaluation. Several anemia classification schemes, including etiologic (Table 10-2), morphologic (Table 10-3), and physiologic (Table 10-5) have been presented. A combined morphologic and physiologic classification scheme based on routine laboratory procedures, including red cell morphologic evaluation, reticulocyte count, and calculated RPI, has also been offered (Figs. 10-2 and 10-3).

Classification and diagnostic schemes for polycythemia and erythrocytosis are presented in Table 10-6 and Figure 10-4, re-

spectively. A diagnostic evaluation involves separating relative and absolute disorders and further differentiating primary and secondary absolute conditions. A number of laboratory tests, many complex, may be required to establish a definitive diagnosis.

Case Studies

For Case Studies 10-1–10-3, answer the following questions:
1. What are this patient's hematologic findings?
2. What is the morphologic classification of this anemia based on your calculations of the MCV and MCHC?
3. What is the physiologic classification of this anemia (*i.e.*, effective or ineffective erythropoiesis) based on your calculation of the RPI?
4. What follow-up laboratory testing could be recommended to assist in the diagnosis?

Case Study 10-1

A 1-year-old child was brought to a clinic. Her mother stated that the child was listless. The following laboratory tests were reported: RBC 3.0×10^{12}/L; Hb 5.0 g/dL; Hct 0.18 L/L; WBC 9.0×10^9/L; WBC differential normal; and reticulocyte count 2.5%.

Case Study 10-2

A nursing student visited the student health laboratory complaining of an excessive, prolonged menstrual period and general fatigue. The following laboratory tests were reported: RBC 2.0×10^{12}/L; Hb 5.5 g/dL; Hct 0.17 L/L; WBC 1.5×10^9/L; and PLT 30.0×10^9/L. RBC morphology on the blood film appeared normal. The reticulocyte count was 0.5%.

Case Study 10-3

A 35-year-old male visited the emergency room complaining of fatigue. He had recently been treated for a respiratory illness. The following laboratory results were reported: RBC 1.7×10^{12}/L; Hb 5.2 g/dL; Hct 0.16 L/L; WBC 7.5×10^9/L; WBC differential normal; and reticulocyte count 22.0%.

Case Study 10-4

A 72-year-old man visited a physician complaining of palpitations, dizziness, and visual disturbances. The following laboratory results were reported: RBC 6.8×10^{12}/L; Hb 20 g/dL; Hct 0.64 L/L; WBC 13.0×10^9/L; PLT 500×10^9/L; WBC differential 75% segmented neutrophils, 11% band neutrophils, 11% lymphocytes, 2% basophils, and 1% eosinophils.
1. Describe this man's hematologic findings.
2. What follow-up laboratory testing could be recommended to assist in the diagnosis?

Review Questions

10-1. An increased MCV is associated with

  A. macrocytic anemia.
  B. microcytic anemia.
  C. normocytic anemia.
  D. all of the above.

10-2. An erythrocyte population with marked variability in size (anisocytosis) can best be identified by a(n)

  A. increased MCV.
  B. decreased MCV.
  C. increased RDW.
  D. decreased RDW.

10-3. An RPI of less than 2.0 is associated with

  A. hypoproliferative anemia.
  B. anemias of maturation disorders.
  C. both A and B.
  D. neither A nor B.

10-4. Inappropriate absolute secondary erythrocytosis may be caused by

  A. pulmonary disease.
  B. renal or extrarenal tumors.
  C. smoker's polycythemia.
  D. all of the above.

10-5. Relative erythrocytosis is caused by a(n)

  A. decrease in plasma volume.
  B. increase in plasma volume.
  C. decrease in red cell mass.
  D. increase in red cell mass.

10-6. A laboratory test that is always useful in the differential diagnosis of relative and absolute erythrocytosis is

  A. hemoglobin electrophoresis.
  B. hemoglobin quantitation.
  C. plasma erythropoietin quantitation.
  D. red cell mass quantitation.

References

1. Berk PD, Goldberg JD, Donovan PB et al: Therapeutic recommendations in Polycythemia Vera Study Group protocols. Semin Hematol 23:132, 1986
2. Bessman JD: Automated Blood Counts and Differentials: A Practical Guide, p 9. Baltimore, The Johns Hopkins University Press, 1986
3. Bessman JD, Gilmer PR, Gardner FH: Improved classification of anemias by MCV and RDW. Am J Clin Pathol 80:31, 1983
4. Beutler E: The red cell indices in the diagnosis of iron deficiency anemia. Ann Intern Med 50:313, 1959
5. Connors DM, Wilson MK: A new approach to the reporting of red cell morphology. J Am Med Technol 3:94, 1986
6. Cotes PM, Dore CJ, Liu Yin JA et al: Determination of serum immunoreactive erythropoietin in the investigation of erythrocytosis. N Engl J Med 315:283, 1986
7. Das Gupta A, Hegde C, Mistri R: Red cell distribution width as a measure of severity of iron deficiency in iron deficiency anaemia. Indian J Med Res 100:177, 1994
8. England JM: Future needs and expected trends in peripheral blood cell analysis: Erythrocyte histograms. Blood Cells 11:61, 1985
9. Erslev AJ, Caro J: Secondary polycythemias: A boon or a burden? Blood Cells 10:177, 1984
10. Erslev AJ, Caro J: Pure erythrocytosis classified according to erythropoietin titers. Am J Med 76:57, 1984
11. Fairbanks VF: Is the peripheral blood film reliable for the diagnosis of iron deficiency anemia? Am J Clin Pathol 55:447, 1971
12. Fairbanks VF: Nonequivalence of automated and manual hematocrit and erythrocytic indices. Am J Clin Pathol 73:55, 1980
13. Figueroa WG: Hematology. New York, John Wiley & Sons, 1981
14. Flynn MM, Reppun TS, Bhagavan NV: Limitations of red blood cell distribution width (RDW) in evaluation of microcytosis. Am J Clin Pathol 85:445, 1986
15. Gilmer PR, Koepke JA: The reticulocyte: An approach to definition. Am J Clin Pathol 66:262, 1976
16. Hillman RS, Finch CA: The Red Cell Manual, 5th ed. Philadelphia, FA Davis, 1985
17. Johnson CS, Tegos C, Beutler E: Thalassemia minor: Routine erythrocyte measurements and differentiation from iron deficiency. Am J Clin Pathol 80:31, 1983
18. Koeffler HP, Goldwasser E: Erythropoietin radioimmunoassay in evaluating patients with polycythemia. Ann Intern Med 94:44, 1981
19. Lloyd EM: How flowcharts improve RBC morphology reporting. MLO 14:49, 1982
20. McClure S, Custer E, Bessman D: Improved detection of early iron deficiency in nonanemic subjects. JAMA 253:1021, 1985
21. Napoli VM, Nichols CW, Fleck SH: A semiquantitative estimate method for reporting abnormal RBC morphology. Lab Med 11:111, 1980
22. Peebles DA, Hochberg A, Clarke TD: Analysis of manual reticulocyte counting. Am J Clin Pathol 76:713, 1981
23. Savage RA: The red cell indices: Yesterday, today, and tomorrow. Clin Lab Med 13:777, 1993

24. Savage RA, Skoog DP, Rabinovitch A: Analytic inaccuracy and imprecision in reticulocyte counting: A preliminary report from the College of American Pathologists Reticulocyte Project. Blood Cells 11:97, 1985

25. Smith JR, Landaw SA: Smoker's polycythemia. N Engl J Med 298:6, 1978

26. Stefanini M, Urbas JV, Urbas JE: Gaisböck's syndrome: Its hematologic, biochemical and hormonal parameters. Angiology 29:520, 1978

27. Wintrobe MM: Anemia: Classification and treatment on the basis of differences in the average volume and hemoglobin content of red corpuscles. Arch Intern Med 54:256, 1934

28. Wu KK, Gibson TP, Freeman RM et al: Erythrocytosis after renal transplantation. Arch Intern Med 132:898, 1973

CHAPTER 11

Anemias of Bone Marrow Failure and Systemic Disorders

Joyce A. Behrens

Objectives

1. Define the following terms with respect to bone marrow and peripheral blood cellularity: aplastic, hypoplastic, myelophthisic, pure red cell aplasia, anemia, pancytopenia, and leukoerythroblastosis.
2. Differentiate between primary and secondary acquired aplastic anemia, and name a minimum of three possible etiologies for secondary aplastic anemia.
3. Discuss Fanconi anemia with respect to its mode of inheritance and its cytogenetic, bone marrow, and peripheral blood abnormalities, including at what point in time they appear. Name a minimum of three other body systems often displaying abnormalities in this disorder.
4. Discuss the effects of the following treatments on bone marrow and peripheral blood laboratory results in patients with aplastic anemia: bone marrow transplantation, immunosuppressive agents (*e.g.*, anti-thymocyte globulin, cyclosporin A), androgens, and blood product support.
5. Differentiate between primary and secondary (acquired) pure red cell aplasia.
6. Describe the laboratory findings in Diamond-Blackfan anemia.
7. Identify the primary etiology for anemia of chronic renal disease. Discuss the expected changes in laboratory results following treatment with erythropoietin, with a kidney transplant, and with renal graft rejection.
8. Name two endocrine organs which, if abnormal, are associated with anemia, and briefly describe the laboratory findings.

Anemia can be the result of an absolute failure of the bone marrow to replace erythrocytes that are either normally destroyed after 120 days or those that are prematurely destroyed, such as by hemolysis. This failure may be the result of a primary defect in the marrow itself, such as occurs in aplastic anemia and pure red cell aplasia. Normal bone marrow cells may also be replaced by metastatic tumor cells (malignant cells that have migrated to the bone marrow from another site). The resulting anemia is called myelophthisic anemia and represents altered hematopoiesis due to the crowding out of the normal marrow.

There also are a number of systemic diseases, including those that affect the renal and endocrine systems, that can result in a secondary decrease in the absolute number of erythroid precursors in the marrow. Here a factor, usually hormonal, is decreased or absent; this factor normally has some erythropoietic stimulatory effect. In these cases the bone marrow is functionally normal; however, anemia may still develop. All of the above causes for anemia will be discussed in this chapter.

ANEMIAS OF BONE MARROW FAILURE

Aplastic Anemia

DEFINITION

Aplastic anemia (AA) is a condition in which there is a peripheral blood pancytopenia, defined as a decrease in all cellular constituents: leukocytes, erythrocytes, and platelets. The bone marrow in AA is, by definition, severely hypoplastic (decreased number of bone marrow cells in all three cell lines) or aplastic (absence of all bone marrow cells); the normal hematopoietic cells are replaced by fat.[11,13,28] The name of this disorder is misleading, as it implies that anemia is the primary problem experienced by these patients; however, their most serious clinical problems relate to neutropenia and thrombocytopenia, so that it might better be called *myeloaplasia*, meaning decreased development of all bone marrow cells. The criteria for laboratory diagnosis of severe AA are listed in Table 11-1. There are milder forms of AA that do not meet these strict criteria and are thus not diagnosed as frank AA, such as hypoplastic anemia secondary to drug toxicity. It is important to note that in AA there are no immature myeloid cells in the peripheral blood. This

TABLE 11-1
Diagnostic Criteria for Severe Aplastic Anemia

BONE MARROW

Cellularity	<25% of normal
	or
	<50% of normal cellularity with <30% hematopoietic cells

Plus Any Two of the Following:

PERIPHERAL BLOOD

Granulocytes	$<0.5 \times 10^9/L$
Platelets	$<20 \times 10^9/L$
Anemia with	<1% reticulocytes (corrected for hematocrit)

TABLE 11-3
Drugs for which Association with Aplastic Anemia, as an Idiosyncratic Reaction, Has Been Well Established on Clinical Grounds

ANTIBACTERIALS
Chloramphenicol
Sulfonamides

ANTI-INFLAMMATORY/ANTIRHEUMATIC AGENTS
Phenylbutazone
Oxyphenbutazone
Gold salts
Indomethacin

ANTICONVULSANTS
Phenytoin
Methoin

DIURETICS
Chlorothiazide and other thiazides

ANTITHYROID DRUGS
Propylthiouracil
Methylthiouracil
Carbimazole
Potassium perchlorate
Thiocyanate

ORAL HYPOGLYCEMIC AGENTS
Chlorpropamide and other sulfonylureas

ANTIMALARIALS
Amodiaquine
Chloroquine
Mepacrine (quinacrine)

From Vincent PC: Drug-induced aplastic anemia and agranulocytosis: Incidence and mechanisms. Drugs 31:52, 1986. Auckland, New Zeland, ADIS Press Limited, with permission

finding, along with the aplastic or hypoplastic marrow, where hematopoietic cells are replaced by fat cells, helps to differentiate AA from a number of other pancytopenic conditions.

AGE INCIDENCE DEMOGRAPHICS

The incidence of AA is low before the age of 1 year, then increases at an intermediate rate until the age of 50, after which the incidence is highest. Marrow aplasia is two to five times more frequent in the Far East than in either North America or Europe.[11]

AA can be divided into primary and secondary types (Table 11-2). The primary group includes Fanconi anemia (an inherited form which is rare) and idiopathic AA, for which there is no known etiology. Forty to seventy percent of the cases in the United States and more than 90% of the cases in Japan[11] are idiopathic. In contrast, secondary AA has a number of identified causative factors and agents (Table 11-3). The secondary types are discussed first in this chapter because they are more easily understood.

Several mechanisms have been implicated as the underlying defect in all forms of AA, whether primary or

TABLE 11-2
Classification of Aplastic Anemia

PRIMARY
Congenital Fanconi anemia
Acquired idiopathic

SECONDARY
Drugs (Table 11-3)
Chemicals (Table 11-3)
Radiation
Immune mechanism
Infection
    Non-A, non-B hepatitis (Hepatitis C)
    Other viral infections
    Miliary tuberculosis
    Brucellosis
    Parasites

secondary. These include a deficiency in the number of bone marrow stem cells, immune suppression of stem cells, or a defect in the stem cells themselves, making them unresponsive to normal hematopoietic growth factors or mitotic stimuli. Damage to the bone marrow microenvironment (those elements within hematopoietic tissue that provide mechanical support for developing hematopoietic cells) has also been implicated in the past[47]; however, this does not seem likely because, as bone marrow transplants have become more successful, they have shown that donor stem cells are usually capable of thriving in the recipient's microenvironment. Whatever the etiology or mechanism, the end result is the same—failure of hematopoietic stem cell growth, resulting in a hypoplastic or aplastic marrow and pancytopenia.

Secondary Aplastic Anemia

ETIOLOGY AND PATHOPHYSIOLOGY

There is extensive literature implicating drugs (Table 11-3), chemicals, radiation, abnormal immune mechanisms, and various other factors as causes of secondary AA.

Drugs and Chemicals. Chloramphenicol, now rarely prescribed, is the classic drug associated with marrow aplasia. Transient marrow hypoplasia after treatment with chloramphenicol is fairly common.[11,25,28] This is associated with the appearance of vacuolated cells in the bone marrow, especially among the erythroid series.[25] Sometimes a more serious persistent marrow aplasia follows chloramphenicol therapy. The incidence of AA is 5- to 40-fold higher in persons who have taken this drug than in persons not exposed to it.[11]

Other drugs and chemicals associated with the development of AA include benzene and benzene derivatives, hydantoins, sulfonamides, and gold preparations.[25,28] Insecticides such as chlordane and chlorophenothane (DDT) have also been cited.[85] Table 11-3 lists drugs associated with idiosyncratic development of AA. Many other drugs, including "innocent" drugs such as aspirin, may be etiologic in an occasional patient.

Radiation. Radiation may damage the stem cells[25] or the hematopoietic microenvironment.[7] Individuals exposed to long-term, low-dose irradiation have an increased incidence of AA. Examples include patients receiving radiation for ankylosing spondylitis, who have a 40-fold increase in the incidence of AA, and American radiologists, with a 20-fold increase in incidence.[11]

High-dose radiation associated with acute exposure—radiotherapy, radioactive isotope administration, or work in unsafe nuclear power plants—can result in rapidly developing bone marrow aplasia and death.[25] After the 1986 Chernobyl (USSR) nuclear accident, 35 individuals who were exposed to high radiation doses were in grave condition with severe marrow aplasia; 11 of these died within 3 weeks of the accident from the complications associated with bone marrow failure as well as of the severe radiation burns they had suffered.[33,82]

Immune Mechanism. There is some support for an autoimmune mechanism as a cause of aplasia, either directly by lymphocytes or by some humoral factor. In 11 of 22 patients with AA who received syngeneic (identical twin) transplants (in which theoretically there should be no rejection of the graft), rejection was experienced. Six of these 11 patients were then conditioned with cyclophosphamide, an immunosuppressive agent, prior to receiving a second infusion of identical twin marrow. In all of these cases engraftment was then successful and permanent, suggesting an immunologic mechanism for AA.[74]

Occasionally, lymphocytes from patients with AA suppress growth of normal marrow cells *in vitro*. To suppress this process *in vivo*, patients have been given antithymocyte globulin (ATG). Thereafter, lymphocytes from the patients no longer suppress *in vitro* growth of their own marrow colony-forming unit–cultures (CFU-C).[11,78]

Humoral inhibitors of stem cell growth have been reported in a few patients whose AA was either idiopathic or associated with systemic lupus erythematosus, quinidine, or cryoglobulinemia.[11]

Miscellaneous Etiologies. Numerous other associations with AA have been observed, most quite rare. Occasionally, infection precedes the syndrome. Most commonly,

this infection is non-A, non-B hepatitis. These patients usually have not had severe hepatitis, and the infection usually has resolved by the time the aplasia develops several months later.[11] This situation is predominantly seen in young adults, and these patients have a poor prognosis, with the disease often being rapidly fatal.[69] Other reported cases have been associated with miliary tuberculosis, brucellosis, and parasitic infestation.[11]

AA is also related to other myeloid stem cell disorders. Twenty-five percent of patients with paroxysmal nocturnal hemoglobinuria (PNH), an acquired clonal disorder (Chap. 18), develop AA. Conversely, 5% to 10% of patients with AA develop PNH. In addition, 1% to 5% of patients who present with AA actually have leukemia. The leukemic cells may release one or more factors that suppress hematopoiesis, causing a hypoplastic marrow with peripheral blood pancytopenia. On the other hand, AA sometimes transforms into acute leukemia (Chap. 34).

CLINICAL PRESENTATION

The symptoms are directly related to pancytopenia.[25,28] If anemia is severe enough, the typical symptoms occur: pallor, weakness, and easy fatigability. Decreased neutrophils result in an increased incidence of bacterial infections; there is no increase in viral infections. Hemorrhage may be seen as a consequence of thrombocytopenia. The lack of a palpable spleen (*i.e.*, a normal spleen) in AA is significant in the diagnosis, because splenomegaly is a common finding in other disorders which demonstrate pancytopenia.

LABORATORY FINDINGS AND CORRELATIONS WITH DISEASE

Peripheral Blood. The patient is anemic, neutropenic, and thrombocytopenic (Fig. 11-1). The total leukocyte count also is decreased.[12,25,28] Table 11-1 summarizes the laboratory criteria for the diagnosis of AA. Lymphocytes are normal to slightly decreased, unless the patient has been on immunosuppressive therapy, in which case lymphocytes may be significantly decreased. The anemia is usually normocytic and normochromic, although occasionally slight macrocytosis is observed. The morphology of the red cells is normal; the reticulocyte count is decreased, and the calculated reticulocyte production index (RPI) is significantly decreased (Chap. 9). Of great significance is that there are no immature cells in the peripheral blood.

Bone Marrow. Both a bone marrow aspirate for evaluation of cell morphology and cell differentiation and a bone marrow biopsy for evaluation of overall marrow structure and cellularity should be performed. The marrow biopsy specimen is usually hypoplastic or aplastic, with increased fat and decreased hematopoietic cells; megakaryocytes generally are notably absent (Fig. 11-2). The principal cells present are lymphocytes and plasma cells. There are no increased numbers of immature cells observed in the marrow, as would be seen, for example, in a patient with pancytopenia and acute leukemia as the etiology. The bone marrow biopsy in patients with AA may have patchy areas of cellularity; thus, occasionally a bone mar-

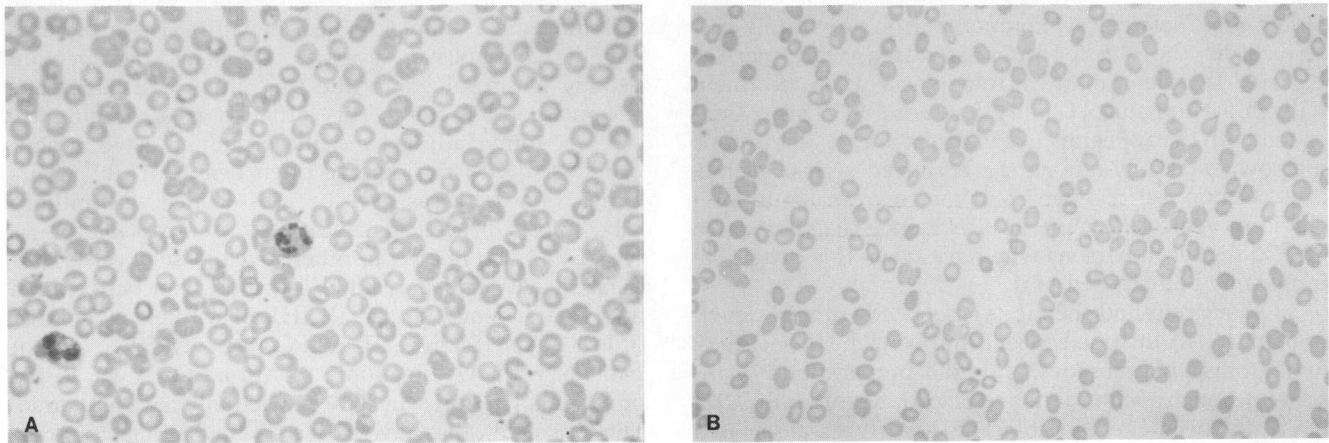

FIGURE 11-1. Normal peripheral blood (**A**) compared with peripheral blood pancytopenia (**B**). Note the lack of leukocytes in (**B**) and obvious scarcity of both red cells and platelets compared with the normal picture.

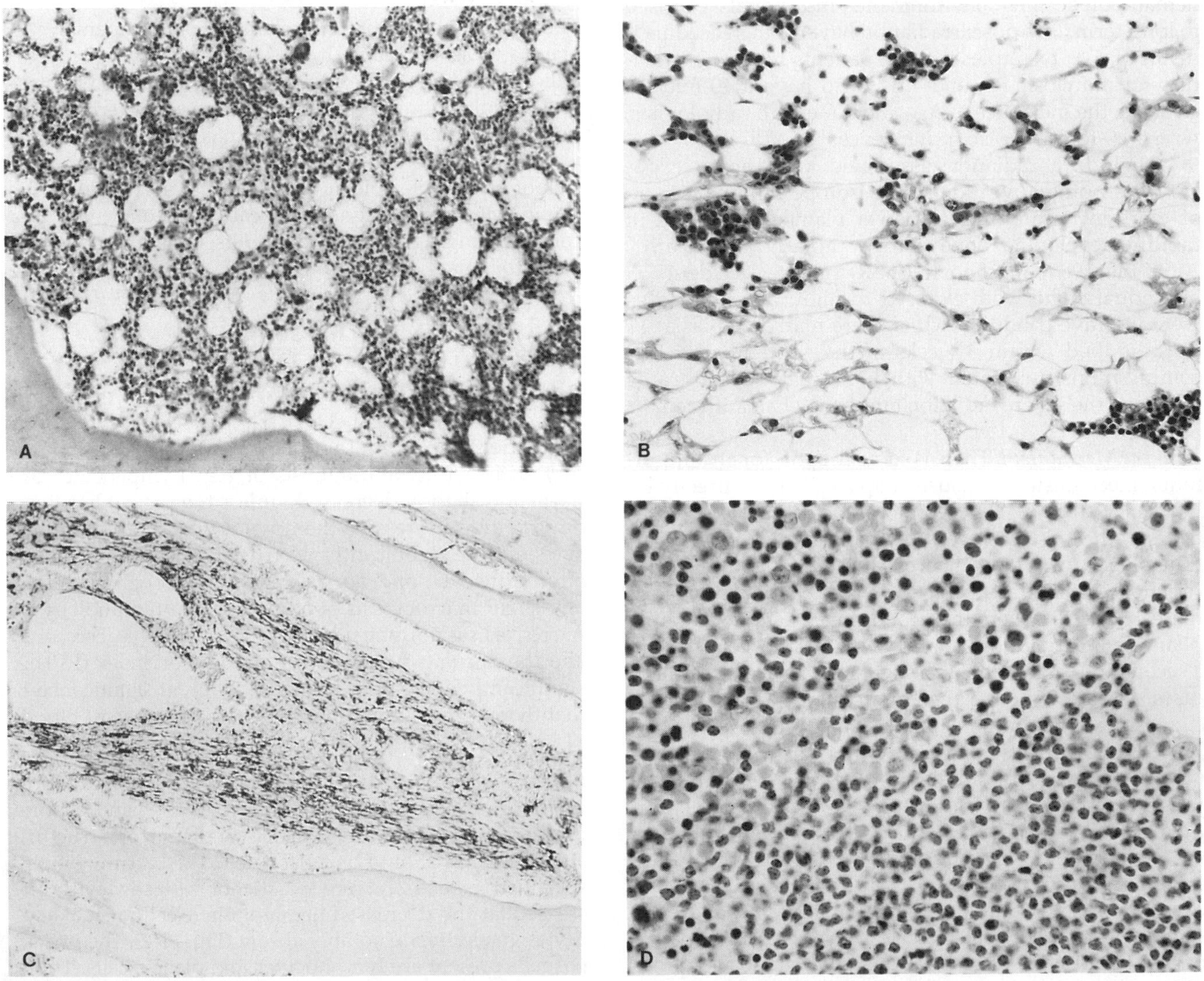

FIGURE 11-2. Comparison of marrow biopsies from (**A**) a normal individual with a normocellular marrow, showing a 1:1 fat to cell ratio; (**B**) an individual with aplastic anemia, showing a hypocellular marrow in which fat has replaced normal hematopoietic cells; the remaining cells are primarily lymphocytes and plasma cells; (**C**) a fibrotic marrow, which is associated with a number of disorders, such as agnogenic myeloid metaplasia; and (**D**) a hypercellular marrow, which is associated with a number of disorders, including leukemia. Note the striking difference among the abnormal marrow structures even though each may cause pancytopenia in the peripheral blood.

row sample indicates some cellularity rather than the hypoplastic or aplastic state defined for AA.

Special Hematology Tests. Hemoglobin F (Hb F) is elevated in some patients,[8,12] and is distributed unevenly in red cells when a Kleihauer-Betke acid elution test (Chap. 15) is performed. In the past it was believed that a high Hb F was associated with a better prognosis,[8] but this view has not been substantiated.[62] Scores for leukocyte alkaline phosphatase (LAP; Chap. 29) are often increased. The Ham acidified serum test (Chap. 18), which is the confirmatory test for paroxysmal nocturnal hemoglobinuria (PNH), also may be positive in AA. (See Differential Diagnosis for an explanation of laboratory differentiation of the two disorders.)

Chemistry. Serum iron generally is elevated and plasma iron clearance delayed because the patient has adequate iron stores and therefore decreased uptake of iron due to a reduction in the number of developing red cells.[12] All of these abnormalities are a reflection of decreased erythropoiesis. Humoral stimulators of hematopoiesis such as erythropoietin (EPO) are usually normal or elevated.[11]

Cytogenetics. Marrow chromosomes are normal in most patients. When abnormalities are found, the diagnosis of a myelodysplastic syndrome should be considered (Chap. 33).[12]

DIFFERENTIAL DIAGNOSIS

Because a number of disorders can cause peripheral blood pancytopenia, acquired AA must be differentiated from them, often by exclusion of all other possibilities, so that appropriate therapy can be given. Table 11-4 lists the disorders most commonly associated with pancytopenia (although they do not always cause pancytopenia) and their distinguishing laboratory characteristics. None of the disorders in Table 11-4 causes a strikingly hypocellular marrow like that of AA. Therefore, the differential diagnosis based on examination of a marrow biopsy usually is not difficult. Figure 11-2 shows a marrow biopsy from a normal individual, termed normocellular, contrasted with marrows that are hypocellular (as seen in AA), fibrotic, and hypercellular.

Physical findings that generally rule out AA include splenomegaly or lymphadenopathy. Radiographic stud-

TABLE 11-4
Differential Diagnosis of Pancytopenia

Condition	Peripheral Blood	Bone Marrow	Splenomegaly	Additional Comments*
Aplastic anemia	No immature leukocytes or erythrocytes; MCV usually normal	Hypoplastic to aplastic (Fig. 11-1)	Absent	LAP score N to ↑; Ham's acidified serum test ±
Acute leukemia	Blasts usually present	Hyperplastic to neoplastic (Fig. 11-1) with immature cells dominant	May be present	
Myelofibrosis	Leukoerythroblastosis often seen; tear drop RBCs prominent	Increased reticulin (Fig. 11-1); may be hypoplastic	Prominent	LAP score variable; usually N to ↑
Megaloblastic anemia	Anemia most prominent MCV > 110 fL	Hypercellular with megaloblastic features	Absent	Serum folate &/or B_{12} ↓
Hairy cell leukemia	Hairy cells usually present	Increased reticulin; characteristic "fried egg" appearance on biopsy because of cells' abundant cytoplasm with hairline projections	Present	Marrow aspirate usually dry tap; malignant cells TRAP+
Paroxysmal nocturnal hemoglobinuria	Anemia most prominent feature; mild to moderate reticulocytosis	Erythroid hyperplasia; may be hypoplastic to aplastic	Absent	Sugar water screening test +; Ham's acidified serum test +; LAP score ↓; hemosiderinuria present
Multiple myeloma	Rouleaux present; anemia most prominent	Plasmacytosis (clonal)	Usually absent	Monoclonal protein in serum; monoclonal light chains in urine
Waldenstrom's macroglobulinemia	Rouleaux present; anemia most prominent	Increased B lymphocytes ("plasmacytoid lymphs")	Often present	IgM monoclonal protein in serum; monoclonal light chains in urine
Lymphoma	Pancytopenia rare	(See Chap. 38)	Usually absent	Lymphadenopathy
Myelodysplastic syndromes	Pancytopenia variable; evidence of dyspoiesis (see Chap. 33)	Hypercellular; dyspoiesis in one or more cell lines	Absent	

*LAP = leukocyte alkaline phosphatase; N = normal; ↑ = increased; ↓ = decreased; TRAP = tartrate-resistant acid phosphatase.

ies of the bone may be necessary to rule out primary or metastatic bone tumors or other focal lesions.

The finding of immature erythrocytes or leukocytes in the peripheral blood also usually rules out AA and indicates any number of disorders, including leukemia, lymphoma, myelofibrosis, and myelodysplastic syndrome (Table 11-4). Usually, the marrow in these disorders is hypercellular.

Table 11-5 summarizes the tests recommended to assist in the diagnosis of AA. The tests most frequently used are most commonly performed to make the initial diagnosis. It is not necessary to perform these tests frequently, unless the patient is undergoing treatment to which the response must be verified.

EFFECTS OF TREATMENT ON LABORATORY RESULTS

Occasionally, a spontaneous remission occurs in AA. For most patients, however, the only cure is bone marrow transplantation from a compatible donor. The ideal donor is syngeneic (an identical twin). Other acceptable donors are allogeneic, with the donor being a human leukocyte antigen (HLA)–matched family member or an HLA-matched but unrelated donor. Patients who undergo bone marrow transplantation have a much more favorable prognosis and survival rate than those for whom no donor can be found, especially in the first 6 months after diagnosis.[13]

The principal problems associated with bone marrow transplantation are failure of sustained marrow engraftment (*i.e.*, rejection) and the development of graft *versus* host disease (GVHD).[74,75] Successful and maintained engraftment is greatly improved if patients receive the transplant early in their disease, prior to any blood product transfusions. If transfusions are necessary because of a life-threatening event, the blood should not come from potential marrow donors in order to avoid sensitization of the patient to minor histocompatibility antigens (for which no immunohematologic typing is available) that

may be present in the donor but not in the recipient.[74] When transfusions are avoided, one study demonstrated that engraftment was achieved in 90% of the patients. Of these successes, 83% were surviving from 9 to 84 months following transplantation. In contrast, engraftment in multiply transfused patients studied during the same time period was 69%, with a survival rate of 54%.[75]

Patients receiving allogeneic transplants require previous conditioning with cyclophosphamide to decrease the risk of rejection.[75] Some groups add irradiation,[74] although the use of radiation carries the risk of future development of a malignancy.[12] Most grafts now are successful with complete hematologic recovery,[74] as evidenced by increasing marrow cellularity followed by a rise in peripheral blood counts within 2 to 4 weeks after engraftment.

Acute and chronic GVHD are still a significant concern. GVHD is understood to be an immune reaction triggered by an incompatibility between the donor and recipient HLA antigens. As its name implies, GVHD is mediated by donor lymphocytes acting against host tissues.[74,75] In the past, methotrexate (MTX) was the agent most frequently used to prevent acute GVHD. The use of another immunosuppressive agent, cyclosporin A (CyA), has proven to be more effective than MTX in reducing the incidence and severity of both acute and chronic GVHD.[6,42,59] Cyclosporine, either alone or in combination with MTX, does improve the success of engraftment.[14a] There is some preliminary evidence that the addition of folinic acid to a combination of MTX and CyA may help patients better tolerate this GVHD prophylactic protocol.[2,42,68]

If acute GVHD does appear, it is usually anywhere from day 10 to day 70 after grafting. Organs attacked include the gut, skin, and liver. Chronic GVHD occurs between 3 to 15 months after grafting, and its forms range from mild to severe. It is treated with prednisone, sometimes in combination with azathioprine, both of which are immunosuppressants. The clinical features of chronic GVHD include a persistent immune deficiency, impaired granulocyte chemotaxis, recurrent bacterial infections, disfiguring skin lesions, and liver dysfunction.[12,74,75] Infectious complications can also occur, the most serious of which is interstitial pneumonia.[12]

For patients who do not have a suitable donor, other modes of therapy for AA are attempted. Most important is blood product support as needed, including both red cell and platelet transfusions. Immunosuppressive therapy is the next mode of treatment usually attempted. This includes the use of either antithymocyte globulin (ATG) or antilymphocyte globulin (ALG). The mechanism of the response in some patients is not clear,[11] but theoretically, these agents are useful when an immune mechanism causes the aplasia.

CyA has also now been successfully used to treat AA patients with no suitable donor. It has proven to be equivalent to the use of ATG, with less toxicity and fewer infectious deaths.[35,73,77] There is a recent report that the addition of recombinant human granulocyte colony-stimulating factor (G-CSF) to CyA may result in stimulation of the bone marrow to produce leukocytes, erythrocytes, and platelets, and patients may actually become transfusion independent.[5] More study is needed, but this may

TABLE 11-5 *Tests Recommended to Assist in Differential Diagnosis of Aplastic Anemia*	
Most frequently required (These tests usually do not need to be repeated frequently)	Complete blood count Platelet count Reticulocyte count (with RPI) Differential Bone marrow biopsy Bone marrow aspirate
Required occasionally	Sucrose hemolysis test Ham's acidified serum test (if sucrose hemolysis test is positive)
Required rarely	Haptoglobin Bilirubin (unconjugated) Serum B_{12} Serum erythropoietin LAP Urine urobilinogen (quantitative) Ferrokinetic studies

prove to be an alternative treatment for patients who lack an HLA-matched marrow donor.

Androgens stimulate erythropoiesis and, to a lesser degree, granulopoiesis and thrombopoiesis. Despite a multi-institutional study that showed no benefit to patients receiving androgens compared with patients who did not,[13] some patients do respond, and therefore androgens continue to be used in the hope of improvement.

Because of the current success of bone marrow transplantation in AA, it is the recommended therapy if a suitable donor is available, especially for patients younger than 40 years of age. For patients over age 40, immunosuppressive therapy is recommended.[74]

PROGNOSIS

Prognosis is dependent on the mode of therapy used. Bone marrow transplants in nontransfused patients result in long-term survival rates as high as 83%; many of these patients have now been followed for more than 12 years and are hematologically normal.[12,74] The prognosis is much poorer for patients for whom a suitable donor cannot be found.[13]

Regardless of the mode of therapy, the survival curves in AA are biphasic, with considerable early mortality rates followed by a much slower decline[12] for those who survive the initial period. Children have a somewhat better prognosis than adults. Long-term survivors of bone marrow transplants can be considered cured.[12]

Primary Aplastic Anemia

PATHOPHYSIOLOGY AND CLINICAL PRESENTATION

Primary (congenital) aplastic anemia is also known as *Fanconi anemia (FA)*. FA is a rare, inherited form of aplastic anemia, first reported in three brothers by Fanconi, after whom the disease was named. It is defined hematologically as a pancytopenic disorder with a hypoplastic to aplastic bone marrow. Inheritance is autosomal recessive.[21,39,43,58] It can be caused by defects in any one of four genes that have now been identified.[20,76]

Prominent congenital abnormalities are usually present in this disorder, and include microencephaly (abnormally small cranial cavity), brown skin pigmentation, short stature, malformations of the thumbs, internal strabismus (crossed eyes), malformations of the kidney, genital hypoplasia, and mental retardation.[63] The phenotype is, however, more variable than previously recognized.[34]

LABORATORY FINDINGS AND CORRELATIONS WITH DISEASE

Hematology. Peripheral blood abnormalities generally do not manifest themselves until 5 to 10 years after birth,[43,58] when anemia, neutropenia, and thrombocytopenia may occur. Both anisocytosis and poikilocytosis are seen. There is a marked increase in Hb F, with a concomitant decrease in Hb A. Osmotic fragility is increased, as is the erythrocyte sedimentation rate (although this may be simply a reflection of the anemia).[43,58] If FA is diagnosed early in life, the bone marrow may initially be described as normocellular. However, with time it invariably becomes hypoplastic and eventually aplastic.[58]

Cytogenetics. These patients usually have multiple chromosomal abnormalities, including ring chromosomes, translocations, dicentric forms, and spontaneous breaks.[21,39,43,58] In contrast to the late appearance of peripheral blood abnormalities years after birth, chromosomal abnormalities can be demonstrated at birth in lymphocytes, myeloid cells, fibroblasts, and other body tissues.[43,58] The diagnosis is confirmed *in vitro* by the unique cellular hypersensitivity of cultured lymphocytes to agents that interfere with DNA synthesis, such as diepoxybutane and mitomycin C.[67,76]

EFFECTS OF TREATMENT ON LABORATORY RESULTS AND PROGNOSIS

Before the advent of androgen therapy, the prognosis of patients with FA was poor, with a life expectancy of 2 to 4 years after the appearance of hematologic symptoms.[39,43,58] The use of androgens to stimulate erythropoiesis, accompanied by corticosteroids, has made it possible to maintain a reasonable Hb level for a period of time,[43] but the disease nevertheless progresses to bone marrow aplasia. Death is most often secondary to hemorrhage or infection and only rarely to the results of severe anemia.[39]

Bone marrow transplantation is a viable possibility, and should be the first consideration for therapy in patients for whom an HLA-matched donor is available.[18,30,46] It can offer long-term survival for FA patients. However, the widespread chromosomal damage in all body tissues still leaves the patient vulnerable to malignant disease.[43] The multiple chromosomal defects, particularly the translocations, are believed to predispose these patients to the development of acute myeloid leukemia (AML) (and rarely, other malignancies).[21,39,43] In fact, the incidence of AML in FA is more than 15,000 times that observed in children in the general population.[3,4] The patient's family also is at increased risk of leukemia, since FA is inherited and carriers thus exist in the family.[21]

Acquired Pure Red Cell Aplasia

Pure red cell aplasia (PRCA) is a rare condition that may be inherited or acquired as a primary or secondary disorder (Table 11-6). The acquired form is seen primarily in individuals older than 40 years of age[49] and is characterized by a severe anemia with normal to slightly decreased peripheral blood leukocyte and platelet counts. In the bone marrow overall cellularity is normal, as are granulopoiesis and thrombopoiesis. However, there is a severe decrease in erythroid elements; sometimes almost no erythroid elements are seen.

PATHOPHYSIOLOGY AND CLINICAL PRESENTATION

The etiology of primary PRCA involves either an idiopathic or an immune mechanism. Some patients have an immunoglobulin inhibitor of erythroid precursors, which is demonstrated by the fact that *in vitro* incubation of a patient's own serum and marrow cells inhibits erythroid

TABLE 11-6
Classification of Pure Red Cell Aplasias

Acquired
  Primary
    Idiopathic
    Immune mechanism
      Immunoglobulin inhibitor to RBC precursors
      Erythropoietin inhibitor
  Secondary
    Benign thymoma
    Drugs
    Chemicals
    Infections
    Hemolytic anemia—aplastic crisis
Congenital
  Diamond-Blackfan anemia

growth. In the absence of the patient's serum the patient's erythroid cells do grow. Patients have increased EPO levels. Much less common with respect to an immune etiology is an inhibitor of EPO; such individuals have little or no EPO.[49,50,79]

Pure red cell aplasia may also be secondary to a variety of etiologic agents (Table 11-6). Probably the most significant association is that with benign thymoma (tumor of the thymus gland).[49,50] Twenty-nine percent of these patients have a remission of their anemia when the thymoma is removed, suggesting a primary relation between the two. The frequency of secondary PRCA associated with thymoma and the frequency of primary PRCA are about the same.

There are a variety of other immunologic associations with PRCA, including the fact that some patients have antinuclear antibodies (Chap. 24), some a spike on protein electrophoresis, and some hypogammaglobulinemia. Other etiologic agents are drugs, chemicals, and infections, and the aplastic crisis of hemolytic anemia. In contrast to the first three etiologies, the aplastic crisis of hemolytic anemia is usually acute and self-limited, requiring no therapy unless the degree of anemia warrants transfusion.[49]

The anemia develops insidiously, and the onset is so gradual that the patient effectively compensates. Thus, by the time a patient presents with symptoms, the anemia usually is severe.[79] The only constant clinical finding is extreme pallor; a significant number of patients develop splenomegaly, hepatomegaly, or both, but these may be consequences of the hemosiderosis that follows the multiple red cell transfusions required for treatment.[49]

LABORATORY FINDINGS AND CORRELATIONS WITH DISEASE

Hematology. In symptomatic patients there is a severe normocytic, normochromic anemia with the reticulocyte count greatly depressed or even 0%. The leukocyte and platelet counts are usually normal, although they may be mildly depressed. The leukocyte differential usually is normal. The bone marrow is normal except for the extreme decrease in or even absence of erythroid precursors.[49,50]

Chemistry. Serum iron and percent transferrin saturation are increased because of the multiple red cell transfusions. EPO levels are increased in most patients as the erythropoietic control mechanism attempts to stimulate erythrocyte production, which is impossible without erythroid precursors.

EFFECTS OF TREATMENT ON LABORATORY RESULTS

A significant number of patients undergo a spontaneous remission, in which hematologic measurements return to normal, sometimes after years of therapy. The mainstay of therapy is red cell transfusion to maintain a reasonable erythrocyte mass. Because of the high incidence of thymomas in these patients, the clinician should search for a thymoma. If one is present and removed, improved clinical and laboratory findings often result. Immunosuppressive therapy has proven beneficial in some patients; therefore, a clinical trial is justified. Androgens have also been effective in stimulating erythropoiesis in some patients.[49,50] If patients do not respond to therapy, such that long-term maintenance with transfusions is necessary, they may eventually succumb to either hepatitis or hemosiderosis, both complications of chronic transfusion therapy.[50]

Diamond-Blackfan Anemia

Diamond-Blackfan anemia (congenital hypoplastic anemia or congenital PRCA) is a rare congenital disorder that was first described in 1938. It is defined as a normochromic, normocytic anemia with normal leukocyte and platelet counts and a marked decrease in marrow erythroblasts. The diagnosis is usually made in infancy or early childhood.[1,19,62]

The etiology of Diamond-Blackfan anemia is unknown, partly because there are so few patients available for study. However, one *in vitro* study, in culture, demonstrated a lack of responsiveness of the patient's marrow sample to added EPO. In other words, the few colony-forming units–erythroid (CFU-E) in the culture were insensitive to erythropoietin stimulation.[62] In at least some patients there may be an immunologic etiology as demonstrated by another study, which showed that patient lymphocytes were able to inhibit *in vitro* erythropoiesis in normal bone marrow, even in the presence of added EPO. Serum from the patients did not inhibit erythropoiesis.[40]

GENETICS AND CLINICAL PRESENTATION

Whether this anemia is congenital (simply present at birth because of some unknown cause) or truly inherited is not clear. However, there is growing evidence that it may be inherited because of reports of a few family members who have the disorder, and the fact that the disorder becomes evident at such an early age.

There rarely are any significant symptoms or physical findings in this disorder. Pallor may be evident at birth and is almost always evident by the age of 1 year. In one study, all patients with Diamond-Blackfan anemia who were more than 14 years of age demonstrated retarded growth, bone age retardation, and failure of secondary sexual maturation.[19] This marked growth retardation may be the result of both intermittent anemia and hemosiderosis; the latter eventually interferes with liver function and endocrine maturation. Characteristically, Diamond-Blackfan patients do not demonstrate renal abnormalities.[19]

LABORATORY FINDINGS AND CORRELATIONS WITH DISEASE

The diagnosis is usually made in infancy, with Hb values ranging from as low as 1.7 g/dL to 9.4 g/dL in a newborn. An increase in nucleated red blood cells, expected because of the severe anemia, is *not* found on the peripheral blood film. The anemia is usually normocytic and normochromic with normal red cell morphology, although occasional poikilocytes have been reported; reticulocytes are less than 1%, and often less than 0.2%. Similarly, the RPI is extremely low, indicating a poor response to the anemia. Red cell survival is normal, and the percentage of Hb F is elevated.[19] Platelet counts are normal, as are the leukocyte count and differential.[19] The bone marrow is cellular with a marked decrease in red cell precursors,[19,40] despite reported elevations in EPO.[48] Those erythroid precursors present are primarily pronormoblasts,[62] with no megaloblastic changes seen. Leukocytes and megakaryocytes are normal in the marrow.

CLINICAL AND LABORATORY DIFFERENTIATION OF DIAMOND-BLACKFAN AND FANCONI ANEMIAS

The reader may find differentiation of the two hereditary forms of bone marrow failure to be somewhat difficult. Table 11-7 is provided to summarize and clarify the principal differentiating factors.

EFFECTS OF TREATMENT ON LABORATORY RESULTS AND PROGNOSIS

Red cell transfusions are one of the mainstays of therapy and may be necessary every 3 to 6 weeks to prevent the symptoms of anemia. Possible complications of treatment with multiple transfusions are hepatitis and hemosiderosis, both of which contribute to liver failure.[19] Occasionally, after months to years of red cell transfusions, patients undergo a spontaneous remission, which may or may not be maintained.[19] Forty to fifty percent of patients respond to corticosteroid therapy,[19,40] supporting a lymphocyte abnormality as the basis for the disorder in some patients.

Recently bone marrow transplantation has been successful in four patients with congenital PRCA, and this is now seen as a potential curative therapy.[54] However, the overall prognosis remains poor,[1,19] with most of the complications being related to the anemia itself or secondary to hemosiderosis.

Myelophthisic Anemia

Myelophthisic anemia is found in many patients with carcinoma and is most often a hypoproliferative anemia; that is, one in which erythropoiesis is decreased with an RPI of less than 2.0 (Chap. 10).[16,31] In some patients the degree of anemia correlates with the tumor burden—the greater the tumor load, the more severe the anemia.[31] In others, however, there is no good correlation between tumor burden and the degree of anemia.[88]

PATHOPHYSIOLOGY

Myelophthisic anemia results when the bone marrow is replaced by abnormal cells[31,53,84]; most often, this term re-

TABLE 11-7
Principal Clinical and Laboratory Factors for Differentiation of Congenital Disorders Causing Bone Marrow Failure

Clinical/Laboratory Features	Fanconi Anemia	Diamond-Blackfan Anemia
Hematologic classification	Aplastic anemia	Pure red cell aplasia
Brown skin pigmentation	Common	Uncommon
Thumb abnormalities	Common	Uncommon
Renal abnormalities	Common	Uncommon
Onset of hematologic abnormalities (years of age)	5 to 10	<1
Bone marrow biopsy	Hypoplastic to aplastic	Cellular
Bone marrow aspirate	Pancytopenia	Marked decrease only in erythroid precursors
Peripheral blood	Pancytopenia	Decrease in RBC; normal WBC and platelets
Cytogenetics	Multiple chromosomal abnormalities in many tissues	No associated abnormalities

fers to replacement by metastatic carcinoma, although some authors include the hematologic malignancies (leukemia and lymphoma) (Parts 7 and 8 of this text) and myelofibrosis (Chap. 35). There also are nonmalignant conditions that can invade the marrow and cause the same picture, including miliary tuberculosis and granulomas.[84,88]

The term *myelophthisic anemia* is sometimes used interchangeably with the term leukoerythroblastic reaction[16,38,84,88]; however, they are not synonymous. A small number of patients with myelophthisic anemia do exhibit a leukoerythroblastic reaction. A leukoerythroblastic reaction describes the simultaneous presence of circulating nucleated red blood cells (NRBC) and immature neutrophils in the peripheral blood, including bands, metamyelocytes, and myelocytes; only rarely are more immature granulocytes encountered.[31,88] The release of immature granulocytes to the peripheral blood is inappropriate; that is, there is generally no evident infection to explain it.

Anemia is not always present in a leukoerythroblastic reaction; if it is, the number of circulating NRBC is much greater than expected for the degree of anemia and, therefore, is considered to be inappropriate. Stippled or polychromatophilic red cells or both may also be present. The mechanism for inappropriate release of immature myeloid and erythroid cells is not fully understood. But in cases of a striking and sustained leukoerythroblastosis, the mechanism may be related to damage to the underlying marrow stroma by invasion of abnormal cells (myelophthisis).

Formerly, it was accepted that if a patient had carcinoma metastatic to the bone marrow, a leukoerythroblastic reaction would invariably occur.[15,16,53] It is now recognized that only a small porportion of patients with proven marrow metastases demonstrate a leukoerythroblastic reaction.[16,53] However, it is true that if leukoerythroblastosis is found in a patient with known metastases, it is likely that marrow metastases have occurred, and that the disease is far advanced, thus forecasting a grave prognosis.[16,84]

In contrast, leukoerythroblastosis may be found in patients with no evidence of malignancy. Diagnoses in these patients range from hemolytic anemia, immune thrombocytopenic purpura, and iron deficiency anemia to infectious mononucleosis.[84] This again proves that a leukoerythroblastic reaction is not synonymous with myelophthisic anemia as was once thought.

DIFFERENTIAL DIAGNOSIS

The carcinomas most likely to metastasize to bone marrow are those of the breast, prostate, lung (especially the small cell or oat cell types), nervous system (neuroblastoma seen in children), adrenal cortex, thyroid, kidney, gastrointestinal tract, genitourinary tract, and malignant melanoma.[16,31,38,53,88] However, carcinoma at any site has the potential of metastasizing to the marrow, possibly causing marrow failure. Marrow biopsy (Chap. 27) is the best method for demonstrating metastatic tumor,[88] because a biopsy provides an overall view of marrow structure, cellularity, and any foreign infiltrates. From 70% to 93% of patients with known marrow involvement will have

a positive biopsy, whereas only 45% have a positive aspirate.[16] However, because there may be false-negative biopsies, it is important to do both a biopsy and an aspirate when searching for metastatic carcinoma in the marrow.

EFFECTS OF TREATMENT ON LABORATORY RESULTS AND PROGNOSIS

Treatment and prognosis depend on the underlying cause of the myelophthisic anemia. See the relevant chapters in Parts 7 and 8 of this text for more information.

ANEMIAS OF SYSTEMIC DISORDERS

A variety of systemic disorders may be associated with anemia. In this section, the anemia of chronic renal disease and the anemia of several endocrine disorders (hypothyroidism, hypopituitarism, adrenal abnormalities, and hypogonadism) will be considered, all of which may be associated with temporary hormonal variations.

Anemia of Chronic Renal Disease

A hypoproliferative anemia that can be severe almost invariably occurs in patients with chronic renal failure (CRF).[17,24,83] Indeed, anemia is almost as frequent a finding as an elevated blood urea nitrogen (BUN) concentration.

PATHOPHYSIOLOGY AND CLINICAL PRESENTATION

The etiology of anemia in CRF is complex. It is related to the etiology of the renal disease itself; the failure of the renal excretory function, with resultant accumulation of waste products in plasma; and the failure of renal production and release of erythropoietin (EPO).[24,45,66] The principal cause is the inadequate marrow response to anemia because of decreased production of EPO.[17,24,26] In fact, if the marrow were stimulated with adequate levels of EPO, very few uremic patients would be anemic, for the marrow could easily compensate with increased production for the slight shortening of red cell survival and the modest blood loss caused by platelet abnormalities.[17,24] However, there is some older evidence that the marrow of some of these patients may not be able to respond normally to any form of EPO,[24,83] suggesting a possible EPO toxin,[83] adding to the complexity of the anemia. More recent studies indicate very good responses to EPO.

The patient may have all the signs and symptoms of anemia, depending on its severity. These symptoms may be the patient's chief complaint at diagnosis, since development of renal failure is slow. One third to one half of patients with CRF experience gastrointestinal or gynecologic bleeding because of abnormal platelet function, and this resultant blood loss contributes to the anemia.[24]

LABORATORY FINDINGS AND CORRELATIONS WITH DISEASE

Hematology. Uremia, the accumulation of waste products, is associated with shortened red cell survival and a resultant mild hemolytic anemia[31,45] in as many as 70% of patients with renal failure.[17] The hematocrit (Hct) usually falls to levels between 0.15 and 0.30 L/L. The anemia is generally normocytic, normochromic with normal indices.[1,23,45] Because of the diseased kidneys, plasma volume is increased, resulting in an artifactually decreased Hct.[24] Thus, Hb and Hct levels are difficult to use as accurate measures of red cell mass.

Although erythrocyte morphology usually is normal, the uremic condition occasionally results in abnormal erythrocyte forms, particularly burr cells (see Fig. 8-8*B*) and possibly some helmet cells and red cell fragments.[17,24] The reticulocyte count usually is normal unless there is a high degree of anemia.[72] Leukocyte counts usually are normal, and platelet counts are normal to slightly elevated. Accumulated waste products may coat platelets, causing abnormal tests of platelet function (Chaps. 56 and 57).

Bone Marrow. The bone marrow in chronic renal failure is characteristically almost normocellular, with normal erythrocyte morphology and maturation. This is misleading, however, because in the context of anemia, a marrow capable of responding normally should display a compensatory increase in erythroid activity.[10,14] In contrast, acute renal failure is often accompanied by erythroid hypoplasia.[60,64]

Chemistry. There is a rough inverse correlation between the degree of renal insufficiency, as measured by the creatinine level, and the Hct. The higher the serum creatinine, the lower the Hct and the more severe the anemia.[24,26,45,66] The degree of shortening of red cell survival is directly proportional to the creatinine level.

Renal disease is associated with a low serum iron but normal total iron binding capacity (TIBC).[24,45] Administration of radiolabeled iron reveals a rapid clearance of iron from the plasma.[45] Iron is believed to be stored preferentially in the liver and spleen rather than in the marrow. This is likely to contribute to the low serum iron. There is depressed marrow utilization of the labeled iron,[17,45] because it does not reappear, as expected, in circulating red cells. Also contributing to low serum iron is the routine loss of blood and iron along with folate in the hemodialysis disposable coils during treatments.[45]

EFFECTS OF TREATMENT ON LABORATORY RESULTS

Transfusions are not indicated for most patients with this disorder because of the risks of hepatitis, acquired immune deficiency syndrome, and volume overload, which increases the risk of pulmonary edema.[45] With good dialysis therapy, erythropoiesis does improve slightly, although it takes several months or even years of treatment for the Hct to rise to reasonable levels.[26] Uremia causes considerable fatigue, but this is relieved by dialysis.

Mass production of recombinant human EPO (r-HuEPO) became a reality in 1987.[27,86] Since then, it has proven to be a safe and highly effective treatment for the anemia of chronic renal disease in almost every patient treated.[7,27,56,70,81] Generally the Hct increases from 0.22 L/L to over 0.35 L/L within 12 weeks.[52] It is essential, however, that adequate iron and folate be present in order to obtain a full response; therefore, monitoring of nutritional status is important.[70]

After successful allotransplantation of a kidney, EPO levels rise to normal with progressive normalization of the Hct.[61] In contrast, just prior to rejection of a renal graft, EPO levels increase and NRBCs may appear in the circulation. This change is probably useful in the diagnosis of chronic renal graft rejection.[61]

Anemia of Endocrine Disorders

It is well known that hormones secreted by endocrine organs play a role in hemopoiesis (Fig. 11-3). Thus, patients with various endocrine abnormalities may be anemic, although the incidence is low. Hormones normally stimulate erythropoiesis by either exerting a direct effect on marrow stem cells; a stimulatory action on EPO production; an augmenting effect on EPO; or an indirect influence on the release of EPO caused by changes in general metabolic rate induced by various hormones.[80] Anemia may develop secondary to interference with the normal action of hormones on red cell production.

Most commonly the anemia seen in endocrine disorders is mild, and red cells are usually normocytic, normochromic, with the marrow showing only decreased erythroid production and normal myeloid and megakaryocyte production.[1,41,51,80] Thus, these anemias are classified as hypoproliferative disorders due to decreased erythropoiesis (RPI <2.0).

HYPOTHYROIDISM

Oxygen (O_2) requirements of the body are influenced by a number of factors, including thyroid function.[80,87] As the body's metabolic rate decreases with diminished thyroid function, its needs for O_2 decrease. Thus, one third to one half of untreated hypothyroid patients are anemic.[80] The incidence of anemia in hypothyroidism may even be underestimated, because there is also a decrease in plasma volume, which may mask a mild anemia.[1,80] This anemia has been called "adaptive," meaning there is a physiologic adjustment to the reduced tissue oxygen requirements.[9,52]

Anemia, when found, is most often a result of the thyroid deficiency alone, but it can be seen in combination with other disorders that may result in anemia, such as iron deficiency (Chap. 13) and pernicious anemia (Chap. 12). Hypothyroidism and pernicious anemia are both thought to have autoimmune mechanisms. Thyroid antibodies occur in a high proportion of patients with pernicious anemia, and a significant number of patients with thyroid disease have antibodies to stomach gastric mucosa,[80] suggesting pernicious anemia.

Laboratory Findings and Correlations with Disease. In patients with hypothyroidism in whom the etiology of anemia is thyroid deficiency alone, the red cells tend to be macrocytic, in spite of normal B_{12} and folate levels.[41] The erythrocytes are normochromic. Acanthocytes may be seen, but they usually are rare and can easily be missed on routine inspection of the blood film. Patients with

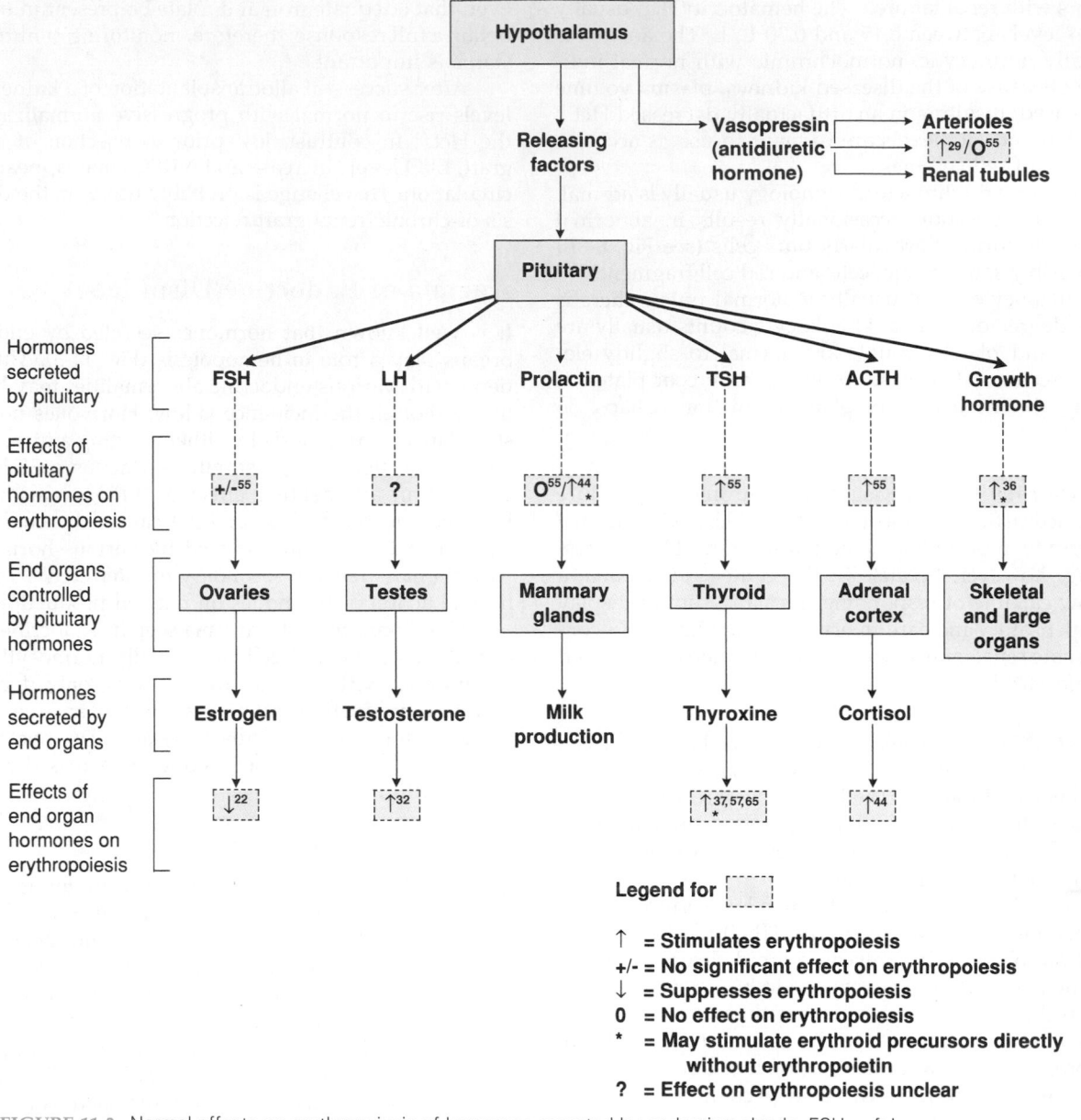

FIGURE 11-3. Normal effects on erythropoiesis of hormones secreted by endocrine glands. FSH = follicle-stimulating hormone; LH = luteinizing hormone; TSH = thyroid-stimulating hormone; ACTH = adrenocorticotropic hormone.

thyroid deficiency characteristically have elevated cholesterol levels.

In most anemias, red cell 2,3-diphosphoglycerate (2,3-DPG) levels are increased, which permits increased delivery of O_2 to the tissues. However, in the anemia of thyroid deficiency, red cell 2,3-DPG levels, as well as the P_{50} (a measure of hemoglobin's affinity for binding oxygen), are normal. Thus, there is no shift in the oxyhemoglobin dissociation curve (Chap. 7), which supports the hypothesis that there is a diminished need for O_2 in these patients and that this may be the etiology of the anemia.

Effects of Treatment on Laboratory Results. When these patients are treated with thyroxin, their MCV falls and stabilizes at a more normal value,[41] whereas their Hb slowly rises.[51] With therapy the Hb may initially fall because of plasma volume normalization, thus creating a relative anemia. Complete hematologic recovery may take as long as 6 months.[1]

ADRENAL ABNORMALITIES

Abnormalities in the secretion of adrenocortical steroids by the adrenal cortex, such as cortisol, have multiple effects on blood cells, most markedly on circulating lymphocytes and eosinophils. Adrenal hormones also have an effect on red cell production, although the mechanism is not understood. The effects are dependent on the type of adrenal abnormality.

Hypoadrenalism results in Addison disease, and hyperadrenalism results in Cushing disease. Patients with

Addison disease, in whom there is a decrease in adrenal production of cortisol, are characteristically anemic. However, with the adrenal insufficiency, there is a reduction in plasma volume,[1,80] and this may mask a mild anemia in these patients. Often, there is also a granulocytopenia and lymphocytosis.[71]

In contrast, patients with Cushing disease have an increased secretion of cortisol accompanied by normal to high normal erythrocyte counts. Rarely, these patients are polycythemic (Chap. 10).[80] Generally, neutrophils and platelets are increased in Cushing disease, whereas lymphocytes and eosinophils demonstrate absolute decreases in their numbers.[1,80]

PITUITARY ABNORMALITIES

A mild to moderate normocytic, normochromic anemia is frequently seen in patients with decreased pituitary function. This may be a result of the deficiency of pituitary hormones, which normally control the thyroid, gonads, or adrenals,[80] among other organ systems. Thus, the anemia is believed to result from a dysfunction in the normal conditioning role that pituitary hormones exert on the secretion of testosterone by the testes, thyroxine by the thyroid gland, and cortisol by the adrenal cortex. Testosterone, thyroxine, and cortisol are the three main hormones produced by pituitary gland end-organs that stimulate erythropoiesis,[32,44,65] as indicated in the last section of Figure 11-3. A number of other hormone deficiencies have had effects on erythropoiesis.

Treatment of anemia in hypopituitarism has included administration of various combinations of pituitary hormones, hormones from the adrenal and thyroid glands, and sex hormones.

HYPOGONADISM

Hypogonadism is characterized by retarded growth and sexual development secondary to a deficiency of the male sex hormone testosterone, which exerts significant influence over the male genital tract. Testosterone is an androgen produced primarily by the testes. In the endocrine disorder of hypogonadism in males, the reduction in testosterone secretion causes erythrocyte values to fall within the female reference range.[1,80]

Androgens, most notably testosterone, have the ability to increase erythropoiesis through increased stimulation of renal EPO production.[1] In contrast to androgens, the female sex hormone estrogen has been shown to suppress erythropoiesis (Fig. 11-3).[22] Therapeutic administration of androgens increases urinary excretion of EPO and increases reticulocyte production, with a subsequent increase in red cell mass.[1,13,80]

CHAPTER SUMMARY

Aplastic anemia (AA) is associated with an absolute failure of the bone marrow. It may be inherited or acquired. It is diagnosed by a hypocellular or aplastic bone marrow in which hematopoietic tissue is replaced by fat. Pancytopenia is seen in the peripheral blood; classically, no immature leukocytes or erythrocytes are found in the blood. Patients with AA are at great risk for infection, bleeding, and signs and symptoms of anemia. The treatment of choice is a bone marrow transplant.

Congenital aplastic anemia is known as Fanconi anemia (FA). The laboratory findings are similar to those in acquired aplastic anemia, except that multiple chromosome abnormalities are also present. These patients are at significant risk for the development of acute leukemia, which is uncommon in acquired AA.

Pure red cell aplasia (PRCA) is acquired or inherited. The granulocytic and megakaryocytic marrow is normocellular; however, erythroid elements are severely decreased and anemia results. Red cell transfusions are a mainstay of therapy, and androgens to stimulate erythropoiesis have been used effectively.

Congenital PRCA is known as Diamond-Blackfan anemia. Laboratory findings are similar to those of acquired PRCA (Table 11-7).

Myelophthisic anemia results when the bone marrow is replaced by abnormal cells in conditions such as metastatic carcinoma. Myelophthisic anemia and leukoerythroblastic reaction are not synonymous. The leukoerythroblastic reaction refers to the presence of both nucleated red blood cells and immature granulocytes in the peripheral blood. A leukoerythroblastic reaction occurs in some but not all patients with a myelophthisic anemia.

Systemic disease, such as chronic renal disease or endocrine disorders, can also cause anemia.

Case Study 11-1

A 25-year-old man was admitted to the hospital in obvious distress. He had multiple, deep soft-tissue abscesses, which were cultured and later grew *Bacillus* sp. A blood culture taken at the same time was likewise positive for *Bacillus*. He had a fever of 99.8°F, but no hepatosplenomegaly or lymphadenopathy. He had had a physical and laboratory evaluation 6 months previously, both of which were normal. At the time of presentation, results of his CBC were as follows: WBC 1.8×10^9/L; RBC 3.07×10^{12}/L; Hb 9.0 g/dL; Hct 0.27L/L; MCV 88 fL; MCH 29.3 pg; MCHC 33.3 g/dL; RDW 13.6; platelets 19×10^9/L; reticulocytes: none seen; manual differential: neutrophils 5% (0.08×10^9/L); lymphocytes 94% (1.7×10^9/L); monocytes 1% (0.02×10^9/L); RBC normocytic, normochromic; platelets markedly decreased; buffy coat preparation: no immature cells seen.

His bone marrow aspirate was markedly hypocellular, consisting primarily of fat cells with a few stromal cells, lymphocytes, and plasma cells. The bone marrow biopsy demonstrated less than 5% cellularity.

1. These peripheral blood and bone marrow results are typical of which of the following disorders: megaloblastic anemia, aplastic anemia, Fanconi anemia, acute leukemia, or myelodysplastic syndrome? Explain.
2. If a bone marrow transplant was successfully given to this patient, what general change would you expect to see in the peripheral blood cell counts and how soon?
3. Are the results of the marrow aspirate sufficient for the physician to make the diagnosis, or is it important to have the biopsy results also? Explain briefly.
4. List a minimum of three possible etiologies for secondary aplastic anemia.

Case Study 11-2

A 25-year-old man was hematologically normal until the age of 10 years, when he was found to have "aplastic anemia." At that time, cytogenetic studies on peripheral blood lymphocytes showed a single chromosomal abnormality. He was then treated for 3 years with androgens and corticosteroids but remained pancytopenic.

At the time of this admission, he complained of acute abdominal pain. Abdominal ultrasound showed a mass behind the right kidney. A laparotomy was performed, an abscess found, and a 30-cm segment of the small bowel was resected. The patient did well on antibiotics for 2 weeks, but suddenly developed a fever with no leukocytosis. Hematologic studies revealed: WBC 1.3×10^9/L; RBC 3.27×10^{12}/L; Hb 11.0 g/dL; Hct 0.33 L/L; MCV 101 fL; MCH 33.6 pg; MCHC 33.3 g/dL; platelets 32×10^9/L; manual differential: neutrophils 62% (0.8×10^9/L); lymphocytes 23% (0.3×10^9/L); monocytes 15% (0.2×10^9/L); RBC normocytic, normochromic; and platelets markedly decreased.

A bone marrow aspirate and biopsy were performed. The marrow was markedly hypoplastic with patchy cellularity; there appeared to be a slight increase in myeloblasts. In contrast, his marrow 6 months before this was essentially aplastic. Cytogenetic studies showed additional chromosomal abnormalities, all translocations or deletions. Thus, it was speculated that the patient was developing an acute leukemia.

1. Are chromosomal (cytogenetic) abnormalities commonly found in secondary acquired aplastic anemia or in congenital aplastic anemia?
2. Based on your answer to number 1, is the disease in this case inherited or acquired?
3. Identify the most likely classification of this man's disease and briefly explain your reasoning.
4. Why would it have been useful, at the time of the original diagnosis, to evaluate the response of this patient's cultured lymphocytes to diepoxybutane, an agent that interferes with DNA?
5. Describe in a few words how a bone marrow biopsy in Fanconi anemia would look beginning with a patient who is younger than 10 years of age, and then following him into adulthood.
6. Do patients with this disease have a significant risk of progression to acute leukemia? What laboratory findings indicated that this was happening in this patient?

Review Questions

For the following questions, choose from these answers:

A. 1, 3
B. 2, 4
C. 1, 2 and 3
D. 4 only
E. All are correct

11-1. The bone marrow in aplastic anemia is characterized as

1. normocellular.
2. showing erythroid and granulocytic hypoplasia.
3. having increased fibrosis in the biopsy.
4. having increased fat in the biopsy.

11-2. Myelophthisic anemia is demonstrated in the bone marrow when there is

1. replacement of myeloid cells by fat.
2. complete absence of all myeloid cells.
3. a leukoerythroblastic reaction in the peripheral blood.
4. replacement of myeloid cells by malignant cancer cells.

11-3. The peripheral blood in aplastic anemia is characterized by

1. neutropenia.
2. thrombocytopenia.
3. leukopenia.
4. immature granulocytes.

11-4. Which of the following is true about Fanconi anemia?

1. The platelet count is normal.
2. Patients are anemic but have a normal absolute neutrophil count.
3. Hematologic cell count abnormalities are present by 1 year of age.
4. The bone marrow eventually becomes aplastic.

11-5. Which of the following laboratory values would be expected in a patient diagnosed with chronic renal failure?

1. Occasional abnormal erythrocytes including burr cells and fragments
2. Abnormal platelet function tests
3. A decreased serum erythropoietin level
4. A microcytic, hypochromic anemia

11-6. A leukoerythroblastic reaction is characterized by the inappropriate release from the bone marrow of

1. nucleated red blood cells.
2. immature lymphocytes.
3. immature granulocytes.
4. platelets.

11-7. Anemia associated with endocrine disorders may result from

1. an increase in erythropoietin.
2. an increase in testosterone.
3. hyperadrenalism (Cushing disease).
4. a decrease in thyroid function (hypothyroidism).

References

1. Adamson JW: Anemia of endocrine disorders. In Lichtman MA (ed): Hematology and Oncology, p 44. New York, Grune & Stratton, 1980
2. Aschan J, Ringd'en O, Sundberg B et al: Methotrexate combined with cyclosporin A decreases graft-versus-host disease, but increases leukemic relapse compared to monotherapy. Bone Marrow Transplant 7:113, 1991
3. Auerbach AD: Fanconi anemia and leukemia: Tracking the genes. Leukemia 6 (Suppl 1):1, 1992
4. Auerbach AD, Allen RG: Leukemia and preleukemia in Fanconi anemia patients. A review of the literature and report of the International Fanconi Anemia Registry. Cancer Genet Cytogenet 51:1, 1991
5. Bacigalupo A, Broccia G, Corda G et al: Antilymphocyte globulin, cyclosporin, and granuloctye colony-stimulating factor in patients with acquired severe aplastic anemia (SAA): A pilot study of the EBMT SAA working party. Blood 85:1348, 1995
6. Bacigalupo A, Maiolino A, Van-Lint MT et al: Cyclosporin A and chronic graft versus host disease. Bone Marrow Transplant 6:341, 1990
7. Bentley SA: Bone marrow connective tissue and the haemopoietic microenvironment. Br J Haematol 50:1, 1982
8. Bloom GE, Diamond LK: Prognostic value of fetal hemoglobin levels in acquired aplastic anemia. N Engl J Med 278:304, 1968
9. Bomford R: Anemia in myxoedema and the role of the thyroid gland in erythropoiesis. Q J Med 7:495, 1938
10. Callen JR, Limarzi LR: Blood and bone marrow studies in renal disease. Am J Clin Pathol 20:3, 1950
11. Camitta BM, Storb R, Thomas ED: Aplastic anemia: Pathogenesis, diagnosis, treatment, and prognosis. N Engl J Med 306:645, 1982
12. Camitta BM, Storb R, Thomas ED: Aplastic anemia: Pathogen-

esis, diagnosis, treatment, and prognosis. N Engl J Med 306:716, 1982

13. Camitta BM, Thomas ED, Nathan DG et al: A prospective study of androgens and bone marrow transplantation for treatment of severe aplastic anemia. Blood 53:504, 1979

14. Caro J, Erslev AJ: Anemia of chronic renal failure. In Beutler E, Lichtman MA, Coller BS et al (eds): Hematology, 5th ed, p 459. New York, McGraw-Hill, 1995

14a. Champlin RE, Horowitz MM, van Bekkum DW et al: Graft failure following bone marrow transplantation for severe aplastic anemia. Blood 73:606, 1989

15. Chen HP, Walz DV: Leukemoid reaction in the bone marrow, associated with malignant neoplasms. Am J Clin Pathol 29:345, 1979

16. Contreras E, Ellis LD, Lee RE: Value of the bone marrow biopsy in the diagnosis of metastatic carcinoma. Cancer 29:778, 1972

17. Desforges JF: Anemia in uremia. Arch Intern Med 126:808, 1970

18. Di-Bartolomeo P, Di-Girolamo G, Olioso P et al: Allogeneic bone marrow transplantation for Fanconi anemia. Bone Marrow Transplant 10:53, 1992

19. Diamond LK, Allen DM, Magill FB: Congenital (erythroid) hypoplastic anemia, a 25 year study. Am J Dis Child 102:403, 1961; Adv Pediatr 22:349, 1976

20. dos-Santos CC, Gavish H, Buchwald M: Fanconi anemia revisited: Old ideas and new advances. Stem Cells 12:142, 1994

21. Dosik H, Hsu LY, Todaro GJ et al: Leukemia in Fanconi's anemia: Cytogenetic and tumor virus susceptibility studies. Blood 36:341, 1970

22. Dukes PP, Goldwasser E: Inhibition of erythropoiesis by estrogens. Endocrinology 69:21, 1961

23. Eklund SG, Johansson SV, Strandberg O: Anemia in uremia. Acta Med Scand 190:435, 1971

24. Erslev AJ: Anemia of chronic renal disease. Arch Intern Med 126:774, 1970

25. Erslev AJ: Aplastic anemia. In Williams WJ, Beutler E, Erslev AJ et al (eds): Hematology, 3rd ed. New York, McGraw-Hill, 1983

26. Eschbach JW, Adamson JW, Cook JD: Disorders of red blood cell production in uremia. Arch Intern Med 126:812, 1970

27. Eschbach JW, Egrie JL, Downing MR et al: Correction of the anemia of end-stage renal disease with recombinant human erythropoietin. N Engl J Med 316:73, 1987

28. Feig SA: Aplastic pancytopenia. In Lichtman MA (ed): Hematology and Oncology, p 156. New York, Grune & Stratton, 1980

29. Fisher JW: Erythropoietin: Pharmacology, biogenesis and control of production. Pharmacol Rev 24:459, 1972

30. Flowers ME, Doney KC, Storb R et al: Marrow transplantion for Fanconi anemia with or without leukemic transformation: An update of the Seattle experience. Bone Marrow Transplant 9:167, 1992

31. Frei E: Hematologic complications of cancer. In Holland JF, Frei E (eds): Cancer Medicine, p 1085. Philadelphia, Lea & Febiger, 1973

32. Fried W, Gurney CW: The erythropoietic-stimulating effects of androgens. Ann NY Acad Sci 149:356, 1978

33. Gale RP, Reisner Y: The role of bone marrow transplants after nuclear accidents. Lancet 1:923, 1988

34. Giampietro PF, Adler-Brecher B, Verlander PC et al: The need for more accurate and timely diagnosis in Fanconi anemia: A report from the International Fanconi Anemia Registry. Pediatrics 91:1116, 1993

35. Gluckman E, Esperou-Bourdeau H, Baruchel A et al: Multicenter randomized study comparing cyclosporine-A alone and antithymocyte globulin with prednisone for treatment of severe aplastic anemia. Blood 79:2540, 1992

36. Golde DW, Bersch N, Li CH: Growth hormone: Species-specific stimulation of erythropoiesis *in vitro*. Science 196:1112, 1977

37. Golde DW, Bersch N, Chopra IJ et al: Thyroid hormones stimulate erythropoiesis *in vitro*. Br J Haematol 37:173, 1977

38. Hansen HH, Muggia FM, Selawry OS: Bone-marrow examination in 100 consecutive patients with bronchogenic carcinoma. Lancet 2:443, 1971

39. Hirschman RJ, Shulman RR, Abuelo JG et al: Chromosomal aberrations in two cases of inherited aplastic anemia with unusual clinical features. Ann Intern Med 71:107, 1969

40. Hoffman R, Zanjani ED, Vila J et al: Diamond-Blackfan syndrome: Lymphocyte-mediated suppression of erythropoiesis. Science 193:899, 1976

41. Horton L, Coburn RJ, England JM et al: The haematology of hypothyroidism. Q J Med 45:101, 1976

42. Hunter AE, Bessell EM, Russell NH: Effective prevention of acute GVHD following allogeneic BMT with low leukaemic relapse using methotrexate and therapeutically monitored levels of cyclosporin A. Bone Marrow Transplant 10:431, 1992

43. Jacobs P, Karabus C: Fanconi's anemia: A family study with 20-year follow-up including associated breast pathology. Cancer 54:1850, 1984

44. Jepson JH, Lowenstein L: The effect of testosterone, adrenal steroids and prolactin on erythropoiesis. Acta Haematol 38:292, 1967; Blood 24:726, 1964; Proc Soc Exp Biol Med 121:1077, 1966; ibid 122:457, 1966; Br J Haematol 15:465, 1968; Arch Intern Med 122:265, 1968

45. Kaye M: The anemia associated with renal disease. J Lab Clin Med 52:83, 1958

46. Kohli-Kuman M, Morris C, DeLaat C et al: Bone marrow transplantation in Fanconi anemia using matched sibling donors. Blood 84:2050, 1994

47. Knospe WH: Aplastic anaemia: A disorder of the bone-marrow sinusoidal microcirculation rather than stem-cell failure? Lancet 1:20, 1971

48. Krantz SB: Annotation: Pure red cell aplasia. Br J Haematol 25:11, 1973; N Engl J Med 291:345, 1974

49. Krantz SB: Diagnosis and treatment of pure red cell aplasia. Med Clin North Am 60:945, 1976

50. Krantz SB: Pure red cell aplasia. In Lichtman MA (ed): Hematology and Oncology, p 45. New York, Grune & Stratton, 1980

51. Larsson SO: Anemia and iron metabolism in hypothyroidism. Acta Med Scand 157:349, 1957

52. Lee GR: The normocytic, normochromic anemias. In Lee GR, Bithell TC, Foerster J et al (eds): Wintrobe's Clinical Hematology, 9th ed, p 902. Philadelphia, Lea & Febiger, 1993

53. Leland J, Macpherson B: Hematologic findings in cases of mammary cancer metastatic to bone marrow. Am J Clin Pathol 71:31, 1979

54. Lenarsky C, Weinberg K, Guinan E et al: Bone marrow transplantation for constitutional pure red cell aplasia. Blood 71:226, 1988

55. Lindemann R, Trygstad O, Halvorsen S: Pituitary control of erythropoiesis. Scand J Haematol 6:77, 1969

56. Macdougall IC: Treatment of renal anemia with recombinant human erythropoietin. Curr Opin Nephrol Hypertens 1:210, 1992

57. Malgor LA, Blanc CC, Klainer E et al: Direct effects of thyroid hormones on bone marrow erythroid cells of rats. Blood 45:671, 1975

58. McDonald R, Goldschmidt B: Pancytopenia with congenital defects (Fanconi's anaemia). Arch Dis Child 35:367, 1960

59. Miller KB, Schenkein DP, Comenzo R et al: Adjusted-dose continuous-infusion cyclosporin A to prevent graft-versus-host disease following allogeneic bone marrow transplantation. Ann Hematol 68(1):15, 1994

60. Morgan T, Innes M, Ribush N: The management of the anae-

mia of patients on chronic haemodialysis. Med J Aust 1:848, 1972

61. Murphy GP, Mirand EZ, Grace JT: Erythropoietin activity in anephric or renal allotransplanted man. Ann Surg 170:581, 1969

62. Nathan DG, Clarke BJ, Hillman DG et al: Erythroid precursors in congenital hypoplastic (Diamond-Blackfan) anemia. J Clin Invest 61:489, 1978

63. Nilsson LR: Chronic pancytopenia with multiple congenital abnormalities. Acta Paediatr 49:518, 1960

64. Pasternack A, Wahlberg P: Bone marrow in acute renal failure. Acta Med Scand 181:505, 1967

65. Popovic WJ, Brown JE, Adamson JW: Thyroid hormone (TH)–stimulated erythropoiesis: Mediation by a β-adrenergic receptor (abstract). Blood 48:979, 1976

66. Radtke HW, Claussner A, Erbes PM et al: Serum erythropoietin concentration in chronic renal failure: Relationship to degree of anemia and excretory renal function. Blood 54:877, 1979

67. Rey JP, Scott R, Muller H: Apoptosis is not involved in the hypersensitivity of Fanconi anemia cells to mitomycin C. Cancer Genet Cytogenet 75:67, 1994

68. Russell JA, Woodman RC, Poon MC et al: Addition of low-dose folinic acid to a methotrexate/cyclosporin A regimen for prevention of acute graft-versus-host disease. Bone Marrow Transplant 14:397, 1994

69. Sandberg T, Lindquist O, Norkrans G: Fatal aplastic anaemia associated with non-A, non-B hepatitis. Scan J Infect Dis 16:403,1984

70. Sanders HH, Rabb HA, Bittle P et al: Nutritional implications of recombinant human erythropoietin therapy in renal disease. J Am Diet Assoc 94:1023, 1994

71. Saphir R: Addison's disease presenting as a lymphocyte dyscrasia. Am J Med 42:855, 1967

72. Shaw AB, Scholes MC: Reticulocytosis in renal failure. Lancet 1:799, 1967

73. Schrezenmeier H, Schlander M, Raghavachar A: Cyclosporin A in aplastic anemia—report of a workshop. Ann Hematolo 65:33, 1992

74. Storb R, Thomas ED, Buckner CD et al: Marrow transplantation for aplastic anemia. Semin Hematol 21:27, 1984

75. Storb R, Thomas ED, Buckner CD et al: Marrow transplantation in thirty "untransfused" patients with severe aplastic anemia. Ann Intern Med 92:30, 1980

76. Strathdee CA, Buchwald M: Molecular and cellular biology of Fanconi anemia. Am J Pediatr Hematol Oncol 14:177, 1992

77. Tong J, Bacigalupo A, Piaggio G et al: Severe aplastic anemia (SAA): Response to cyclosporin A (CyA) *in vivo* and *in vitro*. Eur J Haematol 46:212, 1991

78. Torok-Storb B, Doney K, Sale G et al: Subsets of patients with aplastic anemia identified by flow microfluorometry. N Engl J Med 312:1015, 1985

79. Tsai SY, Levin WC: Chronic erythrocytic hypoplasia in adults. Am J Med 22:322, 1957

80. Tudhope GR: Endocrine diseases. Clin Haematol 1:475, 1972

81. Van Wyck D: Iron management during recombinant human erythropoietin therapy. Am J Kidney Dis 14 (Suppl 1):9, 1989

82. Waldrop MM: The UCLA-Occidental-Gorbachev connection. Science 233:19, 1986

83. Wallner SF, Kurnick JE, Ward HP et al: The anemia of chronic renal failure and chronic diseases: *In vitro* studies of erythropoiesis. Blood 47:561, 1976

84. Weick JK, Hagedorn AB, Linman JW: Leukoerythroblastosis: Diagnostic and prognostic significance. Mayo Clin Proc 49:110,1974

85. Williams DM: Pancytopenia, aplastic anemia, and pure red cell aplasia. In Lee GR, Bithell TC, Foerster J et al (eds): Wintrobe's Clinical Hematology, 9th ed, p 911. Philadelphia, Lea & Febiger, 1993

86. Winearls CG, Pippard MJ, Reid CD et al: Characterization of the anemia of chronic renal disease and the mode of its correction by r-HuEPO. Q J Med 70:113, 1989

87. Zaroulis CG, Kourides IA, Valeri CR: Red cell 2,3-diphosphoglycerate and oxygen affinity of hemoglobin in patients with thyroid disorders. Blood 52:181, 1978

88. Zucker S: Anemia associated with foreign cells in the marrow (myelophthisis). In Lichtman MA (ed): Hematology and Oncology, p 42. New York, Grune & Stratton, 1980

CHAPTER 12

Anemias of Abnormal Nuclear Development

Cheryl A. Lotspeich-Steininger

Objectives

1. Compare vitamin B$_{12}$ and folate with respect to dietary sources (at least four for each), the recommended daily allowance (RDA), serum reference range values, the area of the intestine where absorbed, and their role in DNA synthesis.
2. State three classic laboratory findings in the megaloblastic anemias.
3. Describe the quantitative and morphologic effects of megaloblastic anemias on peripheral blood and bone marrow cells and the effects of treatment on these parameters.
4. Explain the principle, specimen requirements, interpretation, and sources of error and give the reference ranges for the competitive protein-binding radioassay for serum B$_{12}$ and serum and erythrocyte folate and for the Schilling test and food Schilling test.
5. State the expected results—normal, increased, or decreased—for the methylmalonic acid test and the total homocysteine test in both folate and vitamin B$_{12}$ deficiency.
6. List and briefly explain at least four causes each for both acquired vitamin B$_{12}$ and acquired folate deficiency.
7. Differentiate between megaloblastic and megaloblastoid cell maturation in the peripheral blood and bone marrow.
8. List at least three laboratory features that differentiate a megaloblastic macrocytic anemia from a normoblastic macrocytic anemia.
9. Differentiate the congenital dyserythropoietic anemias based on significant peripheral blood, bone marrow, and acidified serum test findings.

The anemias of abnormal nuclear development are a group of disorders in which cell maturation in the bone marrow is abnormal as a result of defective deoxyribonucleic acid (DNA) synthesis. Abnormalities, reflected in both nucleus and cytoplasm, may be seen in erythrocytes, leukocytes, and platelets in the bone marrow and peripheral blood. Characteristic changes in overall cell size, shape, and color are often easily identifiable, as are nuclear abnormalities in size, shape, and chromatin clumping.

The megaloblastic anemias represent a major subgroup of anemias caused by abnormal nuclear development. Classically, these anemias are associated with very large, oval erythrocytes called oval macrocytes and hypersegmented neutrophils (neutrophils with six or more nuclear lobes). The oval macrocytes are usually detected by the classic finding of an increased mean cell volume (MCV) on electronic cell analysis. Megaloblastic anemias are usually acquired disorders caused by vitamin B$_{12}$ or folate deficiency, but a rare case may be an inherited or a drug-induced defect in DNA synthesis. These anemias are characteristically classified as macrocytic, normochromic. They are discussed in detail in this chapter.

The congenital dyserythropoietic anemias (CDAs) are also presented. They are a rare subgroup of anemias of abnormal nuclear development characterized by abnormalities of bone marrow erythrocyte precursors. The CDAs, unlike megaloblastic anemias, virtually always are inherited and are not associated with leukocyte or platelet abnormalities, nor are they related to B_{12} or folate deficiency.

VITAMIN B_{12} AND FOLATE

Since vitamin B_{12} and folate deficiency are the most common causes of megaloblastic anemia, a review of the biochemistry of these compounds, their dietary requirements, and their metabolism is appropriate.

Biochemistry

VITAMIN B_{12}

Vitamin B_{12} belongs to a family of vitamins called cobalamins (Cbl) that have a corrin ring containing cobalt (Fig. 12-1). No other organic compound containing cobalt has been found in nature. This ring is attached to the nucleotide 5,6-dimethylbenzimidazole. The corrin nucleus contains four substituted pyrrole rings and is similar to the porphyrin nucleus of heme (see Fig. 7-3). Vitamin B_{12} is required for a single critical reaction during normal DNA synthesis.

Two chemically active (coenzyme) forms of B_{12} have been identified: adenosylcobalamin (adenosyl-Cbl) and methylcobalamin (methyl-Cbl) (Fig. 12-1). Methyl-Cbl is the one required for normal DNA synthesis and represents approximately 75% of the B_{12} in the plasma. Adenosyl-Cbl represents about 75% of the B_{12} in the liver and most of the B_{12} in erythrocytes and the kidneys.

When cyanide anion (CN^-) is covalently linked to the cobalt atom, cyanocobalamin is formed. This B_{12} form is used to treat B_{12} deficiency.

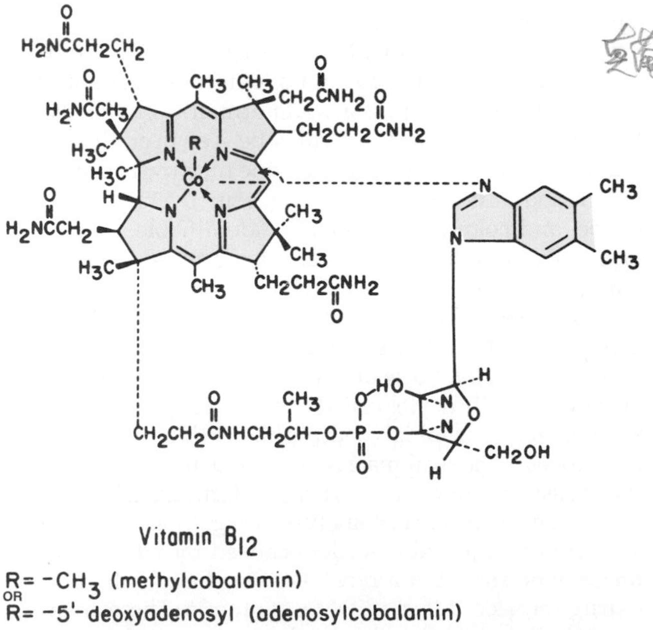

Vitamin B_{12}

R= $^-CH_3$ (methylcobalamin)
OR
R= $-5'$-deoxyadenosyl (adenosylcobalamin)

FIGURE 12-1. The structure of vitamin B_{12}. (From Miller SM: Vitamins. In Bishop ML, Duben-Engelkirk JL, Fody EP [eds]: Clinical Chemistry—Principles, Procedures, Correlations, 2nd ed, p 391. Philadelphia, JB Lippincott, 1992, with permission.)

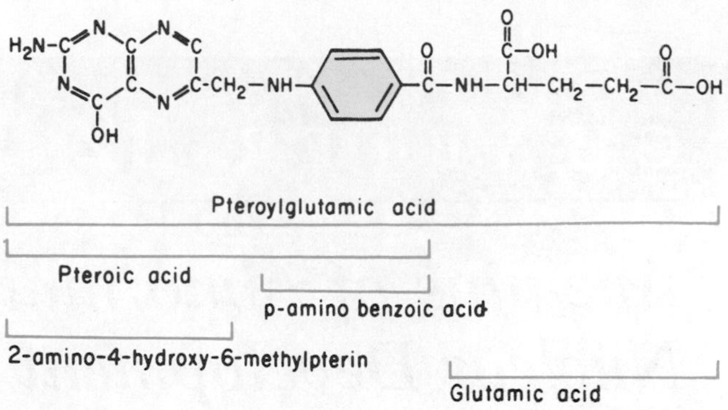

FIGURE 12-2. The structure of folic acid. (From Miller SM: Vitamins. In Bishop ML, Duben-Engelkirk JL, Fody EP [eds]: Clinical Chemistry—Principles, Procedures, Correlations, 2nd ed, p 391. Philadelphia, JB Lippincott, 1992, with permission.)

FOLATE

The folates, also called folacins, represent a family of compounds derived from folic acid, also called pteroylglutamic acid (Fig. 12-2). All folates have a parent compound known as pteroic acid. Pteroic acid is linked by a peptide bond to one molecule of glutamic acid to form the complete folic acid structure. Multiple glutamic acid residues may be conjugated to folic acid forming polyglutamates which are common among food folates. A number of folate analogs, such as tetrahydrofolate (FH_4), are formed by certain structural changes to the parent compound during folic acid metabolism. Folates are required for three reactions that lead to DNA synthesis.

Nutritional Requirements and Absorption

VITAMIN B_{12}

Vitamin B_{12} is produced by microorganisms and certain fungi. Its dietary sources include animal protein products such as meat, liver, kidney, fish, oysters, clams, eggs, cheese, and milk.[38] It is not found in vegetables or fruit. The recommended daily allowance (RDA) for adults is 2.0 μg/day,[83] much less than that for folic acid. During pregnancy, the RDA is 2.5 μg/day. Normally 3 to 5 μg are absorbed daily to meet the normal daily cobalamin turnover rate of about 2 μg/day. The normal liver stores approximately 1 to 10 mg of vitamin B_{12}, an amount adequate for 3 to 6 years if no more is ingested.[38]

Absorption of vitamin B_{12} in the gastrointestinal (GI) tract requires several factors. First, the vitamin must be released from foods by peptic digestion in the stomach, which is facilitated by hydrochloric acid released from the gastric parietal cells. These cells also secrete an important protein called *intrinsic factor (IF)*. In the stomach, IF forms a complex with vitamin B_{12} that is transported through the GI tract. Upon reaching the ileum (the section of the small intestine most distal from the stomach), the complex attaches to mucosal receptors and B_{12} is released from IF and is absorbed into the mucosa. Once in the plasma, vitamin B_{12} is bound by carrier proteins called transcobalamins I, II, and III (TC I, II, III). TC II, the most important of the transcobalamins, is a β globulin synthesized in the liver. TC II transports some B_{12} to storage sites in the liver and tissues and some to the bone marrow. TC II is necessary for transport of cobalamin through cell membranes.

The TC I and III carrier proteins are present in gastric fluid, plasma, amniotic fluid, milk, saliva, and granulocytes. They are called R (rapid) proteins, or R binders, since they migrate faster than IF on zone electrophoresis. R proteins bind biologically active cobalamins and inactive analogs. The physiologic role of the R proteins is not clear, but it is known that they do not assist in ileal B_{12} absorption.[101] TC I binds most B_{12} in the plasma, and this B_{12} is not transported to the marrow. TC I is believed to be synthesized principally by granulocytes. Deficiency of TC II leads to megaloblastic anemia, whereas deficiencies of TC I and III apparently are harmless.

FOLATE

The dietary sources of folate are green leafy vegetables, cauliflower, broccoli, brussel sprouts, liver, kidney, whole grain cereals, yeast, fruit, and dairy products.[47] The RDA for food folate is 200 μg/day for men and 180 μg/day for women.[83] For pregnant women the RDA is 500 μg/day (to reduce the risk of spina bifida) and for lactating women, approximately 270 μg/day.

At any given time the body stores approximately 5 to 10 mg of folate, about half of which is in the liver.[18] This amount is adequate for 3 to 6 months if no additional folate is ingested. Intestinal microflora also produce folates. Note that folate body stores are consumed much more quickly than B_{12} stores (which are normally adequate for several years). Once in the small intestine, enzymes called conjugases remove the excess glutamic acid residues from dietary polyglutamates to produce monoglutamates called methyl-tetrahydrofolates (methyl-FH_4). Such conversion allows folate absorption in the jejunum (the central segment of the small intestine), followed by transport to the liver and bone marrow. Folate is transported in the circulation as 5-methyl-FH_4. Two thirds of plasma folate circulates loosely bound to proteins, including albumin, α_2-macroglobulin, and possibly transferrin. About half the body folate is stored in the liver. Much is also found in the kidneys and erythrocytes. Folate uptake by erythrocytes has been shown to require vitamin B_{12} as a cofactor.[38] Folate is excreted in the bile and urine.

Metabolism

Vitamin B_{12} and folate are integral components in DNA synthesis. Figure 12-3 shows the relationship of folate and B_{12} in DNA synthesis. Initially, the plasma folate monoglutamate 5-methyl FH_4 donates its methyl group to cobalamin (B_{12}) in the presence of methyl transferase to form methylcobalamin. Methylcobalamin transfers the methyl group to homocysteine, forming the amino acid methionine. In the process, FH_4, a polyglutamate, is produced. FH_4 is the primary intracellular form of folate. As serine is converted to glycine, FH_4 is converted to the folate coenzyme 5,10-methylene FH_4, also a polyglutamate, which is part of the rate-limiting reaction in DNA synthesis. As 5,10-methylene FH_4 is converted to dihydrofolate (FH_2), deoxyuridylate (dUMP) is converted to thymidylate (dTTP), in the presence of the enzyme dTTP synthetase. Thymidylate is one of several components required for DNA synthesis (Fig. 12-3). FH_2 is reduced to FH_4 by the enzyme dihydrofolate reductase, thus conserving the supply of FH_4.[18]

A second vitamin B_{12}-dependent reaction involves a step in the process of propionic acid catabolism (Fig. 12-4). Propionic acid is a major metabolic product of intestinal bacteria. One step in the catabolism of this acid involves a reaction in which methylmalonyl coenzyme A (CoA) is converted to succinyl CoA in the presence of the vitamin B_{12} coenzyme adenosyl-Cbl and methymalonyl CoA mutase. If adenosyl-Cbl is not available, methylmalonyl CoA is hydrolyzed to methylmalonic acid (MMA).

THE MEGALOBLASTIC ANEMIAS
Pathophysiology

Vitamin B_{12} deficiency causes defective DNA synthesis that results in megaloblastic peripheral blood and bone marrow changes. An explanation for this mechanism was

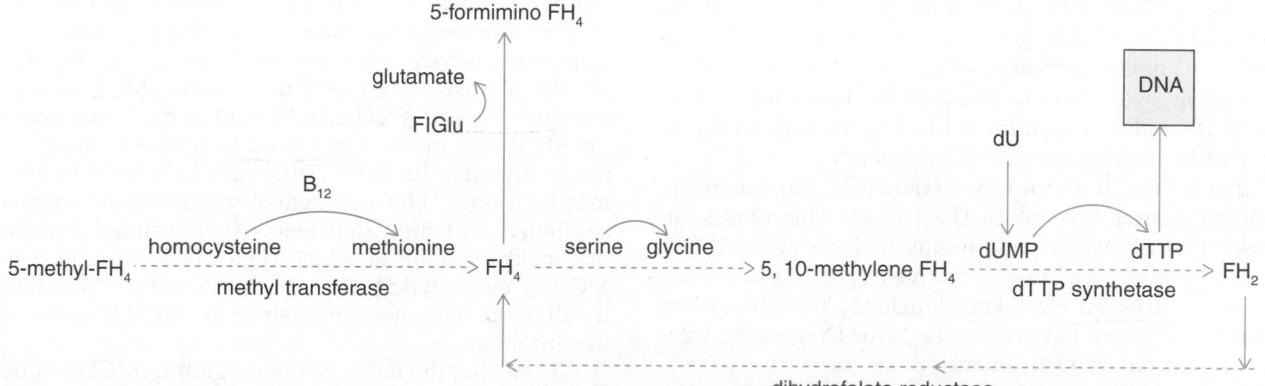

FIGURE 12-3. The interaction of vitamin B_{12} and folate in DNA synthesis. Synthesis of DNA requires vitamin B_{12} and the conversion of folates in the monogluatamate form (5-methyl FH_4) to the polyglutamate form (5,10-methylene FH_4) which is a cofactor in the rate-limiting reaction involving the conversion of dUMP (deoxyuridylate) to dTTP (thymidylate). dTTP is needed for normal DNA synthesis. dU = deoxyuridine; FH_4 = tetrahydrofolate; FH_2 = dihydrofolate; FIGlu = formiminoglutamic acid.

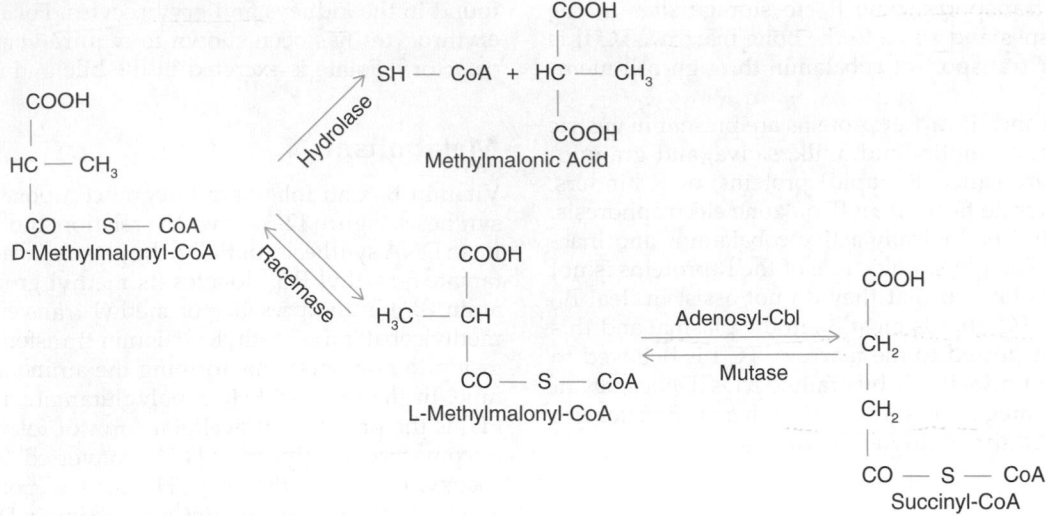

FIGURE 12-4. Adenosylcobalamin (adenosyl-Cbl), a vitamin B_{12} coenzyme, is required for conversion of methylmalonyl-CoA to succinyl-CoA. Methylmalonyl-CoA is a product of the catabolism of propionic acid normally produced by intestinal bacteria. But in the absence of adenosyl-Cbl, the reactions can be reversed and methylmalonyl-CoA is hydrolyzed to methylmalonic acid, which can be quantitated in serum or urine. (From Allen RH, Stabler SP, Savage DG et al: Diagnosis of cobalamin deficiency I: Usefulness of serum methylmalonic acid and total homocysteine concentrations. Am J Hematol 34:90, 1990 John Wiley & Sons, Inc, with permission.)

first proposed in the early 1960s as the "methylfolate trap" hypothesis, which involves the interrelation between B_{12} and folate (Fig. 12-3).[50] More recently, there is evidence in favor of this hypothesis, and it has been suggested that it be renamed the "tetrahydrofolate deficiency" hypothesis, since this name more accurately reflects the defect caused by vitamin B_{12} deficiency, as will be explained.[54]

When B_{12} is deficient, homocysteine cannot be converted to methionine and folate becomes "trapped" in the plasma monoglutamate 5-methyl FH_4 form and cannot be converted to FH_4. FH_4 is necessary for the formation of the polyglutamate 5,10-methylene FH_4, the folate coenzyme required for conversion of dUMP to dTTP, without which DNA synthesis is defective. The trapped 5-methyl FH_4 is, in fact, not trapped in B_{12} deficient cells. Rather it is excreted from cells, accumulates in plasma, and is then lost in the urine.[75]

Also, without FH_4, formiminoglutamic acid (FIGlu) cannot be converted to glutamate, and urinary FIGlu excretion is greatly increased (Fig. 12-3). Quantitation of urine FIGlu was used in the past to detect folate deficiency. It is seldom quantitated today, because it may be elevated in both folate and B_{12} deficiency.

In addition, if vitamin B_{12} is deficient, propionate catabolism cannot take place (Fig. 12-4). This causes increased urinary excretion of methylmalonic acid (MMA). The MMA level provides a sensitive test for B_{12} deficiency that is not affected by folate deficiency (see discussion under Most Useful Laboratory Tests for Diagnosing Vitamin B_{12} and Folate Deficiency).

Because folate and B_{12} are necessary components for DNA synthesis, a deficiency of either, no matter what the source, produces defective DNA synthesis, abnormal cell division, and, if left untreated, eventually megaloblastic anemia.

Peripheral Blood Megaloblastic Changes

It is important to note that in the diagnosis of vitamin B_{12} deficiency in the past, great emphasis was placed on the finding of megaloblastic anemia and the peripheral blood changes to be described. However, it is now well known that B_{12} deficiency can present subtly or atypically or in its early stages without any of these laboratory findings. Often patients with atypical B_{12} deficiency have abnormal nervous system findings without any peripheral blood abnormalities and respond well to B_{12} therapy, so that recognizing these patients is important.[11] (See Total Homocysteine, Comments and Sources of Error later in this chapter.)

Peripheral blood changes in the megaloblastic anemias are very similar no matter what the cause. Macrocytosis characteristically precedes the development of anemia and may even precede it by several years.[12,39] Therefore macrocytosis is an important early clue to the diagnosis of megaloblastic anemias, although many other causes of macrocytosis must also be ruled out (Fig. 12-6). As the disease progresses, usually the MCV increases roughly proportionately. With mild to moderate anemia, the MCV may increase to 110 fL. In severe anemia, it can range from 110 to 130 fL, although values up to 160 fL may be found.[70] However, when megaloblastic anemia is combined with iron deficiency, thalassemia, or inflammatory disease, all of which typically have a decreased MCV, a macrocytic MCV may be "masked," causing it to fall in the reference range, since the MCV is an average (mean) value.

Typically, the mean cell hemoglobin (MCH) value is also increased (from 33 to 38 pg), because hemoglobin content is increased in proportion to cell size. This may reduce or obliterate the normal central pallor of the cells, but the mean cell hemoglobin concentration (MCHC) usually remains normal.

As the megaloblastic anemia becomes more severe, the peripheral blood gradually reflects pancytopenia and a decreased reticulocyte count, even though the bone marrow is generally hypercellular, as a result of ineffective erythropoiesis and erythrocyte destruction in the bone marrow.

HEMATOLOGIC FINDINGS

In the early 1900s, an erythrocyte count as low as 0.086 $\times$ 10^{12}/L was reported[126] for a patient with pernicious anemia. Today, because patients are usually diagnosed much earlier in the course of the disease, severe anemia can be prevented. Reticulocytes are larger than normal, and the reticulocyte production index (RPI) (Chaps. 9 and 10) is often less than 2, indicating inadequate bone marrow response to anemia.

Blood film examination often reveals the classic finding of oval macrocytes with little or no central pallor (Fig. 12-5). Oval macrocytes are large, egg- or oval-shaped erythrocytes. Anisocytosis is also common; usually it leads to an increase in the red cell distribution width (RDW). Oval macrocytes are the most prominent poikilocytes, but tear drops and fragments also may be seen. If anemia is severe, extremely bizarre poikilocytes may be observed (Fig. 12-5) including dumbbell, anvil, cocked hat, and hand mirror forms, among others.[70] In advanced anemia, red cell inclusions may appear, including Howell-Jolly bodies, Cabot rings (rare), and basophilic stippling.

Megaloblasts (large, abnormal, nucleated red cells) in the basophilic, orthochromic, and polychromatophilic stages of maturation may also be present on the blood film, some of which may be binucleated. Megaloblasts have an unusually fine nuclear chromatin structure typical of megaloblastic maturation. Nuclear-cytoplasmic asynchrony—a mature-looking cytoplasm (pink) surrounding an immature nucleus (delicate, fine chromatin)—is characteristic (see Color Plate 12-1). Circulating megaloblasts are more likely to be found in buffy coat preparations (Chap. 3); their finding may eliminate the need for a bone marrow biopsy.

In the early stages, leukocyte counts are usually normal, but they gradually decline as the disorder progresses. In moderate anemia, the leukocyte count has been reported to range from 3.0 to 6.0 $\times$ 10^9/L and in severe anemia, between 1.0 and 3.0 $\times$ 10^9/L.[19] The leukopenia is generally attributable to absolute neutropenia. The platelet count generally declines with the erythrocyte count. It may fall below 100 $\times$ 10^9/L.[86]

Giant neutrophils and bands are common (see Color Plate 12-2). Nuclear hypersegmentation, that is, neutrophils with six to ten lobes, is a classic indicator of megaloblastic anemia (Fig. 12-5). Normal neutrophils have fewer than six lobes. In one large study of patients with megaloblastic anemia, 98% had at least one six-lobed neutrophil on a 100-leukocyte differential compared to 2% of the normal control subjects.[73] Hypersegmentation is one of the first hematologic abnormalities to appear in a developing megaloblastic anemia. In fact, it has been found to be a much more sensitive indicator of megaloblastic hematopoiesis than macrocytic anemia.[73,110] On the other hand, hypersegmentation can be absent, especially in subtle B$_{12}$ deficiency with no hematologic abnormalities. In addition, hypersegmentation is not specific; it can also be found in the myelodysplastic syndromes (Chap. 33) and in some toxic conditions (Chap. 25).

Giant platelets may be found. Platelets may be granule deficient, in which case they stain poorly with Wright stain.

Bone Marrow Megaloblastic Changes

Bone marrow examination is usually not required for the diagnosis of megaloblastic anemias, since the classic peripheral blood findings (increased MCV, oval macrocytes, and hypersegmented neutrophils), chemical analyses, and response to treatment generally provide sufficient diagnostic information. The marrow is usually hypercellular with erythrocyte precursors predominating and a reversed myeloid-erythroid (M:E) ratio (see Color Plate 12-3). The expected adult M:E ratio ranges from 2:1 to 4:1 (Chap. 27) but in megaloblastic anemia, the M:E ratio may range from 1:1 to 1:3. The ratio of megaloblasts to erythroblasts in the marrow increases with the severity of the disease. Megaloblasts are not found in normal bone marrow. They are very large and have characteristically fine chromatin, which is reflected at all stages of maturation. The chromatin has been described as "particulate," in contrast to the clumped chromatin of normal marrow erythroblasts. Early megaloblastic stages have an extremely basophilic cytoplasm. An increased number of mitotic forms is common.

The orthochromic megaloblast, with its distinct nuclear-cytoplasmic asynchrony, is particularly characteristic of megaloblastic anemias (see Color Plate 12-1). It has an abundant, mature-looking pink cytoplasm similar to that of orthochromic erythroblasts, but its nucleus resembles that seen in the less mature polychromatophilic erythroblasts.

Giant metamyelocytes are characteristic, although gi-

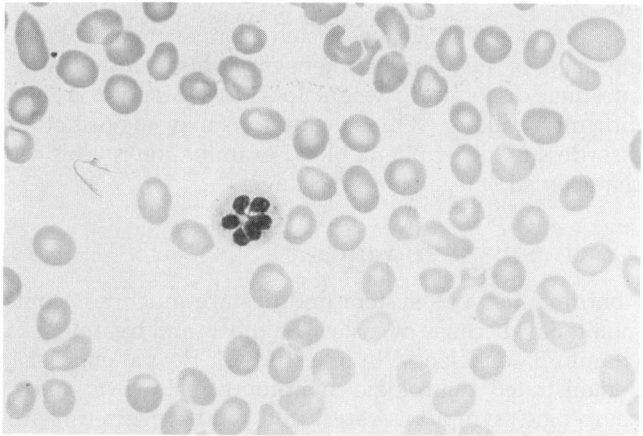

FIGURE 12-5. Peripheral blood film from a patient with pernicious anemia. The neutrophil displays the hypersegmentation (six or more nuclear lobes) typical of this disorder. Red cell morphology displays anisocytosis with some microcytic-looking cells and oval macrocytes that have a characteristic lack of central pallor. A few teardrops and a bizarre red cell are also present. Electronic cell analysis of this sample revealed an MCV of 119 fL. This field of view indicates a platelet deficiency. (Wright stain; original magnification ×400.)

ant leukocyte precursors at all maturation stages are common (see Color Plate 12-2). A giant metamyelocyte contains a nucleus that is enlarged both absolutely and in relation to cell size. Because of the problems in DNA synthesis, its nuclear shape, chromatin structure, and staining characteristics may be bizarre. It is likely that these cells are arrested in a premitotic developmental stage.[122] They probably die in the marrow and are not precursors of peripheral blood hypersegmented neutrophils.

Megakaryocytes are the least affected of the three cell lines, but in severe anemia, they may be reduced in number and display abnormal nuclear shape (extreme lobulation) and immature chromatin patterns (see Color Plate 12-4).[29]

PERNICIOUS ANEMIA

Since pernicious anemia (PA) of adults is the most representative form of megaloblastic anemia and a common cause of vitamin B_{12} deficiency, it is discussed in detail.[44] Other forms of megaloblastic anemia have many features similar to those of PA and are discussed briefly later in the chapter.

Definition and History

PA is associated with vitamin B_{12} deficiency that results from a lack of intrinsic factor (IF) caused by an acquired atrophy of the stomach lining called *achylia gastrica*. In this condition, secretion of IF by the gastric parietal cells is reduced and sometimes eliminated. Without protection by IF, vitamin B_{12} is destroyed in the GI tract before it can be absorbed in the ileum. Gastric atrophy also causes reduction of hydrochloric acid secretion.

PA was probably first described in the early 1800s,[1] although its cause was poorly understood. It was almost always fatal[107] until 1934 when two Boston physicians, George Minot and William Murphy, were awarded the Nobel prize in medicine for demonstrating the successful treatment of PA by a diet rich in liver. The vital ingredient in liver was later shown to be vitamin B_{12}. Soon thereafter, Whipple and his coinvestigators, and in separate studies Minot and his student William Castle, finally began to unravel the cause of this mysterious anemia.[15] It was Castle who first described the gastric protein IF (often called Castle's intrinsic factor) that is vital to vitamin B_{12} absorption.[16]

Demographics and Genetics

PA is most common in people of Scandinavian, British, and Irish descent over 50 years of age, although fewer than 1% of these populations are affected.[35]

In the United States, men and women are equally affected,[70] however in Europe, women seem to be diagnosed more often than men.[21] The peak age of occurrence is 60 years.[25]

It has been noted that patients with PA often have prematurely gray hair and light blue or gray eyes.[10] PA is also somewhat more common in people with blood group A.

Congenital PA is rare and probably inherited as an autosomal recessive trait.[78] The possible genetic origin of PA is suggested by studies that show relatives of PA patients at significantly higher risk of developing PA than the general population.[21,105] Autoantibodies to gastric parietal cells have been found in a significant number of relatives of PA patients when compared to the normal population.[21]

Pathophysiology

The gastritis (inflammation of the stomach lining) associated with PA that suppresses or arrests IF secretion and thus produces B_{12} deficiency may be caused by mucosal damage (mechanical, thermal, or chemical); nutritional deficiency (folate, ascorbate, or iron); endocrine disorders (thyroid, adrenal, or pancreatic); genetic disorders; or autoimmune mechanisms.[37] IF secretion is also decreased or arrested after partial or total excision of the stomach (gastrectomy). In addition, gastritis can be the *result* of PA, since gastrointestinal epithelium has a very high turnover rate and thus becomes vulnerable to the defective DNA synthesis in PA.

Autoimmune disorders have been demonstrated to have an increased incidence among patients with PA, including thyroid disease,[3] diabetes,[21] and hypogammaglobulinemia.[113] It is clear that autoimmune mechanisms are involved in most cases of PA, but the stimulus for the autoimmune changes that lead to PA is still unclear.

Clinical Findings

About half of PA patients develop a sore tongue (glossitis) early in the course of the disease. This is also a result of epithelial vulnerability to abnormal DNA synthesis. Severe glossitis is very painful, and the tongue appears "beefy red." Reappearance of a sore tongue during therapy indicates inadequate treatment. Typically, the tongue becomes very smooth and glazed between attacks of glossitis.

Complaints of weakness stem from anemia. At varying stages of the disorder other symptoms include gastrointestinal discomfort, weight loss due to anorexia, and difficulty walking.[25] Often, symptoms may suggest other disorders until peripheral blood examination reveals the characteristic megaloblastic changes.

Nervous System Findings

Abnormal nervous system findings are much less common today, because of earlier diagnosis and treatment of vitamin B_{12} deficiency. In one study of PA patients, 44% demonstrated neurologic symptoms.[72] However, most neurologic symptoms are mild and reversed with treatment.[4,44]

The neurologic disturbances are caused mostly by the effects of B_{12} deficiency on the brain and spinal cord. These neurologic disturbances include degeneration of peripheral nerves and of myelin. Myelin is a tubular covering of the nerves which acts somewhat like an electrical insulator to speed conduction of nerve impulses. Myelin is synthesized by glial cells which, like epithelial cells, have a high turnover rate and are thus vulnerable to abnormal DNA synthesis.

Degeneration of myelin and peripheral nerves produces the most frequently reported symptom of paresthesias, described as a prickling, tingling, "pins and needles" sensation in the hands and feet.[116] In later stages, degeneration also causes weakness, unsteady gait, clumsiness, decreased sensitivity to vibration, and in severe degeneration, spasticity. Impaired memory is common at this stage.[103] Because multiple nerve pathways are involved, this neurologic disorder is called "subacute combined degeneration." Psychiatric symptoms referred to as *megaloblastic madness* are uncommon, but include hallucinations, maniacal outbursts, paranoia, and schizophrenia.[42] Prompt therapy usually reverses the symptoms.

Laboratory Findings and Correlations with Disease

Exceptions to findings described earlier do occur. For example, studies have shown that the red cell distribution width (RDW) in PA is often normal.[100] Also patients identified early with PA are frequently *not* anemic and 25% to 38% do not have macrocytic erythrocytes.[12,72]

Erythrocyte survival is moderately decreased.[34] There is also intramarrow destruction of megaloblasts. Even normal cells are destroyed early when transfused into these patients,[41] probably in the extravascular system (Chap. 16). Haptoglobin may be decreased and methemalbumin may be increased, suggesting an intravascular component of hemolysis as well.[85]

The bleeding time may be prolonged and blood clot retraction may be poor due to associated thrombocytopenia.[57]

CYTOGENETICS

There are a number of reports of cytogenetic abnormalities in bone marrow cells including chromosome elongation and abnormal gaps or breaks.[67] These abnormalities are only temporary, however, and disappear with appropriate treatment of the disorder.

CHEMISTRY

The serum level of vitamin B_{12} has been reported to range from less than 10 to 110 ng/L (reference range 160–1000 ng/L).[21] Erythrocyte folate is usually reduced, because red cells need B_{12} to absorb folate. The *serum* folate value is usually normal or elevated (see Table 12-3).

In progressive stages of PA, serum iron is usually moderately increased,[21] as are macrophage iron stores and marrow sideroblasts. Plasma total iron-binding capacity may be slightly reduced. Autopsy may reveal a large concentration of iron in the liver, spleen, and kidneys. Such iron overload is caused by ineffective erythropoiesis, which leads to a decrease in iron uptake in red cells. Early destruction of erythrocytes in the bone marrow also increases the level of serum lactate dehydrogenase (LD) in proportion to the degree of anemia. The LD value is usually much higher in PA than in other hemolytic anemias, where it is slightly increased. In PA, the serum LD-1 isoenzyme value is the highest of the five LD isoenzymes,

whereas LD-2 has the greatest serum activity in the other hemolytic anemias.[28] Urine urobilinogen may be elevated, but unconjugated serum bilirubin is usually increased only in severe untreated PA.

Immunology

Because of the simultaneous occurrence of PA and autoimmune disorders in many patients, tests to evaluate both humoral and cell-mediated immunity in patients with PA may reveal a number of abnormalities. In tests of *humoral immunity*, patients may demonstrate serum IgG autoantibodies, including those to IF, parietal cells, and the thyroid.

IF antibodies are produced in approximately 56% of patients with PA.[109,115] Since they are rare in normal subjects, they are a more specific marker for the diagnosis of PA than parietal cell antibodies, which may be found in some healthy people.[71]

There are three types of IF antibodies: blocking antibodies and two types of binding antibodies. Both binding and blocking antibodies may be detected in the laboratory by radioimmunoassay techniques,[93] in which radioactive vitamin B_{12} is used to measure the ability of IF to bind B_{12}.

Blocking IF antibodies are believed to bind with IF and block its vitamin B_{12}-binding site. The test for IF-blocking antibodies is probably the immunologic test of choice in the diagnostic workup for PA patients.

Binding IF antibodies are usually found in conjunction with blocking antibodies. The first type of binding antibody attaches to an antigenic site on IF that is distant from the actual B_{12}-binding site, and binding is not dependent on whether or not IF has complexed with B_{12}. The second type binds to both IF and its complexed B_{12}.

Cell-mediated immunity may also play a role in PA, as evidenced by the transformation of lymphocytes from some patients with PA in the presence of human gastric juice.[23] The fact that human and hog IF concentrates can inhibit leukocyte migration in some PA patients is evidence of cell-mediated immunity to IF.[23]

Differential Diagnosis

A complete blood cell count and a serum vitamin B_{12} level are the only two laboratory evaluations usually necessary to diagnose pernicious anemia. In the past, the Schilling test, which involves administration of a small dose of radioactivity, was popular to assist in the diagnosis. However, its popularity has declined in recent years (see discussion of the Schilling test).

Although macrocytosis usually precedes anemia, as shown in Figure 12-6, the differential diagnosis of macrocytic anemias is complex and macrocytosis is not specific for PA. The early findings of hypersegmentation and oval macrocytes on the blood film may be indicative of a megaloblastic anemia. To confirm the diagnosis of PA in unclear cases, a Schilling test may be done.[17] There are three other conditions shown in Figure 12-6 with the same laboratory results as PA. However, gastric resection can be ruled out by patient history, and ingestion of corrosives and inert IF are rare (see discussion under Other Causes of Acquired Vitamin B_{12} Deficiency). Differentiation of megaloblastic from non-megaloblastic macrocytic anemias (Fig. 12-6) will be addressed later in this chapter.

LABORATORY TESTS FOR VITAMIN B₁₂ AND FOLATE DEFICIENCY

The recommended laboratory tests to assist in the diagnosis and differentiation of B_{12} and folate deficiency are listed in Table 12-1.

Measurement of serum vitamin B_{12}, serum folate, and erythrocyte folate values is often essential to the diagnosis of megaloblastic anemia. The serum B_{12} level is considered a relatively accurate reflection of tissue stores. The erythrocyte folate level indicates tissue folate stores much more accurately than the serum folate value, which is sensitive to recent folate consumption.

A more recent development, the food Schilling test, can be used in those special cases where food-bound B_{12} malabsorption is suspected or the reason for a decreased serum B_{12} cannot be determined; however, it too requires the administration of radioactivity. Other tests that have recently become more practical to perform in the laboratory and are useful diagnostic tools for B_{12} and folate deficiency include serum and urinary methylmalonic acid (MMA) and total homocysteine. The deoxyuridine (dU) suppression test is a more sensitive diagnostic test than the MMA and total homocysteine, but its use is confined to research centers at present. All of these tests will be discussed briefly below.

Serum Microbiologic B₁₂ and Folate Assays. Prior to the 1970s, microbiologic assays were the most common method of measuring serum vitamin B_{12}[2,77] and folic acid,[51] and they are still considered to be the reference methods with which all commercial kit methods must be compared. Microorganisms that require either B_{12} (*Euglena gracilis* or *Lactobacillus leichmannii*[36]) or folic acid (*Lactobacillus casei*) for growth are incubated with patient serum for 48 to 72 hours, after which serum turbidity is measured spectrophotometrically. The results are compared to standards of sera with known concentrations of B_{12} or folic acid to determine the patient's serum concentrations. Although these methods are accurate, sensitive, and specific, they are time-consuming and inaccurate if the patient is taking antibiotics. A

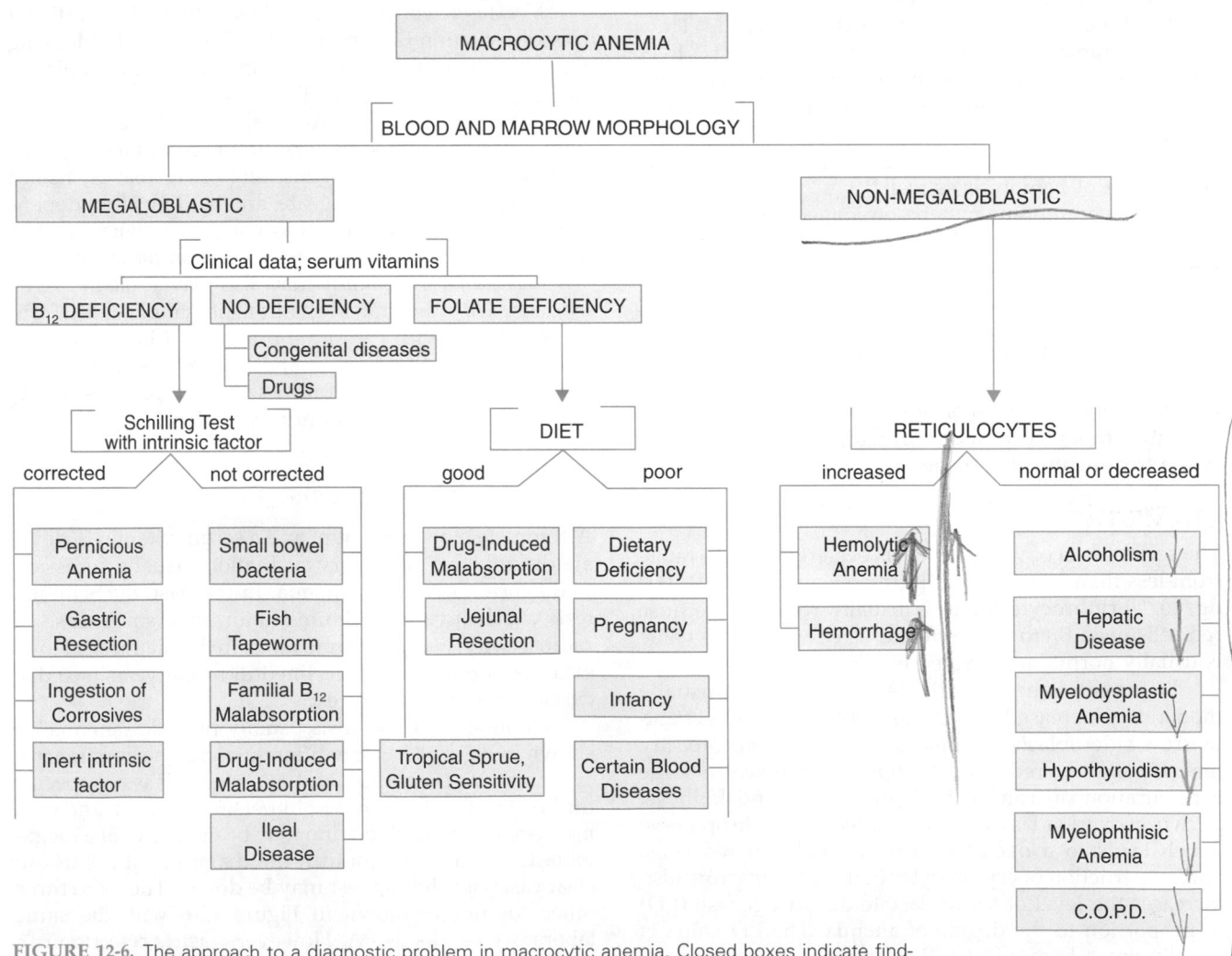

FIGURE 12-6. The approach to a diagnostic problem in macrocytic anemia. Closed boxes indicate findings and open boxes, procedures. C.O.P.D. = chronic obstructive pulmonary disease. (From Lee GR: Megaloblastic and nonmegaloblastic macrocytic anemias. In Lee GR, Bithell TC, Foerster J et al [eds]: Wintrobe's Clinical Hematology, 9th ed, p 772, Philadelphia, Lea & Febiger, 1993, with permission.)

TABLE 12-1
*Recommended Laboratory Tests to Assist
in the Diagnosis and Differentiation
of Vitamin B₁₂ and Folate Deficiency*

Required most frequently	CBC with RBC morphology
	Serum vitamin B_{12}
	Serum folate
	Erythrocyte folate
	WBC differential with count of hypersegmented neutrophils ($\geq$6 nuclear lobes) and RBC morphology check for oval macrocytes
Required occasionally	Plasma total homocysteine
	Serum methylmalonic acid (MMA)
	Deoxyuridine (dU) suppression test*
	Schilling test (if PA† suspected) (absorption of free ^{57}Co-cyanocobalamin)
	IF-blocking antibodies test (if PA† suspected)
Required rarely	Bone marrow examination
	Food Schilling test (if PA† suspected) (absorption of food-bound ^{57}Co-cyanocobalamin)††

The dU suppression test is generally done only in research centers.
†*PA = pernicious anemia.*
††*See text for explanation of the food Schilling test and comparison to the traditional Schilling test.*

reference range reported for one microbiologic B_{12} assay was 200 to 900 pg/mL and for folate, 5 to 16 ng/mL.[61]

Competitive Protein-Binding Radioassay for Serum B_{12} and Serum and Erythrocyte Folate.
Today, competitive protein-binding radioassays are the methods of choice for quantitation of B_{12} and folate because of their technical simplicity and lack of interference from antibiotics or antineoplastic drugs.[30] Only the highlights of these radioassays are presented here. Commercial kits are available for individual and simultaneous measurement of serum B_{12} and serum or erythrocyte folate. The individual kits contain exact procedures. The simultaneous method is described here.

PRINCIPLE. Patient vitamin B_{12} and folate in serum compete for binding sites in the test system with ^{57}Co-labeled cobalamin and ^{125}I-labeled folic acid derivative, respectively. The B_{12} binder is usually nonhuman IF from hog stomach. The folate binder is β-lactoglobulin, a protein that occurs naturally in milk. After incubation and subsequent washing to remove unbound radioactive labels, the sample radioactivity level is measured with a γ-scintillation counter. The lower the patient's serum B_{12} or serum (or erythrocyte) folate value, the more radioactivity remains in the sample. Quantitation is accomplished by comparison with a standard curve.

SPECIMEN AND PATIENT REQUIREMENTS FOR SERUM B_{12} AND FOLATE. Serum is preferred, but EDTA-anticoagulated plasma is acceptable. The patient should fast before any folic acid testing, because recent food intake may increase the serum level of folic acid (but not B_{12}). For serum folate measurement, serum should not be contaminated by cells or hemolysis, since erythrocytes contain about 40 times more folate than the serum. Serum must be protected from light to prevent folate deterioration. It may be stored at 2° to 8°C for up to 3 hours or frozen (−20°C) for longer periods. The specimen must be either boiled

or exposed to an alkaline agent to release the cobalamin and folate from endogenous binding proteins.

SPECIMEN REQUIREMENTS FOR ERYTHROCYTE FOLATE. Whole blood hemolysates for erythrocyte folate assay require EDTA-anticoagulated blood. After the hematocrit is measured, the hemolysate is prepared in ascorbic acid solution (to 100 μL whole blood, 2 mL of ascorbic acid solution, 0.2 g/dL, is added) and incubated 90 minutes to hydrolyze folate polyglutamates. It must be protected from light. Storage is the same as for serum samples.

REFERENCE RANGES. Reference ranges should be established by each laboratory for the selected commercial kits. For fasting adults, the serum vitamin B_{12} reference range as measured by one radioassay is 100 to 700 pg/mL, although the lower limit indicating frank B_{12} deficiency is not well defined.[19,111] The reference range for serum folate is approximately 3 to 16 ng/mL and for RBC folate, 130 to 628 ng/mL.[111] Vitamin B_{12} levels decline significantly with age in healthy adult males.

COMMENTS AND SOURCES OF ERROR. This procedure is generally very sensitive and capable of measuring very low concentrations of B_{12}. The improvement in serum B_{12} assays over the last decade may be one reason for the early identification of B_{12} deficiency in the absence of expected clinical or hematologic findings. On the other hand, in one study, early hematologic relapse (*e.g.*, findings of neutrophil hypersegmentation and oval macrocytes on the blood film) was found in a small but significant number of patients even before the serum B_{12} fell below normal.[74] In that study, the patients' B_{12} values were in the 200 to 400 pg/mL range, within the normal range. Therefore, serum B_{12} measurement cannot be considered 100% sensitive in the detection of B_{12} deficiency nor is it 100% sensitive in predicting hematologic relapse.

B_{12} levels in patients with untreated PA are usually less than 100 pg/mL. In folate-deficient patients, serum folate is usually less than 1.0 ng/mL and RBC folate, less than 100 ng/mL. If results are indeterminate (*i.e.*, B_{12}, 100–400 pg/mL; serum folate, 2.0–3.0 ng/mL),[30] other laboratory or clinical findings may be helpful including serum methylmalonic acid and total homocysteine (see later).[74] Otherwise, serum B_{12} levels should be checked again in a few months.

The nonhuman IF used in this test system must be as nearly pure as possible; otherwise it may contain R binders (transcobalamins I and III), which also bind B_{12} and metabolically inactive B_{12} analogs, causing falsely elevated B_{12} levels.[65]

In procedures in which the binding protein includes both IF and R binders, the R binders are saturated with cobinamide, a B_{12} analog that does not bind to IF. This facilitates blocking of all non-IF vitamin B_{12}-binding sites.

Another procedure that is very specific for cobalamin calls for the use of chicken serum–binding protein with a magnetizable solid-phase separation system.[56] In this procedure, no boiling or pretreatment of the patient sample is required.

Using reliable commercial assays, particularly those with purified IF as the binder or with IF and the nonspecific R-protein sites blocked with "cobinamide," it is reported that the results of B_{12} radioassays are comparable to those obtained by microbiologic assay and that they allow for appropriate diagnosis.[65] Reliable serum and erythrocyte folate radioassays can also provide valuable diagnostic information. However, laboratories should evaluate any kit carefully before it is put into service for reporting patient results.[71]

The Schilling Test.
Although in the past the Schilling test[19,102] was frequently used, it is now generally reserved for only a small number of more complex cases. The decline in popularity has occurred because of the availability of vitamin B_{12} assays

and the problems of disposal of radioactive blood and urine and patient concerns about exposure to radioactivity.

PRINCIPLE. The Schilling test, named for its developer Robert F. Schilling,[125] provides a measure of the body's ability to secrete viable IF and absorb orally administered ^{57}Co-labeled B$_{12}$ in the ileum. Along with the ^{57}Co B$_{12}$, excessive amounts of unlabeled B$_{12}$ are administered to the patient to fill all tissue binding sites. Normal absorption of vitamin B$_{12}$ under such circumstances is reflected by a specified minimum level of urinary excretion of radiolabeled B$_{12}$.

SPECIMEN AND PATIENT REQUIREMENTS. The patient should fast overnight. A 24-hour urine collection is begun immediately upon administration of the labeled B$_{12}$ by mouth.

GENERAL PROCEDURE. A physiologic dose of ^{57}Co-labeled vitamin B$_{12}$ (0.5 to 2.0 μg) is given by mouth, followed by a "flushing dose" of 1000 μg unlabeled B$_{12}$ injected intramuscularly within the next 1 to 2 hours. This dose is given to saturate the liver and tissue binding sites so that, if the labeled B$_{12}$ is absorbed, it will not be completely bound in B$_{12}$-depleted tissues and some will be excreted in the urine.

If results of the initial test are abnormal, the test is repeated 2 to 3 days later. In this phase, IF is administered *with* the ^{57}Co B$_{12}$, to eliminate IF as a variable and to determine whether provision of IF allows for normal (or correction of) B$_{12}$ absorption. The results allow for distinguishing between a deficiency of, or a defect in, IF and a malabsorption syndrome such as that caused by ileal disease or fish tapeworm.

REFERENCE RANGE. Normally more than 8% of the administered dose of ^{57}Co B$_{12}$ is excreted in the initial 24-hour urine specimen. Patients with PA secrete less than 8%, usually about 3%.

INTERPRETATION. Table 12-2 summarizes the possible Schilling test results and their indications. Figure 12-6 provides a more detailed summary of these indications.

If less than 8% of the labeled B$_{12}$ is excreted in the first 24 hours, absorption is abnormal. If administering IF with the B$_{12}$ corrects the malabsorption, then the cause of the deficiency is most likely IF deficiency and the diagnosis of PA is confirmed. It can also indicate the rare case of a defective IF molecule. If administering IF with the B$_{12}$ does not correct the malabsorption,

the possible causes of the malabsorption are listed in Figure 12-6. Food-bound B$_{12}$ malabsorption is another condition in which a low serum vitamin B$_{12}$ level is found but with a *normal* Schilling test result (see Food Schilling Test).

COMMENTS AND SOURCES OF ERROR. Incomplete urine collection is a major source of error.[20] It can lead to false-positive results (that indicate failure to absorb B$_{12}$) by reducing the level of radioactivity measured in the 24-hour urine sample. One recommendation is to assess absorption by measuring the radioactivity in plasma 8 to 12 hours after the test is begun; this indicator is as reliable or more so than 24-hour urine collection.[17a]

Approximately 25% of patients with PA have a secondary intestinal malabsorption disorder that distorts results of the Schilling test performed with IF so it does not show the typical "correction."[30] Thus, lack of test correction after IF administration does not absolutely exclude PA.

If the patient is suffering from renal disease, excretion of labeled B$_{12}$ may be decreased in the first 24-hour urine sample, since excretion may be delayed as long as 72 hours.[70]

Food Schilling Test. When serum B$_{12}$ is decreased but the Schilling test appears normal (Table 12-2), food-bound B$_{12}$ malabsorption may be suspected. In such cases, patients absorb free B$_{12}$ normally (thus the normal Schilling test) but food-bound B$_{12}$ poorly. A test that may help to diagnose this condition is the food Schilling test. It involves the administration of ^{57}Co vitamin B$_{12}$ bound to egg yolk, which is scrambled and fed to the patient. Like the Schilling test, ^{57}Co is measured in a sample from a 24-hour urine collection. Patients with food-bound B$_{12}$ malabsorption have significantly lower egg test results than normal controls.[13]

Serum and Urinary Methylmalonic Acid. Vitamin B$_{12}$ (as the coenzyme adenosyl-Cbl) and the enzyme methylmalonyl CoA mutase are both necessary for conversion of methylmalonyl CoA to succinyl CoA (Fig. 12-4). Without B$_{12}$, methylmalonyl CoA reacts along a different pathway forming increased levels of serum and urinary methylmalonic acid (MMA). Thus, a test for MMA provides a specific test for B$_{12}$ deficiency.[24]

GENERAL PROCEDURE. MMA measurement in both serum and urine can be achieved using a stable-isotope-dilution method.[88] It involves anion exchange using a gas chromatograph and MMA detection by mass spectrometry. Colorimetric and thin layer chromatography methods also exist.

REFERENCE RANGE. The reported reference ranges for serum and urinary MMA are quite variable, depending on the method used and should be calculated by the individual laboratory based on the chosen method. The most important point is that serum and urinary MMA are elevated in most patients with B$_{12}$ deficiency when compared to normal subjects. However, both serum and urinary MMA are normal in patients with folate deficiency.

COMMENTS AND SOURCES OF ERROR. The stable-isotope-dilution method is reported to provide an accurate, precise, rapid, and sensitive assay for serum and urinary MMA.[88]

An increased MMA value has been found to be a reliable diagnostic indicator of cobalamin deficiency, sometimes more reliable than a serum B$_{12}$ level, since it may be elevated even when serum B$_{12}$ is normal.[74] Elevated MMA has been reported to be the first indication of cobalamin deficiency, because it reflects the availability of B$_{12}$ to the tissue.[52] It has been shown to precede the elevation of total homocysteine in early B$_{12}$ deficiency.[74] In folate deficiency, however, serum and urinary MMA are normal; thus MMA is useful in the differentiation of B$_{12}$ and folate deficiency in unclear cases (Table 12-3).

TABLE 12-2
Sample Schilling Test Results for Percent Urinary Excretion of ^{57}Co-Labeled Vitamin B$_{12}$*

Subjects/ Conditions	^{57}Co-Vitamin B$_{12}$ Without IF (%)	^{57}Co-Vitamin B$_{12}$ With IF (%)
Normal	≥8	≥8
Pernicious anemia	<8	≥8 (corrected)
Vitamin B$_{12}$ malabsorption	<8	<8 (not corrected)
Food-bound vitamin B$_{12}$ malabsorption	≥8	≥8 (appears normal)

*A comparison of normal subjects to those with pernicious anemia and malabsorption conditions causing vitamin B$_{12}$ deficiency (see Fig. 12-6). See text for further discussion of these results. Note that the percent urinary excretion depends on the radiolabeled dosage used. The manufacturer's instructions should be consulted for appropriate diagnostic percentages for any given dosage.

TABLE 12-3
Biochemical Differentiation of Vitamin B$_{12}$ and Folic Acid Deficiency

Condition	Serum B$_{12}$	Serum Folic Acid	RBC Folate	Serum or Urinary MMA*	Plasma Total Homocysteine*
Vitamin B$_{12}$ deficiency	Marked decrease	Normal or increased	Moderate decrease	Marked increase	Marked increase
Folic acid deficiency	Normal or decreased	Marked decrease	Marked decrease	Normal	Marked increase
B$_{12}$ and folic acid deficiency	Decreased	Decreased	Decreased	Marked increase	Marked increase

Serum methylmalonic acid (MMA) and plasma total homocysteine may be increased in patients with renal dysfunction.

Total Homocysteine. Homocysteine is a sulfur-containing amino acid that is present in plasma either bound to protein (70%) or in a free form, both of which can be measured together as total homocysteine. Homocysteine is required for DNA synthesis (Fig. 12-3). Both folate and vitamin B$_{12}$ are required for the conversion of homocysteine to methionine.

If either folate or B$_{12}$ is deficient, excess homocysteine is readily exported from the cells into the plasma. Thus measurement of total homocysteine can be valuable in diagnosis of either B$_{12}$ or folate deficiency (although not helpful in differentiation of the two) and the monitoring of effects of treatment on laboratory results (Table 12-1 and 12-3).

SPECIMEN REQUIREMENTS. The method described here requires blood collected in EDTA that is placed immediately on ice and separated within 10 minutes. The plasma must be analyzed immediately or stored at −80°C until analysis. Plasma protein removal is not required in this assay.

GENERAL PROCEDURE. A fully automated method for measurement of plasma total homocysteine has been described, making this metabolite measurement more practical.[90] Readers are referred to the indicated reference for procedure details. The method involves a rapid chromatographic and fluorescence assay using an inexpensive Gilson Model 232-401 programmable sample processor (Gilson Medical Electronics, Inc., Middleton, WI) attached to a high pressure liquid chromatography (HPLC) system and a fluorescence detector.

REFERENCE RANGE. Using this automated method, the reference range was given as 7.3 to 13.0 μmol/L.[90]

COMMENTS AND SOURCES OF ERROR. This method is reported to be highly precise and to have good correlation with two other established although more laborious and time-consuming assays.[8,89]

In cases in which tissue B$_{12}$ is subtly decreased (as evidenced by neuropsychiatric or other abnormalities) but the serum B$_{12}$, hematologic, and other chemical values are *normal*, measurement of homocysteine and MMA may be particularly useful, since they have been found to be elevated in such cases. The tissue B$_{12}$ deficiency and clinical symptoms can be successfully treated with B$_{12}$,[74] and both MMA and homocysteine respond by decreasing within days of treatment with B$_{12}$. However, increased homocysteine is not specific for B$_{12}$ and folate deficiency. It may also be increased in homocysteinuria,[81] renal failure,[123] some malignant states,[64] and in connection with some drugs.[114]

It should also be noted that in early B$_{12}$ deficiency, one study suggested that total homocysteine elevation may often come later than the MMA elevation (discussed earlier).[74] Finally, total homocysteine and MMA are both less sensitive in subtle deficiencies than the deoxyuridine suppression test (see following).[14]

Deoxyuridine (dU) Suppression Test. The deoxyuridine (dU) suppression test is performed using a bone marrow cell sample to detect vitamin B$_{12}$ or folate deficiency.[49,70] The major disadvantages of this test are that it requires bone marrow aspiration, special equipment and materials, and is labor intensive. Thus, its use has been limited to research centers.

GENERAL PROCEDURE. This test measures the lack of 5,10-methylene FH$_4$ at the cellular level that results from either folate or B$_{12}$ deficiency (Fig. 12-3). This is done by adding nonradioactive dU (a dUMP precursor) to a marrow culture and incubating for 1 hour. Subsequently, radioactive ^{3}H-thymidine (a dTTP precursor) is added and incubated for another hour. Normally in cultured bone marrow cells, unlabeled dU is incorporated into DNA and suppresses DNA uptake of the subsequently added ^{3}H-thymidine according to the following reaction:

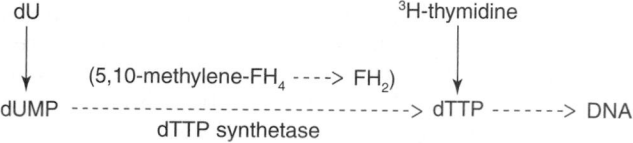

If the DNA takes up a significant amount of radioactive thymidine, then deficient patient conversion from dU to deoxythymidine triphosphate (dTTP) caused by lack of 5,10-methylene FH$_4$ is indicated. Either folate or B$_{12}$ deficiency can result in failure to convert dU to dTTP.

INTERPRETATION. Folate deficiency is identified if the addition of the folate compound 5-methyl FH$_4$ to the marrow culture at the dU incubation stage causes correction of dTTP synthesis. Vitamin B$_{12}$ deficiency is identified by correction with the addition of vitamin B$_{12}$.

COMMENTS AND SOURCES OF ERROR. A highly sensitive test, even more so than MMA or total homocysteine,[14] the dU suppression test is particularly useful for detecting and identifying a deficiency in patients with borderline or nonexistent hematologic changes, or when both serum B$_{12}$ and folate levels are either low or normal.[71]

Serum Blocking–IF Antibodies. Testing for serum blocking–IF antibodies can be very useful for diagnosing PA. The test is rapid, easy to perform, and cost effective.[71] Interested readers may check the indicated references for a description of IF antibody testing.[19,31] These antibodies are found in 50% to 60% of patients with PA. A positive test is fairly specific for PA; the test has only been positive in a few patients without PA. The disadvantage is that the test is negative in about half of the patients with PA.[31]

Plasma Transcobalamin II. Recently, decreased plasma transcobalamin II (TC II) levels have been explored as an early indicator of B_{12} deficiency. An assay for rapid determination has been described.[119] As explained earlier in this chapter, TC II is the only B_{12} binding protein capable of delivering B_{12} from storage sites to cells. Studies of cancer patients revealed some with low plasma TC II levels despite normal plasma B_{12} levels, and this was said to be the first sign of tissue B_{12} depletion or a very early sign of B_{12} malabsorption as shown in AIDS patients.[48] As expected, the lowest TC II levels were found in patients with the highest serum homocysteine levels.[119]

X-Ray or Endoscopic Studies. In cases of suspected PA, x-ray studies or endoscopy may be used to verify gastric atrophy and exclude stomach carcinoma. This ensures appropriate therapy.

Effects of Treatment on Laboratory Results and Prognosis

Treatment most often involves intramuscular injections of vitamin B_{12} (in the hydroxycobalamin form) every 1 to 3 months, although the use of daily 1000 μg doses of oral cobalamin therapy has been shown to be highly successful in Sweden.[5] Oral cobalamin therapy represents a substantial cost savings to the patient, since the cost of administration of the B_{12} injection by a health professional can be very expensive.[68]

If continued as needed throughout life, B_{12} supplementation can provide complete recovery for persons who are not severely affected by neurologic disturbances. Response to initial therapy must be closely monitored with chemical and hematologic tests, and then monitored regularly thereafter. Therapy with the correct agent is very important. If folate is given to treat B_{12} deficiency, the patient's hematologic abnormalities may improve temporarily but not as would be expected with appropriate therapy. Incorrect treatment may actually induce or exacerbate the neurologic abnormalities of a B_{12}-deficient patient.[59]

PERIPHERAL BLOOD AND BONE MARROW

With appropriate therapy the reticulocyte count should increase dramatically within 5 to 7 days, and the RPI should indicate an adequate response to the patient's degree of anemia. Erythroblasts may also appear as a positive sign of effective erythropoiesis. The hematocrit value should also begin to rise within 5 to 7 days and should rise fastest in patients who are severely anemic. Within 1 to 2 months, the hematocrit should be within the reference range, no matter how severe the anemia was at initiation of therapy.[58] In that same period, anisocytosis and poikilocytosis gradually disappear and the MCV should return to normal, although it may rise before it drops, because of reticulocytosis.

The number of neutrophilic leukocytes increases to normal within 7 days. Immature leukocytes may appear in the peripheral blood, causing a temporary left shift which gradually disappears. Usually hypersegmented neutrophils disappear within 2 weeks.[21,82] The platelet count increases and generally is within the reference range within 7 days of initiating therapy.[87]

Transfusion is rarely necessary except in cases of severe anemia, which may lead to (or may have already caused) a potentially fatal myocardial infarction.

Although it is not necessary to perform a bone marrow examination to determine response to therapy, marrow abnormalities are remarkably reduced within 24 hours.[96] Within 6 to 10 hours after initiation of therapy, a significant reduction in megaloblasts is common.[26] Within 1 to 2 days, erythrocyte maturation is normoblastic.[106] The giant metamyelocytes, however, usually do not disappear for at least 7 days.[21]

CHEMISTRY

Serum and urinary MMA and plasma total homocysteine levels should fall toward normal within several days after initiating treatment with vitamin B_{12}.

Serum LD levels should decrease to normal within 1 to 2 weeks. Plasma bilirubin declines to normal within 3 to 4 weeks. Urinary urobilinogen begins to decrease as erythropoiesis levels off to a normal rate.[33]

Plasma iron usually declines within 24 to 48 hours and may even fall below the reference range[43] as accelerated erythropoiesis compensates for the anemia. The serum ferritin level decreases more slowly.

NEUROLOGIC DISORDERS

Neurologic disorders may or may not be reversible with therapy, depending on how long they were present before therapy was instituted. Disturbances present for less than 3 months usually are reversible.[6] Improvement may take months, and any residual manifestations after a year of therapy are most likely irreversible. Spinal cord damage is also usually irreversible.

OTHER CAUSES OF ACQUIRED VITAMIN B_{12} DEFICIENCY

Dietary Deficiency

Dietary deficiency is a rare cause of B_{12} deficiency particularly since normal body stores are sufficient to prevent megaloblastic anemia for several years if no more B_{12} is ingested. Strict vegetarians who avoid meat, eggs, and milk can eventually develop B_{12} deficiency, but this is rare. Infants breast-fed by mothers who are vegans (and asymptomatic) may develop severe anemia.[52]

Food–Vitamin B_{12} Malabsorption

A more common but still atypical cause of B_{12} deficiency is malabsorption due to apparent failure to extract B_{12} bound to food proteins such as egg yolk.[11] This is *not* associated with a failure of the intrinsic factor mechanism as seen in pernicious anemia. Such patients have a normal classic Schilling test but abnormal food Schilling test (Table 12-2). The cause of this malabsorption is believed to be a deficiency of pepsin (a protein-splitting enzyme) and acid in the stomach, both of which are needed to split B_{12} from its protein binder.

Gastrectomy

Total or partial gastrectomy (excision of the stomach) may result in a deficiency of Castle's intrinsic factor, and thus failure to absorb B_{12}. If supplemental parenteral vitamin B_{12} is not provided, B_{12} deficiency will ensue, however it usually does not occur for several years owing to the normally large liver stores of B_{12}.

Intrinsic Factor Molecular Defect

A molecular defect in IF is a rare cause of B_{12} deficiency. The IF in gastric secretions is inert but immunologically normal, it appears normal on chromatography, and its B_{12}-binding affinity is normal; however, it is incapable of facilitating ileal B_{12} absorption.[60]

Small Bowel Bacterial Overgrowth

Healthy persons have either a sterile proximal small bowel or a low concentration of bacterial growth. Two factors normally prevent bacterial overgrowth: (1) normal intestinal peristalsis, which prevents stasis and encourages recirculation of intestinal contents and (2) gastric acid secretion. Some conditions that promote bacterial overgrowth include small bowel diverticulosis, blind loops and pouches, and achlorhydria. Excessive bacterial growth successfully competes for ingested B_{12}, making it unavailable for ileal absorption. Laboratory findings are similar to those in PA, except that correction of absorption is *not* demonstrated in the Schilling test by administration of IF (Fig. 12-6). Treatment with antibiotics usually corrects the problem.

Fish Tapeworm Disease

Diphyllobothrium latum, a common parasite of freshwater fish, especially pike, causes disease in humans. Most often found in Finland, it also occurs in the lakes of north central North America. Fish tapeworm infection is acquired by eating raw or undercooked fish. *D. latum* interferes with B_{12} absorption by competing with IF for binding B_{12}[84]; over time, this results in B_{12} deficiency. Treatment consists of B_{12} administration and eradication of the worms.

Ileal Disease

Because most B_{12} is absorbed in the ileum, ileal resection, bypass,[9] or disease often leads to B_{12} malabsorption.[11] Crohn's disease, also called regional enteritis, is one of the better-known diseases that affects the ileum. Patients with Crohn's disease sometimes develop megaloblastic anemia. Vitamin B_{12} and folate deficiency may occur together in Crohn's disease.

Human Immunodeficiency Virus and Other Causes

Decreased levels of serum B_{12} are common in conjunction with human immunodeficiency virus (HIV) and occur at an early stage.[95] In most patients with HIV, serum B_{12} levels decrease over time, probably due to malabsorption.

This decrease may help to predict those patients whose disease will progress the most rapidly.[95]

In one report, the earliest laboratory indicator of tissue B_{12} deficiency in AIDS patients was a low serum transcobalamin II B_{12} binding protein (which is responsible for B_{12} transport).[48] This parameter was found to be decreased despite normal serum B_{12} and total homocysteine and a normal classic Schilling test. However, the food Schilling test was abnormal in these patients.

Certain drugs, hemodialysis,[92] and normal near-term pregnancy can also cause B_{12} deficiency.

HEREDITARY VITAMIN B_{12} DEFICIENCY (IMERSLUND SYNDROME)

Imerslund syndrome is a rare hereditary disorder that causes B_{12} malabsorption. It usually affects homozygous children during the first 2 years of life causing a megaloblastic anemia and proteinuria. Heterozygotes have decreased B_{12} absorption but are not anemic. Inheritance is probably autosomal recessive.[70] In this disorder there is no IF deficiency or defect, but B_{12} cannot be absorbed, with or without IF. Gastric secretion is normal. The exact defect is not clear, but it is thought to be related to the mechanism of absorption in the ileal mucosa that *follows* the binding of IF with B_{12} to ileal receptors.[70]

Anemia is corrected by B_{12} therapy, but proteinuria persists, perhaps because of an associated renal tubular defect.

FOLATE DEFICIENCY ANEMIA

With the exception of neurologic manifestations, folate deficiency is associated with the same general clinical findings as vitamin B_{12} deficiency. In the unusual case in which neurologic disturbances occur in association with folate deficiency, there is most likely a concurrent B_{12} deficiency or some other disorder.

Laboratory Findings and Correlations with Disease

The hematologic laboratory characteristics are generally the same as those described earlier in this chapter for any megaloblastic anemia.

Biochemical results help to differentiate folate deficiency from B_{12} deficiency (Table 12-3). The serum B_{12} value is usually normal or decreased, the serum folate value is significantly decreased, and erythrocyte folate is also significantly decreased. The following values were reported in studies of folate-deficient patients: serum B_{12}, 50 to 500 pg/mL, mean 190 (below to within the reference range)[21]; serum folate, less than 3 ng/mL (below the reference range)[121]; and RBC folate, less than 100 ng/mL (below the reference range).[55] (See reference ranges under Laboratory Tests for Vitamin B_{12} and Folate Deficiency.)

Other biochemical results are similar to those described for pernicious anemia, because both folate deficiency and PA cause premature erythrocyte destruction in the bone marrow.

In severe folic acid deficiency, the urine concentration of a degradation product of normal histidine metabolism called formiminoglutamic acid (FIGlu) is significantly increased because of the lack of tetrahydrofolate (FH$_4$), which normally reacts with FIGlu to form glutamate and 5-formimino-FH$_4$ (Fig. 12-3).[22] When folate-deficient subjects are given histidine, urinary excretion of FIGlu is increased.[70] Excretion of FIGlu is also increased in vitamin B$_{12}$ deficiency; thus, it cannot be used to differentiate B$_{12}$ from folate deficiency.

Causes of Acquired Folate Deficiency

Folate deficiency may be acquired in many ways; only rarely is it inherited.[66]

DIETARY DEFICIENCY

Dietary folate deficiency occurs much more readily than dietary vitamin B$_{12}$ deficiency, because body stores of folate are smaller. Significant deficiency is indicated by levels of serum folate below 3 ng/mL and of erythrocyte folate below 140 ng/mL.[99] Folate deficiency is one of the most common vitamin deficiencies in the United States. Deficiency may occur within 3 to 6 months if no folate is ingested. It is reported that folate deficiency is the most common dietary deficiency among the elderly.[80] Geographically, it is most common in Southeast Asia and Africa, where diets often consist mostly of starch and grains and are low in animal protein and green leafy vegetables. Destruction of food folate by excessive heat during steaming and boiling can also lead to dietary deficiency. Also B$_{12}$ deficiency can result in clinical symptoms of folate deficiency, since B$_{12}$ is required to produce tetrahydrofolate (FH$_4$), the intracellular form of folate.

ALCOHOLIC CIRRHOSIS

Alcoholic cirrhosis has been reported to cause megaloblastic anemia in about 20% of those afflicted.[62] The MCV is generally greater than 120 fL, which is usually greater than that associated with nonmegaloblastic macrocytic anemia caused by liver disease.[7] Serum folate is reduced, but vitamin B$_{12}$ is normal or increased. Excess alcohol leads to folate deficiency, because alcohol interferes with folate metabolism.[53]

PREGNANCY

Pregnancy may also bring about folate deficiency and megaloblastic anemia because of the developing fetus' requirement for large quantities of folate. Therefore folic acid supplementation, especially in the first trimester, is recommended.

INFANT MALNUTRITION

Infants in developed countries seldom have folate deficiency, in contrast to those in countries plagued with malnutrition.[120] Infants require about 50 μg of folate per day, four to ten times the adult requirement by weight basis.[108]

DRUG-INDUCED FOLATE DEFICIENCY

A number of drugs called folate antagonists or anti-folate medications can impair DNA synthesis. Examples include the antimalarial drug pyrimethamine and chemotherapeutic agent methotrexate.[91] These antagonists inhibit the enzyme dihydrofolate reductase (Fig. 12-3), which is part of the metabolic process of thymidylate and DNA synthesis. Taking drugs that inhibit DNA synthesis by inhibiting purine or pyrimidine synthesis—hydroxyurea and cytosine arabinoside, among others—may cause megaloblastic anemia.

Effects of Treatment on Laboratory Results and Prognosis

These are generally the same as described previously for treatment with B$_{12}$. Treatment of folic acid deficiency usually includes 1 mg of folic acid daily taken orally for 2 to 3 weeks, which should replenish folate stores. Then, if the source of deficiency can be corrected, a normal diet should suffice, but if this is not possible, continued oral administration of about 0.25 to 0.5 mg of folic acid daily is usually prescribed.

CONDITIONS THAT CAUSE BOTH FOLATE AND B$_{12}$ DEFICIENCY
Tropical Sprue and Gluten-Sensitive Enteropathy

Tropical sprue and gluten-sensitive enteropathy both can cause simultaneous B$_{12}$ and folate malabsorption as a result of intestinal atrophy. Patients suffer from steatorrhea (fatty stools), weight loss, weakness, and a wide-ranging nutritional deficiency caused by a general lack of nutrient absorption. Tropical sprue affects the entire small intestine[63] and so causes both B$_{12}$ and folate deficiency; it appears to be caused by some infectious agent and responds to antibiotics[63] and folate therapy.

Gluten-sensitive enteropathy principally affects the proximal intestine.[94] Its two forms are childhood celiac disease and adult nontropical sprue. Affected people have abnormal intestinal sensitivity to gluten, a protein in wheat and other grains.[32]

In childhood celiac disease, anemia usually results from iron deficiency,[27] but sometimes the cause is folate deficiency, and rarely it is B$_{12}$ deficiency. In adult nontropical sprue, most patients experience folate malabsorption and deficiency,[40] but less than half of those diagnosed demonstrate B$_{12}$ deficiency.[21] Therapy includes administration of iron, folate, and in some cases B$_{12}$ depending on the deficiency, and avoidance of dietary gluten.

INHERITED DISORDERS THAT AFFECT DNA SYNTHESIS

Figure 12-3 shows that many components are required in DNA synthesis. A number of inherited disorders impair DNA synthesis. One example is orotic aciduria, a rare hereditary disorder of pyrimidine (cytosine, thymine, and uracil) metabolism that results in a megaloblastic anemia.[104] Most of these patients exhibit physical and mental retardation.

Other inherited disorders that cause defective DNA synthesis include abnormal or defective transcobalamin II and enzyme deficiencies, including methyl transferase and dihydrofolate reductase (Fig. 12-3), among others.

DIFFERENTIAL DIAGNOSIS OF THE MEGALOBLASTIC ANEMIAS

Differential diagnosis of the megaloblastic anemias in the laboratory can be somewhat perplexing at times. The most basic differentiation is usually the cause, whether it be vitamin B_{12} or folate deficiency, or some other, because it indicates the appropriate therapy. A second source of confusion involves distinguishing between megaloblast*ic* and megaloblast*oid* anemias, which have some similar features. Third, megaloblastic anemias must be differentiated from normoblastic, macrocytic anemias. The following sections provide differentiating features in each of these areas.

Differentiation of Vitamin B_{12} and Folic Acid Deficiencies

Although abnormalities in the hematologic findings in these two types of anemia are very similar, serum B_{12} and serum and erythrocyte folate measurements usually help to identify the cause. In cases in which the cause is not clear, serum or urinary MMA and plasma total homocysteine are very useful for differentiation of B_{12} and folate deficiency. Table 12-3 summarizes the results of these five assays in the different disorders. Note that serum folate is often increased in B_{12} deficiency and erythrocyte folate is moderately reduced. This is probably because B_{12} is necessary to act as a cofactor in the transfer of folate into erythrocytes.[112] Also note that serum MMA is increased in B_{12} deficiency but normal in folate deficiency.

Differentiation of Megaloblastic and Megaloblastoid Cell Maturation

Megaloblast*oid* (literally, "resembling megaloblastic") erythrocyte maturation is an abnormal process that is *not* caused by B_{12} or folate deficiency. It is common in malignancies of the myeloid cell lines such as the myeloproliferative disorders (Chaps. 34 and 35) and the dysmyelopoietic (or myelodysplastic) syndromes (DMPS) (Chap. 33). Megaloblastoid morphology (see Color Plate 12-5) generally displays a coarser clumping of the nuclear chromatin in nucleated red cells that makes the parachromatin more prominent than in megaloblastic red cell precursors (see Color Plate 12-1). Recall that the chromatin structure in megaloblastic cells is very delicate in appearance.

Sometimes, abnormal red cell maturation in the DMPS may nonetheless be difficult to distinguish from that seen in megaloblastic anemias. Both may exhibit a macrocytic anemia with oval macrocytes, basophilic stippling, Howell-Jolly bodies, nucleated red cells, and giant platelets in the peripheral blood. Also platelet granulation may be decreased in either disorder.

Distinguishing features include B_{12} and folate levels that are usually normal or increased in the DMPS. Also, the DMPS generally demonstrate abnormal development in other myeloid cell lines such as neutrophils with prominent hypolobulation referred to as pseudo–Pelger-Huët cells, and reflect a left shift on the leukocyte differential, neither of which is typical of megaloblastic anemia. On the other hand, hypersegmentation may occur in both the DMPS and megaloblastic anemias. Also the finding of micromegakaryocytes or megakaryoblasts in the peripheral blood would indicate a megaloblastoid rather than a megaloblastic anemia.

Differentiation of Macrocytic Anemias—Megaloblastic *Versus* Normoblastic

Megaloblastic, macrocytic anemias must be distinguished from normoblastic, macrocytic anemias. In the latter, the red cells show an increase in MCV without the characteristic megaloblastic changes in cell maturation in the bone marrow or peripheral blood.

The oval shape of megaloblastic, macrocytic erythrocytes often distinguishes them from nonmegaloblastic, macrocytic erythrocytes, which are usually round and often thin. Polychromatophilia and reticulocytosis may also occur in the macrocytic, normoblastic anemias but seldom in the megaloblastic anemias. Figure 12-6 provides a flow chart that is useful in the differential diagnosis.

The normoblastic, macrocytic anemias may be caused by reticulocytosis resulting from blood loss or hemolysis. Other normoblastic, macrocytic anemias do not cause reticulocytosis, including those due to liver disease, hypoplastic anemia, acquired sideroblastic anemia and other myelodysplastic syndromes, myelophthisic anemia, and myxedema. Normoblastic macrocytes may also be seen in normal pregnancy and in neonates. Many cytotoxic drugs may also induce normoblastic macrocytosis, including among others, chlorambucil, melphalan, and azathioprine.

In hepatic disease, the macrocytes may appear as target cells or cells with increased central pallor; either feature differentiates the disorder from a megaloblastic anemia.

CONGENITAL DYSERYTHROPOIETIC ANEMIAS

The congenital dyserythropoietic anemias (CDA) are also anemias of abnormal nuclear development, but they are not associated with B_{12} or folate deficiency. They are rare, hereditary disorders characterized by refractory anemia that varies in severity. Other characteristics include abnormalities of bone marrow erythrocyte precursors, including nuclear abnormalities such as karyorrhexis (inability of chromosomes to reform into a nucleus after mitosis resulting in disintegrated, structureless chromatin frag-

TABLE 12-4
Differentiating Features of the Congenital Dyserythropoietic Anemias

Type	Anemia Classification	NRBC Binuclearity, Multinuclearity, and Karyorrhexis	Mode of Inheritance	Acidified Serum Test
I	Slightly macrocytic	Yes	Autosomal recessive	Negative
II	Normocytic	Yes	Autosomal recessive	Positive
III	Normocytic or slightly macrocytic	Yes*	Autosomal dominant	Negative

Multinuclearity may be pronounced, with as many as 12 nuclear lobes in one erythroblast.

ments), multinuclearity, and other bizarre changes. Peripheral blood and bone marrow leukocytes and platelets are not affected in CDA.

Based on cellular morphology, three types of CDA have been defined, types I, II, and III (Table 12-4).[45] Not all the laboratory findings for a given patient may fulfill the criteria for a single category. The disease may first be diagnosed in infancy or adult life.[76] In all three types, the bone marrow generally shows significant erythroid hyperplasia whereas the peripheral blood reticulocyte count usually remains normal.

Type I

Morphologic findings in type I CDA include mild macrocytosis, anisocytosis, and poikilocytosis. Basophilic stippling and Cabot rings may be seen regardless of whether or not the patient has a spleen.[46] The bone marrow demonstrates binucleated erythroblasts (Fig. 12-7), erythroblasts with incompletely separated or multilobulated nuclei, megaloblastoid nuclear chromatin structure, and erythrophagocytosis. A diagnostic feature is the finding of thin, Feulgen-positive, internuclear chromatin bridges joining two erythroblasts.[46]

Type II

Type II CDA is also referred to as hereditary erythroblast multinuclearity with positive acidified serum test (HEM-

PAS).[118] Of the three CDA, type II is the most common, although it is also rare. Its major laboratory diagnostic finding is the abnormal erythrocyte sensitivity to acidified normal serum, which is similar to that seen in paroxysmal nocturnal hemoglobinuria (PNH) (Chap. 18). HEMPAS and PNH can be distinguished by the failure of HEMPAS red cells to lyse in the sugar water screening test (Chap. 18). HEMPAS red cells are also hemolyzed by anti-i and anti-I antibodies. However intravascular hemolysis is not common in type II CDA.

The peripheral blood film commonly reveals anisocytosis, poikilocytosis, and basophilic stippling. Using phase-contrast microscopy, one may detect ghost red cells that reveal irregular dark stretches of thickened membrane believed to represent membrane doubling.[117] This is a significant diagnostic feature. Unlike type I, megaloblastoid bone marrow morphology is not characteristic of type II CDA.

Type III

Type III CDA, probably the first to be reported,[124] is known to have affected about 35 to 40 persons.[79,97] It is characterized by hemolytic anemia, macrocytosis, and megaloblastic erythropoiesis.[98] The most noteworthy feature is the pronounced multinuclearity (up to 12 nuclei per cell) of bone marrow erythroblasts in these subjects. As many as 30% of the red cell precursors may be affected, and they may be gigantic—up to 50 to 60 μm in diameter. Thus their name, gigantoblasts.[69] Table 12-4 provides further details on type III CDA.

CHAPTER SUMMARY

The anemias of abnormal nuclear development, including the megaloblastic anemias and the congenital dyserythropoietic anemias (CDAs), are characterized by abnormal bone marrow cell maturation. Cells in the bone marrow and peripheral blood (and their nuclei) may be abnormal in size, shape, and color. The megaloblastic anemias are characterized by peripheral blood oval macrocytes and hypersegmented neutrophils, an increased erythrocyte MCV, and a decreased hemoglobin, hematocrit, and erythrocyte count. Leukocyte and platelet counts are usually within the reference range.

Most often, megaloblastic anemia is caused by vitamin B_{12} or folate deficiency. Without B_{12} or folate, normal DNA synthesis is interrupted (Fig. 12-3) and megaloblastic erythropoiesis occurs in the bone marrow. This is reflected by a hypercellular marrow

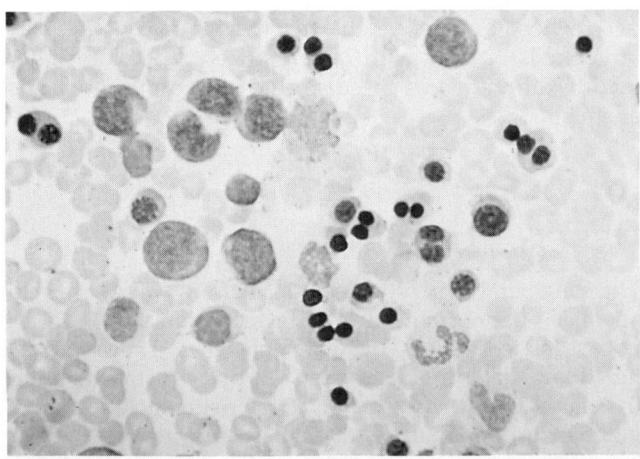

FIGURE 12-7. Bone marrow from a patient with type I CDA contains binucleated erythroblasts associated with the dyserythropoiesis that characterizes this disorder.

containing megaloblasts (very large erythrocyte precursors) that have extremely basophilic cytoplasm and very fine particulate chromatin unlike the clumped chromatin of normal marrow erythroblasts. Megaloblasts often display asynchronous nuclear-cytoplasmic maturation (*i.e.*, an immature nucleus with a mature cytoplasm).

Table 12-1 lists the recommended laboratory tests to assist in the diagnosis and differentiation of vitamin B_{12} and folate deficiency. Figure 12-6 and Table 12-2 summarize the interpretation of the Schilling test results, a test frequently performed in the past, but now used primarily in complicated cases. Since megaloblastic anemia is often *not* the first sign of these disorders, a number of chemical tests that are helpful in the diagnosis are listed in Table 12-1 including serum B_{12}, folate, and methylmalonic acid (MMA) and plasma total homocysteine. Table 12-3 summarizes the expected results of chemical tests in the differential diagnosis.

Megaloblast*oid* cell maturation (observed most frequently in myeloproliferative and myelodysplastic disorders and also in the rare congenital dyserythropoietic anemias [CDA]) can be differentiated from megaloblast*ic* maturation by the coarser clumping of nuclear chromatin in nucleated red cells and the normal or increased B_{12} and folate levels, both characteristic of megaloblast*oid* maturation.

Case Study 12-1

A 63-year-old man, with a 20-year history of non–insulin-dependent diabetes mellitus, reported a recent 27-pound weight loss. His tongue was red and fissured. On neurologic examination, he had decreased vibratory sensation, and his thyroid appeared diffusely enlarged. His complete blood count results were: WBC 8.1×10^9/L; RBC 2.49×10^{12}/L; Hb 10.1 g/dL; Hct 0.31 L/L; MCV 124 fL; MCH 40.5 pg; MCHC 32.7 g/dL; platelets 173×10^9/L. His electronic leukocyte and platelet histograms appeared normal. The red cell distribution width was normal, 14.3%. The red cell histogram was shifted to the right, indicating an increased MCV. The peripheral blood film showed moderate oval macrocytes and hypersegmented neutrophils. Anisocytosis and poikilocytosis were moderate and elliptocytes and target cells were slight. The serum B_{12} value was less than 50 pg/mL and serum folate was 10.3 ng/mL. A Schilling test was performed without intrinsic factor, and 1% ^{57}Co-labeled B_{12} was excreted in the 24-hour urine collection. Upon repeat of the test with IF, 8% was excreted in the 24-hour urine collection. The result of the IF-blocking antibodies test was positive.*

1. Which of the blood count results is abnormal? What does this indicate initially?
2. Is either the serum B_{12} or folate level abnormal?
3. How might the Schilling test results be interpreted?
4. What are IF-blocking antibodies? What does the positive result on the IF-blocking antibodies test indicate?
5. Do the hypersegmented neutrophils or oval macrocytes allow for differentiation between B_{12} and folate deficiency? Are they specific for megaloblastic anemia? What is the minimum number of nuclear lobes necessary for a neutrophil to be considered hypersegmented?
6. Are these results consistent with those generally found in pernicious anemia? Explain.

* This case study is reprinted with permission from Pierre R: Seminar and Case Studies The Automated Differential. Rochester, MN, Mayo Foundation, Medical Education Program. © Coulter Electronics, Inc. Presented as a service by Coulter Electronics, Inc., Hialeah, FL, 1985.

Case Study 12-2

A 41-year-old Palestinian man, born in Bethlehem, was seen in the outpatient clinic of a hospital in Saudi Arabia where he worked as a dietitian. He complained of blood in his stools every morning, especially after drinking some very strong Turkish coffee. Upon sigmoidoscopy, multiple polyps were found in the rectum, colon, and ileum. He was diagnosed with Gardner's syndrome or familial polyposis, which is characterized by multiple benign polyps with malignant potential, lining the mucous membrane of the intestine, particularly the colon. He was treated surgically with a total colectomy and resection of the distal ileum. After surgery, he was told that he would need to take intramuscular injections of vitamin B_{12} every 3 months for the rest of his life to "maintain good health."

Approximately 2 years after surgery, his peripheral blood count and chemistry results were WBC 6.2×10^9/L; RBC 4.33×10^{12}/L; Hb 12.2 g/dL; Hct 0.36 L/L; MCV 82 fL; MCH 27.8 pg; MCHC 33.8 g/dL; platelets 323×10^9/L; the leukocyte differential was normal; stool occult blood was positive; serum vitamin B_{12} 375 pg/mL; serum folate 10 ng/mL; RBC folate 300 ng/mL; serum lactate dehydrogenase 109 IU/L (reference range 100–225 IU/L); total bilirubin 0.6 mg/dL (0.2–1.0 mg/dL); and serum ferritin 28 ng/mL (32–248 ng/mL). Five years later, after continuing problems, the patient was given an ileostomy and is now doing well.

1. Why did this patient need vitamin B_{12} injections for the rest of his life?
2. Without these injections, could the patient develop a megaloblastic anemia? Why or why not?
3. Is the patient anemic 2 years after surgery? If so, is the anemia normocytic, macrocytic, or microcytic?
4. Are any chemistry values abnormal, and if so, do they indicate the possible onset of megaloblastic anemia?
5. Could the erythrocyte size commonly associated with a decreased serum ferritin cause an otherwise macrocytic MCV to become a normocytic MCV in this case? Why or why not?
6. Are the serum ferritin and stool occult blood values likely to be related to each other or to the peripheral blood values in this case? Why or why not?
7. What additional laboratory tests could be recommended in this case to check for early signs of vitamin B_{12} deficiency, even though the serum B_{12} is normal and there are no hematologic indications of a megaloblastic anemia?
8. Based on the laboratory results, does it appear that the patient has been receiving his vitamin B_{12} injections regularly?

Review Questions

12-1. Hypersegmented neutrophils, a classic (although nonspecific) finding in megaloblastic anemia, generally have _____ or more nuclear lobes.

A. 4
B. 6
C. 8
D. 10

12-2. Pernicious anemia is caused by a

A. dietary folate deficiency.
B. dietary vitamin B_{12} deficiency.
C. reduced intrinsic factor secretion in the stomach.
D. defective intrinsic factor molecule.

For the following questions choose from these answers:
A. 1, 3
B. 2, 4
C. 1, 2, and 3
D. 4 only
E. All are correct

12-3. The laboratory findings in megaloblastic anemias may include

1. decreased serum folate.
2. decreased erythrocyte, leukocyte, and platelet counts.
3. decreased serum vitamin B_{12}.
4. asynchronous cell maturation.

12-4. Megaloblastic changes in the peripheral blood may include

1. giant neutrophils with nuclear hypersegmentation.
2. an MCV as high as 130 fL.
3. pancytopenia with increasing severity of anemia.
4. oval macrocytes with increased central pallor.

12-5. Megaloblastic changes in the bone marrow include

1. giant leukocyte precursors, especially metamyelocytes.
2. a hypercellular marrow with leukocyte precursors predominating.
3. nuclear-cytoplasmic asynchrony, especially in orthochromic megaloblasts.
4. an increased ratio of erythroblasts to megaloblasts.

12-6. A *false-positive* Schilling test may be caused by

1. renal disease associated with decreased urine output.
2. neglecting to give the "flushing dose" of unlabeled vitamin B_{12}.
3. incomplete urine specimen collection.
4. urine specimen collection during a 48-hour period.

12-7. The laboratory result(s) that is/are indicative of vitamin B_{12} deficiency include

1. increased serum methylmalonic acid.
2. decreased serum vitamin B_{12}.
3. normal or increased serum folic acid.
4. increased serum total homocysteine.

12-8. In a case of vitamin B_{12} deficiency with severe anemia, the laboratory result(s) within 1 to 2 weeks after appropriate response to treatment with B_{12} injections should include

1. a significant increase in the reticulocyte count.
2. the disappearance of hypersegmented neutrophils.
3. a left shift in the differential which gradually disappears.
4. an increase in the hematocrit to within the reference range.

12-9. Megaloblast*oid* cell maturation may demonstrate _____ which is/are NOT characteristic of megaloblast*ic* maturation.

1. clumping of nuclear chromatin in nucleated red cells
2. hypersegmented neutrophils
3. pseudo–Pelger-Huët cells
4. oval macrocytes

References

1. Addison T: On the Constitutional and Local Effects of Disease of the Suprarenal Capsules. London, S Highly, 1855
2. Anderson BB: Investigations into the Euglena method for the assay of the vitamin B_{12} in serum. J Clin Pathol 17:14, 1964
3. Andrus EC, Wintrobe MM: Hyperthyroidism and pernicious anemia. Johns Hopkins Med J 59:291, 1936
4. Beck WS: Neuropsychiatric consequences of cobalamin deficiency. Adv Intern Med 36:33, 1991
5. Berlin R, Berlin H, Brante G et al: Vitamin B_{12} body stores during oral and parenteral treatment of pernicious anemia. Acta Med Scand 204:81, 1978
6. Bethell FH, Sturgis CC: The relation of therapy in pernicious anemia to changes in the nervous system. Blood 3:57, 1948
7. Bingham J: The macrocytosis of liver disease, I, II. Blood 14:694, 1959; 15:244, 1960
8. Brattström LE, Israelsson B, Jeppsson JO et al: Folic acid—An innocuous means to reduce plasma homocysteine. Scand J Lab Invest 48:215, 1988
9. Buchwald H: Vitamin B_{12} absorption deficiency following bypass of the ileum. Am J Dig Dis 9:755, 1964
10. Callender ST, Denborough MA, Sneath J: Blood groups and other inherited characters in pernicious anaemia. Br J Haematol 3:107, 1957
11. Carmel R: Subtle and atypical cobalamin deficiency states. Am J Hematol 34:108, 1990
12. Carmel R: Macrocytosis, mild anemia, and delay in the diagnosis of pernicious anemia. Arch Intern Med 139:47, 1979
13. Carmel R, Siegel ME: Food cobalamin malabsorption occurs frequently in patients with unexplained low serum cobalamin levels. Arch Intern Med 148:1715, 1988
14. Carmel R, Sinow RM, Karnaze DS: Atypical cobalamin deficiency. Subtle biochemical evidence of deficiency is commonly demonstrable in patients without megaloblastic anemia and is often associated with protein-bound cobalamin malabsorption. J Lab Clin Med 109:454, 1987
15. Castle WB: Current concepts of pernicious anemia. Am J Med 48:541, 1970
16. Castle WB, Heath CW, Strauss MB et al: Observations on the etiologic relationship of achylia gastrica to pernicious anemia. Am J Med Sci 194:618, 1937
17. Chanarin I: How to diagnose (and not misdiagnose) pernicious anaemia. Blood Rev 1(4):280, 1987
17a. Chanarin I: Megaloblastic anaemia, cobalamin, and folate. J Clin Pathol 40:978, 1987
18. Chanarin I: The folates. In Barker BM, Bender DA (eds): Vitamins in Medicine, 4th ed. London, William Heinemann, 1980
19. Chanarin I: The Megaloblastic Anaemias, 2nd ed, p 44. Oxford, England, Blackwell Scientific Publications, 1979
20. Chanarin I, Waters DAW: Failed Schilling tests. Scand J Haematol 12:245, 1974
21. Chanarin I: The Megaloblastic Anaemias. Philadelphia, FA Davis, 1969
22. Chanarin I, Bennett MC: A spectrophotometric method for estimating formimino-glutamic and urocanic acid. Br Med J 1:27, 1962. Nature 196:271, 1962; Proc R Soc Med 57:384, 1964
23. Chanarin I, James D: Humoral and cell-mediated intrinsic factor antibody in pernicious anaemia. Lancet 1:1078, 1974
24. Cox EV, White AM: Methylmalonic acid excretion: An index of vitamin B_{12} deficiency. Lancet 2:853, 1962
25. Cox EV: The clinical manifestations of vitamin B_{12} deficiency in addisonian pernicious anemia. In Heinrich HC (ed): Vitamin B_{12} und Intrinsic Factor, 2nd Europäisches Symposion. Stuttgart, Enke, 1962
26. Davidson LSP, Davis LJ, Innes J: The effect of liver therapy on erythropoiesis as observed by serial sternal punctures in twelve cases of pernicious anaemia. Q J Med 11:19, 1942
27. Dormandy KM, Waters AH, Mollin DL: Folic acid deficiency in coeliac disease. Lancet 1:632, 1963
28. Emerson PM, Wilkinson JH: Lactate dehydrogenase in the diagnosis and assessment of response to treatment of megaloblastic anaemia. Br J Haematol 12:678, 1966
29. Epstein RD: Cells of the megakaryocyte series in pernicious anemia. Am J Pathol 25:239, 1949
30. Fairbanks VF, Klee GG: Biochemical aspects of hematology. In Tietz NW (ed): Fundamentals of Clinical Chemistry, 3rd ed, pp 816—818. Philadelphia, WB Saunders, 1987
31. Fairbanks VF, Lennon VA, Kokmen E et al: Tests for pernicious anemia: Serum intrinsic factor blocking antibody. Mayo Clin Proc 58:203, 1983
32. Falchuk ZM, Gebhard RL, Sessoms C et al: An *in vitro* model of gluten-sensitive enteropathy. J Clin Invest 53:487, 1974
33. Farquharson RF, Borsook H, Goulding AM: Pigment metab-

olism and destruction of blood in Addison's (pernicious) anemia. Arch Intern Med 48:1156, 1931

34. Finch CA: Erythrokinetics in pernicious anemia. Blood 9:807, 1956

35. Friedlander RD: The racial factor in pernicious anemia: A study of five hundred cases. Am J Med Sci 187:634, 1934

36. Gijzen AHJ, deKock HW, Meulendijk PN et al: The need for a sufficient number of low level sera in comparisons of different serum vitamin B_{12} assays. Clin Chim Acta 127:185, 1983

37. Glass GBJ: Antitrophic effects of gastric autoantibodies on parietal and peptic cells. In Glass GBJ (ed): Progress in Gastroenterology, vol 3, p 73. New York, Grune & Stratton, 1977

38. Grant JP: Handbook of Total Parenteral Nutrition, 2nd ed. Philadelphia, WB Saunders, 1992

39. Hall CA: Vitamin B_{12} deficiency and early rise in mean corpuscular volume. JAMA 245:1144, 1981

40. Halsted CH, Reisenauer AM, Romero JJ et al: Jejunal perfusion of simple and conjugated folates in celiac sprue. J Clin Invest 59:933, 1977

41. Hamilton HE, Sheets RF, DeGowin EL: Studies with inagglutinable erythrocyte counts. J Lab Clin Med 51:942, 1958

42. Hart RJ, McCurdy PR: Psychosis in vitamin B_{12} deficiency. Arch Intern Med 128:596, 1971

43. Hawkins CF: Value of serum iron levels in assessing effect of haematinics in the macrocytic anaemias. Br Med J 1:383, 1955

44. Healton EB, Savage DG, Brust JC et al: Neurologic aspects of cobalamin deficiency. Medicine 70(4):229, 1991

45. Heimpel H, Wendt F: Congenital dyserythropoietic anemia with karyorrhexis and multinuclearity of erythroblasts. Blut 31:261, 1976

46. Heimpel H: Congenital dyserythropoietic anemia type I: Clinical and experimental aspects. In Congenital Disorders of Erythropoiesis (Proceedings—Ciba Symposium), p 135. Amsterdam, Elsevier, 1976

47. Herbert V: Recommended dietary intakes (RDI) of folate in humans. Am J Clin Nutr 45:661, 1987

48. Herbert V, Fong W, Gulle V et al: Low transcobalamin II is the earliest serum marker for subnormal vitamin B_{12} (cobalamin) absorption in patients with AIDS. Am J Hematol 34:132, 1990

49. Herbert V, Tisman G, Le-Teng-Go et al: The dU suppression test using ^{125}I-UdR to define biochemical megaloblastosis. Br J Haematol 24:713, 1973

50. Herbert V, Zalusky R: Interrelations of vitamin B_{12} and folic acid metabolism: Folic acid clearance studies. J Clin Invest 41:1263, 1962

51. Herbert V, Baker H, Frank O et al: The measurement of folic acid activity in serum: A diagnostic aid in the differentiation of the megaloblastic anemias. Blood 15:228, 1960

52. Higginbottom MC, Sweetman L, Nyhan WL: A syndrome of methylmalonic aciduria, homocystinuria, megaloblastic anemia and neurologic abnormalities in a vitamin B_{12}-deficient breast-fed infant of a strict vegetarian. N Engl J Med 299:317, 1978

53. Hillman RS, McGuffin R, Campbell C: Alcohol interference with the folate enterohepatic cycle. Trans Assoc Am Physicians 90:145, 1977

54. Hoffbrand AV, Jackson BFA: Correction of the DNA synthesis defect in vitamin B_{12} deficiency by tetrahydrofolate: Evidence in favour of the methyl-folate trap hypothesis as the cause of megaloblastic anaemia in vitamin B_{12} deficiency. Br J Haematol 83:643, 1992

55. Hoffbrand AV, Newcombe FA, Mollin DL: Method of assay of red cell folate activity and the value of the assay as a test for folate deficiency. J Clin Pathol 19:17, 1966

56. Houts TM, Carney JA: Radioassay for cobalamin (vitamin B_{12}) requiring no pretreatment of serum. Clin Chem 27:263, 1981

57. Ingeberg S, Stofferson E: Platelet dysfunction in patients with vitamin B_{12} deficiency. Acta Haematol (Basel) 61:75, 1979

58. Isaacs R, Bethell FH, Riddle MC et al: Standards for red blood cell increase after liver and stomach therapy in pernicious anemia. JAMA 111:2291, 1938

59. Israels MCG, Wilkinson JF: Risk of neurological complication in pernicious anaemia treated with folic acid. Br Med J 2:1072, 1949

60. Katz M, Lee SK, Cooper BA: Vitamin B_{12} malabsorption due to a biologically inert intrinsic factor. N Engl J Med 287:425, 1972

61. Kelleher BP, Walshe KG, Scott JM et al: Microbiological assay for vitamin B_{12} with use of a colistin-sulfate-resistant organism. Clin Chem 33:52, 1987

62. Kimber CL, Deller DJ, Ibbotson RN et al: The mechanism of anemia in chronic liver disease. Q J Med 34:33, 1965

63. Klipstein FA: Tropical sprue. Gastroenterology 54:275, 1968; 68:239, 1975; Blood 45:577, 1975

64. Kredich NM, Hershfield MS, Falletta JM et al: Effects of 2'-deoxycoformycin on homocysteine metabolism in acute lymphoblastic leukemia (abstract). Clin Res 29:541A, 1981

65. Kubasic NP, Ricotta M, Sine HE: Commercially supplied binders for plasma cobalamin (vitamin B_{12}), analysis—"purified" intrinsic factor, "cobinamide"-blocked R protein binder, and nonpurified intrinsic factor R protein binder—compared to microbiological assay. Clin Chem 26:598, 1980

66. Lanzkowsky P: Congenital malabsorption of folate. Am J Med 48:580, 1970

67. Lawler SD, Roberts PD, Hoffbrand AV: Chromosome studies in megaloblastic anaemia before and after treatment. Scand J Haematol 8:309, 1971

68. Lederle FA: Oral cobalamin for pernicious anemia. Medicine's best kept secret? JAMA 265(1):94, 1991

69. Lee GR: The normocytic, normochromic anemias. In Lee GR, Bithell TC, Foerster J et al (eds): Wintrobe's Clinical Hematology, 9th ed, p 885. Philadelphia, Lea & Febiger, 1993

70. Lee GR: Megaloblastic and nonmegaloblastic macrocytic anemias. In Lee GR, Bithell TC, Foerster J et al (eds): Wintrobe's Clinical Hematology, 9th ed, pp 745, 774. Philadelphia, Lea & Febiger, 1993

71. Lindenbaum J: Status of laboratory testing in the diagnosis of megaloblastic anemia. Blood 61:624, 1983

72. Lindenbaum J, Healton EB, Savage DG et al: Neuropsychiatric disorders caused by cobalamin deficiency in the absence of anemia or macrocytosis. N Engl J Med 318(26):1720, 1988

73. Lindenbaum J, Nath BJ: Megaloblastic anaemia and neutrophil hypersegmentation. Br J Haematol 44:511, 1980

74. Lindenbaum J, Savage DG, Stabler SP et al: Diagnosis of cobalamin deficiency: II. Relative sensitivities of serum cobalamin, methylmalonic acid, and total homocysteine concentrations. Am J Hematol 34:99, 1990

75. Lumb M, Deacon R, Perry R et al: Urinary folate loss following inactivation of vitamin B_{12} by nitrous oxide in rats. Br J Haematol 51:235, 1982

76. Maldonado JE, Taswell HF: Type I dyserythropoietic anemia in an elderly patient. Blood 44:495, 1974

77. Matthews DM: Observations on the estimation of serum vitamin B_{12} using *Lactobacillus leichmannii*. Clin Sci 22:101, 1962

78. McIntyre OR, Sullivan LW, Jeffries GH et al: Pernicious anemia in childhood. N Engl J Med 272:981, 1965

79. McKusick VA: Mendelian inheritance in man: Catalogs of autosomal dominant, autosomal recessive, and X-linked phenotypes. In Francomano CA, Antonarakis SE (eds): Autosomal Dominant Phenotypes, 10th ed, vol 1, p 73. Baltimore, Johns Hopkins University Press, 1992

80. Miller SM: Aging and changes in vitamin status. Clin Lab Sci 1(6):342, 1988

81. Mudd SH, Levy HL, Skovby F: Disorders of transsulfuration. In Scriver CR, Beaudet AL, Sly WS et al (eds): The Metabolic Basis of Inherited Diseases, p 693. New York, McGraw-Hill, 1989

82. Nath BJ, Lindenbaum J: Persistence of neutrophil hypersegmentation during recovery from megaloblastic granulopoiesis. Ann Intern Med 90:757, 1979

83. National Academy of Sciences—National Research Council (US), Subcommittee on the Tenth Edition of the RDAs, Food and Nutrition Board, Commission on Life Sciences: Recommended Dietary Allowances, 10th ed. Washington, DC, National Academy Press, 1989

84. Nyberg W, Gräsbeck R, Saarni M et al: Serum vitamin B_{12} levels and incidence of tapeworm anemia in a population heavily infected with *Diphyllobothrium latum*. Am J Clin Nutr 9:606, 1961

85. Owen JA, Carew JP, Cowling DC et al: Serum haptoglobins in megaloblastic anaemia. Br J Haematol 6:242, 1960

86. Paddock FK, Smith KE: The platelets in pernicious anemia. Am J Med Sci 198:372, 1939

87. Rak VK, Varga L, Krizsa F et al: Untersuchung der Thrombocytopoese bei Perniciosa-Kranken. Acta Haematol 34:175, 1965

88. Rasmussen K: Solid-phase sample extraction for rapid determination of methylmalonic acid in serum and urine by a stable-isotope-dilution method. Clin Chem 35(2):260, 1989

89. Refsum H, Helland S, Ueland PM: Radioenzymic determination of homocysteine in plasma and urine. Clin Chem 31:624, 1985

90. Refsum H, Ueland PM, Svardal AM: Fully automated fluorescence assay for determining total homocysteine in plasma. Clin Chem 35(9):1921, 1989

91. Roe DA: Drug-Induced Nutritional Deficiencies. Westport, CT, AVI, 1976

92. Rostand SG: Vitamin B_{12} levels and nerve conduction velocities in patients undergoing maintenance hemodialysis. Am J Clin Nutr 29:691, 1976

93. Rothenberg SP, Kantha KR, Ficarra A: Autoantibodies to intrinsic factor: Their determination and clinical usefulness. J Lab Clin Med 77:476, 1971

94. Rubin CE et al: Biopsy studies on the pathogenesis of coeliac sprue. In Wolstenholme GEW, Cameron MP (eds): Intestinal Biopsy, p 67. Boston, Little, Brown & Co, 1962

95. Rule SAJ, Hooker M, Costello C et al: Serum vitamin B_{12} and transcobalamin levels in early HIV disease. Am J Hematol 47:167, 1994

96. Samson D, Halliday D, Chanarin I: Reversal of ineffective erythropoiesis in pernicious anaemia following vitamin B_{12} therapy. Br J Haematol 35:217, 1977

97. Sandström H, Wahlin A, Eriksson M et al: Intravascular hemolysis and increased prevalence of myeloma and monoclonal gammopathy in congenital dyserythropoietic anaemia type III. European J Haematol 52:42, 1994

98. Sandström H, Wahlin A, Eriksson M et al: Serum thymidine kinase in congenital dyserythropoietic anaemia type III. Br J Haematol 87:653, 1994

99. Sauberlich HF, Skala JH, Dowdy RP: Laboratory Tests for the Assessment of Nutritional Status. Cleveland, CRC Press, 1974

100. Saxena S, Weiner JM, Carmel R: Red blood cell distribution width in untreated pernicious anemia. Am J Clin Pathol 89:660, 1988

101. Schilling RF: Vitamin B_{12}: Assay and absorption testing. Lab Management 20:31, 1982

102. Schilling RF: Intrinsic factor studies. II. The effect of gastric juice on the urinary excretion of radioactivity after the oral administration of radioactive vitamin B_{12}. J Lab Clin Med 42:860, 1953

103. Shulman R: Psychiatric aspects of pernicious anaemia. A prospective controlled investigation. Br Med J 3:266, 1967

104. Smith LH: Hereditary orotic aciduria and pyrimidine auxotrophism in man. Am J Med 38:1, 1965

105. Stamos HF: Heredity in pernicious anemia. Am J Med Sci 200:586, 1940

106. Stasney J, Pizzolato P: Serial bone marrow studies in pernicious anemia. I. Fluctuation in number and volume of nucleated cells. Proc Soc Exp Biol Med 51:335, 1942

107. Sturgis CC: An analysis of the causes of death in 150 fatal cases of pernicious anemia observed since 1927. Trans Assoc Am Physicians 54:46, 1939

108. Sullivan LW, Luhby AL, Streiff RR: Studies of the daily requirement for folic acid in infants and the etiology of folate deficiency in goat's milk megaloblastic anemia. Am J Clin Nutr 18:311, 1966

109. teVelde K, Abels J, Anders GJPA et al: A family study of pernicious anemia by an immunologic method. J Lab Clin Med 64:177, 1964

110. Thompson WG, Cassino C, Babitz L et al: Hypersegmented neutrophils and vitamin B_{12} deficiency. Acta Haematol 81:186, 1989

111. Tietz NW, Blackburn RH (eds): Reference Ranges and General Information. Values used and partially established at the University of Kentucky Medical Center. Lexington, KY, Clinical Laboratories, AB Chandler Medical Center, University of Kentucky, July 1986

112. Tisman G, Herbert V: B_{12} dependence of cell uptake of serum folate: An explanation for high serum folate and cell folate depletion in B_{12} deficiency. Blood 41:465, 1973

113. Twomey JJ, Jordan PH, Jarrold T et al: The syndrome of immunoglobulin deficiency and pernicious anemia. A study of 10 cases. Am J Med 47:340, 1969

114. Ueland PM, Refsum H: Plasma homocysteine, a risk factor for vascular disease: Plasma levels in health, disease, and drug therapy. J Lab Clin Med 114(5):473, 1989

115. Ungar B: Antibody to gastric intrinsic factor in blood donors and hospital patients. Aust Ann Med 17:107, 1968

116. van der Scheer WM, Koek HC: Peripheral nerve lesions in cases of pernicious anaemia. Acta Psychiatr Neurol 13:61, 1938

117. Verwilghen RL: Congenital dyserythropoietic anaemia type II (HEMPAS). In Congenital Disorders of Erythropoiesis (Proceedings—Ciba Symposium), p 151. Amsterdam, Elsevier, 1976

118. Verwilghen RL, Lewis SM, Dacie JV et al: HEMPAS: Congenital dyserythropoietic anaemia (type II). Q J Med 42:257, 1973

119. Vu T, Amin J, Ramos M et al: New assay for the rapid determination of plasma holotranscobalamin II levels: Preliminary evaluation in cancer patients. Am J Hematol 42:202, 1993

120. Walt F, Holman S, Hendrickse RG: Megaloblastic anaemia of infancy in kwashiorkor and other diseases. Br Med J 1:1199, 1956

121. Waters AH, Mollin DL: Observations on the metabolism of folic acid in pernicious anaemia. Br J Haematol 9:319, 1963

122. Wickramasinghe SN, Pratt JR: Myelocyte proliferation in pernicious anaemia. Acta Haematol 44:37, 1970

123. Wilcken DEL, Gupta VJ, Betts AK: Homocysteine in the plasma of renal transplant recipients: Effects of cofactors for methionine metabolism. Clin Sci 61:743, 1981

124. Wolff JA, von Hofe FH: Familial erythroid multinuclearity. Blood 6:1274, 1951

125. Woodson RD: Robert F Schilling—A tribute. Am J Hematol 34:81, 1990

126. Zadek I: Pathogenesis of pernicious anemia: Result of postmortem examination of patients who died during remission. Klin Wochenschr 9:1527, 1929

CHAPTER 13

Anemias of Abnormal Iron Metabolism and Hemochromatosis

William Koss

Objectives

1. Explain the physiologic role of iron and the consequences of iron deficiency and iron overload.
2. List, define, and state the reference ranges for the tests used to evaluate and diagnose anemias with abnormal iron metabolism and the iron overload conditions.
3. Differentiate among iron-depleted and iron-deficient states and iron deficiency anemia based on laboratory tests.
4. Recognize the most common anemias that may present with erythrocyte microcytosis and state how they can be differentiated by laboratory tests.
5. Describe, define and state the significance of a ringed sideroblast.
6. List the hematology-related abnormalities associated with lead toxicity.
7. State the frequency of hereditary hemochromatosis and the laboratory tests useful in screening for this disorder.

Iron is essential to animal and vegetable life.[28] Therefore iron-deficient states and abnormalities related to inadequate iron utilization by cells cause a spectrum of clinical disorders of different severity. However, too much of a good thing is also harmful and excessive accumulations of iron in tissues are toxic. The severity of the damage is directly related to the amount of iron accumulated.

Iron is primarily used for the synthesis of normal, oxygen-carrying hemoglobin (Hb) (Chap. 7). Circumstances that cause reduction in the iron available for Hb synthesis or failure to incorporate iron into heme will cause anemia to develop, with the usual range of signs and symptoms related to a reduced oxygen-carrying capacity. Among the anemias of abnormal iron metabolism is iron deficiency anemia, the most common form of anemia in the United States[30] and worldwide.[27] Another form of anemia related to iron metabolism, the so-called anemia of chronic disease, is also common, probably second only to iron deficiency.[22] These two anemias, plus two other disorders of iron metabolism, sideroblastic anemia and anemia associated with lead intoxication, will be considered in this chapter. Disorders related to abnormal iron accumulation like hemochromatosis will also be discussed.

Synthesis of normally functioning Hb requires that developing erythrocytes have adequate supplies, including the polypeptide chains (*e.g.*, α, β), protoporphyrin IX rings, and iron (Chap. 7). In this chapter, anemias that occur secondary to low availability of the raw material iron will be presented. Three general etiologic mechanisms appear to be involved: (1) deficiency of the raw material (iron deficiency anemia); (2) defective recycling of the macrophage-stored iron (anemia of chronic disease); and (3) defective utilization of iron within the erythroblast (sideroblastic anemia, lead intoxication). These disorders, when typical, differ in their clinical presentations and laboratory features.

LABORATORY TESTS USEFUL IN DIFFERENTIATING DISORDERS OF IRON METABOLISM

Many tests have been used in the differential diagnosis of iron metabolism disorders. Ferritin, free erythrocyte protoporphyrin (FEP), serum iron, total iron binding capacity (TIBC), and percent transferrin saturation are tests used for the direct evaluation of iron status. Red cell morphology, red cell indices, and calculated parameters like the red cell distribution width (RDW) also play important roles. Most recently, measurement of the serum transferrin receptor has been popularized, but its true usefulness requires further evaluation.[4] Table 13-1 provides an overview of laboratory findings in iron deficiency anemia, several other disorders of iron metabolism, and in thalassemia (Chap. 15), which may be confused with iron deficiency because both may present as microcytic, hypochromic anemias. This table should be referred to throughout the chapter as each disorder is discussed.

The following is a brief summary of some laboratory tests used in the differential diagnosis of anemias of abnormal iron metabolism along with the reference ranges. Procedural details for these are beyond the scope of this text.

SERUM FERRITIN

Ferritin is a substance composed of iron bound to a protein called apoferritin. Ferritin is the main storage form of iron in the body.[57] The amount synthesized each day is that required to replace the catabolized ferritin as well as to accommodate any additional iron needed by cells. Serum ferritin differs from intracellular ferritin in some aspects. Serum ferritin has a very low iron content, therefore ferritin does not transport iron, and ferritin's concentration in serum is minimal as compared with the amount present in cells.[46,126]

Serum ferritin concentration reflects the iron stores in body tissues and thus is a good indicator of iron storage status. It is valuable in diagnosing iron deficiency because it is generally the first laboratory test to become abnormal when iron stores begin to decrease.[52] It also becomes abnormal before erythrocyte morphology shows any signs of abnormality. Note in Table 13-1 that, among the disorders listed, serum ferritin is decreased only in iron deficiency anemia. However, an increased serum ferritin level does not exclude the diagnosis of iron deficiency anemia because ferritin is an acute phase reactant,[49] and consequently it is elevated in plasma during the acute phase of an inflammatory process.[125] Recently, the measurement of erythrocyte ferritin has been advocated by some,[41] but its usefulness is unclear at this time.

Principle. Serum ferritin can be measured using radioimmunoassays (RIA), enzyme immunoassays and immunoradiometric assays.

Reference Range. The reference range varies with methodology, age and sex. In men, it is 20 to 250 $\mu g/L$ and in women, 10 to 120 $\mu g/L$.[120] Serum ferritin levels generally increase in women who have reached menopause. Each 1 $\mu g/L$ of ferritin represents approximately 8 mg of iron stored in tissue.[26] Children generally have low ferritin levels, except during the first month of life when reference ranges are 200 to 600 $\mu g/L$. From 1 to 6 months of age they are comparable with those of adult men.[120] Another very important clinical aspect of ferritin is that, in contrast to serum iron, serum ferritin levels do not have diurnal variation and are not influenced by exogenous iron ingestion.[41]

FREE ERYTHROCYTE PROTOPORPHYRIN

Protoporphyrin IX is the porphyrin compound to which ferrous iron is added to form heme needed for Hb synthesis (see Fig. 13-1). Normally, red cells produce slightly more protoporphyrin than is needed; however, when iron is deficient or cannot be properly coupled, protoporphyrin levels build up to several times the normal level as zinc protoporphyrin (ZPP).

Although FEP generally is a very sensitive and valuable early indicator of an iron metabolism disorder, it is not very specific and cannot be used in differentiating iron deficiency,

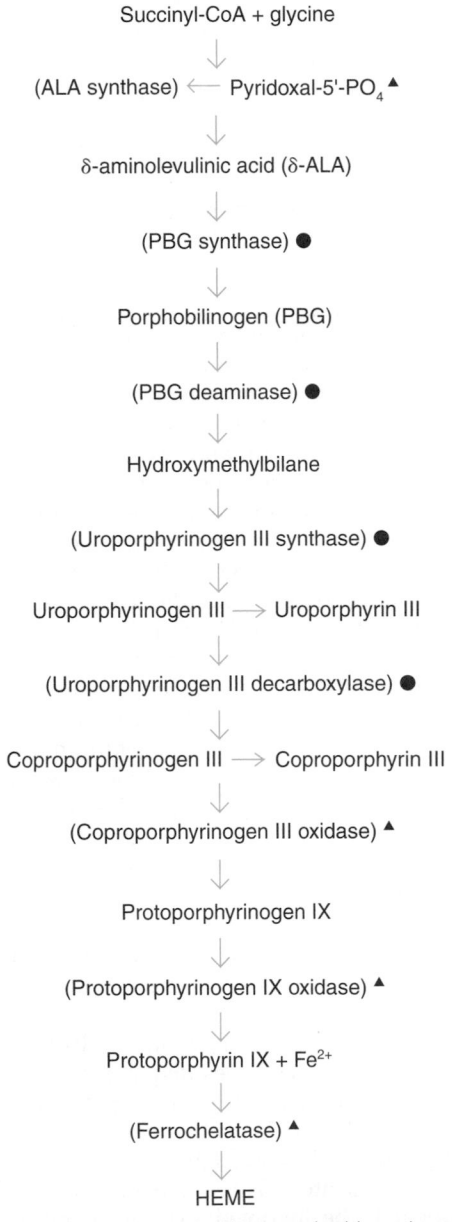

FIGURE 13-1. Heme synthesis. Enzymes in this pathway are denoted by parentheses. PBG synthase is also known as δ-amino levulinic acid dehydratase; ferrochelatase is also known as heme synthase. ▲ = mitochondrial enzyme reaction; ● = cytosolic enzyme reaction. (Modified from Gillen LAF: Hemoglobins, myoglobin, and porphyrins. In Bishop ML, Duben-Von Laufen JL, Fody EP [eds]: Clinical Chemistry—Principles, Procedures, Correlations. Philadelphia, JB Lippincott, 1985, with permission.)

TABLE 13-1
Laboratory Findings in Microcytic, Hypochromic Anemias and Diseases of Abnormal Iron Metabolism

Condition	Serum Ferritin	Transferrin Saturation	Total Iron Binding Capacity	Serum Iron	Free Erythrocyte Protoporphyrin	Marrow Iron	MCV	RDW
Iron deficiency anemia	↓	↓	↑	↓	↑	Absent	↓	↑
Thalassemia minor	N/↑*	N	N	N	N	↑/N	↓	N
Anemia of chronic disease	↑	N	N/↓	↓	↑	↑/N	↓/N	N/↑
Sideroblastic anemia	↑	↑	↓/N	↑	V	↑	V	↑
Lead poisoning	N	N/↑	N	N/↑ (A) N/↓ (C)	↑	V	↓/N	V
Hemochromatosis/Iron overload	↑	↑	N	↑	N	↑	V	V

MCV = mean corpuscular volume; RDW = red cell distribution width; N = normal; V = variable; ↑ = increased; ↓ = decreased; A = adult; C = children.

*When N and ↑ or ↓ appear together, the most frequent occurrence appears first.

Data from Henry JB: Clinical Diagnosis and Management by Laboratory Methods, 18th ed. Philadelphia, WB Saunders, 1991 and Noe DA, Rock RC: Laboratory Medicine: The Selection and Interpretation of Clinical Laboratory Studies. Baltimore, Williams and Wilkins, 1994.

anemia of chronic diseases, and sideroblastic anemias because it may be increased in all three entities (Table 13-1).[60] However, FEP is generally normal in thalassemia.[71,117] Therefore, FEP is helpful in differentiating thalassemia from iron deficiency anemia and the anemia of chronic disease.

There is disagreement about which laboratory test provides the earliest indicator of the onset of a decrease in iron stores. Some believe it is the ferritin level,[41,47] whereas others believe it is the FEP level.[72] However, an elevated FEP can be related to abnormal iron utilization, and consequently it is used clinically as a screening test rather than a confirmatory one.

Principle. Whole blood and free erythrocyte porphyrins may be measured by extraction methods.[103] A hematofluorometric method[93] measures only ZPP. ZPP and FEP measurements are not equivalent because extraction methods measure all porphyrins including those bound to zinc, but for practical purposes there is good correlation between both measurements.[103]

Reference Range. The reference range depends on the method used. Generally, the range for both FEP and ZPP is 17 to 77 μg/dL erythroctyes.[120] The reference range for ZPP may also be expressed as 30 to 70 μmol ZPP/mol of heme.[103]

SERUM IRON

Although the serum iron assay continues to be one of the primary tests used for the differential diagnosis of the common disorders of iron metabolism, it has poor sensitivity for the iron-deficient state. It is particularly helpful in situations where the diagnosis is not apparent from other laboratory tests (Table 13-1).

Principle. The iron measured is iron bound to serum transferrin and excludes iron bound to Hb. Serum ferric iron (Fe^{3+}) is first removed from transferrin by the addition of a chemical such as hydrochloric acid. All iron is then chemically transformed to the reduced ferrous (Fe^{2+}) state by the addition of a chromogenic reagent, such as acid-ferrozine, which results in the formation of a colored complex that can be measured spectrophotometrically. These assays are very sensitive, with an analytical detection level of one part per million.[41,100]

Specimen Requirements. A nonhemolyzed serum sample is required. As a rule, specimens with marked hemolysis should be rejected.[44] Atomic absorption spectrophotometry is most significantly affected by hemolysis. Use of anticoagulated samples may cause erroneous results because of iron chelation (*e.g.*, iron combining with EDTA).[100] Samples should be drawn in the morning, because serum iron levels show diurnal variation and may be approximately 25% lower in the evening.[14,44] The patient should have been fasting for 12 hours and should not have taken any iron-containing medication for 12 to 24 hours before the test.

Reference Range. The reference range is variable with age and sex and also varies slightly with the methodology, with a range of 60 to 175 μg/dL for men and 50 to 170 μg/dL for women.[120]

TOTAL IRON BINDING CAPACITY

The total iron binding capacity (TIBC) measures the amount of iron that the circulating transferrin could bind in a fully saturated state. Therefore, it is an indirect measure of transferrin concentration but expressed as an iron measurement.[41] It is clinically used in combination with an iron measurement to calculate saturation. Serum iron and TIBC are most useful in the evaluation of chronic iron overload as well as acute iron poisoning situations (Table 13-1).[44,100]

Principle. In the TIBC test, the concentration of transferrin is measured indirectly by the addition of ferric (Fe^{3+}) iron to the serum sample. All excess, unbound iron is chemically removed from the specimen, and the remaining sample is then analyzed for iron content using the serum iron method described above. In measuring this iron, the total capacity of transferrin to bind iron is determined.

Specimen Requirements. The requirements are the same as for serum iron determination. However, unlike serum iron, TIBC values are not dependent on the time of day the sample is drawn.

Reference Range. The TIBC reference range for adults is approximately 250 to 425 μg/dL.[120] Serum transferrin concentration may be calculated from the TIBC by using the following equation[44]:

$$\text{Serum transferrin (g/L)} = 0.007 \times \text{TIBC}$$

TRANSFERRIN SATURATION

Transferrin saturation may be calculated only if serum iron and TIBC values are available. It is usually used to diagnose iron deficiency, but with a poor specificity due to the fact that a low saturation may also be seen in the anemia of chronic disease. More importantly, high saturations may be indicative of iron overload (Table 13-1).

Principle. Transferrin saturation values are obtained through the following calculation based on measurements of serum iron and TIBC both in μg/dL:

$$\% \text{ Transferrin saturation} = \frac{\text{Serum iron}}{\text{TIBC}} \times 100$$

Reference Range. The reference range is 20% to 50% saturation in men and 15% to 50% saturation in women.[120]

RED CELL INDICES AND RED CELL DISTRIBUTION WIDTH

Classification of anemias on the basis of the mean corpuscular volume (MCV) and the amount of central pallor of the red cell continues to be popular. However, hypochromia and microcytosis are, in time, very late indicators of an iron-deficient status. Moreover, anemia may be documented in iron deficiency before microcytosis or hypochromia. It has also been reported that morphologic evaluation, even by experts, may not be as accurate and reproducible as expected.[40] Measurement of red cell distribution width (RDW) has been popularized by some investigators as more sensitive and amenable to separate the anemias, although its contribution remains controversial.[17,83,119] Refer to Chapters 9, 10 and 42 for further discussion of RDW.

SERUM TRANSFERRIN RECEPTOR

Maturing nucleated red cells have in their cell membranes an abundant number of transferrin receptors. This allows for the physiologic capture and cell utilization of the iron transported and delivered by transferrin. These receptors normally decrease by shedding from the cell as it matures. Because the number of shed receptors found in serum increases with iron deficiency and decreases with excess iron, assaying for serum transferrin receptor has been suggested to be the most specific and sensitive test for iron deficiency.[44] This assay has only recently been used and its value and role for diagnosis is not yet clear.[4,116]

IRON DEFICIENCY ANEMIA

Pathophysiology and Populations Affected

Iron deficiency may occur by any one or a combination of mechanisms (Table 13-2). The prevalence of iron deficiency varies widely in relation to age, socioeconomic status, the criteria used to establish the diagnosis, and the geographic location.

During infancy and childhood an adequate supply of iron is needed to increase the erythrocyte mass to adult levels. It is not uncommon to find iron deficiency among infants. During the first year of life alone, the total amount of Hb nearly doubles to meet the needs of a body that triples in weight.[105] In children, because of the high de-

TABLE 13-2
Mechanisms of Iron Deficiency

Increased physiologic demand
    Rapid growth: infants, children
    Pregnancy, lactation
Inadequate intake
    Iron-deficient diet
    Inadequate absorption (achlorhydria, decreased absorptive surface)
Blood loss
    Menstrual flow
    Gastrointestinal bleeding
    Hemorrhoids
    Regular blood donation
    Hemolysis

mand for iron, iron reserves are usually low and would be considered depleted by adult standards.[97] The combination of high physiologic demand and low reserves makes infants, in particular, susceptible to iron deficiency anemia. This situation is combined with the low natural availability of iron in the infant's primary source of nutrition, milk. Cow's milk and breast milk contain about 0.5 to 1.0 mg of iron per liter. However, about 50% of the iron in breast milk can be absorbed by an infant as compared with only 10% of the iron in cow's milk.[105] Neither of these, unsupplemented, is an adequate source of iron for a growing infant and recommendations for dietary supplements are available.[105]

Pregnancy presents a special physiologic need for additional nutrients, including iron. In women who eat a good diet and have good prenatal care, red cell mass and plasma volume expand, creating a relative dilutional effect with a decreased Hb value as compared with the nonpregnant state.[108] True anemia in pregnancy is most often the result of iron deficiency; folate is the second most common deficiency. Pregnancy causes an increased iron requirement related to the woman's increasing red cell mass, the fetal needs, and the bleeding that occurs during delivery. The requirement becomes higher as the pregnancy progresses, with a total consumption of about 680 mg of iron per pregnancy.[76] Iron supplementation is required at least during the last half of pregnancy.[76] In addition, iron loss during lactation is approximately the same as iron loss during menstruation.

Another important cause of iron deficiency anemia is an inadequate intake of iron, which may result from a diet low in iron or from the inability to absorb iron (Table 13-2). The normal American diet provides adequate iron for a man or a postmenopausal woman. However, the amount of available iron in the normal diet of a woman of childbearing age is marginal. A variety of factors, including food selection and cooking methods, affect dietary iron levels. For example, iron in the form of heme, from red meats, is more readily absorbed than is nonheme iron from vegetables and iron-enriched grain foods.[90] Food cooked in iron utensils contains more iron than food cooked in Teflon-coated, aluminum, or glass utensils. Even typically iron-rich vegetables, when grown in iron-depleted soil, contribute to iron deficiency.[109]

An additional factor contributing to iron deficiency is achlorhydria (reduced gastric acidity), which may cause inadequate absorption and thus reduced iron stores. Proper gastric acidity is required for the reduction of the ingested Fe^{3+} in vegetables and grains to Fe^{2+}, the absorbable form. Patients who undergo gastric resection have an increased risk of iron deficiency. In addition, malabsorptive syndromes that reduce the available intestinal absorptive surface may cause iron deficiency.

A very important cause of iron deficiency is blood loss (Table 13-2). Iron deficiency anemia is prevalent in women ages 18 to 44 years,[30] presumably because of menstrual loss, which is the largest single contributor to iron deficiency anemia.[80] Iron is tightly conserved by the body in reticuloendothelial (RE) cell stores, and diet is intended to replace the physiologic losses.[45] Thus, when iron deficiency anemia occurs in a man or a postmenopausal woman, it is usually the result of some form of chronic blood loss, most frequently gastrointestinal bleeding. Among possible causes are peptic ulcer disease, neoplastic disease anywhere in the gastrointestinal tract (especially the colon), and hemorrhoids.[9,10] Therefore, establishing the diagnosis of iron deficiency anemia is not as important as identifying the cause of it.

Another important cause of chronic iron loss is regular blood donation, which may cause iron deficiency in the otherwise healthy individual.[115]

Chronic intravascular hemolytic disease causes excess iron loss in the urine in the form of hemoglobinuria.[58] An example is the rare disorder paroxysmal nocturnal hemoglobinuria (PNH; Chap. 18). Also, endurance training may affect iron metabolism and create an iron-deficient state.[25]

The development of iron deficiency anemia is gradual (Table 13-3). An individual with adequate iron stores, as tissue ferritin, is said to be *iron replete.* As the demand for iron increases, for whatever reason, or as iron is lost, the stored iron will be utilized first. In this stage, an individual is said to have depleted iron stores. If conditions continue to produce an increased demand for or loss of iron, deficiency eventually will occur, which may be finally manifested as iron deficiency anemia.[16,62,99] The individual may not exhibit signs or symptoms of iron deficiency until the appearance of frank anemia.

Clinical Presentation and Physical Findings

The presentation of patients with iron deficiency anemia is similar to that of most other forms of anemia and is primarily related to the cause of the anemia as well as the Hb level at the time the patient seeks medical care. Symptoms may include fatigue, breathlessness, and dizziness.[9] These symptoms are related to reduced oxygen delivery to the tissues and so are common to any anemia, regardless of cause. After the appearance of frank anemia, anemia progresses from mild to moderate, and even to severe, before the patient may present to a physician. This is because of the gradual onset that permits compensatory mechanisms to minimize the symptoms until the anemia becomes severe (Chap. 10).[10,109]

TABLE 13-3
Sequential Changes in Development of Iron Deficiency and Iron Overload

Iron Status	Iron Replete (Normal)	Stage 1 (Iron Depleted)	Stage 2 (Iron Deficient Erythropoiesis)	Stage 3 (Iron Deficiency Anemia)	Iron Overload
Serum ferritin (μg/L)	>12	Early: <12	<12	<12	>300
Marrow iron	2–3+	0–1+	0	0	4+
TIBC (μg/dL)	300–360	360	390	410	<300
Serum iron (μg/dL)	65–165	115	Intermediate: <60	<40	>175
Transferrin saturation (%)	20–50	30	<15	<10	>60
Free erythrocyte protoporphyrin (μg/dL)	<50	<50	100	200	<50
Marrow sideroblasts (%)	40–60	40–60	<10	<10	40–60
Hemoglobin	Normal	Normal	Normal	Late: ↓↓↓	Variable
MCV	Normal	Normal	Normal	↓↓↓	Variable
RDW	Normal	Normal	Normal	↑↑↑	Variable
RBC morphology	Normal	Normal	Normal	Microcytic hypochromic	Variable

Adapted from Hillman RS, Finch CA: Red Cell Manual, 5th ed, p 60. Philadelphia, FA Davis, 1985, with permission; and iron overload data from Herbert V: Iron disorders can mimic anything, so always test for them. Blood Rev 3:125, 1992.

Because chronic blood loss is a significant cause of iron deficiency, some patients present with signs and symptoms related to their primary underlying disease.[9,10,62] For example, a man may complain of epigastric pain related to ulcers or a woman may note menorrhagia.

Another frequent clinical finding is pica. Pica is a persistent, compulsive desire to ingest certain food or nonfood substances. Various substances like ice, clay, plaster, or even insects may be craved.[112]

A variety of epithelial changes are common in iron deficiency anemia, particularly disturbances related to the gastrointestinal system, such as angular stomatitis (cracks in the corners of the mouth), tongue abnormalities like soreness and papillary atrophy, and gastritis.[9,10] In some cases, the gastritis progresses to gastric atrophy, which results in achlorhydria. Another interesting epithelial change sometimes encountered is koilonychia, a flattening and spooning of the nails (Fig. 13-2). This appears to be much more common in adults, although it does occur in some iron-deficient infants.[65] Neurologic changes such as those seen in vitamin B_{12} deficiency (Chap. 12) are not found in iron deficiency anemia.

Laboratory Findings and Correlations with Disease

Hematology. The complete blood cell count (CBC) reflects a decreased Hb and hematocrit (Hct) in the late stages of iron deficiency (Table 13-3). The Hb may be markedly decreased (8 g/dL or lower) before the patient complains of anemia-related symptoms.[76] Severe iron deficiency anemia is characterized by a reduced mean corpuscular volume (MCV), mean corpuscular hemoglobin (MCH), and mean corpuscular hemoglobin concentration (MCHC). In one study of 115 patients, all RBC indices were decreased: the average MCV was 75 fL (with a range of 59–80 fL); MCH was 21 pg (range, 15–26 pg); and MCHC was 28 g/dL (range, 22–31 g/dL).[3] On the blood film, erythrocytes appear microcytic and hypochromic (Fig. 13-3). In severe iron deficiency, only the outer rims of the cells are visible, resembling a bagel with little dough. A moderate anisocytosis may be seen and may be reflected by an elevated

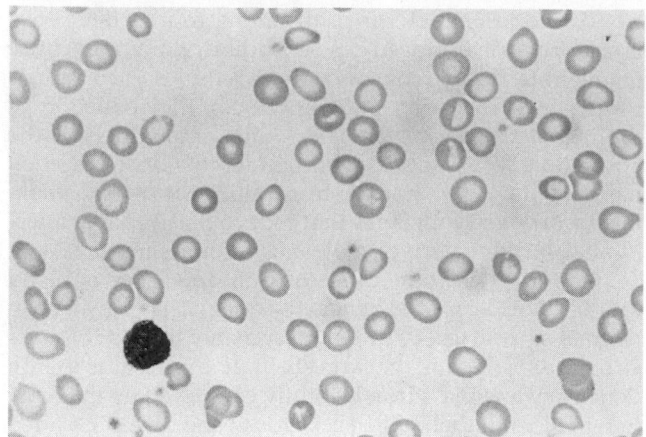

FIGURE 13-3. Anisocytosis with a predominant microcytic, hypochromic erythrocyte population in a case of marked iron deficiency.

RDW. The increasing RDW may be an indicator of impending or overt iron deficiency and may also be useful in the differential diagnosis with thalassemia minor, in which the RDW is either normal or only slightly increased.[94,105] A variety of abnormal erythrocyte shapes (poikilocytes) are also observed on the blood film.[15,76]

Platelet counts are variable. Often, however, the platelet count is increased up to twice the upper limit of the reference range.[114] In such cases, the etiology of the anemia may be related to chronic hemorrhage.[31] Increased platelet counts may also occur in infants.[53] Leukocyte counts usually are within the reference range and are therefore not of particular diagnostic value.[15] The reticulocyte production index (RPI) gradually falls below 2.0 as iron deficiency progresses, because the bone marrow cannot increase erythropoiesis to compensate for the anemia without adequate iron being available.

Bone Marrow. Study of the marrow is rarely necessary to make the diagnosis and is probably the most costly test if performed just for the evaluation of iron status.[41] When it is performed, the sample is stained for Prussian

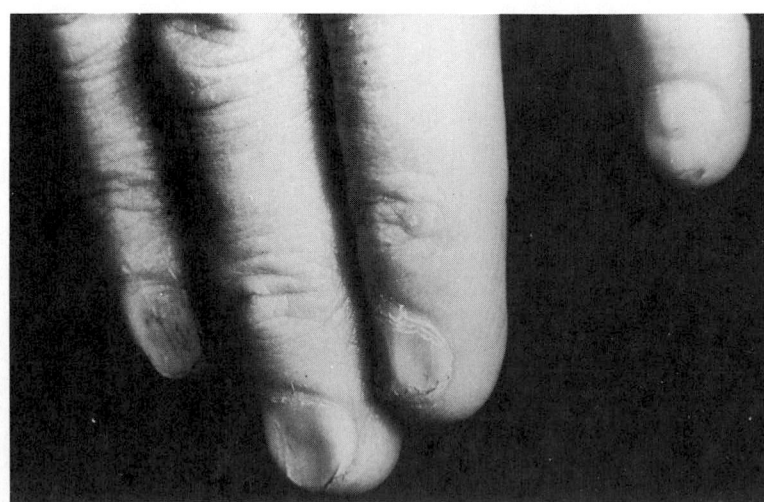

FIGURE 13-2. Koilonychia, the flattened, spooned nails seen in some cases of chronic iron deficiency. (From Hoffbrand AV, Pettit JE: Essential Haematology, 2nd ed, p 33. Oxford, England, Blackwell Scientific Publications Ltd, 1984, duplication with permission.)

blue reactivity to estimate iron stores (Chap. 29). Iron content may be evaluated following different grading scales and the evaluation should be performed from the aspirated material as opposed to the marrow biopsy.[41] Iron stores are severely decreased in the first stage of iron deficiency development (Table 13-3). This simply confirms the deficit of stored iron indicated by the decreased serum ferritin level. Of importance are the marrow sideroblasts (iron-containing nucleated red blood cells [NRBCs]), which are decreased in the second stage of anemia development. Also in established iron deficiency anemia there is usually erythroblastic hyperplasia (an increase in the number of NRBCs).

Chemistry. Chemical analysis of iron status is important to identify the various stages of iron deficiency. Of particular importance are the serum ferritin level and FEP.[32,93] As noted earlier, there is disagreement on whether the serum ferritin or the FEP measurement is the first to indicate the early stages of iron depletion. Ferritin is most commonly used in the diagnosis of iron deficiency. Ferritin and FEP levels become abnormal in the early to intermediate stages (Table 13-3) and much before red cell morphology or Hb levels show any sign of abnormality. However, FEP levels are less often utilized than ferritin and are available most often through reference laboratories.[11,54,92]

Other useful tests of iron status are serum iron, TIBC, and percent transferrin saturation. All of these measurements become abnormal at about the same time as the FEP, although some reports claim that FEP does not increase until 2 to 3 weeks after the decrease in percent transferrin saturation.[47] As iron loss progresses, transferrin saturation and serum iron decrease, whereas the TIBC increases because of the lack of iron available for transport.

Ferritin behaves as an acute-phase reactant and will therefore be elevated during any inflammatory response. When iron deficiency and inflammation are concurrent, ferritin may be elevated, masking the iron deficiency.[87] Therefore, if inflammation is present when iron deficiency is suspected, other measures of iron status must be considered before the diagnosis can be made or excluded.[125]

Differential Diagnosis

Several anemias fall into the category of those with microcytic, hypochromic erythrocytes. Table 13-1 indicates how these anemias may be distinguished. Laboratory tests, although useful, cannot replace the individual patient encounter. Therefore, the number of tests required to establish the diagnosis depends on the particular situation. Appropriate diagnosis is important, because the approach to the disease and the treatment for it varies.

Effects of Treatment on Laboratory Results and Prognosis

Iron deficiency anemia is treated by pinpointing the cause and by giving iron supplements as required. Iron therapy should produce an increase in the reticulocyte count and

RPI (>3) within a few days, reaching a maximum at 7 to 12 days. Hb values increase until the patient's normal level is achieved, usually within 2 months. A dimorphic population of red cells becomes evident as new iron-normal erythrocytes increase in number while the iron-deficient erythrocytes disappear. Both the monitoring of MCV and RDW and the evaluation of the red cell histograms generated by most modern automated cell counters are useful in documenting effective response and patient compliance with medication. Patients should continue iron therapy after hemoglobin levels normalize to reestablish adequate iron stores, which are reflected in normalization of the laboratory indicators of iron status.[10]

If iron therapy does not produce the expected results, patient compliance with the prescribed medication should be ensured, and if confirmed, the diagnosis of iron deficiency should be reevaluated. Continued iron therapy in the absence of iron deficiency can produce iron overload and delay appropriate therapy.

ANEMIA OF CHRONIC DISEASE

Pathophysiology and Populations Affected

Anemia of chronic disease (ACD) is found in association with chronic infections, inflammatory disorders, or malignant diseases. By definition, the anemia is not due to bleeding, hemolysis or marrow replacement by tumor.[21,96] ACD is characterized by decreased iron in the blood in the presence of adequate iron stores. This mild to moderate anemia is common, second only to iron deficiency as a cause of anemia, and in hospital populations, it may be the most common form.[22] Some of the primary disorders producing this form of anemia are listed in Table 13-4. Some investigators take exception to the ACD designation because this anemia may be seen in situations that are not altogether chronic, or as a counterpart, there are several

TABLE 13-4
Causes of Anemia of Chronic Disease

CHRONIC INFLAMMATORY DISEASES

Infectious
    Tuberculosis
    Pulmonary infections, pneumonia
    Pelvic inflammatory disease
    Chronic fungal disease
    Subacute bacterial endocarditis
    Osteomyelitis
    Meningitis
Noninfectious
    Rheumatoid arthritis
    Thermal injury
    Systemic lupus erythematosus

MALIGNANT DISEASES

Carcinoma

Hodgkin disease

Non-Hodgkin lymphoma

Leukemia

Multiple myeloma

chronic conditions in which there is no accompanying anemia.[113]

Several mechanisms may be involved in the pathogenesis of this anemia, which is characterized by the inhibition of iron use despite normal or increased iron stores. Cartwright[21] postulated that at least three possible pathologic processes were responsible for causing the anemia: shortened erythrocyte survival,[19,20] trapping or impaired release of iron from macrophages in the reticuloendothelial system,[78] and impaired bone marrow response to anemia. Later, relative erythropoietin (EPO) deficiency and impaired responsiveness of the bone marrow to EPO were added to the list.[22]

Shortened erythrocyte survival[19] may have several causes,[20] for example, enhanced phagocytic activity of macrophages.[78] The impaired release of iron from storage in macrophages may be related to activated macrophages or monocytes that release cytokines like interleukin-1 (IL-1).[77,96] One effect of IL-1 is stimulation of synthesis of apoferritin (the substance with which iron binds to form ferritin) within macrophages. If apoferritin levels are increased, iron attaching to the apoferritin might be effectively trapped within the macrophages,[69,73] thus reducing the amount of iron circulating to marrow NRBCs. This is reflected in low serum iron and a reduced number of marrow sideroblasts in the presence of adequate to increased storage iron.

Impaired bone marrow response to anemia and defective production or response to EPO are believed to be the primary mechanisms causing ACD.[96] Several cytokines may cause the impaired marrow response to anemia. For example, macrophage-derived tumor necrosis factor-α (TNF-α), when injected into animals, causes anemia that is associated with low serum iron and normal iron stores. The defective production of EPO in some individuals with ACD may be related to cytokines as well.[96]

Clinical Presentation and Physical Findings

By definition, the individual with ACD has some primary infection, inflammation, or malignancy, and the presenting symptoms and physical findings usually are those of the primary disorder. These are quite varied and beyond the scope of this text. Occasionally the primary complaints will be related to the patient's anemia.[39]

Laboratory Findings and Correlations with Disease

Hematology. The anemia is usually mild to moderate, with the Hb perhaps 1 to 2 g/dL below the patient's normal baseline.[21] The anemia is normocytic and normochromic, although there are rare cases showing hypochromia. Microcytosis, which may be seen in about 30% of cases, is not usually as marked as in severe iron deficiency anemia.[20,78] However, mild iron deficiency anemia and anemia of chronic disease may be indistinguishable morphologically. A moderate degree of anisocytosis may occur, but poikilocytosis is minimal unless there are associated factors causing it.[78]

The reticulocyte count may be normal.[39] However, the RPI may be less than 2.0, reflecting the hypoproliferative nature of this anemia (Chap. 10). The leukocyte count and differential and the platelet count vary, depending on the underlying disease.

Bone Marrow. Marrow samples stained with Prussian blue confirm the presence of stored iron in macrophages. The stored iron may commonly be increased. Sideroblasts are relatively few in number, despite ample iron in macrophages.[3] The bone marrow does not show the erythroid hyperplasia expected as a compensatory mechanism in anemia[39]; thus, the categorization of ACD as a hypoproliferative anemia.

Chemistry. Iron studies are particularly useful. Serum iron levels are low, similar to those found in iron deficiency anemia. The TIBC is low in ACD, whereas it is elevated in iron deficiency. The combination of low iron and low TIBC in some cases produces a reduced transferrin saturation. Serum ferritin levels are elevated, in contrast to the low levels in typical iron deficiency.[85] The increased ferritin levels reflect the normal to increased storage iron found in ACD (Table 13-1), but it is also important to remember that ferritin increases in response to an inflammatory process. Free erythrocyte protoporphyrin is also elevated.[60] EPO levels may be either decreased or normal in ACD.[34]

Effects of Treatment on Laboratory Results

Treatment is directed at the primary disease. Iron therapy is avoided because the patient has adequate tissue iron stores, and exogenous iron could cause overload, unless there is an accompanying iron deficiency anemia.[21] Unlike iron deficiency anemia, some of the ACDs may be responsive to EPO treatment, but its use is usually reserved for symptomatic, severely anemic cases. With successful treatment, the laboratory indicators of anemia and abnormal iron metabolism should gradually return to normal, but the time required for this to occur and the degree of improvement depend on the primary disease being treated.

SIDEROBLASTIC ANEMIAS

The sideroblastic anemias are a diverse group of disorders that have the common feature of defective iron utilization in the production of heme for Hb. They are identified by the production of abnormal nucleated red blood cells (NRBCs). These NRBCs have abnormal iron content and pattern distribution. Siderocytes are red cells containing iron granules not yet incorporated into Hb (see Color Plate 13-1), and sideroblasts are NRBCs containing these iron granules. In sideroblastic anemias there is an excessive accumulation of iron in the mitochondria of NRBCs due to the inability to successfully form heme, and consequently Hb. The iron-laden mitochondria often form a ring around the nucleus resulting in the pathognomonic ringed sideroblast (see Color Plate 13-2), which is readily identifiable by examination of a bone marrow aspirate stained with Prussian blue (Chap. 29).

Sideroblasts are separated into three types, sometimes referred to as Types I, II, and III, with Type III being the pathologic ringed sideroblast.[121] The iron in the Type I sideroblast is in the form of ferritin aggregates, and as many as four aggregates can be identified in approximately 50% of the NRBCs in a healthy individual. In some situations when iron is not used effectively for red cell production, the number of ferritin aggregates increases to more than six per cell, creating the Type II sideroblast.[59] In both instances, this ferritin iron is randomly distributed in the cytoplasm and stains weakly with Prussian blue. The Type III pathologic ringed sideroblast of sideroblastic anemia shows larger iron granules, which are deposited within mitochondria and are situated in a ring or collar around the nucleus of the NRBC. For a diagnosis of sideroblastic anemia, at least 15% of the NRBCs must be Type III ringed sideroblasts, according to some investigators.[6,50]

Sideroblastic anemias have the common feature of ringed sideroblasts in the bone marrow, but they differ in regard to etiology and clinical presentation. They are typically classified as hereditary or acquired (Table 13-5). The hereditary form appears to be a group of disorders. The acquired form can be further subdivided into an idiopathic type, which is not reversible, and a reversible type. The idiopathic type includes a form of stem cell disorder associated with myelodysplasias (Chap. 33). The reversible type is associated with many underlying conditions.

Hereditary Sideroblastic Anemia

GENETICS AND PATHOPHYSIOLOGY

This form is relatively uncommon and genetically heterogeneous. The most frequent variety, which affects only men, has an X-linked pattern of inheritance. However, minimal expression of the disorder in carrier females has been observed.[67,74] Autosomal inheritance has been described.[1,18] Also, rare congenital cases with presentation at birth or soon thereafter have been described.[33]

Although the precise nature of the metabolic abnormality remains unclear, defective heme synthesis is likely.

TABLE 13-5
Classification of Sideroblastic Anemias

HEREDITARY

X-linked

Autosomal

ACQUIRED

Idiopathic Acquired Sideroblastic Anemia (IASA)
    Associated with myelodysplastic (dysmyelopoietic)
      syndromes

Reversible
    Alcoholism
    Drugs (isoniazid, chloramphenicol)
    Copper deficiency
    Lead poisoning

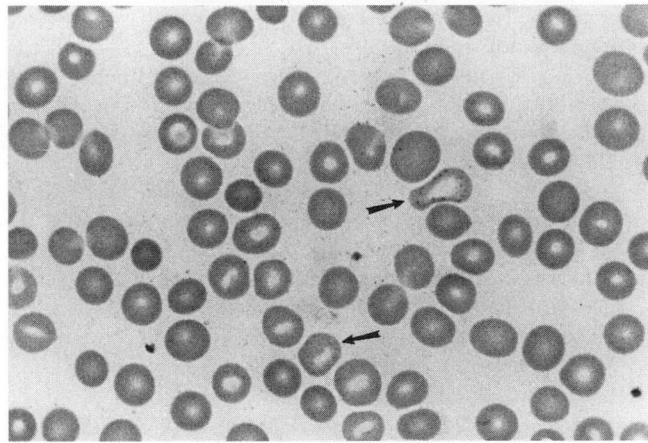

FIGURE 13-4. Dimorphic erythrocyte population, both macrocytic and microcytic, in a case of acquired sideroblastic anemia. Basophilic stippling is seen in several erythrocytes (*arrows*).

Most patients with hereditary sideroblastic anemia have decreased activity of δ-aminolevulinic acid synthase (ALA-S),[74] a mitochondrial enzyme that requires pyridoxal-5'-phosphate, a metabolically active form of vitamin B_6, as a coenzyme (Fig. 13-1). A low level of ALA-S has no diagnostic specificity because it may be observed in other situations.[43]

CLINICAL PRESENTATION AND PHYSICAL FINDINGS

Hereditary forms are, for the most part, manifested early in life. Mild forms may be uncovered late in life.[13,88]

At presentation, patients with hereditary sideroblastic anemia display the usual signs and symptoms of anemia. Patients may also have manifestations of iron overload, including mild to moderate splenomegaly and hepatomegaly, although liver function remains near normal. Late in the disease, cardiac arrhythmias may occur secondary to accumulating iron deposits in myocardial cells.[13]

LABORATORY FINDINGS AND CORRELATIONS WITH DISEASE

Hematology. The anemia is severe, with Hb as low as 6.0 g/dL on the average. Red cell morphology reveals a microcytic, hypochromic picture with anisocytosis, poikilocytosis, target cells, and heavy basophilic stippling. Pappenheimer bodies (iron seen as small irregular, darkstaining granules in red cells when stained with Wright stain) are also seen (Fig. 8-23). A dimorphic population of erythrocytes is common in sideroblastic anemias, including microcytic, hypochromic cells and normocytic, normochromic cells (Fig. 13-4).[67] The leukocyte and platelet counts are usually normal.[13]

Bone Marrow. Examination of the marrow is remarkable because of erythroid hyperplasia with excessive iron stored in macrophages. As many as 40% of the erythroblasts are of the pathologic ringed sideroblast type (see Color Plate 13-2) with rings in the polychromatophilic or orthochromic stage of NRBC maturation.[56] Megaloblastic changes are sometimes observed (Chap. 12).[67]

Chemistry. Iron studies reflect the iron loading in these patients who are unable to use it effectively (see Table 13-1). Ferritin levels are high, consistent with the large amounts of stored iron. In addition, serum iron is high, as is transferrin saturation. The TIBC is generally normal or decreased.

Because the enzymatic defect of hereditary sideroblastic anemia actually affects the production of the Hb porphyrin ring structure, FEP levels may be low or normal. In some circumstances, the dimorphic cell population is also dimorphic with respect to the FEP level; it is within the reference range in normal cells and low in the microcytic, hypochromic cells.[79]

EFFECTS OF TREATMENT ON LABORATORY RESULTS AND PROGNOSIS

About 30% of patients with hereditary sideroblastic anemia respond variably to pyridoxine (a form of vitamin B$_6$) administration. In some patients a remarkable response is observed with reticulocytosis and increasing Hb levels, while serum iron levels decline and FEP levels normalize. Unfortunately, more often than not pyridoxine therapy produces a less than optimal response, with only slight improvement in the Hb level, and in some instances, pyridoxine produces no improvement.[13,67] In individuals whose bone marrow demonstrates megaloblastic changes, folic acid can be added to the treatment regimen.

Some consideration may also be given to the removal of accumulated iron. Although this measure may not improve the patient's hematologic picture, the risk of problems related to iron overload (hemochromatosis) is reduced.[67]

The prognosis is variable and is to some degree dependent on the patient's response to pyridoxine therapy. Some live comfortably for many years.[67] Those who do not respond usually succumb to problems related to iron overload, such as cardiac arrhythmias and hepatic disease.[13]

Idiopathic Acquired Sideroblastic Anemia

PATHOPHYSIOLOGY AND POPULATIONS AFFECTED

The idiopathic type of acquired sideroblastic anemias is a clonal disorder with an abnormal, proliferating erythroid cell line. It most frequently occurs in the adult and elderly population, but occasionally occurs in young adults and children. It may be referred to by a variety of names including refractory anemia with ringed sideroblasts (RARS) and idiopathic acquired sideroblastic anemia (IASA).[50,121] The anemia affects both sexes and is included among the myelodysplastic (dysmyelopoietic) syndromes (Chap. 33) as the anemia may be the result of the clonal growth of a mutated erythroid or hematopoietic precursor cell.[82,86]

Although the mechanism producing IASA is not clear, decreased activity of ALA-S has been found consistently in a number of patients.[74,106] The enzymatic defect appears to be either an increased rate of degradation of ALA-S[2] or an abnormally high requirement for the cofactor pyridoxal-5'-phosphate to maintain active ALA-S.[74] In a few individuals with IASA, low levels of heme synthase (ferrochelatase) have been documented.[12,106] Various chromosomal changes have been identified in 40 to 60% of the patients[102,106]; the most frequently affected chromosomes are 5, 7, 8, 20, and Y. Leukemic transformation, common in the myelodysplastic disorders, occurs in as many as 25% of individuals with IASA.[81,86]

CLINICAL PRESENTATION AND PHYSICAL FINDINGS

The disorder may present with mild symptoms, or most frequently it may be detected as part of a routine examination. The symptoms are the usual ones for anemia.[13,82]

LABORATORY FINDINGS AND CORRELATIONS WITH DISEASE

Hematology. IASA is usually a moderate anemia with Hb in the range of 7 to 10 g/dL.[13] The anemia is normocytic or slightly macrocytic, and a variable number of cells are hypochromic. Dimorphism is evident in these patients, as in the hereditary form of the disease (see Fig. 13-4), although the population of hypochromic cells may be small. Anisocytosis may be marked, as may poikilocytosis, with the presence of some red cell fragments, target cells and occasional basophilic stippling. Pappenheimer bodies, although they may be seen, are inconspicuous as compared with hereditary sideroblastic anemia.

Leukocyte and platelet counts are usually normal, although they may be slightly decreased and part of a pancytopenic picture. Leukocytosis and thrombocytosis as well as morphologic changes in granulocytes that resemble the Pelger-Huët anomaly may also be seen (Chap. 26). In general, granulopoiesis and megakaryocytopoiesis should show minimal if any quantitative or qualitative changes.

Bone Marrow. In contrast to hereditary sideroblastic anemia, ringed sideroblasts are seen at all stages of erythroid maturation and they are usually abundant in number. Some investigators require that 15% or more of all NRBCs must be ringed sideroblasts for a diagnosis of IASA. The stainable iron in macrophages is usually increased.[56] There is usually significant erythroid hyperplasia with a myeloid to erythroid (M:E) ratio approaching at least 1:1, whereas the reference value for normal adults is approximately 2:1 to 4:1. The bone marrow may resemble the erythroleukemic marrow. Megaloblastic changes can also be observed in the marrow.

Chemistry. Iron studies show evidence of iron overload with high transferrin saturation levels which exceed 90% in some patients.[75] Ferritin and serum iron are also increased. FEP is usually moderately increased.

EFFECTS OF TREATMENT ON LABORATORY RESULTS AND PROGNOSIS

Patients are usually followed without treatment if the anemia is mild and asymptomatic. A therapeutic trial of pyridoxine may be attempted, but patients usually do not respond or they respond poorly. Transfusions may be required to support the symptomatic patient, but these should be kept to a minimum to avoid increasing the iron overload. Some of the morphologic features seen in the bone marrow, including more than 30% ringed sideroblasts in association with abnormal granulopoiesis and megakaryocytopoiesis, may be indicative of an accelerated poor prognosis.[50,59]

Acquired Reversible Sideroblastic Anemia

PATHOPHYSIOLOGY AND POPULATIONS AFFECTED

Reversible sideroblastic anemias may be caused by several agents, but they are most commonly associated with drugs. Alcohol-induced sideroblastic anemia is common, but is only one of the erythroid-related abnormalities seen in association with alcoholism.[107,118] The antibiotic chloramphenicol, which is frequently used throughout the world but rarely used in the United States today, and the frequently used antituberculosis drug isoniazid are both associated with sideroblastic anemia. Sideroblastic anemia may also be seen in copper deficiency.[51,74,122] Lead toxicity produces a unique form of sideroblastic anemia discussed later in this chapter.

The mechanisms for the production of reversible sideroblastic anemias for the most part affect heme synthesis. Some variation in the mechanisms occurs, although most drugs and toxins appear to interfere with the activity of either ALA-S or heme synthase or both (Fig. 13-1). Isoniazid, cycloserine, and pyrazinamide (all drugs used in the treatment of tuberculosis) reportedly inhibit reactions requiring pyridoxal-5'-phosphate as a coenzyme,[66] apparently by interfering with the conversion of vitamin B_6 to its active coenzyme form. This, in turn, reduces ALA-S activity and could produce sideroblastic anemia with characteristics similar to those in the hereditary form. Chloramphenicol, another antimicrobial drug, appears to inhibit mitochondrial protein synthesis in general, producing decreases in available ALA-S[110] and heme synthase,[91,95] as well as other mitochondrial enzymes.[48]

Acute ethanol ingestion reduces the activity of several enzymes in the heme synthesis pathway including PBG synthase,[68] uroporphyrinogen decarboxylase, coproporphyrinogen oxidase, and heme synthase (Fig. 13-1).[95] An important alcohol effect may be the one that results from disrupting mitochondrial function. The effects of ethanol on heme synthesis produce sideroblastic anemia in about 30% of hospitalized alcoholics.[64]

CLINICAL PRESENTATION AND PHYSICAL FINDINGS

Presentation is directly related to the agent causing the anemia or the clinical setting associated with the disorder. The signs and symptoms of anemia are usually related to its severity and the time elapsed before the correct diagnosis is made.

LABORATORY FINDINGS AND CORRELATIONS WITH DISEASE

Hematology. The anemia is moderate to severe, with Hb ranging from 6 to 10 g/dL in alcoholics.[64] The blood film characteristics are similar to those in hereditary sideroblastic anemias. The MCV is normal or slightly increased in the alcoholic,[38] and the red cell population is usually dimorphic.[64]

Bone Marrow. The definitive feature of reversible sideroblastic anemias, as with the other sideroblastic anemias, is the characteristic finding of ringed sideroblasts in the bone marrow. In the alcoholic patient the bone marrow may also show megaloblastic changes and vacuoles in the erythrocyte precursors.[64,84]

Chemistry. Nutritional folic acid deficiency is well documented in alcoholics and is responsible for the megaloblastic changes that accompany the sideroblastic changes in these patients. Storage of iron in the marrow is increased. Iron studies reflect the iron overload in the patient (Table 13-1). Transferrin saturation is increased, averaging about 65%.[38] Bilirubin and serum lactate dehydrogenase (LD) may be elevated secondary to ineffective hematopoiesis, which results in hemolysis of NRBCs in the bone marrow.

EFFECTS OF TREATMENT ON LABORATORY RESULTS AND PROGNOSIS

Removal of the offending agent is the principal means of treatment.[122] The administration of pyridoxine and folic acid along with good nutrition aids in reversal of the disorder. In cases in which continued drug therapy is required, supplementary pyridoxine may be helpful, but complete remission will not occur until the offending drug is removed.[55] Disappearance of ringed sideroblasts is usually seen within 2 weeks after the discontinuation of alcohol ingestion.[13]

LEAD INTOXICATION

Pathophysiology and Populations Affected

Lead intoxication occurs in both children and adults. It has long been recognized as a health hazard, and in spite of its being a potentially preventable disorder, it is still a public health problem world wide. Adults acquire lead poisoning most frequently by occupational exposure, while in contrast, children acquire it from ingestion of materials containing lead such as paint chips. The use of improperly glazed pottery for cooking or eating should be considered a source of lead toxicity.[70] Lead is used widely in the electric storage battery, petroleum and paint industries. The ban of lead use in gasoline in the United States has successfully decreased the potential for environmental and occupational exposure to lead in this country.[111]

Three major tissues are affected by lead: the renal, hematopoietic, and central nervous (CNS) systems. The effects on erythropoiesis will be emphasized in this discussion. Lead decreases the activity of several enzymes in the heme synthesis pathway.[12,104] PBG synthase, which converts δ-ALA to PBG, is the first enzyme in the sequence to be affected by lead (see Fig. 13-1). Another enzyme in the pathway profoundly affected by lead is heme synthase (ferrochelatase). As a consequence of the effects on these two enzymes, δ-ALA levels are increased, and PBG levels are normal.[23] This may be useful in distinguishing lead toxicity from acute intermittent porphyria, in which both δ-ALA and PBG are elevated.[13] Similarly, coproporphyrinogen oxidase appears to be inhibited by lead, but to a lesser degree as compared with the previous two enzymes.[13,23]

Lead also appears to have effects on the red cell membrane, possibly by affecting ATPase, thereby interfering with cation exchange. This and some other abnormalities may be conducive to a hemolytic component to the anemia seen with lead toxicity.[8] Synthesis of α- and β-globin chains may be defective in lead poisoning as well.[123]

Clinical Presentation and Physical Findings

Lead toxicity may present with an acute or chronic clinical picture. Damage to kidney and hematopoietic tissues is usually reversible, but CNS damage may sometimes be permanent. In a study of 50 cases of lead poisoning,[29] the most common symptoms were abdominal pain, constipation, vomiting, pain other than abdominal, and muscle weakness. Neurologic and psychologic symptoms were found less frequently. Other than hematologic signs of the disease, the most frequently observed sign of lead toxicity is the so-called *lead line*, a linear blue-black deposit of lead sulfide in the gums near the teeth.[5] Dental caries, abdominal tenderness, and motor disturbances were also reported in 30% to 60% of affected patients.[29]

Laboratory Findings and Correlations with Disease

Hematology. The hematologic changes in lead toxicity are critical because when present, they occur before significant CNS alterations take place.[111] If present, the anemia is typically mild to moderate. The red cells tend to be mildly microcytic and hypochromic.[13] Coarse or fine basophilic stippling is present in the erythrocytes in many cases, but it is not a uniform finding.[124] This pathognomonic stippling is related to inhibition of pyrimidine 5'-nucleotidase activity by lead.[13] The reticulocyte count may be slightly increased, the leukocyte count may be normal or slightly elevated,[29] and platelets are usually normal.

Bone Marrow. Marrow aspirates usually show erythroid hyperplasia. Abnormal siderocytes and sideroblasts are common, but ringed sideroblasts are very uncommon.

Chemistry. Serum iron levels tend to be normal to slightly increased in adults and decreased in children because of the frequently associated iron deficiency anemia.[8,104] Free erythrocyte protoporphyrin is increased in erythrocytes

to a much greater extent than in iron deficiency (Table 13-1). Urinary ALA is elevated, and PBG is normal. Urinary coproporphyrins are increased.[24] In contrast to other iron metabolism disorders, the measurements indicating iron storage status, including serum ferritin and marrow iron, are usually normal in lead intoxication. Transferrin saturation is elevated, and TIBC is normal (Table 13-1).

Children are particularly susceptible to lead intoxication, because they absorb (via the gastrointestinal tract) a greater percentage of lead than adults. Specific criteria to define lead exposure and toxicity have been defined based on whole blood lead values.[104] The ideal specimen to use for diagnosis is venous whole blood collected in an EDTA royal-blue-top tube following metal-free guidelines. Also, a new screening methodology is available utilizing capillary fingerstick collection.[104]

Effects of Treatment on Laboratory Results and Prognosis

Identification and elimination of the source of lead exposure are crucial. Chelation therapy, in which a substance is administered to the patient that chemically binds with lead to cause its urinary excretion, is the treatment of choice. During treatment, urine lead excretion and whole blood lead concentration levels may be monitored.[7,111]

HEREDITARY AND ACQUIRED HEMOCHROMATOSIS/IRON OVERLOAD

Iron which is essential for most living organisms can be fatal when it is accumulated in excess. The lethal effects can be immediate in an accidental or purposeful overdose of medicinal iron or slow as seen in hereditary hemochromatosis and transfusion-related iron overload.[98] The term hemochromatosis is presently used to denote systemic iron overload that may lead to organ injury.[42]

Genetics, Pathophysiology and Populations Affected

Hereditary hemochromatosis is inherited as an autosomal recessive trait and the abnormal gene is tightly linked to the human leukocyte antigen A3 (HLA-A3) locus of the short arm of chromosome 6.[37] The frequency of HLA-A3 is much higher in patients with hemochromatosis than in the normal population. Hemochromatosis may be the most common autosomal recessive disorder in humans. It is estimated that 10% of the United States Caucasian population is heterozygous for the hemochromatosis allele and 0.3% to 0.5% is homozygous. The estimated frequency of hemochromatosis ranges from 1 per 2000 to 2 per 1000 population for Caucasians and lower for other races.[36,37] The clinical expression of the disease is variable and diagnosis of the disease is not as frequent as the estimated frequency of the abnormal gene.

An individual can become overloaded with iron by increased gastrointestinal absorption, which is the primary mechanism in hereditary hemochromatosis, or by parenteral introduction such as that seen with red cell transfusions or iron injections in acquired hemochromatosis.[18] Both hereditary and acquired hemochromatosis cause progressive iron loading of organs.

Clinical Presentation and Physical Findings

The disease, when established, manifests itself between the third and fifth decade, but may occasionally present earlier. Signs and symptoms are related to iron toxicity to the different organs and tissues of the body. Patients present with liver disorders such as cirrhosis, pituitary gland failure, cardiac failure, arthritis, and others. Of importance is that laboratory abnormalities may be present in asymptomatic individuals. Therefore, some investigators advocate screening for this disorder because of its high frequency and the possibility of preventing its devastating complications if identified early.[49]

Laboratory Findings and Correlations with Disease

Serum iron and TIBC with the calculated percent transferrin saturation are very useful in the screening and diagnosis of hemochromatosis. Serum iron concentration, percent transferrin saturation, and serum ferritin level are very high. Bone marrow examination for iron content usually shows increased stainable iron in macrophages, but it is not as reliable as the examination of liver tissue for iron content, especially in the early stages of the disease. Algorithms for establishing the diagnosis of this disorder have been recommended.[89]

Differential Diagnosis

Hereditary hemochromatosis should be distinguished from the other conditions that cause iron overload but are not inherited. Although the iron damage to the tissue may be similar, the other conditions result from excess iron deposition caused by parenteral introduction and without the abnormal gene for hemochromatosis. Individuals requiring lifetime chronic red cell transfusions, such as patients with hemoglobinopathies (Chaps. 14 and 15), are prototype candidates for developing hemosiderosis, which some call "acquired" or secondary hemochromatosis.

Effects of Treatment on Laboratory Results

The treatment for hereditary hemochromatosis is aggressive phlebotomy. With repetitive phlebotomy treatments, the serum iron, percent transferrin saturation, and serum ferritin level decrease as compared to values before treatment. If phlebotomy is contraindicated for medical reasons, the iron can be chelated with medications such as deferoxamine.[35] When the diagnosis is established in a patient, siblings and offspring should be HLA-typed and screened for evidence of iron overload so treatment can be instituted early to delay or prevent a devastating outcome.

CHAPTER SUMMARY

Many patients suffer from anemias secondary to abnormalities of iron metabolism caused either by iron deficiency or by the inability to utilize body iron stores appropriately. The most common form of anemia is iron deficiency anemia, which results from an increased physiologic need for iron, a nutritional deficiency of iron, or a loss of iron stores through bleeding. Iron studies in iron deficiency anemia demonstrate depleted iron stores (Table 13-1).

Anemia of chronic disease is a common mild to moderate anemia accompanying infections, inflammation, and neoplastic disease. Iron appears to be trapped in macrophages where old erythrocytes are catabolized. Therefore, iron is not made available for reutilization in RBC precursors. The effective result is iron deficiency in the presence of adequate iron stores (Table 13-1). The anemia is corrected when the primary disease is resolved.

Sideroblastic anemias are a diverse group of uncommon anemias. The cause may be genetic, idiopathic, drugs, or toxins. The common feature of the sideroblastic anemias is the presence of ringed sideroblasts in bone marrow aspirates stained for iron. A dimorphic erythrocyte population is frequently observed.

Lead intoxication follows exposure to or ingestion of excessive amounts of lead. It produces a picture similar to that of sideroblastic anemia. Anemia is mild to moderate in these patients. Confirmation of elevated lead levels in whole blood is important to the diagnosis.

Hereditary or acquired hemochromatosis (iron overload) can be detected by abnormally high serum iron, transferrin saturation, and ferritin levels.

Case Study 13-1

A 24-year-old black female college student presented with the chief complaint of being tired all the time. She reported that she lived in a dormitory without kitchen facilities and that she did not like the cafeteria food. She did not report unusually heavy menstrual bleeding. Her CBC was reported as follows: WBC 7.8×10^9/L; RBC 4.71×10^{12}/L; Hb 10.3 g/dL; Hct 0.33 L/L; platelets 384×10^9/L; MCV 70 fL; MCH 21.9 pg; and MCHC 31.2 g/dL. The RBC morphology was abnormal, with moderate hypochromia and marked anisocytosis with many small RBCs. Iron studies (with reference ranges in parentheses) revealed serum iron 14 μg/dL (42–135 μg/dL); TIBC 375 μg/dL (250–450 μg/dL); percent transferrin saturation 4% (20%–55%); and serum ferritin 0 μg/L (30–250 μg/L).

1. From the patient's age, sex, and history, what types of anemia might be expected?
2. How do the CBC and red cell morphology influence the differential diagnosis?
3. Do the chemistry findings confirm the suspected diagnosis? Explain.
4. How would this patient's reticulocyte count be expected to respond to a 10-day trial of ferrous sulfate?
5. Could a sound diagnosis have been made on the basis of the ferritin level and CBC alone?
6. Is a bone marrow study necessary in this case?

Case Study 13-2

An 81-year-old man presented with a history of a 1-minute sudden loss of consciousness while driving his car, resulting in a car accident. The patient was on phenytoin (Dilantin) for the control of epilepsy. His physical examination was unremarkable, and he appeared in excellent health for his age. An electrocardiogram showed evidence of a heart arrhythmia that could have been responsible for his loss of consciousness. Significant laboratory values follow (with reference values in parentheses where necessary): WBC 4.4 × 10^9/L; RBC 3.19 × 10^{12}/L; Hb 11.3 g/dL; Hct 0.34 L/L; MCV 105.4 fL; RDW 18.6% (11.0%–15.0%); platelets 227 × 10^9/L; serum B$_{12}$ 1028 pg/mL (250–1100 pg/mL); and serum folate 8.7 ng/mL (3.8–18.0 ng/mL).

The peripheral blood film revealed an apparent double (dimorphic) red cell population consisting of macrocytic RBCs and microcytic, hypochromic RBCs. Mild basophilic stippling was present. Platelets were adequate and morphologically normal. The leukocyte differential showed some reactive lymphocytes but no evidence of immaturity.

After treatment with no improvement, a bone marrow aspirate and biopsy were performed and showed hypercellularity with dyserythropoiesis. Also there was a mild increase of stored iron in macrophages with an accompanying abundant number of ringed sideroblasts at all stages of erythroid maturation.

1. How should this anemia be classified?
2. Is basophilic stippling on the peripheral blood film expected to be found in connection with ringed sideroblasts in the bone marrow?
3. Why was the bone marrow study performed and how are the results helpful?
4. What other tests would have been helpful as part of the bone marrow study?

Review Questions

13-1. A high serum ferritin level, serum iron level, and percent transferrin saturation are most consistent with

   A. iron deficiency anemia.
   B. anemia of chronic disease.
   C. hemochromatosis.
   D. lead poisoning.

13-2. The presence of ringed sideroblasts in the bone marrow is related to

   A. poor iron absorption and a mechanism by which the body retains iron.
   B. defective iron excretion by the body related to an inherited protein defect.
   C. accumulation of iron in mitochondria due to defective iron utilization.
   D. an artifact of the Prussian blue iron stain.

13-3. Which of the following is true concerning ferritin?

   A. It is the most important transport protein for iron.
   B. It is an acute phase reactant and therefore may be normal or elevated in spite of iron deficiency.
   C. It is decreased in cases of hereditary hemochromatosis.
   D. It is only measured by atomic absorption spectrophotometry.

13-4. The typical laboratory findings in iron deficiency anemia are

   A. low serum ferritin, low serum iron, and high percent transferrin saturation.
   B. low serum ferritin, RBC macrocytosis, and high percent transferrin saturation.
   C. low serum ferritin, RBC microcytosis, and low total iron binding capacity (TIBC).
   D. low serum ferritin, RBC microcytosis, and low percent transferrin saturation.

13-5. Which of the following is true concerning anemia of chronic disease?

   A. The erythrocyte population is usually microcytic, hypochromic.
   B. The reticulocyte production index is usually less than 2.0.
   C. Serum ferritin is usually decreased.
   D. Iron stores in the bone marrow are usually decreased.

References

1. Amos RJ, Miller ALC, Amess JAL: Autosomal inheritance of sideroblastic anaemia. Clin Lab Haematol 10:347, 1988
2. Aoki Y, Muranaka S, Nakabayashi K et al: δ-Amino-levulinic acid synthetase in erythroblasts of patients with pyridoxine-responsive anemia: Hypercatabolism caused by the increased susceptibility to the controlling protease. J Clin Invest 64:1196, 1979
3. Bainton DF, Finch CA: The diagnosis of iron deficiency anemia. Am J Med 37:62, 1964
4. Beguin BY, Clemons GK, Pootrakul P et al: Quantitative assessment of erythropoiesis and functional classification of anemia based on measurements of serum transferrin receptor and erythropoietin. Blood 81:1067, 1993
5. Belknap EL: Differential diagnosis of lead poisoning. JAMA 139:818, 1949
6. Bennett JM, Catovsky D, Daniel MT et al: The French–American–British (FAB) co-operative group: Proposals for the classification of myelodysplastic syndromes. Br J Haematol 51:189, 1982
7. Berk PD, Tschudy DP, Shepley LA et al: Hematologic and biochemical studies in a case of lead poisoning. Am J Med 48:137, 1970
8. Beutler E: Hemolytic anemia due to chemical and physical agents. In Williams WJ, Beutler E, Lichtman MA et al (eds): Hematology, 5th ed, p 670. New York, McGraw-Hill, 1995
9. Beveridge BR, Bannerman RM, Evanson JM et al: Hypochromic anemia: A retrospective study and follow-up of 378 inpatients. Q J Med 34:145, 1965
10. Bick RL, Baker WF: Iron deficiency anemia. Lab Med 21:641, 1990
11. Bothwell T: The importance of assessing iron status. Hospital Practice Symposium (Suppl 3):11, April 1991
12. Bottomley SS: Porphyrin and iron metabolism in sideroblastic anemia. Semin Hematol 14:169, 1977
13. Bottomley SS: Sideroblastic anemias. In Lee GR, Bithell TC, Foerster J et al (eds): Wintrobe's Clinical Hematology, 9th ed, p 852. Philadelphia, Lea & Febiger, 1993
14. Bowie EJW, Tauxe WN, Sjoberg WE et al: Daily variation in the concentration of iron in serum. Am J Clin Pathol 40:491, 1963
15. Bridges KR, Seligman PA: Disorders of iron metabolism. In Handin RI, Lux SE, Stossel TP (eds): Blood—Principles and Practice of Hematology, p 1433. Philadelphia, JB Lippincott, 1995
16. Brigden ML: Iron deficiency anemia. Every case is instructive. Postgrad Med 93:181, 1993
17. Brittenham GM, Koepke JA: Red blood cell volume distributions and the diagnosis of anemia. Arch Pathol Lab Med 111:1146, 1987
18. Buchanan GR, Bottomley SS, Nitschke R: Bone marrow delta-aminolevulinate synthetase deficiency in a female with congenital sideroblastic anemia. Blood 55:109, 1980
19. Bush JA, Ashenbrucker H, Cartwright GE et al: The anemia of infection. XX: The kinetics of iron metabolism in the anemia associated with chronic infection. J Clin Invest 35:89, 1956

20. Cartwright GE: The anemia of chronic disorders. Semin Hematol 3:351, 1966

21. Cartwright GE, Lee GR: The anaemia of chronic disorders. Br J Haematol 21:147, 1971

22. Cash JM, Sears DA: The anemia of chronic disease: Spectrum of associated diseases in a series of unselected hospitalized patients. Am J Med 87:638, 1989

23. Chisolm JJ: Disturbances in the biosynthesis of heme in lead intoxication. J Pediatr 64:174, 1964

24. Chisolm JJ: Screening techniques for undue lead exposure in children: Biological and practical considerations. J Pediatr 79:719, 1971

25. Cook J: The effect of endurance training on iron metabolism. Semin Hematol 31:146, 1994

26. Cook JD: Clinical evaluation of iron deficiency. Semin Hematol 19:6, 1982

27. Cook JD, Skikne BS, Lynch SR et al: Estimates of iron sufficiency in the US population. Blood 68:726, 1986

28. Crosby WH: Physiology and pathophysiology of iron metabolism. Hospital Practice Symposium (Suppl 3):7, April 1991

29. Dagg JH, Goldberg A, Lochhead A et al: The relationship of lead poisoning to acute intermittent porphyria. Q J Med 34:163, 1965

30. Dallman PR, Yip R, Johnson C: Prevalence and causes of anemia in the United States, 1976 to 1980. Am J Clin Nutr 39:437, 1984

31. Dincol K, Askoy M: On the platelet levels in chronic iron deficiency anemia. Acta Haematol (Basal) 41:135, 1969

32. Dine MS, Oski FA: What is the best test for iron deficiency? Pediatrics 72:909, 1983

33. Dolan G, Reid MM: Congenital sideroblastic anemia in two girls. J Clin Pathol 44:464, 1991

34. Douglas SW, Adamson JW: The anemia of chronic disorders: Studies of marrow regulation and iron metabolism. Blood 45:55, 1975

35. Edwards CQ: Hemochromatosis and other iron storage disorders. In Lee GR, Bithell TC, Foerster J et al (eds): Wintrobe's Clinical Hematology, 9th ed, p 872. Philadelphia, Lea & Febiger, 1993

36. Edwards CQ, Griffen LM, Goldgar D et al: Prevalence of hemochromatosis among 11,065 presumably healthy blood donors. N Engl J Med 318:1355, 1988

37. Edwards CQ, Griffen LM, Kushner JP: Disorders of excess iron. Hospital Practice Symposium (Suppl 3):30, April 1991

38. Eichner ER, Hillman RS: The evolution of anemia in alcoholic patients. Am J Med 50:218, 1971

39. Erslev AJ: Anemia of chronic disease. In Williams WJ, Beutler E, Lichtman MA et al (eds): Hematology, 5th ed, p 518. New York, McGraw-Hill, 1995

40. Fairbanks VF: Is the peripheral blood film reliable for the diagnosis of iron deficiency anemia? Am J Clin Pathol 55:447, 1971

41. Fairbanks VF: Laboratory testing for iron status. Hospital Practice Symposium (Suppl 3):17, April 1991

42. Fairbanks VF, Baldus WP: Iron overload. In Williams WJ, Beutler E, Lichtman MA et al (eds): Hematology, 5th ed, p 529. New York, McGraw-Hill, 1995

43. Fairbanks VF, Dickson RE, Thompson M: Hereditary sideroblastic anemia. Hospital Practice Symposium (Suppl 3):53, April 1991

44. Fairbanks VF, Klee GG: Biochemical aspects of hematology. In Burtis CA, Ashwood ER (eds): Tietz' Textbook of Clinical Chemistry, 2nd ed, p 1974. Philadelphia, WB Saunders, 1994

45. Finch C: Regulators of iron balance in humans. Blood 84:1697, 1994

46. Finch CA, Bellotti V, Stray S et al: Plasma ferritin determination as a diagnostic tool. West J Med 145(5):657, 1986

47. Finch CA, Cook JD: Iron deficiency. Am J Clin Nutr 39:471, 1984

48. Firkin FC: Mitochondrial lesions in reversible erythropoietic depression due to chloramphenicol. J Clin Invest 51:2085, 1972

49. Gambino R: Routine screening for iron status. Hospital Practice Symposium (Suppl 3):41, April 1991

50. Goasguen JE, Bennett JM: Classification and morphologic features of the myelodysplastic syndromes. Semin Oncol 19:4, 1992

51. Goodman JR, Hall SG: Accumulation of iron in mitochondria of erythroblasts. Br J Haematol 13:335, 1967

52. Green R: Disorders of inadequate iron. Hospital Practice Symposium (Suppl 3):25, April 1991

53. Gross S, Keefer V, Newman AJ: The platelets in iron-deficiency anemia. I: Response to oral and parenteral iron. Pediatrics 34:315, 1964

54. Guyatt GH, Oxman AD, Ali M et al: Laboratory diagnosis of iron-deficiency anemia: An overview. J Gen Intern Med 7:145, 1992

55. Haden HT: Pyridoxine-responsive sideroblastic anemia due to antituberculosis drugs. Arch Intern Med 120:602, 1967

56. Hall R, Losowsky MS: The distribution of erythroblast iron in sideroblastic anaemias. Br J Haematol 12:334, 1966

57. Halliday JW, Powell LW: Ferritin and cellular iron metabolism. Ann New York Acad Sci 526:101, 1988

58. Hartmann RC, Jenkins DE, McKee LC et al: Paroxysmal nocturnal hemoglobinuria: Clinical and laboratory studies relating to iron metabolism and therapy with androgen and iron. Medicine 45:331, 1966

59. Hast R: Sideroblasts in myelodysplasia: Their nature and clinical significance. Scand J Haematol 36 (Suppl 45):53, 1986

60. Hastka J, Lassere J-J, Schwarzbeck A et al: Zinc protoporphyrin in anemia of chronic disorders. Blood 81:1200, 1993

61. Henry JB: Clinical Diagnosis and Management by Laboratory Methods, 18th ed. Philadelphia, WB Saunders, 1991

62. Herbert V: Iron disorders can mimic anything, so always test for them. Blood Rev 3:125, 1992

63. Hillman RS, Finch CA: Red Cell Manual, 5th ed, p 60. Philadelphia, FA Davis, 1985

64. Hines JD, Cowan DH: Studies on the pathogenesis of alcohol-induced sideroblastic bone-marrow abnormalities. N Engl J Med 283:441, 1970

65. Hogan GR, Jones B: The relationship of koilonychia and iron deficiency in infants. J Pediatr 77:1054, 1970

66. Holtz P, Palm D: Pharmacological aspects of vitamin B_6. Pharmacol Rev 16:113, 1964

67. Horrigan DL, Harris JW: Pyridoxine-responsive anemia: Analysis of 62 cases. Adv Intern Med 12:103, 1964

68. International Union of Biochemistry Nomenclature Committee: Enzyme Nomenclature 1984. Orlando, Academic Press, 1984

69. Klasing KC: Effect of inflammatory agents and interleukin 1 on iron and zinc metabolism. Am J Physiol 247:R901, 1984

70. Klein M, Namer R, Harpur E et al: Earthenware containers as a source of fatal lead poisoning. N Engl J Med 283:669, 1970

71. Koenig HM, Lightsey AL, Schanberger JE: The micromeasurement of free erythrocyte protoporphyrin as a means of differentiating alpha thalassemia trait from iron deficiency anemia. J Pediatr 86:539, 1975

72. Koller ME, Romslo I, Finne PH et al: The diagnosis of iron deficiency by erythrocyte protoporphyrin and serum ferritin analyses. Acta Paediatr Scand 67:361, 1978

73. Konijn AM, Hershko C: Ferritin synthesis in inflammation. 1: Pathogenesis of impaired iron release. Br J Haematol 37:7, 1977

74. Konopka L, Hoffbrand AV: Haem synthesis in sideroblastic anaemia. Br J Haematol 42:73, 1979

75. Kushner JP, Lee GR, Wintrobe MM et al: Idiopathic refractory sideroblastic anemia. Medicine 50:139, 1971

76. Lee GR: Iron deficiency and iron deficiency anemia. In Lee GR, Bithell TC, Foerster J et al (eds): Wintrobe's Clinical Hematology, 9th ed, p 808. Philadelphia, Lea & Febiger, 1993

77. Lee GR: The anemia of chronic disease. Semin Hematol 20:61, 1983

78. Lee GR: The anemia of chronic disorders. In Lee GR, Bithell TC, Foerster J et al (eds): Wintrobe's Clinical Hematology, 9th ed, p 840. Philadelphia, Lea & Febiger, 1993

79. Lee GR, MacDiarmid WD, Cartwright GE et al: Hereditary X-linked, sideroachrestic anaemia: The isolation of two erythrocyte populations differing in Xg^a blood type and porphyrin content. Blood 32:59, 1968

80. Lennartsson J, Bengtsson C, Hallberg L et al: Characteristics of anaemic women: The population study of women of Goteborg 1968–1969. Scand J Haematol 22:17, 1979

81. Lewy RI, Kansu E, Gabuzda T: Leukemia in patients with acquired idiopathic sideroblastic anemia: An evaluation of prognostic indicators. Am J Hematol 6:323, 1979

82. Lichtman MA: Myelodysplastic disorders. In Williams WJ, Beutler E, Lichtman MA et al (eds): Hematology, 5th ed, p 257. New York, McGraw-Hill, 1995

83. Lin C-K, Lin J-S, Chen S-Y et al: Comparison of hemoglobin and red blood cell distribution width in the differential diagnosis of microcytic anemia. Arch Pathol Lab Med 116:1030, 1992

84. Lindenbaum J, Lieber CS: Hematologic effects of alcohol in man in the absence of nutritional deficiency. N Engl J Med 281:333, 1969

85. Lipschitz DA, Cook JD, Finch CA: A clinical evaluation of serum ferritin as an index of iron stores. N Engl J Med 290:1213, 1974

86. List AF, Jacobs A: Biology and pathogenesis of the myelodysplastic syndromes. Semin Oncol 19:14, 1992

87. Lorier MA, Herron JL, Carrell RW: Detecting iron deficiency by serum tests. Clin Chem 31:337, 1985

88. Losowsky MS, Hall R: Hereditary sideroblastic anaemia. Br J Haematol 11:70, 1965

89. Ludwig J, Batts KP, Moyer TP et al: Liver biopsy diagnosis of homozygous hemochromatosis: A diagnostic algorithm. Mayo Clin Proc 68:263, 1993

90. Lynch SR, Dassenko SA, Morck TA et al: Soy protein products and heme iron absorption in humans. Am J Clin Nutr 41:13, 1985

91. Manyan DR, Arimura GK, Yunis AA: Chloramphenicol-induced erythroid suppression and bone marrow ferrochelatase activity in dogs. J Lab Clin Med 79:137, 1972

92. Marie B, Cals MJ, De Jaeger C et al: Indicators of iron status in nonanemic elderly subjects: Influence of sex and age. Clin Chem 40:1779, 1994

93. Marsh WL, Nelson DP, Koenig HM: Free erythrocyte protoporphyrin (FEP). I: Normal values for adults and evaluation of the hematofluorometer. II: The FEP test is clinically useful in classifying microcytic RBC disorders in adults. Am J Clin Pathol 79:655, 1983

94. McClure S, Custer E, Bessman JD: Improved detection of early iron deficiency in nonanemic subjects. JAMA 253:1021, 1985

95. McColl KEL, Thompson GG, Moore MR et al: Acute ethanol ingestion and haem biosynthesis in healthy subjects. Eur J Clin Invest 10:107, 1980

96. Means RT Jr, Krantz SB: Progress in understanding the pathogenesis of the anemia of chronic disease. Blood 80:1639, 1992

97. Milman M, Cohn J: Serum iron, serum transferrin and transferrin saturation in healthy children without iron deficiency. Eur J Pediatr 143:96, 1984

98. Nathan D: An orally active iron chelator. N Engl J Med 332:953, 1995

99. National Center for Health Statistics: Diet and Iron Status, A Study of Relationships, United States, 1971–74. Vital and Health Statistics, series 11. Data from the National Health Survey, No. 229. Hyattsville, MD, National Center for Health Statistics, DHHS publication No. (PHS) 83-1679, 1982

100. National Committee for Clinical Laboratory Standards: Determination of Serum Iron and Total Iron-Binding Capacity, Proposed Standard. NCCLS Publication H17-P. Villanova, PA, NCCLS, 1990

101. Noe DA, Rock RC: Laboratory Medicine: The Selection and Interpretation of Clinical Laboratory Studies. Baltimore, Williams and Wilkins, 1994

102. Nowell PC: Chromosome abnormalities in myelodysplastic syndromes. Semin Oncol 19:25, 1992

103. Nuttall DL: Porphyrins and disorders of porphyrin metabolism. In Burtis CA, Ashwood ER (eds): Tietz' Textbook of Clinical Chemistry, 2nd ed, p 2073. Philadelphia, WB Saunders, 1994

104. Nuttall KL: Evaluating lead exposure in the laboratory. Lab Med 26:118, 1995

105. Oski FA: Iron deficiency in infancy and childhood. N Engl J Med 329:190, 1993

106. Pasanen AVO, Vuopio P, Borgstrom GH et al: Haem biosynthesis in refractory sideroblastic anaemia associated with the preleukaemic syndrome. Scand J Haematol 27:35, 1981

107. Pierce HI, McGuffin RG, Hillman RS: Clinical studies in alcoholic sideroblastosis. Arch Intern Med 136:283, 1976

108. Pritchard JA: Changes in the blood volume during pregnancy and delivery. Anesthesiology 26:393, 1965

109. Reynolds RD, Lewis JP: Blood-loss anemias and the iron-deficient states. In Koepke JA (ed): Laboratory Hematology, p 11. New York, Churchill Livingstone, 1984

110. Rosenberg A, Marcus O: Effect of chloramphenicol on reticulocyte δ-aminolaevulinic acid synthetase in rabbits. Br J Haematol 26:79, 1974

111. Sassa S, Kappas A: Disorders of heme production and catabolism. In Handin RI, Lux SE, Stossel TP (eds): Blood—Principles and Practice of Hematology, p 1473. Philadelphia, JB Lippincott, 1995

112. Sayetta RB: Pica: An overview. Am Fam Phys 33(5):181, 1986

113. Schilling R: Anemia of chronic disease: A misnomer. Ann Intern Med 115:572, 1991

114. Schloesser LL, Kipp MA, Wenzel FJ: Thrombocytosis in iron-deficiency anemia. J Lab Clin Med 66:107, 1965

115. Simon TL, Hunt WC, Garry PJ: Iron supplementation for menstruating female blood donors. Transfusion 24:469, 1984

116. Skikne BS, Flowers CH, Cook JD: Serum transferrin receptor: A quantitative measure of tissue iron deficiency. Blood 75:1870, 1990

117. Stockman JA, Weiner LS, Simon GE et al: The measurement of free erythrocyte porphyrin (FEP) as a simple means of distinguishing iron deficiency from beta-thalassemia trait in subjects with microcytosis. J Lab Clin Med 85:113, 1975

118. Tenner S, Rollhauser C, Butt F et al: Sideroblastic anemia: A diagnosis to consider in alcoholic patients. Postgrad Med 92:147, 1992

119. Thompson WG, Meola T, Lipkin M Jr et al: Red cell distribution width, mean corpuscular volume, and transferrin saturation in the diagnosis of iron deficiency. Arch Intern Med 148:2128, 1988

120. Tietz NW: Clinical Guide to Laboratory Tests, 3rd ed. Philadelphia, WB Saunders, 1995

121. Travis WD, Pierre RV: Preleukemia/dysmyelopoietic syndrome. Lab Med 16:147, 1985

122. Verwilghen R, Reybrouck G, Callens L et al: Antituberculous drugs and sideroblastic anaemia. Br J Haematol 11:92, 1965

123. White JM, Harvey DR: Defective synthesis of α- and β-globin chains in lead poisoning. Nature 236:71, 1972

124. White JM, Selhi HS: Lead and the red cell. Br J Haematol 30:133, 1975

125. Witte DL: Can serum ferritin be effectively interpreted in the presence of the acute-phase response? Clin Chem 37(4):484, 1991

126. Witte DL, Angstadt DS, Davis SH et al: Predicting bone marrow iron stores in anemic patients in a community hospital using ferritin and erythrocyte sedimentation rate. Am J Clin Pathol 90(1):85, 1988

CHAPTER 14

Anemias of Abnormal Globin Development— Hemoglobinopathies

Robbi Safko

Objectives

1. Define hemoglobinopathy and abnormal hemoglobin (Hb) variants.
2. Interpret the scientific designation of any abnormal Hb variant.
3. Give several examples of the Mendelian inheritance pattern of hemoglobinopathies.
4. List and briefly define five molecular and five functional abnormalities of abnormal Hb variants and give an example of each.
5. List the most useful laboratory tests for the diagnosis of hemoglobinopathies, and explain their principles, interpretation of results, and common sources of error.
6. List the order of Hb migration, from anode (positive electrode) to cathode (negative electrode), of the normal and common abnormal Hb variants on cellulose acetate (alkaline pH) and citrate agar (acid pH) electrophoresis.
7. State the approximate reference range for Hbs A, A_2 and F, and list several conditions in which Hb F is increased.
8. List and differentiate the significant laboratory findings in sickle cell disease and sickle cell trait.
9. Discuss the laboratory findings unique to each of the following hemoglobinopathies and state the results of the solubility test for each: Hbs CC, AC, SC, DD, SD, EE, O-Arab and C-Harlem.
10. Identify the classic laboratory finding in unstable Hb disease.
11. List the most useful laboratory tests for the diagnosis of unstable Hbs, and explain their principles, interpretation of results, and common sources of error.

Hemoglobinopathies are conditions caused by qualitative structural abnormalities of the globin polypeptide chains that result from alteration of the DNA genetic code for those chains. The disorders may or may not cause clinical or laboratory abnormalities. Understanding hemoglobinopathies depends on understanding the basic structure of the hemoglobin (Hb) molecule (Chap. 7).

These abnormalities cause the production of abnormal Hbs known as *abnormal hemoglobin variants*. Table 14-1 explains the basic terminology of hemoglobinopathies. Hereditary abnormalities of the β-globin chain are the most common causes of hemoglobinopathies. For example Hb S, the most common variant, is caused by a β-chain abnormality. Abnormalities of the α-, γ-, and δ-chains are much less frequent but do occur. When Hb variants are produced the patient is said to have a *hemoglobinopathy*. Thalassemias (Chap. 15), in contrast, are conditions caused by a *quantitative* abnormality in globin chain production (*i.e.*, reduced or no production). Hemoglobinopathies and thalassemias are found worldwide. Figure 14-1 shows the overall geographic distribution of the more common hemoglobinopathies and thalassemias.

TABLE 14-1
Basic Hemoglobinopathy Terms

Term	Definition	Example
Hemoglobin variant	The abnormal hemoglobin caused by a globin chain structural abnormality	Hb S
Hemoglobinopathy	The condition diagnosed when the presence of a variant is confirmed in the blood by laboratory tests	Sickle cell disease (Hb SS) Sickle cell trait (Hb AS)
Qualitative globin chain abnormality	An abnormality in the *amino acid sequence* of the globin chain, not in the amount of globin produced	Substitution for one or more amino acids in globin chain with other amino acids Deletion of amino acids from globin chain Addition of extra amino acids to globin chain
Structural globin chain abnormality	Abnormalities in globin chain composition that produce hemoglobin variants	

GENETICS OF ABNORMAL GLOBIN CHAIN PRODUCTION

Inheritance of Hb variants follows Mendelian patterns (Fig. 5-7). A person who has two Hb variants (*e.g.*, Hb SC) is said to be doubly heterozygous, having inherited a different abnormal variant from each parent. Another category of double heterozygosity is the combination of an abnormal globin chain and thalassemia.

By convention, genotypes for Hb inheritance always indicate the Hb of greater concentration first. For example, when Hb S is inherited from one parent and Hb A from the other, Hb A is present in higher concentration, so the genotype is written Hb AS.

NOMENCLATURE

Hb variants have both a common name and a scientific designation. The common names generally refer to the associated morphology (*e.g.*, Hb S for sickle cells, Hb C for intracellular crystals) or to the city, district, province, or hospital where they were discovered (*e.g.*, Hb Gun Hill, Hb Constant Spring). The M Hbs have been so designated because they are associated with the presence of methemoglobinemia.

The scientific designation denotes (1) the affected polypeptide chain, (2) the sequential amino acid number(s) affected, (3) the helix number involved, and (4) the nature of the abnormality (amino acid substitution, deletion, addition, or globin chain fusion). Table 14-2 lists the scientific designations of major β-chain variants.

The primary Hb structure consists of amino acids in a specified sequence, 1 to 141 for α-chains and 1 to 146 for β-chains. The secondary Hb structure is divided into eight rigid helical segments (A through H) that contain groups of amino acids (Fig. 7-2). There are also seven nonhelical segments (*e.g.*, NA, AB, CD) that lie between the eight helical segments to provide flexibility and allow physical bending of the globin chain (Fig. 7-2). Thus, the scientific designation of Hb S is $\beta^{6(A3)Glu \rightarrow Val}$. This is interpreted as a β-chain variant affecting the sixth sequential amino acid position, which is the third position in the A helical segment. The variant is caused by a substitution

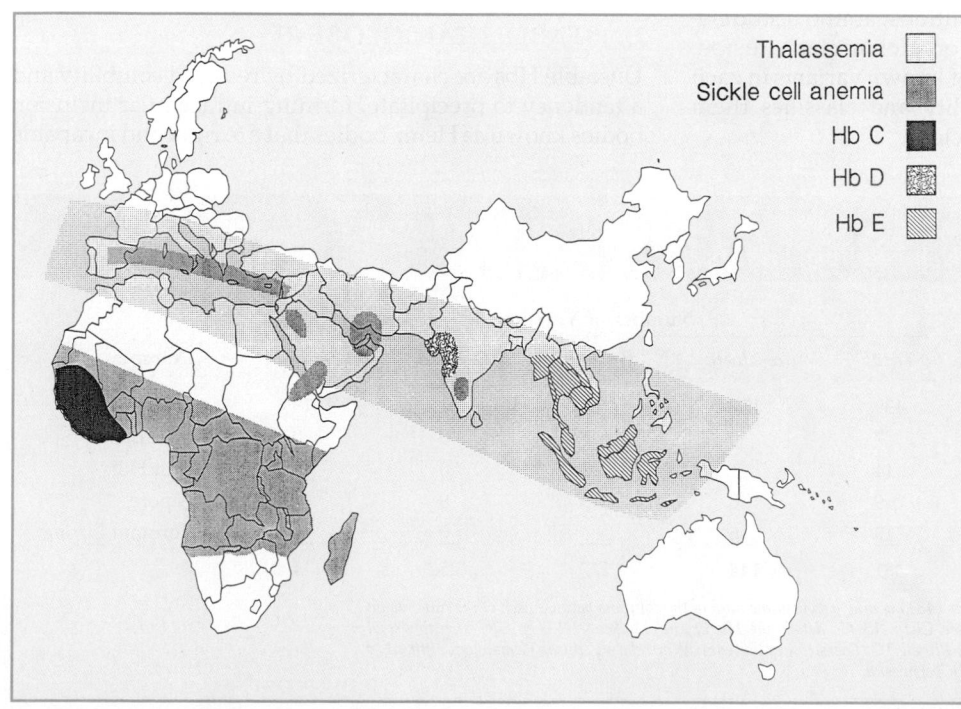

FIGURE 14-1. The geographic distribution of the more common structural hemoglobin abnormalities and the thalassemias. (From Hoffbrand AV, Pettit JE: Essential Haematology, 2nd ed. London, Blackwell Scientific Publications, 1984, with permission.)

Thalassemia

Sickle cell anemia

Hb C

Hb D

Hb E

TABLE 14-2
Common Names and Scientific Designations of the Well-Known Abnormal Hemoglobin Variants

Molecular Abnormality	Hemoglobin Common Name	Affected Chain	Amino Acids Affected	Helical Numbers Affected	β-Chain Substitution	Scientific Designation
Amino acid substitution	S	β	6	A3	Glu $\rightarrow$ Val	$\beta^{6(A3)Glu\rightarrow Val}$
	C	β	6	A3	Glu $\rightarrow$ Lys	$\beta^{6(A3)Glu\rightarrow Lys}$
	D-Los Angeles D-Punjab	β	121	GH4	Glu $\rightarrow$ Gln	$\beta^{121(GH4)Glu\rightarrow Gln}$
	E	β	26	B8	Glu $\rightarrow$ Lys	$\beta^{26(B8)Glu\rightarrow Lys}$
	O-Arab	β	121	GH4	Glu $\rightarrow$ Lys	$\beta^{121(GH4)Glu\rightarrow Lys}$
Amino acid deletion	Gun Hill	β	91–95	F7-FG2	NA	$\beta^{91-95\ (F7-FG2)\ Leu\ His\ Cys\ Asp\ Lys\rightarrow 0}$
Amino acid elongation	Constant Spring	α	NA	NA	NA	$\alpha^{+31c\ (142\ Gln)}$
Globin chain fusion	Lepore-Baltimore	$\delta\beta$	NA	NA	NA	$\delta^{(1-50)}\beta^{(86-146)}$

Key: Asp, asparagine; Cys, cysteine; Gln, glycine; Glu, glutamic acid; His, histidine; Leu, leucine; Lys, lysine; Pro, Proline; Thr, threonine; Val, valine; NA, not applicable.

in that position of valine (Val) for the normal glutamic acid (Glu).

CLASSIFICATION OF HEMOGLOBINOPATHIES

The hemoglobinopathies may be classified according to molecular or functional abnormalities.

Classification by Molecular Abnormality

From a molecular or structural standpoint, Hb variants may result from a single amino acid substitution in the α- or β-chain (the most common form of hemoglobinopathy), multiple amino acid substitutions, amino acid deletions, globin chain elongation, or globin chain fusion. Table 14-3 lists the total number of known variants in each category of molecular abnormality and classifies them according to which chain is affected.

Classification by Functional Abnormality

Some Hb variants cause a number of abnormal conditions (Table 14-4), whereas others produce no detectable clinical disability.

AGGREGATION

Hemoglobins that aggregate and have reduced solubility are capable of polymerizing or crystallizing (Hbs S and C, respectively) within the red cell. This causes distortion of cell shape, decreased "deformability," and consequent susceptibility to hemolysis.

UNSTABLE HEMOGLOBINS

Unstable Hbs are characterized by reduced solubility and a tendency to precipitate, forming intracellular inclusion bodies known as Heinz bodies that are rigid and incapable

TABLE 14-3
Molecular Abnormalities of Hemoglobin Variants

Abnormality	Number of Variants					Examples
	Total	α-Chain	β-Chain	γ-Chain	δ-Chain	
Single amino acid substitution	439	137	242	17	43	S, C, D, E
Two amino acid substitutions	7	0	7	0	0	C-Harlem
Deletion	14	1	13	0	0	Gun Hill
Fusions*	9	0	9	8	1	Lepore
Elongated Chains	12	6	6	0	0	Constant Spring
TOTALS*	481	144	277	25	44	

* The total number of abnormal hemoglobins (481) is nine less than the sum of the columns because each of the nine fusion hemoglobins is recorded in two columns (see Chap. 15 for details on Hb Lepore). Lukens JN, Lee GR: The abnormal hemoglobins: General principles. In Lee GR, Bithell TC, Foerster J et al (eds): Wintrobe's Clinical Hematology, 9th ed, p 1025. Philadelphia, Lea & Febiger, 1993, with permission.

TABLE 14-4
Functional Classification of Hemoglobin Variants

Functional Abnormality	Clinical Condition	Example
None	None	Hb G-Philadelphia
Aggregation with reduced solubility	Hemolytic anemia: painful crisis (homozygous state)	Hb S
Unstable	Hemolytic anemia: (heterozygous state)	Hb Köln Hb Gun Hill
Methemoglobinemia	Cyanosis	Hb M
Increased oxygen affinity	Erythrocytosis	Hb Chesapeake
Decreased oxygen affinity	Cyanosis or mild hemolytic anemia	Hb Kansas

Modified from Lukens JN, Lee GR: The abnormal hemoglobins: General principles. In Lee GR, Bithell TC, Foerster J et al (eds): Wintrobe's Clinical Hematology, 9th ed, p 1043. Philadelphia, Lea & Febiger, 1993, with permission.

of traversing the splenic microcirculation. Affected red cells lose membrane and eventually are trapped and destroyed in the spleen. These Hbs are also sensitive to heat (*i.e.*, 50°C) in vitro. Hbs Köln and Gun Hill are examples of unstable Hbs. Unstable Hbs may or may not have altered oxygen affinity; others may cause methemoglobinemia.

METHEMOGLOBINS

This abnormality is associated with five variants of Hb M, all of which cause iron to remain permanently in the oxidized (ferric; Fe^{3+}) form referred to as methemoglobin (Chap. 7). Because methemoglobin cannot bind oxygen, cyanosis results.

OXYGEN AFFINITY

Increased Hb oxygen affinity is associated with some variants (*e.g.*, Hb Gun Hill). When release of oxygen to the tissue from Hb is decreased, decreased oxygen tension in the tissues results in increased production of erythropoietin and erythrocytes (erythrocytosis). Some of these variants also are unstable.

Hbs with *decreased oxygen affinity* also occur (*e.g.*, Hb Kansas) and some are unstable. Because these Hbs release more oxygen per gram of Hb, slight anemia may occur. Some variants do not cause detectable symptoms or signs. Others may cause cyanosis owing to decreased Hb oxygen saturation.

See Table 14-5 for a summary of molecular abnormalities associated with each group of functional abnormalities.

GENERAL LABORATORY FINDINGS

Laboratory findings vary from no detectable abnormalities to striking alterations, depending on which Hb variant is involved. Patients who are homozygous for the more common β-chain variants (Hbs S, C, D-Los Angeles, and E) may demonstrate anemia. Target cells are often found on the peripheral blood film. Heinz bodies are characteristic of the unstable Hbs.

MOST USEFUL LABORATORY TESTS FOR DIAGNOSING HEMOGLOBINOPATHIES

The most significant laboratory tests for diagnosis of the hemoglobinopathies are outlined in Table 14-6. Two of the most commonly used tests include (1) the solubility test for sickling Hbs and (2) hemoglobin electrophoresis, for variant identification on cellulose acetate at alkaline pH and by citrate agar at acid pH.

Two other forms of more specialized electrophoresis include isoelectric focusing and globin chain electropho-

TABLE 14-5
Functional Characteristics of Hemoglobin Variants

Abnormality	Amino Acid Substitutions				Deletions	Fusion	Elongated Chains
	α-Chain	β-Chain	δ-Chain	γ-Chain			
None or unknown	84	84	14	42	1	6	5
Aggregation	0	7	0	0	0	0	0
Unstable	17	45	2	1	3	0	2
Methemoglobin	2	5	0	2	0	0	0
Increased oxygen affinity	24	49	1	0	2	3	1
Decreased oxygen affinity	3	17	0	0	0	0	0
Unstable/increased oxygen affinity	4	23	0	0	7	0	4
Unstable/decreased oxygen affinity	3	12	0	0	1	0	0
TOTAL	137	242	17	45	14	9	12

From Lukens JN, Lee GR: The abnormal hemoglobins: General principles. In Lee GR, Bithell TC, Foerster J et al (eds): Wintrobe's Clinical Hematology, 9th ed, p 1044. Philadelphia, Lea & Febiger, 1993, with permission.

TABLE 14-6
Recommended Laboratory Tests
for Diagnosis of Hemoglobinopathies

Tests	Comments
MOST FREQUENTLY REQUIRED	
Complete blood count	
RBC morphology evaluation	
Solubility test	
Hb electrophoresis, cellulose acetate (pH 8.4–8.6)	
Hb electrophoresis, citrate agar (pH 6.0–6.2)	To distinguish or identify some abnormal Hbs detected on cellulose acetate electrophoresis
Supravital stain for Heinz bodies	To screen for unstable Hb; not a specific test because it also indicates G6PD and related deficiencies
Hb F quantitation	Alkali denaturation to quantitate Hb F in 2%–40% range
Hb A_2 quantitation	Column chromatography
OCCASIONALLY REQUIRED	
Heat denaturation test	To screen for unstable Hb
Isopropanol precipitation test	To screen for unstable Hb
Globin chain electrophoresis, acid or alkaline pH	To differentiate Hbs S, D, G, and Q, or Hbs A_2, C, E, and O-Arab
Isoelectric focusing	To detect an Hb present in a small percentage; to screen for or confirm hemoglobinopathies in newborns
RARELY REQUIRED	
P_{50} quantitation	To screen for abnormal Hb oxygen affinity
2,3-DPG quantitation	To screen for 2,3-DPG deficiency or abnormal Hb oxygen affinity

resis. Isoelectric focusing is electrophoresis in a pH gradient (a medium with a pH range, *e.g.*, 3 to 10). It is performed in most newborn screening laboratories in the United States. Globin chain electrophoresis at acid or alkaline pH is a more specialized test performed when a high degree of specificity is needed that is not possible with routine electrophoresis.

The alkali denaturation test for fetal hemoglobin (Hb F) quantitation is useful to help identify conditions in which Hb F is characteristically elevated, such as sickle cell anemia (Hb SS) and Hb S–thalassemia conditions, and to differentiate hemoglobinopathies from thalassemias.

Hb A_2 quantitation (Chap. 15) may be performed to rule out the possibility of thalassemia or the doubly heterozygous Hb S–thalassemia conditions. Hb A_2 is usually normal in Hb SS and AS, but increased in Hb S–thalassemia and other thalassemic syndromes.

Tests for unstable Hbs such as Heinz body staining can also be diagnostic. All of the foregoing laboratory procedures will be described in some detail in the following.

Solubility Test

The solubility test[34,44,57,64] is a screening test for the detection of sickling hemoglobin (*e.g.*, Hb S). It gives rapid results, is inexpensive, and has a high degree of accuracy, although it is not specific for Hb S. Several prepackaged kits are available.

PRINCIPLE AND SPECIMEN REQUIREMENTS. Red cells are lysed by saponin, allowing Hb to escape. Sodium dithionite binds and removes oxygen from the test environment. Hb S polymerizes in the resulting deoxygenated state and forms a precipitate in a high-molarity phosphate buffer solution. The precipitate consists of tactoids, which are liquid crystals. The tactoids refract and deflect light, making the solution turbid.

Whole blood, collected in ethylenediaminetetraacetic acid (EDTA), heparin or sodium citrate, is recommended. Store at 4°C until testing, but do not store for more than 3 weeks. Some procedures call for whole blood; others require packed erythrocytes. The cells should be separated just before the test is performed.

REAGENTS. Kits are available with prepackaged supplies and reagents. The National Committee for Clinical Laboratory Standards (NCCLS) sickle solubility procedure[64] provides instructions for laboratory reagent preparation.

QUALITY CONTROL. A positive and a negative control[64] should be run with each set of tests. The positive control specimen should contain approximately 30% to 45% Hb S and have a Hb value of 12 ± 2 g/dL. The negative control should have normal adult percentages of Hb A and A_2 and no Hb S.

PROCEDURE. The manufacturer's instructions should be followed closely. The following procedure is an example of one that requires packed red cells.

1. Label three 12×75-mm test tubes: Patient, Neg. control, Pos. control.
2. Pipet 2 mL working solution at room temperature into each tube. Add 10 μL packed erythrocytes. Mix and wait 5 minutes.
3. Observe specimen for turbidity by holding tube 2.5 cm in front of newsprint or a reader card with thin black lines, or by placing the tube in a special reading rack designed for this test.

INTERPRETATION OF RESULTS. Figure 14-2 shows the results of a positive control (*A*), negative control (*B*) and a positive patient sample (*C*). Turbidity indicates the presence of sickling Hb, regardless of the genotype (*e.g.*, SS, AS, S–thalassemia). If the solution is clear and lines are visible through it, the result is reported as negative.

This test is not specific for Hb S. It is positive in the presence of other abnormal Hbs, such as Hb Barts and Hb I, and some unstable Hbs, such as Hb Sabine. Hb C-Harlem,[5,6] Hb C-Ziguinchor[33] and Hb S-Travis[58] also cause a positive result. These last three Hbs have the same amino acid substitution abnormality as Hb S, but each also has an additional unique β-chain substitution.

The solubility test is used only for screening purposes. Normally, it should be performed after electrophoresis (at alkaline pH) to determine whether a Hb band that travels in the Hb S or Hb C position is a sickling Hb. The test may be performed as a quick screening procedure before electrophoresis in a laboratory where only a few electrophoresis requests are received each

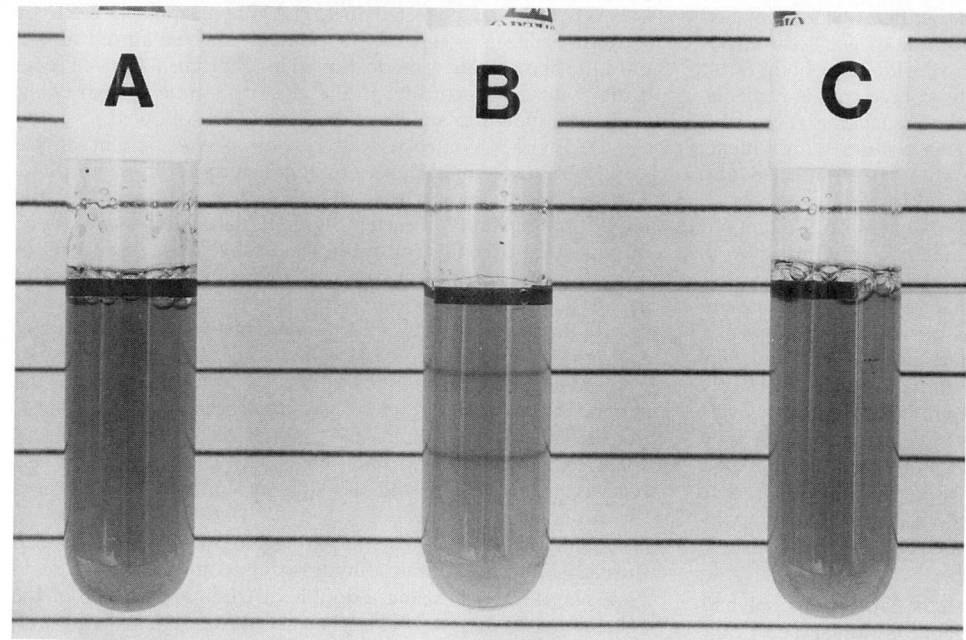

week; however, specimens should not be stored for more than 10 days before hemolysate preparation for electrophoresis.

COMMENTS AND SOURCES OF ERROR. When performing this test, keep the following points in mind: (1) a positive solubility test must always be confirmed by electrophoresis at alkaline pH, and sometimes at acid pH; (2) blood from infants younger than 6 months of age should not be tested by this method because production of the abnormal β-chain that causes Hb S may not yet be functioning at full capacity; and (3) all solutions must be at room temperature before use for testing. Reagents are usually stored in the refrigerator.

If whole blood is used instead of packed erythrocytes, false-positive or false-negative results may occur (Table 14-7). The use of 10 × 75-mm test tubes may cause a false-negative result because the smaller tube diameter may allow the reader to see the black lines even if the solution is turbid. Also a recent transfusion may cause a false-negative result because of the dilution of Hb S by the normal blood.

Hemoglobin Electrophoretic Procedures

Electrophoresis is the migration of charged particles, such as various Hbs, in an electrical field. Particles with a positive charge migrate toward the negatively charged electrode called the cathode. Particles with a negative charge migrate toward the positively charged electrode called the anode. Particle velocity is controlled by five factors: the net charge on the particle, the size and shape of the particle, the strength of the electrical field, chemical and physical properties of the supporting medium (*e.g.*, cellulose acetate or citrate agar for Hb electrophoresis), and the electrophoretic temperature.

Specimen Requirements. Venous blood may be collected in EDTA, heparin, sodium citrate, acid-citrate–dextrose (ACD) or citrate–phosphate–dextrose (CPD).[13,63] Whole blood should be stored at 4°C for no longer than 10 days before the hemolysate is prepared.

Hemolysate Preparation Using Water and Organic Solvent

PROCEDURE
1. Centrifuge whole blood at a relative centrifugal force (RCF) of 1500 to 2000 × *g* for 10 minutes to separate cells and plasma.
2. Remove plasma with a disposable pipet.
3. Wash cells three times with 0.85% NaCl solution (normal saline) and remove final wash solution.

TABLE 14-7
Sources of Physiologic and Technical Errors in the Solubility Test for Sickling Hemoglobin

FALSE-POSITIVE RESULTS

Erythrocytosis

Hyperglobulinemia*

Extreme leukocytosis*

Hyperlipidemia*

More blood added to reagent than called for by test procedure

Deteriorated reagent

FALSE-NEGATIVE RESULTS

Anemia (Hb < 7 g/dL)*

Patient recently transfused with normal blood

Holding tube too close to card when reading results

Testing blood from infant younger than 6 months

Deteriorated reagent

Use of 10- × 75-mm test tubes

* These false-positive or -negative results may be avoided by using packed erythrocytes instead of whole blood and following appropriate methods for use of packed erythrocytes in this test.

4. Lyse cells by adding six volumes of distilled water to washed cells and a half volume (half the volume of washed cells) of toluene, chloroform, or carbon tetrachloride. One of the latter two solvents is preferred if 1 mL or less of red cells is available, because the hemolysate appears as the top layer after centrifugation with these solvents, but at the bottom with toluene. (Caution: These organic solvents are toxic if inhaled and should be handled under a fume hood.)

5. Shake vigorously by hand or by vortex mixer until bright red uniform mixture appears (approximately 5 minutes).

6. Centrifuge 25 minutes at approximately 1500 to 2000 × g. (The calculation for converting relative centrifugal force to revolutions per minute is provided in Appendix D).

7. If toluene is used, remove top toluene and cell stroma layers with a suction apparatus. If carbon tetrachloride or chloroform is used, clear hemolysate solution will be at the top.

8. Filter hemolysate through a layer of Whatman 1 filter paper.

9. Hemolysate may be stoppered and stored at 3° to 5°C after addition of 2 or 3 drops of 3% KCN per 5 mL hemolysate to convert methemoglobin to cyanmethemoglobin (methemoglobin could interfere with test interpretation).

COMMENTS AND SOURCES OF ERROR. The organic solvents used in this procedure may produce denaturation and precipitation of Hb Barts, Hb H, and other unstable Hbs. Only water should be used to lyse red cells if unstable Hbs are suspected, and the solution should be centrifuged at 2000 × g for 30 minutes to remove stroma. If turbidity remains, filter through two layers of Whatman 1 filter paper.

Hemolysate Preparation Using Hemolysate Reagent

PROCEDURE. The method using a hemolysate reagent is faster, easier (e.g., for large-scale screening), and useful when only a small sample can be obtained, as from an infant, but it is not very reproducible and not adequate for tests requiring larger amounts of hemolysate or stroma-free hemolysate. Either saponin or EDTA hemolyzing reagent may be used. They are available commercially.

Prepare hemolysate following the hemolyzing reagent manufacturer's instructions. The Centers for Disease Control and Prevention (CDC)[13] recommends 3 drops hemolysate reagent for every 50 μL washed red cells. Add 1 drop 3% KCN. The NCCLS standard[63] states that blood taken by skin puncture (e.g., for an infant) may be drawn directly into saponin or EDTA hemolyzing reagent to prepare a hemolysate for electrophoresis.

Cellulose Acetate Hemoglobin Electrophoresis. Cellulose acetate electrophoresis[7,13,35,63,76] is a relatively simple method for detection and preliminary identification of both normal and abnormal Hbs, particularly Hbs A, F, S and C. It provides for sharp band resolution in a short time. Abnormal Hbs found on cellulose acetate require confirmation by other methods (e.g., solubility test, citrate agar electrophoresis). When either Hb F or A$_2$ appears to be elevated, it must be quantitated by other methods.

A small quantity of red cell hemolysate is placed on a cellulose acetate membrane. The membrane is then placed between the cathode (negative pole) and anode (positive pole) of an electrophoretic chamber. An electrical field is created in the chamber through the use of a power supply, and a current is generated through a buffer at alkaline pH. Hb molecules have a net negative charge at alkaline pH and migrate on the membrane toward the anode. Owing to variations in the amino acid content of different Hbs, the net charge on each Hb type is unique, and this determines each Hb's rate of mobility in the electrical field.

Whole blood collected in EDTA, heparin, ACD, CPD or sodium citrate is acceptable. Specimens may be stored at 4°C until the hemolysate is made, but no longer than 10 days. Procedures will vary according to the electrophoretic system being used. Manufacturer's instructions should be followed.

A Hb A$_1$FSC control as well as a normal A$_1$A$_2$ patient sample should be run with each set of patient samples on every plate. The patterns of unknown samples should be compared with the known samples run on each individual plate because variations in current, buffer lots, or application may cause variations in migration rate with each run. Precision should be rechecked occasionally using duplicate samples.

Plates are stained, cleared,[63] and scanned with densitometer to semiquantitate separated Hb bands. The densitometer uses a photometer to measure absorption or concentration of the stained Hbs separated by electrophoresis. Because the concentration of various Hbs differs, the amount of light absorbed will vary from one fraction to another. (*Note*: Carbonic anhydrase released from red cells will also stain as a narrow band close to the application point.)

If a Hb variant appears to be migrating in a position nearer the cathode than carbonic anhydrase, a second cellulose acetate plate should be run using a double or triple application of the specimen and a control. This plate should be stained with Ponceau S and then with o-toluidine dihydrochloride counterstain for a few minutes until desired color appears; it is then rinsed with 5% acetic acid. The counterstain stains Hb fractions purple, whereas nonheme protein remains pink or red. Specimen results must be compared with the control specimen. Commonly, counterstaining is used to differentiate Hb G$_2$ from carbonic anhydrase. Hb G$_2$, an α-chain variant, appears as a bluish purple band that migrates only a short distance (between application point and carbonic anhydrase). Other α-chain variants may migrate in a similar position.

INTERPRETATION OF RESULTS. Interpretation of results is based on known migration patterns of various Hbs (Fig. 14-3) and by comparison with controls. Hb percentages may be calculated based on densitometry results.

REFERENCE RANGES. Hb A$_1$, 97%; Hb A$_2$, 2% to 3.5%; Hb F, at birth 60% to 90%, 1% after 1 year of age. Each laboratory should determine its own reference ranges.

COMMENTS AND SOURCES OF ERROR. Definitive diagnosis of abnormal Hbs cannot be made on the basis of electrophoresis performed at a single pH. Citrate agar electrophoresis at acid pH provides another method to confirm the presence of certain variants. The solubility test is always performed as a confirmatory measure when a Hb band migrates in the S position on cellulose acetate.[63]

Errors may result from use of unacceptable reagents, equipment, or samples, including buffers of incorrect pH or ionic strength or ones that are contaminated or cloudy; use of sample wells, applicator tips, blotters, or cellulose acetate plates contaminated with dirt, blood, or other proteins; and use of hemolysates that are old or discolored, contain red cell stroma, or are bacterially contaminated, all of which may cause poor separation, artifacts, or smearing of Hb bands.

Technical errors include (1) improper loading of plates into buffer, which can cause trapped air or peeling; improper sample application, or improper blotting that leaves plates excessively wet or dry; (2) lack of contact between buffer and cellulose acetate; (3) excessive heat during electrophoresis (this can be controlled by placing ice in the center compartments [not the buffer] or by reducing voltage); (4) application points that are too close to the anode; (5) any delay in sample application, applying current to plate or staining after electrophoresis; and (6) failure to remove leukocytes from specimen with increased leukocyte count, which may lead to migration of a band that is

Hemoglobin Electrophoresis

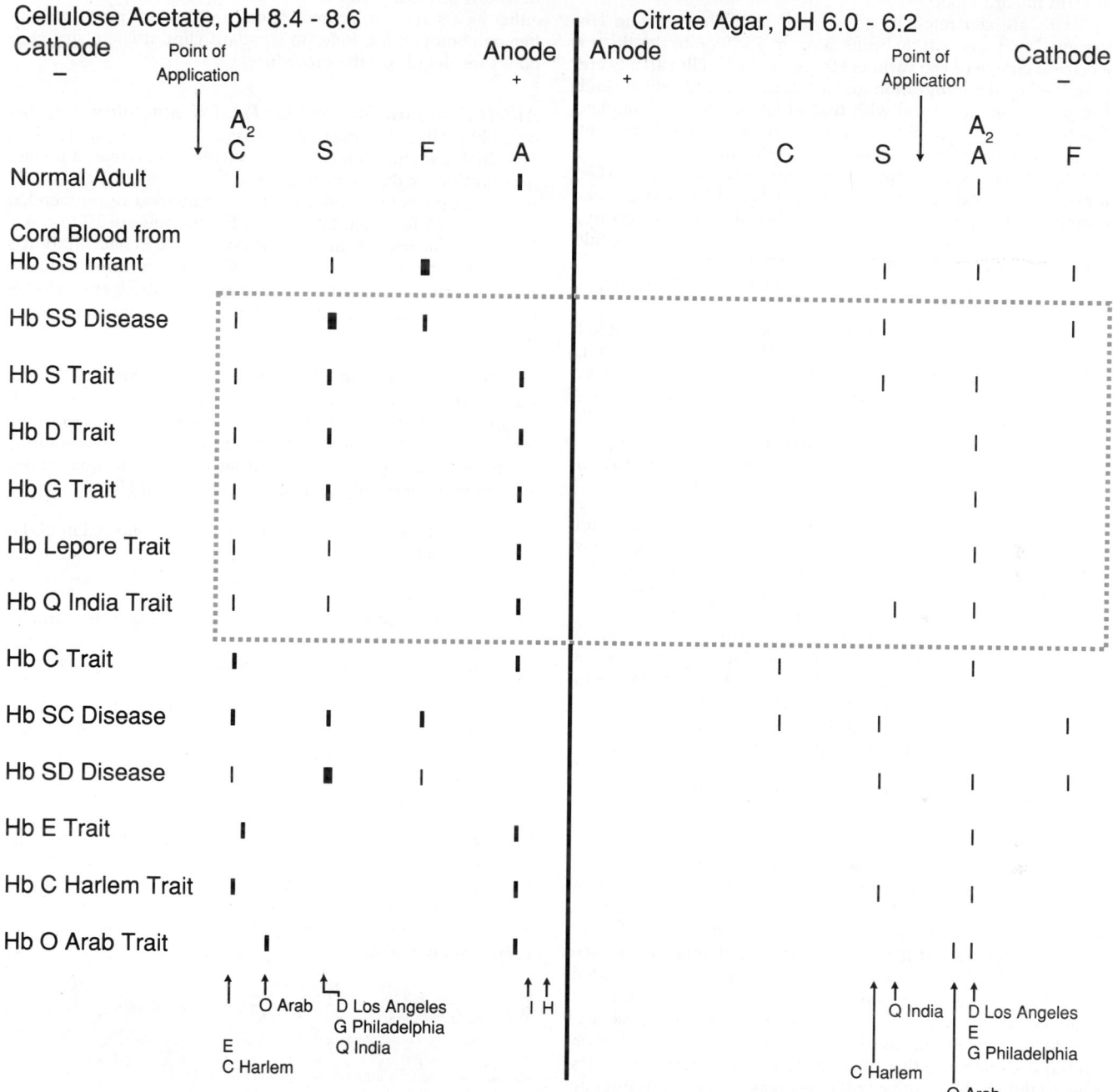

FIGURE 14-3. Hemoglobin migration patterns on cellulose acetate and citrate agar electrophoresis for major hemoglobinopathies. Note points of sample application and locations of anodes and cathodes for each method. *Box* around patterns in cellulose acetate electrophoresis indicates hemoglobins that are indistinguishable from Hb S at alkaline pH but distinguishable on citrate agar at acid pH. Hb I and Hb H (migration patterns not shown) both migrate faster on cellulose acetate than all other hemoglobins depicted.

much faster than any known Hb variant. This band is thought to be leukocyte-derived myeloperoxidase.

Blood of poorly controlled diabetic patients may show a band of glycosylated Hb that appears slightly toward the anode from Hb A.

Citrate Agar Hemoglobin Electrophoresis. Citrate agar electrophoresis[13,40,57,62] is routinely performed at acid pH as a comple-

ment to cellulose acetate electrophoresis, which is performed at alkaline pH. It differentiates some Hb variants that migrate together on cellulose acetate. For example, it is used to differentiate Hb S from D and G, all of which migrate similarly on cellulose acetate. Citrate agar is also used to differentiate Hb C from C-Harlem, E, and O-Arab, which also migrate together on cellulose acetate (Fig. 14-3).

This procedure is useful for detecting small amounts of

either Hb A or F in the presence of large amounts of the other and in revealing small amounts of adult Hbs A and S present at birth in cord blood.

Hbs are separated based on the interactions among Hb variants, agar, and citrate buffer ions, in addition to the altered electrical charge of the various Hbs at acid pH. Hb variants are identified by their migration toward the anode and cathode and comparing the migration with that of known control samples. The test is strictly qualitative: the percentage of each Hb present cannot be determined accurately using this method.

Specimen requirements are similar to those stated earlier for cellulose acetate electrophoresis. The NCCLS standard[62] recommends that specimen Hb levels be checked and, if necessary, diluted with distilled water to about 0.5 to 1.0 g/dL for adult samples or 4 g/dL for umbilical cord blood.

Manufacturer's instructions should be followed for the specific procedure.

Each new lot of agar plates should be tested to ensure good separation of known control samples. If Hb O-Arab is suspected, a Hb O-Arab control should be run if one is available. Strict adherence to expiration dates is required. Plates made in-house are usually acceptable for 1 month when stored at 4°C. A Hb A₁FSC control should be run on each plate with patient samples.

Figure 14-3 shows the migration pattern of normal Hbs and some common variants on citrate agar at acid pH.

COMMENTS AND SOURCES OF ERROR. Cellulose acetate and citrate agar electrophoresis together confirm the presence of Hbs S, C, O and several others. Other Hbs (*e.g.*, Hb D-Los Angeles and Hb G-Philadelphia) cannot be defined solely by these two methods. Globin chain electrophoresis may be required.

When using the citrate agar method, Hb mobilities are more affected by concentration and state of the Hb, small changes in buffer composition, electrical conditions, and other factors than in other methods. Therefore, use of controls is imperative.

Many of the same technical errors that may occur in performing cellulose acetate electrophoresis also apply to citrate agar.

Agar-impregnated cellulose acetate is an alternative to the medium described in the foregoing.[62,78]

Globin Chain Electrophoresis.

Over 450 Hb variants have been identified up to the present time, so there are many that migrate together on both routine cellulose acetate and citrate agar electrophoresis. Globin chain electrophoresis[13,39,77,82] provides another method that can be used to differentiate the variants (Table 14-6). In this procedure, 2-mercaptoethanol is added to the hemolysate to separate globin chains from heme, and urea is added to separate the α- and non−α-chains. Subsequently, the sample containing free globin chains is electrophoresed on cellulose acetate at either alkaline or acid pH. Heme migrates toward the anode (positive pole), whereas globin chains migrate at varying speeds toward the cathode.

Since globin chain electrophoresis is not performed in most routine hematology laboratories, it will not be described here. Details may be found in the indicated references.

Isoelectric Focusing.

Isoelectric focusing (IEF)[19,43] is a modified, more advanced form of electrophoresis in which the support medium along which proteins migrate has a pH gradient or pH range of approximately 3 to 10.

Because of its amino acid composition, a protein such as Hb can be either negatively or positively charged (*i.e.*, proteins are amphoteric). However, at a certain environmental pH, a protein has no net charge and, when this occurs, the protein ceases to move. This is the protein's isoelectric point or pI. Therefore, proteins can be separated into discrete bands based on differences in pI.

IEF is particularly useful in situations where small percentages of Hbs need to be detected. It is used in almost all of the newborn screening laboratories throughout the United States either as a screening procedure or confirmatory procedure for hemoglobinopathies. Refer to standard clinical chemistry textbooks for details on the procedure.

Alkali Denaturation Test for Fetal Hemoglobin.

Fetal hemoglobin (Hb F) is increased in several conditions (Table 14-8). The alkali denaturation test[3,42,65,83] provides accurate and precise quantitation of the percentage of Hb F in blood, particularly when it appears to be elevated. It is the method recommended by the NCCLS for quantitation of Hb F in the range of 2% to 40%.[65] Radioimmunoassay is more accurate when Hb F concentration is less than 2%, and column chromatography is more accurate when it is greater than 40%.[65] Quantitation of Hb F by densitometry of samples electrophoresed on cellulose acetate is *not* satisfactory.

PRINCIPLE. Hb F resists the denaturation exhibited by other Hbs at alkaline pH. After a specified period, denaturation is stopped by addition of saturated ammonium sulfate, which lowers the pH and precipitates any denatured Hb. The test solution is filtered, leaving Hb F in solution that can be quantitated spectrophotometrically as a percentage of total Hb.

SPECIMEN REQUIREMENTS. Whole blood collected in EDTA is recommended.

REAGENTS

1. Cyanmethemoglobin (Drabkin's) reagent, available commercially (Chap. 9).
2. Sodium hydroxide reagent (1.25 mol/L), available commercially.
3. Saturated ammonium sulfate (4.06 mol/L at 20°C). To 550 g ammonium sulfate add distilled water to approximately 1 L. Mix. Store in glass bottle at 20° to 25°C. Solution is stable up to 3 months. Undissolved crystals should always be present at bottom of bottle.

QUALITY CONTROL. A specimen known to be normal and one with confirmed elevation of Hb F should be run with each batch of specimens tested. An elevated Hb F control may be prepared by mixing umbilical cord blood and normal adult blood of the same ABO group. It is not clear how long Hb F preparations are stable.

TABLE 14-8
Conditions Commonly Associated with Increased Levels of Hb F

Condition	Comments
Infancy	Newborns have 60% to 90% Hb F
Hemoglobinopathies	Particularly Hb SS
Unstable hemoglobins	
Doubly heterozygous conditions	SC, SD, Hb S−thalassemia, Hb C−thalassemia
Thalassemia	See Chap. 15
Hereditary persistence of fetal hemoglobin	See Chap. 15
Aplastic anemia	Some cases
Leukemia	Some cases
Pregnancy	Some cases

PROCEDURE. The following recommended NCCLS procedure[65] should be performed at room temperature.

1. Prepare hemolysate (as described in the section on hemoglobin electrophoretic procedures) using water and toluene.
2. Determine hemolysate Hb concentration using standard cyanmethemoglobin method (Chap. 9). Acceptable concentration is 8 to 12 g/dL.
3. Based on the Hb concentration of the hemolysate, calculate the amount of hemolysate to be added to 10 mL of cyanmethemoglobin reagent to make an approximately 0.5 g/dL solution. If hemolysate Hb concentration is 8.0 g/dL, add 0.6 mL hemolysate to reagent. For each additional Hb 1 g/dL, decrease the amount of hemolysate added by 0.05 mL. For example, for hemolysate Hb of 12.0 g/dL, add 0.4 mL hemolysate to 10 mL reagent.
4. Pipette 3.0 mL diluted hemolysate into each of three 17 × 100-mm tubes, two labeled *Test* and one labeled *Total*.
5. At 15- or 30-second intervals, timed with a stopwatch, add 0.2 mL of sodium hydroxide reagent to each tube labeled *Test*. Mix well with vortex mixer.
6. Add 0.2 mL water to tube labeled *Total*.
7. Exactly 2 minutes after adding sodium hydroxide, add 2.0 mL saturated ammonium sulfate reagent to each tube (both tubes labeled *Test* and tube labeled *Total*).
8. After 5 minutes, filter contents of all three tubes through two layers of Whatman 42 (or 1) 7-cm filter paper folded into 5-cm short-stemmed funnels. Collect filtrates into clean, properly labeled tubes. Filtrates must be absolutely clear.
9. Prepare a blanking solution by mixing 3.0 mL cyanmethemoglobin reagent with 0.2 mL sodium hydroxide reagent and 2.0 mL ammonium sulfate reagent. Filter through two layers of filter paper as described for patient samples. Blank spectrophotometer at 540 nm.
10. Pipette 1 mL filtrate labeled *Total* into 4 mL distilled water; label *Diluted Total*.
11. Measure absorbance (A) at 540 nm of the two test filtrates and of the diluted total.
12. Calculate fraction of Hb F as a percentage:

$$\text{Hb F}(\%) = \frac{A_{\text{test}}}{A_{\text{diluted total}} \times 5} \times 100$$

(A = absorbance; 5 is the additional dilution factor).

REFERENCE RANGE. After 1 year of age, the reference range is about 1%.[3] Each laboratory should determine its own population reference range.

COMMENTS AND SOURCES OF ERROR. Difference between duplicate tests for each specimen must not exceed 0.5% Hb F for values less than 5%; 1% Hb F for values 5% to 15%; or 2% Hb F for values greater than 15%.[65]

Other acceptable methods exist for use with small samples, such as that described by Singer and coworkers[81] or the NCCLS.[65]

Possible sources of error in this procedure are poor technique (*e.g.*, of pipetting and mixing); allowing more or less than 2 minutes reaction time; spectrophotometric errors (Chap. 9); filtrate turbidity; using outdated reagents or incorrect reagent concentrations; and using poor-quality filter paper.

SYSTEMATIC LABORATORY DIAGNOSIS OF HEMOGLOBINOPATHIES

Figure 14-4 provides a basic systematic flow chart of laboratory testing for the hemoglobinopathies. The chart begins with electrophoresis on cellulose acetate and the test sequence thereafter is based on the preliminary results on cellulose acetate. This chart is also useful in selecting appropriate test procedures for differentiating thalassemia from hemoglobinopathies.

VARIANTS CAUSED BY β-CHAIN SUBSTITUTIONS

The β-globin chain amino acid substitutions are the most common cause of hemoglobinopathies (Table 14-5). The best known are single substitutions and include Hbs S, C, D-Los Angeles, and E. Each affects millions of people worldwide.

Sickle Cell Anemia

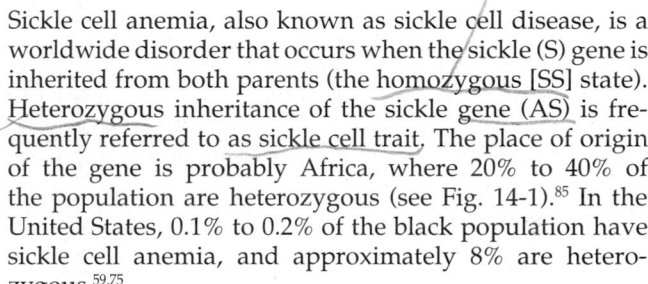

DEMOGRAPHICS AND GENETICS

Sickle cell anemia, also known as sickle cell disease, is a worldwide disorder that occurs when the sickle (S) gene is inherited from both parents (the homozygous [SS] state). Heterozygous inheritance of the sickle gene (AS) is frequently referred to as sickle cell trait. The place of origin of the gene is probably Africa, where 20% to 40% of the population are heterozygous (see Fig. 14-1).[85] In the United States, 0.1% to 0.2% of the black population have sickle cell anemia, and approximately 8% are heterozygous.[59,75]

Hb S results from a point mutation for the sixth amino acid in the β-chain in which one nucleotide base is substituted for another (GAG becomes GUG). As a result, valine is substituted for glutamic acid (see Table 14-2). Otherwise, Hb S is structurally the same as Hb A. Researchers have proposed that the Hb S gene mutation has provided resistance, but not immunity, from the malarial parasite *Plasmodium falciparum*, which is transmitted by mosquitoes.[2] When a red cell containing *P. falciparum* undergoes the sickling process, the parasite dies.[31] Geographic areas where *P. falciparum* is found coincide closely with areas where large numbers of persons carry the Hb S gene (*e.g.*, Africa).[38] The molecular events resulting from the Hb S mutation include production of intramolecular hydrophobic bonds in Hb, which are responsible for the insoluble characteristics of Hb S. The amino acid substitution causes a loss of negatively charged ions on the molecule. Thus Hb S migrates slower than Hb A toward the positive pole in electrophoresis at alkaline pH (see Fig. 14-3).

PATHOPHYSIOLOGY

When oxygenated, Hb S is fully soluble. Sickling occurs when oxygen decreases at the tissue level. When oxygen is released from the Hb molecule, a conformational change occurs, which results in polymerization of the Hb molecule and leads to the formation of tactoids or crystals, which cause the cell to become rigid (Fig. 14-5). Sickle cells impede blood flow to tissues and organs, resulting in tissue death, organ infarction, and pain.

Hemolysis is common. Sickled red cells are prematurely destroyed by the phagocytic system (extravascular hemolysis), especially the spleen, and by their inability to traverse the microcirculation (intravascular hemolysis).

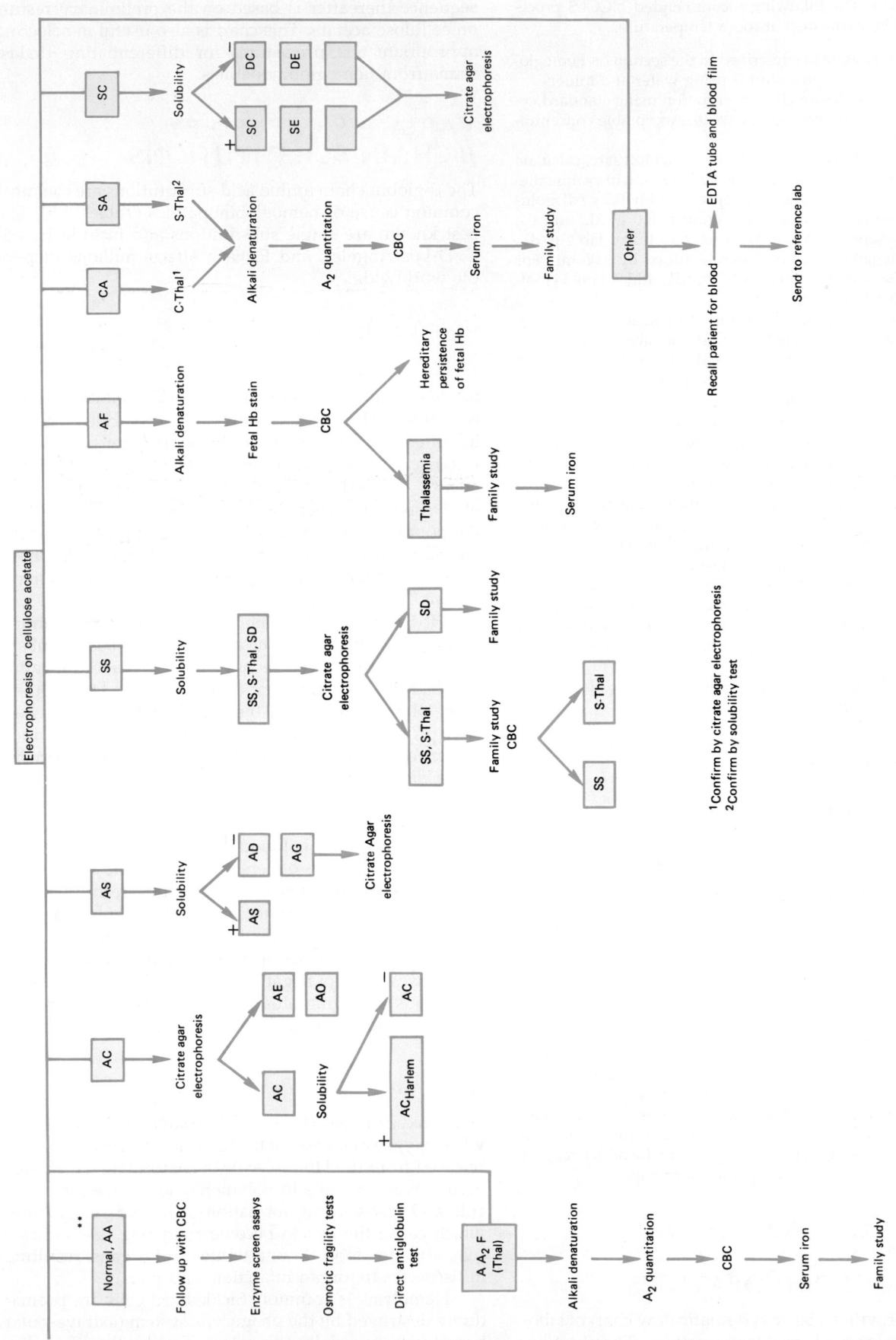

FIGURE 14-4. Flowchart for laboratory diagnosis of hemoglobinopathies.

*Does not include cord blood specimens
**If clinically indicated

¹Confirm by citrate agar electrophoresis
²Confirm by solubility test

202

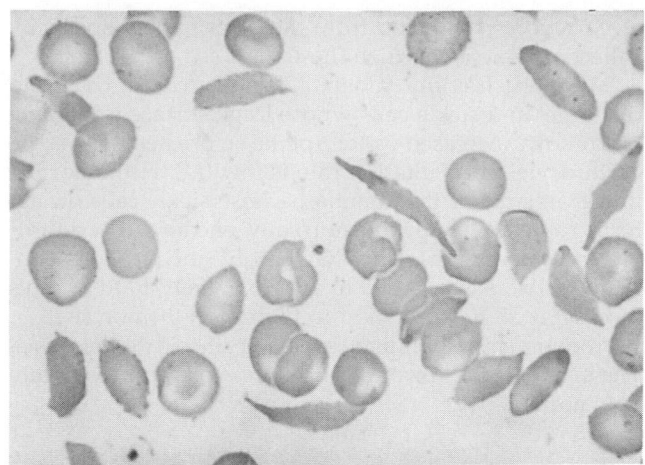

FIGURE 14-5. Peripheral blood film from patient with Hb SS, sickle cell anemia.

The bone marrow responds by increasing erythropoiesis. As a result, the marrow spaces widen and the bone cortex thins. Extramedullary hematopoiesis (*e.g.*, in the liver) may be observed in severe cases.

SYMPTOMS AND SICKLE CELL CRISES

Among sickle cell anemia patients aged 10 through 20 years, growth and sexual maturation generally lag behind that of normal adolescents. Symptoms can be severe. Every organ in the body is affected, and symptoms include pain of many types. Chronic hemolysis causes fatigue, weakness, pallor, and other symptoms of anemia. Many symptoms are associated with sickle cell crises.

Painful sickle cell crises occur in patients of all ages. Any situation that produces excessive deoxygenation of the red cells may cause a crisis (*e.g.*, infection, dehydration, violent exercise, obstetric delivery, and high altitude [flying in unpressurized aircraft]). Low-grade fever is often found in association with crises.

Vasoocclusive crises occur when rigid sickle cells increase blood viscosity. Sickle cells are associated with development of microthrombi, vascular occlusions, and microinfarctions in the joints and extremities as well as in major organs, which can cause organ failure.

Infectious crises are a primary cause of death in sickle cell anemia.[52] *Streptococcus pneumoniae* is the major infectious agent among children. This may be partially attributed to abnormal splenic function.[80] Susceptibility to infection is also caused by depression of immune function.[32]

The first sites affected by decreased blood flow are frequently the small bones of the hands and feet at age 6 to 9 months. The condition is referred to as hand–foot syndrome or dactylitis. Affected patients experience painful swelling of the backs of the hands and feet. This swelling may be the first sign of sickle cell anemia. Infarctions of the small bones may cause fingers to grow to varying lengths. During puberty, affected sites include the femurs and humeri. The abnormally thin bone cortex is especially vulnerable to wearing and fracture.

In *bone, joint and other crises*, pain may occur in the joints of arms and legs where sickle cells accumulate, in shafts of bones as sickle cells occlude the bone marrow

sinusoids, and in the lungs, which are the site of frequent infarcts in adults owing to sickle cell accumulation. Pulmonary infarcts can lead to severe chest or abdominal pain.

Splenic sequestration crises occur when sickle cells become trapped in the splenic microcirculation. The spleen enlarges as more cells are trapped, leading to hypovolemia (decreased blood volume), which may cause shock and even death. This usually occurs in children before the age of 6 years.

Aplastic crises are thought to be caused by infection and fever. They result in a temporary (usually 5 to 10 days), but significant, reduction in erythrocyte count, Hb, Hct, reticulocyte count, and bone marrow erythroblasts. Leukocytes and platelets may or may not be affected.

ORGANS AFFECTED BY SICKLE CELL ANEMIA

Liver and Spleen. Sickle cell sequestration in the liver sinusoids may cause hepatomegaly and liver malfunction in children and adults. It can also result in jaundice and hyperbilirubinemia. Splenomegaly and abnormal splenic function may begin in early infancy (after 6 months of age). Later in childhood, splenic infarction and fibrosis occur because of vascular occlusion. Eventually, the spleen atrophies and becomes nonfunctional. This is referred to as autosplenectomy. In contrast, patients with Hb S–thalassemia or Hb SC disease usually exhibit splenomegaly.

Kidneys. Infarcts may also occur in the kidneys, resulting in hematuria and failure of urine-concentrating ability.

Heart and Lungs. Iron deposition in the heart, mostly attributable to the frequent transfusions patients require, may lead to heart failure. Cardiomegaly may appear in early childhood. Infarctions in the lung tissue can occur because of infections and sickle cell occlusion.

Skin. An ulcer or scar on the leg, particularly the ankle, is common. It usually appears during adolescence.

Charache and colleagues[15] have published a valuable reference on management and therapy of sickle cell crises and organ involvement in sickle cell anemia.

LABORATORY FINDINGS

Peripheral Blood. Anemia is usually severe (Hb is 5 to 9 g/dL) and of the normocytic, normochromic type. It appears at about 6 to 9 months of age when the abnormal β-chains forming Hb S are first produced. Anisocytosis is common and the most important poikilocyte is the sickle cell (Fig. 14-5). Sickle cells must always be investigated and reported to the physician, even if they are seen only in an occasional microscopic field. Target cells usually are abundant. Ovalocytes and fragments (schistocytes) may also be seen. The red cell distribution width (RDW) is increased.

Cells that have transformed several times back and forth between the normal and sickle state generally become irreversibly sickled and appear as dense elliptocytes with areas where the Hb has pulled away from the cell membrane. Other findings include polychromasia, nucleated red cells (1 to 100 per 100 leukocytes), reticulocytosis (8.1% to 16.5%), and basophilic stippling. Howell-Jolly and Pappenheimer bodies indicate a nonfunctional spleen (autosplenectomy).

Leukocytosis (10 to 30 × 10^9/L) and neutrophilia are common. If infection is present, a left shift may occur, causing immature leukocytes to appear in the peripheral blood. Thrombocytosis is also common (mean 440 × 10^9/L).[30] This is due to the fibrotic spleen, which cannot pool one-third of the peripheral blood platelets as a normal spleen does. The megathrombocyte number is increased, especially during marrow infarcts.[17] During vasoocclusive crisis, total platelet and megathrombocyte numbers may decrease.[30]

Special Hematologic Tests. All patients with Hb S in their genotype (*e.g.*, Hb SS, AS, S–thalassemia, SC and SD) have a positive solubility screening test (see Fig. 14-2).

Hb electrophoresis is performed to confirm the presence of Hb S. Quantitative Hb electrophoresis results for Hb SS disease are shown in Table 14-9 in comparison with results found in other hemoglobinopathies. Quantitation of Hb S by densitometry reveals 80% to 90% Hb S. Hb F may be increased but usually by no more than 10%. Occasionally Hb F is as high as 20%. Hb A$_2$ is usually normal. If Hb A$_2$ or Hb F is increased, the possibility of a thalassemic condition interacting with Hb S should be investigated. Hb F should be quantitated by alkali denaturation and Hb A$_2$ by ion-exchange microchromatography (Chap. 15).

Hbs D-Los Angeles (also called D-Punjab), G-Philadelphia, and Q-India all migrate in the same position as Hb S on cellulose acetate (pH 8.4; see Fig. 14-3). Citrate agar electrophoresis (pH 6.0) helps separate Hb S from these other Hbs.

Diagnosis of sickle cell anemia in a fetus may be made as early as the second trimester of pregnancy by electrophoresis of blood from the placenta, but specimen collection may jeopardize the fetus.

Osmotic fragility (Chap. 17) is decreased, owing to the target and sickle cells whose large surface to volume ratio allows increased water uptake before hemolysis. The erythrocyte sedimentation rate is low (*i.e.*, in the normal range) in spite of the anemia because sickle cells do not form rouleaux (rouleaux normally encourages erythrocyte sedimentation). The ^{51}Cr half-life of red cells containing Hb S is shortened to approximately 10 to 20 days (normal is 28 days), owing to their early hemolysis.

Bone marrow biopsy reveals erythroid hyperplasia. The myeloid to erythroid (M:E) cell ratio is approximately 1:1 (normal, 3:1).

Chemistry. The generally increased values of lactate dehydrogenase, unconjugated (indirect) bilirubin, and urobilinogen, and the decreased serum haptoglobin level, all reflect the hemolytic component of sickle cell disease.

EFFECTS OF TREATMENT ON LABORATORY RESULTS

The primary goal of treatment is prevention of crises by avoiding situations that precipitate them. If a crisis does occur, the patient is hydrated, pain is alleviated with analgesics such as aspirin, and infection is treated with appropriate antibiotics. Patients are kept warm, because exposure to cold may precipitate a crisis. Excessive sweating should be avoided because dehydration precipitates a crisis. Response to treatment may be crudely indicated on the blood film by a decrease in the number of sickle cells. Transfusions may be required when physical signs and symptoms warrant, although patients usually tolerate a Hb value as low as 6.5 g/dL.[14]

Patients whose quality of life is poor may need repeated packed cell transfusions to maintain the Hb S level below 30%. After a cerebrovascular accident (*e.g.*, brain

---

TABLE 14-9
Results of Cellulose Acetate Electrophoresis (pH 8.6) for Major Hemoglobinopathies

Hemoglobinopathy	Hemoglobins*						Degree of Clinical Abnormality†
	A (%)	F (%)	S (%)	C (%)	D (%)	E (%)	
Hb CC		1–7		>90			Mild
Hb AC	50–60	<2		40–50			None
Hb SC		1–7	50	50			Moderate to severe
Hb SS		1–10	80–90				Severe
Hb AS	55–70	<2	30–45				None or mild
Hb DD		<2			95		None
Hb AD	50–65	<2			35–50		None
Hb EE		1–5				95	Mild
Hb AE	60–80					20–40	None

* These are general figures to allow comparison of major differences in the percentages of hemoglobin in the various disorders. Patients diagnosed with one of these conditions may have percentages slightly different from those shown. The numbers do not add up to 100 in some cases because there are approximations and also because Hb A$_2$ (%), which may account for a small amount of the total hemoglobin in some disorders, is not shown in the table.
† Indicates whether patients experience any clinical signs or symptoms of illness.

hemorrhage leading to a stroke), transfusions must be continued for several years to prevent another stroke.[14] Preoperatively, transfusions are required to raise the Hb A level to more than 50% with a Hct of 0.30 to 0.35 L/L.[24]

Many substances have been tested as antisickling agents, but none has proved to be totally satisfactory, and research in this area is ongoing.[1] Cyanate has been used successfully for treatment by *in vitro* exposure of erythrocytes to cyanate, after which they are reinfused into the patient. This treatment increases the Hb level and red cell survival time without causing toxic side effects.[49] Urea has also been studied because it is believed to prevent or reverse gelation of sickle cells. However, its benefit has not been proven.[1]

Nitrogen mustard is too toxic to administer *in vivo*; however, it may be useful in the treatment of red cells *in vitro* for reinfusion to prevent sickling.[15,72] Clinical trials are needed to prove or disprove its benefits.

Additional substances currently under long-term investigation fall into the category of cell membrane modifiers. They include zinc,[69] procaine hydrochloride,[67] cetiedil and piracetam.[1] Further studies are needed to evaluate all these agents.

One report on treatment of children with sickle cell anemia states that no chemical compound has satisfactorily met the criteria of efficiency, safety, and dependability and that pain control must still be provided.[79]

Bone marrow transplantation may be an alternative for selected patients.[46] However, it is difficult to find a matching marrow donor, and the problems of graft-versus-host disease cause significant rates of morbidity and mortality. If these problems can be overcome in the future, this treatment may be a viable alternative in special cases for whom there are virtually no other treatment choices.

PROGNOSIS

In the past, sickle cell anemia caused a shortened life span. As a result of genetic counseling of partners who carry the sickle gene, prenatal diagnosis, and education in the prevention of crises and in proper nutrition, life expectancy and quality of life have been improved to the point where some patients live a relatively normal and relatively long life.

The finding of Howell-Jolly bodies or pits or vacuoles in red cells on careful observation of the blood film may be an early indication of immunodeficiency.[71] Prophylactic penicillin and vaccines are helping to prevent infections and reduce deaths.

Training parents to palpate the abdomen to monitor spleen size allows early detection of acute splenic sequestration crises and prevention of death owing to hypovolemic shock.

Sickle Cell Trait

DEFINITION AND DEMOGRAPHICS

Sickle cell trait is the heterozygous (AS) state of sickle cell disease. The nomenclature for Hb S in sickle cell trait is $\alpha_2\beta_1\beta_2^{6Glu\rightarrow Val}$. Because Hb A is present in higher percentages than Hb S, Hb A compensates for Hb S, and

these patients usually have no symptoms. The disorder may go undetected, but patients may experience the painful crises described for Hb SS if they encounter situations that cause extreme tissue hypoxia, such as those caused by severe respiratory infection or exposure to extreme cold.

Among American blacks, the incidence of sickle cell trait is approximately 8%.[59,75] In some African tribes, the incidence is much higher. It is found in the same geographic areas as sickle cell anemia.

LABORATORY FINDINGS

Table 14-10 summarizes the differential laboratory and clinical features of Hb SS and Hb AS.

Peripheral Blood. Anemia is generally not present. Red cell morphology is usually normal, with the possible exception of a few target cells and an occasional sickle cell.

Special Hematologic Tests. The solubility test is positive. Results of Hb electrophoresis for heterozygous patients are shown in Tables 14-9 and 14-10. Hb A levels should always be higher than Hb S in sickle cell trait.

Urinalysis. On rare occasions, hematuria may be present. In occasional patients, the kidneys may fail to concentrate urine, causing hyposthenuria.

PROGNOSIS

Patients have a normal life span and quality of life. Treatment is rarely required.

TABLE 14-10

Differential Laboratory and Clinical Features of Hb SS and Hb AS Compared with the Normal Adult

Feature	Hb SS	Hb AS	Normal Adult
Anemia	+++	−/+	—
Anemia classification*	N/N	N/N	—
Hb S (%)†	80–95	20–40	0
Hb A (%)†	0	60–80	97
Hb F (%)†	0.5–10	<2	<2
Hb A₂ (%)†	2.0–3.5	2.0–3.5	2.0–3.5
Solubility test for sickling Hb	+	+	—
Peripheral blood sickle cells	++	+/−	—
β/α-Chains	1/1	1/1	1/1
Splenomegaly	−	−/+	—
Painful crises	+++	−/+	—
Hematuria	+	Rare	—
Hemolytic episodes	++	−/+	—

* *N/N, normocytic, normochromic.*
† *Percentages are based on cellulose acetate electrophoresis (alkaline pH). The percentages given are general guidelines. In reality, the results associated with any given case may vary from these ranges.*

Hb S–Thalassemia

Hb S–thalassemia is a doubly heterozygous condition in which the mutant genes for both Hb S and thalassemia are inherited by a single individual. This condition is discussed in Chapter 15.

Hb C Disease

The abnormal variant Hb C results from an amino acid substitution of lysine for glutamic acid at position 6 of the β-chain. This is technically written as $\beta^{6Glu\rightarrow Lys}$. Persons may be homozygous (Hb CC) or heterozygous (Hb AC) for this variant.

Hb CC tends to crystallize when dehydrated (hence, the name crystal Hb or Hb C). The cells most vulnerable to intracellular crystallization are older erythrocytes (approaching 120 days of age) because they tend to lose water as they age. Thus, older red cells containing Hb C are more rigid than normal cells. Fragmentation may occur in the microcirculation, resulting in the production of microspherocytes. Hb C crystals are also produced in the microcirculation and are removed by the spleen. If the spleen is defective or nonfunctional, Hb C crystals are seen on the peripheral blood film (Fig. 14-6).

Hb C is the second most common Hb variant after Hb S in the United States. It is associated with the black race and is found mostly in Africa (Fig. 14-1). Homozygous Hb CC disease is estimated to affect 22 of every 100,000 American blacks.[59]

Persons with Hb CC disease commonly exhibit splenomegaly, which may cause abdominal pain. Hb CC, however, does not generally cause any other clinical abnormalities, and many patients have no symptoms, even though they may have mild hemolytic anemia.

LABORATORY FINDINGS

Peripheral Blood. There is a mild to moderate normocytic, normochromic anemia with numerous (40% to 90%) tar-

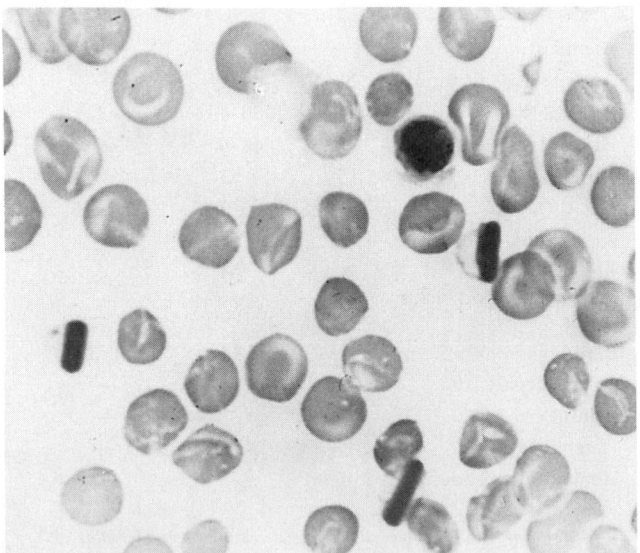

FIGURE 14-6. Peripheral blood film showing Hb C crystals and prominent target cells.

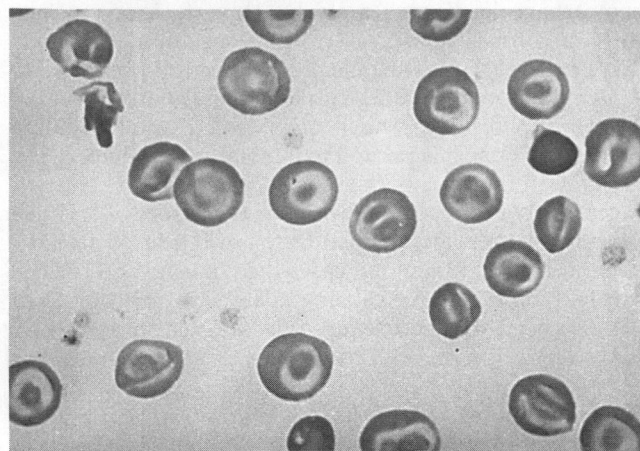

FIGURE 14-7. Peripheral blood film from patient with Hb SC disease. Note SC crystal in *upper left corner* of field. Prominent target cells and characteristic "pocketbook" cells are also present.

get cells and a few spherocytes (Fig. 14-6). Hexagonal or rod-shaped crystals may occasionally be observed on the blood film, especially after splenectomy. These crystals are usually intracellular, elongated, and have parallel sides with both ends blunt. Hb CC crystals are significantly different from Hb SC crystals (Figs. 8-20 and 14-7). The Hb concentration ranges from 8 to 12 g/dL. The reticulocyte level is usually between 4% and 8%. Some patients do not experience anemia. The MCV and MCH are normal; MCHC is increased.

Red cell survival is decreased,[45] an effect attributed to early destruction by the spleen of red cells containing rigid Hb C crystals.

Special Hematologic Tests. Hb electrophoresis results for Hb CC disease are shown in Table 14-9. Characteristically, most Hb is Hb C; Hb F is increased in some instances and there is no Hb A. Hb C migrates with Hb A_2, E and O-Arab on cellulose acetate (alkaline pH). It may be separated from all three by citrate agar (acid pH), because Hb C migrates farther toward the anode (positive pole) than the other variants in this medium (Fig. 14-3). Column chromatography may also be used to separate and quantitate Hb C and Hb A_2 when both are present in one specimen.[41]

PROGNOSIS

Patients generally are asymptomatic and treatment is not required.

Hb C Trait (Hb AC)

Heterozygous Hb C (Hb AC) is found in about 3% of American blacks and is common in West Africans.[4] It produces no symptoms and no anemia. The red cells are slightly hypochromic, and approximately 40% are target cells. Results of Hb electrophoresis are shown in Table 14-9 and Figure 14-3. The percentage of Hb A is higher than that of Hb C. The presence of microspherocytes along with a smaller percentage of Hb C suggests the possible presence of Hb C–α-thalassemia.

Hb SC Disease

The incidence of Hb SC in American blacks is less than 1%, but it is one of the most common variants in Africa.[59] Persons who have Hb SC disease are said to be doubly heterozygous, because they inherited two Hb variants. Hb SC disease differs from Hb SS disease in that clinical symptoms are milder (although similar) and complications are fewer.

Significant symptoms first occur during the teenage years, including anemia and joint, abdominal, and skeletal pain caused by sickle cell vasoocclusion. Splenomegaly occurs in childhood and continues into adulthood, in contrast to the pattern in sickle cell anemia. In some cases, aseptic necrosis of the head of the femur can cause lameness. Diseases of the retina may result from blood viscosity that is higher than in sickle cell anemia. The concentration of sickle cells is higher in Hb SC than in sickle cell anemia because the Hct is higher in Hb SC than Hb SS disease. The resulting high blood viscosity can cause death.

LABORATORY FINDINGS

Peripheral Blood. Anemia may or may not be present. When present, it is usually mild and classified as normocytic, normochromic. Target cells generally are present (Fig. 14-7). In addition, folded, so-called pocketbook cells characteristic of Hb SC, an occasional spherocyte, and rare sickle cells may be found (Fig. 14-7). Hb SC crystals, which have fingerlike projections ("Washington monument" projections) and usually protrude outside the cell membrane, can be found with careful searching (see Fig. 14-7 and Fig. 8-20).

Special Hematologic Tests. Results of the solubility test are positive. Hb electrophoresis on cellulose acetate (alkaline pH) reveals about equal amounts of Hb S and Hb C (Table 14-9). Hb F ranges from normal to 7%, and no Hb A is produced, for no normal β-chains are produced.[66]

TREATMENT AND PROGNOSIS

Therapy for Hb SC disease is similar to that for Hb S disease when crises occur. One of the most critical periods is pregnancy owing to the high blood viscosity and possibility of sickle crises. During childbirth, patients receive sodium bicarbonate to avoid acidosis. After childbirth, the mother may receive heparin to prevent the formation of thrombi.[50]

The life span of the patient with Hb SC is normal. All patients are encouraged to have their retinas examined regularly for lesions, which can be detected early, before major damage or vision loss occurs.

Hb D

There are at least six β-chain variants and one α-chain variant classified as Hb D that migrate in the same position as Hb S on cellulose acetate (alkaline pH), but do not cause sickling.[54] Both homozygous (Hb DD) and heterozygous (Hb AD) conditions have been reported. Hb D may also be found in combination with Hb S or thalassemia. Many variants are named for the place where

they were discovered, such as Hb D-Los Angeles (also known as Hb D-Punjab) in which glycine (Gln) is substituted for glutamic acid (Glu) in position 121 of the β-chain ($\alpha_2\beta_2^{121Glu\rightarrow Gln}$).

Hb D-Punjab is found principally in Pakistan and northwest India (Fig. 14-1). The frequency in India is estimated to be 3%.[50] Hb D-Los Angeles is probably the most common Hb D variant in the United States. In general, Hb D is rare.

No clinical abnormalities are associated with the heterozygous state. Homozygous Hb D often is associated with splenomegaly, but patients are otherwise clinically normal.

LABORATORY FINDINGS

Peripheral Blood. Homozygous Hb D disease usually is associated with mild hemolytic anemia and concomitant decreases in red cell parameters. Indices are normal, but numerous flat target cells are seen on the blood film. The heterozygous state is not associated with hematologic abnormalities.

Special Hematologic Tests. In the homozygous state, cellulose acetate electrophoresis (alkaline pH) reveals 95% Hb D, which migrates in the same position as Hb S, and normal Hb A_2 and F. In the heterozygous state, there is less than 50% Hb D (the remainder being Hbs A, A_2, and F; see Table 14-9). On citrate agar electrophoresis (acid pH), Hb D migrates toward the cathode in the same position as Hbs A and A_2 whereas Hb S migrates toward the anode (Fig. 14-3). Results of the solubility test are negative in either state.

Hb SD

Hb SD is a doubly heterozygous condition. Hb S has been found in association with at least 9 of the 16 Hb D and Hb G variants (Hb G migrates with S and D on cellulose acetate [alkaline pH] and includes both α- and β-chain variants).[56] Only Hb SD-Los Angeles produces a clinical abnormality, a condition similar to mild sickle cell anemia.

Citrate agar electrophoresis is the definitive test for separation and verification of Hbs S, D, and G. Results of the solubility test are positive, but the citrate agar electrophoresis results separate Hb S from Hb D and Hb G (Fig. 14-3).

Hb E

Hb E is a β-chain variant in which lysine is substituted for glutamic acid in position 26 ($\alpha_2\beta_2^{26Glu\rightarrow Lys}$). Both homozygous (Hb EE) and heterozygous (Hb AE) states exist.

Hb E is the second most common abnormal Hb variant in the world, affecting an estimated 30 million people.[27,29] It occurs with the greatest frequency in Southeast Asia (Fig. 14-1), and has also been reported in American blacks.[50] Hb E frequently occurs in combination with β-thalassemia, causing a condition clinically similar to β-thalassemia major.

Neither Hb EE nor Hb AE is associated with clinical abnormalities, except possibly splenomegaly associated with the homozygous state.

LABORATORY FINDINGS

Peripheral Blood. Laboratory findings for Hb E disorders are similar to those described for Hb D disorders. Hb EE disease causes mild microcytic, normochromic hemolytic anemia. Red cell survival time is slightly decreased. Hb E is unstable. There are usually many target cells on the peripheral blood film.

Heterozygous Hb E may cause an elevated red cell count and target cells. Red cell survival is normal, and patients are not anemic.

Special Hematologic Tests. Hbs E, C, O-Arab and A_2 migrate closely on cellulose acetate (alkaline pH), although Hb E migrates slightly faster than C and A_2 (Fig. 14-3). Typically, in homozygous persons, Hb E represents 92% to 98% of the Hb, and the amount of Hb F is normal or slightly increased (see Table 14-9). Hb E may be differentiated from Hb C and O-Arab on citrate agar electrophoresis at acid pH, for Hb E migrates with Hb A on this medium (Fig. 14-3). Hbs that migrate with Hb A_2 on cellulose acetate at alkaline pH must always be suspected when the Hb A_2 value estimated by densitometry is greater than 10%. Hb A_2 rarely exceeds 10%, even when it is elevated in thalassemias.

In the heterozygous state (Hb AE), the concentration of Hb E is usually near 20% to 40%. This is high enough to indicate that there is a variant in the Hb A_2 position, but lower than the 40% to 50% found more frequently in the heterozygous Hb C state (Hb AC). This may be because Hb E is unstable, a certain amount may be lost during specimen processing for electrophoresis.

Hb O-Arab

Hb O-Arab is a β-chain variant caused by the same type of substitution as in Hb C: glutamic acid is replaced by lysine—but the substitution point is amino acid 121 instead of 6 ($\alpha_2\beta_2^{121Glu\rightarrow Lys}$).

Hb O-Arab is rare. It is found in Israel, Bulgaria, Egypt, Rumania, Jamaica, Kenya and in 0.4% of black Americans. Persons with Hb O-Arab are clinically normal, except for some homozygous persons who have splenomegaly. Heterozygotes are asymptomatic. If Hb O-Arab is inherited in conjunction with Hb S, a severe clinical condition results that is similar to that seen with Hb SS.

Homozygotes (HbOO) demonstrate a mild hemolytic anemia with many target cells. Because Hb O-Arab migrates with Hbs A_2, C, and E on cellulose acetate, citrate agar electrophoresis is required for the differential diagnosis because only Hb O-Arab moves just slightly away from the point of application toward the cathode on this medium (Fig. 14-3).

MULTIPLE AMINO ACID SUBSTITUTIONS

Hb C-Harlem

Hb C-Harlem (also known as Hb C-Georgetown) is a β-chain variant caused by two amino acid substitutions. One occurs at amino acid 6 and is identical with the Hb S substitution. The other occurs at position 73, where aspartic acid is replaced by asparagine ($\alpha_2\beta_2^{6Glu\rightarrow Val;73 Asp\rightarrow Asn}$). Hb C-Harlem, Hb C-Ziguinchor and Hb S-Travis are among the few Hbs that cause a positive solubility test owing to the same substitution as that for Hb S (in addition to another in the β-chain).

Hb C-Harlem is rare and occurs in both homozygous and heterozygous states. Double heterozygosity for Hbs S and C-Harlem is also possible.

The clinical picture for homozygotic persons is unclear, because few have been identified.[6] Heterozygotes are asymptomatic. Patients with Hb SC-Harlem have a clinical picture similar to that of Hb SC disease.

Results of the solubility test are positive in the presence of Hb C-Harlem in any genetic state. On cellulose acetate (alkaline pH), there is a band in the Hb C position. On citrate agar, Hb C-Harlem migrates with Hb S (Fig. 14-3).

α-CHAIN SUBSTITUTIONS

Hb G-Philadelphia

Hb G-Philadelphia is the only α-chain variant of significance in the United States. It results from the replacement of asparagine by lysine in position 68 of the α-chain ($\alpha_2^{68Asn\rightarrow Lys}\beta_2$). It is found among West Africans and is the third most common variant among American blacks after Hbs S and C.[75]

The homozygous form of this disorder is not compatible with life, because the condition prevents production of normal α-chains necessary for production of oxygen-carrying Hb. Heterozygotes are asymptomatic.

Hb G-Philadelphia migrates on cellulose acetate (ranging from 25% to 40%) in the Hb S position (Fig. 14-3), but results of the solubility test are negative. Citrate agar provides further evidence that the variant is not Hb S because Hb G-Philadelphia migrates with Hb A. Globin chain electrophoresis is important for confirmation, because at alkaline pH, the abnormal α-chain moves farther toward the cathode than most other Hbs. In addition, these patients have both normal and abnormal forms of Hbs A_2 and F. The abnormal variants result from the abnormal α-chains produced. Typically, the abnormal Hb A_2, known as Hb G_2, migrates as a minor, faint band toward the cathode (*i.e.*, backward from the point of application, in the opposite direction from all other Hbs on cellulose acetate [alkaline pH]). It is identified by using an *o*-toluidine or *o*-dianisidine counterstaining procedure (see under the cellulose acetate Hb electrophoresis procedure) that takes only a few minutes.

OTHER VARIANTS

Hb I

The Hb I variant is rare. It affects either the α- or β-chain at various positions; usually lysine is replaced by glutamic acid. Hb I migrates between Hb Barts and Hb H, all of which migrate farther toward the anode than Hb A on cellulose acetate (alkaline pH) (Fig. 14-3). Hb I and Hb H are best differentiated on cellulose acetate electrophoresis at pH 7.0, at which Hb H migrates but Hb I does not.[74,77] Hb I, when present, constitutes approximately 25% of the total Hb.

Hb Barts and Hb H

These two variants are found in patients with α-thalassemia who produce fewer α-chains than normal. Hb Barts occurs in the newborn infant and consists of four γ-chains. Hb Barts is replaced gradually during the first months of life by Hb H (as γ-chain production switches normally to β-chain production). Hb H consists of four normal β-chains. Both variants migrate farther toward the anode than Hb A on cellulose acetate (alkaline pH) (Fig. 14-3).

AMINO ACID DELETION
Hb Gun Hill

Hb Gun Hill has a deletion of five β-chain amino acids (β 91 to 95). The Hb structure is altered so that no heme can bind to the β-chain at the normal point of contact between heme and globin. This is caused by unequal crossing-over between the β-chain genes and production of two β-chains of unequal length.[10] The result is an unstable Hb, which produces mild hemolytic anemia. On cellulose acetate (alkaline pH) Hb Gun Hill migrates close to the Hb A_2 position. On citrate agar, it migrates with Hb A or between Hb A and Hb S.

ELONGATION OF THE POLYPEPTIDE CHAIN
Hb Constant Spring

Hb Constant Spring or Hb CS (not to be confused with the doubly heterozygous Hb SC disease) has an elongated α-chain. Thirty-one amino acids are added to the end of the chain. This is caused by replacement of a terminator codon, which normally stops amino acid addition, with a codon for glutamine, which results in the addition of 31 amino acids before another terminator codon is reached. Because the α-chain is affected, the clinical picture resembles α-thalassemia.[10] Often, Hb CS is inherited in a double heterozygous condition (Hb H Constant Spring) (Chap. 15).

Hb CS is prevalent among Greeks and Chinese. Homozygotes have mild microcytic, hemolytic anemia and 3% to 5% Hb CS. On cellulose acetate (alkaline pH), Hb CS migrates slower than Hb A_2. To rule out the possibility of a nonheme protein migrating in this position, the cellulose acetate should be counterstained for a few minutes with o-toludine or o-dianisidine (see cellulose acetate Hb electrophoresis procedure). Hb CS stains purple; nonheme protein remains pink. Hb CS heterozygotes have little or no anemia, red cells are microcytic, and target cells may be observed.[20]

UNSTABLE HEMOGLOBIN DISEASE

Unstable Hb disease (congenital Heinz body hemolytic anemia) is very rare, although over 125 unstable variants have been identified.[55] The pattern of inheritance is autosomal dominant. Only heterozygotes exist; apparently homozygous fetuses do not survive. In addition to being unstable, some variants have other functional abnormalities, as shown in Table 14-11. Molecular abnormalities that result in Hb instability are frequently those that disrupt contact between heme and globin, alter amino acids involved in the interface between α- and β-chains, or significantly change the shape or structure of the globin molecule. Regardless of the abnormality, the result is denaturation and precipitation of globin chains. Precipitation of globin in erythrocytes leads to formation of Heinz bodies, which cling to the membrane and are removed as the cells pass through the spleen. This predisposes the cells to hemolysis.

Severity of disease depends on the variant. Clinical

TABLE 14-11
Examples of Unstable Hemoglobin Variants and Their Other Functional Abnormalities*

Variant	Decreased Oxygen Affinity	Increased Oxygen Affinity	Methemoglobin Formation	Degree of Hemolytic Disease
Caribbean	X			Moderate to mild
Hope	X			Moderate to mild
Seattle	X			Moderate to mild
Hammersmith	X			Severe
Köln		X		Moderately severe
Gun Hill		X		Moderate to mild
Freiburg			X	Moderate to mild
St. Louis			X	Moderately severe
Tübingen			X	Moderate to mild

* A complete list of the clinical classifications of unstable hemoglobins is available in reference 55.
From Lukens JN, Lee GR: Unstable hemoglobin disease. In Lee GR, Bithell TC, Foerster J et al (eds): Wintrobe's Clinical Hematology, 9th ed, pp 1055, 1057. Philadelphia, Lea & Febiger, 1993.

findings may be severe or moderate, but most commonly they are mild, or nonexistent. Hb Köln, the most commonly reported unstable Hb,[55] causes only a moderately severe hemolytic anemia which is improved by splenectomy.

Laboratory Findings

Peripheral Blood. The Hb ranges from less than 7 g/dL in the most severe forms to normal in some mild forms. Reticulocytosis is common, although it may or may not be adequate to compensate for the degree of red cell destruction. Usually, the MCHC is decreased, sometimes as low as 25 g/dL. This may be so because (1) unstable Hb is partially heme deficient; (2) some Hb is lost when Heinz bodies are removed by the spleen; or (3) the Hb in Heinz bodies is not measured by standard hemoglobinometry.[55]

The blood film reveals anisopoikilocytosis with some hypochromic cells, polychromatophilia, and basophilic stippling. Fragments and spherocytes may be seen in severe disease. Bite cells (keratocytes [see Fig. 17-6]) formed by splenic removal of Heinz bodies may also be seen.

Heinz bodies—a classic finding in this disorder—consist of denatured globin seen in red cells after supravital staining (Fig. 14-8A). They are not visible on Wright-stained blood films because they have the same charge as normal Hb. Usually Heinz bodies appear during hemolytic episodes or after splenectomy. One report asserts that the Heinz bodies of unstable Hb disease are larger and are found in younger cells than those associated with glucose-6-phosphate dehydrogenase (G6PD) deficiency (Chap. 17).[73]

Hemoglobin Electrophoresis. Routine Hb electrophoresis may or may not identify unstable Hbs. Some migrate with Hb A, some slower, and some faster. Hb Köln migrates slower than Hb A. On average, unstable Hbs that affect the β-chain represent 25% of the total Hb whereas those that affect the α-chain represent only about 12%.[55] Hbs A_2 and F may be increased in association with β-chain variants.

Special Hematologic Tests. The chromium-51 half-life (Chap. 16) of erythrocytes that contain unstable Hb correlates with the severity of disease (2 days in severe disease, 6 to 16 days in moderate disease, and 9 to 23 days in mild disease; normal ^{51}Cr half-life is approximately 28 days).[47] Increased oxygen affinity has been observed in at least 35 unstable variants and decreased affinity in at least 14.[54] Results of the heat denaturation test and isopropanol precipitation test are positive for almost all unstable Hbs, although the latter test is plagued with false-positive results. The only way to confirm unstable Hb is by peptide analysis, which is performed only in very specialized centers. This study is not necessary if the patient can be managed without knowing the exact identity of the unstable Hb.

Treatment and Prognosis

For patients with mild unstable Hb disorders, the aim of treatment is prevention of hemolytic crises. In some cases of moderately severe disease, splenectomy may be considered to reduce hemolysis. Splenectomy is not helpful in severe cases, apparently because the liver also phagocy-

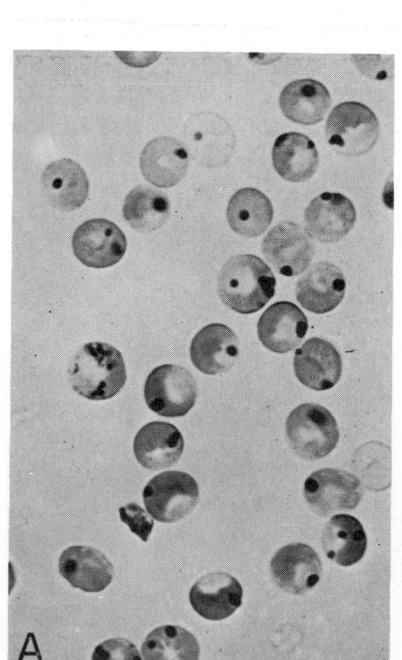
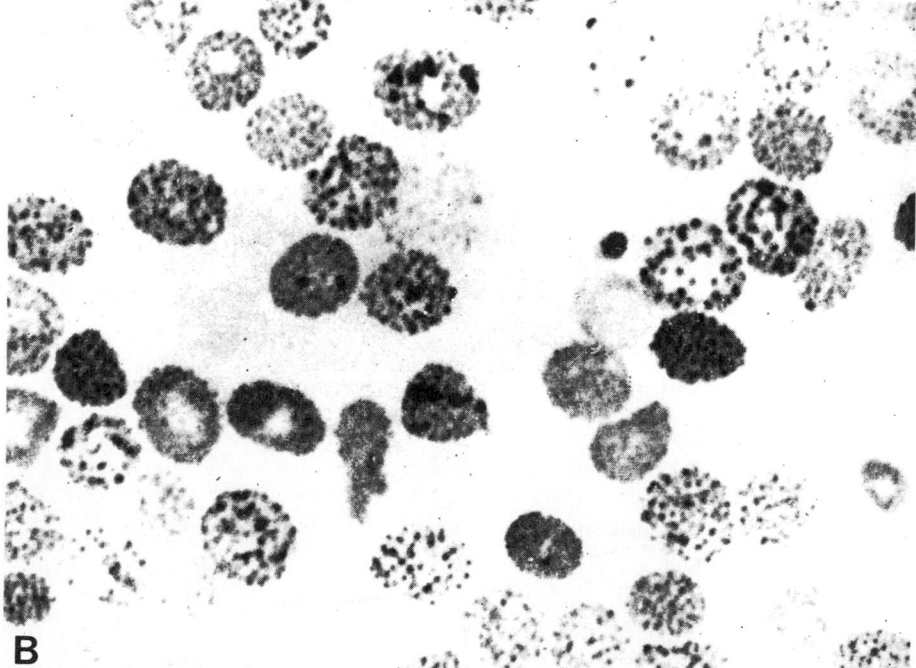

FIGURE 14-8. (**A**) Heinz bodies associated with unstable hemoglobin disease (crystal violet stain) (Reprinted by permission from Beutler E et al: Estimation of small percentages of hemoglobin. Nature 184:1877, ©1959 MacMillan Journals Limited.) (**B**) Hb H inclusion bodies from a patient with Hb H disease precipitated and stained with brilliant cresyl blue. (Reprinted by permission from Dittman WA et al: Hemoglobin H associated with an uncommon variant of thalassemia trait. Blood 15:975, 1960.)

tizes the severely damaged red cells.[48,84] Prognosis is still unclear, because unstable variants are rare.

MOST USEFUL LABORATORY TESTS FOR DIAGNOSING UNSTABLE HEMOGLOBINS

Many unstable Hbs are not detected by electrophoresis.[23] Tests specifically designed to detect unstable Hbs include the Heinz body-staining technique, the heat denaturation test, and the isopropanol precipitation test.

Heinz Body-Staining Technique

PRINCIPLE AND SPECIMEN REQUIREMENTS. Heinz bodies (Fig. 14-8*A* and see Fig. 8-26) result from denaturation and precipitation of unstable Hb. Denatured Hb precipitates in erythrocytes, forming small inclusion bodies that adhere to the membrane. These inclusions are visible in vitro after supravital staining,[12,13,21,28,68] but not on Wright-stained films. Formation of Heinz bodies may be induced in normal red cells by treating them with highly oxidative substances, such as acetylphenylhydrazine, and incubating them for a long period. Fresh whole blood anticoagulated with EDTA or heparin is required.

REAGENTS
1. **Saline, normal, 0.85%**
2. **Sodium citrate (Na$_3$C$_6$H$_5$O$_7$·2H$_2$O), 3 g/dL**: Add 3.0 g sodium citrate to distilled water up to 100 mL.
3. **Brilliant cresyl blue stain, 1 g/dL**: Mix 0.5 g brilliant cresyl blue (water soluble) in 40.0 mL normal saline and add 10.0 mL 3 g/dL sodium citrate solution.

QUALITY CONTROL. A negative control test should be run using a normal blood specimen drawn at the same time as the patient's specimen. A positive control test may be run if a specimen is available.

PROCEDURE
1. Label three 13- × 100-mm tubes: Patient, Negative control, and Positive control (if available).
2. Mix stain thoroughly before using and filter a small amount through Whatman 42 or 44 filter paper just before using it.
3. Mix whole blood and add 2 drops blood to 3 drops filtered stain in respective tubes and mix. Incubate at 37°C.
4. Make blood films from each tube after 20 minutes, 1 hour, and 2 hours.
5. Cover tubes and let stand overnight at room temperature. Make blood films at 24 hours.
6. Examine films from each time interval with oil immersion microscopy.

INTERPRETATION OF RESULTS. Heinz bodies, which may be single or multiple in any given cell, appear refractile (Fig. 14-8*A*). They may be round, oval, or serrated, and they stain pale blue with brilliant cresyl blue or deep purple with crystal violet. They vary from 1 to 4 μm and usually appear eccentrically, either near or attached to the cell periphery.

Normal, nonoxidized red cells should show no Heinz body formation, or at most, only rare Heinz bodies. Red cell populations that contain unstable Hb from splenectomized persons contain significant numbers of Heinz bodies that become visible early in the incubation process. Red cells with unstable Hb from patients who still have their spleen may have to be induced to form Heinz bodies by treating them with highly oxidative substances and long incubation.

COMMENTS AND SOURCES OF ERROR. Heinz bodies may not circulate in patients with unstable Hb unless the patient has been splenectomized.

Heinz bodies are not specific indicators of unstable Hb; red cell enzyme deficiencies (*e.g.*, G6PD) may also cause Heinz body formation if red cells are exposed to oxidant drugs (Chap. 17).

Heinz bodies and Hb H inclusions (Fig. 14-8*B*) are both stained with brilliant cresyl blue. Table 14-12 provides some clues to differentiating the two, although it is not always possible.

The isopropanol precipitation test or heat denaturation test should be run to confirm the results of a Heinz body screening test.

Heat Denaturation Test

PRINCIPLE. For the heat denaturation test,[37,51,60] washed red cells are hemolyzed with water, a phosphate buffer is added, and the mixture is allowed to incubate at 50°C for 3 hours. Many unstable Hbs are heat-sensitive and their partial denaturation causes the appearance of a flocculent precipitate within 1 hour of incubation, whereas normal blood shows little, if any, precipitate.

SPECIMEN. Use fresh whole blood anticoagulated with EDTA or heparin. A normal control blood sample should be collected at the same time as the patient's blood.

REAGENT. Phosphate buffer, pH 7.4: 0.1 mol/L NaH$_2$PO$_4$ (13.8 g NaH$_2$PO$_4$·2H$_2$O in 1 L distilled water); 0.1 mol/L Na$_2$HPO$_4$ (anhydrous) (14.2 g in 1 L distilled water). Add 19.2 mL 0.1 mol/L NaH$_2$PO$_4$ to 80.8 mL 0.1 mol/L Na$_2$HPO$_4$. Mix and let stand 10 minutes. Adjust pH if necessary.[1]

QUALITY CONTROL AND PROCEDURE
1. A normal blood sample serves as a negative control.
2. Add 1 mL patient blood and 1 mL control blood to separate 16- × 100-mm tubes.
3. Wash cells four times with 0.85% saline. Discard each supernatant wash. Add 5 mL distilled water to each tube and mix to lyse erythrocytes.
4. Add 5.0 mL phosphate buffer and mix. Centrifuge tubes at 3000 rpm for 10 minutes.
5. Transfer upper 2 mL clear supernatant from each tube to clean, labeled tube. Incubate at 50°C for 60 minutes.

TABLE 14-12

*General Distinguishing Features of the Hb H and Heinz Body Inclusions Stained Supravitally with Brilliant Cresyl Blue**

Feature	Heinz Bodies	Hb H Inclusions
Staining characteristics	Pale blue	Greenish blue
Number per cell	One or more	Multiple
Cell location	Eccentric	Cover the cell
Associated disorders	Unstable Hb, G6PD deficiency	Hb H

In some cases, the two may be indistinguishable because this is only a screening test. Refer to Figures 14-8A and B for photomicrographic comparison of the two inclusions and to Figure 8-28 for comparison of these inclusions to stained reticulocytes.

6. Record appearance of test and control solutions at 60 minutes.
7. Incubate for an additional 120 minutes and observe again.

INTERPRETATION OF RESULTS. Normal control should show little if any precipitation. Positive results are indicated by copious flocculent precipitate after 60 minutes and even greater precipitation after 3 hours.

COMMENTS AND SOURCES OF ERROR. If only a small amount (%) of abnormal Hb is present, or if it is relatively insensitive to heat, results may be negative.

Quantitative results may be obtained by running duplicate patient and control specimens, one of which is heated for each. The specimens are then centrifuged, and the supernate is read in a spectrophotometer. Calculation of the percentage of unstable Hb present in a sample based on absorbance (A) readings as follows[9, 22]:

$$\% \text{ Unstable Hb} = \frac{A_{(unheated)} - A_{(heated)}}{A_{(unheated)}} \times 100$$

Isopropanol Precipitation Test

PRINCIPLE. Only the principle of this test will be discussed. Please see the indicated reference for full details of this procedure.[11] Nonpolar solvents in a Hb solution cause the internal-bonding forces of the Hb molecule to weaken and the molecule's stability to decrease. Thus, in a 17% isopropanol solution incubated at 37°C, stability of normal Hb is borderline, and it begins to precipitate after approximately 40 minutes. The presence of an unstable Hb results in rapid precipitation, usually apparent within 5 minutes, and heavier flocculation after about a 20-minute incubation.

THE M HEMOGLOBINS

Seven Hb variants are designated as Hb M because they are associated with the presence of methemoglobin and congenital cyanosis. They include Hb M Boston, Hb M Iwate, Hb M Saskatoon, Hb M Hyde Park, Hb M Milwaukee, Hb M Osaka, and Hb M Fort Ripley.[53] The α-, β-, or γ-chains may be affected. Amino acid substitutions within the Hb M molecule prevent protection of iron from oxidation. Hence, Hb M contains iron in the ferric (Fe^{3+}) state (methemoglobin) and is incapable of carrying oxygen.

The pattern of inheritance is autosomal dominant. Hb M is found worldwide but is particularly prevalent in the Japanese. The homozygous state is apparently not compatible with life. Heterozygotes, however, live a relatively normal life.

Affected individuals have a lavender blue (cyanotic) skin color that can be differentiated from the blue-gray color of cyanotic heart disease. In some cases, the fingers are clubbed at birth. Cyanosis is usually observed during the first day of life of babies with the α-chain variants; cyanosis is transient during the first weeks of life for babies with the γ-chain variants; whereas infants with β-chain variants do not demonstrate cyanosis until after the third to sixth month of life (after the γ- to β-chain switch).

Laboratory Findings

The blood is characteristically brown. Some Hb M β-chain variants cause mild hemolytic anemia.[70] In addition,

methemoglobin causes globin chain precipitation, so Heinz bodies may be seen *in vitro*.

A pH of 7.1 is recommended for electrophoresis.[50] It is also recommended that all Hb in the specimen be oxidized to methemoglobin by adding potassium ferricyanide before performing electrophoresis. Doing so ensures that any migration differences observed are due to an amino acid substitution in the globin chains, rather than to differences in the iron states.[50] Hb M migrates slightly cathodal to (*i.e.*, slightly slower than) Hb A on cellulose acetate. Hb M accounts for 15% to 30% of the total Hb in Hb M γ-chain heterozygotes and 40% to 50% in Hb M β-chain heterozygotes.[53]

Spectrophotometric analysis of specimens is recommended for identification and quantitative analysis of Hb M.[50,53] Determining the absorption spectrum peaks of diluted hemolysates at various wavelengths and comparing them with the spectrum of normal hemolysates allows identification of Hb M variants.[25,26] Each variant has a unique absorption maximum and each is abnormal.[50] Ultimately, Hb M must be confirmed by globin chain amino acid studies, which usually are performed by specialized laboratories.

Treatment and Prognosis

Treatment generally is not necessary. The condition must be diagnosed properly so that inappropriate treatment is avoided. For example, the presumptive diagnosis may be cyanotic heart disease (because of skin color) until laboratory tests reveal Hb M.

HEMOGLOBINS WITH INCREASED OXYGEN AFFINITY

Certain alterations in the Hb molecule result in decreased delivery of oxygen to the tissues (*i.e.*, increased affinity of Hb for oxygen). Many of these variants cause secondary erythrocytosis. Inheritance appears to be autosomal dominant and most patients are heterozygotes.

The first Hb variant with increased affinity for oxygen was described in 1966[18] and named Hb Chesapeake. At least 80 such variants have now been identified (see Table 14-5),[54] although all do not cause erythrocytosis. Hb Chesapeake is an α-chain variant in which arginine is replaced by leucine in position 92.

Laboratory Findings

The Hb value usually ranges from normal to 20 g/dL.[10] The leukocyte and platelet counts are usually normal. Some of these variants can be identified on either cellulose acetate or citrate agar electrophoresis, but a few cannot. The level of erythrocyte 2,3-diphosphoglycerate (2,3-DPG) should also be measured to rule out the possibility of abnormal oxygen affinity secondary to 2,3-DPG deficiency, which itself causes increased Hb oxygen affinity when Hb structure is normal. The steps required for identification of abnormal oxygen affinity Hbs are outlined elsewhere.[16]

The P_{50} (partial pressure of oxygen at which hemogobin is half saturated) is usually decreased in these patients (*i.e.*, it takes less oxygen pressure than normal for Hb to be half saturated with oxygen). This shifts the oxyhemoglobin dissociation curve to the left (Fig. 7-5).

Treatment and Prognosis

Most patients with high oxygen affinity Hbs live a normal life and require no treatment. The patient and family must be educated about the disorder to avoid unnecessary treatment of the erythrocytosis as a misdiagnosed myeloproliferative disorder (*i.e.*, polycythemia vera; Chap. 35).

HEMOGLOBINS WITH DECREASED OXYGEN AFFINITY

Twenty-eight Hb variants have been identified that have decreased affinity for oxygen.[54] In some patients, the Hb oxygen affinity is so low that it causes cyanosis. In others, decreased oxygen affinity causes increased release of oxygen to the tissues and resultant decreases in the number of red cells, and the patient appears anemic. The best-known variant in this group is Hb Kansas, which is caused by a single amino acid substitution in position 102 of the β-chain, where asparagine is replaced by threonine. The oxyhemoglobin dissociation curve is shifted significantly to the right and the P_{50} is greatly increased.

These variants may be stable or unstable. Stable variants usually cause cyanosis. Unstable variants frequently cause a mild hemolytic anemia. Cyanosis and normal arterial oxygen tension together are indicative of the presence of Hb with decreased oxygen affinity. Most of these unusual Hbs may be detected by starch gel electrophoresis (alkaline pH).[53]

CHAPTER SUMMARY

Hemoglobinopathies involve structural abnormalities in the α-, β-, γ-, or δ-chains, which may or may not cause clinical disorders. The abnormalities range from amino acid substitutions and deletions to chain elongation or fusion of two different chains.

Sickle cell anemia is the best known hemoglobinopathy. It is characterized by moderate to severe normocytic, normochromic anemia, sickle cells on the blood film (see Fig. 14-5), a band migrating in the Hb S position on electrophoresis (see Fig. 14-3), and a positive solubility test (see Fig. 14-2). It causes severe clinical abnormalities.

There are hundreds of abnormal Hb variants (see Tables 14-3 through 14-5), and a number of laboratory tests are necessary to identify them (see Table 14-6). Tests include cellulose acetate electrophoresis (alkaline pH), citrate agar electrophoresis (acid pH), globin chain electrophoresis (alkaline and acid pH), and isoelectric focusing (pH gradient). The solubility test is required to confirm any Hb band migrating in the Hb S position on cellulose acetate. Special techniques for Hb A_2 and Hb F quantitation may be useful in detecting patients who are doubly heterozygous for both a hemoglobinopathy and thalassemia.

Unstable Hbs such as Hb Köln may also cause significant clinical abnormalities. By using the procedures described in the foregoing, as well as the Heinz body stain, heat denaturation test, and isopropanol precipitation test, the clinical laboratory may assist in confirming the presence of unstable Hbs.

Hb variants with an abnormal affinity for oxygen (increased or decreased) are identified by routine methods but may also require oxygen affinity studies including quantitation of P_{50}.

Case Study 14-1

A 12-year-old black boy was admitted to the hospital for the first time with fever, cough, and pain in the upper chest area. These symptoms had been present for 1 week. For years he had been troubled with recurring chronic ulcers in the lower tibial region (near the ankle). A 10-year-old brother had a similar illness, which was characterized by recurring attacks of fever and chronic ulceration of the legs. One sister had died 10 days earlier of unknown causes. The patient's father, mother, and four additional siblings were alive and well.

A blood count revealed the following data: WBC 22.0×10^9/L; RBC 1.4×10^{12}/L; Hb 4.0 g/dL. The differential cell count revealed 80% neutrophils, 17% lymphocytes, and 3% monocytes. On examination of erythrocyte morphologic appearance, a significant number of elongated red cells with points and many target cells were found, and the cells appeared normocytic, normochromic.

1. Identify any abnormal hematologic results. What disorder might be indicated by these abnormalities? Explain.
2. What screening test could be recommended?
3. If the screening test is positive, what test should be performed next? What result is expected to confirm the positive screening test? Describe the appearance of the results.
4. What is the most likely cause of the elevated leukocyte count in patients with this disorder?

Case Study 14-2

A 22-year-old black woman had developed a productive cough (a cough that brought forth sputum or mucus) 3 days before being admitted. The cough brought up yellow sputum that was not associated with chest pain, fever or chills. On admission, the patient complained of pain in the shoulders, arms and lower back.

Hematologic data included the following: WBC 9.0×10^9/L; RBC 3.78×10^{12}/L; Hb 11.0 g/dL; Hct 0.33 L/L; MCV 87 fL; MCH 29.1 pg; MCHC 33.6 g/dL. The differential count revealed 79% neutrophils, 12% lymphocytes, 4% monocytes, 4% eosinophils and 1% basophils. Platelet number and appearance were normal, and there was slight polychromasia. Abnormal erythrocyte morphologic appearance included an occasional unusual-looking pointed crystal, pocketbook cells, target cells and slight spherocytes.

Cellulose acetate electrophoresis (alkaline pH) indicated a moderately heavy band that migrated close to or in the Hb A_2 position and another moderately heavy band in the Hb S position when compared with the control.

1. What laboratory procedure would be recommended first in this situation to begin the diagnostic workup?
2. From the results obtained on cellulose acetate electrophoresis, name all of the Hbs that could possibly be present.
3. What test should be used to confirm the results on cellulose acetate? How could the Hbs identified in question 2 be distinguished by the results of such a test?

Review Questions

14-1. Abnormal hemoglobins are most often caused by

    A. amino acid substitutions.
    B. amino acid deletions.
    C. globin chain elongations.
    D. globin chain fusions.

14-2. The most common cause of hemoglobinopathies is an abnormality in the _____ globin chain.

    A. α-
    B. β-
    C. γ-
    D. δ-

14-3. Laboratory values that could be found in a patient with sickle cell anemia (Hb SS) disease include all of the following *except*

    A. 85% Hb S on cellulose acetate electrophoresis.
    B. 7% Hb A_2 on cellulose acetate electrophoresis.
    C. normocytic, normochromic anemia.
    D. hemoglobin 6.0 g/dL.

14-4. A false-positive sickle solubility test can be caused by

    A. a hemoglobin lower than 7 g/dL.
    B. holding the test tube too close to the card reader when determining the results.
    C. testing blood from an infant younger than 6 months of age.
    D. extreme leukocytosis when using a whole blood sample.

14-5. Cellulose acetate hemoglobin electrophoresis is run at a(n)

    A. alkaline pH.
    B. acid pH.
    C. pH gradient.
    D. alkaline and acid pH.

14-6. The condition(s) associated with increased levels of Hb F is (are)

    A. infancy.
    B. hemoglobinopathies.
    C. thalassemia.
    D. all of the above.

14-7. Two Hbs that migrate together on cellulose acetate electrophoresis at alkaline pH are

    A. A_1 and A_2.
    B. A_1 and E.
    C. S and C.
    D. S and D.

14-8. The migration speed of Hbs on cellulose acetate at alkaline pH from fastest to slowest is

    A. H, A_2, F, S, A_1.
    B. A_2, F, S, A_1, H.
    C. H, A_1, F, S, A_2.
    D. A_2, S, F, A_1, H.

References

1. Aluoch JR: The treatment of sickle cell disease. A historical and chronological literature review of the therapies applied since 1910. Trop Geogr Med 36:Sl, 1984
2. Arends T, Bemski G, Nagel RL: Genetical, Functional and Physical Studies in Hemoglobins, pp 2, 8, 46, 175. Paris, S Karger, 1971
3. Betke K, Marti HR, Schlicht I: Estimation of small percentages of foetal haemoglobin. Nature 184:1877, 1959
4. Boggs DR: The frequency of heterozygosity for S and C hemoglobins in western Pennsylvania. Blood 44:699, 1974
5. Bookchin RM, Nagel RL, Ranney HM et al: Hemoglobin C Harlem: A sickling variant containing amino acid substitutions in two residues of the β-polypeptide chain. Biochem Biophys Res Commun 23:122, 1966
6. Bookchin RM, Davis RP, Ranney HM: Clinical features of hemoglobin C Harlem, a new sickling hemoglobin variant. Ann Intern Med 68:8, 1968
7. Briere RO, Galias T, Balsakis JG: Rapid qualitative and quantitative hemoglobin fractionation. Cellulose acetate electrophoresis. Am J Clin Pathol 44:695, 1965
8. Brosious EM, Morrison BY, Schmidt RM: Effects of hemoglobin F levels, KCN, and storage on the isopropanol precipitation test for unstable hemoglobins. Am J Clin Pathol 66:878, 1976
9. Brown BA: Hematology: Principles and Procedures, 6th ed, pp 171-2. Philadelphia, Lea & Febiger, 1993
10. Bunn HF, Forget BG, Ranney HM: Human Hemoglobins, pp 31, 152–154, 166, 167, 178, 221, 225, 226, 268, 277, 279, 290. Philadelphia, WB Saunders, 1977
11. Carrell RW, Kay R: A simple method for the detection of unstable haemoglobins. Br J Haematol 23:615, 1972
12. Cartwright GE: Diagnostic Laboratory Hematology. New York, Grune & Stratton, 1963
13. Centers for Disease Control: Laboratory Methods for Detecting Hemoglobinopathies, p 129. Atlanta, Centers for Disease Control, 1984
14. Charache S, Lubin B, Reid CD (eds): Management and Therapy of Sickle Cell Disease. NIH Publication 85-2117. Bethesda MD, National Institutes of Health, 1985
15. Charache S, Dreyer R, Zimmerman I et al: Evaluation of extracorporeal alkylation of red cells as a potential treatment for sickle cell anemia. Blood 47:481, 1976
16. Charache S: Haemoglobins with altered oxygen affinity. Clin Haematol 3:357, 1974
17. Charache S, Page DL: Infarction of bone marrow in the sickle cell disorders. Ann Intern Med 67:1195, 1967
18. Charache S, Weatherall DJ, Clegg JB: Polycythemia associated with a hemoglobinopathy. J Clin Invest 45:813, 1966
19. Council of Regional Networks for Genetic Services (CORN), National Newborn Screening Report—1991, 1994
20. Dacie J: The Hemolytic Anemias, vol 1, pp 1–3. London, Churchill Livingstone, 1985
21. Dacie JV, Lewis SM: Practical Haematology, 6th ed. New York, Churchill Livingstone, 1984
22. Dacie JV, Lewis SM: Practical Haematology, 5th ed. New York, Churchill Livingstone, 1975
23. Dacie JV, Grimes AJ, Meisler A et al: Hereditary Heinz body anaemia. A report of studies on 5 patients with mild anaemia. Br J Haematol 10:388, 1964
24. Daniel SJ, Morris RC, Liu PI: Transfusion therapy in sickle cell disease. Ala Med 55:18, 1986
25. Drabkin DL: Spectroscopy, photometry and spectrophotometry. In Glasser O (ed): Medical Physics, vol 2, p 1039. Chicago, Year Book Medical Publishers, 1950
26. Dubowski KM: Measurement of hemoglobin derivatives. In Sunderman FW, Sunderman FW Jr (eds): Hemoglobin. Its Precursors and Metabolites, p 49. Philadelphia, JB Lippincott, 1964
27. Fairbanks VF, Gilchrist GS, Brimhall B et al: Hemoglobin E trait reexamined: A cause of microcytosis and erythrocytosis. Blood 53:109, 1979
28. Fertman MH, Fertman MB: Toxic anemia and Heinz bodies. Medicine 34:131, 1955
29. Flatz G: Hemoglobin E: Distribution and population dynamics. Humangenetik 3:189, 1967
30. Freedman ML, Karpatkin S: Elevated platelet count and megathrombocyte number in sickle cell anemia. Blood 46:579, 1975
31. Friedman MJ: Erythrocytic mechanism of sickle cell resistance to malaria. Proc Natl Acad Sci USA 75:1994, 1978
32. Gavrilis P, Rothenberg SP, Guy R: Correlation of low serum

IgM levels with absence of functional splenic tissue in sickle cell disease syndromes. Am J Med 57:542, 1974

33. Goossens M, Garel MC, Auvinet J et al: Hemoglobin C-Ziguinchor $\alpha A_2\beta^{62}1(A_3)$glu·val$\beta^{58}$(E2)pro·arg: The second sickling variant with amino acid substitutions in 2 residues of the β-polypeptide chain. FEBS Lett 58:149, 1975

34. Greenberg MS, Harvey HA, Morgan C: A simple and inexpensive screening test for sickle hemoglobin. N Engl J Med 286:1143, 1972

35. Helena Laboratories, Beaumont TX: Hemoglobin Electrophoresis Procedure Using Cellulose Acetate Plate in Alkaline Buffer, 1985

36. Helena Laboratories, Beaumont TX: Titan IV Citrate Hemoglobin Electrophoresis Procedure, 1983

37. Huehns ER: Disease due to abnormalities of hemoglobin structure. Annu Rev Med 21:157, 1970

38. Huehns ER, Shooter EM: Human haemoglobins. J Med Genet 22:48, 1965

39. Huisman THJ, Jonxis JHP: The Hemoglobinopathies: Techniques of Identification, p 201. New York, Marcel Dekker, 1977

40. Huisman THJ, Jonxis JHP: The hemoglobinopathies: Techniques of identification. Clin Biochem Anal 6:1, 1977

41. Huisman THJ: Chromatographic separation of hemoglobins A_2 and C. Clin Chim Acta 40:159, 1972

42. International Committee for Standardization in Haematology: Recommendations for fetal haemoglobin reference preparations and fetal haemoglobin determination by the alkali denaturation method. Br J Haematol 42:133, 1979

43. Isolab Inc, Akron OH: Isoelectric Focusing—IEF Informational, 1993

44. Itano HA: Solubilities of naturally occurring mixtures of human hemoglobin. Arch Biochem Biophys 47:148, 1953

45. Jensen WN, Schoefield RA, Agner R: Clinical and necropsy findings in hemoglobin C disease. Blood 12:74, 1957

46. Johnson FL: Bone marrow transplantation in the treatment of sickle cell anemia. Am J Pediatr Hematol Oncol 7:254, 1985

47. Jones RT, Koler RD, Duerst M et al: Hemoglobin Casper G8$\beta^{106Leu\rightarrow Pro}$: Further evidence that hemoglobin mutations are not random. In Brewer GJ (ed): Hemoglobin and Red Cell Structure and Function, vol 28, p 79. New York, Plenum Press, 1972

48. Koler RD, Jones RT, Bigley RH et al: Hemoglobin Casper $\beta^{106(G8)Leu\rightarrow Pro}$, a contemporary mutation. Am J Med 55:549, 1973

49. Langer EE, Stamatoyannopoulos G, Hlastala MP et al: Extracorporeal treatment with cyanate in sickle cell disease: Preliminary observations in four patients. J Lab Clin Med 87:462, 1976

50. Lehmann H, Huntsman RG: Man's Haemoglobins, 2nd ed, pp 164–172, 178–181, 269, 304–306, 310, 311, 404, 413–416. Philadelphia, JB Lippincott, 1974

51. Lehmann H, Huntsman RG: Man's Haemoglobins, p 293. Philadelphia, JB Lippincott, 1966

52. Lukens JN: Hemoglobinopathies S, C, D, E, and O and associated diseases. In Lee GR, Bithell TC, Foerster J et al (eds): Wintrobe's Clinical Hematology, 9th ed, p 1071. Philadelphia, Lea & Febiger, 1993

53. Lukens JN: Methemoglobinemia and other disorders usually accompanied by cyanosis. In Lee GR, Bithell TC, Foerster J et al (eds): Wintrobe's Clinical Hematology, 9th ed, pp 1266, 1267. Philadelphia, Lea & Febiger, 1993

54. Lukens JN, Lee GR: The abnormal hemoglobins: General principles. In Lee GR, Bithell TC, Foerster J et al (eds): Wintrobe's Clinical Hematology, 9th ed, pp 1028, 1044. Philadelphia, Lea & Febiger, 1993

55. Lukens JN, Lee GR: Unstable hemoglobin disease. In Lee GR, Bithell TC, Foerster J et al (eds): Wintrobe's Clinical Hematology, 9th ed, pp 1054, 1055, 1058. Philadelphia, Lea & Febiger, 1993

56. McCurdy PR: Hemoglobin S-G (S-D) syndrome. Am J Med 57:665, 1974

57. Milner PF, Gooden HM, General RT: Rapid citrate agar electrophoresis in routine screening for hemoglobinopathies using a simple hemolysate. Am J Clin Pathol 64:58, 1975

58. Moo-Penn WF, Schmidt RM, Jue DL et al: Hemoglobin S Travis: A sickling hemoglobin with two amino acid substitutions (β6[A3] glutamic acid·valine and β142 [H20] alanine·valine). Eur J Biochem 77:561, 1977

59. Motulsky AG: Frequency of sickling disorders in US blacks. N Engl J Med 288:31, 1973

60. Motulsky AG, Stamatoyannopoulos G: Drugs, anesthesia, and abnormal hemoglobins. Ann NY Acad Sci 151:807, 1968

61. Nalbandian RM, Nichols BM, Camp FR et al: Dithionite tube test—a rapid, inexpensive technique for the detection of hemoglobin S and non-S sickling hemoglobin. Clin Chem 17:1028, 1971

62. National Committee for Clinical Laboratory Standards: Citrate agar electrophoresis for confirming the identification of variant hemoglobins; Tentative Guideline. NCCLS document H23-T. Villanova, PA, NCCLS, 1988

63. National Committee for Clinical Laboratory Standards: Detection of abnormal hemoglobin using cellulose acetate electrophoresis, 2nd ed; Approved Standard. NCCLS document H8-A2. Villanova, PA, NCCLS, 1994

64. National Committee for Clinical Laboratory Standards: Solubility test to confirm the presence of sickling hemoglobins; Approved Standard. NCCLS document H10-A. Villanova, PA, NCCLS, 1986

65. National Committee For Clinical Laboratory Standards: Quantitative measurement of fetal hemoglobin by the alkali denaturation method; Approved Guideline. NCCLS document H13-A. Villanova, PA, NCCLS, 1989

66. Nelson DA, Davey FR: Erythrocytic disorders. In Henry JB (ed): Clinical Diagnosis and Management by Laboratory Methods, 17th ed, p 679, 685. Philadelphia, WB Saunders, 1984

67. Palek J, Liu A, Liu D et al: Effect of procaine HCl on ATP: Calcium-dependent alterations in red cell shape and deformability. Blood 50:155, 1977

68. Papayannopoulou T, Stamatoyannopoulos G: Stains for inclusion bodies. In Schmidt R et al (eds): The Detection of Hemoglobinopathies. Cleveland, CRC Press, 1974

69. Prasad AS, Ortega J, Brewer GJ et al: Trace elements in sickle cell disease. JAMA 235:2396, 1976

70. Pulsinelli PD, Perutz MF, Nagel RL: Structure of hemoglobin M-Boston, a variant with a five-coordinated ferric heme. Proc Natl Acad Sci USA 70:3870, 1973

71. Rodgers DW, Serjeant BE, Serjeant GR: Early rise in pitted red cell count as a guide to susceptibility to infection in childhood sickle cell anemia. Arch Dis Child 57:338, 1982

72. Roth EF Jr, Wenz B, Lee HB et al: Pathophysiological aspects of sickle cell vaso-occlusion. Prog Clin Biol Res 240:245, 1987

73. Schmid R, Brecher G, Clemens T: Familial hemolytic anemia with erythrocyte inclusion bodies and a defect in pigment metabolism. Blood 14:991, 1959

74. Schmidt RM, Brosious EM: Basic laboratory methods of hemoglobinopathy detection. DHEW Publication (CDC) 76-8266, Atlanta, Centers for Disease Control, 1975

75. Schneider RG, Hightower B, Hosty TS et al: Abnormal hemoglobins in a quarter million people. Blood 48:629, 1976

76. Schneider RG, Schmidt RM: Electrophoretic screening for abnormal hemoglobins. In Schmidt RM (ed): Abnormal Hemoglobins and Thalassemia—Diagnostic Aspects. New York, Academic Press, 1975

77. Schneider RG: Differentiation of electrophoretically similar hemoglobins—such as S, D, G, and P; or A₂, C, E, and O—by electrophoresis of the globin chains. Clin Chem 20:1111, 1974

78. Schneider RG, Hosty TS, Tomlin G et al: Identification of hemoglobins and hemoglobinopathies by electrophoresis on cellulose acetate plates impregnated with citrate agar. Clin Chem 20:74, 1974

79. Scott RB: Advances in the treatment of sickle cell disease in children. Am J Dis Child 139:1219, 1985

80. Seeler RA, Metzger W, Mufson MA: *Diplococcus pneumoniae* infections in children with sickle cell anemia. Am J Dis Child 123:8, 1972

81. Singer K, Chernoff AI, Singer L: Studies on abnormal hemoglobins. I. Their demonstration in sickle cell anemia and other hematologic disorders by means of alkali denaturation. Blood 6:413, 1951

82. Ueda S, Schneider RG: Rapid differentiation of polypeptide chains of hemoglobin by cellulose acetate electrophoresis of hemolysates. Blood 34:230, 1969

83. White JM: Fetal hemoglobin: Whole blood quantitation and intracellular distribution. In Schmidt RM et al (eds): The Detection of Hemoglobinopathies. Cleveland, CRC Press, 1974

84. White JM, Dacie JV: The unstable hemoglobins—molecular and clinical features. In Brown EB, Moore CV (eds): Progress in Hematology, vol 7, p 69. New York, Grune & Stratton, 1971

85. Williams WJ, Beutler E, Erslev AJ et al (eds): Hematology, 3rd ed, pp 509, 586, 593. New York, McGraw-Hill, 1983

Anemias of Abnormal Globin Development—Thalassemias

J. Lynne Williams

Objectives

1. Describe the demographics of the thalassemias, explaining the connection with malaria.
2. Define thalassemia and briefly discuss the abnormality in common forms and variants.
3. Briefly define the genetic terms used to describe the thalassemias.
4. Discuss the pathophysiology of thalassemia and its consequences.
5. List the laboratory tests performed in the diagnostic workup for thalassemia and describe results indicative of the disease, including the appearance of the peripheral blood film.
6. Discuss the nomenclature of the α- and the β-thalassemias and relation to their molecular pathology.
7. Describe the pathophysiology and laboratory findings for the clinical phenotypes of the α- and the β-thalassemias.
8. State the cause of hereditary persistence of fetal hemoglobin (HPFH), and compare the laboratory results in HPFH with those of $\delta\beta$-thalassemia.
9. List two special tests used to diagnose and differentiate the thalassemias.

The thalassemias are a diverse group of genetic disorders characterized by a quantitative reduction in synthesis of one or more of the globin chains of the hemoglobin tetramer (Fig. 7-1). The thalassemias as a group are the most common single-gene disorders known.

HISTORY

In 1925, thalassemia was first described by Cooley and Lee in a case of severe anemia occurring early in life that was associated with splenomegaly and bone changes.[15] The term thalassemia is derived from a Greek term meaning "the sea," because the early patients identified were all of Mediterranean background.[85] Between 1925 and 1940, the clinical features of thalassemia were described, and between 1940 and 1950, the genetic basis of the disorder was recognized. By 1960, it was obvious that the term *thalassemia* encompasses multiple genetic disorders. Since 1960, steady progress has been made in elucidating the structural basis of the thalassemias, and in the past few years it has become possible to clone and sequence the globin genes for numerous patients with thalassemia.[78] As a result, a wide spectrum of specific molecular defects has now been pinpointed, and the remarkable heterogeneity of these syndromes is evident.[36,78]

DEMOGRAPHICS

Although the thalassemias have been found sporadically in virtually every ethnic group and geographic region, they occur with particularly high frequency from the shores of the Mediterranean and Africa through the Middle East, the Indian subcontinent, Burma and Southeast Asia (Fig. 14-1).[70,80] This geographic distribution follows that of malaria, and it was suggested that thalassemia

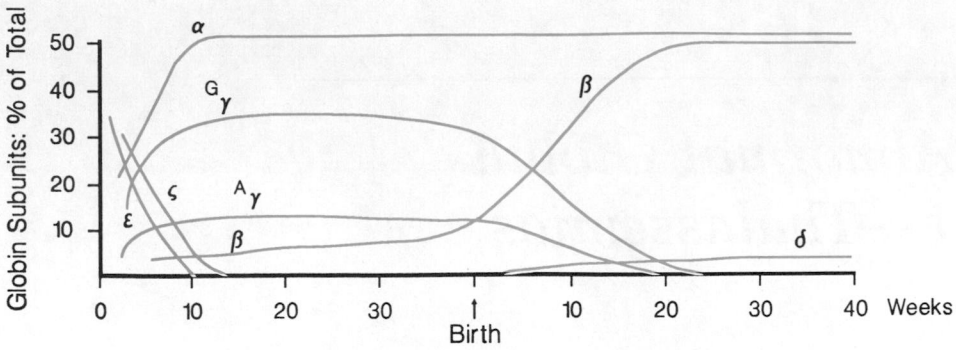

FIGURE 15-1. Changes in globin subunits during human development from embryo to early infancy. (Adapted from Bunn HF, Forget BG: Hemoglobin: Molecular, Genetic and Clinical Aspects. Philadelphia, WB Saunders, 1986, with permission.)

exerted a protective effect against *Plasmodium falciparum*.[22,25] The protective effect may be the result of parasitized thalassemic cells being more prone to ingestion by macrophages. Also, the low concentration of hemoglobin in thalassemic cells provides a protective effect in that hemoglobin is an essential nutrient for malarial parasites.[56a] However, thalassemic red cells apparently do not alter the *rate* of parasite invasion and growth.[49]

DEFINITIONS AND NOMENCLATURE

Discussion of the classification, genetic basis, and pathophysiology of the thalassemias depends on a thorough understanding of the structure and biosynthesis of the human hemoglobins, thus the reader should review Chapter 7. Table 7-2 summarizes the globin structure of the normal human hemoglobin variants and Figure 15-1 shows the changes in globin chain production during human development. Table 15-1 provides a summary of common genetic terms and definitions used to describe the thalassemias.

The thalassemias are inherited, quantitative defects in the synthesis of one or more globin chains, with the individual syndromes usually classified according to the particular globin chain for which synthesis is suppressed. Thus the major subtypes are α-, β-, γ-, δ-, $\delta\beta$- and $\varepsilon\gamma\delta\beta$-thalassemia. It is also useful to subclassify the syndromes according to whether synthesis of the affected chain is

TABLE 15-1
Summary of Genetic Terms and Definitions Used in the Thalassemias

Terms to Describe Thalassemias	Genetic Representations	Definition of Terms
Genes for globin production	Chromosome 11 Chromosome 16	$^{G}\gamma$, $^{A}\gamma$, β, δ, ε α, ζ
α-Genes (genetic representation)	4 $\alpha\alpha/\alpha\alpha$	Normal number of α-genes; two inherited from each parent
α-Gene deletions	$--/--$ $--/-\alpha$ $--/\alpha\alpha$ $-\alpha/-\alpha$ $-\alpha/\alpha\alpha$	(4–α-gene deletion) (3–α-gene deletion) (2–α-gene deletion; both deletions inherited from one parent) (2–α-gene deletion; one deletion inherited from each parent) (1–α-gene deletion)
Nonfunctional α-genes	$\alpha\alpha^{T}$	α-Genes are present, but one or more may be nonfunctional
β-Genes	2 β/β	Normal number of β-genes; one inherited from each parent
Reduced β-chain production	β^{+}	+ Indicates decrease, but not total deficit, of β-chain production by that gene
No β-chain production	β^{0}	0 Indicates no β-chain production by that gene
δ- and β-gene deletions	$(\delta\beta)^{0}$	Both δ- and β-globin genes deleted from chromosome 11
Hb Lepore designation	$(\delta\beta)$Lepore	Nonhomologous meiotic crossing over between δ- and β-globin genes on chromosome 11 (Fig. 15-5)

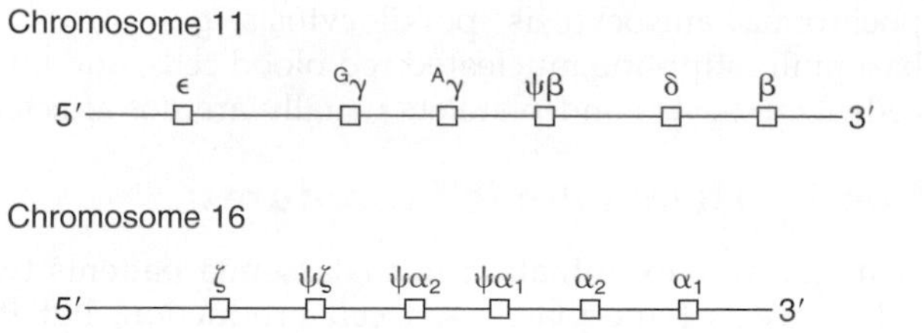

Chromosome 11

Chromosome 16

FIGURE 15-2. Human globin gene arrangement on chromosomes 11 and 16.

partially reduced (*e.g.*, β^+-thalassemia) or is totally absent (*e.g.*, β^0-thalassemia).

The most common forms of thalassemia are due to partial reduction or total absence of synthesis of structurally normal globin chains. However, the abnormal hemoglobin variant known as Hb Lepore (composed of fused δ- and β-chains) is produced in reduced amounts and is thus phenotypically a form of $\delta\beta$-thalassemia; similarly Hb Constant Spring (an α-chain variant) is associated with an α-thalassemia phenotype.

In addition, there is a group of hereditary disorders characterized by persistence of fetal hemoglobin (Hb F) production into adult life (hereditary persistence of fetal hemoglobin [HPFH]), which in some cases may be associated with extremely mild forms of thalassemia. Many populations in which thalassemia is common also have a high prevalence of abnormal hemoglobin variants, thus it is not uncommon for a hemoglobinopathy (Chap. 14) and thalassemia to be found in the same individual.[80]

GENETIC CONTROL OF GLOBIN SYNTHESIS

The genetic information for the production of the seven different globin chains is encoded on chromosomes 11 (ε, $^G\gamma$, $^A\gamma$, δ, β) and 16 (ζ, α). Figure 15-2 illustrates one of each pair of homologous chromosomes, thus depicting half of the full component of functional genes (haplotype) that direct specific globin chain synthesis. The chromosome ends designated as 3' and 5' aid in discussion of locations on the chromosomes.

Chromosome 11, containing the so-called "β-gene cluster," contains one functional β-gene, one functional δ-gene, two functional γ-genes, and a single $\psi\beta$-gene. The genes designated with ψ are pseudogenes and are nonfunctional.[65,83] The two γ-genes, denoted $^A\gamma$ and $^G\gamma$, code for polypeptide chains which differ only at amino acid position 136, with an alanine on the $^A\gamma$- and a glycine on the $^G\gamma$-chains. At birth, the ratio of molecules containing $^G\gamma$-chains to those containing $^A\gamma$-chains is about 3:1; this ratio varies widely in the trace amounts of Hb F present in normal adults, or in those with HPFH.

Chromosome 16 has the α-gene cluster with two functional α-genes, one ζ-gene, and three pseudogenes. The coding regions (exons) of the two α-genes have identical nucleotide sequences and thus code for identical proteins.[43,44] However their relative output (transcription product) is not the same; it appears that the production of α_2 messenger RNA (mRNA) is two to three times that of α_1.[60]

The thalassemia syndromes are caused by the inheritance of one or more pathologic alleles of the globin genes. These genetic lesions are classified as deletional mutations (*i.e.*, segments of the chromosome containing the gene in question have been deleted) or nondeletional mutations (*i.e.*, the gene is intact, but nonfunctional). Nondeletional mutations are often point mutations (*i.e.*, a change in a single base pair in the DNA molecule) that result in impaired transcription, processing, or translation of globin mRNA which is required for the production of globin chains.[36,78,83] Specific examples will be summarized in each section.

The regulation of the globin gene clusters is also of major relevance to an understanding of the thalassemias. There is increasing evidence that deletions or mutations involving regulatory regions of globin genes may result in defective expression of the gene(s) and reduced mRNA and protein output, accounting for at least some forms of thalassemia. One regulatory region on most genes contains "upstream promoter elements" at the 5'-end of the coding sequences, which are required for optimal transcription during which DNA produces mRNA.[56] In addition, there are several enhancer sequences, similar to the upstream promoter elements, that are important for the spatial apposition of the promoter sequences on particular genes.[2]

Upstream (toward the 5'-end of the chromosome) in both the α- and β-gene clusters, there is another particularly important control element called the locus-activating region (LAR).[33] This region is important for organizing the entire gene cluster into a transcriptionally active conformation that is available for gene expression.

PATHOPHYSIOLOGY— GENERAL PRINCIPLES

The primary lesion in all forms of thalassemia is reduced or absent synthesis of one or more globin chains. The immediate consequence of this is the reduced production of functioning hemoglobin tetramers and, as a result, microcytic, hypochromic red blood cells, characteristic of virtually all patients with thalassemia.

The second consequence is the imbalance of globin chain biosynthesis. Apparently there is no compensatory regulatory mechanism to down-regulate (reduce) synthesis of one globin chain when the synthesis of its "partner" globin chain is reduced. Thus, unpaired α-globin chains continue to accumulate in β-thalassemia, and likewise β-globin chains in α-thalassemia. Free or unpaired α-chains are incapable of forming a viable hemoglobin tetramer, are highly insoluble, and tend to precipitate in the cytosol. Free β- or γ-chains tend to form homotetramers of β_4 (known as Hb H) or γ_4 (known as Hb Barts) which, although they remain soluble in the cytosol of the cell, have extremely high oxygen affinity and are useless as oxygen carriers for the tissue.[82]

Thus, thalassemias cause symptomatology both by the underproduction of hemoglobin as well as by the accumulation of unpaired globin subunits. In the severe forms of thalassemia, it is the behavior of the unpaired globin chains accumulating in relative excess that is the major source of morbidity and mortality.[78]

The spectrum of clinical expression of the thalassemia syndromes can range from clinically undetectable (in mild forms of the disease) to severe, life-threatening, transfusion-dependent conditions. The most prevalent and clinically important thalassemias are those resulting in reduced expression of the α- or β-globin chains. Because α-chains are shared by both fetal and adult hemoglobins, defective α-chain production (α-thalassemia) is manifest in both fetal and adult life. Recall that in the normal fetus, for the majority of the gestational period (from the 3rd month on) and at birth, the predominant circulating hemoglobin is Hb F ($\alpha_2\gamma_2$). Hb F is slowly replaced by adult Hb A ($\alpha_2\beta_2$), so that infants do not depend on normal amounts and function of Hb A until they are 4 to 6 months of age. Thus, infants with β-thalassemia are asymptomatic until this time because they have normal α- and γ-chains for Hb F production .[87]

LABORATORY FINDINGS AND CORRELATION WITH DISEASE

Table 15-2 lists the tests performed in the diagnostic workup for thalassemia. Some generalizations may be made concerning laboratory characteristics of all thalassemias.

Hematology

The various thalassemia syndromes include at least some of the following hematologic characteristics in varying degrees. In most forms of thalassemia, erythrocyte indices indicate a microcytic, hypochromic anemia. The hemoglobin (Hb) and hematocrit (Hct) values are variable, and the erythrocyte count is usually elevated relative to the degree of anemia. The reticulocyte count is also variable and reflects the response of the bone marrow to anemia. Erythrocyte abnormalities may include microcytosis, hy-

---

TABLE 15-2
Recommended Tests for Laboratory Diagnosis of Thalassemia

MOST FREQUENTLY REQUIRED

CBC (with red cell indices)
Red cell morphology evaluation
Serum ferritin
Hemoglobin electrophoresis, cellulose acetate
Hb F quantitation (alkali denaturation)
Hb A$_2$ quantitation (column chromatography)
Brilliant cresyl blue Hb H inclusion body test
Reticulocyte count

OCCASIONALLY REQUIRED

WBC differential
Serum iron
TIBC
Transferrin saturation (%)
Hemoglobin electrophoresis, citrate agar

NOT ROUTINELY REQUIRED

Bone marrow examination
DNA analysis
α/β-Globin chain analysis

---

pochromia, anisocytosis, poikilocytosis, polychromasia, basophilic stippling, nucleated red blood cells, and target cells. Leukocytes and platelets usually are not affected.

Special Hematologic Procedures

Bone marrow examination in thalassemia patients typically reveals hyperplastic red cell production, but it is seldom necessary for diagnosis. Determination of the production ratio of α/β-globin chain biosynthesis or DNA analysis may be required for reliable diagnosis of extremely mild forms of the disease (see "Silent Carrier" state of α-thalassemia).

Hemoglobin electrophoresis on cellulose acetate at alkaline pH reveals variable results, depending on the type of thalassemia involved, and is discussed under the individual syndromes. Citrate agar electrophoresis at acid pH serves two major purposes: Hb F, which is often elevated in β-thalassemia, is effectively separated from Hb A, and hemoglobin variants may migrate differently in this medium, permitting tentative identification. The quantities of Hb A$_2$ and Hb F, and the presence of Hb H inclusions in erythrocytes can be diagnostic as well.

Knowledge of a patient's transfusion status is important for correct interpretation of electrophoresis results. Blood samples taken soon after transfusion contain both the patient's and the transfused red cells, thus an abnormal hemoglobin fraction may be decreased or not detected on hemoglobin electrophoresis as long as normal transfused cells continue to circulate.

Concurrent iron deficiency in thalassemia is known to lower the concentrations of Hb A$_2$ and Hb H[57,80] as well as serum iron and iron stores. This may mask the diagnosis of heterozygous β-thalassemia and Hb H disease, respectively. Additionally, Hb H inclusions may be more difficult to detect in red cells by supravital staining. If a subject is iron deficient, iron stores should first be repleted; then diagnostic tests for thalassemia may be performed.

The acid elution slide test for Hb F is sometimes useful for differentiating thalassemia from HPFH. In most thalassemias, Hb F occurs heterogeneously (*i.e.*, some cells contain Hb F and some do not), whereas there is a homogeneous distribution pattern in pancellular HPFH.

Chemistry

Iron studies are often beneficial, particularly because thalassemia can morphologically mimic iron deficiency states (see Table 15-9). Differentiation of the two disorders is discussed later in this chapter. Among transfusion-dependent thalassemic patients, testing for iron overload is important, as overload can and does occur in transfusion-dependent thalassemia major and (occasionally) thalassemia intermedia.[63] The possibility of iron overload is indicated by the persistence of serum iron levels in excess of 160 μg/dL and transferrin saturation greater than 60%.[29]

Testing in Early Infancy

Although most persons with thalassemia require no treatment, those who are transfusion dependent usually develop severe anemia during the first year of life.[82] Proper evaluation of infant hematologic parameters requires knowledge of the normal differences between infant and adult values. At birth, a normal infant's red cells are macrocytic, but the mean corpuscular volume (MCV) subsequently begins to fall. At 10 months of age, the lower limit of the MCV reference range is 70 fL, which should not be confused with pathologic microcytosis. This gradually rises to adult levels (80 to 100 fL) by approximately 12 years of age. Hb F is not diagnostic of β-thalassemia in infants, because it is normally elevated in the first year of life.

α-THALASSEMIA

Nomenclature and Molecular Pathology

Normally, four α-globin genes are inherited, two from each parent (Fig. 15-2); consequently, the genetics of α-thalassemia are more complicated than that of β-thalassemia. The normal genotype for the α-locus is designated αα/αα. The various forms of α-thalassemia result from a decrease in number of α-chains produced, owing to a deletion or mutation affecting one, two, three or all four α-globin genes (Table 15-3).

There are two main groups of α-thalassemia haplotypes, α^0 and α^+. The α^0-thalassemias (formerly called α-thalassemia 1) are haplotypes in which both linked α-globin genes on chromosome 16 are deleted, and thus no α-chains are produced from an affected chromosome (−−). The α^+-thalassemias (formerly called α-thalassemia 2) are haplotypes in which only one of the linked pair of α-globin genes is deleted (−α) or nonfunctional ($\alpha^T\alpha$; see later discussion).

At least 14 different mutations that delete both α-genes causing α^0-thalassemia and abolishing α-chain production from the affected chromosome, have been described.[83] Deletion of the α-globin locus-activating region,

leaving the α-globin genes intact, has also been documented as a cause of α^0-thalassemia.[27,45]

The α^+-thalassemias are divided into deletion and nondeletion types. In the deletion type, the most common of the two, the genetic nomenclature −α is used to signify a single α-gene deletion. If both genes are intact (i.e., nondeletion), the nomenclature $\alpha^T\alpha$ is used, with the superscript T indicating that the gene is thalassemic (Table 15-1). The nondeletion mutants are presumably nonfunctional or dysfunctional genes that are incapable of normal α-chain synthesis.[61] Examples of nondeletion α-thalassemias include those resulting from mutations that interfere with the translation of mRNA needed for the production of globin chains, interfere with the translation start signal, or inactivate either the initiator or stop codon[28] (see Hb H–Constant Spring disease).

Misalignment and reciprocal crossover between the duplicated α-globin gene segments at meiosis can give rise to chromosomes with either single (−α) or triplicated (ααα) α-globin genes (Fig. 15-3).[17,24] And finally, more than a dozen mutations resulting in structural hemoglobin variants have been described which produce an α-thalassemia phenotype by a variety of mechanisms (the so-called thalassemic hemoglobinopathies).[1,67] Some of these variant hemoglobins are so unstable that they can be considered to be equivalent to an α-gene deletion. Because expression of the α_2 gene is two to three times greater than that of the α_1 gene, lesions of the α_2 gene result in a greater phenotypic effect, and are thus likely to produce more serious clinical effects.

Pathophysiology

Interactions of the various α-thalassemia haplotypes results, phenotypically, in one of four broad categories, corresponding to 3, 2, 1 or 0 functional α-globin genes (Table 15-3). The silent carrier state (−α/αα), resulting from the heterozygous state for deletion or nondeletion

TABLE 15-3
Genotypes of α-Thalassemia

α-Chain Genes (Chromosome 16)*	Genotype	Genotypic Description	Disorder
-■-■- -■-■-	−−/−−	Homozygous α^0 thal	Barts hydrops fetalis
-■-■- -□-■-	−−/−α	Heterozygous α^0 thal/ α^+ thal	Hb H disease
-■-■- -□-cs-	−−/$\alpha^{cs}\alpha$	Heterozygous α^0 thal/ Constant Spring	Hb H/Constant Spring disease
-■-■- -□-□-	−−/αα	Heterozygous α^0 thal	α-Thalassemia minor
-□-■- -□-■-	−α/−α	Homozygous α^+ thal	α-Thalassemia minor
-□-■- -□-□-	−α/αα	Heterozygous α^+ thal	Silent carrier (no disorder)
-□-□- -□-□-	αα/αα	Normal	None

* Four α-globin chain genes (open squares) normally are present on the chromosome 16 pair. Gene deletions that cause α-thalassemia are shown as black rectangles.
(Modified from Fishleder AJ, Hoffman GC: A practical approach to the detection of hemoglobinopathies. Part I. The introduction and thalassemia syndromes. Lab Med 18:369, 1987, with permission.)

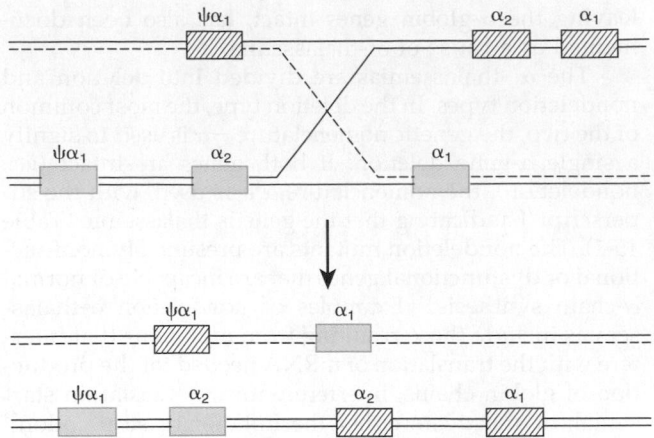

FIGURE 15-3. Mechanism of unequal crossover that gives rise to the α^+ thalassemia ($-\alpha$) and triplicated ($\alpha\alpha\alpha$) haplotypes.

forms of α^+-thalassemia, is essentially normal. α-Thalassemia minor (or α-thalassemia trait) results from either homozygosity for α^+-thalassemia ($-\alpha/-\alpha$) or heterozygosity for α^0-thalassemia ($--/\alpha\alpha$); both are characterized by mild hematologic changes but no clinical abnormality.

The two major clinical phenotypes of the α-thalassemias are Hb H disease, a moderately severe hemolytic condition resulting from the compound heterozygous state for α^0- and α^+-thalassemia ($--/-\alpha$), and the lethal Barts hydrops fetalis syndrome, homozygosity for α^0-thalassemia ($--/--$). A significantly reduced rate of α-chain synthesis in fetal life results in an excess of γ-chains, forming γ_4 tetramers, or Hb Barts. In adult life, the excess of β-chains form β_4 tetramers, or Hb H. Because both Hb homotetramers are relatively soluble, they do not precipitate to any significant degree in the red cell precursors, and there is relatively little ineffective erythropoiesis. Thus, the α-thalassemia phenotypes are predominantly due to the combined effect of a hypochromic anemia and the ineffective oxygen-carrying capacity associated with synthesis of Hb H and Hb Barts. However, Hb H does tend to precipitate and form inclusions as the mature red cells age in the circulation, resulting in a mild degree of hemolysis in Hb H disease.[78]

Barts Hydrops Fetalis

GENETICS, DEMOGRAPHICS AND PATHOPHYSIOLOGY

Barts hydrops fetalis (homozygous α^0-thalassemia) occurs almost exclusively in Southeast Asians and Filipinos, in whom the α^0-haplotype is relatively prevalent.[82] The α-globin genes are usually totally absent; no α-globin is produced, so that no physiologically useful Hb accumulates beyond the embryonic stage. The disorder is lethal, and infants are usually stillborn or die within hours of birth. Hb Barts (γ_4), the predominant Hb at delivery in these infants, has an extraordinarily high oxygen affinity. Thus it binds oxygen delivered to the placenta, but releases almost none of it to developing fetal tissues. As a result, severe hypoxia occurs at the tissue level, causing profound edema, congestive heart failure and death. Survival into the third trimester of fetal life is attributed to

the presence of Hb Portland ($\zeta_2\gamma_2$), a normal embryonic hemoglobin, that is capable of delivering oxygen to the tissues. Infants with the disease who are liveborn are underweight and edematous, with marked hepatosplenomegaly owing to extreme extramedullary erythropoiesis in response to the profound hypoxia. Obstetric complications may lead to significant morbidity and mortality for the mothers of these infants.

LABORATORY FINDINGS AND CORRELATIONS WITH DISEASE

Anemia in these infants is usually severe (Hb levels in cord blood vary from 4.0 to 10.0 g/dL), with markedly microcytic, hypochromic red cells. The blood film shows red cells with gross thalassemic changes, including marked anisopoikilocytosis, hypochromia, variable reticulocytosis and numerous nucleated red cell precursors.

Hb electrophoresis (alkaline pH) of cord blood hemolysates shows approximately 80% Hb Barts, with about 20% embryonic Hb Portland and little or no Hb H (Fig. 15-4). There is no Hb A. This condition can be diagnosed prenatally by performing DNA analysis on a chorionic biopsy specimen at about 8 to 10 weeks' gestation.[59]

Hb H Disease

GENETICS, DEMOGRAPHICS AND PATHOPHYSIOLOGY

Hb H (β_4) disease usually results from coinheritance of α^+- and α^0-thalassemia alleles ($--/-\alpha$), with α-chain production only 25% to 30% of normal, but there are nondeletional forms ($--/\alpha^T\alpha$) as well. Family studies tend to show that one parent has heterozygous α^0-thalassemia and the other has heterozygous α^+-thalassemia (Table 15-3). Hb H disease is widespread in Southeast Asia, parts of the Middle East, and in the Mediterranean island populations.[75,82] Both Hb H disease and Barts hydrops syndrome are rare in African Americans, as chromosomes having deletions of both α-genes are rare in this population.[36]

In spite of the decreased synthesis of α-chains, Hb A always constitutes the major component. The concentration of Hb H is variable, usually from 5% to 30%; however, concomitant iron deficiency may reduce this value. Hb H tends to precipitate in older red cells, which are removed prematurely from the circulation by the spleen. The result is a lifelong, mild to moderate hemolytic anemia owing to the instability of Hb H and the inability of the marrow to adequately compensate for the hemolysis. The severity of anemia depends on the degree of imbalance of the α/β-chain ratio. The association of mental retardation and Hb H disease has been reported.[84]

LABORATORY FINDINGS AND CORRELATIONS WITH DISEASE

In the adult steady state, Hb levels vary from 8.9 to 12.7 g/dL and the red cell indices are decreased.[70] There is a reticulocytosis of approximately 5%, but the reticulocyte response is inadequate for the degree of anemia, a consistent finding in chronic anemia.

Lane	Hb	Origin	CA	CS	C Harlem O Arab E C A₂	G D Lepore S	F	A	Portland	Barts	H
1	Barts								I	I	(I)$^\Delta$
2	H		I		I			I		(I)*	I
3	H/Constant Spring		I	I	I			I		(I)*	I
4	α Thal minor		I		I			I			
5	α Thal (silent carrier)		I		I			I			
6	AA₂ (normal)		I		I			I			

FIGURE 15-4. Relative electrophoretic mobilities of hemoglobins on cellulose acetate, pH 8.4, of various α-thalassemia syndromes. (*Lane 1*) Barts hydrops fetalis cord blood (Δ, Hb H may or may not be present). Carbonic anhydrase (*CA*) and Hb A₂ are not detectable at birth. (*Lane 2*) Hb H disease (adult) (*, Hb Barts is present in ~10% of adult patients). (*Lane 3*) Hb H/Constant Spring (CS) (adult) (*, Hb Barts may or may not be present). (*Lane 4*) α-Thalassemia minor pattern in an adult is the same as that of a normal adult (Hb Barts = 2% to 10% at birth). (*Lane 5*) α-Thalassemia silent carrier (adult); the pattern is the same as in a normal adult (Hb Barts = 1% to 2% at birth). (*Lane 6*) Normal adult pattern.

On the peripheral blood film, red cells are microcytic, hypochromic with anisopoikilocytosis. The electronically measured red cell distribution width (RDW) is increased.[8] Almost all red cells have Hb H inclusions, which are visible microscopically when erythrocytes are incubated and supravitally stained with brilliant cresyl blue (BCB), a redox dye that causes the precipitation of Hb H in vitro. Individual inclusions appear similar to Heinz body inclusions, which are associated with precipitation of abnormally oxidized Hb. However, Hb H inclusions (see Figs. 8-29 and 14-8*B*) generally occur in multiples and cover the cell surface, producing a golf-ball-like appearance, whereas Heinz bodies (see Fig. 14-8*A*) are usually eccentrically located and are relatively few per cell.

Hb electrophoresis (alkaline pH) in affected neonates shows about 25% to 40% Hb Barts (γ_4), but as β-chain synthesis replaces γ during the first few months of life, Hb Barts is gradually replaced by Hb H (β_4). Electrophoresis of adult specimens shows Hbs A, H and A₂, with a trace amount of Hb Barts in approximately 10% of patients (Fig. 15-4). The Hb F level is normal, whereas the Hb A₂ levels are nearly always reduced.[70] Hb H levels can vary widely, from 2% to 40%.[82]

Hb H may occasionally occur in certain acquired disorders such as erythroleukemia,[6] acute[58] or chronic granulocytic leukemia,[7] sideroblastic anemia,[88] and other myeloproliferative disorders.[72] In these cases, the Hb H level has been reported to be between 5% and 70% of the total Hb.[80]

TREATMENT AND PROGNOSIS

Most individuals with Hb H disease require no therapy; their growth, development and life expectancy are usually normal. However, intercurrent infections should be treated promptly, and oxidant drugs should be avoided, because of potential further deleterious effects on hemoglobin solubility.

Hb H–Constant Spring Disease

GENETICS, DEMOGRAPHICS AND PATHOPHYSIOLOGY

Hb H–Constant Spring (Hb H/CS) disease has a phenotype similar to that of Hb H disease. It may be caused by compound heterozygous inheritance of Hb Constant Spring (Hb CS) and α^0-thalassemia ($--/\alpha^{CS}\alpha$; Table 15-3). Hb Constant Spring is an α-globin mutant in which a nucleotide change causes a mutation in the normal terminator codon. As a result, polyribosomes continue to read through the usual translation stop site until another terminator codon is reached.[13] This causes more than the normal number of amino acids to be added to the globin chain. Three other variants have been reported with similar characteristics.[1] These mutations, which differ only at amino acid 142 (the normal α-chain terminator codon), all extend the variant α-globins by 31-amino acid residues. These α-chain variant mRNAs are synthesized at a very low rate, and variant α-chains are present in only minute amounts, thus producing the thalassemic phenotype.

The haplotype containing the Hb CS allele ($\alpha^{cs}\alpha$) is particularly common in Southeast Asia, as is the α^0-thalassemia haplotype. Thus Hb H/CS occurs frequently in Orientals and has been observed in Mediterranean populations. It represents up to 40% of all Hb H-like syndromes in Southeast Asians.[70]

Individuals who are homozygous for Hb CS ($\alpha^{cs}\alpha/\alpha^{cs}\alpha$) would be expected to be hematologically similar to α-thalassemia minor ($--/\alpha\alpha$ or $\alpha-/\alpha-$). However, they have been found to resemble individuals with Hb H disease more closely ($--/\alpha-$)

LABORATORY FINDINGS AND CORRELATIONS WITH DISEASE

The peripheral blood and blood film findings in Hb H/CS are very similar to those previously described for Hb H disease. Hb electrophoresis at alkaline pH reveals Hbs

H, A, A_2, little or no Barts, and approximately 1.5% to 2.5% Hb CS (Fig. 15-4). Because the percentage of Hb CS is small, it may be missed, and hemolysate should be applied heavily to the electrophoretic support medium when it is suspected.[21]

In the homozygous state for Hb CS ($\alpha^{cs}\alpha/\alpha^{cs}\alpha$), the hemoglobin consists of about 5% to 6% Hb CS, normal levels of Hb A_2, and trace amounts of Hb Barts. The remainder is Hb A. The heterozygous state for Hb CS ($\alpha^{cs}\alpha/\alpha\alpha$) shows no hematologic abnormality, with a normal hemoglobin pattern except for the presence of about 0.5% Hb CS.[46]

TREATMENT AND PROGNOSIS

Hemolysis may be more severe with Hb H/CS than with the typical three–α-gene deletion Hb H disease. Treatment and prognosis are generally the same in both conditions.[70]

α-Thalassemia Minor

GENETICS, DEMOGRAPHICS AND PATHOPHYSIOLOGY

α-Thalassemia minor (also known as α-thalassemia trait) has two genotypic forms: heterozygous α^0-thalassemia ($--/\alpha\alpha$) and homozygous α^+-thalassemia ($-\alpha/-\alpha$). The result in either form is a decrease in α-chain synthesis. Both forms are common in Southeast Asians, Chinese and Filipinos.[41] Homozygous α^+-thalassemia is common in African Americans (3.0%), whereas the heterozygous α^0 form is rare.[16] Neither condition produces clinical disease.

LABORATORY FINDINGS AND CORRELATIONS WITH DISEASE

The hematologic findings are the same for both genotypes. Erythrocytes typically are microcytic and slightly hypochromic with decreased MCV and MCH levels; the MCHC is normal to slightly decreased. Target cells and other poikilocytes are common. Hct and Hb levels are usually at the lower limit of the reference range, although in some cases there may be mild anemia. The erythrocyte count is usually above 5.5×10^{12}/L, with the RDW normal or only slightly increased.[37,74]

Newborns with α-thalassemia minor exhibit 5% to 15% Hb Barts in cord blood samples.[12,23,47,62,76,81] Thus Hb electrophoresis may be helpful in diagnosing α-thalassemia minor in newborns. However, Hb Barts disappears after the first few months of life and is not replaced by a similar amount of Hb H; thereafter, the electrophoretic pattern is normal (Fig. 15-4). The presence of sufficient Hb H to be detected by electrophoresis usually requires the deletion of three of the four α-globin genes ($--/-\alpha$).[78] Hb H may be detectable microscopically in an occasional cell after incubation with brilliant cresyl blue (BCB), as described earlier, and this is often used as a diagnostic test for α-thalassemia minor. A modified BCB inclusion body test can be used to enhance the precipitation of Hb H, often causing the inclusions to be more visible (see procedure later in this chapter).[34] A negative test result does not, however, absolutely exclude either form of α-thalassemia minor. A definitive diagnosis can be made by DNA analysis, but the test expense usually is not justified for this benign disorder.[36] DNA analysis can be important, however, in determining specific genotypes for purposes of genetic counseling.

DIFFERENTIAL DIAGNOSIS

Microcytosis in the presence of normal Hb A_2 and Hb F levels is suggestive of α-thalassemia minor, particularly when other family members are similarly affected. It has been proposed that a Hct of less than 0.31 L/L in women and children, or less than 0.37 L/L in men, may indicate a concomitant secondary disorder.[31] Microcytosis with decreased iron stores may indicate iron deficiency alone or thalassemia with coincident iron deficiency anemia.

The Silent Carrier

GENETICS AND DEMOGRAPHICS

The silent carrier form of α-thalassemia, heterozygous α^+-thalassemia ($-\alpha/\alpha\alpha$), is common in Southeast Asians, Chinese and Filipinos. Approximately 28% of African Americans have heterozygous α^+-thalassemia.[16] The silent carrier state is benign and is often discovered only during family studies.

LABORATORY FINDINGS AND CORRELATIONS WITH DISEASE

There are no consistent hematologic manifestations for the silent carrier state. The blood count and blood film are normal, or very minimally abnormal; the red cells are generally not microcytic. One to two percent Hb Barts may be found in affected infants at birth, but the electrophoresis pattern is normal in adults (Fig. 15-4). Rare Hb H inclusions may be found using the modified BCB inclusion body test,[34] but similar to α-thalassemia minor, the silent carrier state cannot be ruled out on the basis of a negative BCB result. A definitive diagnosis can be made reliably only by DNA analysis.

A summary of hematologic data on α-thalassemia is presented in Table 15-4.

β-THALASSEMIA

Nomenclature and Molecular Pathology

In contrast with the α-globin genes, there is only a single β-globin gene present per haploid β-gene cluster in humans (Fig. 15-2). Its analogue, the δ-globin gene, produces only about 1/50th the amount of globin chains. Historically, the β-thalassemias were divided into two clinically significant states, trait (thalassemia minor) and disease (thalassemia major) in contrast to the four α-thalassemia states.

Most individuals with β-thalassemia trait carry one normal and one thalassemic β-globin gene, and are essentially in good health, with red cell microcytosis, but mild or minimal anemia. Individuals with β-thalassemia major generally carry two thalassemic genes, and have a severe, transfusion-dependent hemolytic anemia. However, gradations of severity exist, and the term β-thalassemia intermedia has been applied to a clinical phenotype of interme-

TABLE 15-4
Hematologic Features of α-Thalassemia

Diagnosis	Genotype*	Red Cell Morphology	Hemoglobin Electrophoresis	Mean Globin Chain Synthesis Values in Reticulocytes (α/β Ratio)*	Anemia	Life Expectancy
Hb Barts Hydrops Fetalis	$--/--$	↓ MCV and MCH, ↑ NRBC	Hb Barts (80%)† Hb Portland	0:1	Severe	Fatal
Hb H Disease	$--/-\alpha$	↓ MCV and MCH, +++ Hb H inclusions‡	Hb A Hb H (2% to 40%) ± Hb Barts ↓ Hb A$_2$	0.40:1	Moderate	Normal
α-Thalassemia Minor						
Heterozygous α^0 or homozygous α^+ thalassemia	$--/\alpha\alpha$ $-\alpha/-\alpha$	↓ MCV and MCH, ++ Hb H inclusions‡	Normal	0.77:1	None or mild	Normal
Silent Carrier						
Heterozygous α^+ thalassemia	$-\alpha/\alpha\alpha$	Normal or sl ↓ MCV and MCH, ± Hb H inclusions‡	Normal	0.88:1	None	Normal

* Normal genotype is ($\alpha\alpha/\alpha\alpha$) and normal α/β ratio is 1:1.
† Cord blood sample
‡ Modified brilliant cresyl blue Hb H inclusion body test
Key: ↑, elevated; ↓, depressed; +++, marked; ++, moderate; ±, occasional or none.
(Modified from Todd D: Thalassemia. Pathology 16:5, 1984, with permission.)

diate severity between the trait and the disease, in which significant anemia occurs but chronic transfusion therapy is not absolutely required. Thalassemia minima has been used to describe the "silent carrier" state of heterozygous β-thalassemia which causes no detectable clinical or hematologic abnormalities. These four clinical types of β-thalassemia each include many genotypes, some of which overlap between two groups (Table 15-5).

Many different mutations cause β-thalassemia and its related disorders. These various haplotypes can be inherited in a multitude of genetic combinations, resulting in the extreme heterogeneity reported for these clinical syndromes.[78] Nondeletion mutations are the most common, and have been reported to affect every step in the pathway of globin gene expression, including transcription, processing of the mRNA precursor, translation of mature mRNA, and posttranslational integrity of the polypeptide chain. Large deletions removing one or more genetic loci (as seen in the α-thalassemias) are rare. Most of the genetic mutations that have been mapped in individuals with β-thalassemia are due to point mutations affecting one or a few DNA nucleotide bases. Although more than 125 point mutations causing β-thalassemia have been mapped, about 15 account for the vast majority of affected patients, with five or six mutations accounting for more than 90% of the cases in a given ethnic group or geographic area.[36] Further details concerning specific molecular alterations can be found in a number of recent reviews.[36,78,83]

Pathophysiology

In β-thalassemia there is unbalanced globin chain synthesis owing to a reduced biosynthesis of β-chains. In homozygotes for β^0-thalassemia (β^0/β^0), β-globin synthesis is absent; β-globin synthesis is reduced to 5% to 30% of normal levels in β^+-thalassemia homozygotes (β^+/β^+) or β^+/β^0 thalassemia compound heterozygotes.[82] Synthesis of Hb A ($\alpha_2\beta_2$) is markedly reduced or absent, resulting in microcytic, hypochromic red cells. Hb F production in utero is normal; it is only when the switch from γ- to β-chain production occurs that the clinical manifestations of β-thalassemia first appear, during the fourth to sixth month after birth. γ-Chain synthesis may be partially reactivated, resulting in an increased proportion of Hb F in the patient. In β-thalassemia heterozygotes, there is an elevated level of Hb A$_2$, owing to both the relative decrease in Hb A and to an absolute increase in the output of δ-chains. However, the increased δ- and γ-chains are insufficient to replace β-chain production.

The excess α-chains produced as a consequence of decreased β-chain biosynthesis are very unstable. If the imbalance is relatively minor, unpaired α-chains are simply removed by proteolysis during erythroid maturation; however, if the degradation process is overwhelmed by massive imbalance, excess free α-chains precipitate to form inclusion bodies. These cause oxidative membrane damage within the red cell starting with the earliest hemoglobinized precursor and throughout the erythroid matu-

TABLE 15-5
Classifications of β-Thalassemias and Their Genotypes

Classification	Genotype
Normal	β/β
THALASSEMIA MAJOR	
Homozygous β^0	β^0/β^0
Homozygous β^+ (Mediterranean [severe] form)	β^+/β^+
Double heterozygous β^0/β^+	β^0/β^{+*}
Homozygous $(\delta\beta)^{\text{Lepore}*}$	$(\delta\beta)^{\text{Lepore}}/(\delta\beta)^{\text{Lepore}}$
THALASSEMIA INTERMEDIA	
Double heterozygous β^0/β^{+*}	β^0/β^+
Homozygous $(\delta\beta)^{\text{Lepore}*}$	$(\delta\beta)^{\text{Lepore}}/(\delta\beta)^{\text{Lepore}}$
Homozygous β^+ (mild form)	β^+/β^+
Homozygous $(\delta\beta)^0$	$(\delta\beta)^0/(\delta\beta)^0$
Double heterozygous β^0 or $\beta^+/(\delta\beta)^0$	$\beta^0/(\delta\beta)^0$ or $\beta^+/(\delta\beta)^0$
Double heterozygous β^0 or $\beta^+/(\delta\beta)^{\text{Lepore}}$	$\beta^0/(\delta\beta)^{\text{Lepore}}$ or $\beta^+/(\delta\beta)^{\text{Lepore}}$
Double heterozygous $(\delta\beta)^0/(\delta\beta)^{\text{Lepore}}$	$(\delta\beta)^0/(\delta\beta)^{\text{Lepore}}$
Heterozygous β^0†	β^0/β
Double heterozygous β^0/β^{sc}	β^0/β^{sc}
THALASSEMIA MINOR	
Heterozygous β^0 or β^+†	β^0/β or β^+/β
Heterozygous $(\delta\beta)^0$	$(\delta\beta)^0/\beta$
Heterozygous $(\delta\beta)^{\text{Lepore}}$	$(\delta\beta)^{\text{Lepore}}/\beta$
THALASSEMIA MINIMA	
Heterozygous β^{SC}	β^{SC}/β

Key: β, gene with normal β-chain production; β^+, gene with decreased β-chain production; β^0, gene with no β-chain production.
* Some overlap between thalassemia intermedia and thalassemia major.
† Overlap between intermedia and minor; sc, silent carrier.

ration pathway; severe erythrocyte dysfunction and destruction of immature developing erythroblasts within the bone marrow (ineffective erythropoiesis) occur as a result. The erythrocytes that do survive erythropoiesis still contain inclusion bodies, and are removed prematurely by macrophages in the spleen, liver and bone marrow, producing a hemolytic anemia.

Thus the anemia and other clinical symptomatology of this disease are caused by three separate effects: (1) ineffective erythropoiesis (impaired production of new red cells); (2) hemolysis (a shortened survival of the few red cells produced); and (3) reduced hemoglobinization of the red cells (reducing the oxygen-carrying capacity of the red cells that do survive).

The profound deficit in oxygen-carrying capacity in the severe forms of the disease stimulates high levels of erythropoietin in an unsuccessful attempt to compensate by erythroid hyperplasia. Ineffective erythropoiesis precludes success, and the result is a massively enlarged erythron, but very few erythrocytes actually being supplied to the circulation. Profound anemia persists, resulting in erythroid hyperplasia and, occasionally, extramedullary erythropoiesis. Massive bone marrow expansion exerts numerous adverse effects on the growth, development and function of critical organ systems (*e.g.*, skeletal deformities and pathologic fractures).

Homozygotes (or double heterozygotes) with the severe form of the disease show increased intestinal absorption of iron that is related to the erythroid hyperplasia, in spite of adequate or increased total body storage iron. The increased absorption causes a steady accumulation of iron, first in macrophages of the liver and spleen, but later in the parenchymal cells, the endocrine glands, the pancreas and the myocardium.[78] This leads to dysfunction of these organs.

The β-thalassemias occur most frequently in the Middle East, Africa, Southeast Asia, India and Indonesia (Fig. 14-1).[18] The hematologic laboratory features and severity of anemia differentiating the β-thalassemias are summarized in Table 15-6.

β-Thalassemia Major

GENETICS, DEMOGRAPHICS, PATHOPHYSIOLOGY AND PHYSICAL FINDINGS

β-Thalassemia major, also known as Cooley's anemia, is due to inheritance of two β-thalassemia alleles, one on each copy of chromosome 11. Four genotypes associated with β-thalassemia major are summarized in Table 15-5. The most common causes of β-thalassemia major are homozygous β^0/β^0 or (severe) β^+/β^+; double heterozygous β^0/β^+; or homozygous Hb Lepore.

Hb Lepore is composed of two normal α-chains and two abnormal non–α-chains formed by fusion of the NH_2-terminal (beginning) of a normal δ-chain and the COOH-terminal (end) of a normal β chain.[4] This abnormal hemoglobin is caused by unequal crossing-over between misaligned δ- and β-globin gene loci during meiosis, which creates two abnormal chromosomes (Fig. 15-5). The Lepore chromosome resulting from this event contains only the two γ-genes and the fused δβ gene (*i.e.*, no "normal" δ- or β-genes). The anti-Lepore chromosome, which contains the remaining portions of the δ- and β-genes as a reciprocal fusion product (a βδ-gene) or anti-Lepore, also contains intact δ- and β-globin genes.

Three different Lepore Hbs have been described (Baltimore, Boston and Hollandia), each differing in the point at which crossing-over occurs, with Hb Lepore–Boston being the most common. All Lepore Hbs are ineffectively synthesized, presumably because they are under the control of the δ-globin gene promoter, which normally maintains transcription at only about 2% of the level of the β-globin gene.[78] The result is a β-thalassemia phenotype, with the presence of 5% to 15% Hb Lepore. In contrast, some chromosomes with the anti-Lepore gene have a normal, intact β-globin gene that can produce normal β-globin chains and sometimes prevent the β-thalassemia phenotype.

Infants with thalassemia major are well at birth, but severe anemia develops within the first year of life. They fail to thrive and, in the absence of adequate transfusions,

TABLE 15-6
Summary of Pertinent Hematologic Features of β-Thalassemia

Diagnosis	Erythrocyte Count	Erythrocyte Morphology	Hemoglobin Electrophoresis*	Mean Globin Chain Synthesis Values in Reticulocytes (β/α Ratio)†	Anemia	Life Expectancy (Yr)
Thalassemia Major	↑	↓ MCV and MCH, ++ stippling, +++ NRBC, +++ targets	↑ Hb, F, variable Hb A₂, ± Hb A‡	0–0.3/1	Severe	20–30
Thalassemia Intermedia	↑	↓ MCV and MCH, + stippling, ± NRBC, ++ targets	N/ ↑ Hb F, variable Hb A₂, ± Hb A‡	0–0.4/1	Moderate	Normal
Thalassemia Minor	↑	↓ MCV and MCH, + stippling, + targets	N/ ↑ Hb F, variable Hb A₂, variable Hb A	0.5/1	None to mild	Normal
Thalassemia Minima	Normal	Normal or slight ↓ MCV and MCH, ± stippling, ± targets	Normal	0.88/1	None	Normal

Key: ↑, elevated; ↓, depressed; +++, marked; ++, moderate; +, slight; ±, occasional or none.
* See Table 15-7.
† Normal β/α ratio is 1:1.
‡ Hb A is absent in genotypes containing only β⁰, (δβ)⁰, or (δβ) Lepore genes.
(Modified from Todd D: Thalassemia. Pathology 16:5, 1984, with permission.)

develop the typical features of Cooley's anemia. Bone marrow expansion in an attempt to compensate for excessive ineffective erythropoiesis causes marked skeletal deformities with frontal bossing (Fig. 15-6), cheek bone and jaw protrusions, distortions of ribs and vertebrae, and pathologic fractures of long bones. Often forward protrusion of the upper teeth and overbite lead to dental and orthodontic problems. Without adequate treatment, there is progressive cardiomegaly, and other complications arise such as gallstones, chronic leg ulcers, and hypersplenism. Growth and sexual development are retarded, and intercurrent infections are common.[70] The extreme erythrocytic hyperplasia often results in folate deficiency. Extramedullary erythropoiesis may cause hepatosplenomegaly, and later development of iron overload contributes to hemosiderosis and hepatic failure. If affected children are maintained on an adequate transfusion program, they grow and develop normally and have no abnormal physical signs.

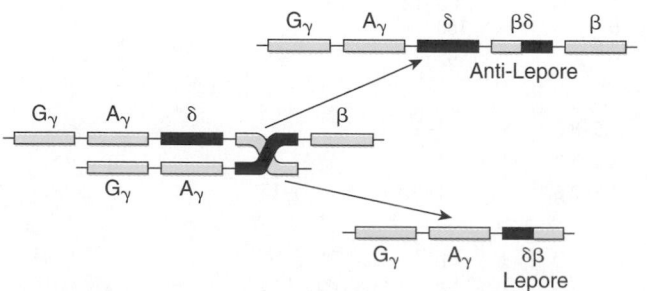

FIGURE 15-5. The abnormal crossing-over mechanism involved in the generation of the Lepore and anti-Lepore hemoglobins. (From Stamatoyannopoulos G, Nienhaus AW, Leder P et al [eds]: The Molecular Basis of Blood Diseases, 2nd ed. Philadelphia, WB Saunders, 1994, with permission.)

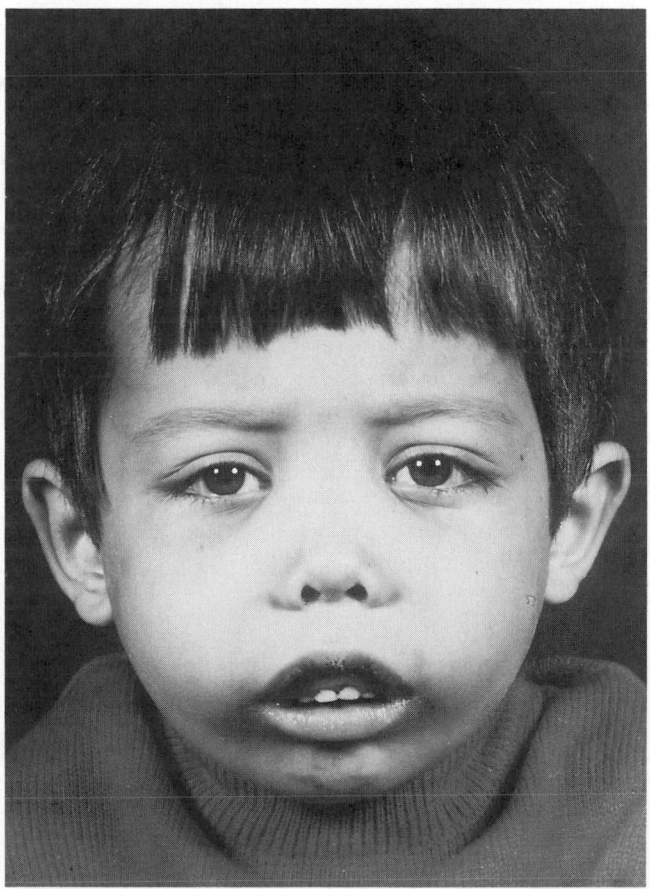

FIGURE 15-6. The facial appearance of a child with β-thalassemia major. The skull is bossed, with prominent frontal and parietal bones, and the maxilla is enlarged. (From Hoffbrand AV, Pettit JE: Essential Haematology, 2nd ed. London, Blackwell Scientific, 1984, with permission.)

LABORATORY FINDINGS AND CORRELATIONS WITH DISEASE

Peripheral Blood and Bone Marrow. Without transfusion, Hb values range between 2.5 and 6.5 g/dL. RBC morphology is strikingly abnormal, with microcytosis, hypochromia and extreme anisopoikilocytosis (Fig. 15-7). Numerous nucleated red cells, target cells and basophilic stippling are typical. In spite of the severe anemia and erythroid hyperplasia, the reticulocyte response is inadequate. This lower than expected reticulocytosis is reflective of the ineffective erythropoiesis that does not allow for adequate compensation of the severe anemia. Leukocytes characteristically are increased whereas the platelet count is generally normal. The bone marrow is hypercellular, showing marked erythroid hyperplasia.

Special Hematologic Tests. The pretransfusion Hb electrophoresis pattern (cellulose acetate, alkaline pH) in thalassemia major consists almost entirely of Hb F. Hb A_2 may be absent or the level may be reduced, normal, or slightly elevated (Table 15-7). In homozygous β^0-thalassemia (β^0/β^0) no β-chain synthesis occurs, so Hb A is absent. In the severe Mediterranean form (β^+/β^+) and in the β^0/β^+ form of thalassemia major, Hb A may be detected once the switch from γ- to β-chain production is complete a few months after birth. Transfusions will confound the estimation of the patient's own hemoglobin production ability.

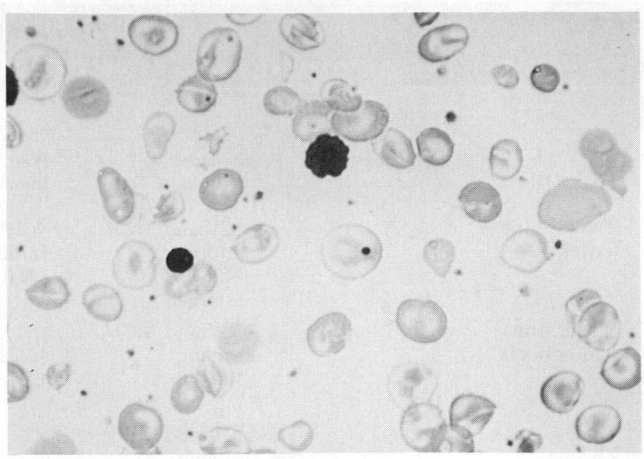

FIGURE 15-7. Peripheral blood film shows the morphologic appearance of red blood cells in homozygous β^0-thalassemia (Cooley's anemia). There is marked variation in erythrocyte size and shape. Note microcytosis and hypochromia. Target cells and nucleated red cells are present. (From the American Society of Hematology Slide Bank, 2nd ed. Seattle, 1977, used with permission.)

In homozygous Hb Lepore [$(\delta\beta)^{Lepore}/(\delta\beta)^{Lepore}$], approximately 8% to 30% of the Hb on electrophoresis at alkaline pH is Hb Lepore; the remainder is Hb F (see Table 15-7). Hbs A and A_2 characteristically are absent

TABLE 15-7
Hemoglobin Electrophoretic Results on Cellulose Acetate (Alkaline pH) in Various β-Thalassemia Syndromes

Genotype	Hb A (%)	Hb A_2 (%)	Hb F (%)	Hb Lepore (%)
NORMAL				
β/β	97	2.5–3.2	<1	
THALASSEMIA MAJOR				
β^0/β^0	0	1.0–5.9	>94	
β^+/β^+ (severe Mediterranean form)	Present	2.4–8.7	20–90	
β^0/β^+	Present	0.6–3.4	>75	
$(\delta\beta)^{Lepore}/(\delta\beta)^{Lepore}$	0	0	70–92	8–30
THALASSEMIA INTERMEDIA				
β^+/β^+ (mild form)	Present	5.4–10.0	30–73	
β^0/β	Present	>3.2	1.5–12	
$(\delta\beta)^0/(\delta\beta)^0$	0	0	100	
$(\delta\beta)^0/(\delta\beta)^{Lepore}$	0	0	92	8
THALASSEMIA MINOR				
β^+ or β^0/β	>90	3.5–8.0	1–2	
$(\delta\beta)^0/\beta$	<90	2.5–3.0	5–20	
$(\delta\beta)^{Lepore}/\beta$	Present	1.2–2.6	1–3	5–15
THALASSEMIA MINIMA				
β^{sc}/β	97	<3.2	<1	

Key: β^+, reduced β-chain production; β^0, no β-chain production; $(\delta\beta)^0$, deletion of δ- and β-genes; $(\delta\beta)^{Lepore}$, nonhomologous meiotic crossing-over between δ- and β-globin genes on chromosome 11; sc, silent carrier.

(Modified from Lukens JN: The thalassemias and related disorders: Quantitative disorders of hemoglobin synthesis. In Lee GR, Bithell TC, Foerster J et al [eds]: Wintrobe's Clinical Hematology, 9th ed, p 1119. Philadelphia, Lea & Febiger, 1993, with permission.)

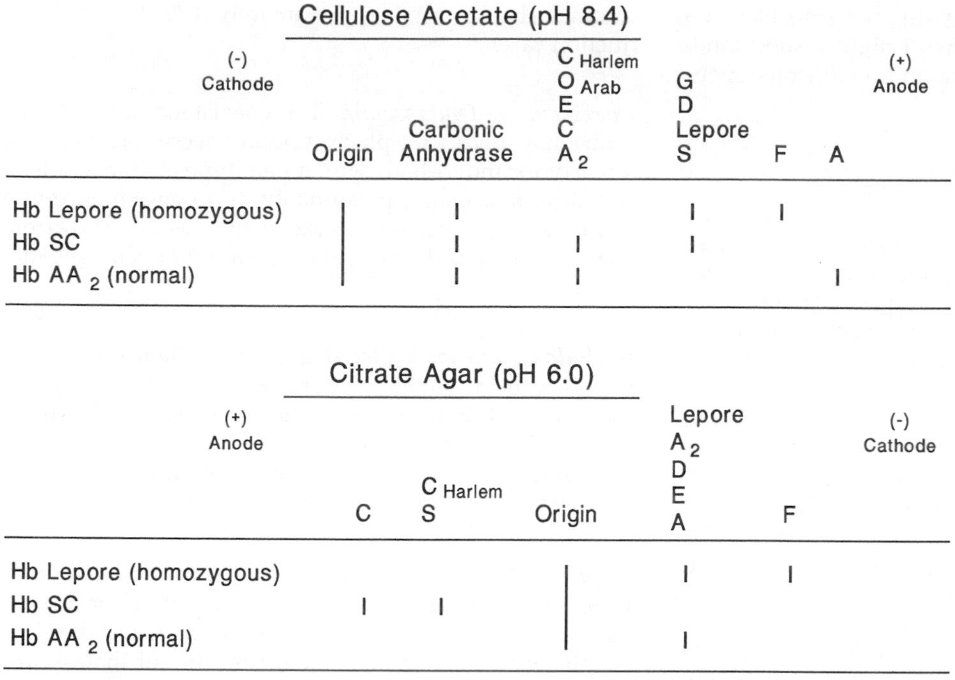

Cellulose Acetate (pH 8.4)

	Origin	Carbonic Anhydrase	C Harlem / O Arab / E / C / A_2	G / D / Lepore / S	F	A
	(-) Cathode					(+) Anode
Hb Lepore (homozygous)	|	I		I	I	
Hb SC	|	I	I	I		
Hb AA_2 (normal)	|	I	I			I

Citrate Agar (pH 6.0)

	C	C Harlem / S	Origin	Lepore / A_2 / D / E / A	F	
	(+) Anode					(-) Cathode
Hb Lepore (homozygous)			|	I	I	
Hb SC	I	I	|			
Hb AA_2 (normal)			|	I		

FIGURE 15-8. Differentiation of hemoglobins Lepore and S using cellulose acetate electrophoresis, pH 8.4, and citrate agar electrophoresis, pH 6.0. Note that both hemoglobins migrate to the same position on cellulose acetate, but are separated on citrate agar.

because normal β and δ chains are not produced. Hb Lepore migrates to the same position as Hb S on cellulose acetate electrophoresis at alkaline pH (Fig. 15-8). Hb Lepore produces a negative result for the solubility test for sickling hemoglobins (Chap. 14); however, this is not definitive for Hb Lepore. Citrate agar electrophoresis (acid pH) is required to differentiate Hb Lepore from Hb S. Hb Lepore migrates to the Hb A position on this medium, whereas Hb S migrates in the opposite direction, toward the anode (Fig. 15-8).

Note that Hbs Lepore and D migrate to the same position on both cellulose acetate (alkaline pH) and citrate agar (acid pH) electrophoresis. However, recall that Hb Lepore usually represents from 8% to 30% of the total Hb, whereas Hb D is usually 35% to 50% in the heterozygous (AD) state and approximately 95% in the homozygous (DD) state (see Table 14-9). Hbs Lepore and D may be definitively identified by globin chain electrophoresis (Chap. 14).

The acid elution technique for qualitative analysis of Hb F (see procedure later in this chapter) is helpful to differentiate the thalassemia major disorders (which all have increased Hb F) from hereditary persistence of fetal hemoglobin (HPFH). Thalassemia major syndromes generally reveal a heterogeneous distribution of Hb F in the red cells.[70] HPFH, in contrast, reveals a homogeneous distribution, with all cells containing Hb F.

Although not a particularly useful test in the diagnosis, the osmotic fragility of red cells (Chap. 17) is markedly decreased in thalassemia major. Some red cells do not even hemolyze in water owing to the large surface/volume ratio characteristic of target cells, which are common in these syndromes.

Chemistry. The hemolytic process associated with ineffective erythropoiesis results in a mild elevation of unconjugated bilirubin. Urine urobilinogen and fecal urobilin may also be increased. Lactate dehydrogenase (LD) levels are elevated as a consequence as well, and haptoglobin and hemopexin are reduced or absent. Serum ferritin and iron are elevated, and transferrin is often fully saturated owing to the iron overload problem in these disorders.

Other Special Tests. Routine and reliable prenatal diagnosis of the β-thalassemia major syndromes can be obtained by performing direct DNA analysis of a chorionic villus biopsy specimen obtained at 8 to 10 weeks' gestation. Chorionic villus sampling (CVS) will probably replace amniocentesis because it provides relatively large amounts of material for study and affords earlier diagnosis.[59]

EFFECTS OF TREATMENT ON LABORATORY RESULTS AND PROGNOSIS

In all cases of thalassemia major, the treatment and prognosis are generally the same. Without treatment, death usually occurs in the first or early second decade of life.[82] The mainstay of therapy is packed red cell transfusions. Hypertransfusion programs (to maintain Hb levels higher than 9 to 10 g/dL) and supertransfusion programs (to maintain Hb levels higher than 12 g/dL) have both been successful at restoring normal patterns of growth and development, and suppressing ineffective erythropoiesis while ameliorating the anemia, and reducing the gastrointestinal absorption of iron.[78] Transfusion hemosiderosis is now the major cause of late morbidity and mortality in thalassemia major. Because there is no physiologic way to induce significant excretion of iron, pharmacologic removal by the administration of an iron-chelating agent such as deferoxamine can be used to help forestall iron overload. Without chelation, death occurs in the second or third decade of life, principally due to hemosiderosis-induced heart disease. Therapy with nightly subcutaneous deferoxamine extends survival in transfusion-dependent thalassemia patients.[78]

NOVEL THERAPEUTIC APPROACHES

Allogeneic bone marrow transplantation has been used selectively for severe cases of β-thalassemia major. Risks associated with this procedure, including failure to engraft, have caused many clinicians to approach this procedure with caution.[68] Excess α-chain production underlies all the manifestations of β-thalassemia. Thus, any mechanism that reduces the excess of α-chains should reduce the clinical severity of the disease.

A novel approach to therapy that is still under investigation involves attempts to increase γ-chain synthesis by reactivation of γ-globin gene expression.[42,73] The γ-chains can then combine with the α chains to form Hb F. The drugs that have shown the greatest ability to augment Hb F production to date have all been antileukemia drugs with uncertain potentials for causing secondary malignancies if administered over long periods. Obviously long-term administration of cytotoxic compounds will never be an ideal therapeutic option, and research continues for more specific and less toxic agents to achieve this goal.

A major focus of current research involves the possibility of correcting the defect by gene therapy.[3,79] The success of this approach depends on two factors: (1) being able to deliver the gene into the pluripotent hematopoietic stem cells and integrating it into the genome so the gene will persist in the hematopoietic system, and (2) regulating the gene so that it will be expressed at a high level in the erythropoietic lineage.

Thalassemia Intermedia

Thalassemia intermedia describes certain β-thalassemias that are clinically milder than most thalassemia major syndromes, but are more severe than the thalassemia minor conditions. This classification is a clinical distinction, not a genetic one. The genetic defects are variable, and there is overlap between thalassemia intermedia and thalassemia major and minor (Table 15-5). It is the severity of the disorder which ultimately differentiates the subgroups.

In thalassemia intermedia, impairment of β-chain synthesis is less than that usually seen in thalassemia major, or the relative α-chain excess is reduced. This may be due to a variety of conditions discussed briefly below.

Mild β-Thalassemia Mutations. Homozygous β^+ (β^+/β^+) thalassemia can be caused by "mild" β^+-thalassemia alleles that result in the phenotype of thalassemia intermedia. The "mild form" of the β^+/β^+ genotype is common in Africans and African Americans and is associated with β^+-thalassemia alleles that cause less impairment of β-chain synthesis (approximately 50% of normal production rate) than seen with the β^+/β^+ genotype causing thalassemia major that is characteristic of individuals of Mediterranean background (approximately 10% of normal production rate).[82]

Coexistent α-Thalassemia. The coexistence of α-thalassemia may modify the phenotype and decrease the clinical severity for individuals with a genotype characteristic of β-thalassemia major, presumably as a consequence of a decrease in the total α-chain excess that results. The extent of amelioration is dependent on the number of α genes deleted.

β-Thalassemia with Elevated γ-Chain Synthesis. Coinheritance of a genotype characteristic of β-thalassemia major and HPFH, or one of the other less well-defined causes of a sustained production of γ-chains into adult life, results in a net decrease in α-chain excess, and a lessening of the clinical severity of β-thalassemia.

Triplicated α-Globin Genes with β-Thalassemia Trait. When the $\alpha\alpha\alpha$ haplotype is inherited with β^+ or β^0 trait, the extent of α-chain excess is compounded, and the clinical phenotype is often changed from that of thalassemia minor to thalassemia intermedia.

CLINICAL FINDINGS

Thalassemia intermedia presents with a wide spectrum of disability. At the mild end, growth and development of affected children may be relatively normal. At the severe end, patients may present with anemia later than is usual in the transfusion-dependent forms of β-thalassemia major, but growth and development may be compromised without some transfusion support. Clinical findings are similar to, but less severe than, those of thalassemia major; they may include pallor and moderate splenomegaly. Whether or not these individuals receive regular transfusions, they generally still develop progressive iron overload owing to the increased absorption of dietary iron secondary to marrow hyperactivity.

LABORATORY FINDINGS AND CORRELATIONS WITH DISEASE

Peripheral Blood and Bone Marrow. The peripheral blood picture is similar to that of thalassemia major, but the anemia is not as severe. Hb values range from 6 to 10 g/dL in untransfused patients. Generally these levels are sustained, and patients do not need to receive transfusions routinely. Erythrocytes are microcytic and hypochromic, with marked anisopoikilocytosis. Target cells, basophilic stippling and nucleated red cells are usually present on the peripheral blood film. The marrow shows significant erythroid hyperplasia.

Special Hematologic Tests. Hb electrophoresis at alkaline pH reveals a variety of patterns, depending on the genotype of the individual, and thus serves as an initial screening procedure (Table 15-7). Again, the distinction of β-thalassemia intermedia from β-thalassemia major or minor is based primarily on clinical presentation and transfusion requirements.

EFFECTS OF TREATMENT ON LABORATORY RESULTS AND PROGNOSIS

Treatment for thalassemia intermedia is supportive rather than active, and most individuals have a normal life span. Chelation therapy with deferoxamine may be necessary in individuals with significant iron overload.

Thalassemia Minor

Inheritance of a single β-thalassemia allele (thalassemia minor) is rarely associated with any clinical disability, and the abnormality is discovered only on performing a blood examination. This generally asymptomatic β-thalassemia disorder produces little or no anemia, although peripheral blood erythrocyte morphology is abnormal. The syndromes producing the phenotype of thalassemia minor are indistinguishable, clinically and hematologically, except when Hb Lepore is found on Hb electrophoresis (see Table 15-5). Usually no treatment is required, and affected individuals have a normal life span.

HETEROZYGOUS β⁰- OR β⁺-THALASSEMIA

This condition, also called β-thalassemia trait or high-Hb A₂ thalassemia, is caused by the combination of a normal β-gene and either a β^0 or a β^+ gene (β^0/β or β^+/β). Clinically, there seem to be no distinguishing features between the two genotypes, but differentiation can be accomplished by special DNA studies, if necessary. Hb electrophoresis usually shows an elevated Hb A₂ level (see Table 15-7).

LABORATORY FINDINGS AND CORRELATIONS WITH DISEASE

Peripheral Blood and Bone Marrow. Hb values of individuals with β-thalassemia minor are usually 1 or 2 g/dL lower than that seen in normal persons of the same age and sex (mean Hb concentration for men 12.9 g/dL[50,51,64] and for women, 10.9 g/dL[51,64]). The peripheral blood film shows microcytic, hypochromic red cells, with anisopoikilocytosis, target cells and basophilic stippling (Fig. 15-9). Unlike thalassemia major and intermedia, nucleated red cells are generally not present. The reticulocyte count may be slightly elevated if anemia is present. The bone marrow shows slight erythroid hyperplasia.

Special Hematologic Tests. Hb electrophoresis for β^0 or β^+/β characteristically shows an elevated Hb A₂ to about twice the normal level, although concomitant iron deficiency will reduce the Hb A₂, sometimes into the normal range.[74] Approximately half of all thalassemia minor patients have a slightly elevated Hb F.[18] Special stains for erythrocyte inclusions are negative. It is important to perform chemical analysis to differentiate the microcytosis of β-thalassemia minor from that of iron deficiency (see Differentiation of Iron Deficiency and Thalassemia and Table 15-9).

Thalassemia Minima (Silent β-Thalassemia Trait)

Thalassemia minima describes a form of β-thalassemia in which no clinical or laboratory abnormality is usually detected. The disorder is discovered accidentally or during family studies. The genotype (β^{sc}/β) indicates the silent form (sc denotes silent carrier) of an abnormal β-globin gene (Table 15-7).[80]

HEREDITARY PERSISTENCE OF FETAL HEMOGLOBIN AND δβ-THALASSEMIA

Hereditary persistence of fetal hemoglobin (HPFH) is characterized by either deletion or inactivation of the δ and β structural gene complex, with continued synthesis of γ chain production into adult life, preventing significant clinical abnormalities. HPFH describes a heterogeneous group of inherited disorders characterized by increased levels of Hb F in adults, in the absence of the usual clinical and hematologic features of thalassemia.[82] There are two morphologically defined categories of HPFH: (1) pancellular, in which there is uniform distribution of Hb F among all red cells, as determined by the acid elution slide test, and (2) heterocellular, in which only a subpopulation of red cells contains increased Hb F.

Specific clinical and hematologic characteristics of HPFH vary among ethnic groups, owing to differences in the causative genetic mutations.[14,78,86] In general, heterozygotes have normal RBCs, a near normal MCH and Hct, a slightly elevated RBC count, and 15% to 35% Hb F on Hb electrophoresis. Homozygotes have 100% Hb F on electrophoresis, with slightly microcytic, hypochromic red cells. The red cell count is elevated as a compensatory measure for the increased oxygen affinity of Hb F, which causes a left shift in the oxygen dissociation curve (Fig. 7-5).

The δβ-thalassemia disorders are those in which there is reduced $(\delta\beta)^+$ or absent $(\delta\beta)^0$ output of δ and β chains from the affected chromosomes.

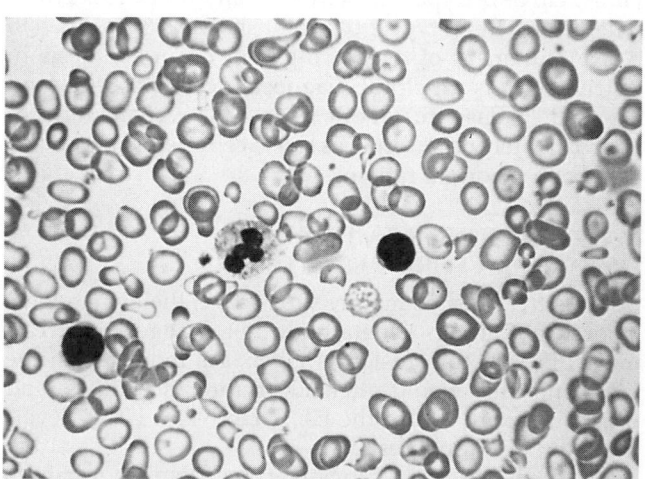

FIGURE 15-9. The morphologic appearance of red blood cells in heterozygous β-thalassemia (β-thalassemia trait) demonstrates microcytosis and varying degrees of hypochromia and poikilocytosis. Target cells and basophilic stippling are common findings. (From the American Society of Hematology Slide Bank, 2nd ed. Seattle, 1977, used with permission.)

The $(\delta\beta)^0$-thalassemias usually result from deletions involving the β-gene cluster, which remove the β and δ genes, but which leave either one or both of the γ-globin genes intact.[78] They produce a phenotype that is similar to the phenotype of deletion forms of HPFH, as there is increased output of γ-chains from the γ-locus, but to a lesser extent. As a result, individuals show abnormal red blood cell morphology and a variable anemia. Indeed, it has been proposed that $\delta\beta$-thalassemia and HPFH represent varying degrees of the same genetic phenomenon, with HPFH producing a milder phenotype owing to a greater output of γ-chains. It is not known why such similar genetic lesions result in different phenotypes.

The homozygous state for $\delta\beta$-thalassemia $[(\delta\beta)^0/(\delta\beta)^0]$ is clinically milder than Cooley's anemia (β^0/β^0), and is one form of thalassemia intermedia. Only Hb F is present (see Table 15-7); the red cells are microcytic, hypochromic, and the individual generally has a Hb concentration of 8 to 11 g/dL. Heterozygotes $[(\delta\beta)^0/\beta)]$ are clinically and hematologically similar to β-thalassemia minor, though the Hb F is higher (5% to 20% range), and the Hb A_2 is normal or slightly reduced.

THALASSEMIA WITH ABNORMAL HEMOGLOBIN VARIANTS

There are numerous well-documented cases of the double heterozygous condition in which thalassemia is associated with an abnormal hemoglobin variant.[82] A common feature is the presence of microcytic, hypochromic red cells.[10] When the same type of globin chain is affected in such double heterozygous subjects, the percentage of variant hemoglobin is usually greater than when it occurs in the simple heterozygous state. For example, when sickle hemoglobin (Hb S) (a β-chain variant) coexists with β-thalassemia, the Hb S concentration in red cells is higher than that of Hb A. However in the simple heterozygous AS state, the Hb A concentration is higher than that of Hb S.

Conversely, when the affected globin chains are different (*e.g.*, when α-thalassemia is inherited with a β-chain structural variant) the β-chain Hb variant is present in lower amounts than when it is found in the simple heterozygous state.[70] This is believed to be due to a higher affinity of α-chains for normal β-chains than variant β-chains. Therefore the α-chains that are synthesized combine preferentially with normal β-chains, thereby increasing the Hb A concentration.[78]

Hb S–β-Thalassemia

The doubly heterozygous condition Hb S–β-thalassemia is associated with clinical features similar to, although not as severe as, those of sickle cell anemia. Hb S–β^0-thalassemia (with no production of Hb A) is clinically more severe than Hb S–β^+-thalassemia, and is similar in severity to sickle cell anemia. The Hb S–β^+-thalassemias are classified as type 1 (clinically severe and hematologically abnormal, although less so than Hb S–β^0) and type

2 (causes only a mild anemia and patients are asymptomatic).

GENETICS, DEMOGRAPHICS AND CLINICAL FINDINGS

Hb S–β-thalassemia is a common double heterozygous sickling disorder among African Americans (1 in 1667 births), second only to the double heterozygous Hb SC disease (1 in 833 births).[53] It is also prevalent in people of Greek, Turkish, Indian, North African, Mediterranean and Rumanian ancestry.[86] Both Hb S–β^0 and Hb S–β^+ may be seen in any of these groups.

In Hb S–β^0-thalassemia, many of the same findings and crises that occur in sickle cell anemia occur, although the disease is somewhat milder. Unlike Hb SS disease, splenic infarction usually does not occur. Table 15-8 provides a comparison of the clinical findings in Hb S–β^0- and Hb S–β^+-thalassemia with those in a normal individual.

LABORATORY FINDINGS AND CORRELATIONS WITH DISEASE

In severe Hb S–β^0-thalassemia the Hb ranges from 5 to 10 g/dL, and the reticulocyte count between 10% and 20%. Erythrocytes are microcytic, hypochromic with marked anisopoikilocytosis, a high RDW, basophilic stippling, and many target cells and sickle cells on the peripheral blood film (Fig. 15-10). In Hb S–β^+-thalassemia type 1, the Hb ranges from 7 to 10 g/dL; sickle cells may be found, and the reticulocyte count may be normal or slightly decreased. In Hb S–β^+-thalassemia type 2, there is little or no anemia, and there are few red cell abnormalities. Decreases in MCV and MCH may be the only clues to the abnormality.

The solubility test for sickling Hb is positive, and the percentage Hb S on cellulose acetate electrophoresis is always higher than that of Hb A. Hbs A_2 and F levels are characteristically elevated. Note that in sickle cell (Hb SS) disease, the Hb F level is also increased, but the Hb A_2 level is usually normal. Hb S–β^0-thalassemia shows no Hb A; Hb S–β^+ type 1 usually has only up to 15% Hb A, whereas Hb S–β^+ type 2 typically shows 20% to 30% Hb A. Measurement of α- and β-globin chain synthesis in reticulocytes is a helpful diagnostic tool. Hb S–β^0- and Hb S–β^+-thalassemias both have a β/α chain ratio of approximately 0.5:1, whereas sickle cell anemia and sickle trait have a normal ratio of 1:1.[10]

EFFECTS OF TREATMENT ON LABORATORY RESULTS

Because treatment is mainly supportive, the hematologic laboratory findings generally do not change with treatment unless a transfusion is given. As indicated in the foregoing, this would alter all erythrocyte values, and proportionately reduce the Hb S, Hb F and Hb A_2 levels found on electrophoresis.

Patients with mild Hb S–β^+ type 2 live a normal life and require little medical attention. Because this condition is so variable, those with Hb S–β^+ type 1 and Hb S–β^0 may also live full lives with proper medical care, or they may have severe anemia and recurrent sickling crises.

TABLE 15-8
Differential Laboratory and Clinical Features
of Hb S–β⁰-Thalassemia and Hb S–β⁺-Thalassemia

	Normal Adult	Hb S–/β⁰-Thalassemia	Hb S–β⁺-Thalassemia*
Anemia	−	+++	+/+++
Anemia classification†	−	M/H	M/H
Hb S (%)‡	0	80–95	55–75
Hb A (%)‡	97	0	5–30
Hb F (%)‡	<1	≤5–20§	≤5–20§
Hb A₂ (%)‡	2.5–3.2	>3.5	>3.5
Solubility test‖	−	+	+
Peripheral blood sickle cells	−	+	+/−
β/α chains	1/1	0.5/1	0.5/1
Splenomegaly	−	++	−/++
Painful crises	−	+++	−/+++
Hematuria	−	+/−	−/+
Hemolytic episodes	−	++	−/++

Key: −, none or negative; +/−, occasional or none; + slight; ++, moderate; +++, marked.
* Hb S–β⁺-thalassemia actually comprises two groups, types 1 and 2 (see text).
† M/H, Microcytic, hypochromic.
‡ Percentages are based on cellulose acetate electrophoresis (alkaline pH). The percentages given are general guidelines.
In reality, the results associated with any given case may vary from these ranges.
§ Fetal hemoglobin levels of 20% are also seen with Hb S—hereditary persistence of fetal hemoglobin (HPFH).
‖ Solubility test for sickling hemoglobin (Chap. 14).

Bone marrow transplantation may be a therapeutic alternative for those most severely affected.

UNUSUAL FORMS OF THALASSEMIA

There are many rare and unusual forms of thalassemia[19,20,30,35,70,80] that may be inherited including the $\varepsilon\gamma\delta\beta$-thalassemias, γ-thalassemias, and δ-thalassemias. Refer to the foregoing referenced texts for details on these disorders.

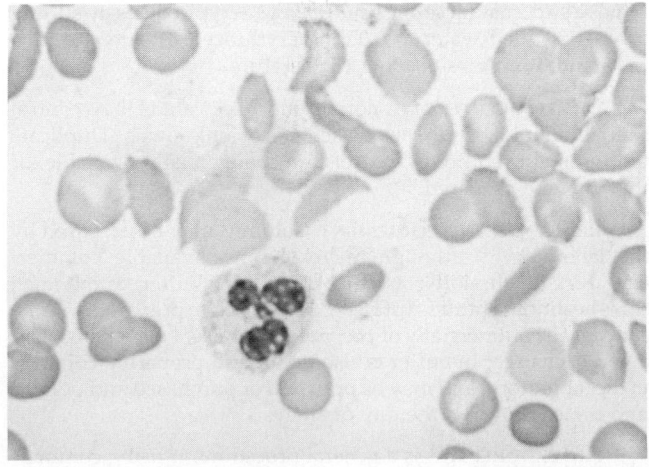

FIGURE 15-10. Peripheral blood film from a patient with Hb S–β⁰-thalassemia.

DIFFERENTIATION OF IRON DEFICIENCY ANEMIA AND THALASSEMIA

Presenting symptoms, physical findings, and the morphologic appearance of erythrocytes in the severe thalassemia disorders are generally so distinctive that there should be no confusion with iron deficiency. When microcytic indices are first detected, without such abnormal morphology or clinical findings, iron deficiency is often the first condition considered because it is more common. However, unsuspected or mild thalassemia minor should be ruled out in these situations.

Laboratory tests for the differentiation of iron deficiency and thalassemia are summarized in Table 15-9. The results of the erythrocyte count and RDW are distinctly different,[37,74] as are serum ferritin,[29,32,52] serum iron, total iron-binding capacity and transferrin saturation.[69] Iron studies are discussed in Chapter 13.

The zinc protoporphyrin/heme (ZPP/H) ratio is a measurement of iron status that is increased in chronic iron deficiency,[39] but normal in thalassemia minor (Table 15-9). Thus, the ZPP/H ratio is useful in differentiating the two disorders. ZPP is the substance that builds up in red cells when ferrous iron (Fe²⁺) is deficient or not available for binding with protoporphyrin IX to make heme (see Fig. 13-1). Excess ZPP may be the result of iron deficiency caused by a variety of conditions (e.g., poor diet or excessive blood loss). The ZPP test may be used in place of the previously used free erythrocyte protoporphyrin (FEP) test, in which acid extraction removes the zinc,

TABLE 15-9
Laboratory Tests to Differentiate Iron Deficiency and Thalassemia Minor

	Erythrocyte Count ($\times 10^{12}$ cells/L)	RDW	Serum Ferritin	Serum Iron	Total Iron-Binding Capacity	Transferrin Saturation (%)	ZPP/H
Thalassemia minor	>5.5	Normal or sl ↑	Normal or sl ↑	Normal	Normal	Normal	Normal
Iron deficiency	<5.5	↑	↓	↓	↑	↓	↑

Key: sl, slight; ↑, elevated; ↓, depressed; ZPP/H, zinc protoporphyrin/heme ratio.

leaving FEP in the test solution. Now, ZPP may be measured directly with a hematofluorometer. The increase in the ZPP/H ratio in iron deficiency may be the first biochemical change that is readily measurable following a decline in iron status.[40]

Thalassemia minor may also have to be differentiated from other disorders of iron metabolism (see Table 13-1).

MOST USEFUL LABORATORY TESTS FOR DIAGNOSING THALASSEMIA

The laboratory tests that are beneficial in diagnosing thalassemia are summarized in Table 15-2. They are discussed briefly in this section.

Hemoglobin Electrophoresis

Electrophoresis on cellulose acetate medium at alkaline pH is a useful screening procedure for separating normal and abnormal hemoglobin variants (Chap. 14) and the hemoglobins of the thalassemia syndromes such as Hbs H, Barts, Constant Spring and Lepore (see Figs. 15-4 and 15-8). Electrophoresis at alkaline pH should not be the sole diagnostic test for thalassemia trait. The Hb A_2 elevation associated with β-thalassemia trait may be suspected from careful inspection of the electrophoresis strip, but it must be confirmed quantitatively. The electrophoretic pattern in α-thalassemia minor and silent carrier α-thalassemia is normal except in newborns.[71]

Citrate agar electrophoresis at acid pH is useful in differentiating some abnormal hemoglobins that migrate together on cellulose acetate (*e.g.*, Hb Lepore and Hb S; see Fig. 15-8).

Quantitation of Hb F

There are numerous situations in which the quantitation of Hb F (Chap. 14) is beneficial to further categorize certain thalassemia conditions. Significantly elevated Hb F levels are seen in many forms of β-thalassemia (see Table 15-7) as well as pancellular HPFH. Moderate or slight elevations in Hb F generally are seen in thalassemia minor conditions and the heterocellular forms of HPFH.

Quantitation of Hb A_2 by Microchromatography[54]

Very small amounts of Hb A_2 (up to about 3.5%) are found in normal adults. Elevated levels of Hb A_2, usually 4.0% to 8.0%, generally indicate β-thalassemia trait, but in some persons, homozygous β-thalassemia may be indicated. Hb A_2 may also be slightly elevated in association with Hb S trait or sickle cell anemia, unstable hemoglobin variants, and megaloblastic anemias.

Decreased Hb A_2 may be found in iron deficiency anemia, Hb H disease, δ- and $\delta\beta$-thalassemia trait, many forms of HPFH, and Hb Lepore trait. Patients with β-thalassemia trait who are also iron deficient may have a Hb A_2 level in the normal range.

Hb A_2 by Microchromatography

PRINCIPLE. In ion-exchange chromatography, the interaction of charged groups on the anion-exchange medium with charged groups on the hemoglobin molecules results in separation of different hemoglobin fractions. At a pH above 8.5, the majority of hemoglobins bind to the anion-exchange support medium. At pH 8.3, Hb A_2 is eluted from the column; the remaining hemoglobins are eluted when a buffer of lower pH (*e.g.*, 7.0) is passed through. The separated hemoglobins may be quantitated by spectrophotometry.

SPECIMEN REQUIREMENTS AND PREPARATION. EDTA blood samples are required (may be stored at 4°C up to 10 days). To prepare the specimen, centrifuge sample, remove plasma, and wash erythrocytes once in isotonic saline. Centrifuge again and remove supernatant saline solution. Lyse erythrocytes by adding 0.4 mL distilled water to 0.05 mL erythrocytes. Vortex to mix. Let stand 5 minutes at room temperature.

QUALITY CONTROL. A normal and an elevated Hb A_2 control sample should be run with each set of unknowns. Duplicate testing is not required. Controls are commercially available, or they may be prepared.[31,66]

REAGENTS AND EQUIPMENT. Columns may be prepared by the laboratory,[54] although microcolumns, available commercially, are much more convenient. The stock buffer, from which three additional buffers (pH 8.5, 8.3 and 7.0) are prepared, may be purchased commercially or prepared in-house.[54] A suspension of anion exchanger in buffer is also required if preparing columns in the laboratory, and may be prepared or purchased and poured into the columns on the day of analysis.

PROCEDURE. This is a general procedure. If using commercially purchased equipment and reagents, follow package insert instructions.

1. Set up columns containing pH 8.5 buffer and anion-exchange medium vertically in racks. Some procedures may require allowing columns to stand for a short period to drain.
2. Remove excess pH 8.5 buffer from top of column by aspiration using a Pasteur pipette, leaving a small residual layer of buffer (about 0.05 mL) to make the next step easier.
3. Using another Pasteur pipette, carefully apply 0.05 mL hemolysate to top of column, being careful not to disturb exchange medium. If hemolysate is dilute, use 0.1 mL. Allow hemolysate to soak into the top 5 mm of the column.
4. Fill reservoir with 6 mL pH 8.3 buffer. Collect approximately 6 mL of the effluent dripping from the bottom of the column into a 10-mL volumetric flask. This takes approximately 1 hour and represents fraction I. Final drops of effluent appear colorless. Dilute to 10-mL volume with distilled water.
5. Add 6 mL of pH 7.0 buffer to top of column. Collect this 6-mL effluent, which contains all remaining hemoglobin, in a 25-mL volumetric flask and designate as fraction II. Dilute to 25-mL volume with distilled water. A small amount of red-brown color may remain at the top of the column. This is normal, but no red bands should remain in the ion exchange column.
6. Mix and measure absorbance of fractions I and II at 415 nm using pH 7.0 buffer as a blank.

CALCULATIONS

$$\text{Hb A}_2 \text{ (\% of total)} = \frac{\text{A fraction I}}{\text{A fraction I} + (2.5 \times [\text{A fraction II}])} \times 100\%$$

where A fraction I = Absorbance (at 415 nm) of Hb A_2 eluate (after diluting to 10-mL volume)

A fraction II = Absorbance (at 415 nm) of eluate (after diluting to 25-mL volume) containing all other hemoglobins after Hb A_2 has been eluted. (Multiplying by a factor of 2.5 corrects for the difference in dilution volumes between fractions I and II.)

REFERENCE RANGE. Each laboratory must establish its own reference range. As a guideline, results for normal adults established by the CDC National Hemoglobinopathy Laboratory are 1.8% to 3.5%.[11]

COMMENTS AND SOURCES OF ERROR

1. Hemoglobin A_2 must be measured with considerable precision, because the diagnosis of β-thalassemia trait may hinge on the determination of a Hb A_2 value only 1% to 2% above the reference range.
2. When slow-moving hemoglobin fractions such as Hb S are present, this procedure must be modified slightly. Commercial kits are available for the quantitation of Hb A_2 when variants such as Hb S are present (see item 8).[5,9]
3. Other methods may be used to measure Hb A_2, including elution from segments cut from cellulose acetate followed by spectrophotometry. Measurements are also possible using densitometric scanning of electrophoretic strips, but these methods may suffer from considerable imprecision.[26]
4. If reagents prepared by the laboratory are too acidic, the pH should not be adjusted with a base, as this will cause salts to form and strip the hemoglobin from the column. In this situation, the reagent should be prepared again from scratch.
5. Inaccurate pH adjustment of anion-exchange medium and buffers, and bubbles in the slurry, will cause erroneous results.
6. Overloading columns with hemolysate sample may cause incomplete Hb A_2 separation.
7. Insufficient hemolysate sample may make visual collection of Hb A_2 fraction impossible.
8. Hbs A_2, S, S-G hybrid, C, E, D and O (O-Arab) may coelute

(i.e., be removed from the column in a single fraction) using some microchromatographic procedures. Any measured values for Hb A_2 of 10% or more should be assumed to indicate the presence of one or more of these other Hbs and investigated further. The Sickle-Thal Quik Column (Helena Laboratories, Beaumont TX) is designed for quantiation of Hb A_2 in the presence of Hbs A, F, S and numerous other abnormal Hb variants.

Brilliant Cresyl Blue Test for Hb H Inclusions

In Hb H disease, α-thalassemia trait, and silent carrier α-thalassemia, the redox dye BCB can be used to induce precipitation of intrinsically unstable Hb H.[9,34] Because inclusion-containing cells may be rare in both the trait and silent forms of α-thalassemia, a modified procedure that enhances the development of Hb H inclusions is described.

Brilliant Cresyl Blue Stain for Hb H

PRINCIPLE. Cells containing an unstable hemoglobin, such as Hb H, normally are removed promptly from the circulation by the reticuloendothelial system. When relatively young erythrocytes containing sufficient Hb H to form inclusions are released to the circulation, they are diluted in a population of cells with more nearly balanced globin chain synthesis and a normal life span.

When a blood sample is centrifuged to separate plasma and cells, the red cells taken from just below the buffy coat consist primarily of young, buoyant cells. These young cells are the most capable of forming the typical Hb H inclusions if α-thalassemia is in fact present. Hb H inclusions, if present, are stained by BCB and may be viewed microscopically on blood films after special staining.

SPECIMEN REQUIREMENTS AND REAGENTS. A fresh whole blood specimen anticoagulated with EDTA is required.

For 1% BCB solution, combine sodium citrate, 0.4 g; normal saline, 100 mL; and BCB, 1 g. Filter before using. Solution must be stored in a dark bottle.

QUALITY CONTROL. A significant number of reticulocytes should be visible on the patient specimen. If there are no reticulocytes, the specimen may not have been concentrated properly during preparation.

PROCEDURE

1. Fill four microhematocrit tubes with blood and seal. Spin in microhematocrit centrifuge for 5 minutes. Score and break tubes approximately 3 mm above and 5 mm below the plasma-cell interface. Safely discard the end pieces.
2. Expel contents of the four tube sections into a 12- $\times$ 75-mm test tube. Add 1 to 1-1/2 drops of BCB stain to test tube and mix. Incubate at 37°C for 30 minutes.
3. Fill one microhematocrit tube with BCB-cell mixture. Balance this tube with an empty tube in microhematocrit centrifuge and spin for 5 minutes. Score and break tube approximately 4 mm below BCB–cell meniscus.
4. Expel cells and small amount of BCB solution onto microscope slide and mix. Remove buffy coat if it is expelled onto the slide.
5. Make a wedge preparation blood film. Let dry. Examine approximately 50,000 red cells under 100$\times$ oil immersion lens (approximately 200 fields containing 250 red cells per field; adjust according to each film reviewed). Count the number of cells with inclusions and report as number per 50,000 cells reviewed.

INTERPRETATION OF RESULTS. Hemoglobin H inclusions, consisting of denatured β-globin chains, typically appear as small, multiple, irregularly shaped greenish blue bodies with a pitted pattern similar to that of golf balls (Figs. 8-29 and 14-8*B*). They usually are fairly uniformly distributed throughout the erythrocyte.

Almost all red cells contain inclusions in Hb H disease, whereas few to several cells may contain inclusions in α-thalassemia trait. Rare cells, perhaps as few as 1 in 50,000, may be positive in silent carrier α-thalassemia. Negative BCB results do not necessarily exclude the trait or silent forms of α-thalassemia.

COMMENTS AND SOURCES OF ERROR
1. Hb H inclusions must be distinguished from reticulocytes on the specimen film. Reticulocytes have a bluish purple, irregular, granular or filamentous pattern (Fig. 8-29).
2. If conditions favor Heinz body formation (Chap. 14; Figs. 8-29 and 14-8*A*), these red cell inclusions can be differentiated from Hb H inclusions, as Heinz bodies are larger, are fewer and most often appear eccentrically along the membrane of the red cell.
3. Hb H is not entirely specific to α-thalassemia because rare patients with erythroleukemia, granulocytic leukemia, or other myeloproliferative disorders have also been described with this abnormality.
4. Each BCB dye lot must be tested against red cells known to contain Hb H because individual lots of dye vary in their ability to produce satisfactory preparations.

Acid Elution Slide Test (Kleihauer–Betke Stain) for Hb F

Frequently the intracellular distribution of Hb F is used to differentiate thalassemias with increased Hb F from pancellular HPFH. In thalassemia there is nonuniform (heterogeneous) distribution of Hb F from cell to cell (*i.e.*, some cells contain Hb F and some do not). In pancellular HPFH, all erythrocytes show nearly uniform (homogeneous) retention of Hb F.

It is important to recognize that a heterogeneous distribution of Hb F may also be found in sickle cell anemia and other hemoglobinopathies, as well as in acquired aplastic anemia (Chap. 11), owing to the elevated Hb F concentration in these disorders.

Acid Elution of Hb F

PRINCIPLE. All hemoglobins, with the exception of Hb F, are eluted from red cells on a blood film by citric acid–phosphate buffer at acid pH (3.3 to 3.5). Following the elution procedure, blood films are stained with Ehrlich's acid hematoxylin and counterstained with erythrosin (eosin B; 0.1% w/v). Slides are then examined microscopically under high, dry magnification.[9,11,38]

SPECIMEN REQUIREMENTS. Either EDTA-anticoagulated blood or blood obtained by microcollection may be used.

QUALITY CONTROL. A known normal sample and a known sample of HPFH should be run with each set of slides. If a known HPFH sample cannot be obtained, an abnormal control is prepared by mixing 1 drop normal adult blood with 1 drop fresh cord blood, which must be ABO blood group compatible.

PROCEDURE
1. Incubate citric acid–phosphate buffer in Coplin jar covered with Parafilm for 30 minutes at 37°C.
2. Dilute patient sample, normal, and abnormal control 1 : 1 with normal saline.
3. Make thin blood films using the patient, normal, and abnormal control specimens. Allow to air dry for 10 to 60 minutes.
4. Fix blood films in 80% (v/v) ethyl alcohol for 5 minutes. Rinse gently with distilled water.
5. Incubate slides in 37°C citric acid–phosphate buffer (see step 1) for 6 minutes. Occasionally lift slides up and down to provide gentle agitation during incubation.
6. After 6 minutes, remove slides, rinse with distilled water, and air dry. Stain in acid hematoxylin for 3 minutes. Rinse with distilled water, then blot edge of glass slide on absorbent material to remove as much water as possible. Counterstain with erythrosin for 3 minutes. Rinse with distilled water and air dry.
7. Examine using light microscopy under high, dry magnification.

INTERPRETATION OF RESULTS. Cells containing Hb F will be stained bright pink to red, whereas normal adult cells that do not contain Hb F appear as "ghost cells" (only the outer cell membrane is visible).

COMMENTS AND SOURCES OF ERROR
1. The elution time and pH of the citric acid–phosphate buffer must be carefully controlled.
2. High, dry magnification should be used to examine as much of the stained slide as possible. It is actually more difficult to focus on the acid-eluted and stained specimen using oil immersion microscopy, owing to the faint appearance of the ghost cells.
3. Kits are available commercially (Sigma Diagnostics, St. Louis MO) that measure the distribution of Hb F in red cells. Such kits may help standardize the procedure, particularly in laboratories where this test is performed infrequently.
4. There are instances when the differentiation of HPFH and thalassemia may be difficult, even in laboratories with personnel experienced in looking at samples from patients with these disorders.

SPECIAL LABORATORY PROCEDURES FOR DIAGNOSING THALASSEMIA

Specialized testing, including globin chain synthesis and DNA analysis, may be performed to identify thalassemia and to elucidate specific genotypes when a conclusive diagnosis cannot be made by routine laboratory tests. On a case-by-case basis, the physician, with the help of laboratory personnel, must decide whether the benefit of a complete diagnosis warrants the expense of further specialized testing.

Globin chain synthesis studies reveal the ratio of β- to α-globin chains. This is accomplished by incubating reticulocytes with a radioactive amino acid, usually [^{14}C]leucine. The globin chains synthesized by the reticulocytes during the incubation period incorporate the radioactive amino acid. The radioactive β- and α-globin chains are then precipitated, separated by column chromatography, and the fractions counted for radioactivity. The rate of synthesis for each chain is calculated to determine the production ratio of β- to α-chains.[11] Table 15-6 shows the results of β/α ratio calculations for the β thalassemias.

DNA analysis is also useful (Chap. 31), both in the postnatal and prenatal diagnosis of some thalassemias. The procedure requires special equipment and reagents, as described elsewhere.[11] DNA analysis may be required in special situations when a patient's genotype is necessary for accurate diagnosis or for genetic counseling purposes.

CHAPTER SUMMARY

The thalassemias are a heterogeneous group of hereditary disorders found worldwide. They result from varied genetic mutations that lead to a quantitative reduction in globin chain synthesis. The α- and β-thalassemias are the most prevalent and result from a decrease in the synthesis of α- and β-globin chains, respectively.

The primary cause of α-thalassemia is gene deletion; however, nondeletion types have been described. Major hematologic features of the α-thalassemias are summarized in Table 15-4.

The β-thalassemias are classified as β^0 and β^+. In β^0-thalassemia, no β-globin chains are produced by the mutant gene, whereas in β^+-thalassemia, some β-globin chains are produced. Unlike α-thalassemia, most β-thalassemias are not due to gene deletion, but to point mutations in the DNA genetic code. Laboratory findings for some of the β-thalassemias are summarized in Tables 15-6 and 15-7. Additionally, thalassemias and hemoglobinopathies may coexist (*e.g.*, Hb S–β^0-thalassemia; see Table 15-8).

Synthesis of other globin chains may also be impaired. Hereditary persistence of fetal hemoglobin (HPFH) is a condition caused by deletion or inactivation of the β- and δ-gene complex. It results in persistence of Hb F synthesis throughout adult life, but is usually not associated with a thalassemia phenotype. The γ-chain synthesis in HPFH is able to compensate for the absence or decrease of β- and δ- globin production. In the $\delta\beta$-thalassemias, there is also decreased or absent β- and δ-globin synthesis, but the increase in γ-chain production is not as great as seen in HPFH; therefore, a thalassemic phenotype results.

Most thalassemias can be diagnosed by doing a few carefully selected laboratory procedures (see Table 15-2). Differentiation of thalassemia minor and iron deficiency through laboratory studies (see Table 15-9) is also important for appropriate patient therapy.

Treatment of symptomatic thalassemia generally consists of red cell transfusion with the regular provision of chelating agents to help control iron overload. The vast majority of thalassemias are benign and do not require treatment.

Case Study 15-1

A 22-year-old Italian man was hospitalized with a broken leg. He had always been in good health; this was his first hospitalization. Laboratory tests were ordered and the results (and corresponding reference ranges for this laboratory) were as follows: WBC 7.4 × 10⁹/L (4.0–10); RBC 6.35 × 10¹²/L (4.7–6.1); Hb 13.3 g/dL (13.5–17.5); Hct 0.40 L/L (0.41–0.53); MCV 63 fL (82–100); MCH 21.0 pg (27–33); MCHC 32.0 g/dL (31–35); serum iron 110 μg/dL (65–165); TIBC 320 μg/dL (300–360); percentage transferrin saturation 34% (20–50); Hb electrophoresis on cellulose acetate (alkaline pH), Hb A 92.2% (more than 95); Hb F 2.1% (less than 1.0); Hb A₂ 5.7% (1.8–3.5).

1. Identify all abnormal laboratory results. What condition might these results suggest? Why?
2. What would be the expected red cell morphology on the Wright-stained peripheral blood film?
3. Does this condition require treatment?

4. What is the life expectancy of this patient?
5. If the mother of this man's children were heterozygous for β-thalassemia (β^0/β), what are the predicted chances that their offspring will inherit normal β-genes or be homozygous or heterozygous for β-thalassemia?

Case Study 15-2

A 17-year-old Southeast Asian girl presented with a chronic, moderate, microcytic, hypochromic anemia. She had an enlarged spleen, but was otherwise physically normal. Her reticulocyte count was increased to 5%. There was no anemia in her father's history, but her mother had a very mild microcytic anemia with no associated clinical disabilities.

1. A complete blood count has already determined that the patient was moderately anemic. Because this probably is a hereditary disorder and the patient is Southeast Asian, what laboratory test might next be ordered?
2. Given the suspected diagnosis of an α-thalassemia syndrome, what is the probable genotype of this patient and why (see Table 15-4)?
3. What are the most probable genotypes of the mother and father?
4. Considering the patient's suspected genotype, what results would be expected of the laboratory test recommended in answer no. 1?

Case Study 15-3

A 21-year-old black man was seen for pain and stiffness of 13 weeks' duration in the right knee. He stated that at 2 years of age he was diagnosed with sickle cell anemia when he was hospitalized for swelling of his ankles and wrists. He was successfully treated with analgesics and blood transfusions. Since then, he had continued to have similar problems of varying severity.

Arthralgia (joint pain) was his main complaint for many years, but he had also suffered from back and chest pain and severe headaches. He had never experienced abdominal pain. Exertion, minor infection, and exposure to cold seemed to precipitate these symptoms. Other symptoms included shortness of breath and difficulty climbing stairs.

Family history revealed that four of seven siblings were dead. One was known definitely to have died from anemia; another was said to have "a touch of" sickle cell anemia. His mother was in good health, but nothing was known of his father.

A blood count revealed the following data: WBC 5.2 × 10⁹/L; Hb 7.0 g/dL; Hct 0.22 L/L; MCV 84 fL; MCH 26.9 pg; MCHC 31.8 g/dL; platelets 440 × 10⁹/L. Reticulocytes were 5.8%. Erythrocyte morphology showed a rare sickle cell and moderate target cells and anisocytosis. Three nucleated red cells per 100 WBC were present, and the results of the differential count were normal.

Cellulose acetate electrophoresis revealed 21% Hb A, 70% Hb S, and Hbs F and A₂. Hb F (by alkali denaturation) was 4.9% and Hb A₂ (by microchromatography) was 4.1%.

1. Are hemoglobin abnormalities indicated by electrophoresis, alkali denaturation, or microchromatography results? Explain.
2. Which of the following hemoglobinopathies exhibit an increase in Hb F or A₂ values: sickle cell trait, sickle cell disease, sickle C (Hb SC) disease, or Hb S-thalassemia?
3. Based on your answer to question 2 and other laboratory findings, what is the most likely diagnosis in this case? Explain.
4. Are the MCV and MCH generally consistent with the diagnosis given in answer to question 3?
5. If no Hb A had been found on cellulose acetate electrophoresis

but Hbs S, F and A$_2$ were increased as in this patient's case, what would the most likely diagnosis be? Why?

Review Questions

15-1. The genetic defect that characterizes most thalassemias is

    A. abnormal incorporation of iron into heme.
    B. decreased production of normal globin chains.
    C. excessive production of porphyrins.
    D. increased production of abnormal globin chains.

15-2. Barts hydrops fetalis is lethal because

    A. Hb Barts cannot bind oxygen.
    B. the excess α-globin chains form insoluble precipitates.
    C. Hb Barts cannot release oxygen to tissues.
    D. microcytic red cells become trapped in the placenta.

15-3. The Hbs that are composed of four γ-chains (γ_4) and four β-chains (β_4) are, respectively,

    A. Hbs H and C.
    B. Hbs H and Barts.
    C. Hbs Barts and H.
    D. Hbs Barts and S.

For the following questions choose from these answers:
    A. 1, 3
    B. 2, 4
    C. 1, 2 and 3
    D. 4 only
    E. All are correct

15-4. Homozygous β-thalassemias can be confused with iron deficiency because both have

    1. decreased serum ferritin.
    2. decreased serum iron.
    3. decreased percentage transferrin saturation.
    4. microcytic, hypochromic RBC.

15-5. Hb(s) that migrate with Hb S on cellulose acetate at alkaline pH is(are)

    1. Hb Constant Spring.
    2. Hb Barts.
    3. Hb H.
    4. Hb Lepore.

15-6. The abnormally increased Hb electrophoresis value(s) that would usually *exclude* the possibility of α-thalassemia is(are)

    1. Hb A$_2$
    2. Hb H
    3. Hb F
    4. Hb Barts

15-7. If a value of 11% Hb A$_2$ is obtained using microchromatography

    1. Hbs C, E or O Arab might be in the specimen.
    2. the same test procedure should be repeated.
    3. the test should be repeated using a different method.
    4. the results should be reported.

15-8. Hb H inclusion bodies may

    1. be found in β-thalassemia.
    2. be seen on Wright-stained blood films.
    3. appear eccentrically near the red cell membrane.
    4. make red cells look like "pitted golf balls."

15-9. In the blood film slide test for Hb F,

    1. an acid buffer elutes all Hbs except Hb F.
    2. cells with Hb F stain bright pink.

    3. cells without Hb F appear as "ghost cells."
    4. blood films should be fixed in ethyl alcohol.

References

1. Adams JG III, Coleman MB: Structural hemoglobin variants that produce the phenotype of thalassemia. Semin Hematol 27:229, 1990
2. Antoniou M, DeBoer E, Habets G et al: The human β-globin gene contains multiple regulatory regions: Identification of one promoter and two downstream enhancers. EMBO J 7:377, 1988
3. Apperley JF, Williams DA: Gene therapy: Current status and future directions. Br J Haematol 75:148, 1990
4. Baglioni C: The fusion of two peptide chains in hemoglobin Lepore and its interpretation as a genetic deletion. Proc Natl Acad Sci USA 48:1880, 1962
5. Baine RM, Brown HG: Evaluation of a commercial kit for microchromatographic quantitation of hemoglobin A$_2$ in the presence of hemoglobin S. Clin Chem 27:1244, 1981
6. Beaven GH, Coleman PN, White JC: Occurrence of haemoglobin H in leukaemia: A further case of erythroleukaemia. Acta Haematol 59:37, 1978
7. Beaven GH, Stevens BL, Dance N et al: Occurrence of haemoglobin H in leukaemia. Nature 199:1297, 1963
8. Bessman JD: New parameters on automated hematology instruments. Lab Med 14:488, 1983
9. Brown BA: Special hematology procedures. In Brown BA: Hematology: Principles and Procedures, 6th ed, pp 160-63, 168-171. Philadelphia, Lea & Febiger, 1993
10. Bunn HF, Forget BG: Hemoglobin: Molecular, Genetic and Clinical Aspects. Philadelphia, WB Saunders, 1986
11. Centers for Disease Control: Laboratory Methods for Detecting Hemoglobinopathies. Division of Host Factors, Center for Infectious Diseases, Centers for Disease Control, Atlanta GA, 1984
12. Charache S, Conley CL, Doeblin TD et al: Thalassemia in black Americans. Ann NY Acad Sci 232:125, 1974
13. Clegg JB, Weatherall DJ, Milner PF: Haemoglobin Constant-Spring—a chain termination mutant? Nature 234:337, 1971
14. Conley CL, Weatherall DJ, Richardson SN et al: Hereditary persistence of fetal hemoglobin. A study of 79 affected persons in 15 Negro families in Baltimore. Blood 21:261, 1963
15. Cooley TB, Lee P: A series of cases of splenomegaly in children with anemia and peculiar bone changes. Trans Am Pediatr Soc 37:29, 1925
16. Dozy AM, Kan YW, Embury SH et al: α-Globin gene organisation in blacks precludes the severe form of α-thalassemia. Nature 280:605, 1979
17. Embury SH, Miller JA, Dozy AM et al: Two different molecular organizations account for the single α-globin gene of the α-thalassemia-2 genotype. J Clin Invest 66:1319, 1980
18. Fairbanks VF: Hemoglobinopathies and Thalassemias. Laboratory Methods and Case Studies. New York, BC Decker, 1980
19. Fearon ER, Kazazian HH, Waber PG et al: The entire β-globin gene cluster is deleted in a form of $\gamma\delta\beta$-thalassemia. Blood 61:1269, 1983
20. Fessas P, Stamatoyannopoulos G: Absence of haemoglobin A$_2$ in an adult. Nature 195:1215, 1962
21. Fishleder AJ, Hoffman GC: A practical approach to the detection of hemoglobinopathies: Part I. The introduction and thalassemia syndromes. Lab Med 18:368, 1987
22. Friedman MJ: Oxidant damage mediates variant red cell resistance to malaria. Nature 280:245, 1979
23. Friedman SH, Atwater J, Gill FM et al: α-Thalassemia in Negro infants. Pediatr Res 8:955, 1974

24. Goosens M, Dozy AM, Emburt SH et al: Triplicated α-globin loci in humans. Proc Natl Acad Sci USA 77:518, 1980

25. Haldane JBS: The rate of mutation of human genes. Hereditas 35(suppl):267, 1949

26. Hamilton SR, Miller ME, Jessop M et al: Comparison of microchromatography and electrophoresis with elution of hemoglobin (Hb A_2) quantitation. Am J Clin Pathol 71:388, 1979

27. Hatton CSR, Wilkie AOM, Drysdale HC et al: alpha Thalassemia caused by a large (62kb) deletion upstream of the human α-globin gene cluster. Blood 76:221, 1990

28. Higgs DR, Vickers MA, Wilkie AOM et al: A review of the molecular genetics of the human α-globin gene cluster. Blood 72:1081, 1989

29. Hillman RS, Finch CA: Red Cell Manual, 5th ed. Philadelphia, FA Davis, 1985

30. Huisman THJ, Reese MB, Gardiner MB et al: The occurrence of different levels of $^A\gamma$ chain and of the $^A\gamma$T variant of fetal hemoglobin in newborn babies from several countries. Am J Hematol 14:133, 1983

31. Huntsman RG, Carrell RW, White JM: Recommendations for selected methods for quantitative estimation of Hb A_2 and for Hb A_2 reference preparation. International Committee for Standardization in Haematology. Br J Haematol 38:573, 1978

32. Hussein HS, Hoffbrand AV, Leulicht M et al: Serum ferritin levels in β-thalassaemia trait. Br Med J Clin Res 2:920, 1976

33. Jarman AP, Wood WG, Sharpe JA et al: Characterization of the major regulatory element upstream of the human α-globin gene cluster. Mol Cell Biol 11:4679, 1991

34. Jones JA, Broszeit HK, LeCrone CN et al: An improved method for detection of red cell hemoglobin H inclusions. Am J Med Technol 47:94, 1981

35. Kan YW, Forget BG, Nathan DG: gamma-beta-Thalassemia: A cause of hemolytic disease of the newborn. N Engl J Med 286:129, 1972

36. Kazazian HH: The thalassemia syndromes: Molecular basis and prenatal diagnosis in 1990. Semin Hematol 27:209, 1990

37. Klee GG, Fairbanks VF, Pierre RV et al: Routine erythrocyte measurements in diagnosis of iron deficiency anemia and thalassemia minor. Am J Clin Pathol 66:870, 1976

38. Kleihauer E, Braun H, Betke K: Demonstration van fetalem Hamoglobin in den Erythrocyten eines Blutausstrichs. Klin Wochenschr 35:637, 1957

39. Labbe RF, Lamon JM: Porphyrins and disorders of porphyrin metabolism. In Tietz NW (ed): Fundamentals of Clinical Chemistry, 3rd ed, p 839. Philadelphia, WB Saunders, 1987

40. Labbe RF, Rettmer RL: Zinc protoporphyrin: A product of iron-deficient erythropoiesis. Semin Hematol 26:40, 1989

41. LeCrone CN, Detter JC: Screening for hemoglobinopathies and thalassemia. J Med Technol 2:389, 1985

42. Ley TJ, DeSimone J, Anagnou NP et al: 5-Azacytidine selectively increases γ-globin synthesis in a patient with β-thalassemia. N Engl J Med 307:1469, 1982

43. Liebhaber SA, Goossens M, Kan YW: Homology and concerted evolution at the α_1 and the α_2 loci of human α-globin. Nature 290:26, 1981

44. Liebhaber SA, Goossens MJ, Kan YW: Cloning and complete nucleotide sequence of human 5'-α-globin gene. Proc Natl Acad Sci USA 77:7054, 1980

45. Liebhaber SA, Griese E-U, Cash FE et al: Inactivation of human α-globin gene expression by a de novo deletion located upstream of the α-globin gene cluster. Proc Natl Acad Sci USA 81:9431, 1990

46. Lie-Injo LE, Ganesan J, Clegg JB et al: Homozygous state for Hb Constant Spring (slow-moving Hb X components). Blood 43:251, 1974

47. Lopez CG, Lie-Injo LE: alpha-Thalassemia in newborns in West Malaysia. Hum Heredity 21:185, 1971

48. Lukens JN: The thalassemias and related disorders: Quantitative disorders of hemoglobin synthesis. In Lee GR, Bithell TC, Foerster J et al (eds): Wintrobe's Clinical Hematology, 9th ed, p 1102. Philadelphia, Lea & Febiger, 1993

49. Luzzatto L: Malaria and the red cell. In Hoffbrand AV (ed): Recent Advances in Haematology, p 109. Edinburgh, Churchill Livingstone, 1985

50. Malamos B, Fessas P, Stamatoyannopoulos G: Types of thalassaemia-trait carriers as revealed by a study of their incidence in Greece. Br J Haematol 8:5, 1962

51. Mazza U, Saglio G, Cappio FC et al: Clinical and haematological data in 254 cases of β-thalassaemia trait in Italy. Br J Haematol 33:91, 1976

52. Mehta BC, Pandya BG: Iron status of β-thalassaemia carriers. Am J Hematol 24:137, 1987

53. Motulsky AG: Frequency of sickling disorders in US blacks. N Engl J Med 288:31, 1973

54. National Committee for Clinical Laboratory Standards: Chromatographic (microcolumn) determination of hemoglobin A_2; Approved Standard. NCCLS document H9-A.Villanova, PA, NCCLS, 1989

55. Nienhuis AW, Anagnou NP, Ley TJ: Advances in thalassemia research. Blood 63:738, 1984

56. Nienhuis AW, Maniatis T: Structure and expression of globin genes in erythroid cells. In Stamatoyannopoulos G, Nienhuis AW, Leder P et al (eds): The Molecular Basis of Blood Disease. Philadelphia, WB Saunders, 1995

56a. Nurse GT: Iron, the thalassaemias, and malaria. Lancet 2:938, 1979

57. O'Brien RT: The effect of iron deficiency on the expression of hemoglobin H. Blood 41:853, 1973

58. Old J, Longley J, Wood WG et al: Molecular basis for acquired haemoglobin H disease. Nature 269:524, 1977

59. Orkin SH: Prenatal diagnosis of hemoglobin disorders by DNA analysis. Blood 63:249, 1984

60. Orkin SH, Goff SC: The duplicated human α-globin genes: Their relative expression as measured by RNA analysis. Cell 24:345, 1981

61. Orkin SH, Old J, Lazarus H et al: The molecular basis of α thalassemia: Frequent occurrence of dysfunctional loci among non-Asians with Hb H disease. Cell 17:33, 1979

62. Pearson HA, McPhedran P, O'Brien RT et al: Comprehensive testing for thalassemia trait. Ann NY Acad Sci 232:135, 1974

63. Pippard MJ, Callender ST, Warner GT et al: Iron absorption and loading in β-thalassaemia intermedia. Lancet 2:819, 1979

64. Pootrakul P, Wasi P, Na-Nakorn S: Haematological data in 312 cases of β-thalassaemia trait in Thailand. Br J Haematol 24:703, 1973

65. Pressley L, Higgs DR, Clegg JB et al: Gene deletions in α-thalassaemia prove that the 5'H locus is functional. Proc Natl Acad Sci USA 77:3586, 1980

66. Schmidt RM, Brosious EM, Wright JM: Preparation and use of a quality control hemolysate for microchromatographic determinations of Hb A_2. Am J Clin Pathol 67:215, 1977

67. Steinberg MH, Adams JG III: Thalassemic hemoglobinopathies. Am J Pathol 113:396, 1983

68. Thomas ED: Marrow transplantation for non-malignant disorders. N Engl J Med 312:46, 1985

69. Tietz NW (ed): Textbook of Clinical Chemistry. Philadelphia, WB Saunders, 1986

70. Todd D: Thalassemia. Pathology 16:5, 1984

71. University of Washington, Department of Laboratory Medicine: Handbook of Diagnostic Tests for Intrinsic Hemolytic Disorders and Thalassemia. Seattle, University of Washington, 1988

72. Veer A, Kosciolek BA, Bauman AW et al: Acquired hemoglo-

bin H disease in idiopathic myelofibrosis. Am J Hematol 6:199, 1979

73. Veith R, Galanello R, Papayannopoulou T et al: Stimulation of F-cell production in patients with sickle-cell anemia treated with cytarabine or hydroxyurea. N Engl J Med 313:1571, 1985

74. Walford DM, McPherson K, Deacon R: Discrimination between iron deficiency and heterozygous thalassaemia. Lancet 1:323, 1979

75. Wasi P, Na-Nakorn S, Pootrakul S: The α-thalassaemias. Clin Haematol 3:383, 1974

76. Wasi P, Na-Nakorn S, Pootrakul S et al: alpha- And beta-thalassemia in Thailand. Ann NY Acad Sci 165:60, 1969

77. Weatherall DJ: Bone marrow transplantation for thalassemia and other inherited disorders of hemoglobin. Blood 80:1379, 1992

78. Weatherall DJ: The thalassemias. In Stamatoyannopoulos G, Nienhaus AW, Leder P et al (eds): The Molecular Basis of Blood Diseases, 2nd ed. Philadelphia, WB Saunders, 1994

79. Weatherall DJ: Gene therapy in perspective. Nature 349:275, 1991

80. Weatherall DJ (ed): The Thalassemias. Edinburgh, Churchill Livingstone, 1983

81. Weatherall DJ: Abnormal haemoglobins in the neonatal period and their relationship to thalassaemia. Br J Haematol 9:265, 1963

82. Weatherall DJ, Clegg JB: The Thalassaemia Syndromes, 3rd ed. Oxford, Blackwell Scientific, 1981

83. Weatherall DJ, Clegg JB, Higgs DR et al: The hemoglobinopathies. In Shriver CR, Beauder AL, Sly WS et al (eds): The Metabolic Basis of Inherited Diseases. New York, McGraw-Hill, 1994

84. Weatherall DJ, Higgs DR, Bunch C et al: Hemoglobin H disease and mental retardation. N Engl J Med 305:607, 1981

85. Whipple DJ, Bradford WL: Mediterranean disease—thalassemia (erythroblastic anemia of Cooley): Associated pigment abnormalities simulating hemochromatosis. J Pediatr 9:279, 1936

86. Wood WG, MacRae IA, Darbre PD et al: The British type of non-deletion HPFH: Characterization of developmental changes in vivo and erythroid growth in vitro. Br J Haematol 50:401, 1982

87. Wood WG, Weatherall DJ, Hart GH et al: Hematologic changes and hemoglobin analysis in β-thalassemia heterozygotes during the first year of life. Pediatr Res 16:286, 1982

88. Yoo D, Schechter GP, Amigable AN et al: Myeloproliferative syndrome with sideroblastic anemia and acquired hemoglobin H disease. Cancer 45:78, 1980

CHAPTER 16

Introduction to Anemias of Increased Erythrocyte Destruction

Loretta Nemchik

Objectives

1. Discuss three methods of classifying hemolytic anemias.
2. Define extravascular and intravascular hemolysis, and briefly describe the sites and mechanisms involved in each.
3. Describe the process of intravascular and extravascular red cell catabolism.
4. Identify three laboratory tests that can be used to screen for the presence of a hemolytic anemia and describe the expected results.
5. Identify five laboratory tests that are strongly indicative of an intravascular hemolytic anemia and describe the expected results.

Anemias may result from either decreased erythrocyte production or increased erythrocyte loss or destruction. When the rate of destruction exceeds the bone marrow's capacity to produce red cells, anemia results. Because a normal bone marrow can increase its rate of production by as much as six to eight times normal, the red cell life span must be significantly shortened for anemia to develop. The term *hemolytic anemia* or *anemia of increased destruction* should be reserved for cases in which the rate of erythrocyte destruction is accelerated and the bone marrow, in spite of its increased erythrocyte production, is not capable of keeping up with the destruction.[11] The term implies both increased erythrocyte destruction and production.

Some anemias result from a combination of decreased production and increased destruction. In megaloblastic anemias (Chap. 12) and thalassemias (Chap. 15), decreased production is the major underlying problem. Because many of the developing red cells are very abnormal

(dyserythropoietic), there is even increased destruction of the cells before they leave the bone marrow (ineffective erythropoiesis). The red cells in other anemias, such as those associated with iron deficiency and chronic disease (Chap. 13), may also have a somewhat shortened life span. All of these anemias are said to have a hemolytic component, but because hemolysis is not the primary underlying cause, they should not be called hemolytic anemias.[42]

CLASSIFICATION

Hemolytic anemias may be classified according to several schemes (Table 16-1). Traditional classifications have included inherited and acquired disorders. Others have categorized hemolytic anemias according to the type of red cell defect—intrinsic or extrinsic. An intrinsic defect is one in which the red cells themselves are defective. In other words, the patient's red cells would not survive normally when transfused into a normal recipient. Normal red cells have a normal life span when transfused into a patient who has an intrinsic red cell defect. Extrinsic red cell defects result from abnormal environmental factors that damage normal red cells. Normal red cells have a shortened life span when transfused into a patient with an extrinsic red cell defect, but such a patient's red cells would survive normally if given to a normal recipient.

Most inherited hemolytic anemias are due to intrinsic red cell defects (see Table 16-1). These defects may affect any part of the cell–the membrane (Chap. 17), metabolic systems (*i.e.*, enzyme deficiencies; Chap. 17), or hemoglobin molecule (*i.e.*, hemoglobinopathies; Chap. 14). Some inherited anemias are evident in infancy, whereas others do not become evident until adulthood.[28]

Most extrinsic hemolytic anemias are acquired. Red cells coated with antibodies or complement (Chap. 19), or damaged by some abnormal environmental factor (Chap. 18) or by liver or renal disease have a shortened life span, which may result in anemia. Prolonged sequestration of red cells in an enlarged spleen (hypersplenism) can cause significant extravascular red cell destruction.

Abetalipoproteinemia and lecithin-cholesterol acyltransferase (LCAT) deficiency (Chap. 17) are examples of inherited disorders in which hemolysis is due to an extrinsic defect. These extremely rare disorders cause ab-

TABLE 16-1
Classification of Hemolytic Anemias

INTRINSIC HEMOLYTIC ANEMIAS

Hereditary

    Membrane defects

        Hereditary spherocytosis

        Hereditary elliptocytosis

        Hereditary pyropoikilocytosis

    Enzyme defects

        G6PD deficiency

        Pyruvate kinase deficiency

        Glutathione reductase deficiency

    Hemoglobinopathies

        Hemoglobin SS, CC, SC, and S–β-thalassemia

Acquired

    Paroxysmal nocturnal hemoglobinuria

EXTRINSIC HEMOLYTIC ANEMIAS

Hereditary

    LCAT deficiency

    Abetalipoproteinemia

Acquired

    Immune mediated

    Mechanical, thermal, chemical damage

    Infectious agents

    Hypersplenism

    Secondary to liver or renal disease

    Secondary to hypertension

normalities in plasma lipids, which result in a red cell membrane defect and subsequent hemolysis.

Another proposed method of classifying hemolytic anemias combines the mean corpuscular volume (MCV) with the red cell distribution width (RDW).[5] This method places hemolytic anemias in several categories and appears, however, to be most useful in the diagnosis and differentiation of microcytic anemias.[16,34]

SITES OF ERYTHROCYTE HEMOLYSIS

Extravascular Sites

Most destruction of both normal and abnormal red cells occurs in the organs of the reticuloendothelial system (RES), which include the spleen, lymph nodes, bone marrow, and liver. Most RES cells are fixed or free macrophages. The liver's RE cells are called Kupffer cells. There are also scavenger cells in the lungs called alveolar macrophages that can destroy red cells. The endothelial cells lining the sinuses in the liver, bone marrow, spleen, and lymph nodes are also considered part of the RES, as are circulating monocytes. Some hematologists now use the term *mononuclear phagocyte system* (MPS) for the RES, but the terms RES and MPS may be used interchangeably.[1] The term *extravascular hemolysis* is used to describe red cell destruction that occurs by phagocytosis of intact or

fragmented red cells in the RES with release of hemoglobin into the macrophages. Most hemolytic diseases are characterized by extravascular hemolysis.

In an immune reaction, red cells in the circulation may become coated with immunoglobulin. Subsequently, the complement system cascade is activated, which leads to generation of an intermediate complement component known as C3b (Chap. 19). Cells coated with immunoglobulin and complement may be destroyed by the liver Kupffer cell macrophages because they have receptors for the complement component C3b. Attachment of C3b to the red cell surface is generally associated with extravascular hemolysis in the liver.

Severely damaged red cells that enter the circulation may also be destroyed by the Kupffer cell macrophages. Clearance of red cells correlates with the extent of shape alteration. In one study, 50% to 80% of cells that were extreme forms of echinocytes and stomatocytes were cleared by the liver. Cells that were only mildly altered and retained their disk shape were cleared (*i.e.*, destroyed), principally by the spleen.[10]

Because of the unique structure of the spleen (see Fig. 6-8), most destruction of normal, senescent (older than 120 days) and abnormal red cells occurs in this organ. Conditions causing decreased red cell flexibility will affect their passage through the spleen. Decreased flexibility can occur if the cell membrane has been altered. Pieces of membrane may be removed by macrophages, which recognize antibodies or complement attached to the red cell surface. Erythrocytes that contain inclusion bodies (Chap. 8) are too rigid to pass easily through the spleen. In a process known as *pitting*, splenic macrophages remove the inclusions along with a piece of the red cell membrane and adjacent hemoglobin while leaving the red cell intact. Cells may also be rigid and, therefore, less flexible because of poor hemoglobin solubility (*e.g.*, deoxygenated Hb S; see Chap. 14). Difficulty in squeezing through the walls of the splenic sinuses can cause further damage. Eventually the cell is trapped and phagocytized (Chap. 6).

If the spleen is enlarged, the splenic circulation is even more sluggish than normal. Cells with very mild abnormalities may lyse more readily than they would in a normal spleen. Increased splenic hemolysis causes further splenic enlargement.[25] Liver disease can cause both erythrocyte membrane abnormalities[9] and splenic congestion. As the abnormal red cells attempt to pass through the congested spleen, they are subject to damage, which eventually leads to hemolysis and more splenic enlargement.[26]

Intravascular Sites

When erythrocytes are severely damaged in the circulation, they may be destroyed without phagocytic cell involvement. This *intravascular hemolysis* results in release of hemoglobin directly into the plasma. Intravascular hemolysis accounts for only a small portion of normal 120-day-old erythrocyte destruction.

Intravascular hemolysis may be the predominant mode of hemolysis in some immune hemolytic anemias in which complement is involved (Chap. 19). Intravascular hemolysis that is complement mediated involves more complement components than those associated with extravascular hemolysis, in which the final component leading to red cell destruction is generally C3b. When complement is further activated in intravascular hemolysis, a complex known as *C5b6789*, otherwise known as the *membrane attack unit* or *terminal complex*, is ultimately formed (Chap. 19). This complex is so named because it is capable of penetrating the red cell surface, causing formation of a transmembrane pore. This damage may result in leakage of hemoglobin and other cellular components or osmotic swelling owing to excessive permeability to water and electrolytes, both of which produce intravascular hemolysis. One example of this mechanism is found in hemolytic transfusion reactions caused by major ABO incompatibility (Chap. 19).

Intravascular hemolysis may also be the predominant mode of hemolysis in extrinsic acquired hemolytic anemias (see Table 16-1 and Chap. 18). There are several types of mechanical damage that can cause intravascular hemolysis. In microangiopathic hemolytic anemias (MAHA), which classically demonstrate red cell frag-

ments on the blood film, red cells may be ruptured, for example, as they pass through diseased vessels, small vessels blocked by fibrin strands, a diseased cardiac valve, or a defective prosthetic valve. Malarial infestation, *Clostridium* septicemia, and severe kidney or liver disease may also cause intravascular hemolysis and anemia. Rare cases of intravascular hemolysis are caused by exposure to chemicals, physical trauma, and severe burns (Chap. 18).

ERYTHROCYTE CATABOLISM

Extravascular Hemolysis

When an erythrocyte is phagocytosed in the extravascular system, the hemoglobin molecule is broken down into heme and globin in the phagocytic cell (Fig. 16-1). The globin chains are catabolized, and the amino acids are returned to the amino acid pool to be used again. Iron is released from heme, bound to the protein carrier molecule transferrin, and recycled. The enzyme heme oxygenase opens the heme molecule to produce carbon monoxide and *biliverdin*. Biliverdin is immediately reduced to *biliru-*

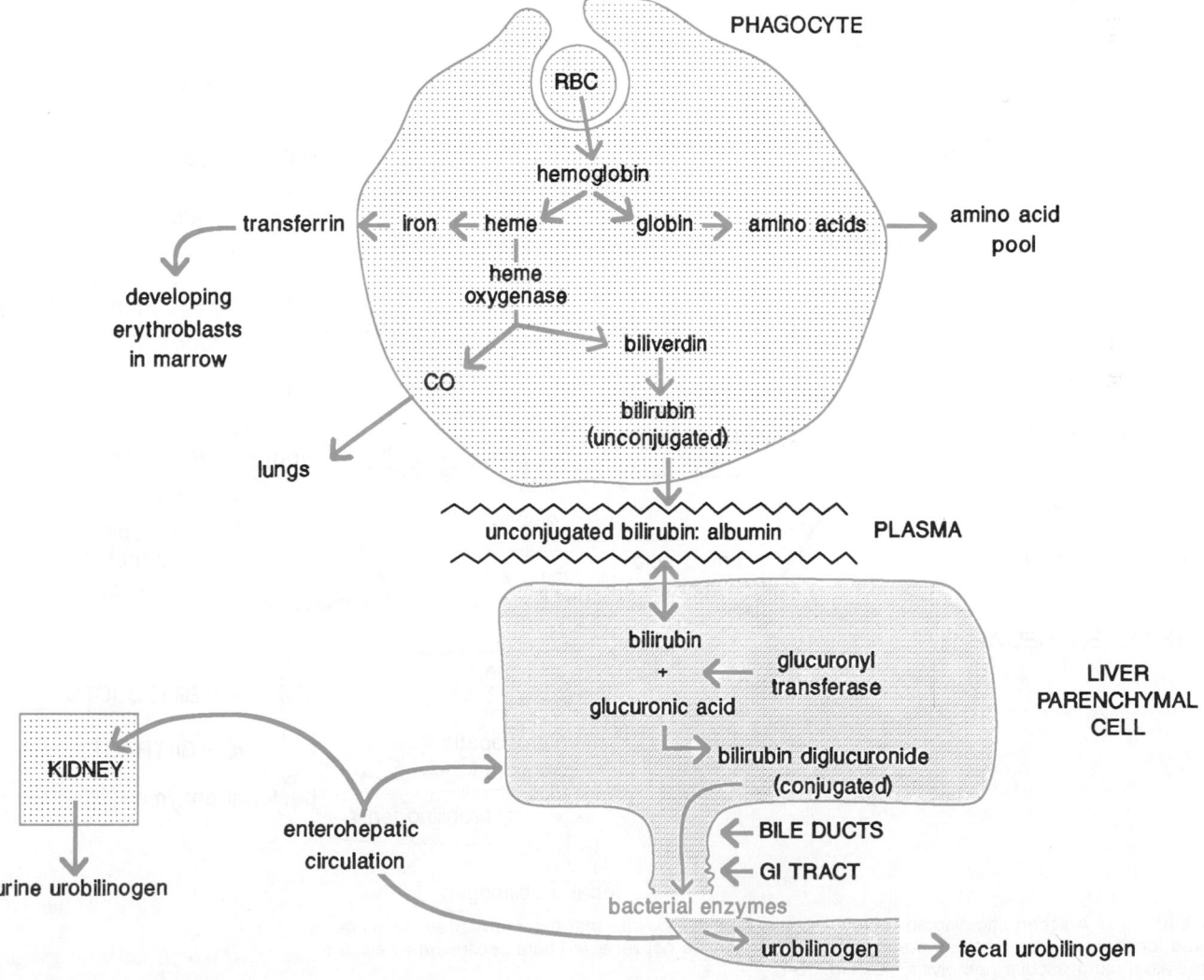

FIGURE 16-1. A schematic diagram of extravascular hemolysis.

bin, and released carbon monoxide is subsequently exhaled from the lungs. Bilirubin is released from the phagocytic cell into the plasma, where it binds to albumin and is carried to the liver. At this stage, it is termed *unconjugated (or indirect) bilirubin*. It is insoluble in water but highly soluble in fat. If the albumin-binding capacity is exceeded, unconjugated bilirubin is deposited in tissues that have a high lipid content.

Unconjugated bilirubin dissociates from albumin and passes across the hepatocyte membrane into the liver parenchymal cells. About 40% of this bilirubin flows back into the plasma, which accounts for the increase in unconjugated bilirubin in hemolytic anemias.[2] In the liver, bilirubin is conjugated with glucuronic acid, by the enzyme glucuronyl transferase, to form bilirubin diglucuronide. This form of bilirubin, called *conjugated (or direct) bilirubin*, is soluble in water but poorly soluble in lipids.

Conjugated bilirubin is excreted from the liver into the bile ducts by an active transport mechanism. The ducts direct the bile into the duodenum. In the terminal ileum and colon, the conjugated bilirubin is converted by bacterial enzymes into a group of pigments called *urobilinogens*. Most urobilinogen is excreted in the stool; some is reabsorbed into the enterohepatic circulation, but most returns again to the gastrointestinal tract. A small portion of urobilinogen is excreted into the urine.[29]

Intravascular Hemolysis

In intravascular hemolysis (or excessive extravascular hemolysis), free hemoglobin may be released directly into the plasma, where it typically exists in α-β-dimers (Fig. 16-2). The free hemoglobin is bound to the plasma protein *haptoglobin*. The hemoglobin–haptoglobin complex is transported to the liver, where heme catabolism proceeds in the parenchymal cells along the extravascular pathway of degradation. Once haptoglobin releases hemoglobin in the liver, it is destroyed; haptoglobin is not recycled.[8] Therefore, the haptoglobin level may be used as an indicator of the degree of intravascular hemolysis, although it may also be depleted in extravascular hemolysis.

The hemoglobin–haptoglobin complex is too large to pass the kidney's glomerulus; however, when the haptoglobin-binding capacity is exceeded, free hemoglobin may be detected in the plasma, causing hemoglobinemia, or filtered by the kidney into the urine, causing hemoglobinuria. Hemoglobinemia and hemoglobinuria are findings unique to intravascular hemolysis (*i.e.*, they are

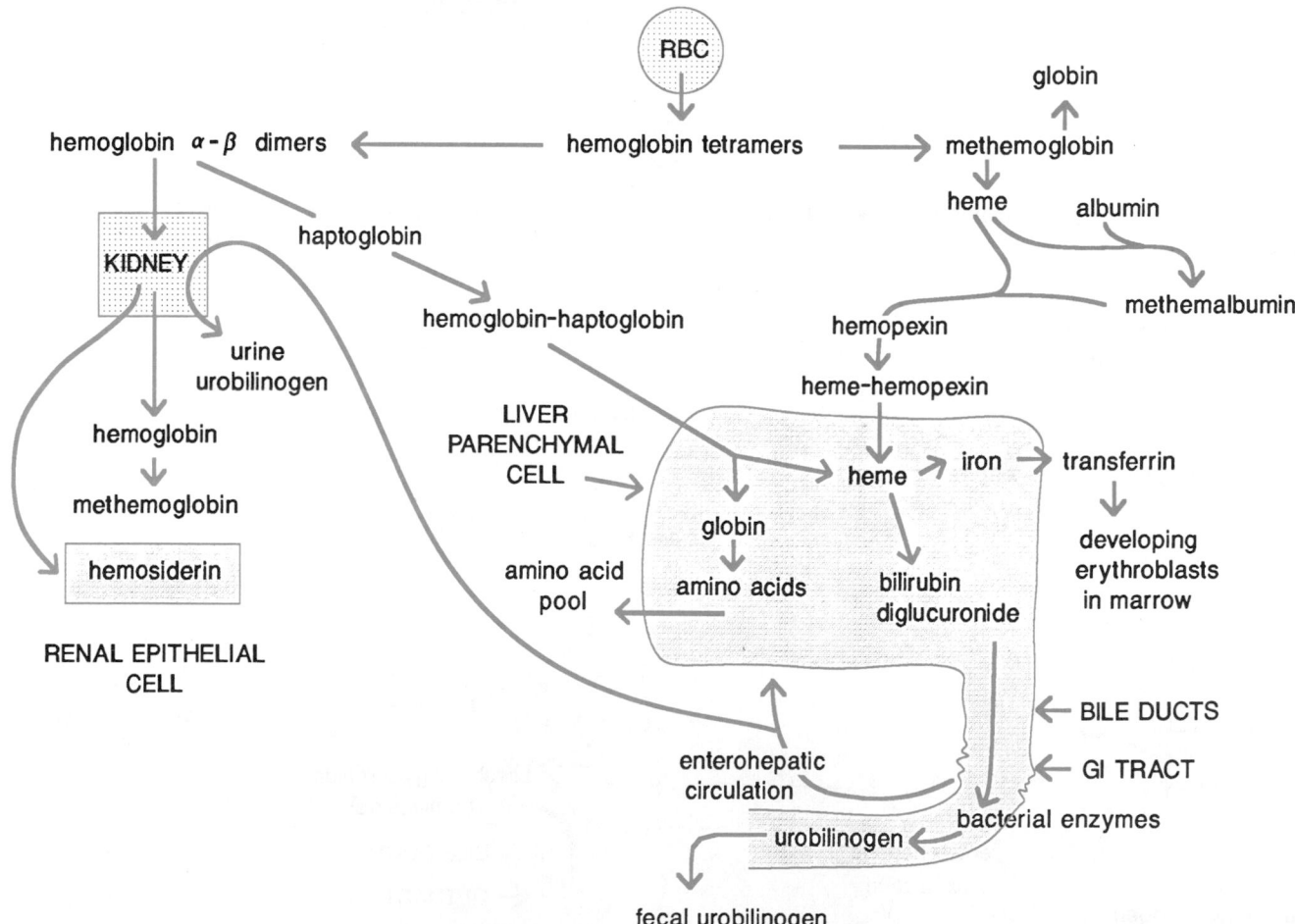

FIGURE 16-2. A schematic diagram of intravascular hemolysis. Note that the intermediate steps required for the conversion of heme to conjugated bilirubin are not repeated here because they are the same as in extravascular hemolysis (see Fig. 16-1).

not associated with extravascular hemolysis). A certain amount of free hemoglobin is reabsorbed by the proximal tubules and degraded into bilirubin, but a portion of the iron is left in the renal epithelial cells as ferritin or hemosiderin.[37] Because renal epithelial cells are not capable of recycling iron, hemosiderinuria results within a few days as these cells are naturally sloughed into the urine, another finding unique to intravascular hemolysis. In severe hemolytic states, the maximum rate of reabsorption is exceeded and free hemoglobin passes into the urine, resulting in hemoglobinuria and methemoglobinuria.[35]

In the plasma, some free hemoglobin can be taken up by the liver and some is oxidized to methemoglobin, from which the heme molecule and globin chains are readily extracted (see Fig. 16-2). Free heme is bound to the plasma protein *hemopexin*. Unlike haptoglobin, hemopexin may return to the circulation once it serves its function of delivering the heme molecule to the liver; however, in severe hemolysis, hemopexin is also increasingly catabolized. The hemopexin level is not as indicative of hemolysis as the haptoglobin level while the haptoglobin level is decreasing. However, once the haptoglobin level reaches 0 mg/dL, a falling hemopexin level may be an indicator of continued severe hemolysis. In severe hemolysis, when sufficient hemopexin is not available, the free heme is oxidized and bound to albumin to form *methemalbumin*. This complex remains in the plasma until more hemopexin is produced and made available by the liver.

The heme from the heme–hemopexin complexes and hemoglobin–haptoglobin complexes is converted to bilirubin in the liver, conjugated with glucuronic acid, and excreted as urobilinogen through the gastrointestinal tract.[8,18]

LABORATORY FINDINGS AND CORRELATIONS WITH DISEASE

In a patient with the usual complaints related to anemia, the presence of jaundice, splenomegaly, or occasionally dark urine suggests a hemolytic process. To establish hemolysis, laboratory data must show that both erythrocyte destruction and production are increased without evidence of blood loss. Table 16-2 summarizes the laboratory findings in hemolytic anemias. The results of tests indicated in Table 16-2 for initial screening purposes are used in the decision to order more specific tests, which may be necessary to pinpoint the exact cause of the hemolysis and anemia.

Note, as indicated in Table 16-2, that the findings of free hemoglobin and methemalbumin or a decreased hemopexin level in the plasma and hemoglobin and hemosiderin in the urine are strongly suggestive of an intravascular hemolytic anemia.

Table 16-3 summarizes the characteristics of important iron-containing compounds evaluated in the workup for hemolysis.

TABLE 16-2
Laboratory Findings in Hemolytic Anemias

Sample	Results	Method of Detection
Plasma or serum	↑ Free hemoglobin†	Visual/chemical
	↑ Methemoglobin	Visual/chemical
	+ Methemalbumin†	Visual/chemical
	↑ Unconjugated bilirubin*	Visual/chemical
	↓ Haptoglobin	Nephelometry
	↓ Hemopexin†	Radial immunodiffusion
	↑ Lactate dehydrogenase (LD)	Chemical
Urine	+ Urobilinogen	Dipstick
	+ Free hemoglobin†	Dipstick/visual
	+ Methemoglobin	Dipstick/visual
Urine sediment	+ Hemosiderin†	Prussian blue stain
	+ Ferritin	Prussian blue stain
Bone marrow	Erythroid hyperplasia	Microscopic evaluation of Wright-stained concentrate
Whole blood	↓ RBC, Hb, Hct*	Automated counter
	↑ MCV (sometimes)*	Automated counter
	↑ Reticulocyte count*	Reticulocyte stain or flow cytometer
Blood film	Polychromasia and morphology specific to underlying disease*	Microscopic evaluation of Wright-stained blood film
Feces	−Occult blood*	Chemical

Key: ↑, elevated; ↓, decreased; +, positive result; −, negative result.
* Tests recommended for initial screening. Other tests may be performed, as indicated, based on results of initial screening tests.
† Results particularly indicative of intravascular hemolysis.

TABLE 16-3
Important Iron-Containing and Related Compounds Commonly Evaluated in the Hemolysis Workup

Compound	Function	Laboratory Assessment	Reference Values
Ferritin	Main storage form of iron, therefore reflects tissue iron stores	Serum concentration	12–250 μg/L
Transferrin	Transport of iron to erythroid marrow	Serum concentration	220–400 mg/dL
Hemoglobin	O_2, CO_2 transport to and from tissues	Whole blood concentration as cyanmethemoglobin	14–16 g/dL
Methemoglobin	Iron oxidized to Fe^{3+}	Spectrophotometric analysis	0 g/dL or % of total hemoglobin
Myoglobin (muscle hemoglobin)	Involved in skeletal muscle function	Semiquantitative urine assay (performed in cases of suspected muscle necrosis)	Negative
Hemosiderin	Storage form of iron	Urine, Prussian blue stain on sediment	Negative
Haptoglobin*	Carrier for free hemoglobin in plasma	Immunologic analysis, nephelometry	30–190 mg/dL

* Haptoglobin itself is not composed of iron.

Hematology

Complete Blood Count (CBC)

The mean corpuscular volume (MCV) may help limit the diagnostic possibilities. MCV varies, depending on the presence or absence of extreme reticulocytosis or red cell fragmentation. In hemolytic anemias, the degree of reticulocytosis and macrocytosis may correspond to the duration and degree of anemia. On the other hand, if the reticulocyte count is increased in response to acute hemorrhage or compensated hemolysis, the reticulocytes are only 5% to 8% larger than the mature erythrocytes, generally resulting in a normal MCV.[27] For cases in which the MCV is normal, the presence of an elevated red cell distribution width (RDW) may prove useful in identifying the presence of reticulocytes.[36] The decrease in hemoglobin, hematocrit, and red blood cell count reflect the degree of anemia. Increased leukocyte and platelet counts are typically associated with increased erythropoiesis, but are more prominent in acute hemorrhage than in hemolysis. A decreased platelet count is a valuable clue to the recognition of microangiopathic hemolytic anemias, such as disseminated intravascular coagulation (DIC; Chap. 18).

Peripheral Blood Film

Blood film evaluation may provide specific clues to the type of hemolytic anemia present. Polychromasia or polychromatophilic shift cells and nucleated red cells represent a response to an increased level of erythropoietin that is due to either blood loss or hemolysis. The finding of spherocytes, microspherocytes, target cells, sickle cells, echinocytes, elliptocytes, schistocytes, ghost cells, agglutination, parasites, or other inclusions may reveal the underlying disorder causing hemolysis. The presence of normal red cell morphology also helps exclude certain possibilities. Most hemolytic anemias have normal leukocyte morphology, although occasionally abnormalities, such as erythrophagocytosis or the findings associated with septicemia, may point to a specific problem. These findings permit appropriate selection of special tests for diagnosis.

Reticulocyte Count

The reticulocyte count is the most useful test in the initial evaluation for hemolysis.[39] An increased reticulocyte count—and particularly an increased reticulocyte production index (RPI; Chap. 9)—support the suspicion that a case of anemia is due to increased loss or destruction of erythrocytes, rather than to decreased production. An increased reticulocyte count and RPI may be seen following hemorrhage and following treatment for nutritional anemias, so these conditions must be excluded. An increased reticulocyte count and anemia may also be seen in conjunction with gastrointestinal blood loss, so this condition must also be excluded (see Urinalysis section, Occult Blood).

In several conditions reticulocytopenia may confuse the picture. Occasionally, reticulocytes are not released from the bone marrow, resulting in the paradox of a hyperplastic marrow with a peripheral blood reticulocytopenia. Patients who experience an acute hemolytic episode may not show the expected reticulocytosis for 4 or 5 days. Abnormal reticulocytes, such as those produced in pyruvate kinase (PK) deficiency (a hereditary hemolytic anemia; Chap. 17), may escape the bone marrow, but be destroyed quickly in other areas of the RES. Consequently, the expected reticulocytosis may not always be observed in a PK-deficient patient with an intact spleen.[15] In any of these examples, the expected signs of increased production are absent while there is truly a hemolytic process present.

In the absence of blood loss, the RPI is a sensitive and specific indicator of hemolysis. If hemolysis is recent or chronic but mild, the RPI is expected to be two to four times the basal level. However, if hemolysis is chronic but moderate or severe, the RPI may be in the range of four to eight times the basal value.[28]

It should be recognized that the reticulocyte count remains elevated after hemolysis stops, until the anemia is corrected, so reticulocyte counts should not be used to determine the need for therapy in hemolytic anemias, although they may be useful in determining the response to therapy in nutritional anemias (Chap. 12).[4]

Bone Marrow Examination

Bone marrow examination should reveal erythroid hyperplasia with a myeloid-to-erythroid (M/E) ratio of approximately 0.5:1 instead of the usual 2:1 to 4:1. Cellularity is best judged on a biopsy section, rather than an aspirate (Chap. 27). However, if the clinical setting and laboratory data suggest that a hemolytic anemia is present, bone marrow study usually is not required.[31]

Hemostasis

A syndrome that is associated with both abnormal coagulation and hemolytic anemia is disseminated intravascular coagulation (DIC; Chaps. 18 and 52). DIC may actually be both the cause and result of certain hemolytic disorders. The coagulation pathway may be activated *in vivo* in cases of mechanical hemolysis (*e.g.*, abnormal blood vessel structures that damage erythroctyes) because of the presence of substances in erythrocyte stroma that promote coagulation. The resulting DIC then causes deposition of fibrin in vessels, which further damages erythrocytes. Severe hemolytic transfusion reactions may occasionally be complicated by DIC, which results from interaction of the complement and coagulation systems.[6]

Prolongation of the prothrombin time (PT) and partial thromboplastin time (PTT), and decreased fibrinogen (Chap. 49) along with the presence of D-dimer (Chap. 50) are important coagulation laboratory findings in the diagnosis of hemolytic anemia owing to DIC. Tests for D-dimer are important because the presence of D-dimer is specifically diagnostic of intravascular fibrin formation.

Chemistry

Much of the laboratory workup for hemolysis involves chemistry and urinalysis. Readers should refer to appropriate texts for details on the procedures discussed below.

Increased *unconjugated bilirubin* in plasma (see Fig. 16-1) is either an indicator of hemolysis or of liver disease. There is normally a low level of unconjugated bilirubin (1 mg/dL of serum), which comes from the small amount of normal daily extravascular erythrocyte senescence and from the minute quantity of hemoglobin that is shed when the nucleus is extruded from developing erythrocytes in the bone marrow. Total bilirubin levels reflect both the rate of erythrocyte destruction and liver function. Therefore, an increased total bilirubin can represent increased production from hemolysis, decreased hepatic clearance, or a combination of both. The unconjugated bilirubin fraction is elevated in increased extravascular and intravascular hemolysis. With normal liver function, chronic hemol-

ysis cannot elevate the unconjugated bilirubin to more than 4 mg/dL.[4] In hypoproliferative anemias (Chap. 11), the unconjugated bilirubin is usually less than 0.4 mg/dL; in ineffective erythropoiesis (*e.g.*, megaloblastic anemias), it is usually higher than 0.7 mg/dL.[21]

Bilirubin concentration depends on red cell turnover. Other influences on bilirubin concentration include the patient's plasma volume, the concentration of albumin in the patient's plasma, and the presence of substances that can compete with bilirubin for binding with albumin.[4] Because a decrease in unconjugated plasma bilirubin concentration is the earliest indicator of a decreased rate of hemolysis, repeated determinations are useful indicators of the need for therapy (or lack thereof).[4]

Serum haptoglobin is the plasma protein that binds free hemoglobin. Serum haptoglobin measurement is useful for identifying hemolytic disorders, especially now that simple and sensitive analytic techniques such as nephelometry are available. Levels below 25 mg/dL (reference range 30 to 190 mg/dL or 0.4 to 2.4 g/L) are highly specific for identifying hemolytic disorders. Haptoglobin is usually absent when intravascular red cell destruction reaches two times the normal minimal rate.[7] It may also be depleted in some extravascular hemolytic disorders such as sickle cell anemia. The lowest haptoglobin values are found in cases of malfunctioning prosthetic cardiac valves, and consistently low values are associated with immune hemolytic anemias (Chap. 19). Haptoglobin determination may be especially helpful for confirming the presence of intravascular hemolysis in patients whose hemoglobinemia is undetectable.[33]

Because haptoglobin is an acute phase reactant, it may be increased in cases of inflammatory diseases such as systemic lupus erythematosus and rheumatoid arthritis, in neoplastic disease, and in infections. A patient with both a hemolytic anemia and one of these diseases may have a normal haptoglobin level. Therefore, failure to document a reduction in haptoglobin does not rule out hemolysis, although absence of haptoglobin does confirm it.[28,38]

Hemopexin is the plasma protein that carries free heme and can be measured in the laboratory by radial immunodiffusion methods. It is expected to be decreased in hemolytic states, but this is not uniformly so as it is most often decreased only in severe hemolysis. The presence of hemopexin–heme complexes in the plasma (which gives plasma a coffee-brown color) is strongly suggestive of intravascular hemolysis. Hemopexin is greatly decreased with severe hemolysis following cardiac surgery and, in some conditions, is associated with extravascular hemolysis, including thalassemia major and Hb SS (sickle cell) disease. It is minimally to moderately decreased in pernicious anemia, paroxysmal nocturnal hemoglobinuria, hereditary spherocytosis and autoimmune hemolytic anemia. The degree of depletion is proportional to the concentration of free heme in the plasma and to the severity of hemolysis. Similar to haptoglobin, hemopexin is an acute-phase reactant (although a weak one); therefore, it may be mildly increased with an inflammatory stimulus such as that found in infections.

Plasma hemoglobin (Hb), unlike total red cell Hb, is usually measured as oxyhemoglobin because plasma Hb levels that indicate hemolysis in hemolytic anemias are too low to be detected by the cyanmethemoglobin method.[24] A plasma Hb concentration of 10 to 40 mg/dL imparts a visible red tinge to the plasma. However the cyanmethemoglobin reaction is only used to detect levels in excess of 100 mg/dL. The measurement of plasma Hb as oxyhemoglobin is performed at 415 nm[20] (the Soret band of maximal absorbance). Because of the narrow absorption peak of oxyhemoglobin at 415 nm, the spectrophotometer must have a very narrow bandpass; that is, a 1-nm spectral resolution is required. The spectrophotometer must also be accurately calibrated for wavelength. In contrast, the cyanmethemoglobin method requires only a 10-nm spectral resolution because of the broad absorption peak of cyanmethemoglobin at 540 nm.

The oxyhemoglobin method is also recommended over another method called the benzidine reaction[17,19,41] because the former is more accurate although less sensitive than the latter. Although the benzidine reaction is capable of detecting free Hb when the level is less than 100 mg/dL, the presence of a hydrogen peroxide inhibitor in normal plasma can cause plasma Hb concentrations measured by this method to be underestimated by about 50%.[17] When plasma Hb has been oxidized to form methemoglobin, the heme readily dissociates and binds to albumin (see Fig. 16-2). Both *methemoglobin* and *methemalbumin* impart a brownish color to the plasma, which may mask hemoglobinemia.[12] Methemalbumin circulates for a long time and is useful for confirming that moderate to severe hemolysis occurred several days earlier.[8] Hemoglobinemia, methemoglobinemia, and methemalbuminemia usually occur only when there is significant intravascular hemolysis; however, their absence does not rule out intravascular hemolysis.[28]

Lactate dehydrogenase (LD) serum levels are often increased in hemolytic anemias, although not as much as those in megaloblastic anemias. In hemolytic anemias, isoenzyme LD-2 predominates, in megaloblastic anemias, it is isoenzyme LD-1. Increased total LD is a rather nonspecific finding, for it occurs in myocardial infarction, liver disease, and also ineffective erythropoiesis.[28] A normal LD level indicates almost certainly that hemolytic anemia can be ruled out.[40]

Additional red cell enzyme activity studies have also been recommended to establish the presence or absence of hemolytic anemia.[22]

Urinalysis may reveal hemoglobinuria and methemoglobinuria when there is severe intravascular hemolysis and haptoglobin-binding capacity is saturated.[35] The urine may be red or brown, depending on the oxidation state of heme. Free hemoglobin gives a positive urine dipstick (*e.g.*, Multistix) reaction. Microscopic urine examination is necessary to exclude the presence of intact red cells, which lyse in hypotonic urine and also cause a positive test result for hemoglobinuria, but do not necessarily indicate *in vivo* hemolysis.[21]

Hemosiderinuria, the presence of hemosiderin (an insoluble form of storage iron) in the urine, is a valuable sign of current or recent intravascular hemolysis.[12] A Prussian blue stain of urine sediment reveals the presence of iron in renal epithelial cells that have been shed into the urine. Hemosiderinuria is especially useful to document mild intravascular hemolysis.[12] Iron remains in the urine sediment for several days after hemoglobinuria ends.[35]

Hemosiderinuria may also be caused by frequent red cell transfusions which result in transfusion-induced hemosiderosis (iron overload; Chap. 13). However most patients who require many transfusions are already known to have a severe hemolytic anemia. Patients with hereditary hemochromatosis (an iron metabolism disorder characterized by abnormal iron deposition in the tissues causing a bronze skin pigmentation) may occasionally show increased urinary iron excretion, but this condition is readily distinguished from hemolytic anemia by other clinical and laboratory findings. Serum iron is normal in transfusion-induced hemochromatosis, but it is increased in hereditary hemochromatosis.[12]

Increased *urine urobilinogen* reflects increased intravascular or extravascular hemolysis (see Figs. 16-1 and 16-2), but the urine urobilinogen level is also affected by liver and kidney function[14] and by urine pH,[30] so it may not accurately reflect the degree of heme degradation. Because unconjugated bilirubin is insoluble in water, it is not present in the urine. Bilirubinuria (conjugated bilirubin in the urine) would be seen in hemolytic anemia only if the patient also had liver disease and increased serum levels of conjugated bilirubin.

In the past, quantitation of fecal urobilinogen was used as an indicator of the rate of heme degradation. Today it is seldom used because of various factors that are difficult to control and, therefore, likely to cause inaccurate results.[14,29]

A test for *occult* (present but not visible to the unaided eye) *blood* in the stool can be performed easily and quickly using a chemical reaction. It is helpful to differentiate hemolysis from gastrointestinal (GI) blood loss, both of which cause anemia and reticulocytosis. A positive test result for stool occult blood can actually be useful to *exclude* the diagnosis of hemolysis because it should be negative in hemolytic anemias, whereas it is positive in cases of gastrointestinal blood loss.

ERYTHROKINETICS

Red Cell Survival Studies

Determination of erythrocyte survival by erythrokinetic studies is rarely necessary to document hemolysis as the cause of an anemia. However, a brief explanation of the procedure is provided here because it may be useful in obscure cases whose other laboratory findings are equivocal and in determining the exact site of erythrocyte destruction.

The International Committee for Standardization in Haematology has published the reference method for red cell survival studies.[23] Approximately 10 mL of the patient's blood is anticoagulated with sterile acid citrate dextrose (ACD). A calculated amount of radioactive chromium (^{51}Cr) in the form of chromate ion ($^{51}CrO_4^{2-}$) diluted in normal sterile saline is added to the erythrocytes and incubated for 15 minutes, either at room temperature or in a 37°C water bath to allow red cell binding of ^{51}Cr. The cells are washed twice in sterile isotonic saline to remove unattached ^{51}Cr, are resuspended, and are administered intravenously to the patient.

An EDTA-anticoagulated blood sample is taken 10 minutes, 60 minutes, and 24 hours after the labeled cells are injected. Further samples are taken on three different days between days

2 and 7, and then twice weekly until the blood radioactivity is minimal. A precisely measured volume of each sample is lysed, transferred to a counting tube, and gently mixed, and the radioactivity is counted on a well-type scintillation counter.

The radioactivity levels of all subsequent samples are compared on a percentage basis with the day 0, 100% sample (usually the 60-minute sample) to determine the percentage of radioactivity remaining in the circulating blood. These percentages are plotted on semilogarithmic paper against the number of days into the study to determine average red cell half-life, abbreviated as $T_{1/2}$, which is the number of days that have passed when 50% of the radioactive red cells have disappeared, while 50% remain in circulation (Fig. 16-3). Since normal erythrocyte life span is approximately 120 days, the half-life would be expected to be 60 days, but the rate of elution of ^{51}Cr from erythrocytes is considered to be 1% per day, which causes a reduction in the expected half-life value. Additionally, because the patient sample is a random peripheral blood sample, the red cells vary in age from 0 to 120 days. Consequently, the reference range for erythrocyte half-life using this method is 25 to 32 days.

A half-life of 20 to 25 days suggests mild hemolysis, 15 to 20 days, moderate hemolysis, and fewer than 15 days, severe hemolysis (see Fig. 16-3). Measuring radioactivity over the spleen, liver, and heart may be useful in determining whether the spleen is a major source of erythrocyte destruction.[32] This test may be performed in conjunction with an erythrocyte production study, using radioactive iron to determine whether significant extramedullary erythropoiesis is occurring (Chap. 6).[3] Results of the two studies may aid in determining the major role of the spleen (*i.e.*, erythrocyte production or destruction) and whether splenectomy would have therapeutic value.

This test is logistically complex, requires a number of days to complete, requires that the patient be in a physiologic steady state (no change in the rate of hemolysis, no transfusions, no change in blood volume), exposes the patient to ionizing radioactivity, and is expensive. It is available only in specialized centers. In most cases, the hemoglobin concentration and RPI are sufficient to estimate the rate of hemolysis; measurement of erythrocyte life span would only confirm and quantify what is already evident from clinical findings and simpler laboratory determinations.[28]

Plasma Iron and Erythrocyte Iron Turnover

Measurements of plasma iron turnover and erythrocyte iron turnover use radiolabeled iron to evaluate total erythropoiesis and effective erythropoiesis, respectively. These tests have many of the same disadvantages as the ^{51}Cr red cell survival studies. Because the results correspond well with more readily available procedures (*e.g.*, the RPI and the bone marrow examination for hypercellularity), these more sophisticated tests are rarely indicated.

CHAPTER SUMMARY

Hemolytic anemias occur when the erythrocyte's life span is shortened and the bone marrow's capacity to produce erythrocytes is exceeded by erythrocyte destruction. Hemolytic anemias may be inherited or acquired. Most inherited ones result from intrinsic erythrocyte defects. Acquired hemolytic anemias are usually due to extrinsic abnormalities that damage erthrocytes.

Most phagocytosis of both normal and abnormal erythrocytes occurs extravascularly in the spleen. Erythrocytes with extreme abnormalities may be destroyed in the liver or bone marrow. Abnormal erythrocyte destruction may also occur intravascularly. Characteristic laboratory findings are found in Table 16-2.

Case Study 16-1

An 8-year-old boy first presented with acute rheumatic fever and congestive heart failure and was treated with digitallis and penicillin. At age 14 years he underwent mitral valve replacement with a prosthetic valve and was treated with oral iron therapy because his hematocrit level was 0.29 L/L.

At age 24 he was admitted to the hospital with a 6-week history of coughing up blood, shortness of breath, and massive ankle edema. He was a heavy smoker and consumed about a pint of alcohol daily. Physical examination revealed massive hepatomegaly and jaundice. The physician was unable to hear the expected clicking of the prosthetic valve. Echocardiography showed poor motion of the valve, suggesting the presence of an infection or clot, or both. Radiography showed massive lung hemorrhage.

Laboratory data were as follows: WBC 8.7×10^9/L; RBC 3.25×10^{12}/L; Hb 9.1 g/dL; Hct 0.29 L/L; MCV 88 fL; MCHC 32.0 g/dL; and platelets 70×10^9/L. Results of the differential cell count were 90% neutrophils, 1% bands, 6% lymphocytes and 3% monocytes; neutrophils displayed moderate toxic granulation and marked vacuoles. Red cell morphology showed marked anisocytosis with macrocytes and microcytes; moderate poikilocytosis with target cells, schistocytes, echinocytes, and microspherocytes; moderate hypochromia and moderate polychromasia. Results of coagulation studies were prothrombin time 19.4 seconds (reference range 10 to 14 seconds), partial thromboplastin time more than 150 seconds (reference range 28 to 35 seconds).

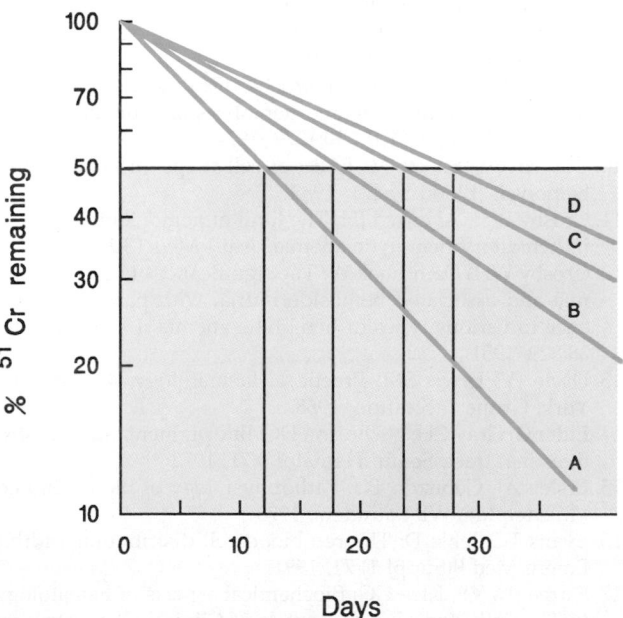

Days

FIGURE 16-3. Chromium-51 (^{51}Cr) erythrocyte survival study: The time required for one-half of the radioactivity to disappear from the circulation is expressed as erythrocyte half-life ($T_{1/2}$). Normal $T_{1/2}$ is about 28 days when measured by ^{51}Cr survival methods. Decreasing $T_{1/2}$ corresponds to an increasing severity of hemolysis and an increasingly shortened erythrocyte survival time. The four patient studies on this graph represent (*A*) severe hemolysis, (*B*) moderate hemolysis, (*C*) mild hemolysis, and (*D*) normal (no hemolysis). In this example, the respective half-lives were (*A*) 12 days, (*B*) 18 days, (*C*) 23 days, and (*D*) 27 days.

There are several possible causes for this patient's anemia. Most patients with artificial valves have some hemolysis, but iron supplementation is usually sufficient to prevent anemia. Alcohol abuse and the increased erythropoiesis secondary to chronic hemolysis can lead to folate deficiency anemia. Liver disease may be associated with macrocytic anemia.

1. Are the red cell distribution width (RDW) and reticulocyte count expected to be normal, increased, or decreased in this case?
2. What red cell morphologic findings suggest that the anemia is due to hemolysis?
3. How is the clot or infection in the prosthetic mitral valve related to hemolysis?
4. What might the coagulation study results indicate? What other laboratory results in chemistry, urinalysis, and coagulation would support the preliminary diagnosis of hemolytic anemia?

Case Study 16-2

A 54-year-old woman was seen in the emergency room of a large metropolitan hospital complaining of fever, acute respiratory distress and abdominal pain. She had been previously diagnosed with advanced cervical cancer and had been experiencing diarrhea for 2 days. Laboratory data were as follows: leukocyte count, increased; Hb, 5.5 g/dL; and Hct, 0.11 L/L; the plasma had a reddish tinge. In spite of massive blood transfusions the patient died. An autopsy revealed a perforation of the large intestine and blood cultures were positive for *Clostridium perfringens*.

1. What is indicated by the reddish tinge in the plasma?
2. What is the most likely explanation for the low Hb and Hct? Do they match according to the rule of three (Chap. 9)? Explain.
3. What additional hematology or chemistry studies could have been done to confirm the cause of the low Hb and Hct, and what results would be expected?

Review Questions

16-1. In the absence of blood loss, the laboratory result most useful in the initial diagnosis of a hemolytic anemia is a(n)

A. increased reticulocyte count.
B. increased total bilirubin level.
C. decreased Hb and Hct.
D. increased lactate dehydrogenase.

16-2. The laboratory test that is abnormal because of intravascular hemolysis, but usually normal with increased extravascular hemolysis is

A. fecal urobilinogen.
B. urine urobilinogen.
C. reticulocyte count.
D. plasma hemoglobin.

16-3. The substance that is present in the urine in increased amounts if extravascular hemolysis is increased but there is no intravascular hemolysis is

A. methemoglobin.
B. urobilinogen.
C. hemoglobin.
D. hemosiderin.

16-4. A decrease in the concentration of _____ in plasma is the earliest indicator of a decreased rate of hemolysis.

A. haptoglobin
B. unconjugated bilirubin
C. hemopexin
D. methemalbumin

16-5. If an intravascular hemolysis is suspected, but hemoglobinemia is not detected visually or spectrophotometrically, the first test that could be recommended that may confirm the suspicion is

A. serum hemopexin.
B. serum lactate dehydrogenase.
C. serum haptoglobin.
D. urine free hemoglobin.

16-6. Hemolytic anemia is **not** indicated by a(n)

A. positive urine hemosiderin.
B. positive fecal occult blood.
C. increased plasma unconjugated bilirubin.
D. decreased serum haptoglobin.

References

1. Beck WS: Reticuloendothelial (mononuclear phagocyte) system, lymphatic system, and spleen. In Beck WS (ed): Hematology, 4th ed. Cambridge MA, MIT Press, 1985
2. Berk PD, Howe RB, Bloomer JR et al: Studies of bilirubin kinetics in normal adults. J Clin Invest 48:2176, 1969
3. Berlin NI: Erythrokinetics. In Williams WJ, Beutler E, Erslev AJ, Lichtman MA (eds): Hematology, 3rd ed. New York, McGraw-Hill, 1983
4. Berlin NI, Berk PD: Quantitative aspects of bilirubin metabolism for hematologists. Blood 57:983, 1981
5. Bessman JD, Gilmer PR, Gardner FH: Improved classification of anemias by MCV and RDW. Am J Clin Pathol 80:322, 1983
6. Brozovic M: Acquired disorders of blood coagulation. In Bloom AL, Thomas DP (eds): Haemostasis and Thrombosis. Edinburgh, Churchill Livingstone, 1981
7. Brus I, Lewis SM: The haptoglobin content of serum in haemolytic anaemia. Br J Haematol 5:348, 1959
8. Bunn HF: Erythrocyte destruction and hemoglobin catabolism. Semin Hematol 9:3, 1972
9. Cooper RA, Kimball DB, Durocher JR: Role of the spleen in membrane conditioning and hemolysis of spur cells in liver disease. N Engl J Med 290:1279, 1974
10. Cosgrove P, Sheetz M: Effect of cell shape on extravascular hemolysis. Blood 59:421, 1982
11. Crosby WH, Akeroyd JH: The limit of hemoglobin synthesis in hereditary hemolytic anemia. Am J Med 13:273, 1952
12. Crosby WH, Dameshek W: The significance of hemoglobinemia and associated hemosiderinuria, with particular reference to various types of hemolytic anemia. J Lab Clin Med 38:829, 1951
13. Dacie JV, Lewis SM: Practical Haematology, 4th ed. New York, Grune & Stratton, 1968
14. Elder G, Gray CH, Nicholson DC: Bile pigment fate in gastrointestinal tract. Semin Hematol 9:71, 1972
15. Erslev AJ, Gabuzda TG: Pathophysiology of Blood, 2nd ed. Philadelphia, WB Saunders, 1979
16. Evans TC, Jehle D: The red blood cell distribution width. J Emerg Med 9(Suppl 1):71, 1991
17. Fairbanks VF, Klee GG: Biochemical aspects of hematology. In Tietz NW (ed): Fundamentals of Clinical Chemistry, 3rd ed, pp 805-806. Philadelphia, WB Saunders, 1987
18. Gillen LAF: Hemoglobins, myoglobin, and porphyrins. In Bishop ML, Duben-Von Laufen JL, Fody EP (eds): Clinical Chemistry—Principles, Procedures, Correlations. Philadelphia, JB Lippincott, 1985
19. Hanks GE, Cassell M, Ray RN et al: Further modification of the benzidene method for measurement of hemoglobin in plasma. J Lab Clin Med 56:486, 1960
20. Harboe M: A method for determination of hemoglobin in

plasma by near-ultraviolet spectrophotometry. Scand J Clin Lab Invest 11:66, 1959

21. Hillman RS, Finch CA: Red Cell Manual, 5th ed. Philadelphia, FA Davis, 1985

22. Ideguchi H, Ishikawa A, Futata Y et al: A comprehensive scheme for the systematic investigation of hemolytic anemia. Ann Clin Lab Sci 24:412, 1994

23. International Committee for Standardization in Haematology: Recommended method for radioisotope red cell survival studies. Br J Haematol 45:659, 1980

24. International Committee for Standardization in Haematology: Recommendations for haemoglobinometry in human blood. Br J Haematol 13(Suppl):68, 1967

25. Jacob HS, MacDonald RA, Jandl JH: Regulation of spleen growth and sequestering function. J Clin Invest 42:1476, 1963

26. Jandl JH: The anemia of liver disease: Observations on its mechanism. J Clin Invest 34:390, 1955

27. Karnad A, Poskitt TR: The automated complete blood count: Use of the red blood cell volume distribution width and mean platelet volume in evaluating anemia and thrombocytopenia. Arch Intern Med 145:1270, 1985

28. Le Celle PL, Lichtman MA: Anemia with reticulocytosis: Hemolytic disorders. In Lichtman MA (ed): Hematology for Practitioners. Boston, Little, Brown & Co, 1978

29. Lester R, Schumer W, Schmid R: Intestinal absorption of bile pigments. IV. Urobilinogen absorption in man. N Engl J Med 272:939, 1965

30. Levy M, Lester R, Levinsky N: Renal excretion of urobilinogen in dogs. J Clin Invest 47:2117, 1968

31. Lichtman MA: An approach to the diagnosis of reduced blood cell counts. In Lichtman MA (ed): Hematology for Practitioners. Boston, Little, Brown & Co, 1978

32. Macpherson AIS, Richmond J, Stuart AE: The Spleen. Springfield, IL, Charles C Thomas, 1973.

33. Marchand A, Galen RS, Van Lente F: The predictive value of serum haptoglobin in hemolytic disease. JAMA 243:1909, 1980

34. Miller WM: Anemia in women ages 20 to 89 years: Rationale and tools for differential diagnosis. Clin Ther 15:192, 1993

35. Pimstone N: Renal degradation of hemoglobin. Semin Hematol 9:31, 1972

36. Roberts GT, Badawi SB: Red blood cell distribution width index in some hematological diseases. Am J Clin Pathol 83:222, 1985

37. Sears DA, Anderson PR, Foy AL et al: Urinary iron excretion and renal metabolism of hemoglobin in hemolytic diseases. Blood 28:708, 1966

38. Simmons A: Technical Hematology, 3rd ed. Philadelphia, JB Lippincott, 1980

39. Tabbara IA: Hemolytic anemias. Diagnosis and management. Med Clin North Am 76:649, 1992

40. Van Lente F, Marchand A, Galen RS: Diagnosis of hemolytic disease by electrophoresis of erythrocyte LDH isoenzymes on cellulose acetate or agarose. Clin Chem 27:1453, 1981

41. Vanzetti G, Valente D: A sensitive method for determination of hemoglobin in plasma. Clin Chim Acta 11:442, 1965

42. Yip R, Mohandas N, Clark M et al: Red cell membrane stiffness in iron deficiency. Blood 62:99, 1983

CHAPTER 17

Hereditary Anemias of Increased Destruction

Dianne M. Hansen

Objectives

1. Identify the membrane defects and mechanism of hemolysis in the hereditary erythrocyte membrane disorders.
2. Compare the peripheral blood film and clinical findings in hereditary spherocytosis, hereditary elliptocytosis, and hereditary pyropoikilocytosis.
3. Describe the principle of the osmotic fragility test and its application in the diagnosis of hereditary spherocytosis.
4. Briefly explain the mechanisms of hemolysis in the two most common hereditary erythrocyte enzymopathies.
5. List the most commonly used diagnostic tests for pyruvate kinase deficiency and glucose-6-phosphate dehydrogenase (G6PD) deficiency and describe their principles and expected results.
6. Identify the major genetic variants of the G6PD enzyme.
7. Define abetalipoproteinemia and lecithin-cholesterol acyltransferase deficiency and describe the most significant peripheral blood film finding in each disorder.

There are three major categories of hereditary disorders causing anemias that are due to abnormal erythrocyte destruction. Of these, intrinsic erythrocyte membrane structural abnormalities and erythrocyte enzymopathies are the most common and best understood. Extrinsic plasma constituent abnormalities are a rare cause of hereditary hemolytic anemia.

HEREDITARY ERYTHROCYTE MEMBRANE ABNORMALITIES

The erythrocyte membrane skeleton is responsible for preserving red cell shape and integrity. The normal membrane is composed of equal amounts of lipid and protein (Chap. 6). Membrane abnormalities that result in hemolytic anemia often are due to alterations in one or more structural proteins. Membrane lipid content and cation transport abnormalities may also be involved. These structural defects, in turn, lead to loss of membrane surface area, increased rigidity, fragmentation, or deformation. Such abnormal red cells become trapped in the spleen and are prematurely destroyed. Disorders characterized as erythrocyte membrane abnormalities include hereditary spherocytosis, hereditary elliptocytosis, hereditary pyropoikilocytosis, and hereditary stomatocytosis.

The Normal Erythrocyte Membrane

In order to understand the hereditary erythrocyte abnormalities, some knowledge of the normal erythrocyte membrane is required (Fig. 17-1). Several groups of proteins are important to red cell membrane structure.[29,53,54] These proteins may be generally classified as integral or peripheral. The integral proteins span the membrane, touching both the inner and outer surfaces. The most abundant integral protein is glycophorin. The peripheral proteins are attached to the integral proteins on the inner (cytoplasmic) side of the membrane. Spectrin is the most abundant peripheral protein, and it is composed of α and β chains twisted to form a heterodimer. Spectrin heterodimers are joined together as tetramers and more complex two-dimensional structures. Another peripheral protein known as actin facilitates binding of spectrin tetramers. The spectrin-actin linkage, which maintains the erythrocyte's biconcave shape, is mediated by a third peripheral protein, protein 4.1.

In addition, the spectrin-actin protein skeleton is attached to the inner surface of the membrane by two linkages.[54] Protein 4.1 binds spectrin to the integral membrane protein glycophorin C. Another integral membrane protein, band 3, is linked to β spectrin through ankyrin and protein 4.2.[29]

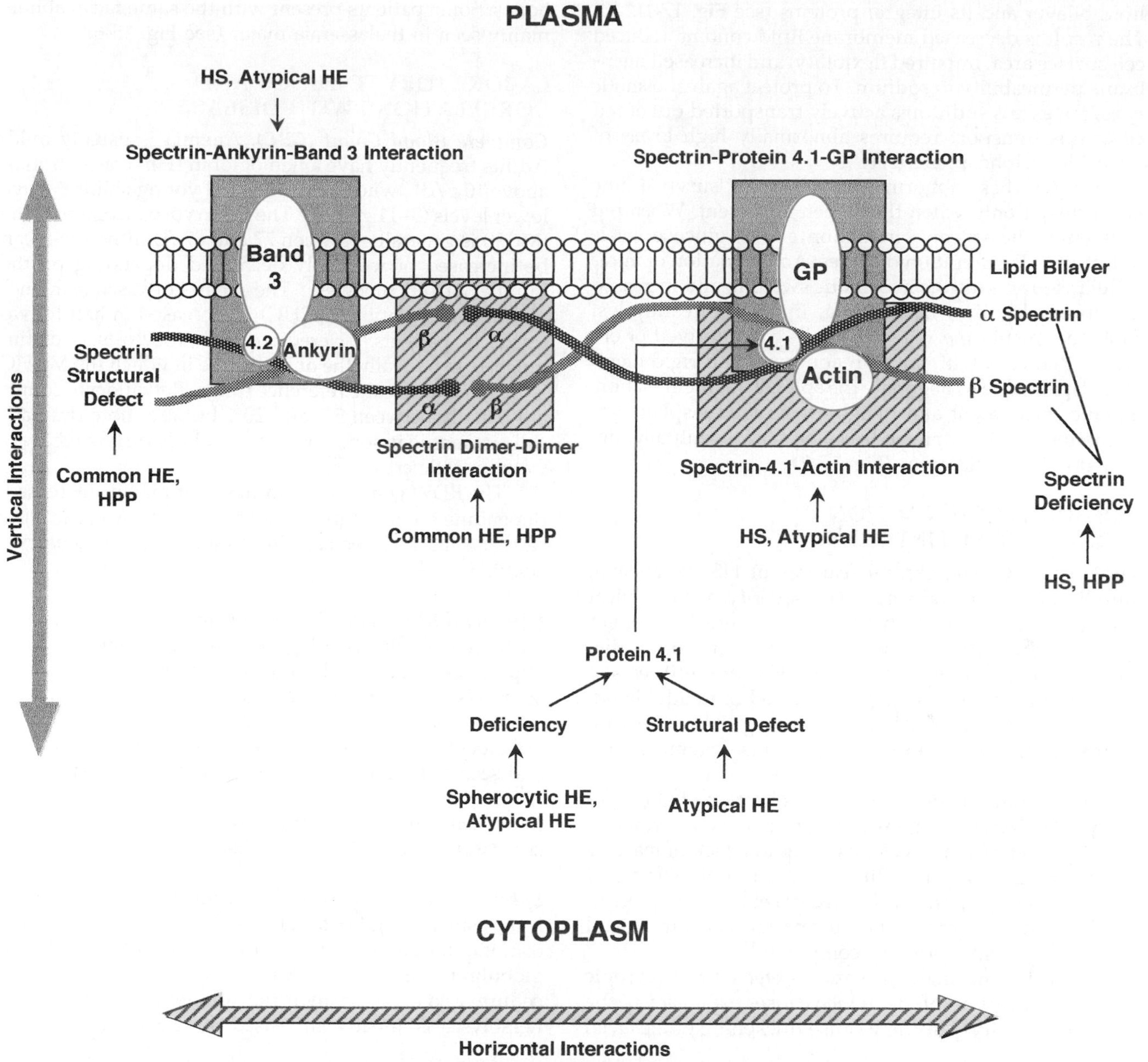

PLASMA

HS, Atypical HE
↓

Spectrin-Ankyrin-Band 3 Interaction   **Spectrin-Protein 4.1-GP Interaction**

Band 3   **GP**   **Lipid Bilayer**

Spectrin Structural Defect   **4.2** **Ankyrin**   β   α   **4.1**   **α Spectrin**

                                                                                   α   β   **Actin**   **β Spectrin**

↑
Common HE, HPP

Spectrin Dimer-Dimer Interaction   **Spectrin-4.1-Actin Interaction**   **Spectrin Deficiency**

↑   ↑   ↑
Common HE, HPP   **HS, Atypical HE**   **HS, HPP**

Vertical Interactions

Protein 4.1

Deficiency   **Structural Defect**

↑   ↑
Spherocytic HE,   **Atypical HE**
Atypical HE

CYTOPLASM

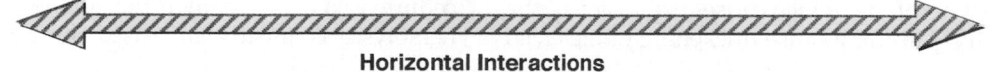

Horizontal Interactions

FIGURE 17-1. Vertical and horizontal interactions of erythrocyte membrane proteins. Defects in vertical interactions are seen in hereditary spherocytosis. The principle lesions in hereditary elliptocytosis and hereditary pyropoikilocytosis involve horizontal membrane protein interactions. GP = glycophorin. (Modified from Palek J, Jarolim P: Clinical expression and laboratory detection of red blood cell membrane protein mutations. Semin Hematol 30:249, 1993, with permission.)

Hereditary Spherocytosis

DEFINITION

Hereditary spherocytosis (HS) is a hemolytic disorder characterized by numerous microspherocytic erythrocytes seen on the blood film.

GENETICS AND PATHOPHYSIOLOGY

Inheritance of HS is usually autosomal dominant, and therefore it is found in heterozygotes. The homozygous state appears to be incompatible with life.[34] Several cases are often found in one family. In 25% of cases, neither parent is affected[38]; this may be the result of a spontaneous mutation, reduced penetrance of the dominant gene, or a recessive form of the disease.[37] HS is the most common hemolytic anemia in people of northern European extraction (incidence 1 in 5000).[37]

The basic abnormality in HS is a defect in red cell membrane protein composition. The membrane protein defects in HS are heterogeneous, involving deficiencies or dysfunctions of spectrin, ankyrin, band 3, and protein 4.2.[29,42,48,66] However, a common feature exists among HS RBCs. There appears to be a weakening of the "vertical" interactions of the membrane skeleton. These membrane protein defects facilitate the uncoupling of the overlying lipid bilayer and its integral proteins (see Fig. 17-1).[46,49,50] The result is decreased membrane lipid content, reduced cell surface area, impaired flexibility, and increased membrane permeability to sodium. To protect against osmotic lysis, the excess sodium is actively transported out of red cells; this transport requires abnormally high levels of adenosine triphosphate (ATP).

Despite these abnormalities, the cells' survival time is shortened only when the spleen is present. When red cells enter the spleen, circulation slows, glucose levels fall, and ATP generation declines. Accumulation of intracellular sodium results in osmotic swelling and increased membrane rigidity. In addition, lipids are readily lost from the membrane when red cells are deprived of energy.[37] Red cells with such an abnormal and rigid membrane are unable to negotiate the splenic microcirculation. Splenic entrapment and phagocytosis causes spherocyte formation, further splenic trapping, and eventually, destruction of erythrocytes (Fig. 17-2).

CLINICAL PRESENTATION AND PHYSICAL FINDINGS

Three characteristic clinical features of HS are anemia, jaundice, and splenomegaly. The severity of the clinical course varies, typically being more severe in younger patients[41] and with autosomal recessive forms of the disease.[29] Patients usually present with HS before 10 years of age, but mild cases may not be detected until adulthood. Increased metabolism of bile pigment (*e.g.*, bilirubin) from increased red cell hemolysis may cause pigment gallstones.

An uncommon but serious complication of HS, especially in children, is aplastic crisis in which peripheral blood pancytopenia develops owing to a lack of marrow cell production. The resulting anemia can be severe and life threatening. These self-limited crises are often precipitated by viral infections. Leg ulceration is common and may be a patient's primary complaint.[59]

Skeletal abnormalities may be detected from chronic bone marrow hyperplasia, which causes expansion of the medullary cavity. This may cause thickening of the facial bones. Some patients present with the same facial abnormality seen in thalassemia major (see Fig. 15-6).

LABORATORY FINDINGS AND CORRELATIONS WITH DISEASE

Complete Blood Count (CBC). Anemia is usually mild. Adults frequently have a hemoglobin (Hb) concentration above 10 g/dL, whereas infants and young children have lower levels (8–11 g/dL).[38] The mean corpuscular volume (MCV) is generally between 77 and 87 fL, although it can be increased or markedly decreased depending on the number of reticulocytes.[36] The mean corpuscular hemoglobin concentration (MCHC) is increased in half to two thirds of patients.[37] Hereditary spherocytosis is distinguished as basically the only disease in which the MCHC is elevated above the reference range. Reticulocyte counts are usually between 5% and 20% but are more dramatically increased in some cases, particularly during recovery from aplastic crisis.[34,41]

The RDW generally is normal[2] but may be increased, depending on the degree of reticulocytosis. Aplastic crisis causes a marked decrease in Hb and a low reticulocyte count.

Peripheral Blood Film. Numerous microspherocytes seen on the blood film (see Fig. 8-6) are characteristic. They appear small and dark and lack central pallor. Anisocytosis is prominent owing to a mixture of microspherocytes and large polychromatophilic cells (reticulocytes). Poikilocytosis other than the spherocytes is not common and seen only in more severe forms of the disease.

Bone Marrow. The bone marrow displays erythroid hyperplasia. An aplastic crisis causes marrow hypoplasia.

Special Hematology Tests. The confirmatory test for HS is the osmotic fragility test. Red cells in HS have increased osmotic fragility (see procedure below). The direct antiglobulin test is negative. Another special diagnostic procedure used occasionally is the autohemolysis test. Autohemolysis is greatly increased in HS; however, this

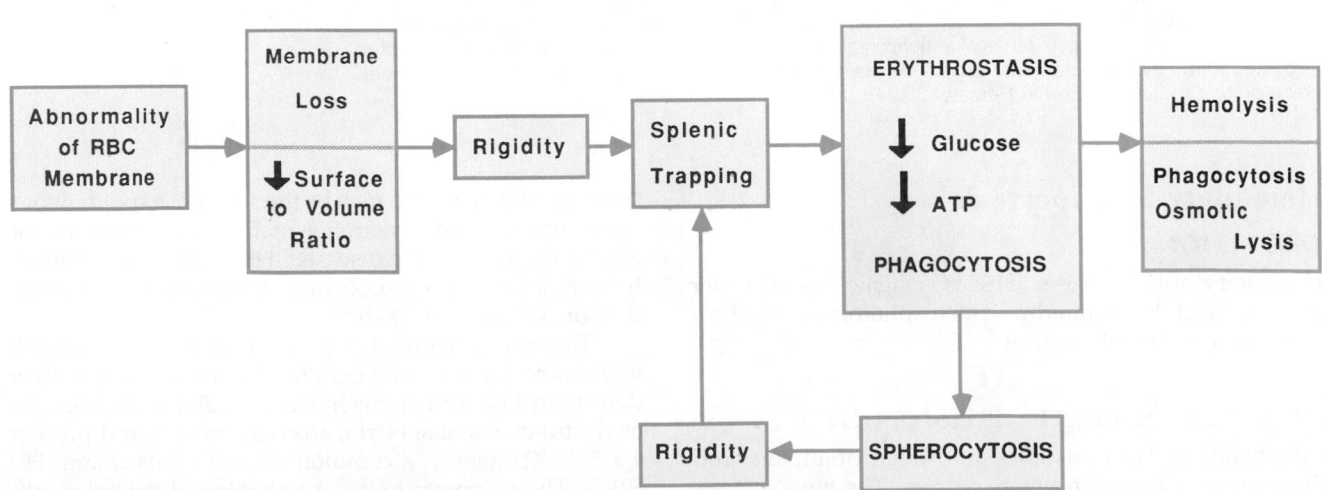

FIGURE 17-2. Pathophysiology of spherocyte formation and red cell destruction in hereditary spherocytosis.

phenomenon does not occur if either glucose or ATP is added to the test system. Other disorders do not yield the same results. The autohemolysis test is discussed in a later section on pyruvate kinase deficiency, for which it is more applicable to the diagnosis.

Chemistry. Other laboratory findings common to hemolytic processes support the diagnosis of HS. A slight to moderate rise in unconjugated (indirect) bilirubin, elevated fecal urobilinogen, and decreased haptoglobin levels may be observed. The intravascular hemolytic indicators of hemoglobinemia, hemoglobinuria, and hemosiderinuria do *not* appear in HS. In cases for which diagnosis is in doubt, analysis of red cell spectrin by radioimmunoassay may be useful.[54] The degree of spectrin deficiency appears to correlate with the degree of spherocytosis and the clinical severity of the disease.[1]

MOST USEFUL LABORATORY TESTS FOR DIAGNOSING HEREDITARY SPHEROCYTOSIS

The most useful diagnostic test for HS is the osmotic fragility test, but other tests (Table 17-1), including the incubated osmotic fragility and the direct antiglobulin test, may be helpful. Step-by-step procedures for these tests may be found in the references provided and in some cases, in manufacturer's test kit enclosures.

Osmotic Fragility Test[19]

PRINCIPLE. Osmotic fragility reflects the shape of erythrocytes. The test involves the mixture of patient's red cells with various concentrations of sodium chloride (saline; NaCl). When red cells are placed in isotonic solution (0.85% NaCl) there is no movement of water into or out of the cells. However, when red cells are placed in increasingly hypotonic solutions (*e.g.,* decreasing concentrations of NaCl; solutions that cause water to flow across the cell membrane into the cell) more and more water will move into the cells, eventually causing most cells to rupture or hemolyze.

Because of their decreased surface area-to-volume ratio, spherocytes have a more limited capacity to take up fluid in hypotonic solutions and therefore lyse at higher concentrations

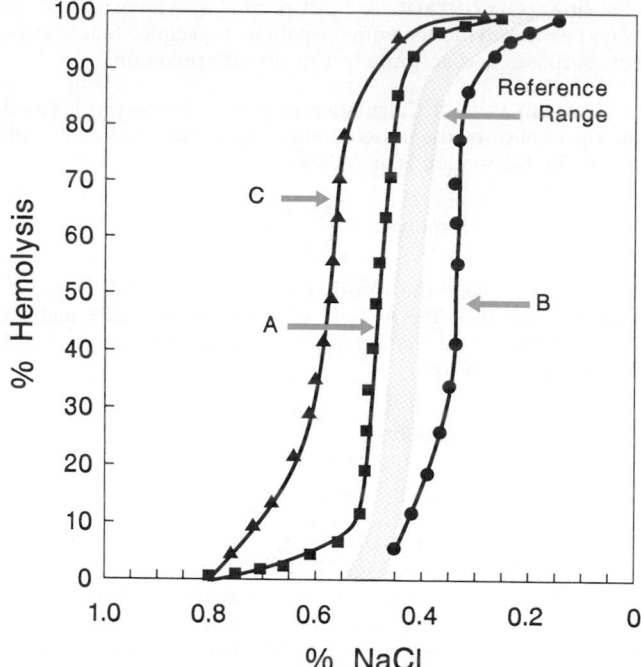

FIGURE 17-3. Results of erythrocyte osmotic fragility test under various conditions. Curve A shows the increased osmotic fragility of cells in hereditary spherocytosis. Curve B shows the decreased fragility of target cells in thalassemia. Curve C shows the markedly increased fragility in hereditary spherocytosis when the incubated osmotic fragility test is used. Compare each curve to the reference range.

of NaCl than normal biconcave red cells. This behavior is referred to as increased osmotic fragility. On the other hand, cells that are hypochromic or flatter and have a high surface area-to-volume ratio (*e.g.,* hypochromic cells in iron deficiency, target cells in thalassemia and sickle cell anemia, and sickle cells themselves) have decreased osmotic fragility (Fig. 17-3). They have a greater capacity to take up fluid in hypotonic solution and lyse at lower concentrations of NaCl than normal cells.

SPECIMEN REQUIREMENTS. Fresh heparinized blood is preferred. Fifteen to twenty milliliters of defibrinated whole blood, prepared by placing whole blood into a flask with glass beads, may also be used. Anticoagulants containing oxalates are undesirable because they alter pH. The test should be set up within 2 hours of collection or within 6 hours if the specimen is refrigerated.

REAGENTS. The various saline concentrations may be prepared in the laboratory or purchased prepackaged. Saline concentrations already prepared by a manufacturer (*e.g.,* the osmotic fragility kit produced by Becton Dickinson, Rutherford, NJ) may be preferable for ease of use, time savings, and more reliable results. However, due to the low frequency in use of this test, outdating of these kits before they are ever used may prove to be costly for some laboratories.

GENERAL PROCEDURE. The test is performed by suspending red cells in a series of saline (NaCl) solutions ranging from 0.85% to 0.0% (water) and incubating for 30 minutes at room temperature. After each test suspension is centrifuged, the absorbance of each supernatant is measured at 540 nm. Using this absorbance, percent hemolysis is calculated by comparing each test solution to the 0.85% and 0.0% NaCl solutions (see Calculations). More details on this procedure may be found in many laboratory procedure manuals.

TABLE 17-1
Recommended Laboratory Tests to Assist in Diagnosis of Hereditary Spherocytosis

MOST FREQUENTLY REQUIRED

CBC with MCHC

Peripheral blood film examination

Osmotic fragility test

Reticulocyte count

OCCASIONALLY REQUIRED

Autohemolysis test

Direct antiglobulin test

Serum unconjugated (indirect) bilirubin

Serum haptoglobin

RARELY REQUIRED

Bone marrow examination

QUALITY CONTROL. A fresh normal specimen should always be run and plotted with the patient's specimen for comparison purposes and accurate test result interpretation.

CALCULATIONS. Calculation of percent hemolysis is based on absorbance of the supernatant of each NaCl concentration ($A_{x\%}$). The calculation is as follows:

$$\% \text{ Hemolysis} = \frac{A_{x\%} - A_{0.85\%}}{A_{0.0\%} - A_{0.85\%}} \times 100\%$$

For example, if the absorbance of the 0.20% NaCl supernatant ($A_{0.20\%}$) is 0.77, the $A_{0.00\%}$ (100% hemolysis) is 0.89, and the $A_{0.85\%}$ is 0.05, the calculation of percent hemolysis for the 0.20% NaCl test suspension is

$$\% \text{ Hemolysis} = \frac{0.77 - 0.05}{0.89 - 0.05} \times 100\%$$

$$= 85.7\%$$

Percent hemolysis is plotted against NaCl concentration on linear graph paper (see Fig. 17-3). Note that the denominator should represent the largest amount of change in absorbance of all the test solutions because complete hemolysis is expected in 0.00% NaCl, which is pure water. All other NaCl concentrations are compared to complete hemolysis to obtain their percent hemolysis. The 0.85% absorbance is subtracted from the numerator and denominator to correct for any *minimal* incidental hemolysis that might result from specimen handling rather than true osmotic fragility. Neither normal nor abnormal erythrocytes should lyse in 0.85% isotonic saline.

REFERENCE RANGE. The reference range at 20°C is shown in Table 17-2. In clinically normal subjects, hemolysis begins around 0.45% and generally is complete between 0.35% and 0.30% NaCl.

Incubated Osmotic Fragility. In mild forms of HS, osmotic fragility may be normal. To detect these mild forms, including

TABLE 17-2
Reference Ranges for Osmotic Fragility at 20°C

NaCl (%)	Hemolysis* (%)
0.00	100
0.10	100
0.20	100
0.30	97–100
0.35	90–97
0.40	50–90
0.45	0–45
0.50	0–5
0.55	0
0.60	0
0.65	0
0.70	0
0.85	0

* Hemolysis normally begins around 0.45% and generally is complete between 0.35% and 0.30% NaCl.

those in family members who do not demonstrate a clinical disorder, a test variation calls for measurement of the osmotic fragility following sterile incubation of specimens for 24 hours at 37°C, which enhances osmotic fragility if HS is present. The patient and normal control specimens can be either sterile defibrinated whole blood or sterile heparinized whole blood. Following 24-hour incubation, the test is performed with saline solutions using the same procedure as that for the unincubated osmotic fragility. Figure 17-3 demonstrates the increased fragility found in HS when the incubated method is used.

COMMENTS AND SOURCES OF ERROR. There are many factors that can cause a false increase in the percent hemolysis and osmotic fragility. It is important to obtain the blood sample with a minimum of stasis and trauma, and the test must be performed as soon as possible after the specimen is obtained. Saline solutions must be chemically pure, dilutions must be accurate, and the temperature and pH (7.4) must be kept constant.[31] In the incubated osmotic fragility test, the major source of error is bacterial contamination. To avoid this, heparinized specimens must be unopened prior to incubation. If defibrinated whole blood is to be used, flasks with beads should be plugged with sterile cotton and sterilized before being used. While incubating blood, the flask should remain plugged with sterile cotton.

If plasma color is abnormal (*e.g.*, jaundiced or lipemic) it may be necessary to replace plasma with isotonic saline prior to testing to avoid test interference. When a decreased hemoglobin level and poikilocytosis are both present in a specimen, these conditions may cause decreased osmotic fragility, most likely because of the decreased hemoglobin.

Occasionally the highest absorbance reading will occur in either the 0.30%, 0.20%, or 0.10% NaCl test solution (it is normal to have 100% hemolysis in 0.30% NaCl). If this happens, use the highest absorbance reading obtained in place of the 0.00% reading in the denominator of the calculation.

Increased osmotic fragility is characteristic of HS but may also be seen in other acquired hemolytic anemias that typically have spherocytes (*e.g.*, hemolytic disease of the newborn and autoimmune hemolytic anemia).[44] A greater increase in the incubated osmotic fragility is seen in HS than in other anemias.

Microcapillary[31] and automated[20] methods are also available for osmotic fragility testing.

Direct Antiglobulin Test. Because the laboratory findings in HS are similar to those in immune hemolytic anemias, the direct antiglobulin test (DAT) is useful in the differential diagnosis. The DAT detects antibody on the red cell surface, so a negative result rules out immune-mediated hemolytic anemias and is expected in HS. The DAT procedure can be found in immunohematology textbooks.

EFFECTS OF TREATMENT ON LABORATORY RESULTS

The usual treatment for HS is splenectomy, which removes the agent of red cell destruction and prevents complications such as aplastic crisis and gallbladder disease. Splenectomy should be delayed as long as possible, because the spleen is important in the developing immune system, particularly in adolescence. Splenectomized patients have a normal life expectancy.

Following splenectomy, spherocytes persist on the peripheral blood film, and Howell-Jolly bodies become a more prominent feature. Spiculated cells may also be present.[66] Reticulocyte counts decrease to high normal levels; and if anemia was present, hemoglobin increases, usually to normal ranges. Leukocytosis and thrombocytosis are expected after splenectomy. Bilirubin levels decrease but may remain in the high normal range.[37] The osmotic fragility curve becomes less shifted than before splenectomy.[63]

Hereditary Elliptocytosis

DEFINITION

Hereditary elliptocytosis (HE) is a heterogeneous group of disorders characterized by large numbers of elliptical erythrocytes on the blood film (see Fig. 8-7).

DEMOGRAPHICS AND PATHOPHYSIOLOGY

HE is only about one fifth as common as hereditary spherocytosis[23] and is found in all racial groups.[38] Inheritance is generally autosomal dominant.

Studies indicate that the membrane structural defect in HE involves spectrin or proteins with which spectrin closely associates.[17] Spectrin is quantitatively normal but structurally abnormal in HE. Common HE is typically caused by an alteration in the horizontal interaction of spectrin dimers (see Fig. 17-1), resulting in impaired ability to self-associate into spectrin tetramers.[45] A second defect is related to abnormal spectrin–actin–protein 4.1 interactions. The degree of hemolysis in HE may correlate with the severity of the molecular defect (*e.g.*, abnormal spectrin heterodimer self-association or abnormal spectrin structure).[16]

Factors that determine the elliptical shape of red cells are only beginning to be understood. Since bone marrow erythroblasts and circulating reticulocytes are normal in shape, red cells appear to acquire the elliptical shape as they age in the circulation. Rearrangement of protein-protein contacts in the red cell membrane may occur as HE red cells flow through the microcirculation or are subjected to shear stress.[49] Whereas normal red cells resume a biconcave shape when shear stress has ceased, the elliptical shape becomes permanent in HE. The mechanism of hemolysis is known to involve membrane loss, decreased red cell "deformability," and shortened red cell survival due to splenic destruction.

CLINICAL PRESENTATION AND PHYSICAL FINDINGS

The clinical severity of common HE varies considerably, ranging from an asymptomatic carrier to a severe, life-threatening hemolysis. Hemolysis is present in 10% to 15% of affected individuals. When present, hemolyis is usually mild and is accompanied by anemia, jaundice, and splenomegaly.

LABORATORY FINDINGS AND CORRELATIONS WITH DISEASE

Routine Hematology. The red cells in HE are normocytic and normochromic. Characteristically, the Hb value is greater than 12 g/dL and the reticulocyte count is less than 4%.[60]

The peripheral blood film reveals greater than 25% elliptocytes and oval erythrocytes (see Fig. 8-7).[34,44] At least

three types of HE have been described based on red cell morphology and clinical presentation: common HE, spherocytic HE, and stomatocytic HE.[37,48] Common HE, the most prevalent form, reveals typical HE red cell morphology. Hemolysis ranges from nonexistent to moderate. Spherocytic HE accounts for approximately 10% to 20% of cases, and the blood shows a significant number of elliptocytes that are more rounded than those found in typical HE and variable numbers of microspherocytes. Stomatocytic HE is characterized by the presence of ovalocytes, some of which have a longitudinal slit in the middle (a stomatocyte). This form of HE is prevalent in parts of Southeast Asia, presumably because it offers some protection against invasion by malarial parasites.[47]

Special Hematologic Tests. The osmotic fragility test and autohemolysis test usually are normal. In cases of spherocytic HE, values of these test results are increased. Bone marrow erythroblasts are normal in shape. Erythroid hyperplasia correlates with the degree of compensation for hemolysis.

Chemistry. Increased serum unconjugated bilirubin and fecal urobilinogen and decreased serum haptoglobin levels can be observed when hemolysis is present.

EFFECTS OF TREATMENT ON LABORATORY RESULTS

In most cases no treatment is necessary. People with moderately severe hemolytic disease may benefit from splenectomy, which ameliorates anemia and restores a normal reticulocyte count, but elliptocytosis persists on the peripheral blood film. Other forms of poikilocytes may increase because they are not removed by the spleen.

Hereditary Pyropoikilocytosis

GENETICS AND PATHOPHYSIOLOGY

Hereditary pyropoikilocytosis (HPP) is an extremely rare hemolytic disorder characterized by extreme anisocytosis and micropoikilocytosis including schistocytes (Fig. 17-4).[37,48,67] Inheritance is autosomal recessive and the disorder characteristically occurs in black children.

In HPP, the red cell membrane structural abnormality is related to both a quantitative decrease in and structural abnormality of red cell spectrin. As in hereditary elliptocytosis (HE), spectrin heterodimers fail to self-associate, which leads to a decrease in spectrin tetramers (see Fig. 17-1).[48] Evidence indicates that the molecular defect is similar in HPP and HE, although in HE, spectrin is quantitatively normal. In HPP, the defect in heterodimer association and structurally abnormal spectrin is greater than in HE, causing a greater degree of hemolysis.[16] The instability of the red cell membrane in HPP leads to both extreme morphologic abnormalities and thermal instability of the cells. As in HS, the mechanism of hemolysis appears to be related to membrane loss and rigidity. HPP red cells are also characterized by elevated calcium content with increased inflow and reduced outflow of calcium, but this abnormality appears to be secondary to the membrane structural defect.

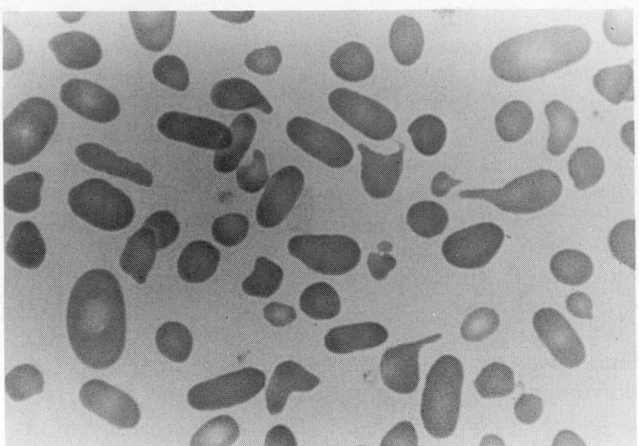

FIGURE 17-4. Blood film demonstrates hereditary pyropoikilocytosis. Note microspherocytes, fragments, elliptocytes, and bizarre forms. (From McKenna RW, Hoffman GC, Horwitz CA, Ward PCJ: Laboratory approach to the diagnosis of hemolytic anemias. Workshop manual. Chicago, IL, American Society of Clinical Pathologists, 1984, with permission. Photomicrograph by Robert W. McKenna.)

CLINICAL PRESENTATION AND PHYSICAL FINDINGS

HPP presents in infancy or early childhood with severe, often transfusion-dependent hemolytic anemia. In addition, jaundice, splenomegaly, and gallbladder disease may be present.

LABORATORY FINDINGS AND CORRELATIONS WITH DISEASE

Routine Hematology. The most striking feature is extreme microcytosis. The MCV often is between 25 and 55 fL.[65] Hemoglobin is decreased in proportion to the degree of hemolysis. Reticulocyte counts are elevated, but the reticulocyte production index depends on the ability of the patient's bone marrow to respond to anemia.

There is striking anisocytosis and micropoikilocytosis with budding red cells, microspherocytes, fragments, elliptocytes, and other bizarre forms (Fig. 17-4). Polychromasia is also present.

Special Hematologic Tests. Suspected HPP red cells should be tested for thermal sensitivity. In contrast to normal cells, which fragment at temperatures above 49°C, red cells in HPP fragment at temperatures as low as 45° to 46°C. HPP is also characterized by an increased osmotic fragility, especially after incubation, and a markedly elevated autohemolysis test result.

EFFECTS OF TREATMENT ON LABORATORY RESULTS

Hemolysis is reduced but not always corrected by splenectomy. Abnormal red cell morphology remains following splenectomy.[67]

Hereditary Stomatocytosis (Hydrocytosis) and Hereditary Xerocytosis

GENETICS AND PATHOPHYSIOLOGY

Hereditary stomatocytosis, also known as hydrocytosis, and hereditary xerocytosis are a heterogeneous group of red cell membrane disorders. They are characterized by mild to moderate hemolytic anemia, altered membrane permeability to cations, and most commonly, autosomal dominant inheritance.

Red cell water content is dependent on the cellular concentration of sodium and potassium cations. Red cells in hereditary stomatocytosis are characterized by increased permeability and flux (flow into and out of the cell) of both sodium and potassium, resulting in increased water content and swollen cells. There is a net increase in cellular sodium and a net decrease in potassium. The defect in sodium permeability is greater than that of potassium, causing a net *increase* in cellular cation concentration, which stimulates the entry of water into the cells to maintain osmotic equilibrium. These cells swell and take on the appearance of stomatocytes (from the Greek word *stoma*, "mouth") on the peripheral blood film (*i.e.*, they have a slit- or mouthlike area of central pallor; see Fig. 8-10). Stomatocytes have an increased volume and a decreased surface-to-volume ratio, leading to decreased ability to deform and increased splenic destruction.

More commonly, however, the efflux (outflow) of potassium is greater than the influx (inflow) of sodium. In this condition, there is a net *decrease* in cellular cation concentration, which stimulates the movement of water out of the cells. The cells become dehydrated and are known as xerocytes (from the Greek word *xeros*, "dry"). Xerocytes have an increased surface-to-volume ratio, so the peripheral blood film reveals the presence of target cells[55,64] and cells with Hb concentrated at one pole of the cell. The cells are not very deformable and are subject to reticuloendothelial destruction.

The structural basis for these membrane abnormalities is poorly understood. There is some evidence that hereditary stomatocytosis is associated with a deficiency of a band 1 protein, but no mutations of this protein have been detected.[46,55] Hemolysis is related to decreased red cell deformability and osmotic lysis in the spleen.[40]

CLINICAL PRESENTATION AND PHYSICAL FINDINGS

The clinical features of hereditary stomatocytosis and xerocytosis are similar to those of other chronic hemolytic anemias. The degree of hemolytic anemia is usually mild but varies both within and between families.[44]

LABORATORY FINDINGS AND CORRELATIONS WITH DISEASE

Routine Hematology. Hemoglobin is rarely less than 8 to 10 g/dL. Reticulocytosis is usually moderate (10%–20%), but variations range from normal to as high as 45%. The MCV usually is increased in both conditions, and the

MCHC is generally decreased in stomatocytosis and increased in xerocytosis.

In some cases of hereditary stomatocytosis, 10% to 50% of circulating red cells are stomatocytes. Target cells predominate in hereditary xerocytosis; some cells demonstrate the concentrated area of Hb toward one pole of the cell.

Special Hematologic Tests. Osmotic fragility is increased when stomatocytes persist, due to the decreased cellular surface-to-volume ratio. On the other hand, osmotic fragility is decreased when the target cells of xerocytosis predominate.[40] Autohemolysis (see procedure later in this chapter) is increased and may or may not be corrected by the addition of glucose.[35]

Chemistry. Increased serum unconjugated bilirubin and decreased serum haptoglobin reflect the degree of hemolysis. Confirmatory tests include abnormal red cell cation content and increased cation transport; these tests are performed by a special chemistry or reference laboratory.

EFFECTS OF TREATMENT ON LABORATORY RESULTS

Splenectomy has proven beneficial in correcting hemolysis in patients with hereditary stomatocytosis. Those with hereditary xerocytosis generally do not benefit from splenectomy, presumably because xerocytes are being destroyed in areas other than the spleen.

HEREDITARY ERYTHROCYTE ENZYMOPATHIES

Normal erythrocyte metabolism in the Embden-Meyerhof pathway (EMP) and pentose phosphate pathway (PPP) is discussed in detail in Chapter 6. A number of hereditary enzymopathies cause abnormalities in these pathways.

About 90% of the energy for red cell metabolism is produced by anaerobic glycolysis through the EMP, which produces the ATP necessary for normal cell function and survival. Enzymopathies in this pathway are numerous and are referred to collectively as congenital nonspherocytic hemolytic anemias. Many lead to varying degrees of hemolytic anemia. The most common, pyruvate kinase (PK) deficiency, is discussed in detail. Other enzymopathies of this pathway are extremely rare.

The PPP is responsible for aerobic glycolysis, which generates about 10% of the red cell's energy. This pathway generates reduced nicotinamide adenine dinucleotide phosphate (NADPH), which is required for oxidized glutathione (GSSG) reduction. Reduced glutathione (GSH) protects enzymes and Hb from oxidation. Enzyme deficiencies of this pathway result in build-up of hydrogen peroxide, oxidative denaturation of hemoglobin, and hemolysis, usually as a result of oxidant stress which can be caused by certain drugs and foods. The most common enzymopathy of the PPP is glucose-6-phosphate dehydrogenase (G6PD) deficiency, which is discussed in detail later in this chapter.

Pyruvate Kinase Deficiency

DEFINITION

Itself a rare disorder, pyruvate kinase (PK) is the most common enzyme deficiency of the EMP. The disease results in mild to moderately severe hemolytic anemia.

GENETICS AND PATHOPHYSIOLOGY

Although most cases are found in people of northern European origin, PK deficiency occurs worldwide. It is inherited as an autosomal recessive trait. PK genetic mutants are numerous, and most people with hemolytic anemia are homozygous or doubly heterozygous for two mutant genes.[58,61] Those who are heterozygotes generally demonstrate about half the normal PK activity and do not have anemia or other hematologic changes.[57] Acquired PK deficiency occurs in some cases of hematologic malignancies and dyserythropoietic syndromes.[43,62]

PK catalyzes the formation of pyruvate from phosphoenol-pyruvate (PEP) and is accompanied by the transformation of adenosine diphosphate (ADP) to ATP (see Fig. 6-7). Thus, PK deficiency leads to a marked reduction in ATP production, which is necessary for maintenance of the membrane sodium-potassium pump. Potassium and water are lost from the cell, resulting in cell shrinkage, distortion of shape, and spiculation. Irreversible membrane injury resulting from potassium loss and an increase in membrane calcium causes decreased deformability and premature destruction in the spleen.

Reticulocytes derive their energy principally through mitochondrial oxidative phosphorylation rather than glycolysis. As mitochondria are lost during maturation, reticulocytes are very vulnerable to the effects of their glycolytic defect and are destroyed in the spleen.

Metabolic intermediates, such as 2,3-diphosphoglycerate (2,3-DPG) accumulate in PK deficiency as a result of the block in glycolysis. The cellular concentration of 2,3-DPG may exceed two to three times normal.[32] This increase in 2,3-DPG is responsible for a shift to the right in the oxyhemoglobin dissociation curve (see Fig. 7-5), and the ability of red cells to release oxygen more readily to the tissues to compensate for anemia.

CLINICAL FEATURES AND PHYSICAL FINDINGS

The clinical features of PK deficiency are highly variable. Some newborns require exchange transfusion; others have fully compensated hemolytic anemia and experience no symptoms. The disease is usually detected in infancy or early childhood, but occasionally it is not detected until adulthood. The signs and symptoms are those associated with chronic hemolysis including anemia, splenomegaly, jaundice, and gallstones.

LABORATORY FINDINGS AND CORRELATIONS WITH DISEASE

Routine Hematology. Hemoglobin ranges widely from 6 to 12 g/dL.[43] Red cells generally are normocytic and normochromic, although the MCV may be elevated when reticulocytosis is marked. Before splenectomy reticulocyte counts range from 2.5% to 15%.[35] Following splenectomy reticulocyte counts increase; counts as high as 56% are not uncommon.[57] Leukocytes and platelets are generally normal.

There are no prominent morphologic features. As indicated earlier, occasional spiculated cells (echinocytes) may be seen. Polychromasia, poikilocytosis, and variable numbers of nucleated red cells may be found. Microspherocytes usually are not present.

Chemistry. Serum unconjugated bilirubin is moderately elevated and haptoglobin levels are decreased. Erythrocyte glycolytic intermediates such as 2,3-DPG and PEP are increased, whereas ATP, lactate, and pyruvate, which require PK for production, are decreased.

Special Hematologic Tests. Results of the osmotic fragility test are normal, but the incubated fragility test may show variable degrees of abnormality. Autohemolysis is discussed in the next section. Heinz bodies are not present, and the result of the direct antiglobulin test is negative.

MOST USEFUL LABORATORY TESTS FOR DIAGNOSING PYRUVATE KINASE DEFICIENCY

Readers should refer to the references provided for detailed procedures for performing the following tests.

PK Fluorescent Spot Test and Quantitative PK assay. The PK fluorescent spot test[3,4] is the recommended screening test for PK deficiency (reagents available from Sigma Chemical Company, St. Louis, MO). An abnormal spot test result must be confirmed by the quantitative PK assay.[11]

PRINCIPLE AND SPECIMEN REQUIREMENTS. Both the qualitative and quantitative methods involve the same reactions. In the spot test, the reaction mixture (containing PEP, fluorescent NADH, and lactate dehydrogenase [LD], incubated with the patient hemolysate) is spotted on filter paper at timed intervals (*e.g.*, 0, 10, 20, and 30 minutes). After allowing the spots to dry for 10 to 15 minutes, they are observed in a dark room under long-wave ultraviolet light for expected disappearance of fluorescence. The test is based on the following reactions:

$$PEP + ADP \overset{PK}{\to} ATP + Pyruvate$$

$$Pyruvate + \underset{(fluorescent)}{NADH} \overset{LD}{\to} Lactate + \underset{(nonfluorescent)}{NAD}$$

PK in the patient's red cells is required to catalyze the conversion of PEP to pyruvate. Then fluorescent NADH reacts with pyruvate in the presence of the LD enzyme and is converted to nonfluorescent NAD with the formation of lactate.

Loss of fluorescence of NADH under ultraviolet light usually occurs within 10 to 20 minutes and indicates normal PK activity. PK-deficient erythrocytes fail to complete this reaction, and fluorescence persists at 30 minutes and for as long as 45 to 60 minutes. In the quantitative assay, the change in absorbance of the reaction mixture is measured spectrophotometrically at 340 nm to quantitate PK activity.

Whole blood anticoagulated with EDTA, heparin, or acid-citrate-dextrose (ACD) solution is acceptable. Red cell hemolysates are prepared for analysis.

REFERENCE RANGE. PK activity is reported in units (U) per liter, and the reference range is highly dependent on the method

used. It is higher for infants than adults. Most PK-deficient people have 5% to 25% of the normal mean activity. Heterozygous carriers have approximately half the normal activity.[57,58]

COMMENTS AND SOURCES OF ERROR. Spots must be dry before examining with ultraviolet light. Wet spots will quench (decrease) fluorescence and could cause a false-negative (*i.e.,* normal PK) result.

Leukocytes contain about 300 times as much PK as red cells and must be completely removed from the sample before the hemolysate is prepared. Platelets also have a very high PK level and must also be completely removed. In addition, a recent transfusion provides normal cells that may obscure PK deficiency until the donor cells are removed from circulation in 3 to 4 months. Finally, reticulocytes contain higher levels of PK, and test results may be normal for some time following a hemolytic episode.

Autohemolysis Test. This test[19] is sometimes used to screen for PK deficiency and G6PD deficiency, each of which produces a different test result. A third result is obtained using cells from patients with hereditary spherocytosis (HS), but the osmotic fragility test should be the principal diagnostic tool used to investigate HS.

PRINCIPLE AND SPECIMEN REQUIREMENTS. The autohemolysis test measures the spontaneous lysis of red cells incubated at 37°C for 48 hours.[19] During this time, depletion of glucose and ATP results in membrane loss and spherocyte formation. Glucose or ATP added to the blood may protect against autohemolysis partially or completely. Sterile, defibrinated blood is the specimen of choice. The procedure and quality control are discussed elsewhere.[19]

REFERENCE RANGE. Normal red cells incubated under these conditions exhibit 0.2% to 2.0% hemolysis. With the addition of glucose, 0% to 0.9% hemolysis is seen; or with ATP, 0% to 0.8% is seen.

COMMENTS AND SOURCES OF ERROR. Dacie[19] describes three patterns of autohemolysis.

1. *Type I:* Autohemolysis is slightly to moderately increased but is partially corrected by glucose. This is seen in G6PD deficiency, hereditary elliptocytosis, and unstable hemoglobin disease.
2. *Type II:* Autohemolysis is greatly increased and glucose has no effect; however, ATP corrects the hemolysis. This is associated with pyruvate kinase deficiency.
3. *Hereditary spherocytosis:* Autohemolysis is greatly increased but can be corrected with either glucose or ATP. This pattern has also been found in triose phosphate isomerase deficiency.

The autohemolysis test is tedious, neither sensitive nor specific, and is very vulnerable to bacterial contamination, so it is not used widely today.[24]

EFFECTS OF TREATMENT ON LABORATORY RESULTS

PK deficiency is treated with transfusions in severe cases of hemolytic anemia and by exchange transfusions to prevent neonatal hyperbilirubinemia. Although it is not curative, splenectomy is indicated for patients who require regular blood transfusions. Following splenectomy, the Hb value increases by 1 to 2 g/dL in most patients,[43] reticulocyte counts are markedly increased, and echinocytes are more prevalent on the peripheral blood film.[33]

Glucose-6-Phosphate Dehydrogenase Deficiency

DEFINITION, HISTORY AND GENETICS

G6PD deficiency is the most common red cell enzymopathy associated with hemolysis.[6] The disorder results from the inheritance of any one of a large number of abnormal genes that code for the G6PD enzyme. The course of the disorder varies from episodic hemolysis induced by drugs and other oxidant stresses to severe, chronic nonspherocytic hemolytic anemia. G6PD deficiency was discovered in the 1950s after it was observed that some black soldiers receiving the antimalarial drug primaquine developed hemolytic anemia.[21]

G6PD deficiency is an X-linked inherited disease, so it is fully expressed in men with the genetic abnormality. In women it is fully expressed only in homozygotes. Because of X chromosome inactivation (Lyon hypothesis) in which one of the two X chromosomes of each cell is believed to be inactive, heterozygous women have two populations of erythrocytes. One population has normal enzyme activity (the genetically defective X chromosome was inactivated), and the other population is G6PD deficient (the normal X chromosome was inactivated).[56] Most heterozygous women are clinically normal and have a normal G6PD level; however, due to the random nature of X-chromosome inactivation, some heterozygous women may be extremely G6PD deficient.[10,36]

VARIANTS, DEMOGRAPHICS, AND PATHOPHYSIOLOGY

G6PD deficiency is most common in West Africa, the Mediterranean, the Middle East, and Southeast Asia. Black people often have a mild deficiency (10%–60% of normal activity), Orientals have a more severe deficiency, and Mediterraneans the most severe.

There are over 400 genetic variants of the G6PD enzyme,[10] which generally are named for the geographic region in which they are prevalent (*e.g.,* G6PD Canton). Many G6PD variants can be classified according to enzyme activity, electrophoretic mobility, and clinical mani-

festations.[7,8] This chapter focuses on two well known variant groups in addition to a group of variants that produces similar laboratory findings.

The normal G6PD enzyme, designated as G6PD B, is found in all white people and most black people. A variant with normal G6PD activity called G6PD A is prevalent among blacks and differs from G6PD B by a single amino acid substitution. The G6PD A and B enzymes differ in electrophoretic mobility due to the amino acid composition. The variant G6PD A− (the minus sign indicates deficient enzyme activity) is the most common one associated with hemolysis. It is electrophoretically identical to G6PD A but has only 5% to 15% of the normal enzyme activity.[8] G6PD A− is found in 11% of American black men,[8] whereas about 25% of American black women are carriers.[13]

Among Caucasians, the most common abnormal variant is G6PD Mediterranean, which affects 1 in 1000 people in Mediterranean regions.[23] The electrophoretic mobility of G6PD Mediterranean is identical to that of G6PD B, but its catalytic activity is often less than 1% of normal.[8] In addition, there is a large group of variants that expresses chronic hereditary nonspherocytic hemolytic anemia. These variants are rare and occur sporadically among various ethnic groups.

Oxidative denaturation of Hb is the major contributor to the hemolytic process in G6PD deficiency.[61] G6PD is necessary for converting glucose-6-phosphate (glucose-6-P) to 6-phosphogluconate (6-PG) and for the subsequent production of NADPH and reduced glutathione (GSH) (see Figs. 6-7 and 17-5). GSH protects enzymes and Hb against oxidation by detoxifying hydrogen peroxide and free radicals. Hydrogen peroxide is generated in small amounts during normal red cell metabolism and in larger amounts when an oxidant drug interacts with oxyhemoglobin.

Normal red cells exhibit sufficient G6PD activity to maintain adequate GSH levels. When G6PD is deficient, red cells cannot generate sufficient GSH to detoxify hydrogen peroxide. Hemoglobin is then oxidized to methemoglobin (Hb with iron in the oxidized Fe^{3+} state). Heme is liberated from globin, and globin denatures, forming

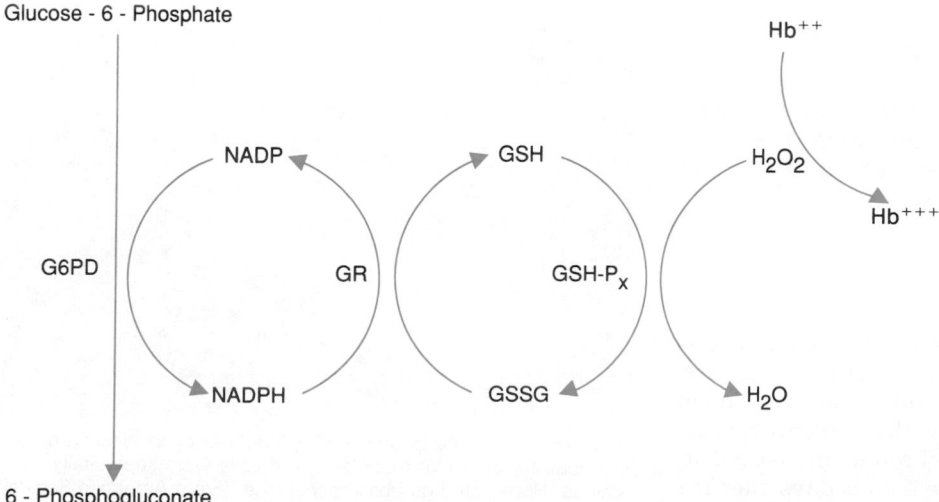

Glucose - 6 - Phosphate

6 - Phosphogluconate

FIGURE 17-5. Pentose phosphate pathway (hexose monophosphate shunt) where glucose-6-phosphate dehydrogenase (G6PD), nicotinamide-adenine dinucleotide phosphate (NADPH), and reduced glutathione (GSH) are necessary to detoxify hydrogen peroxide (H_2O_2) generated in erythrocytes and to keep hemoglobin in a reduced state (Hb^{++}). In G6PD deficiency, inadequate production of NADPH results in accumulation of oxidized glutathione (GSSG) and H_2O_2, oxidation of hemoglobin (Hb^{+++}), Heinz body formation, and hemolysis. GR = glutathione reductase; GSH-Px = glutathione peroxidase.

Heinz bodies. Heinz bodies attach to membrane sulfhydryl groups, inducing cell rigidity. At this point, red cells can no longer traverse the splenic microcirculation and lysis occurs.

Numerous drugs and chemicals are known to induce hemolysis in G6PD-deficient individuals. They include primaquine, phenylhydrazine (has been used to treat polycythemia vera), nitrofurantoin (an antibacterial used to treat urinary tract infections), nalidixic acid (an antimicrobial for gram-negative organisms), sulfanilamide (an antibacterial compound), methylene blue (used to treat methemoglobinemia), and naphthalene (formerly used as an antiseptic in diarrhea of typhoid fever).[5]

CLINICAL PRESENTATION AND PHYSICAL FINDINGS

The clinical features of G6PD deficiency vary, depending on the degree of oxidant stress, the race of the person, and the genetic variant involved. People who inherit the G6PD A− variant are not anemic, and hemolysis occurs more commonly with infections and only intermittently in association with the neonatal period, diabetic acidosis, or exposure to oxidant drugs.

The degree of hemolysis varies from asymptomatic to life-threatening episodes accompanied by abdominal pain, shock, and intravascular hemolysis resulting in hemoglobinuria, jaundice, and pallor. Because G6PD activity declines as cells age, hemolysis in G6PD-deficient black men is limited to older cells. Hemolysis usually subsides as the reticulocyte response increases, even if drug administration or infection persists, since reticulocytes have a nearly normal G6PD content.

With G6PD Mediterranean, G6PD levels are grossly deficient in red cells of *all ages*. Patients with this variant, like those with G6PD A−, commonly experience hemolysis that is initiated by infection. Hemolysis following oxidant stress in association with drugs is more common and more severe than that found in G6PD A−, and it is not self-limited. G6PD Mediterranean is occasionally associated with severe, potentially fatal hemolytic episodes following ingestion of fava beans (favism). Favism is not associated with G6PD A−. Patients with G6PD Mediterranean occasionally require transfusion when hemolysis is severe. G6PD Mediterranean is occasionally associated with hemolytic disease of the newborn.

Some of the rare types of G6PD deficiency are associated with chronic hereditary nonspherocytic hemolytic anemia. The deficiency of enzyme activity may be so great that chronic hemolysis occurs even without exposure to oxidants or stress.[9]

LABORATORY FINDINGS AND CORRELATIONS WITH DISEASE

Routine Hematology. In most cases Hb concentrations are decreased only following episodes of oxidant stress. Acute hemolysis is followed by a sudden decrease in Hb concentration of 3 to 4 g/dL below the reference range.[36] Anemia is normocytic and normochromic, and the reticulocyte count should begin to rise 4 to 5 days after the onset of hemolysis.

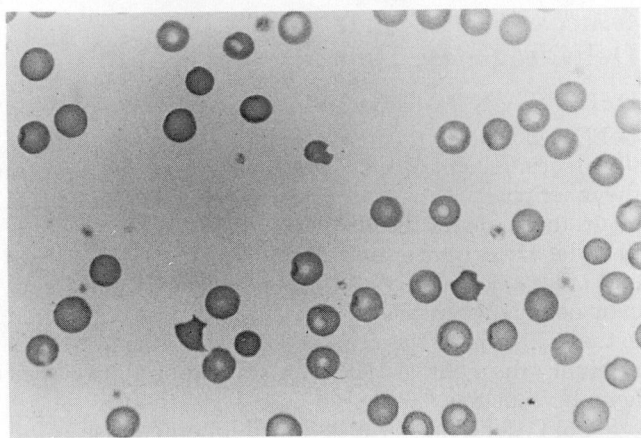

FIGURE 17-6. Bite cells in G6PD deficiency. (From McKenna RW, Hoffman GC, Horwitz CA, Ward PCJ: Laboratory approach to the diagnosis of hemolytic anemias. Workshop manual. Chicago, IL, American Society of Clinical Pathologists, 1984, with permission. Photomicrograph by Patrick CJ Ward.)

Even during hemolytic episodes, morphologic changes are neither striking nor specific. Polychromasia, poikilocytosis, and some spherocytes may be observed. "Bite" cells are often seen during acute hemolytic episodes (Fig. 17-6). The bites in these cells probably represent the recent pitting of Heinz bodies by the spleen (see Special Hematologic Tests following). Bite cells are not diagnostic of G6PD deficiency and occur in acute oxidant hemolysis associated with unstable hemoglobins, in GSH deficiency, and in normal individuals following exposure to oxidizing agents.[32]

Chemistry. Signs of intravascular hemolysis include increased plasma Hb and serum bilirubin levels, a decreased serum haptoglobin level, hemoglobinuria, hemosiderinuria, and increased urinary and fecal urobilinogen.

Special Hematologic Tests. Heinz bodies, which represent denatured Hb, cannot be seen by Romanowsky stains, but they may be observed through the use of a supravital staining procedure (Fig. 17-7; Chap. 14). Patients with

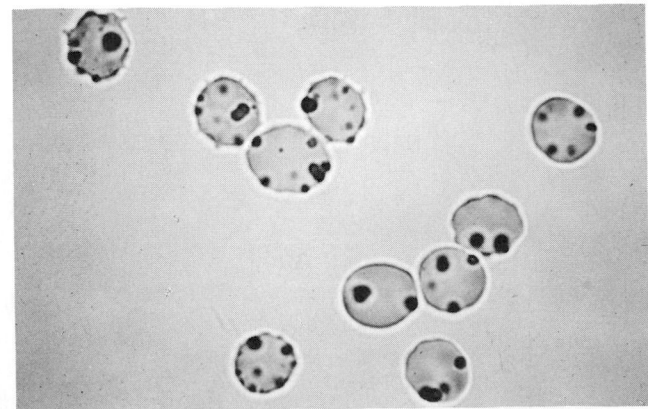

FIGURE 17-7. Heinz bodies in G6PD deficiency as visualized microscopically on a film made after red cells were supravitally stained. Note pitted golf ball appearance. (From American Society of Hematology Slide Bank, 2nd ed. Seattle, ASH, 1977.)

G6PD deficiency develop Heinz bodies in their red cells during hemolytic episodes, although Heinz bodies are not specific for G6PD deficiency.

Results of the direct antiglobulin test are negative, and it is often used to rule out immune-mediated hemolysis.

MOST USEFUL LABORATORY TESTS FOR DIAGNOSING G6PD DEFICIENCY

Table 17-3 lists tests that may assist in the diagnosis of G6PD deficiency. The following discussion includes three screening methods, a quantitative procedure for measuring G6PD enzyme activity, and a summary of the advantages and disadvantages of each. Readers should refer to references provided for exact test procedures.

G6PD Fluorescent Spot Test.
The G6PD fluorescent spot test[3,4,11] (reagents available from Sigma Chemical Company, St. Louis, MO) is the recommended screening test for G6DP deficiency.

PRINCIPLE AND SPECIMEN REQUIREMENTS. The basic reaction, which requires the G6PD enzyme, involves the reduction of NADP to NADPH and the conversion of G6P (glucose-6-phosphate) to 6-PG (6-phosphogluconate) (see Fig. 6-7, *D* and *E*). The reaction is as follows:

$$G6P + \underset{\text{(nonflourescent)}}{NADP} \xrightarrow{G6PD} \underset{\text{(flourescent)}}{NADPH} + 6PG$$

Blood is added to reagent, and after brief incubation, the mixture is spotted on filter paper at timed intervals (*e.g.*, 0, 5, and 10 mintues). After allowing the spots to dry for 10 to 15 minutes, they are observed in a dark room for fluorescence of NADPH under long-wave ultraviolet light. Blood with a normal G6PD level shows fluorescence. Whole blood anticoagulated with EDTA, heparin, or ACD is required. Red cell hemolysates are prepared for analysis.

QUALITY CONTROL. A normal control specimen should be run along with the patient's sample for comparison purposes to ensure that the test system is working properly. Normal saline may be used to simulate a negative control. Fluorescence should not be observed in the negative control.

INTERPRETATION OF RESULTS. Normal G6PD activity should cause strong fluorescence (similar to that from the normal control) within 10 minutes. A partial deficiency causes fluorescence only half as strong as that from the normal control. With severe deficiency, no fluorescence is observed (similar to the negative control).

COMMENTS AND SOURCES OF ERROR. Spots must be dry before examining with ultraviolet light. Wet spots will quench (decrease) fluorescence and could cause a false-positive (*i.e.,* G6PD-deficient) result. Hemoglobin can also quench fluorescence; therefore, if a patient's hematocrit (Hct) is greater than 0.50 L/L, half the usual amount of specimen should be used; on the other hand, if the Hct is less than 0.20 L/L, the amount of specimen should be doubled.

Use of outdated reagents may cause erroneous results. If abnormal or questionable results are obtained with this test, a quantitative assay for G6PD should be performed for verification (see following).

This test is highly specific, simple to perform, and inexpensive. In heterozygous women, the result may be normal. During acute hemolysis in patients with G6PD deficiency, the fluorescent spot test may be normal because of increased levels of G6PD in reticulocytes and younger red cells; these should be separated by removing the top portion of the erythrocyte population after centrifugation of the sample.[28] Otherwise, it is necessary to delay testing for 2 to 4 months or to utilize a more sensitive method.

In addition, measurement of G6PD activity and other enzymes in red cells can be affected by the presence of leukocytes and platelets which may contain these enzymes in greater concentration. Results are more accurate if the buffy coat is removed before testing or if the blood if filtered through cotton wool to remove the leukocytes.[12,22]

Methemoglobin Reductase Test

PRINCIPLE. This screening test indirectly detects NADPH generation by G6PD.[14,15] In the test, methemoglobin is reduced to hemoglobin by transfer of a hydrogen ion from NADPH to methemoglobin with methylene blue as the facilitator. G6PD-deficient cells lack this ability.

SPECIMEN REQUIREMENTS. Fresh whole blood is required.

COMMENTS AND SOURCES OF ERROR. This test is very sensitive and can detect G6PD deficiency even in the presence of hemolysis.[14] False-positive results occur if blood is stored more than a few hours.[5] A modification of this procedure has been developed for detecting the percentage of affected cells in female heterozygotes.[26]

Ascorbate-Cyanide Test

PRINCIPLE. This test measures the ability of normal cells with G6PD to detoxify hydrogen peroxide.[30] Hb is oxidized to methemoglobin by hydrogen peroxide generated by the interaction of ascorbate and oxyhemoglobin. Cyanide is used in the test system as a catalase inhibitor, since RBC catalase is an enzyme that also detoxifies hydrogen peroxide and would interfere with specific measurement of the glutathione peroxidase system. In the absence of adequate G6PD activity, the reaction mixture develops a brown color owing to methemoglobin formation. The control specimen and normal patient specimens should remain red.

TABLE 17-3
Recommended Laboratory Tests to Assist in Diagnosis of G6PD Deficiency

MOST FREQUENTLY REQUIRED
CBC
Peripheral blood film examination
Reticulocyte count
Erythrocyte enzyme screen
Heinz body stain

OCCASIONALLY REQUIRED
Serum unconjugated (indirect) bilirubin
Serum haptoglobin
Urine hemoglobin
Direct antiglobulin test
Erythrocyte enzyme assay

RARELY REQUIRED
Bone marrow examination
Autohemolysis test

SPECIMEN REQUIREMENTS. EDTA-, heparin- or ACD-anticoagulated blood from the patient and a normal control is required. EDTA is the preferred anticoagulant.

COMMENTS AND SOURCES OF ERROR. This screening test is very sensitive and easy to perform. It will detect G6PD deficiency even in heterozygous women and in black men during hemolytic episodes (when G6PD is elevated because of reticulocytes). However, it is nonspecific, and the result may be positive in pyruvate kinase deficiency, paroxysmal nocturnal hemoglobinuria, and in people who have unstable hemoglobins.[24]

Quantitative G6PD Assay

PRINCIPLE. The assay[4,11] (reagents available from Sigma Chemical Company, St. Louis, MO) is identical in principle to the fluorescent spot test. However, this test is quantitative for G6PD activity because the exact change in absorbance caused by the reaction, which correlates directly with G6PD activity, is measured spectrophotometrically at 340 nm.

REFERENCE RANGE. The reference range for G6PD activity is dependent on the method used. It is usually reported in units (U) per gram of Hb. Individuals with the G6PD A− variant show 10% to 60% of normal enzyme activity, whereas those with G6PD Mediterranean and chronic nonspherocytic hemolytic anemia have less than 10% of normal activity.[36]

COMMENTS AND SOURCES OF ERROR. Results may be normal in heterozygotes and black men during hemolytic episodes. Attention must be paid to leukocyte and reticulocyte removal to prevent falsely elevated results. Again, this can be achieved by centrifugation and removal of the buffy coat and the top quarter (¼) of red cells. Normal donor cell G6PD activity in transfused blood may obscure G6PD deficiency. Tests for G6PD deficiency must, in this case, be delayed 3 to 4 months to allow normal donor cells to be cleared from the circulation.

EFFECTS OF TREATMENT ON LABORATORY RESULTS

There is no specific treatment for hemolysis due to G6PD deficiency. In most cases, it is sufficient to avoid exposure to potential sources of oxidant stress. This includes vigorous treatment of infection and withdrawal of offending medications. Following treatment, the Hb level rises, the appearance of the peripheral blood film returns to normal, and Heinz bodies disappear. In variants that demonstrate chronic nonspherocytic hemolytic anemia, treatment such as exchange transfusion in newborns and transfusion during aplastic crisis may be necessary. Splenectomy generally is not helpful.

HEREDITARY PLASMA CONSTITUENT ABNORMALITIES

In this group of disorders, red cell survival is affected by abnormalities in lipid metabolism. Since there is a passive transfer of lipids between plasma and the red cell membrane, the lipid composition of the red cell membrane depends on the lipid composition of plasma. Therefore, disorders associated with abnormalities in lipid metabolism, including abetalipoproteinemia and lecithin-cholesterol acyltransferase (LCAT) deficiency, may cause red cell membrane defects.

Abetalipoproteinemia

DEFINITION AND GENETICS

Abetalipoproteinemia, also known as hereditary acanthocytosis, is a very rare but serious disorder caused by the absence of apolipoprotein B (Apo B) in the blood. Apo B is a major protein component of all lipoproteins except high density lipoproteins (HDL). Thus the serum levels of Apo B–containing lipoproteins are severely decreased to absent (see Laboratory Findings for details). Inheritance is autosomal recessive. The disease is characterized by acanthocytosis of red cells.

PATHOPHYSIOLOGY

Recent studies have linked the molecular defect in abetalipoproteinemia to a deficiency in microsomal triglyceride transfer protein (MTP). MTP is a necessary component for the assembly and secretion of Apo B–containing lipoproteins from the liver and intestine.[27,51]

The relationship between abnormal plasma lipid content and acanthocyte formation is not well understood. An increase in membrane rigidity appears to be the cause of a slightly increased rate of red cell destruction. Decreased deformability of the acanthocyte membrane results from an increase in sphingomyelin (a rigid layer) over lecithin (a more fluid layer).[18] Red cell membrane cholesterol is normal or only slightly increased, and phospholipid is normal or slightly decreased.

CLINICAL FEATURES AND PHYSICAL FINDINGS

The findings in this disease include malabsorption of fat, retinitis pigmentosa (a degenerative condition of the retina), neurologic damage, mental retardation, and growth failure.

Hemolytic anemia is not a serious problem in abetalipoproteinemia, but complications due to nervous system and gastrointestinal disorders usually lead to early death.

LABORATORY FINDINGS AND CORRELATIONS WITH DISEASE

Routine Hematology. Anemia, when present, is mild, and red cell indices are normal. The reticulocyte percentage is normal or slightly increased.

Red cells are normocytic and normochromic. The most striking feature is the presence of large numbers of acanthocytes with irregular, pointed projections, some of which are long and spindly.

Chemistry. Serum lipids are markedly decreased. Plasma triglyceride levels are decreased, and plasma cholesterol is usually less than 50 mg/dL,[18] which is three to five times lower than the reference range. The Apo B–containing lipoproteins, including low density lipoproteins (LDL), very low density lipoproteins (VLDL), and chylomicrons, are decreased to absent. The expected serum chylomicrons after a fatty meal are not found. Fasting serum contains only high density lipoproteins (HDL) since they do not contain Apo B.

EFFECTS OF TREATMENT ON LABORATORY RESULTS

There is no definitive therapy for abetalipoproteinemia; treatment of hemolysis usually is unnecessary.

Lecithin-Cholesterol Acyltransferase Deficiency

Familial LCAT deficiency is a rare inherited disorder characterized by mild normocytic, normochromic anemia. The disorder has been found only in Scandinavian families. Renal disease and corneal opacities are other features of the disease. Plasma LCAT deficiency leads to a reduction in plasma cholesterol esters and an increase in free cholesterol in the plasma. Prominent target cell formation results from increased red cell membrane cholesterol. Both hemolysis and decreased erythropoiesis have been implicated in the pathogenesis of anemia. The latter may be due to concurrent renal disease.[34]

CHAPTER SUMMARY

Hereditary hemolytic anemias involving red cell membrane and enzyme defects and plasma constituent abnormalities generally are characterized by normocytic, normochromic anemia, which is usually mild. They are also characterized by findings common to extravascular hemolytic processes (*e.g.*, increased unconjugated serum bilirubin).

Red cell membrane structural defects involve either quantitative protein deficiencies or qualitative defects in the protein structures themselves. Hemolysis results from loss of membrane surface area, increased membrane rigidity, and premature destruction by the spleen. Hereditary spherocytosis (HS), the most common disorder of this group, is characterized by microspherocytes on the blood film and an increased osmotic fragility. An increased MCHC is a classic finding almost unique to HS.

Hereditary elliptocytosis (HE) is the second most common red cell membrane disorder, and anemia is present in only 10% to 15% of cases. The blood film characteristically reveals more than 25% elliptocytes. Hereditary pyropoikilocytosis (HPP) is a rare membrane disorder accompanied by severe anemia, extreme poikilocytosis and microcytosis, and red cell thermal sensitivity.

The membrane structural defect in hereditary stomatocytosis may involve altered membrane permeability to cations. Most commonly, target cells are prevalent.

Enzyme deficiencies can occur in the red cell metabolic pathways. The most common are pyruvate kinase (PK) deficiency in the Embden-Meyerhof pathway and glucose-6-phosphate dehydrogenase (G6PD) deficiency in the pentose phosphate pathway. PK deficiency may cause varying degrees of hemolysis. Persistence of test specimen fluorescence in the popular PK spot screening test indicates a PK deficiency. Quantitative PK assays provide a definitive diagnosis. G6PD deficiency is an X-linked disorder that causes abnormal G6PD enzyme variants. Absence of fluorescence in the G6PD fluorescent spot screening test indicates a G6PD deficiency. The methemoglobin reductase test is another very sensitive G6PD screening assay. The quantitative G6PD assay provides a definitive diagnosis.

Plasma constituent abnormalities such as abetalipoproteinemia and LCAT deficiency are rare disorders resulting from abnormalities in lipid metabolism. Acanthocytosis of red cells and decreased serum lipids are found in abetalipoproteinemia, and LCAT deficiency is characterized by prominent target cell formation.

Case Study 17-1

A 13-year-old white boy was in apparent good health until he developed a severe case of influenza. He was seen by his family physician and complained of continued fatigue. Physical examination revealed pallor, mild jaundice, and splenomegaly. He had no previous history of anemia. Mild hyperbilirubinemia in the newborn period required phototherapy. The patient's brother was abnormally jaundiced at birth, but was now in reasonable health. His mother had undergone splenectomy for a hematologic disorder. The complete blood count revealed Hb 5.2 g/dL; Hct 0.19 L/L; RBC 1.8 × 10¹²/L; MCV 78 fL; MCH 28.9 pg; and MCHC 37.0 g/dL. The reticulocyte count was 0.4%. The peripheral blood film revealed numerous microspherocytes and no polychromasia. The result of the direct antiglobulin test was negative and total bilirubin was 1.9 mg/dL (reference range <0.2–1.0 mg/dL).

1. What is indicated by the peripheral blood film and other laboratory data?
2. Combining the laboratory data and the family history, what hereditary disorder is suggested?
3. What specific laboratory test could be recommended and what results are expected?
4. How do you explain the severe anemia and low reticulocyte count when the patient previously had been well?
5. What might family studies reveal?

Case Study 17-2

A 6-year-old black boy was thought to be suffering from an acute hemolytic episode following a viral infection. The patient's older brother suffers from G6PD deficiency. The complete blood count revealed Hb 6.2 g/dL; Hct 0.19 L/L; RBC 2.2 × 10¹²/L; MCV 86 fL; MCH 28.2 pg; and MCHC 33.0 g/dL. The reticulocyte count was 22%. The ascorbate-cyanide test demonstrated early formation of a brown color while the control remained red. The result of the G6PD fluorescent spot test was positive for fluorescence, as was the normal control.

1. Identify and explain the discrepancy in the G6PD screening tests.
2. Identify the possible solution to the discrepancy.
3. Calculate the reticulocyte production index (RPI; Chap 9). Does the indicated bone marrow response seem adequate?
4. What test could be performed to clarify the results of these two discrepant screening tests?

Review Questions

17-1. Which of the following statements concerning the osmotic fragility test is true?

A. Increased osmotic fragility is seen only in hereditary spherocytosis.
B. The presence of target cells can cause an increase in osmotic fragility.
C. Incubating the osmotic fragility test at 37°C for 24 hours can enhance the osmotic fragility in hereditary spherocytosis.
D. Specimens for testing are normally stable for a few days.

For questions 17-2, 17-3, and 17-4 choose from these answers:

A. 1, 3
B. 2, 4
C. 1, 2, and 3
D. 4 only
E. All are correct

17-2. The following results were obtained for an osmotic fragility test on a specimen incubated for 24 hours at 37°C using NaCl dilutions prepared in the laboratory: 100% hemolysis was detected in all of the following NaCl dilutions: 0.00%, 0.10%, 0.20%, 0.30%, 0.40%, and 0.50%. The other dilutions of NaCl and their respective percent hemolysis (%H) were as follows: 0.60% NaCl, 90%H; 0.70% NaCl, 50%H; 0.80% NaCl, 25%H; 0.85% NaCl, 15%H. Which of the following statements about these results is/are true?

1. Hemolysis in normal saline dilution (0.85%) may indicate a possible error in saline concentration.
2. 37°C should not have been used as the incubation temperature.
3. Incubation temperature and pH or bacterial contamination may be sources of error in these results.
4. The test results are valid and indicate increased osmotic fragility.

17-3. A possible source of error in quantitative enzyme assays for G6PD or PK is

1. hemolysate contamination with leukocytes that contain higher G6PD and PK enzyme activity than red cells.
2. recent transfusion which may obscure a G6PD or PK enzyme deficiency.
3. hemolysates containing a high number of reticulocytes that have high G6PD and PK enzyme activity.
4. hemolysate contamination with platelets that have high G6PD and PK enzyme activity.

17-4. Which of the following statements about the ascorbate-cyanide test is/are true?

1. The reaction mixture of enzyme-deficient specimens turns red.
2. The test is specific for G6PD deficiency.
3. The test cannot detect G6PD deficiency in heterozygous women.
4. The test is based on the ability of normal cells to detoxify hydrogen peroxide.

References

1. Agre P, Asimos A, Casella JF et al: Inheritance pattern and clinical response to splenectomy as a reflection of erythrocyte spectrin deficiency in hereditary spherocytosis. N Engl J Med 315:1579, 1986
2. Bessman JD, Gilmer PR, Gardner FH: Improved classification of anemias by MCV and RDW. Am J Clin Pathol 80:322, 1983
3. Beutler E: A series of new screening procedures for pyruvate kinase deficiency, glucose-6-phosphate dehydrogenase deficiency, and glutathione reductase deficiency. Blood 28:553, 1966
4. Beutler E: Red Cell Metabolism: A Manual of Biochemical Methods, 3rd ed. Orlando, Grune and Stratton, 1984
5. Beutler E: Hemolytic Anemia in Disorders of Red Cell Metabolism. New York, Plenum, 1978
6. Beutler E: Red cell enzyme defects as nondiseases and as diseases. Blood 54:1, 1979
7. Beutler E: Glucose-6-phosphate dehydrogenase deficiency. In Stanbury JB, Wyngaarden JB, Fredrickson DS et al (eds): The Metabolic Basis of Inherited Disease, 5th ed, p 1629. New York, McGraw-Hill, 1982
8. Beutler E: Glucose-6-phosphate dehydrogenase deficiency. In Williams WJ, Beutler E, Erslev AJ et al (eds): Hematology, 4th ed, p 591. New York, McGraw-Hill, 1990
9. Beutler E: Glucose-6-phosophate dehydrogenase deficiency. N Engl J Med 324:169, 1991
10. Beutler E: G6PD deficiency. Blood 84:3613, 1994
11. Beutler E, Blume KG, Kaplan JC et al: International Committee for Standardization in Haematology: Recommended methods for red-cell enzyme analysis. Br J Haematol 35:331, 1977
12. Beutler E, Blume KG, Kaplan JC et al: International Committee for Standardization in Haematology: Recommended screening test for glucose-6-phosphate dehydrogenase (G-6-PD) deficiency. Br J Haematol 43:465, 1979
13. Brewer GJ: Inherited erythrocyte metabolic and membrane disorders. Med Clin North Am 64:579, 1980
14. Brewer GJ, Tarlov AR, Alving AS: Methemoglobin reductase test: A new simple in vitro test for identifying primaquine-sensitivity. Bull WHO 22:633, 1960
15. Brewer GJ, Tarlov AR, Alving AS: The methemoglobin reduction test for primaquine type sensitivity of erythrocytes: A simplified procedure for detecting a specific hypersusceptibility to drug hemolysis. JAMA 180:386, 1962
16. Coetzer T, Lawler J, Prchal JT et al: Molecular determinants of clinical expression of hereditary elliptocytosis and pyropoikilocytosis. Blood 70:766, 1987
17. Cooper RA: Hereditary elliptocytosis and related disorders. In Williams WJ, Beutler E, Erslev AJ et al (eds): Hematology, 3rd ed, p 553. New York, McGraw-Hill, 1983
18. Cooper RA, Jandl JH: Acanthocytosis. In Williams WJ, Beutler E, Erslev AJ et al (eds): Hematology, 3rd ed, p 556. New York, McGraw-Hill, 1983
19. Dacie JV, Lewis SM: Practical Hematology, 6th ed. New York, Churchill Livingstone, 1991
20. Danon D: A rapid micromethod for recording red cell osmotic fragility by continuous decrease of salt concentration. J Clin Pathol 16:377, 1963
21. Dern RJ, Weinstein IM, LeRoy GV et al: The hemolytic effect of primaquine. J Lab Clin Med 43:303, 1954; 44:171, 1954
22. Echler G: Determination of glucose-6-phosphate dehydrogenase levels in red cell preparations. Am J Med Tech 49:259, 1983
23. Erslev AJ, Gabuzda TG: Pathophysiology of Blood, 3rd ed. Philadelphia, WB Saunders, 1985
24. Fairbanks VF, Fernandez MN: The identification of metabolic errors associated with hemolytic anemia. JAMA 208:316, 1969
25. Foo LC, Rekhraj V, Chiang GL et al: Ovalocytosis protects against severe malaria parasitemia in Malayan aborigines. Am J Trop Med Hyg 45:271, 1992
26. Gall JC, Brewer GJ, Dern RJ: Studies of glucose-6-phosphate dehydrogenase activity of individual erythrocytes. The methemoglobin elution test for identification of females heterozygous for G6PD deficiency. Am J Hum Genet 17:359, 1965
27. Gregg RE, Wetterau JR: The molecular basis of abetalipoproteinemia. Curr Opin Lipidol 5:81, 1994
28. Herz F, Kaplan E, Scheye ES: Diagnosis of the erythrocyte glucose-6-phosphate dehydrogenase deficiency in the Negro male despite hemolytic crisis. Blood 35:90, 1970
29. Iolascon A, Miraglia del Giudice E, Camascella C: Molecular pathology of inherited erythrocyte membrane disorders: Hereditary spherocytosis and elliptocytosis. Haematologica 77:60, 1992
30. Jacob HS, Jandl JH: A simple visual screening test for glucose-6-phosphate dehydrogenase deficiency employing ascorbate and cyanide. N Engl J Med 274:1162, 1966
31. Jandl JH, Cooper RA: Hereditary spherocytosis. In Williams WJ, Beutler E, Erslev AJ et al (eds): Hematology, 3rd ed, p 547. New York, McGraw-Hill, 1983
32. Keitt AS: Diagnostic strategy in a suspected red cell enzymopathy. Clin Hematol 10:3, 1981
33. Leblond PF, Lyonnais J, Delage J: Erythrocyte populations in pyruvate kinase deficiency anaemia following splenectomy. I. Cell morphology. Br J Haematol 39:55, 1978

34. Lukens JN: Hereditary spherocytosis and other hemolytic anemias associated with abnormalities of the red cell membrane and cytoskeleton. In Lee BR, Bithell TC, Foerster J et al (eds): Wintrobe's Clinical Hematology, 9th ed, p 965. Philadelphia, Lea & Febiger, 1993

35. Lukens JN: Hereditary hemolytic anemias associated with abnormalities of erythrocyte anaerobic glycolysis and nucleotide metabolism. In Lee GR, Bithell TC, Foerster J et al (eds): Wintrobe's Clinical Hematology, 9th ed, p 990. Philadelphia, Lea & Febiger, 1993

36. Lukens JN: Glucose-6-phosphate dehydrogenase deficiency and related deficiencies involving the pentose phosphate pathway and glutathione metabolism. In Lee GR, Bithell TC, Foerster J et al (eds): Wintrobe's Clinical Hematology, 9th ed, p 1006. Philadelphia, Lea & Febiger, 1993

37. Lux SE, Becker PS: Disorders of the red cell membrane skeleton: hereditary spherocytosis and hereditary elliptocytosis. In Scriver CR, Baudet AB, Sly US et al (eds): The Metabolic Basis of Inherited Disease, 6th ed, p 2367. New York, McGraw-Hill, 1989

38. Lux SE, Wolfe LC: Inherited disorders of the red cell membrane skeleton. Pediatr Clin North Am 27:463, 1980

39. McCormick JB: Microcapillary technic for red blood cell osmotic fragility. Am J Clin Pathol 46:392, 1966

40. Mentzer WC, Smith WB, Goldstone J et al: Hereditary stomatocytosis: Membrane and metabolism studies. Blood 46:659, 1975

41. Miale JB: Laboratory Medicine: Hematology, 6th ed. St Louis, CV Mosby, 1982

42. Miraglia del Giudice E, Iolascon A, Pinto L et al: Erythrocyte membrane protein alterations underlying clinical heterogeneity in hereditary spherocytosis. Br J Haematol 88:52, 1994

43. Miwa S: Pyruvate-kinase deficiency and other enzymopathies of the Embden-Meyerhof pathway. Clin Hematol 10:57, 1981

44. Nelson DA: Erythrocytic disorders. In Henry JB (ed): Clinical Diagnosis and Management by Laboratory Methods, 17th ed. Philadelphia, WB Saunders, 1984

45. Nurse GT, Coetzer TL, Palek J: The elliptocytoses, ovalocytosis, and related disorders. Baillieres Clin Haematol 5:187, 1992

46. Palek J, Jarolim P: Clinical expression and laboratory detection of red blood cell membrane protein mutations. Semin Hematol 30:249, 1993

47. Palek J, Lambert S: Genetics of the red cell membrane. Semin Hematol 27:290, 1990

48. Palek J, Lux SE: Red cell membrane skeletal defects in hereditary and acquired hemolytic anemias. Semin Hematol 20:189, 1983

49. Palek J, Sahr KE: Mutations of the red blood cell membrane proteins: From clinical evaluation to detection of the underlying genetic defect. Blood 80:308, 1992

50. Peters LL, Lux SE: Ankyrins: Structure and function in normal cells and hereditary spherocytes. Semin Hematol 30:85, 1993

51. Rader DJ, Brewer HB Jr: Abetalipoproteinemia. New insights into lipoprotein assembly and vitamin E metabolism from a rare genetic disease. JAMA 18:270, 1993

52. Schilling RF: Hereditary spherocytosis: A study of splenectomized persons. Semin Hematol 13:169, 1976

53. Shohet SB, Lux SE: The erythrocyte membrane skeleton: Pathophysiology. Hospital Practice 19:89, 1984

54. Smedley JC, Bellingham AJ: Current problems in haematology 2: Hereditary spherocytosis. Clin Pathol 44:441, 1991

55. Stewart GW: The membrane defect in hereditary stomatocytosis. Baillieres Clin Haematol 6:371, 1993

56. Sullivan DW, Glader BE: Erythrocyte enzyme disorders in children. Pediatr Clin North Am 27:449, 1980

57. Tanaka KR, Paglia DE: Pyruvate kinase deficiency. Semin Hematol 8:367, 1971

58. Tanaka KR, Zerez CR: Red cell enzymopathies of the glycolytic pathway. Semin Hematol 27:165, 1990

59. Taylor ES: Chronic ulcer of the leg associated with congenital hemolytic jaundice. JAMA 112:1574, 1939

60. Torlontano G, Fontana L, DeLaurenzi A et al: Hereditary elliptocytosis. Haematological and metabolic findings. Acta Haematol 48:1, 1972

61. Valentine WN: Hemolytic anemia and inborn errors of metabolism. Blood 54:549, 1979

62. Valentine WN, Tanaka KR, Paglia DE. Pyruvate kinase and other enzyme deficiency disorders of the erythrocyte. In Scriver CR, Baudet AB, Sly US et al (eds): The Metabolic Basis of Inherited Disease, 6th ed, p 2341. New York, McGraw-Hill, 1989

63. Weed RI, Bowdler AJ: Metabolic dependence of the critical hemolytic volume of human erythrocytes: Relationship to osmotic fragility and autohemolysis in hereditary spherocytosis and normal red cells. J Clin Invest 45:1137, 1966

64. Wiley JS, Gill FM: Red cell calcium leak in congenital hemolytic anemia with extreme microcytosis. Blood 47:197, 1976

65. Wiley JS, Ellory JC, Shuman MA et al: Characteristics of the membrane defect in the hereditary stomatocytosis syndrome. Blood 46:337, 1975

66. Wolfe LC, John KM, Falcone JC et al: A genetic defect in the binding of protein 4.1 to spectrin in a kindred with hereditary spherocytosis. N Engl J Med 307:1367, 1982

67. Zarowsky HS, Mohandas N, Speaker CB et al: A congenital haemolytic anaemia with thermal sensitivity of the erythrocyte membrane. Br J Haematol 29:537, 1975

CHAPTER 18

Acquired Nonimmune Anemias of Increased Destruction

Susan J. Leclair

Objectives

1. Define microangiopathic hemolytic anemia (MAHA) and the characteristic poikilocyte associated with it.
2. List two peripheral blood film findings and the expected effects on the reticulocyte count and RDW in association with hemolysis that is being compensated by the bone marrow.
3. List and briefly define the three major presentations of MAHA, identify the general age of the population usually affected by each, and summarize the hematologic and other significant laboratory values associated with each.
4. Identify the disorder associated with MAHA that is characterized by abnormal coagulation and platelet function tests, and list five of the expected abnormalities in these tests.
5. Briefly define hemangioma, malignant hypertension, march hemoglobinuria, and cardiac and large vessel abnormalities; state their relationship to MAHA; and state at least one significant hematologic and one chemical laboratory result for each.
6. Define paroxysmal nocturnal hemoglobinuria (PNH), identify the most common age affected, and summarize its hematologic and other significant laboratory values.

7. State the principle of the sugar water screening test and the Ham's acidified serum test, discuss the interpretation of results for each test, and state at least two sources of error for each.

The erythrocyte, despite its remarkable resilience, can be damaged and destroyed by various conditions that are neither inherited (Chap. 17) nor immune mediated (Chap. 19). This chapter deals with a number of situations in which such a hemolytic event can occur.

MICROANGIOPATHIC HEMOLYTIC ANEMIA

Microangiopathic (*i.e.*, pertaining to a small blood vessel disease) hemolytic anemia (MAHA) is a term used to describe the hemolytic anemia found in disorders in which there is a disturbance of the microvascular environment causing red cell fragmentation and thus hemolytic anemia.[3] These disorders are many and varied, and appear to be associated with changes in the small vessels that are the result of (1) fibrin deposition, an activity that follows vessel injury (Chap. 48); (2) severe systemic hypertension (high blood pressure); or (3) vessel abnormalities.[17]

A general discussion of MAHA will be presented first, followed by specific details about MAHA in several of its associated primary disorders, which are also called fragmentation syndromes. The primary disorders displaying MAHA to be included in this chapter are disseminated intravascular coagulation (DIC); thrombotic thrombocytopenic purpura (TTP); hemolytic uremic syndrome (HUS); and abnormalities of small blood vessel structure such as hemangiomas and those found in malignant hypertension or malignant disease.[1] March hemoglobinuria, the last fragmentation syndrome to be discussed, is rare and interestingly does not show peripheral blood evidence of fragmentation. Table 18-1 presents a comparison of hematologic and other laboratory values associated with the major presentations of MAHA discussed in this chapter and also includes a comparison with paroxysmal nocturnal hemoglobinuria (PNH). PNH is a disorder caused by an acquired intracorpuscular mechanism of RBC injury and is presented later in this chapter. The reader is encouraged to refer to Table 18-1 throughout the reading of this chapter.

TABLE 18-1
*Comparison of Hematologic and Other Laboratory Values Associated
with the Major Presentations of MAHA and PNH*

Disease	Most Common Age Affected	Red Blood Cells	WBC/Platelets	Coagulation/ Platelet Function Tests	Other
Microangiopathic hemolytic anemia (MAHA)	Any age	Anisocytosis; schistocytes; reticulocytosis; NRBCs; polychromasia; RDW ↑	WBC V PLT N/↓	Variable depending on primary disease state	Variable depending on primary disease state
Disseminated intravascular coagulation (DIC)	Any age	See MAHA	WBC V PLT ↓	PT, APTT, TT—prolonged; some coagulation factor levels ↓; FDP ↑; D-dimer ↑; PLT adhesion &/or aggregation may be abnormal	LD-1, LD-3 ↑; haptoglobin ↓. In active hemolysis: plasma Hb ↑; hemoglobinuria
Thrombotic thrombocytopenic purpura (TTP)	Young adults (peak third decade of life)	See MAHA	WBC ↑ PLT ↓	Usually within reference ranges except FDP may be sl ↑	LD ↑; haptoglobin ↓; unconj bili ↑; hemoglobinuria
Hemolytic uremic syndrome (HUS)	Infants and young children	Burr cells and see MAHA	WBC N/↑ PLT N/↓	Usually within reference ranges	Plasma Hb ↑/ ↑ ↑ ↑; haptoglobin ↓; unconj bili N/↑; BUN & creatinine ↑. Urinalysis: protein, WBCs, RBCs, & casts present; hemoglobinuria; hemosiderinuria
Paroxysmal nocturnal hemoglobinuria (PNH)	Third to fifth decades of life	Marked anisocytosis; NRBCs; inadequate reticulocytosis	WBC ↓ PLT N/↓	Usually within reference ranges	LAP ↓; sugar water test +; Ham's test +. In active hemolysis: LD ↑; haptoglobin ↓; unconj bili ↑; hemoglobinuria; hemosiderinuria

↑ = *Increased;* ↑ ↑ ↑ = *markedly increased;* ↓ = *decreased; V = variable; NRBCs = nucleated red blood cells; RDW = red cell distribution width; WBC = white blood cells; PLT = platelets; PT = prothrombin time; APTT = activated partial thromboplastin time; TT = thrombin time; FDP = fibrin(ogen) degradation products; sl = slight; LD = lactate dehydrogenase; unconj bili = unconjugated bilirubin; BUN = blood urea nitrogen; LAP = leukocyte alkaline phosphatase; + = positive; Ham's test = Ham's acidified serum test; N = normal.*

Pathophysiology

Erythrocytes undergo several different types of circulatory stress. Arterial blood pressure, cardiac output, pH, and variations in tonicity (osmotic tension in plasma) are among the more prominent circulatory stresses.[7] The shear force caused by arterial blood pressure is sufficient to fragment red cells that are caught by endothelial projections or have partially penetrated the endothelial cells of the vessel wall.[4] Abnormal deposition of fibrin, atheromas (deposits of yellowish fatty plaque on arterial walls occurring in atherosclerosis), anatomic defects, and malignancy may reduce the vessel lumen diameter, causing a localized increase in blood pressure.[28] The combination of this abnormal increase in the force of the moving cells and the smaller vessel cross-sectional area causes injury and subsequent fragmentation of the red cells.[8] The physical findings in these cases are related to the primary disease, whereas signs and symptoms of fatigue, weakness, pallor, dizziness, and jaundice are related to the degree of anemia.

Laboratory Findings and Correlations with Disease

Peripheral Blood. The peripheral blood picture varies with the primary inciting event and the ability of the patient's bone marrow to compensate for hemolysis. As a result, the anemia may range from nonexistent to severe. Anisocytosis and schistocytes (red cell fragments; Fig. 8-12) are a characteristic finding, regardless of the Hct value. Generally, the number of schistocytes is an indication of the extent of hemolysis.

If hemolysis is active and the bone marrow competent, compensation results in a reticulocytosis, which is seen on the peripheral blood film as anisocytosis with a subpopulation of larger-than-normal cells and polychromasia. The RPI is usually greater than 3 in a hemolytic disorder if the bone marrow is capable of compensating for red cell destruction. If hemolysis is brisk and the marrow is attempting to compensate, nucleated red blood cells (NRBCs) may be seen in the peripheral blood, although not to the extent that they can be found in some hereditary hemoglobinopathies (Chap. 14). Occasionally, microspherocytes may also be observed.

Because of the anisocytosis that may be present, the erythrocyte mean corpuscular volume (MCV) represents the average of larger reticulocytes, smaller fragments, spherocytes, and normocytes, which yields an overall MCV in the low to normal range. Bessman and others[2] have developed interpretations of the relationship of MCV, red cell distribution width (RDW; Chap. 10), and the red cell histogram that have led to a more comprehensive analysis of the red cell populations found in these abnormal states. The RDW indicates the degree of actual red cell size variability and is generally increased in MAHA. It is more sensitive than the MCV in the diagnosis of MAHA.

Leukocyte counts vary with the primary disease state, although moderate leukocytosis is not uncommon. Thrombocytopenia may be found, since several disease states associated with MAHA present with a consumption coagulopathy during which platelets and other coagulation factors are consumed at a faster rate than they can be replenished.

Bone Marrow. Examinations of aspirates or biopsy specimens are not diagnostic and typically show erythroid hyperplasia (an increase in the number of normal, maturing RBCs) and occasionally hyperplasia of the megakaryocyte line. If the latter is present, the megakaryocytes may appear to be somewhat immature.

Coagulation. The results of coagulation tests are variable depending on the primary disorder. Coagulation, fibrinolysis, and platelet function tests are generally abnormal in DIC but normal in the other primary disorders discussed in this chapter. Coagulation tests must be performed to determine whether intravascular coagulation has initiated hemolysis. Decreases in several components of the coagulation system, including factors I, V, and XIII (Chap. 48), are common in DIC if the coagulopathy is moderate to severe. If it is mild, tests that reflect actual clotting and clot degradation *in vivo* or tests of the fibrinolytic system are useful for DIC detection. The importance of evaluation of the coagulation system cannot be overemphasized, since it is essential for the determination of the patient's exact diagnosis.

Other Laboratory Findings. Other important findings in many conditions demonstrating MAHA include increased plasma hemoglobin, decreased serum haptoglobin values, and a slight to moderate increase in unconjugated bilirubin (Table 18-1). Urinary findings include occasional hemoglobinuria and hemosiderinuria.

Most Useful Laboratory Tests for Diagnosing Microangiopathic Hemolytic Anemia

Initially, the tests required to assist in the diagnosis include a complete blood count and a microscopic evaluation of the peripheral blood film, including observation of erythrocyte morphology, specifically to evaluate the number of schistocytes (*e.g.*, occasional, few, frequent, many; Chap. 8). Although daily blood counts may monitor hemolysis, generally, daily microscopic observations of the blood film are neither necessary nor helpful unless other complications arise. Bone marrow examination rarely, if ever, is necessary to make the diagnosis.

Effects of Treatment on Laboratory Results

Since this condition is secondary to an underlying disorder, prognosis and treatment are linked to that disorder. Since one of the more common causes of MAHA is preeclampsia/eclampsia (a serious condition occurring in pregnancy associated with hypertension, edema, and/or proteinuria), there are times when treatment may be difficult. Regardless of cause, however, the hemolytic component of the syndrome must be adequately monitored. If appropriate treatment for the underlying cause is effective, anemia should diminish gradually until the erythrocyte count and Hb and Hct values return to normal. The RDW returns to normal as the schistocyte and spherocyte populations decline and the erythrocytes become more uniform. The reticulocyte count should be performed periodically (not daily) to check for bone marrow compensation. Haptoglobin, plasma Hb, and urinary Hb levels are useful for diagnosis but not very useful in follow-up, because they are not particularly good indicators of the degree of hemolysis or marrow compensation.

MAHA in Disseminated Intravascular Coagulation (DIC)

When there is extensive damage to vessel endothelium or exposure to compounds that initiate clotting (*e.g.*, thromboplastic substances such as various proteolytic enzymes or tissue fluid from damaged tissue in burns, injuries, or surgery), DIC may follow.[37] As a direct result of fibrin deposition along and across the vessel lumen, erythrocytes can be fragmented or destroyed as they are pushed through the vessel by the action of blood pressure and rapidly flowing circulation (Fig. 18-1). DIC with MAHA may occur at any age because it is strictly dependent on the primary disorders that can cause it, which are many. For further discussion of the pathophysiology of this condition, see Chapter 52.

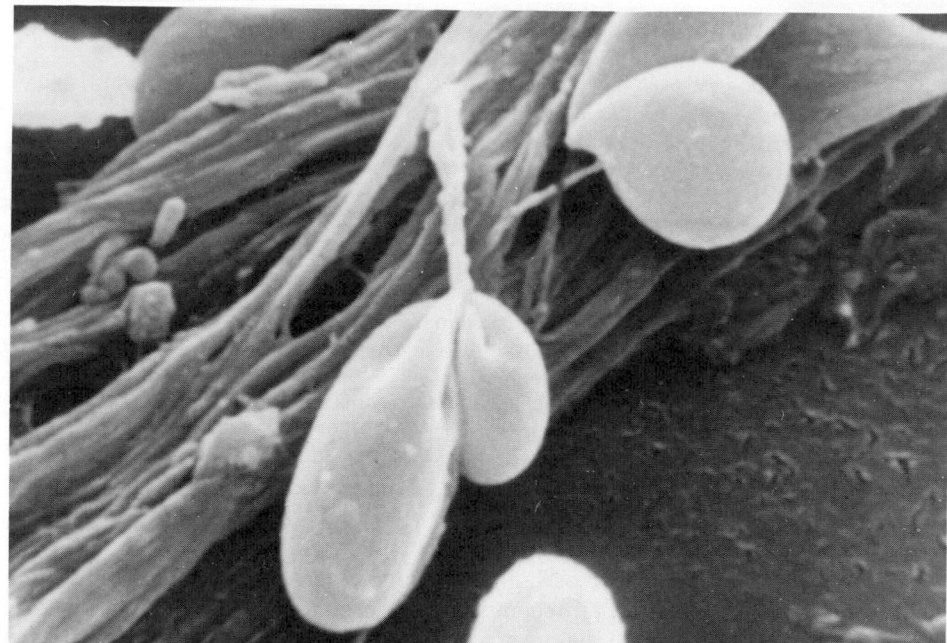

FIGURE 18-1. Classic scanning electron micrograph of the so-called hanged red cell, which helped to clarify the pathogenesis of schistocyte formation in patients with inappropriate fibrin deposition (×5200). Dense fibrin band in background formed from accumulations of finer strands, some of which are still evident. (From Bull BS, Kuhn IN: The production of schistocytes by fibrin strands. Blood 35:104, 1970, with permission.)

LABORATORY FINDINGS AND CORRELATIONS WITH DISEASE

Peripheral Blood. Since DIC can range from mild to severe forms, the peripheral blood findings vary according to the degree of active hemolysis. In acute DIC there are signs of red cell destruction and signs of bone marrow compensation, as described in the general discussion of MAHA. Schistocytes are common but are a relatively insensitive indicator of DIC. Subtle alterations due to compensation are found in erythrocyte numbers and morphology and in the reticulocyte count. The presence of reticulocytes, microspherocytes, and unusually shaped or fragmented erythrocytes affects the MCV. The Hb and Hct levels depend on the extent of hemolysis, the amount of dehydration, and the duration of the coagulopathy.

Thrombocytopenia is an early and consistent finding that is due to platelet consumption by excessive coagulation. The leukocyte count varies depending on the ability of marrow to respond appropriately to the causative agent or event. Granulocytopenia may be a sign of the inability of the marrow to compensate. Other abnormal findings in the leukocytes, particularly in cases of DIC associated with bacterial sepsis, might include toxic granulation, Döhle bodies, and an increase in the number of immature granulocytes (*i.e.,* a shift to the left; Chap. 25).[34]

Bone Marrow. Marrow examination is generally not diagnostic but is rather to ascertain the state of the compensatory mechanism. In most patients with DIC, the marrow reflects erythroid hyperplasia with some megakaryocytic hyperplasia. After prolonged episodes of DIC, the marrow may become "exhausted" and mimic a hypoplastic state in which it becomes hypocellular (Chap. 11).

Coagulation and Fibrinolysis. Table 18-1 provides a summary of the abnormal coagulation and fibrinolysis test results found in DIC. These tests are required to correctly identify acute and chronic DIC. The reader is referred to Chapter 52 for a discussion of DIC and to other chapters on coagulation laboratory procedures in the Hemostasis section of this textbook.

Chemistry. Chemical blood findings are important in chronic DIC because intravascular hemolysis is often undetectable because of adequate compensation by the marrow. In these cases, chemical abnormalities are more helpful than hematologic parameters. Increased levels of serum lactate dehydrogenase (isoenzymes 1 [LD-1] or 3 [LD-3]) and decreased levels of haptoglobin are important findings in suspected chronic DIC and would also be expected in acute DIC. Hemoglobinemia and hemoglobinuria occur during active periods of hemolysis.

EFFECTS OF TREATMENT ON LABORATORY RESULTS

Because DIC is the result of a primary disease state, treatment of the underlying cause must be initiated before any resolution is likely. If treatment is successful, abnormal laboratory findings should return to normal and schistocytes should disappear from the peripheral blood film.

MAHA in Thrombotic Thrombocytopenic Purpura (TTP)

In contrast to DIC, which has no age preference, and to hemolytic uremic syndrome, which is more common in children, TTP is most often seen in young adults (peak incidence is in the third decade of life). TTP is characterized by fever, hemorrhagic signs such as petechiae, neurologic signs such as seizures (and coma in some cases), and renal disease.[26] Hemolytic anemia is a consistent finding. TTP shows striking pathology in the gray matter of the cerebral cortex and medulla of the brain secondary to vascular occlusions. These occlusions show extensive platelet aggregation, leading to excessive platelet consumption. Although many causes have been proposed, those cited most frequently are inappropriate immune response, complications during pregnancy, decrease in prostaglandin formation, and stimulation by oral contraceptives and other drugs.[12,21]

LABORATORY FINDINGS AND CORRELATIONS WITH DISEASE

Peripheral Blood. Typically, the Hb value in TTP is below 10 g/dL. Initial values below 5 g/dL are not uncommon. Reticulocytosis is brisk, and NRBCs are present on the peripheral blood film. Large numbers of schistocytes are characteristic. Significant poikilocytosis includes bizarre and distorted forms. Thrombocytopenia is common; values can be as low as $10 \times 10^9/L$ (Fig. 18-2). Granulocytosis is common, and counts may exceed $20 \times 10^9/L$. Immature granulocytic forms may be present.

Coagulation. In contrast to DIC, the coagulation system and platelet function test results are usually within reference ranges in TTP with a few exceptions.[16] Fibrin degradation products (FDP) are often increased and the platelet release reaction may be deficient.

Bone Marrow. As with DIC, a bone marrow examination is not necessary for the diagnosis of TTP. Typically, however, the marrow shows erythroid hyperplasia, and it may also demonstrate an increase in megakaryocytes.

Chemistry. Intravascular hemolysis is the most likely cause of anemia in TTP, since plasma Hb and unconjugated bilirubin levels are elevated and the haptoglobin level is decreased.

EFFECTS OF TREATMENT ON LABORATORY RESULTS

TTP is a serious, progressive, and rapidly fatal disease unless intervention with correct therapy occurs. Therapy includes the use of platelet inhibitors such as aspirin, dextran, and sulfinpyrazone; plasma exchange transfu-

TABLE 18-2
Conditions Associated with Pregnancy That May Cause a Microangiopathic Hemolytic Anemia

During Pregnancy
  Pre-eclampsia
    Hemolytic anemia with elevated liver enzymes and
      low platelet count (HELLP syndrome)*
  Eclampsia
  Hypertension
  Thrombotic thrombocytopenic purpura (TTP)
  Pyelonephritis
Post partum
  Thrombotic thrombocytopenic purpura (TTP)
  Hemolytic uremic syndrome (HUS)

  * HELLP syndrome is a subset of severe pre-eclampsia.

sion; or high-dose corticosteroids.[20,36] Splenectomy and heparin therapy may be used if the concurrent presence of DIC has been confirmed. Most patients achieve a complete and long-lasting remission. With an effective therapeutic approach, some abnormal values begin to revert toward normal within 48 hours (*e.g.*, platelet counts increase and schistocytes disappear within 2 days).

MAHA in Hemolytic Uremic Syndrome (HUS)

Hemolytic uremia, first described in 1955,[11] is a syndrome of infants and young children that involves acute intravascular hemolysis and renal failure. HUS has also been reported in women during normal pregnancy, particularly in the postpartum period.[31] Table 18-2 provides a summary of some conditions that may occur in pregnancy and cause MAHA.

HUS involves hemolytic anemia of the microangiopathic type and variable amounts of platelet destruction. Although the inciting event is not clearly defined, mild febrile illnesses, certain immunizations, bone marrow transplantation, illicit drug use, and gastrointestinal disturbances have been implicated.[6,18,38] The onset of symptoms usually is acute. Typical signs and symptoms include pallor, increased blood pressure, vomiting, diarrhea, abdominal pain, and dark colored urine. The condition often progresses to either oliguria or anuria (decreased or complete suppression of urinary excretion, respectively). Hepatomegaly is common; splenomegaly is not. Although there are some neurologic signs, such as drowsiness and convulsions, they are neither as frequent nor as severe as those seen in TTP. Skin lesions that are purpuric (patches of purplish discoloration) and ecchymotic (large black and blue marks) may be caused by either a low platelet count, ingestion of aspirin during the initial stages of the illness, or a combination of both.

LABORATORY FINDINGS AND CORRELATIONS WITH DISEASE

Peripheral Blood. The Hb value is severely decreased, sometimes as low as 4 g/dL. The leukocyte count may be elevated with a predominance of neutrophils. Throm-

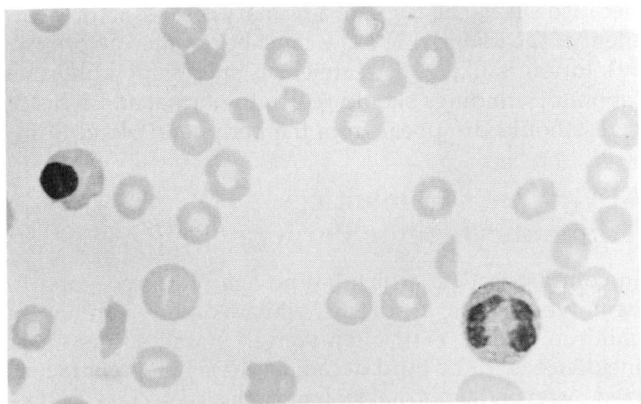

FIGURE 18-2. Peripheral blood from a patient with thrombotic thrombocytopenic purpura shows helmet cells, schistocytes, spherocytes, immature forms (note nucleated erythrocyte), and severe depletion of platelet number. (From Kapff CT, Jandl JH: Blood: Atlas and Sourcebook of Hematology. Boston, Little, Brown, & Co, 1981, with permission.)

bocytopenia, when present, seems to be in proportion to the severity of the anemia. The peripheral blood film shows schistocytes, characteristic burr cells (Fig. 8-8*B*), and when compensation is occurring, moderate to marked polychromasia, indicating a reticulocytosis.

Coagulation. As in TTP, coagulation test results are usually within reference ranges in HUS.

Chemistry. The hemolytic portion of HUS causes a marked elevation of plasma Hb values. In many cases, the plasma appears pink to the unaided eye. Haptoglobin is decreased and methemoglobin is present. Serum bilirubin values may be slightly elevated. The uremic portion of HUS is demonstrated by other findings, such as extreme elevations of blood urea nitrogen (BUN) and serum creatinine. As with most cases of renal failure, urinalysis will reveal many abnormalities (Table 18-1).

EFFECTS OF TREATMENT ON LABORATORY RESULTS

The increase in the recovery rate of children appears to be correlated with the increase in the treatment quality of the renal failure aspect of HUS. Current therapy includes conservative management of fluid, electrolytes, and blood gases together with a precise control of blood pressure.[5] Some more severely affected children may require peritoneal dialysis or hemodialysis. Laboratory values return toward normal after therapy has been established. Presently, therapy for the hemolytic component of the disease is somewhat controversial.

MAHA in Disorders with Abnormal Small Blood Vessel Structure

Hemangiomas (benign tumors of the blood vessels) and malignant hypertension both cause abnormal small blood vessel structures that are associated with MAHA. Hemangiomas are found most often in the skin and liver. The proposed explanation for the hemolytic process is that local coagulation initiated by the presence of an abnormal vessel structure causes red cell fragmentation.

Malignant hypertension is a rapidly progressive form of high blood pressure associated with severe vascular damage.[24] This damage may cause a MAHA. Uremic changes in the form of peripheral blood burr cells may be noted (Fig. 18-3) in this condition.

A number of patients suffering from malignant disease have also been observed to have acute hemolytic episodes that are considered to be MAHAs. In most of the cases studied, hemolysis appears to have been initiated by localized coagulation caused by the presence of abnormal vessel endothelium or tumor production of mucin.[33] Patients with carcinoma of the stomach, breast, or lung are more likely to have vessel abnormalities than those with other forms of carcinoma. Again, as with most MAHAs, the erythrocyte fragmentation usually results from shearing of the cells as they are caught on fibrin strands produced in the coagulation process.

LABORATORY FINDINGS AND CORRELATIONS WITH DISEASE

Peripheral Blood. With hemangiomatous lesions, the hemolysis is chronic and mild, whereas with malignant hypertension the process is more acute. The Hb may drop abruptly to about 10 g/dL or less. Thrombocytopenia is present. Evaluation of leukocytes and any immature red cells in the peripheral blood is difficult because it must take into account the possibility of an underlying disease process, which could be myelophthisis (replacement of the bone marrow) in the case of disseminated malignancy.

Coagulation. Some patients have a consumptive coagulopathy, demonstrable by abnormal results of coagulation studies.

Chemistry. Hemolysis is confirmed by the presence of elevated indirect (unconjugated) bilirubin levels, elevated LD-1 and LD-2 isoenzymes, and decreased haptoglobin levels.

EFFECTS OF TREATMENT ON LABORATORY RESULTS

Standard treatment of hemangiomas involves irradiation of the tumor site or surgical removal if possible, either of which should end red cell fragmentation. There is no standard therapy for MAHA in patients with carcinoma and usually their prognosis is poor, with survival around 1 to 2 months. In cases of hypertension, treatment with appropriate drug intervention should be sufficient to end erythrocyte fragmentation; however, treatment should include an appreciation of the possibility that antihypertensive agents such as α-methyldopa (Chap. 19) can initiate autoimmune hemolytic anemia.[29]

Stress or March Hemoglobinuria

A rare form of hemolysis occurs in susceptible people (usually young adults) who engage in extremely stressful exercise, typically involving forceful contact of some or all of the body with a hard surface. It is believed that the

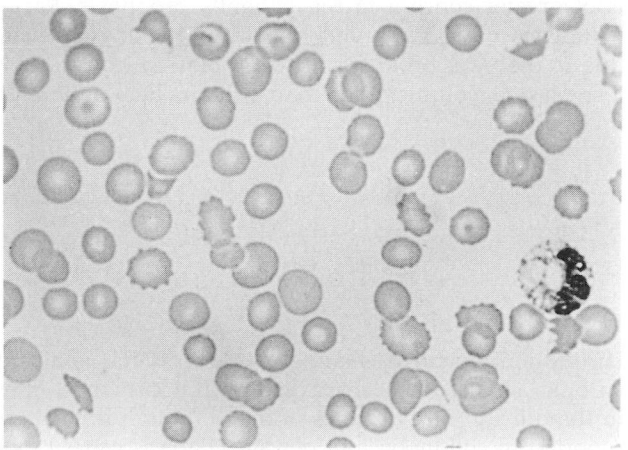

FIGURE 18-3. The peripheral blood picture of a patient suffering from malignant hypertension shows both fragmentation and burr cells, indicating uremic changes. Note vacuolated, nearly destroyed appearance of granulocyte, which has almost no granules. (From Kapff CT, Jandl JH: Blood: Atlas and Sourcebook of Hematology. Boston, Little, Brown, & Co, 1981, with permission.)

activity causes mechanical injury to erythrocytes, although schistocytes are not usually seen on the blood film. This transient hemolysis has been seen in soldiers after prolonged forced marches and in competitive long-distance runners. Complaints include passage of red or dark urine, which usually lasts for only a few hours after exercise.

The peripheral blood may show polychromatophilia after recurrent episodes of hemolysis. Schistocytes are *not* a common finding.

CARDIAC AND LARGE VESSEL ABNORMALITIES

Not uncommonly, patients who have aortic valvular disease such as aortic stenosis or a cardiovascular prosthesis develop a form of red cell fragmentation.[35] Several mechanisms have been proposed for this hemolysis, including direct mechanical injury, abnormal turbulence, fibrin deposition, and autoimmune antibody formation.

The peripheral blood in this anemia has no distinctive features. Patients have signs and symptoms that relate to the red cell damage. Normal erythropoietic response to the hemolysis may compensate for the anemia. If hemolysis is compensated, the peripheral blood numbers and picture (except for reticulocytosis) may be normal. Patients who usually have an MCV in the high normal range may have macrocytic cells in association with a reticulocytosis. If hemolysis is significant, the peripheral blood picture and other laboratory findings are similar to those of a microangiopathic hemolytic process (Fig. 18-4). The rise in plasma bilirubin, especially the unconjugated fraction, parallels the severity of the hemolysis.

If the hemolysis is severe enough to suggest the necessity for surgical intervention, replacement or repair of the anatomic lesion, whether valve, patch, or rupture, must be considered. Until that decision is made, bed rest and other palliative therapy are recommended. Only after the cause is corrected will hemolysis diminish.

MISCELLANEOUS EXTRACORPUSCULAR MECHANISMS OF INJURY

Infections and Infestations

Hemolysis can occur as a complication of exposure to a variety of infectious agents. Malaria, caused by any of the four species (*Plasmodium vivax*, *P. malariae*, *P. falciparum*, *P. ovale*; Chap. 8), results in a hemolytic process initiated by the direct invasion of erythrocytes by the parasite. Anemia may be mild to severe and persists for some time after successful treatment of the infestation.[40] Infection with *Toxoplasma gondii*, occasionally contracted from domestic cats, has been associated with hemolytic events in children and adults.[25]

Hemolytic episodes have also been associated with infections of various species of *Clostridium*, *Staphylococcus*, and *Streptococcus*, and many gram-negative bacilli.[27] The mechanisms of these episodes are unclear, but they may be secondary to the activation of so-called T antigens on the red cell surface.

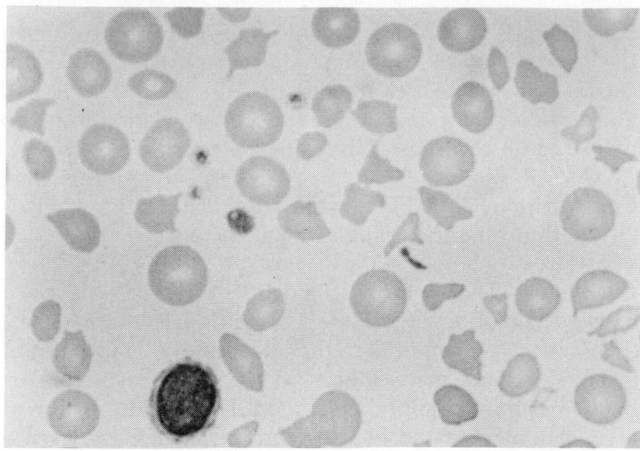

FIGURE 18-4. A typical representation of the mechanical injury that may be induced by prosthetic valves or great vessel abnormalities. (From Kapff CT, Jandl JH: Blood: Atlas and Sourcebook of Hematology. Boston, Little, Brown, & Co, 1981, with permission.)

Exposure to Chemicals and Toxins

Hemolytic anemias also have been reported as complications of spider bites, bee stings, snake venom, and arsine poisoning. Again, the mechanisms are unclear. A well known complication of hemodialysis has been the onset of a hemolytic event. Probable causes of this include oxidizing compounds used to purify water supplies or contaminants in the water.

Thermal Injury

Because mature erythrocytes are extremely fragile and sensitive to changes in osmotic pressure and mechanical injury, exposure to elevated temperatures caused by burns results in fragmentation and membrane loss. Thus, schistocytes and microspherocytes are found on the peripheral blood film immediately after a burn (see Fig. 8-15). Hemoglobinemia and hemoglobinuria are common the first day after a thermal injury. The morphologic damage seen in burn victims is self-limited and eventually resolves. The renal aspect of the hemolysis (Chap. 16) is of greater concern in the patient's prognosis. Rarely hemolysis may occur several days after the thermal event due to the infusion of fresh frozen plasma (to replenish lost plasma volume) that may contain hemolytic antibodies.

ACQUIRED INTRACORPUSCULAR MECHANISMS OF INJURY

Paroxysmal Nocturnal Hemoglobinuria

PATHOPHYSIOLOGY

Paroxysmal nocturnal hemoglobinuria (PNH) is a rare, chronic, acquired hemolytic disease. It occurs most often in the third to fifth decades of life, although it has been reported in childhood and old age. PNH is caused by a defect of insidious (gradual and subtle) onset, which arises from a mutation in a single bone marrow precursor that results in an abnormal clone of bone marrow stem cells affecting erythrocytes, leukocytes and platelets.

Many different biochemical and membrane abnormalities have been demonstrated in the cells of patients with PNH. Recent evidence suggests that the defect in PNH involves the inability to produce the first enzyme necessary for the synthesis of glycosylphosphatidylinositol (GPI) anchor.[23,41,42] The GPI anchor is required for linkage or "anchoring" of some proteins (*e.g.*, decay accelerating factor [DAF], glycophorin A, and acetylcholinesterase [AChE]) to cell membranes. These proteins and others requiring the GPI anchor for membrane linkage are either absent or found in greatly reduced numbers on PNH cells. DAF protects normal erythrocytes from complement attack[19]; therefore its deficiency is probably one factor in the hemolysis seen in PNH.

All erythrocytes, granulocytes, and platelets from the PNH clone possess an abnormal sensitivity to complement (Chap. 19) causing patients to experience hemolysis and also causing increased lysis of PNH granulocytes and platelets. The abnormal sensitivity of PNH erythrocytes to complement can be demonstrated in the laboratory by exposing them to acidified plasma or a low ionic strength environment, which results in complement-mediated lysis (see Most Useful Laboratory Tests for Diagnosing PNH following).

In the erythrocyte line, cells appear to demonstrate three different types of complement sensitivity. PNH I erythrocytes react normally in the presence of complement, whereas PNH II cells are three to five times more susceptible to lysis. The PNH III cell population reacts most strongly on average, with 15 to 25 times more susceptibility to lysis. Patients generally appear to have a mixture of two of the cell subcategories, the combination of PNH I and PNH III being most common.

Patients with PNH may exhibit chronic extravascular hemolysis and hemoglobinuria which occur chiefly at night, when blood pH falls (acidifies) slightly. Exercise, which also causes a slight reduction in blood pH, has been associated with hemolysis in these patients, but the association of acid pH with hemolysis is still unclear.

CLINICAL SIGNS AND SYMPTOMS

The clinical signs and symptoms are wide ranging, since the abnormal cell populations vary and thus the degree of hemolysis varies. The hemolysis may be asymptomatic, or rarely, very severe. Hemoglobinuria is only found in about one quarter of the patients with PNH. Typically, patients present with weakness, slight jaundice, abdominal pain of unknown origin, and splenomegaly. Hepatomegaly is unusual.

LABORATORY FINDINGS
AND CORRELATIONS WITH DISEASE

Peripheral Blood. The hematologic findings are variable in severity and presentation. The Hb level may drop below 6 g/dL.[9] Red cells can vary from macrocytic, normochromic to microcytic, hypochromic if there is increased urinary iron loss. The typical finding is one of unusually severe anisocytosis relative to the level of anemia present. Relative reticulocytosis does occur but it is usually inadequate for true compensation. NRBCs may be found in the peripheral blood. Leukopenia is common,

with neutropenia and relative lymphocytosis. There is some speculation that neutropenia may be the result of a shift from the circulating pool to the marginating granulocyte pool (Chap. 22). Thrombocytopenia does occur, but the platelet life span appears to be normal.

Bone Marrow. Marrow examination is not necessary for diagnosis. Most commonly, the marrow demonstrates normoblastic hyperplasia with some decrease in the megakaryocyte number. One complication of PNH is the progression of the disease into aplastic anemia, in which case marrow examination is valuable for demonstrating the replacement of normally cellular areas with fat, which results in pancytopenia.[30] Another complication is the progression of PNH to acute myelogenous leukemia.[15,22]

Chemistry. Some biochemical defects have been noted in the granulocytes and erythrocytes. Decreased leukocyte alkaline phosphatase (LAP; Chap. 29) has been found in PNH neutrophils. Acetylcholinesterase (AChE) enzyme activity is decreased in both PNH erythrocytes and granulocytes. It is probable that like the erythrocytes, there are two or more populations of leukocytes, one with normal enzyme content and one with decreased enzyme content.[10]

MOST USEFUL LABORATORY TESTS
FOR DIAGNOSING PNH

The diagnosis of PNH is based on two tests that amplify the PNH erythrocyte's abnormal sensitivity to complement (*i.e.*, the membrane-puncturing capability of activated complement; Chap. 19). These tests include the so-called sugar water screening test[13,14] and the more specific Ham's acidified serum test.

Because PNH erythrocytes are more sensitive to complement than their normal counterparts, they readily undergo hemolysis in these tests. The phenomenon occurs in the absence of any antibody.

Sugar Water Screening Test

PRINCIPLE. Whole blood is incubated in a low ionic strength solution which promotes binding of complement components, particularly C3 (Chap. 19) to the erythrocyte surface.[13,14] This environment strains the ability of erythrocytes to remain intact. Normal erythrocytes do not hemolyze under these conditions, but erythrocytes from patients with PNH, which are extremely sensitive to complement-mediated lysis, do hemolyze.

SPECIMEN. Venous blood is collected by mixing 9 parts whole blood with one part 0.109M sodium citrate (or 0.1M sodium oxalate). A normal specimen should be drawn in the same manner for use as a control.

REAGENTS. To make sugar water solution, add 9 to 10 g commercial granulated sugar to 100 mL of distilled water. The pH should be 7.4 ± 0.1. Prepare fresh.

QUALITY CONTROL. A fresh normal control sample should be tested as a negative control along with the patient sample. Before the test is performed, a small amount of the normal sample and the patient's sample should be centrifuged and the plasma checked for hemolysis due to traumatic venipuncture, which would cause a false-positive test result. Hemolyzed specimens cannot be used for testing.

PROCEDURE

1. Pipette 4.5 mL sugar water solution into each of two 13 × 100-mm test tubes; label one *Control* and one *Patient*.
2. Add 0.5 mL well-mixed control and 0.5 mL patient whole blood to respective tubes. Cover with Parafilm and invert both tubes gently to mix.
3. Incubate both tubes at room temperature for 30 minutes. Then centrifuge tubes at 1200 to 1500 × *g* for 5 minutes to sediment red cells.
4. Observe supernatant for hemolysis.

INTERPRETATION OF RESULTS. If a patient's supernatant shows hemolysis, the result is positive and indicates the possibility of PNH as well as other hemolytic states. A normal control sample must yield a negative result, otherwise the test is invalid and should be repeated.

COMMENTS AND SOURCES OF ERROR

1. If result is negative, no further testing is necessary because this test is quite sensitive for PNH.
2. The sugar water screening test is not very specific (*i.e.*, a positive result does not necessarily indicate PNH). Therefore, if the result is positive, it must be confirmed by performing Ham's acidified-serum test (see following).
3. Blood for this test should not be collected in heparin or EDTA, nor should defibrinated specimens be used, because all of these types of specimens may cause erroneous results.
4. False-negative results may be due to (A) lack of complement in the plasma or serum (it is therefore imperative to use fresh samples to ensure complement activity); (B) use of sugar water solution at the wrong pH (pH should be 7.4 ± 0.1); or (C) recent massive transfusion of the patient with normal erythrocytes.
5. False-positive results may be due to (A) traumatic venipuncture during which the specimen was hemolyzed; (B) a severely anemic specimen; or (C) a specimen from a patient with an immune hemolytic anemia, although hemolysis in this case is usually much less prominent than in PNH.

Ham Acidified Serum Test

PRINCIPLE. Erythrocytes in PNH are abnormally sensitive to complement-mediated lysis in acidified serum. Several combinations of patient and normal serum and cells are mixed and some are acidified to maximize the hemolytic effect associated with PNH.

SPECIMEN. A defibrinated whole blood sample is required from the patient and a normal ABO-compatible control sample is also required. The control specimen may be defibrinated or allowed to clot in a test tube at room temperature. Patient samples, however, should be defibrinated and processed in the following manner, since PNH red cells are especially susceptible to lysis:

1. Place 10 glass beads in a small Erlenmeyer flask. Using a syringe, collect a 10-mL blood sample and immediately place in the prepared flask allowing blood to flow gently down the side of the flask.
2. Gently rotate the flask until the noise of the beads on the glass is no longer heard. This takes about 10 minutes. The fibrin will collect on the beads leaving a mixture of free serum and red cells for testing, which must be decanted to a centrifuge tube.
3. Centrifuge patient and control sample at 1500 × g for 5 minutes and separate serum and cells.
4. Heat inactivate a small amount of the control serum at 56°C for 30 minutes to destroy complement.

PROCEDURE

1. Set up eight 12 × 75-mm tubes, as shown in Table 18-3. Serum is added in 0.5-mL quantities; cells and 0.2 N hydrochloric (HCl) acid are added in 0.05-mL quantities.
2. Mix and incubate for 60 minutes at 37°C.
3. Centrifuge at 800 × g for 2 minutes and observe each supernatant for hemolysis. If hemolysis is observed, procedures are described in other textbooks of hematology for quantitation of percent hemolysis.

TABLE 18-3
Ham's Acidified Serum Test*

Constituents	Test Tube No.							
	1	*2*	*3*	*4*	*5*	*6*	*7*	*8*
Control fresh serum	X	X			X	X		
Patient fresh serum			X					X
Control heat-inactivated serum				X			X	
Patient erythrocytes	X	X	X	X				X
Control erythrocytes					X	X	X	
HC1, 0.2N		X	X	X		X	X	
	Lysis Patterns							
Lysis pattern in PNH	− / TRACE	+ / + + +	+	−	−	−	−	− / TRACE
Lysis pattern in hereditary spherocytosis	−	+	+	+	−	−	−	−
Normal specimen	−	−	−	−	−	−	−	−

* Mixtures of control and patient specimen with heat-inactivated serum and 0.2 N HCl for the Ham's test. Expected pattern of hemolysis is indicated for PNH and for hereditary spherocytosis. No hemolysis is expected with a normal, ABO-compatible control specimen.
X = Add serum to tube in 0.5-mL quantites, add cells and 0.2 N HCl in 0.05-mL quantities; − = negative; + = slight hemolysis; + + + = marked hemolysis.

QUALITY CONTROL. Several quality control features are built into this test. Note in Table 18-3 that tubes 4 and 7 contain heat-inactivated serum and therefore should not demonstrate lysis, even with cells from PNH patients, since complement is not available (except for patients with hereditary spherocytosis, see Comments). Tubes 5 and 6 should not show lysis because they contain normal serum and cells; the HCl in tube 6 should not cause lysis of normal cells. If any tubes expected not to exhibit hemolysis do show it, the test results are invalid and the test should be repeated, taking care to follow the procedure.

INTERPRETATION. Table 18-3 demonstrates the lysis pattern in PNH when this procedure is followed. Note that tubes 1 and 8 may have a trace of hemolysis or none. Hemolysis is often stronger with patient cells, normal serum, and HCl, than with patient cells, patient serum, and HCl.

The lysis pattern for hereditary spherocytosis (HS) is also shown in Table 18-3. The differential result is in tube 4. Spherocytes will hemolyze in acidified serum without complement; thus if hemolysis occurs in tube 4, HS may be indicated. PNH cells do not hemolyze without complement, so the result in tube 4 will be negative in PNH.

COMMENTS AND SOURCES OF ERROR. False-negative results may occur if fresh serum is not used. Heat inactivation of serum must be complete (*i.e.*, 56°C for 30 minutes) to prevent erroneous results.

In addition to PNH, results of the Ham test may be positive in aplastic anemia, leukemia, and myeloproliferative disorders.[9] It is positive in 60% of cases[39] of the rare type II form of congenital dyserythropoietic anemia known as hereditary erythroblastic multinuclearity with positive acidified-serum test (HEMPAS; Chap. 12). Fortunately, PNH and HEMPAS can be differentiated because in HEMPAS, lysis never occurs with the patient's own acidified serum (tube 3), only with acidified control serum (tube 2). Also, the result of the sugar water screening test is positive in PNH but negative in HEMPAS.

DIFFERENTIAL DIAGNOSIS

The diagnosis of PNH is difficult to make with any one procedure or symptom. Laboratory tests and symptoms must demonstrate idiopathic intravascular hemolysis with or without hemoglobinuria, pancytopenia with or without hypocellularity in the bone marrow, recurrent thrombotic episodes, and unexplained abdominal pain or headache in association with hemolytic episodes. A positive Ham test result is also important for making the diagnosis.

EFFECTS OF TREATMENT ON LABORATORY RESULTS

There is no definitive therapy for PNH except for bone marrow transplantation. Other treatments have been used in various situations including hormone therapy, infusions of washed red cells, oral iron therapy, anticoagulants, and antimicrobials.[32] Management should be conservative and given as needed. Treatment should be based on the degree and frequency of hemolytic episodes. As a result, laboratory values may retain many abnormalities throughout the course of the disease although, in some patients, over time, laboratory values have returned to normal. The median survival is aproximately 10 years. Prognosis is difficult to predict because some patients appear to achieve complete clinical remission; others re-

main in a chronic hemolytic state with an increased possibility of thrombotic events; some progress into more malignant states; and still others enter an aplastic state that leads to hemorrhage and infection, either of which may be fatal.[15,22,30]

ACQUIRED INTRACORPUSCULAR DEFECTS

Some anemias have a hemolytic component that results from defective erythropoiesis and / or the abnormal environment to which the erythrocytes are exposed. These include anemias associated with nutritional deficiencies (*e.g.*, iron [Chap. 13] and folate deficiencies [Chap. 12]), abnormalities in plasma constituents (*e.g.*, Waldenström macroglobulinemia and multiple myeloma [Chap. 39]), severe liver disease, and certain acquired secondary enzymopathies.

CHAPTER SUMMARY

The major causes of acquired extracorpuscular defects (see Table 18-1) associated with microangiopathic (small blood vessel disease) hemolytic anemia (MAHA) include disseminated intravascular coagulation (DIC); thrombotic thrombocytopenic purpura (TTP); hemolytic uremic syndrome (HUS); vessel abnormalities due, for example, to malignant hypertension and hemangiomas; and mechanical injury by forceful bodily contact with a hard surface (march hemoglobinuria).

Acquired extracorpuscular defects may also be associated with cardiac and large vessel abnormalities such as those associated with mechanical injury from a heart valve prosthesis or aortic damage, and miscellaneous other mechanisms of injury (infections, toxins, and heat). Although hemolysis is important as a major complication of acquired extracorpuscular defects, discovering hemolysis is less important than determining the etiology. Proper therapy generally involves correction of the primary disorder rather than direct treatment of the hemolysis. In addition to the complete blood count, laboratory profiles of these patients should include studies of the coagulation system and renal or liver function testing as a way of discriminating among the various primary causes.

Paroxysmal nocturnal hemoglobinuria (PNH) is categorized as an acquired intracorpuscular injury. PNH cells are derived from a mutation in a clone of bone marrow stem cells and are abnormally sensitive to complement. In an acid or low ionic strength environment, PNH cells bind complement, particularly the C3 component, and hemolyze through complement mediation. Differential laboratory diagnosis of PNH is best accomplished using the sugar water screening test and the more specific Ham acidified serum test (see Table 18-3).

Case Study 18-1

A 4-year-old boy complaining of fever, vomiting, and sore throat was seen in the pediatric outpatient clinic. He lived out of state and had been visiting his grandparents for the month. His grandmother gave no pertinent medical history except that he had experienced some kidney trouble in the past year and that his appetite was poor but had gotten worse in the last few days.

The child was pale and listless. He had a temperature of 39°C (normal, 37°C), his throat was red and inflamed with occasional white patches, and his cervical lymph nodes were palpable, all indicative of an infection. Small ecchymoses (blue-black hemorrhagic areas on the skin) were present on his thigh and upper arms and his mucous membranes were pale, both indicating some type of bleeding problem. The child was unable to produce a urine specimen.

The CBC results were WBC 11.0 × 10⁹/L; RBC 3.41 × 10¹²/L; Hb 9.0 g/dL; Hct 0.30 L/L; MCV 88 fL; MCH 26.3 pg; MCHC 30.0 g/dL; and platelets 125 × 10⁹/L. The differential count revealed 64% neutrophils, 2% bands, 27% lymphocytes, 3% monocytes, and 4% eosinophils. RBC morphology showed some cells were normocytic and some microcytic with slight hypochromia. There was moderate poikilocytosis, with few schistocytes and moderate burr cells.

1. For a 4-year-old boy, are the CBC and differential results normal (refer to Tables 9-1 and 24-3)?
2. How could the variability in the red cell morphology be explained?
3. Are the poikilocytes significant in this case; why or why not?
4. Which of the MAHAs is particularly associated with the finding of burr cells? Is it usually found in young children?
5. For the MAHA identified in question 3, are there any significant urinalysis or chemistry results? If so, list the tests and their expected findings.
6. What is the expected result of coagulation and platelet function tests in this MAHA? Would you recommend that any be done?
7. Assuming that the diagnosis of this MAHA is correct, what is the prognosis for this child?
8. A throat culture taken at the time of his presentation grew β-hemolytic *Streptococcus pyogenes*. Does this result have any relation to the child's present condition?

Case Study 18-2

A 28-year-old woman in her 30th week of pregnancy was admitted to the emergency room with a spontaneous abortion and vaginal bleeding. Recent history suggested pre-eclampsia as a possible cause. The admission CBC results were WBC 22.0 × 10⁹/L; RBC 2.81 × 10¹²/L; Hb 9.0 g/dL; Hct 0.30 L/L; MCV 94.6 fL; MCH 31.3 pg; MCHC 33.0 g/dL; and platelets 142 × 10⁹/L. The differential count revealed 89% neutrophils, 2% bands, and 9% lymphocytes. RBC morphology showed a normocytic, normochromic presentation with schistocytes and burr cells. Chemistry values of interest included a blood urea nitrogen of 90 mg/dL and elevated alanine aminotransferase (ALT), an enzyme that is found in high amounts in the liver and kidney. ALT is occasionally elevated in pre-eclampsia, particularly in severe cases causing the syndrome known as hemolytic anemia with elevated liver enzymes and low platelet count (HELLP).

1. Are problems such as pre-eclampsia in pregnancy known to cause microangiopathic hemolytic anemia (MAHA)?
2. What laboratory result(s) indicates hemolysis in this case?
3. Is there any relationship between the elevated alanine aminotransferase and the suggested diagnosis of pre-eclampsia? Explain briefly.
4. Since TTP is another condition associated with pregnancy that may cause a MAHA, what laboratory value in this case differentiates TTP from HELLP?

Review Questions

18-1. A common peripheral blood finding in ALL microangiopathic hemolytic anemias is

A. many NRBCs.
B. thrombocytopenia.
C. neutrophilia.
D. schistocytes.

18-2. Disseminated intravascular coagulation (DIC) differs from thrombotic thrombocytopenic purpura in that DIC is usually characterized by

A. significant numbers of schistocytes.
B. a brisk reticulocytosis.
C. decreased coagulation factor levels.
D. significant thrombocytopenia.

18-3. The expected laboratory values in a pediatric patient with hemolytic uremic syndrome would include a/an _____ plasma haptoglobin level and a/an _____ blood urea nitrogen level.

A. decreased, increased
B. decreased, decreased
C. increased, increased
D. increased, decreased

18-4. A false-negative sugar water screening test might be caused by

A. use of an ABO-incompatible control.
B. use of a 2-day-old specimen.
C. traumatic patient venipuncture.
D. all of the above.

18-5. When performing a Ham's acidified serum test, the test combination that should demonstrate hemolysis and helps to confirm a diagnosis of paroxysmal nocturnal hemoglobinuria is

A. patient RBC + control heat-inactivated serum + HCl.
B. control RBC + control heat-inactivated serum + HCl.
C. patient RBC + control fresh serum + HCl.
D. control RBC + control fresh serum + HCl.

References

1. Antman KH, Skarin AT, Mayer RJ et al: Microangiopathic hemolytic anemia and cancer: A review. Medicine 58:377, 1979
2. Bessman JD, Gilmer PR, Gardner FH: Improved classification of anemia by MCV and RDW. Am J Clin Pathol 80:332, 1983
3. Brain MC, Dacie JV, Hourihane OB: Microangiopathic haemolytic anaemia: The possible role of vascular lesions in pathogenesis. Br J Haematol 8:358, 1962
4. Bull BS, Kuhn IN: The production of schistocytes by fibrin strands. Blood 35:104, 1970
5. Carvalho ACA: Bleeding in uremia—A clinical challenge. N Engl J Med 308:38, 1983
6. Cleary TG: *Escherichia coli* that cause hemolytic uremic syndrome. Infect Dis Clin North Am 6(1):163, 1992
7. Cokelet GR: Rheology and hemodynamics. Ann Rev Physiol 42:311, 1980
8. Cokelet GR, Meiselman JH, Brooks DE: Erythrocyte Mechanics and Blood Flow, vol 13. New York, Alan R Liss, 1980
9. Conrad ME, Barton JC: The aplastic anemia-paroxysmal nocturnal hemoglobinuria syndrome. Am J Hematol 7:61, 1979
10. Dockter ME, Morrison M: Paroxysmal nocturnal hemoglobinuria erythrocytes are two distinct types: Positive or negative for acetylcholinesterase. Blood 67:540, 1986
11. Gasser WC, Gautier E, Spek A et al: Hamolytisch-uramische Syndrome: Bilaterale Nierenrindennekrosen bei akuten erworbenen hamolytischen Anamien. Schweiz Med Wochenschr 85:905, 1955
12. Gross AS, Thompson FL, Arzubiaga MC et al: Heparin-associated thrombocytopenia and thrombosis (HATT) presenting with livedo reticularis. Int J Dermatol 32(4):276, 1993
13. Hartmann RC, Jenkins DE Jr: The "sugar water" test for paroxysmal nocturnal hemoglobinuria. N Engl J Med 275:155, 1966

14. Hartmann RC, Jenkins DE Jr, Arnold AB: Diagnostic specificity of sucrose hemolysis test for paroxysmal nocturnal hemoglobinuria. Blood 35:462, 1970

15. Hirsch VJ, Neubach PA, Parker DM et al: Paroxysmal nocturnal hemoglobinuria: Termination in acute myelomonocytic leukemia and reappearance after leukemic remission. Arch Intern Med 141:525, 1981

16. Hoffman M, Monroe DM, Roberts HR: Platelet activation in patients with thrombotic thrombocytopenic purpura. Am J Hematol 42(2):182, 1993

17. Jubelirer SJ: Primary pulmonary hypertension. Its association with microangiopathic hemolytic anemia and thrombocytopenia. Arch Intern Med 151(6):1221, 1991

18. Juckett M, Perry EH, Daniels BS, Weisdorf DJ: Hemolytic uremic syndrome following bone marrow transplantation. Bone Marrow Transplant 7(5):405, 1991

19. Kinoshita T, Medof ME, Silber R et al: Distribution of decay-accelerating factor in the peripheral blood of normal individuals and patients with paroxysmal nocturnal hemoglobinuria. J Exp Med 162:75, 1985

20. Kolodziej M: Case report: High-dose intravenous immunoglobulin as therapy for thrombotic thrombocytopenic purpura. Am J Med Sci 305(2):101, 1993

21. Kovacs MS, Soong PY, Chin-Yee IH: Thrombotic thrombocytopenia purpura associated with ticlopidine. Ann Pharmacother 27(9):1060, 1993

22. Krause JR: Paroxysmal nocturnal hemoglobinuria and acute nonlymphocytic leukemia. Cancer 51:2078, 1983

23. Lida Y, Takeda J, Miyata T et al: Characterization of genomic PIG-A gene: A gene for glycosylphosphatidylinositol-anchor biosynthesis and paroxysmal nocturnal hemoglobinuria. Blood 83(11):3126, 1994

24. Linton AL, Gavras H, Cleadle RI et al: Microangiopathic haemolytic anaemia and the pathogenesis of malignant hypertension. Lancet 1:1277, 1969

25. Michelson AD, Lammi AT: Haemolytic anaemia associated with acquired toxoplasmosis. Aust Paediatr 20:333, 1984

26. Moschcowitz E: An acute febrile pleiochromic anemia with hyaline thrombosis of the terminal arterioles and capillaries: An undescribed disease. Arch Intern Med 36:89, 1925

27. Myers KA, Marrie TJ: Thrombotic microangiopathy associated with *Streptococcus pneumoniae* bacteremia: Case report and review. Clin Infect Dis 17(6):1037, 1993

28. Nordstrom B, Strang P: Microangiopathic hemolytic anemias (MAHA) in cancer. A case report and review. Anticancer Res (Greece) 13(5D):1845, 1993

29. Physician's Desk Reference, 49th ed. Oradell, NJ, Medical Economics, 1995

30. Rosse WF: Paroxysmal nocturnal haemoglobinuria in aplastic anaemia. Clin Haematol 7:541, 1978

31. Rozdzinski E, Hertenstein B, Schmeiser T et al: Thrombotic thrombocytopenic purpura in early pregnancy with maternal and fetal survival. Ann Hematol 64(5):245, 1992

32. Saraya AK, Saxena A, Dhot PS et al: Metronidazole: A potential therapeutic agent in paroxysmal nocturnal hemoglobinuria. Am J Hematol 47(2):150, 1994

33. Satoh K, Imai H, Yasuda T et al: Sclerodermatous renal crisis in a patient with mixed connective tissue disease. Am J Kidney Dis 24(2):215, 1994

34. Siegal T, Seligsohn U, Aghai E et al: Clinical and laboratory aspects of disseminated intravascular coagulation (DIC): A study of 118 cases. Thromb Haemostas 39:122, 1978

35. Smith RE, Berg D: Occult paravalular leak in a clinically normal St Jude's mitral valve presenting with life-threatening microangiopathic hemolytic anemia. J Cardiovasc Surg 32(10):56, 1991

36. Snyder HW Jr, Mittelman A, Oral A et al: Treatment of cancer chemotherapy-associated thrombotic thrombocytopenic purpura/hemolytic uremia syndrome by protein A immunoadsorption of plasma. Cancer 71(5): 19982, 1993

37. Spero JA, Lewis JH, Hasiba U: Disseminated intravascular coagulation. Thromb Haemostas 43:28, 1980

38. Tumlin JA, Sands JM, Someren A: Hemolytic-uremic syndrome following "crack" cocaine inhalation. Am J Med Sci 299(6):366, 1990

39. Verwilghen RL, Lewis SM, Dacie JV et al: HEMPAS: Congenital dyserythropoietic anaemia (type II). Q J Med 42:257, 1973

40. Woodruff AW, Ansdell VE, Pettitt LE: Cause of anaemia in malaria. Lancet 1:1055, 1979

41. Yeh ET, Kamitani T, Chang HM: Biosynthesis and processing of the glycosylphosphatidylinositol anchor in mammalian cells. Semin Immunol 6(2):73, 1994

42. Yu J, Magarajan S, Veda E et al: Characterization of alternatively spliced PIG-A transcripts in normal and paroxysmal nocturnal hemoglobinuria cells. Braz J Med Biol Res 27(2):195, 1994

CHAPTER 19

Acquired Immune Anemias of Increased Destruction

Catherine Sherry

Objectives

1. Define acquired immune hemolytic anemia, antigen and antibody.
2. Define complement, C3b, and C5b6789 and briefly explain their hemolytic role in acquired immune hemolytic anemia.
3. Identify and discuss the principal causes of acquired alloimmune and autoimmune hemolytic anemias.
4. Describe hemolytic disease of the newborn (HDN) and list its significant laboratory findings.
5. Define and differentiate the two types of hemolytic transfusion reactions and list their significant laboratory findings.
6. Describe warm and cold antibody autoimmune hemolytic anemia and differentiate warm from cold antibodies.
7. Define paroxysmal cold hemoglobinuria and describe the Donath-Landsteiner antibody.
8. Describe the three mechanisms postulated for drug-induced hemolytic anemia.

In the normal immune system, the presence of a foreign antigen (one not recognized as the body's own) results in the production of a protein called an antibody that is specific for the antigen as a self-defense mechanism.

Immune hemolytic anemia is characterized by accelerated destruction or hemolysis of red cells with foreign antigens by antibodies. The resultant anemia is due to the function, or in some cases malfunction, of the body's immune system.

Alloantibodies develop when a person is exposed to antigens that are found in the same species (*e.g.*, human species), but are not present on the exposed person's cells. In some cases, the normal process that prevents formation of antibodies to the host's own antigens is impaired, and the immune system produces antibodies called *autoantibodies* that react with the host's own cell or tissue antigens.

A third type of antibody is induced in some persons by certain drugs. These antibodies may resemble autoantibodies but they demonstrate several modes of formation and cell destruction, which will be described in this chapter.

The anemias caused by any of these mechanisms are all acquired (*i.e.*, they are never inherited). They are called acquired immune hemolytic anemias and are classified as alloimmune, autoimmune, or drug-induced (Table 19-1). In all of these hemolytic disorders, the bone marrow must increase red cell production to compensate for increased destruction, so an erythroblastic hyperplasia in the marrow may be expected in all cases of adequate response. Bone marrow examination usually is not required to diagnose an acquired immune hemolytic anemia.

HEMOLYSIS IN ACQUIRED IMMUNE HEMOLYTIC ANEMIAS

In the acquired immune hemolytic anemias (AIHA), hemolysis may occur in the vascular system or in the extravascular reticuloendothelial system, depending on the disorder. When hemolysis is caused by an immune mechanism, however, other components are involved in the process.

Role of Complement

The complement system plays an important role in AIHA. It consists of enzymatic proteins that interact to mediate certain effects of the body's inflammatory response to tissue injury or exposure to foreign substances. The com-

TABLE 19-1
Classification of Immune Hemolytic Anemias

ALLOIMMUNE

Hemolytic disease of the newborn (HDN)

Hemolytic transfusion reaction

AUTOIMMUNE

Warm-antibody
  Primary (idiopathic)
  Secondary
    Chronic lymphocytic leukemia (CLL)
    Lymphoma
    Systemic lupus erythematosus
    Viral infections
    Immune deficiency disease

Cold-antibody
  Primary
    Idiopathic cold agglutinin syndrome; Raynaud's phenomenon
  Secondary cold agglutinin syndrome
    Mycoplasma pneumoniae
    Infectious mononucleosis (Epstein-Barr virus)
    Lymphoproliferative disease

Paroxysmal cold hemoglobinuria (PCH)
  Primary (idiopathic)
  Secondary
    Syphilis
    Viral disease
      Mumps, measles, chicken pox, infectious mononucleosis

DRUG-INDUCED

Hapten (drug-adsorption) mechanism

Immune complex (innocent bystander) mechanism
  α-Methyldopa (autoimmune/unknown) mechanism

---

plement system also interacts with the coagulation, fibrinolytic, and kinin systems (Chap. 48).

Two pathways of reaction are involved in the sequential activation of complement components, the classic pathway and the alternate pathway. The classic pathway (Fig. 19-1) is activated when immunoglobulin G (IgG) or IgM antibodies complex with antigens. This pathway, the one associated with autoimmune hemolytic anemias, is defined in some detail in this chapter. The alternate (Properdin) complement pathway is activated by certain cells, particles, or microorganisms without the presence of antibodies. Because the alternate pathway is a nonimmune mechanism of defense against these foreign elements,[27,31] it is beyond the scope of this chapter.

Complement components are symbolized as C1 to C9.[2] The C1 molecule is a unique component with three subunits designated as C1q, C1r, and C1s, all of which are stabilized by the presence of calcium in the molecule. The C1 component is also known as the recognition unit, since it initiates the complement cascade by recognizing IgG or IgM antibodies on cell surfaces (see Fig. 19-1).

Activated components in the fluid phase (*i.e.*, not attached to a cell or particle surface) are designated by a bar over the component number (*e.g.*, $\overline{C4a}$). Activated components bound to cell surfaces do not have such an indicator. When a complement component is activated, complement fragments are produced. These are indicated by lower case letters as suffixes, for example, C2a (see Fig. 19-1).

Extravascular Hemolysis in AIHA

In an immune reaction, cells in circulation may become coated with immunoglobulin (antibodies). Subsequently, the complement system cascade is initiated, leading to generation of an intermediate component known as C3b. C3b is bound to the cell surface, and this attachment generally is associated with extravascular red cell destruction in the liver. Destruction of immunoglobulin and complement-coated cells by liver Kupffer cell macrophages may be attributed to Kupffer cell receptors for the complement component C3b.

The complement system (see Fig. 19-1) is initiated as a result of activation of two antibody-binding sites close to each other on the red cell surface. These two sites may be activated by attachment of a single IgM antibody or, less effectively, by two IgG antibodies. When activated, these sites fix complement, beginning with the C1q component. Generally speaking, activated C1 acts on C4, converting it to an active state. Activated C4 along with C1 converts C2 to an active form. Finally, the combination of activated C4 and C2, termed C4b2a (or C3 convertase), cleaves C3 into C3b and $\overline{C3a}$. C3b remains attached to the red cell membrane and is responsible for hepatic hemolysis. $\overline{C3a}$, however, is released to the plasma, where it acts as an anaphylatoxin, which serves as a mediator of inflammation by inducing mast cell degranulation and histamine release.

COMPLEMENT SYSTEM CONTROL

A serum enzyme called C3b inactivator (see Fig. 19-1) readily cleaves C3b into $\overline{C3c}$ and C3d if membrane interaction or cell destruction does not occur rapidly. C3d, once bound to the red cell membrane, actually prevents cell destruction because it does not bind to macrophage receptor sites; it also appears to prevent the further attachment of C3b to the membrane, thus preventing complement-mediated extra- or intravascular destruction.

C4 inactivator and C1s inhibitor also serve to control and limit complement system activity. In addition, the C4b2a component is unstable, which provides another control mechanism.[27]

Complement-mediated hemolysis is limited by the same components as those associated with extravascular hemolysis. One further regulating component is the instability of the C4b2a3b enzyme complex,[27] also known as C5 convertase (see Fig. 19-1), which is needed for generation of the membrane attack unit.

Intravascular Hemolysis in AIHA

Intravascular hemolysis that is complement mediated involves more complement components than those associated with extravascular hemolysis. As described above, the final component leading to extravascular red cell destruction is generally C3b. However, when the C3b com-

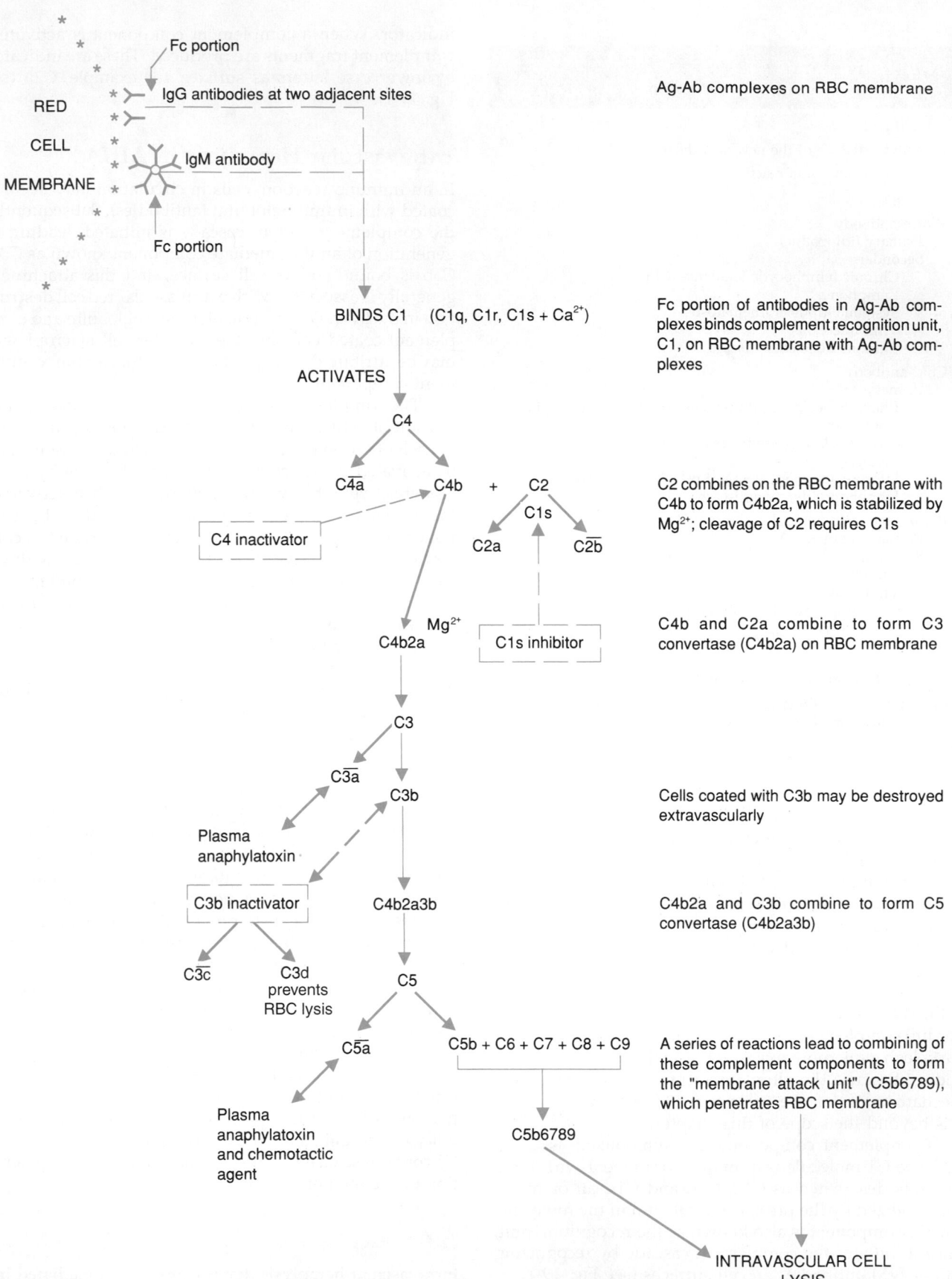

FIGURE 19-1. In the classic complement pathway, either two IgG antibodies or one IgM antibody combines with antigens on the RBC membrane, forming antigen-antibody (Ag-Ab) complexes. The Fc portion of the antibodies may then bind the complement component C1, thus activating the complement cascade. Activated components in the fluid phase which are *not* attached to a cell surface are designated by a bar over the component number. Other components are attached to a cell surface.

ponent is further activated, a series of reactions leads to formation of C5b6789, otherwise known as the membrane attack unit or terminal complex (see Fig. 19-1). This complex is so named because it is capable of penetrating the red cell surface by forming a transmembrane pore. This damage may result in leakage of hemoglobin and other cellular components or osmotic swelling due to excessive permeability to water and electrolytes, both of which result in intravascular hemolysis. One example of this mechanism is found in hemolytic transfusion reactions resulting from ABO incompatibility.

ALLOIMMUNE HEMOLYTIC ANEMIA

Alloantibodies are produced when an individual is exposed to antigens of another individual of the same species that are not already present on the exposed individual's cells. Alloantibodies do not react with the immunized person's own antigens. Alloimmune hemolytic anemias are characterized by the presence of alloantibodies and are most commonly associated with either hemolytic disease of the newborn (HDN) or hemolytic transfusion reactions.

Hemolytic Disease of the Newborn

DEFINITION, HISTORY, AND PATHOPHYSIOLOGY

Hemolytic disease of the newborn (HDN), also known as erythroblastosis fetalis, is an anemia caused by destruction of an infant's red cells when a maternal antibody that is specific to an antigen on the infant's red cells crosses the placenta. Antibodies to Rh, ABO, and Kell antigens, among others, can cause HDN.[33]

In 1940 Landsteiner and Wiener[21] discovered the Rh system of red cell antigens. It was thought that the Rh antigens might account for the observation of maternal antibodies in a newborn with erythroblastosis fetalis reported in 1939 by Levine and Stetson.[24] This was later confirmed by others.[22]

Transplacental passage of small amounts of fetal blood to the mother is relatively common, even during normal pregnancy. The mother's system may be stimulated to produce antibodies by the passage of incompatible fetal red cells. The resulting antibody crosses back into the fetal circulation, and the fetus' red cells are destroyed. The most severe effects of such an event have been associated with Rh incompatibilities, although ABO incompatibilities can produce HDN with milder symptoms.

CLINICAL PRESENTATION, SYMPTOMS, AND PHYSICAL FINDINGS

The affected infant is anemic and jaundiced with hepatosplenomegaly. The degree of jaundice parallels the severity of the anemia. Infants most adversely affected may develop central nervous system deficits, such as bilirubin encephalopathy (brain damage) also known as kernicterus, and as a result, mental retardation. Some infants may be stillborn.

The infant's initially acceptable skin color becomes paler as the anemia increases, and then icteric (yellow) as hemolysis continues. Edema and ascites may occur owing to heart failure. Lethargy and hypotonicity as well as hypoxia due to the severe anemia may occur in more severely affected infants.

LABORATORY FINDINGS AND CORRELATIONS WITH DISEASE

Cord Blood Hematology. Cord blood shows a normal or decreased hemoglobin level (compared to newborn reference ranges), reticulocytosis, and an increased number of nucleated red cells (hence the term *erythroblastosis fetalis*).[1] Red cell macrocytosis and polychromatophilia are prominent due to the increased rate of erythropoiesis in response to antibody-mediated hemolysis.

Chemistry. The bilirubin levels in cord blood may be slightly to significantly elevated, depending on the severity of hemolysis. A progressively increasing plasma bilirubin level seen within 48 to 72 hours after birth indicates the extent of hemolysis as well as the inability of the infant's immature liver enzyme system to conjugate and excrete bilirubin. Hyperbilirubinemia is due to unconjugated bilirubin.

Immunohematology. In HDN due to anti-Rh antibodies, the infant's red cells react positively in the direct antiglobulin test (DAT), previously called the Coombs' test, which detects antibody-coated red cells. In ABO disease, negative or weakly reactive DAT results may be found. This may be due to the small number of A and B antigens on cord blood cells (when compared to adult cells). See standard immunohematology texts for further details.

Prenatal antibody detection tests on the mother's serum (indirect antiglobulin test) and amniotic fluid analysis for bilirubin may predict the onset of HDN in the infant. However, widely varying antibody levels have been observed in women who deliver unaffected babies.[13]

EFFECTS OF TREATMENT ON LABORATORY RESULTS—PROGNOSIS

If the severity of the disease indicates, intrauterine exchange transfusions are performed from about the 26th week of gestation until delivery. This replaces the fetus' antibody-coated red cells with donor cells that do not carry the antigen that the mother's antibody is attacking; however, it carries maternal risks and a high risk of fetal mortality. With this procedure, results of the DAT soon become weak or negative, anemia is corrected, and a significant reduction in plasma bilirubin level is observed. In less severe cases, exchange transfusion may be performed as soon as the infant is born. In mild cases, phototherapy (exposure of the infant to natural sunlight or fluorescent light) reduces bilirubin levels by oxidizing bilirubin to biliverdin and then to colorless bilirubin precursors. Phototherapy is quite effective.

More important, however, is *prevention* of HDN due to anti-Rh antibodies. This is accomplished by passive immunization of Rh-negative mothers (those who have not already developed anti-Rh antibodies during a previous pregnancy or from receiving a transfusion of incompatible Rh-positive blood) by administering anti-Rh antibodies in the form of commercially prepared Rh_o immunoglobulin, also known as Rh_o IgG. This treatment is administered to Rh-negative mothers immediately following amniocentesis, abortion, during the course of prenatal care and after delivery of an Rh-positive baby. Rh_o IgG is administered to prevent the baby's Rh-positive cells from stimulating an immune response that could adversely affect future fetuses. This program has reduced anti-Rh HDN significantly.

Babies born severely affected by anti-Rh antibodies have a 10% to 20% chance of surviving. Infants with mild to moderate disease who are promptly treated have excellent survival rates.[17]

Hemolytic Transfusion Reactions

DEFINITION, HISTORY AND PATHOPHYSIOLOGY

A hemolytic transfusion reaction results from the transfusion of red cells bearing antigens that are foreign to the recipient's immune system. Recognition of hemolytic transfusion reactions followed the discovery of the ABO blood group system by Landsteiner in 1900 and the subsequent identification of other blood group systems such as Rh and Kell.

If antibodies to the antigens introduced by transfusion are already present in a patient's plasma (*e.g.*, ABO antibodies), there is an immediate intravascular destruction of the transfused cells called an *immediate hemolytic transfusion reaction.* However, if the antibodies are not already present in the plasma, they soon develop through a secondary immune response causing a more gradual, less clinically serious extravascular destruction of antibody-sensitized red cells called a *delayed hemolytic transfusion reaction.*

Immediate Hemolytic Transfusion Reactions. If the ABO system is involved, anti-A and anti-B antibodies of the IgM type cause immediate intravascular destruction of the transfused red cells. This occurs through the activation of two antibody-binding sites close to each other on the red cell surface which fix complement and activate the complement cascade (see Fig. 19-1). Thus the membrane attack unit is formed, which causes intravascular hemolysis and the release of hemoglobin and incompatible red cell stroma-antibody complexes to the circulation. The subsequent release of mediators of the inflammatory response, cytokines, contributes to the production of renal and respiratory failure.[5]

Delayed Hemolytic Transfusion Reactions. Sometimes the hemolytic process does not begin for 2 to 14 days. Such reactions are most often associated with IgG antibodies, which are less effective in activating antibody-binding sites and less potent than IgM. When the incompatibility involves recipient IgG antibodies, such as anti-Rh antibodies, which do not bind complement, or Duffy- or Kidd-system antibodies with sublytic complement activation properties (*i.e.*, antibodies that activate complement to a small extent but not to the point of actual cell lysis by generation of the membrane attack unit), extravascular hemolysis may result. This is due to sequestration of the C3b-sensitized, transfused red cells either by the liver Kupffer cells (anti-Duffy or anti-Kidd antibodies) or the spleen (anti-Rh antibodies). Destruction of IgG-coated cells may not be as severe as that associated with IgM- and complement-coated cells.

CLINICAL PRESENTATION, SYMPTOMS, AND PHYSICAL FINDINGS

Initial symptoms of a transfusion reaction are facial flushing, anxiety, nausea, clammy skin, chest pain, and back and leg pain.

Hypotension, fever, and increased respiratory and pulse rates may occur. In serious cases, renal failure and disseminated intravascular coagulation (DIC; Chaps. 18 and 52) may develop.

LABORATORY FINDINGS AND CORRELATIONS WITH DISEASE

By examining the plasma of a carefully drawn blood specimen, hemoglobinemia may be visually observed as a pink color in the plasma, particularly in severe cases involving the ABO system, in which immediate intravascular destruction of the transfused red cells occurs. The positive DAT demonstrates the sensitization or coating of the transfused cells with IgG antibodies such as anti-Rh_o. Hemoglobin (Hb) and urobilinogen in the urine and subsequent hyperbilirubinemia may be observed.

When severe intravascular hemolysis occurs, the Hb and hematocrit (Hct) may not correlate by the usual "rule of three" (Chap. 9). This is because the whole blood Hb measurement includes Hb inside the red cells *and* that which is free in the plasma, whereas the Hct measurement is based only on intact red cells. For example, an affected individual might have a Hb of 9.8 g/dL and a Hct of 0.20 L/L (20%).

Intravascular hemolysis can activate the coagulation system, which results in depletion of fibrinogen, factor VIII, and platelets. This is demonstrated by low levels of these factors in plasma, a prolonged prothrombin time (PT), and a prolonged partial thromboplastin time (PTT). The D-dimer may be found in plasma and this is specific evidence for intravascular coagulation and fibrinolysis (Chap. 50).

EFFECTS OF TREATMENT ON LABORATORY RESULTS—PROGNOSIS

The best treatment is prevention. ABO transfusion reactions are due to human error in blood typing or in clerical aspects of the transfusion. Treatment of an immediate transfusion reaction is usually focused on treating the hypotension and preventing renal failure by infusing a diuretic or a drug that increases renal blood flow. Reversal of abnormal laboratory test findings should occur as the patient's condition improves.

With delayed transfusion reactions, treatment is usually unnecessary. With time, the spherocytes seen on the blood film disappear as the damaged and hemolyzed cells are destroyed in the reticuloendothelial system.

If the amount of incompatible transfused blood is minimal or the antigen-antibody system involved has a weak reactivity, the prognosis is favorable with treatment.

AUTOIMMUNE HEMOLYTIC ANEMIA

The autoimmune hemolytic anemias (AIHA) include warm-antibody AIHA, cold-antibody AIHA (cold agglutinin syndrome), and paroxysmal cold hemoglobinuria (PCH) (see Table 19-1).

In these disorders, the normal mechanism that prevents formation of antibodies to the host's own antigens is flawed, and the immune system produces antibodies called autoantibodies that react with the host's own cell or tissue antigens.

Warm-Antibody Autoimmune Hemolytic Anemia

DEFINITION AND PATHOPHYSIOLOGY

Warm-antibody AIHA occurs when the patient's own immune system produces anti–red cell antibodies that react most effectively in the laboratory at warm temperatures (37°C) (Table 19-2).[9] The approximate incidence of the disorder is one in 80,000 persons. Approximately 75% of all AIHA is classified as warm-antibody type.[15]

These autoantibodies usually are IgG, although some may be IgM or IgA. IgG warm autoantibodies do not bind complement. Red cell destruction occurs as a consequence of adherence of the red cell–bound autoantibodies to Fc receptors on monocytes and macrophages and the subsequent phagocytosis and cytotoxic lysis of red cells.[10] The autoantibodies are called incomplete because they do not cause direct agglutination of red cells. By binding to red cell surfaces, they cause extravascular destruction of red cells, principally in the spleen (see Table 19-2).

IgM incomplete warm autoantibodies bind complement which may lead to formation of the membrane attack unit and intravascular lysis. The warm-antibody AIHAs are categorized as primary or idiopathic if the specific cause is unknown and secondary if the patient has another disease complicated by hemolytic anemia (see Table 19-1).[11] Recent research based on newer and more accurate methods indicates that 30% of these anemias are primary whereas 70% are secondary to some other disorder.[14]

CLINICAL PRESENTATION, SYMPTOMS, AND PHYSICAL FINDINGS

This disease is seen in both sexes but slightly more often in women. It may be acquired at any age, although the frequency of onset is higher after 40 years of age. The course may be very mild, with gradually developing symptoms, or acute with fulminating symptoms. Physical findings commonly include progressive weakness, occasional acute fever, pain, hemoglobinuria, mild jaundice, hepatosplenomegaly, and lymphadenopathy.

TABLE 19-2

Delineation of Common Antibodies and Other Key Features of the Acquired Autoimmune Hemolytic Anemias

	Warm Antibody	Cold Antibody	Paroxysmal Cold Hemoglobinuria
Optimal reaction temperature	37°C	0°–4°C (antibody binds to cell) 10°–30°C (hemolysis takes place)	0°–4°C (antibody binds to cell) 37°C (hemolysis takes place)
Thermal amplitude*	20–37°C	0–32°C	<15°C
Immunoglobulin type	Usually IgG†	Usually IgM‡	IgG (Donath-Landsteiner auto-antibody)
Antibody type	Incomplete††	Complete†† (agglutinin)	Hemolysin
Mechanism of antibody production	Immune response	Naturally occurring and immune response	Immune response
Complement (C') activation	Does not bind C'	Binds C'	Binds C'
Protein structure	Polyclonal	Monoclonal or polyclonal	Polyclonal
Blood group specificity	Rh, Kell, others	Ii	Pp
Primary mechanism of cell destruction	Extravascular, principally splenic	Extravascular, principally hepatic	Principally intravascular
Severity of disease	Often severe	Often mild	Distinct episodes of severity
Treatment	Steroids, splenectomy, immunosuppressants	Avoid cold	Avoid cold
Transfusion requirements	Transfusions contraindicated	Rarely needed	Could be required

* Thermal amplitude refers to the temperature range in which antibody binds to the red cell surface.
† Occasionally IgM or IgA. IgM does bind complement.
‡ Occasionally IgG.
†† Incomplete antibodies do not cause direct agglutination of cells, whereas complete antibodies do.

LABORATORY FINDINGS AND CORRELATIONS WITH DISEASE

Hemoglobin values vary with the severity of hemolysis. Red cells are often macrocytic, but there is marked anisocytosis. Spherocytes indicate the hemolytic process. Marked reticulocytosis is evident as the marrow tries to compensate for the hemolysis. With a competent marrow, the reticulocyte production index (RPI) should be greater than 3.0. Thrombocytopenia may also occur. The serum unconjugated bilirubin value is moderately increased. Hemoglobinemia and hemoglobinuria may be seen in severe cases.

The DAT is positive in the majority of cases, confirming the presence of IgG antibodies with or without complement on the red cells. The indirect antiglobulin test may also demonstrate autoantibody in the serum when there is active hemolysis. Warm autoantibodies usually have a specificity for Rh antigens, although Kell and a number of other blood group specificities have been described.[7]

EFFECTS OF TREATMENT ON LABORATORY RESULTS—PROGNOSIS

For secondary warm-antibody AIHA, treating the underlying disease may reverse the hemolytic process. Transfusion as a treatment for severe anemia may be fraught with problems, from difficulty in accurate blood typing to finding a compatible blood unit in the presence of blood group–specific autoantibodies. Successful treatment with corticosteroids, which act to inhibit the clearance of IgG-sensitized red cells and suppress antibody synthesis, results in increased hemoglobin values. Intravenous administration of immune globulins has sometimes been useful. Splenectomy for patients who do not respond to corticosteroids may result in hematologic improvement, since the spleen is the major site of sequestration of IgG-sensitized cells.

Prognosis varies depending on the severity of the hemolytic episodes and the nature of the underlying disease in the secondary form.

Cold-Antibody Autoimmune Hemolytic Anemia (Cold Agglutinin Syndrome; Raynaud's Phenomenon)

DEFINITION, HISTORY AND PATHOPHYSIOLOGY

Humans normally have a small and harmless amount of cold autoantibody, including anti-I, anti-H, and anti-IH. However most people who have cold agglutinin syndrome, also known as cold agglutinin disease, develop a pathologic form of anti-I antibody that leads to complement-mediated hemolysis in the temperature range of 10° to 30°C. The pathologic anti-I antibodies bind avidly to red cells at cold temperatures (0°–10°C) *in vivo* and *in vitro* and react optimally in the laboratory from 0° to 4°C.

These cold-reacting antibodies were identified by Landsteiner[20] and Wiener[34] and were later found to be related to hemolytic anemia and Raynaud's phenomenon, a vascular disorder that causes pain in the extremities on exposure to cold temperatures. They are less common than warm antibodies.

Pathologic cold anti-I autoantibodies are usually IgM antibodies (see Table 19-2). Because of their ability to bind and activate complement (*e.g.*, C3b), destruction of red cells is primarily extravascular in the liver, due to Kupffer cell C3b receptors. To a lesser extent, complement-mediated intravascular hemolysis may occur, as may hemolysis due to red cell shape changes caused by cold agglutinins.

Cold-antibody AIHA or cold agglutinin syndrome is categorized as primary (idiopathic) or secondary. In the latter, infectious agents constitute the major precipitating disorder (see Table 19-1).[30]

CLINICAL PRESENTATION, SYMPTOMS, AND PHYSICAL FINDINGS

Primary cold agglutinin disease is most common in elderly people, but the secondary form is seen in all ages, depending on the incidence of the underlying disease. When the patient is exposed to cold, red cell agglutinates occur that obstruct the capillary circulation, causing numbness, pain, and blue or red skin discoloration. This circulatory abnormality is known as acrocyanosis (blue-gray discoloration of extremities) or Raynaud's phenomenon. It usually involves exposed body parts, the tip of the nose, ear lobes, or fingers. Gangrene may develop in the extremities in severe cases.

In primary disease, the physical findings in addition to acrocyanosis include anemia, and at times, mild jaundice, which are the result of hemolysis. In acute episodes, hemoglobinuria and renal failure may ensue. In secondary disease the underlying disease dictates the physical findings.

LABORATORY FINDINGS AND CORRELATIONS WITH DISEASE

Hematology. Hemoglobin values decrease as hemolysis increases and may, in fact, vary seasonally with the temperature. Reticulocytes proliferate in relation to hemolysis. Leukocyte and platelet numbers generally are normal. Of importance is the effect of these cold agglutinins on laboratory procedures. Clumping of red cells while preparing blood films or when using an automated cell counter can result in erroneous values if it is not detected. Classically, the MCV for these samples is artefactually elevated, and the MCH and MCHC appear entirely unrealistic. To overcome this problem, the blood sample should be warmed for at least 15 minutes at 37°C, and the equipment and reagents should be prewarmed if possible.

Other Laboratory Findings. Bilirubin levels are mildly increased. Haptoglobin and complement levels may be decreased as hemolysis progresses. Mild hemoglobinemia may be observed.

A cold agglutinin screening test is helpful in the diagnosis. If the patient's serum agglutinates normal red cells at 20°C, the serum cold agglutinin must be titered at 4°C and the thermal amplitude (the range of temperatures over which these antibodies attach to red cells) must be determined (see standard immunohematology texts for procedures). For patients experiencing hemolysis, the cold agglutinin titer at 4°C is usually over 1000, whereas that for healthy subjects is generally under 64. Pathologic anti-I antibodies have a broad thermal amplitude (0°–32°C), whereas normal anti-I antibodies in healthy persons have a thermal amplitude of 0° to 22°C. The higher thermal amplitude of pathologic anti-I antibodies is significant because complement is most hemolytic at temperatures of 22°C and higher, thus pathologic anti-I antibodies are capable of causing hemolysis.

At 37°C, the agglutinating property of cold agglutinins is characteristically reversed. This is why blood samples from these patients require warming before being analyzed. At room temperature, the astute technologist handling the blood sample may provide the diagnosis by observing the clumping phenomenon seen along the tube walls.

Cold agglutinins show specificity for the I antigen of adult cells in most cases or for the i antigen of fetal or cord red cells. The DAT is usually positive when a polyspecific antiglobulin serum is used that detects both complement and antibodies on the red cell surface. Complement is actually the only component being detected on the red cell, as demonstrated by a positive result with anti-C3–specific antiglobulin serum and a negative result with reagents lacking anti-C3.

EFFECTS OF TREATMENT ON LABORATORY RESULTS—PROGNOSIS

For patients with secondary cold agglutinin syndrome, keeping them warm and treating any underlying disease is the best therapy, since infectious disease and the related hemolytic process are ordinarily of limited duration. For persons who have the idiopathic syndrome, steroid therapy and immunosuppressive therapy with alkylating agents such as chlorambucil may be effective in normalizing test results. Plasmapheresis to remove intravascular IgM antibodies may benefit acutely ill patients.

Transfusion to correct anemia is technically difficult, since blood typing and cross-matching results are affected by the presence of cold agglutinins. Blood should be warmed prior to transfusion in order to avoid intravascular agglutination. The prognosis is variable, depending on the underlying disease.

Paroxysmal Cold Hemoglobinuria

DEFINITION, HISTORY, AND PATHOPHYSIOLOGY

Paroxysmal cold hemoglobinuria (PCH), the rarest form of AIHA, is similar to cold-antibody AIHA. It is caused by binding of the Donath-Landsteiner (D-L) autoantibody to the patient's red cells following exposure to cold, which results in intravascular hemolysis and gross hemoglobinuria.

PCH was one of the first hemolytic anemias to be described and correlated to cold exposure. A causative "autolysin" was suggested by Donath and Landsteiner in 1904. The autoantibody responsible for PCH is still called the D-L antibody and is demonstrated by the Donath-Landsteiner test. It has been suggested that genetic

factors controlling immune responsiveness may dictate who will develop this disease, which represents less than 1% of acquired AIHAs.[16]

The D-L autoantibody is an IgG antibody (as opposed to the IgM type found in cold-antibody AIHA), which is also a powerful hemolysin (see Table 19-2). Both idiopathic[3] and secondary PCH have been described. PCH may be secondary to viral diseases, particularly among children and less commonly secondary to advanced syphilis (see Table 19-1).[8,35] This antibody shows specificity for the Pp blood group system.[23] It binds to red cells at temperatures below 15°C in the presence of complement, then hemolyzes them upon warming to 37°C.

CLINICAL PRESENTATION, SYMPTOMS, AND PHYSICAL FINDINGS

After exposure to varying degrees and periods of cold, the patient may present with headache, vomiting, pain in the abdomen and extremities, severe chills and fever, and significant hemoglobinuria. Following the attack, patients often pass dark brown or black urine and complain of weakness. Patients are often free of symptoms between attacks, and the duration of symptoms during and after exposure is limited. Physical findings may include mild jaundice and hepatosplenomegaly.

LABORATORY FINDINGS AND CORRELATIONS WITH DISEASE

In a severe hemolytic attack, hemoglobin values drop rapidly as hemoglobinuria is observed. Red cell morphology is generally normal, although microspherocytes, polychromasia, and nucleated red blood cells may be noted in children. Leukopenia develops after an attack followed by leukocytosis. Immature leukocytes and phagocytosis of red cells may be observed on the blood film.

The result of the Donath-Landsteiner test is positive.[25] Refer to standard immunohematology texts for the procedure.

Urine contains hemoglobin and methemoglobin, giving it a dark red, brown, or almost black appearance, as serum haptoglobin becomes saturated with hemoglobin from lysed cells. The DAT is positive at the time of attack if a complement-specific (*i.e.*, non–gamma globulin) antiserum is used and the test is performed at a cold temperature. Cells are coated by inactivated complement components. The serum unconjugated bilirubin level may be mildly elevated after the attack.[37]

EFFECTS OF TREATMENT ON LABORATORY RESULTS—PROGNOSIS

In secondary PCH, successful treatment of the syphilis or viral infection most often relieves the symptoms. The short duration of viral diseases usually precludes specific therapy. In both instances, laboratory test values return to normal. In idiopathic primary disease, however, avoidance of cold is the preventive therapy of choice. Although results of the D-L test may continue to be positive, attacks and their associated abnormal laboratory test results are minimized by avoiding the cold.

DRUG-INDUCED IMMUNE HEMOLYTIC ANEMIA

In some people, certain drugs provoke abnormal antibody production that causes immune hemolytic anemia. These antibodies may resemble autoantibodies.[29] Three principal modes of formation and cell destruction are involved: (1) the hapten or drug adsorption mechanism; (2) the immune complex or "innocent bystander" mechanism; and (3) the α-methyldopa or autoimmune (unknown) mechanism. These mechanisms are shown graphically in Figure 19-2 and summarized in Table 19-3. Recent attempts to unify these concepts have proposed that all drug-related, immune cytopenias are initiated by interaction of the drug or its metabolites with constituents of the red cell membrane, resulting in an antigenic structure which produces drug dependent and/or drug independent antibodies.[32]

Hapten (Drug Adsorption) Mechanism

DEFINITION, HISTORY, AND PATHOPHYSIOLOGY

A *hapten* is a low molecular weight substance (less than 5000 daltons) that rarely stimulates antibody production. However molecules of some drugs or their metabolites are haptens that can stimulate production of an antibody causing drug-induced immune hemolytic anemia.

Increasing use of large doses of antibiotics such as penicillin led to the development of this type of hemolytic anemia. This mechanism is also associated with some cephalosporins such as cephalothin, a drug used to treat some bacterial infections and as a penicillin substitute.

A drug or one of its metabolites adsorbs nonspecifically to the red cell surface and induces production of an antibody specific for the drug. The antidrug antibody then combines with the drug attached to the red cell (see Fig. 19-2). The antibody is usually IgG, warm reactive, and does not bind complement. The IgG-coated red cells are then subject to extravascular, mainly splenic, destruction (see Table 19-3).[26]

Low levels of antipenicillin antibody have been found in normal persons, but about 3% of all patients who receive large doses of penicillin develop a positive DAT reaction. Of these, sensitization is more common following intramuscular penicillin therapy; only a small number who are receiving massive intravenous doses on a long-term basis develop overt hemolytic anemia.

CLINICAL PRESENTATION

Abnormal clinical findings develop only while under treatment with the offending drug for an underlying dis-

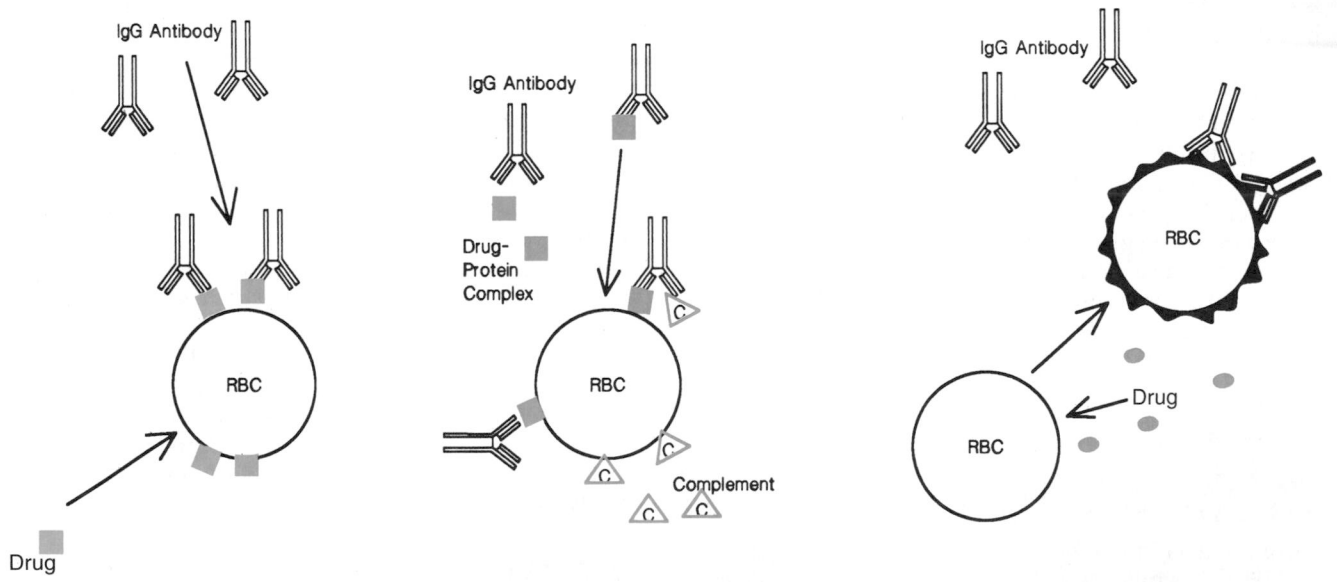

Hapten Type
Drug Adsorption Mechanism
e.g., Penicillin

Innocent Bystander Type
Immune Complex Mechanism,
e.g., Phenacetin, Stibophen

Apha-Methyldopa Type
Autoimmune/Unknown Mechanism,
e.g., Alpha-Methyldopa, Levodopa

FIGURE 19-2. The three mechanisms of drug-induced immune hemolytic anemia. In the *drug adsorption mechanism*, a drug (hapten) is adsorbed to the red cell membrane. This stimulates antidrug-antibody production, and this antibody complexes to the drug on the red cell surface leading to extravascular hemolysis. In the *immune complex mechanism*, a drug-protein complex in the plasma stimulates antibody production, and antibody binds to the drug-protein complex while it is still in the plasma. This complex binds nonimmunologically, or perhaps immunologically, with complement to "innocent" red cells leading to intravascular hemolysis. In the α-methyldopa type, production of autoantibody specific for Rh antigens on the red cell surface is induced by the drug circulating in the plasma. These antibodies bind to the cell surface but the drug does not.

TABLE 19-3
Summary of Mechanisms Causing Drug-Induced Immune Hemolytic Anemias

Mechanism	Drug Type	Antibody Type and Specificity	DAT* Result (Polyspecific)	Hemolysis
Hapten (drug adsorption)	Penicillin (large doses), streptomycin, cephalothin	IgG to drug	+	Extravascular, mainly splenic; develops slowly; severe in rare cases; stops with removal of drug
Innocent bystander (immune complex)	Stibophen (small doses), phenacetin	IgM or IgG to drug	+	Intravascular, acute hemolysis; stops 1 to 2 days after removal of drug
α-Methyldopa (autoimmune/unknown)	α-Methyldopa (dose-related), levodopa, mefenamic acid	IgG to Rh antigens	+	May develop slowly in a few patients after 3 months or more of therapy; less than 1% of patients on methyldopa experience hemolysis; stops several days to a week after removal of drug

* *Direct antiglobulin test performed using polyspecific antiserum.*

ease. If hemolysis ensues, the typical symptoms of anemia develop.

LABORATORY FINDINGS AND CORRELATIONS WITH DISEASE

The most significant finding is the positive DAT. The patient's red cells react strongly with anti-IgG antiglobulin reagent. Eluates from these red cells fail to react with normal red cells but do react with drug-coated cells. Because normal people may have low levels of antipenicillin antibody, high titers must be demonstrated in order to implicate the drug as a cause of hemolysis.

An abrupt decrease in hemoglobin level followed by a gradual increase in reticulocyte count and RPI can be expected, along with an increased serum unconjugated bilirubin level. Thrombocytopenia and neutropenia have been reported, suggesting that the development of penicillin-coated myeloid precursor cells may be suppressed by antipenicillin antibodies.[28]

EFFECTS OF TREATMENT ON LABORATORY RESULTS—PROGNOSIS

Removal of the offending drug ordinarily reverses the hemolytic process, and the DAT result becomes negative over a period of a few days to weeks. If necessary, a drug that has previously induced hemolytic anemia can be given again if the patient is monitored carefully for the appearance of a secondary immune response.

Immune Complex (Innocent Bystander) Mechanism

DEFINITION, HISTORY, AND PATHOPHYSIOLOGY

The drugs in this mechanism cause the formation of immunogenic antigen–antibody complexes in the plasma which bind complement and settle on the red cell surface leading to intravascular hemolysis. It was previously thought that the red cell was an "innocent bystander," because this complex was not binding specifically to a red cell antigen (see Fig. 19-2). However, it is now proposed that some of these immunogenic complexes do have specificity for certain red cell antigens.[19]

The innocent bystander type of hemolytic anemia was described in 1954 in a patient with schistosomiasis who was treated with the drug stibophen. Other drugs that may act in a similar manner are quinidine, quinine, sulfonamides, and phenacetin.[36]

The drugs involved in this immune hemolytic mechanism are small molecules that in themselves are not immunogenic, but once they are bound firmly to a carrier plasma protein, the resulting complex is capable of eliciting an immune response. This complex then induces antidrug antibody production and binds with the antibody in the plasma. In the second step of this mechanism, the drug-protein-antibody complex binds nonimmunologically, or perhaps immunologically, to the red cell surface. The antibodies are either IgM or IgG and have the ability to bind complement, which results in intravascular hemolysis (see Table 19-3). Often complement may be found alone on the red cell surface, owing to dissociation of the drug-protein-antibody complex after complement fixation occurs (see Fig. 19-2).

CLINICAL PRESENTATION

The common symptoms of hemolysis occur when the drug is being administered. The acute onset of symptoms in the face of the underlying disease for which the drug was prescribed dictate the physical findings.

LABORATORY FINDINGS AND CORRELATIONS WITH DISEASE

A decrease in hemoglobin occurs as intravascular hemolysis proceeds. Hemoglobinemia is apparent. Spherocytosis, leukopenia, and thrombocytopenia may be observed in some cases. The rapid hemolysis results in hemoglobinuria, and renal failure is a common finding. A prolonged

PTT result and low factor VIII and fibrinogen levels reflect an intravascular coagulation process as well. Results of the DAT are positive when polyvalent or complement-specific reagents are used. Serum unconjugated bilirubin rises as hemolysis progresses.

EFFECTS OF TREATMENT ON LABORATORY RESULTS—PROGNOSIS

Immediate removal of the offending drug may be the only therapy required. Steroids may be helpful when hemolysis is severe. Abnormal test results gradually become normal after the drug is removed, but the DAT may remain positive for up to 2 months, owing to the firm attachment of inactivated complement to red cells. Renal failure indicates a poor prognosis.

α-Methyldopa or Autoimmune (Unknown) Mechanism

DEFINITION, HISTORY, AND PATHOPHYSIOLOGY

In this AIHA, a drug induces the formation of an IgG antibody with specificity for Rh red cell antigens (rather than for the drug itself), which may result in hemolysis (see Fig. 19-2). In 1966, the first reports were published of significant numbers of patients who had received α-methyldopa (Aldomet) for hypertension and developed a positive DAT result and in some cases, a hemolytic anemia.[6] Since then, other drugs with similar modes of action have been recognized including levodopa and mefenamic acid. However, α-methyldopa is the most common cause of drug-induced hemolytic anemia.

Hemolytic disease occurs in about 1% of patients who take α-methyldopa.[36] The autoantibody is produced only after several months of continuous therapy. The drug does not bind to the red cell surface, and appears to induce an immune process in which it does not participate.[16] The capacity of α-methyldopa to inhibit normal suppressor T-cell function[18] resulting in uncontrolled B-cell autoantibody production may be the cause of this disorder; however, this is still uncertain.[12]

CLINICAL PRESENTATION

The course of the disease is rather insidious; hemolysis may start from 18 weeks to 4 years after therapy begins.[36] Symptoms and physical findings are those associated with anemia.

LABORATORY FINDINGS AND CORRELATIONS WITH DISEASE

Hematologic studies show decreased hemoglobin, a compensatory increase in reticulocytes, and moderate numbers of spherocytes. The antibody is similar in activity to those of the warm-antibody autoimmune type and has specificity for Rh antigens (see Table 19-3). Bilirubin (total and unconjugated) levels are moderately elevated.

Although the DAT is positive with anti-IgG sera in approximately 15% of patients who have been taking the drug for at least 3 months,[36] most show no evidence of overt hemolysis.

EFFECTS OF TREATMENT ON LABORATORY RESULTS—PROGNOSIS

Removal of α-methyldopa rapidly stops the hemolytic process. Corticosteroid therapy is sometimes useful, and transfusions may be necessary for severe cases. Results of the DAT are negative within a few months after the drug is discontinued. A number of patients so affected often have other autoantibodies (*e.g.,* antinuclear antibody [ANA] or rheumatoid factor; Chap. 24).[4]

CHAPTER SUMMARY

The combination of decreased hemoglobin and a positive result on the direct antiglobulin test (DAT) may suggest an anemia of increased red cell destruction. The role of isoimmune antibodies (produced after exposure to foreign antigens from an individual of the same species) or autoimmune antibodies (abnormally produced against the host's own antigens) as causative agents should be considered. These antibodies are associated with acquired immune hemolytic anemia (see Table 19-1).

Immune hemolysis is associated with both intravascular and extravascular hemolysis. The hemolytic process involves not only antibodies and antigens, but also the complement system (see Fig. 19-1). Extravascular hemolysis is often associated with the formation of complement component C3b on the red cell surface. Intravascular hemolysis is ultimately caused by the complement membrane attack unit C5b6789, formed on the red cell surface, which penetrates the surface and causes cell lysis.

Hemolysis due to alloantibodies is more common than that due to autoantibodies. Alloimmune hemolytic anemia is seen in HDN and transfusion reactions, which may be immediate or delayed for 2 to 14 days. Immediate transfusion reactions often occur with IgM anti-A and anti-B isoantibodies, which cause intravascular hemolysis when incompatible blood is transfused. Delayed transfusion reactions commonly occur with IgG antibodies that usually cause hemolysis.

In the autoimmune hemolytic anemias, a disturbance of the normal immune system occurs in which antibodies to the host's own antigens are produced. The antibodies may be either warm reacting (37°C) or cold reacting (0°–10°C); the latter causes cold agglutinin disease (see Table 19-2). Paroxysmal cold hemoglobinuria (PCH) is a rare autoimmune disorder caused by an autoantibody to the Pp blood group system.

The three mechanisms of drug-induced immune hemolytic anemia are shown in Figure 19-2.

Case Study 19-1

On a cold February day, a 6-year-old boy was brought to the emergency room by his frantic mother because he had passed red urine and looked very pale. He was a normal, active boy, and in fact had played out in the snow the day before. He had had the "flu" for 1 week about 10 days before this episode. He had not received any medication except acetaminophen. On admission his CBC values were WBC 12.2 × 10⁹/L; RBC 3.0 × 10¹²/L; Hb 8.0 g/dL; Hct 0.22 L/L; PLT 350 × 10⁹/L. The differential cell count was neutrophils 40%; bands 10%; lymphocytes 43%; monocytes 7%. The reticulocyte count was 0.9% but rose significantly within 1 week.

1. Do the Hb and Hct values match?
2. What is the most likely cause of the red urine?
3. What patient history might be significant in the passing of red urine?
4. What diagnoses might the physician consider?

5. What additional tests could be recommended to help the physician determine the diagnosis?
6. What treatment might the physician prescribe?

Case Study 19-2

A male adult patient blood sample was analyzed on routine admission using an automated cell counter. The results were WBC 7.1 × 10⁹/L; RBC 3.2 × 10¹²/L; Hb 13.5 g/dL; Hct 0.36 L/L; MCV 112.5 fL; MCH 42.2 pg; MCHC 37.5 gs/dL.
1. Do the Hb and Hct values match?
2. Do the RBC and Hb values match?
3. Identify the abnormal results and their implications.
4. What simple thing could the laboratory scientist do to investigate this?
5. Are the WBC and Hb results *accurate*?
6. Can anything be done to obtain accurate results for this patient?

Review Questions

19-1. Complement plays a direct role in acquired immune hemolytic anemia by

A. coating the Kupffer cells of the liver.
B. preventing the formation of antigen-antibody complexes.
C. forming the "membrane attack unit."
D. controlling fibrinolysis.

19-2. Complement combines with antibodies causing immune hemolysis that is

A. extravascular.
B. intravascular.
C. both A and B.
D. none of the above.

19-3. Warm autoantibodies that cause hemolytic anemia are usually _____ antibodies.

A. anti-Rh
B. anti-ABO
C. anti-I
D. anti-P

19-4. Patients with Raynaud's phenomenon may have _____ reacting antibodies and a falsely _____ MCV.

A. cold; decreased
B. cold; increased
C. warm; decreased
D. warm; increased

19-5. Grossly abnormal erythrocyte indices with a low RBC count may indicate the presence of _____ antibodies.

A. warm reacting
B. cold reacting
C. Donath-Landsteiner
D. IgG

19-6. For a specimen like that described in question 19-5, the blood count should be performed again following 15 minutes of specimen

A. cooling to room temperature.
B. refrigeration at 4°C.
C. incubation at 37°C.
D. None of the above is recommended.

19-7. In the α-methyldopa mechanism of drug-induced immune hemolytic anemia, the antibodies produced are specific for

A. α-methyldopa.
B. penicillin.
C. ABO antigens.
D. Rh antigens.

References

1. Allen FH, Diamond LK: Erythroblastosis Fetalis. Boston, Little, Brown & Co, 1957
2. Austen KF, Becker EL, Biro CE et al: Nomenclature of complement. Bull WHO 39:935, 1968
3. Bird GW, Wingham J, Martin AJ et al: Idiopathic nonsyphilitic paroxysmal cold hemoglobinuria in children. J Clin Pathol 29:215, 1976
4. Breckenridge A, Dollery CT, Worlledge SM et al: Positive direct Coombs' tests and antinuclear factor in patients treated with methyldopa. Lancet 2:1265, 1967
5. Capon SM, Goldfinger D: Acute hemolytic transfusion reaction, a paradigm of the systemic inflammatory response: New insights into pathophysiology and treatment. Transfusion 15:513, 1995
6. Carstairs KC, Breckenridge A, Dollery CT et al: Incidence of a positive direct Coombs' test in patients on α-methyldopa. Lancet 2:133, 1966
7. Charles LT: Resolving incompatibilities in patients with warm reactive autoantibodies. J Med Technol 35:291, 1986
8. Colley EW: Paroxysmal cold haemoglobinuria after mumps. Br Med J 1:1552, 1964
9. Dacie JV: Autoimmune hemolytic anemia. Ann Intern Med 135:1293, 1975
10. Engelfriet CP, Overbeeke MAM, von dem Borne AEG: Autoimmune hemolytic anemia. Semin Hematol 29:3, 1992
11. Foerster J: Autoimmune hemolytic anemias. In Lee GR, Bithell TC, Foerster J et al (eds): Wintrobe's Clinical Hematology, 9th ed, p 1171. Philadelphia, Lea & Febiger, 1993
12. Garratty G, Arndt P, Prince HE et al: The effect of methyldopa and procainamide on suppressor cell activity in relation to red cell autoantibody production. Br J Haematol 84:310, 1993
13. Hadley AG: *In vitro* assays to predict the severity of hemolytic disease of the newborn. Trans Med Rev 9:302, 1995
14. Issit PD: Applied Blood Group Serology, 3rd ed, p 514. Miami, Montgomery Scientific Publications, 1985
15. Issit PD: Applied Blood Group Serology, 3rd ed, p 540. Miami, Montgomery Scientific Publications, 1985
16. Issit PD: Applied Blood Group Serology, 3rd ed, p 548. Miami, Montgomery Scientific Publications, 1985
17. Kanto WP Jr, Marino B, Godwin AS et al: ABO hemolytic disease: A comparative study of clinical severity and delayed anemia. Pediatrics 62:365, 1978
18. Kirtland HH III, Mohler DN, Horwitz DA et al: Methyldopa inhibition of suppressor lymphocyte functions. N Eng J Med 302:825, 1980
19. Kleinman S et al: Positive direct antiglobulin test and immune hemolytic anemia in patients receiving procainamide. N Engl J Med 311:809, 1984
20. Landsteiner K, Levine P: On the cold agglutinins in human serum. J Immunol 12:441, 1926
21. Landsteiner K, Wiener AS: An agglutinable factor in human blood recognized by immune sera for Rhesus blood. Proc Soc Exp Med 43:220, 1940
22. Levine P, Katzin EM, Burnham L: Isoimmunization in pregnancy; its possible bearing on etiology of erythroblastosis foetalis. JAMA 116:825, 1941
23. Levine P, Celano MJ, Falkowski F: The specificity of the

antibody in paroxysmal cold hemoglobinuria (PCH). Transfusion 3:278, 1963

24. Levine P, Stetson KE: An unusual case of intragroup agglutination. JAMA 113:126, 1939

25. Mackenzie GM: Paroxysmal hemoglobinuria. A review. Medicine 8:159, 1929

26. Marchand A: Immune hemolytic anemia: Classification, manifestation, and mechanisms of destruction. Diag Med 5:51, 1982

27. Muller-Eberhard HJ: Complement. Ann Rev Biochem 44:697, 1975

28. Murphy MF, Riordan T, Minchinton RM et al: Demonstration of an immune-mediated mechanism of penicillin-induced neutropaenia and thrombocytopaenia. Br J Haematol 55:155, 1983

29. Petz LG: Drug-induced autoimmune hemolytic anemia. Trans Med Rev 7:242, 1993

30. Pruzanski W, Schumak KW: Biologic activity of cold-reacting autoantibodies. N Eng J Med 297:538, 1977

31. Ruddy S, Gigli I, Austen KF: The complement system of man. N Eng J Med 287:489, 545, 592, 642, 1972

32. Salama A, Mueller-Eckhardt C: Immune mediated blood cell dyscrasias related to drugs. Semin Hematol 29:54,1992

33. Weinstein L: Irregular antibodies causing HDN. Obstet Gynecol Surv 31:581, 1976

34. Wiener AS, Unger LJ, Cohen L et al: Type-specific cold autoantibodies as a cause of acquired hemolytic anemia and hemolytic transfusion reactions: Biologic test with bovine red cells. Ann Intern Med 44:221, 1956

35. Wishart MM, Davey MG: Infectious mononucleosis complicated by acute haemolytic anemia with a positive D-L reaction. J Clin Pathol 26:332, 1973

36. Worledge SM: Immune drug induced hemolytic anemia. Semin Hematol 6:181, 1969

37. Worledge SM, Rousso C: Studies on the serology of paroxysmal cold hemoglobinuria (PCH) with special reference to its relationship with the P blood group system. Vox Sang 10:293, 1965

CHAPTER 20

Anemias of Blood Loss

Kathleen M. Mugan

Acute Blood Loss
Pathophysiology
Clinical Presentation and Symptoms
Laboratory Findings and Correlations with Disease
Effects of Treatment on Laboratory Results

Chronic Blood Loss
Pathophysiology

Clinical Presentation and Symptoms
Laboratory Findings and Correlations with Disease
Effects of Treatment on Laboratory Results

Case Studies 20-1 and 20-2

Objectives

1. Briefly discuss the pathophysiology of acute and chronic blood loss.
2. Differentiate acute from chronic blood loss based on laboratory data.
3. List two laboratory tests that are useful in monitoring the treatment of blood loss and describe the expected results.

Bleeding is defined as an injury that allows blood to escape from the vessels into surrounding tissue or into the environment. The anemias caused by acute and chronic bleeding are often given less significance than their frequency or clinical seriousness would suggest. Chronic blood loss leading to iron deficiency, together with acute bleeding, makes up almost one half of all anemias in the United States.[5] This percentage is even higher in the hospitalized population, in which there are large numbers of trauma, post-surgical and obstetric patients. If extensive, uncompensated, or untreated, acute blood loss (hemorrhage) can quickly lead to shock and death. Iron deficiency anemia (primarily caused by chronic blood loss[6]; Chap. 13) has been called one of the most common maladies of humankind[1] and is responsible for tremendous morbidity throughout the world. Since blood transfusions and other treatment decisions are frequently based on laboratory analysis, it is important to understand the physiology and laboratory findings associated with these common and clinically important anemias.

ACUTE BLOOD LOSS

Pathophysiology

To understand the body's response to acute blood loss, it is helpful to have a basic understanding of the heart's requirement for an adequate blood volume. The amount of blood which returns to the heart after circulating red blood cells deliver oxygen to the tissues—the *venous return*—is partly responsible for the strength of the next heart beat. If not enough blood returns to the heart to stimulate the heart beat, a potentially serious chain of events is initiated. The amount of blood pumped from the heart, known as the *cardiac output*, drops. As the cardiac output drops, many cells throughout the body have inadequate oxygen delivery (perfusion). As oxygen levels fall, the cells cannot make new adenosine triphosphate (ATP), the biologic energy for cells that is normally made by aerobic glycolysis in the tricarboxylic acid (Krebs') cycle. ATP is needed to maintain the cellular ion pumps. Without these pumps, extracellular sodium enters the cells causing them to swell and eventually be destroyed by lysis.[2]

Hemorrhage of more than 20% of the total blood volume, a leading cause of disrupted oxygen perfusion and subsequent cell death, is a serious medical emergency. Blood loss can occur from a variety of conditions including trauma, obstetric problems, ruptured aneurysm (a sac formed by the dilation of the wall of an artery, a vein, or the heart), injured spleen, gastrointestinal (GI) disorders, and surgical procedures. If the various compensatory mechanisms (to be discussed) fail, or if the loss is too great, acute bleeding can result in circulatory shock and death. The greatest immediate danger in acute blood loss is overall blood volume depletion rather than the reduced oxygen-carrying capacity of fewer red blood cells. If there is an insufficient volume of blood in the vessels to maintain pressure against the walls, the vessels collapse and blood does not return to the heart to initiate beating.[4]

When a blood volume decrease is detected, the body's most immediate goal is to continue to provide oxygen to the heart and brain. Several complex, multi-organ compensatory mechanisms exist to help maintain cardiac output and blood pressure. The average human body contains approximately 5 L of blood. A small blood loss of 10% (500 mL) or less of the total volume generally produces no observable effect; even blood donors rarely experience lightheadedness. As the amount of blood lost increases, the symptoms become more severe, as seen in Table 20-1. Note that a loss of 40% to 50% of the total blood volume will usually result in shock and death.

As blood volume decreases, the outward pressure exerted on the vessels also decreases. Receptors in the carotid arteries detect lowered arterial pressure and stimulate the brain to signal the adrenal gland to release epinephrine and norepinephrine. These hormones are re-

TABLE 20-1

Symptoms Related to Degree of Blood Loss for a Normal Adult with a 5000-mL Blood Volume

Blood Loss		
(%)	*(mL)*	**Symptoms**
10	500	Usually none Occasional lightheadedness
20	1000	Increased heart rate with exercise Hypotension when standing
30–40	≥1500	Decreased cardiac output and blood pressure Rapid pulse, gasping for air Cold, clammy skin
40–50	2500	Compensatory mechanisms fail Unconsciousness, severe shock and death

Data from Hillman RS: Acute blood loss anemia. In Beutler E, Lichtmann MA, Coller BS et al (eds): Williams' Hematology, 5th ed, p 705. New York, McGraw-Hill, 1995, with permission.

sponsible for venous and arteriole vasoconstriction (vessel narrowing), increasing the heart rate, and improving heart contraction strength.[7] Venous constriction increases the venous return by "squeezing" blood from pooled areas such as the hepatic and splenic sinuses and the large veins of the lower body. This enhanced venous return helps the heart maintain the cardiac output, making up for the blood that was lost.[3] Also there is vasoconstriction of arterioles in the kidneys, skin, and muscles which diverts blood, with its critical oxygen-carrying capacity, to the heart and brain.[7]

Another mechanism to keep blood pressure from falling when blood volume decreases is a shift of fluid from the extravascular spaces to the inside of the blood vessels. This is accomplished in several ways. First, the reduced volume of blood exerts less outward pressure on the vessels. Second, the osmolarity of the blood is increased by the norepinephrine-induced release of glucose into the blood from the liver. Third, the oxygen-sensitive kidneys induce increased sodium and water reabsorption by way of the renin-angiotensin-aldosterone system and antidiuretic hormone (ADH). Lowering the outward vessel pressure, increasing the blood osmolarity, and reducing urine production all contribute to the vessels drawing in even more fluid and further expanding the blood volume.[7,8]

Impairment of oxygen delivery causes the body to switch to the less effective anaerobic glycolysis for ATP production, which produces lactic acid and eventually metabolic acidosis (decreased blood pH). Acidosis causes additional compensation by increasing the breathing rate and stimulating the increased production of 2,3-diphosphoglycerate (2,3-DPG) in red cells, which reduces hemoglobin's affinity for oxygen. This allows more oxygen to be delivered from the red cells to the tissues.[7]

If bleeding continues, the brain stem becomes underperfused and loses its control of the compensatory mechanisms. Blood pressure then drops because there is not enough venous return to initiate adequate cardiac output.

At this point there is major cell and organ failure. Bleeding must be contained and volume restored if the patient is to live.

Clinical Presentation and Symptoms

The symptoms of acute bleeding vary substantially depending on the amount and how fast the blood is lost. If the blood loss is gradual, thus allowing time (20–60 hours)[4] for the fluid from the extravascular spaces to replace the volume lost, symptoms will be much less severe than if the loss is immediate. Animal studies have shown that primates can survive with hematocrits as low as 0.06 L/L if intravascular volume is maintained at normal levels.[9] The severity of symptoms also depends on the age and cardiac health of the individual. Whereas a young, healthy person can sustain a relatively low blood volume, an older person or one with heart disease cannot mount the cardiac and vascular compensation mechanisms previously discussed. (See Table 20-1 for symptoms of acute blood loss and advancing shock.) When there is less blood, the body tries to aerate and circulate it more quickly by increasing heart and respiration rates. Cold, pale skin results from blood being diverted from the skin.

Laboratory Findings and Correlations with Disease

During the first few hours following an acute bleeding episode, there is usually no reduction in the hemoglobin (Hb) or hematocrit (Hct) until the volume is replaced by extravascular refill or by the addition of intravenous fluids. At first glance, it is difficult to understand how a patient could lose 20% to 30% of their blood volume and have normal hematology values. To illustrate, think of performing a Hct on a full tube of blood anticoagulated with EDTA. Now picture decanting 30% of the blood. The percentage of the blood that is composed of red cells (Hct) would be the same as in the full tube. Now imagine adding saline to replace the 30% that had been discarded, mixing and performing a Hct again; the Hct would be reduced by 30%. Until volume replacement is started, the degree of blood loss must be assessed on clinical signs.

Within 3 to 4 hours after an acute hemorrhage, the Hb and Hct values may begin to decrease, but they will not reach their minimum levels for several days. Also within 3 to 4 hours of hemorrhage, the leukocyte count will usually rise (up to 30×10^9/L) due to epinephrine, causing cells to demarginate from the vessel lining (Chap. 22), and to increased bone marrow release. (See Table 20-2 for laboratory data expected in acute blood loss.)

Lowered oxygen perfusion stimulates erythropoietin (EPO) release, which has several mechanisms to increase the number of circulating red blood cells. EPO causes immature red cells to be released from the bone marrow earlier than expected, which produces a reticulocyte response within several hours after an acute blood loss.[5] EPO also stimulates stem cells to increase the number of erythroid precursors and eventually the number of circulating erythroid cells. As there is no reserve of mature red cells available, it takes 2 to 5 days for the bone marrow

TABLE 20-2
Laboratory Data in Anemias of Blood Loss

	Acute Blood Loss	Chronic Blood Loss Leading to Iron Deficiency
Erythrocytes	Normocytic, normochromic anemia with polychromasia	Microcytic, hypochromic anemia with ↓ MCV, MCH, and MCHC
Leukocytes	Leukocytosis with a left shift (bands and metamyelocytes)	Usually normal
Platelets	Thrombocytosis	Often thrombocytosis
Reticulocytes	↑ to 15% (maximum 10 days after bleeding epidode)	Usually normal or ↓ at diagnosis; ↑ to 10% with iron therapy
Iron studies	Serum ferritin may be ↓ from lost iron	↓ Serum ferritin, ↓ serum Fe, ↑ TIBC
Bone marrow	Erythroid hyperplasia	Small RBC precursors with scant, ragged cytoplasm; absent iron stores
Others	If caused by acute DIC, PT, PTT, and TT usually prolonged; abnormal arterial blood gases	↑ RDW; ↑ FEP; extreme anisocytosis after therapy producing a bi-modal red cell histogram

TIBC = total iron binding capacity; RDW = red cell distribution width; FEP = free erythrocyte protoporphyrin; DIC = disseminated intravascular coagulation; PT = prothrombin time; PTT = partial thromboplastin time; TT = thrombin time.

to produce and release these new red cells.[4] In cases of severe blood loss, nucleated red blood cells may be released to the peripheral blood. If the marrow has adequate iron stores, the reticulocyte count reaches a maximum of 15% in 10 days with the reticulocyte production index (RPI) being greater than 3, an indication of an adequate bone marrow response to anemia (Chap. 9).[6] Bleeding that is not visually evident (*e.g.*, a broken femur or ruptured spleen) may cause an elevated bilirubin from increased internal breakdown of red cells. Unless more specific tests for hemolysis are performed such as haptoglobin or urine hemoglobin, internal bleeding could be mistaken for hemolysis.[5]

Effects of Treatment on Laboratory Results

The initial treatment for acute blood loss is volume replacement with either crystalloids such as saline, or colloids such as albumin, or both.[7] As fluid is replaced in the vessels, the Hb and Hct drop accordingly. Once volume has been restored, assessment for possible transfusion is made. This decision is based on the arterial blood gases to assess peripheral oxygenation, degree of anemia, symptoms, and any additional risk factors such as cardiac or circulatory diseases. Transfusions should be avoided, if possible. Surgical bleeding can sometimes be treated by reinfusing autologous blood. If autologous blood is not available, the amount of allogeneic blood transfused should be limited to that required to relieve symptoms.[8]

Once bleeding is under control, the patient may be given iron to replace what was lost if iron stores are found to be inadequate. Using available iron, the bone marrow can make new red cells. The reticulocyte count should go up dramatically, causing polychromasia to appear on the peripheral blood film. The leukocyte count should return to normal within a few days of a bleeding episode. The Hb, Hct, and all other laboratory values should return to normal within 1 to 2 months.

CHRONIC BLOOD LOSS
Pathophysiology

Chronic blood loss involves smaller volumes of blood escaping from the vessels over a longer period of time. The bone marrow can keep up with this type of loss until iron stores have been exhausted. If bleeding continues, chronic blood loss will result in iron deficiency anemia (Chap. 13). In contrast to acute blood loss in which the volume depletion is the main concern, reduced oxygen-carrying ability is the principal problem in chronic blood loss.

Most iron for Hb production is recycled from the 1% of senescent red cells destroyed by the spleen daily. Chronic red cell loss removes iron from the body thus requiring the body to use, and eventually deplete, stored iron for production of new red cells. Chronic blood loss arises most often from GI bleeding due to ulcers, gastritis, parasites, hemorrhoids, or malignancies and in women, from menstruation and childbirth. One pregnancy can cause the loss of iron equivalent to that of 2 L of blood.[4]

The body compensates for chronic blood loss in some of the same ways it does for acute bleeding by (1) increasing the heart rate; (2) redistributing blood away from the skin; (3) increasing the level of red cell 2,3-DPG, thus reducing Hb affinity for oxygen; and (4) increasing iron absorption.

Clinical Presentation and Symptoms

The reduction in Hb oxygen affinity and other compensatory mechanisms allow an otherwise healthy individual to have quite a low Hb level before symptoms appear. The symptoms are those of any anemia and may not be evident until several months after the bleeding has started. Melena (stool containing dark red or black blood) may be seen with GI bleeding. Other symptoms include pallor, fatigue, inability to concentrate, increased heart rate, headache, and pica (the desire to eat unusual things such as dirt, clay, ice, or cardboard).[4]

Laboratory Findings and Correlations with Disease

Since chronic blood loss leads to iron deficiency, the hematologic findings are the same as those described in Chapter 13 and will only be summarized here in Table 20-2. A decreased serum ferritin and increased total iron-binding capacity (TIBC; Chap. 13), is the earliest indication of chronic blood loss. The Hb, Hct, and red cell count decrease later if chronic blood loss continues without treatment. A positive stool occult blood is also useful in diagnosing GI bleeding.

Effects of Treatment on Laboratory Results

Once the underlying condition is controlled and bleeding is stopped, treatment with oral iron therapy should produce reticulocytosis (5%–10%) within 5 to 10 days.[6] If the patient does not respond to iron therapy with reticulocytosis and a rise in Hb, iron should be discontinued and another cause for the anemia considered. Harmful iron overload can result if anemia resulting from inflammation or chronic disease is treated with iron. Patients with a Hb of less than 7 g/dL may require transfusions, but this should be avoided unless the patient exhibits severe signs of anemia or has evidence of an inability to compensate adequately.[8] Oral iron must be given for a long enough time (up to 12 months) to renew the iron stores.[6]

Once the patient starts to make normal-sized red cells (or has been transfused), a bimodal red cell curve will be evident on the red cell histogram from an automated blood counter (Chap. 42). This dimorphic picture results from normal red cells produced under the influence of the iron therapy being mixed with the microcytic, hypochromic cells. This will also be reflected in an elevated red cell distribution width (RDW).

CHAPTER SUMMARY

Acute and chronic blood loss represent two of the most common and clinically important anemias throughout the world. A significant acute blood loss is a medical emergency with restoration of blood volume and control of bleeding being critical to survival.

During the first few hours after acute blood loss, Hb and Hct values generally remain steady owing to vasoconstriction and other compensatory mechanisms designed to keep blood flowing to the heart and brain. Blood volume must be restored by a shift of extravascular fluid into the vessels, by administration of intravenous electrolyte and/or colloid solutions, or finally with red cell transfusions. A normocytic, normochromic anemia develops with polychromasia and elevated absolute reticulocyte count and RPI.

Chronic blood loss occurs slowly over a longer period of time and is most often associated with excessive gastrointestinal or menstrual bleeding. As the iron stores are depleted, chronic blood loss leads to iron deficiency anemia. The typical laboratory findings are microcytic, hypochromic anemia with decreased serum ferritin and iron and increased TIBC and FEP. Once bleeding is controlled, and iron supplementation begun, the bone marrow will produce and release increased numbers of normal red cells, increasing the reticulocyte count, RPI, RDW, and eventually the Hb and Hct. It can take months for the body to replace iron stores to previous levels.

Case Study 20-1

A CBC was performed on a 68-year-old black male who went to his doctor complaining of recent fatigue. The Hb was 8.0 g/dL; MCV 70 fL; RDW 15.7; peripheral blood film red cell morphology was reported as microcytic and hypochromic.
1. Are these results consistent with chronic blood loss?
2. What is the most common anemia to be expected with this blood picture?
3. What is the most likely cause of the anemia?
4. List two laboratory procedures that could be recommended to confirm the diagnosis.

Case Study 20-2

A patient with a gunshot wound was brought to the emergency room by friends who said the patient had lost "a lot of blood." The CBC collected at admission had a Hb of 14.0 g/dL and a Hct of 0.43 L/L. The patient's bleeding was controlled, and he was stabilized with intravenous fluid replacement. Eight hours after admission the Hb was 9.2 g/dL and the Hct was 0.27 L/L.
1. Are these laboratory values consistent with the patient's clinical condition or was there probably a mistake made in collection or testing of the blood?
2. What would be the expected reticulocyte count at admission and 10 days later?
3. Is it important to calculate the reticulocyte production index (RPI) to assess this patient's recovery after about 10 days? Explain.

Review Questions

20-1. The most immediate problem facing the patient with an acute blood loss of 30% of total blood volume is

    A. loss of oxygen carrying ability.
    B. left shift of oxygen dissociation curve.
    C. shifting of blood away from the skin.
    D. reduced blood volume.

20-2. At the time of diagnosis of chronic blood loss, the red blood cells may usually be described as

    A. microcytic, hypochromic.
    B. microcytic, hyperchromic.
    C. normocytic, normochromic.
    D. macrocytic, hypochromic.

20-3. The laboratory values that would be expected for a patient 5 days after successful treatment for acute or chronic blood loss include a(n)

    A. normal CBC and reticulocyte count.
    B. leukopenia and thrombocytopenia.
    C. increased reticulocyte count with polychromasia.
    D. increased reticulocyte count and increased serum ferritin.

20-4. The laboratory values that would be expected within the first 2 hours following acute blood loss are

    A. a marked decrease in the Hb and Hct.
    B. a normal Hb and Hct.
    C. a marked increase in the Hb and Hct.
    D. any of the above.

References

1. Baker WF, Bick RL: Iron deficiency anemia. In Bick RL: Hematology: Clinical and Laboratory Practice, p 257. St Louis, Mosby, 1993

2. Dronen SC, Birrer P: Shock. In Tintinalli JE, Krome RL, Ruiz E (eds): Emergency Medicine: A Comprehensive Study Guide, 3rd ed, p 132. New York, McGraw-Hill, 1992

3. Guyton AC: Textbook of Medical Physiology, 8th ed. Philadelphia, WB Saunders, 1991

4. Hillman RS: Acute blood loss anemia. In Beutler E, Lichtman MA, Coller BS et al (eds): Williams' Hematology, 5th ed, p 704. New York, McGraw-Hill, 1995

5. Hillman RS, Finch CA: Red Cell Manual, 6th ed, p 69. Philadelphia, FA Davis, 1992

6. Lee GR: Iron deficiency and iron-deficiency anemia. In Lee GR, Bithell TC, Foerster J et al (eds): Wintrobe's Clinical Hematology, 9th ed, p 808. Philadelphia, Lea & Febiger, 1993

7. Littleton M: Shock. In Rea RE (ed): Trauma Nursing Manual, 2nd ed, p IV-3. Chicago, Award Printing, 1988

8. Stowell CP: When to pull the trigger: Making the decision to transfuse red blood cells. Lab Med 26:56, 1995

9. Wilkerson DK, Rosen AL, Sehgal LR et al: Limits of cardiac compensation in anemic baboons. Surgery 103:665, 1988

CHAPTER 21

Systematic Laboratory Evaluation of Erythrocyte Abnormalities

John A. Koepke

The preceding chapters in this section on nonmalignant erythrocyte abnormalities have included detailed discussions of the various types of anemia. With this knowledge in hand, this chapter seeks to put these preceding chapters into perspective. It brings these discussions together for a global understanding of how to evaluate erythrocyte abnormalities from a laboratory standpoint when a disorder is first discovered but has not yet been diagnosed. Both physician and laboratory scientist should have a systematic (and hopefully similar) approach to laboratory evaluation of erythrocyte abnormalities, and they should work together for the patient's benefit.

The value of laboratory studies in the diagnosis of disease is probably best exemplified by the close relationship between hematologic examinations and clinical anemia. Indeed the identification of hematologic abnormalities frequently uses the laboratory characterization of the disorder as the name of the condition. Think, for example, of macrocytic or microcytic anemias, sickle cell anemia, pyruvate kinase deficiency, and many others.

Anemia may result from decreased synthesis of hemoglobin and erythrocytes, increased destruction of erythrocytes, or acute or chronic blood loss. As discussed in Chapter 10, the most useful classification, from a laboratorian's point of view, is based on the red cell measurements, particularly mean corpuscular volume (MCV) and mean corpuscular hemoglobin concentration (MCHC). Dr. Maxwell Wintrobe's pioneering work with the red cell indices was very important in the development of laboratory hematology and in guiding our approach to these problems.[11] These studies are reinforced by the evaluation of red cell morphology on the stained peripheral blood film.

THE PHYSICIAN'S ROLE IN THE DIAGNOSTIC PROCESS

The cause of anemia is identified by integrating clinical information with the results of laboratory studies. The patient's physician plays a key role in evaluating clinical information obtained from the medical history and physical examination, and incorporating erythrocyte measurements, including the reticulocyte count, and sometimes serum iron or ferritin measurements, and bone marrow examination when necessary.[3]

The exact diagnosis may not always be obvious to the physician. More than likely the doctor will note that the patient is somewhat pale and in the subsequent history taking, will seek to discover the possible cause of the anemia. Table 21-1 lists some clues in the patient's history that may suggest specific causes of anemia and, in turn, indicate laboratory tests that may be useful in the diagnostic process.

Similarly, the physical examination may reveal significant clues to the cause of anemia. Table 21-2 lists some of these signs, which the physician will try to identify. Again, other definitive studies may be suggested.

Why does the physician order a blood count in the first place? What can be learned from it? In some cases if the count is to be used as a screening procedure, will the rapid report of a normal or abnormal count suffice? Or is the count being requested to monitor some aspect of the patient's condition? How do anemias affect the composition and morphology of the peripheral blood cells?

The definitive diagnosis of anemia depends, to a greater or lesser extent, on laboratory studies.[4,8–10,12] For many years blood films have been carefully examined in an effort to discover the cause of anemia as well as many other hematologic and systemic disorders. With the development of increasingly sophisticated automated hematologic analyzers, which can, within a minute or two, provide an accurate and precise blood count (including the differential leukocyte count), there has been a tendency to forget the importance of the blood film examination.

It is very useful to use the instruments to make an initial sort of the specimens, separating normal from possibly abnormal specimens. Flagging systems have been developed that can perform this function quite accepta-

TABLE 21-1
Patient History and the Cause of Anemia: Examples of Some Common Associations

History	Associated Anemia
Chronic hepatic, renal, or other diseases (*e.g.,* cancer)	Anemia of chronic disease
Alcoholism	Folate deficiency
Vegetarian diet	Iron deficiency
Bleeding (gastrointestinal, menorrhagia, multiple pregnancies)	Iron deficiency
Exposure to toxic chemicals	Hypoplastic or aplastic anemia
Chronic drug therapy	Megaloblastic, hypoplastic, or aplastic anemia

bly; when such systems are used properly, only flagged specimens require evaluation of the blood film. When trying to find the cause of anemia, very useful clues can be obtained from the blood film by (1) the morphologic review of red cells; (2) the search for concomitant abnormalities in the leukocyte or platelet population; or (3) the finding of evidence such as red cell rouleaux or protein abnormalities.[6]

TABLE 21-2
Physical Signs and the Cause of Anemia: Examples of Some Common Associations

Physical Signs	Associated Anemia
Jaundice (skin, sclerae)	Hemolytic anemia, anemia associated with chronic liver disease
Leg ulcers (black patient)	Sickle cell anemia
Spooned nails	Iron-deficiency anemia
Dark line at base of teeth	Lead toxicity
Neurologic deficit	Megaloblastic (vitamin B_{12}) anemia
Lymph node enlargement	Anemia secondary to lymphoma, leukemia, or infection
Spleen enlargement	Hemolytic anemia, chronic liver disease, leukemia, lymphoma
Liver enlargement	Hemolytic anemia, metastatic carcinoma
Prominent forehead (frontal bossing)	Thalassemia, sickle cell anemia
Bone tenderness	Anemia secondary to myeloma or metastatic carcinoma
Bluish skin color	Methemoglobinemia
Oriental or Mediterranean ethnicity	Thalassemia syndromes

LABORATORY EVALUATION OF ANEMIA

Systematic Approach

About 30 years ago, Dr. William R. Best presented a systematic and logical way to use the laboratory efficiently. He developed a hemolytic anemia "tree" and a hemolysis "tree."[2] (Today the decision tree method is called an *algorithm.*) Figure 21-1 shows a more complete anemia algorithm, which serves as a tool for efficiently arriving at a possible diagnosis by obtaining key laboratory data in a step-by-step fashion. Each question is contingent on the answer to the preceding question, which is also a decision point in the physician's diagnostic thinking. This system, with its many branches, forms a logical approach to the diagnosis of the cause of anemia. The roots of the tree are the basic measurements (hemoglobin, hematocrit, and red cell count) that establish the presence or absence of anemia.

Blood Cell Counting

The basic hematologic laboratory study is the so-called complete blood count (CBC). This study, in all its many variations, includes some measurement of red cells, leukocytes, and platelets. In investigating anemia we may quantitate only the red cell population, or we may measure the oxygen-carrying capacity of the red cells by quantitating hemoglobin. The leukocyte count may be amplified with a differential leukocyte count, performed either with an instrument or by examining a Romanowsky-stained blood film. Thus the blood count may be performed in many different ways.

With the development of rapid, precise, and accurate hematology instruments, blood counts are now even more common. Any evaluation of cost *versus* benefit of care for the patient usually includes scrutiny of this test, since it is so widely used. But its popularity is well justified because so many diseases produce identifiable, if at times nonspecific, changes in the blood count.

The blood count is, in reality, a *panel* of measurements or studies. In the diagnosis of anemia, the hemoglobin and the MCV are the most important parameters. Several measurements of the erythrocytes (*e.g.,* the MCHC or the RDW[1]), better serve as quality control checks within the laboratory and need not be routinely reported.[5]

Conceivably blood cell counting could be revamped to meet patient care needs better. There is a basic premise for the most efficient use of currently available instrumentation. That is, if a carefully chosen set of quantitative and qualitative parameters are found to be within a prescribed set of limits, additional studies probably are not necessary and significant abnormalities are not likely to be found on a blood film. If such studies are not done, significant savings can be realized and laboratory scientists' efforts can be devoted to more useful work.[5]

If anemia is present, the next logical question is whether it represents a hemolytic or a nonhemolytic process. The reticulocyte count, which is a count of the red cells most recently released from the bone marrow, has served as a simple yet useful test to answer this question.

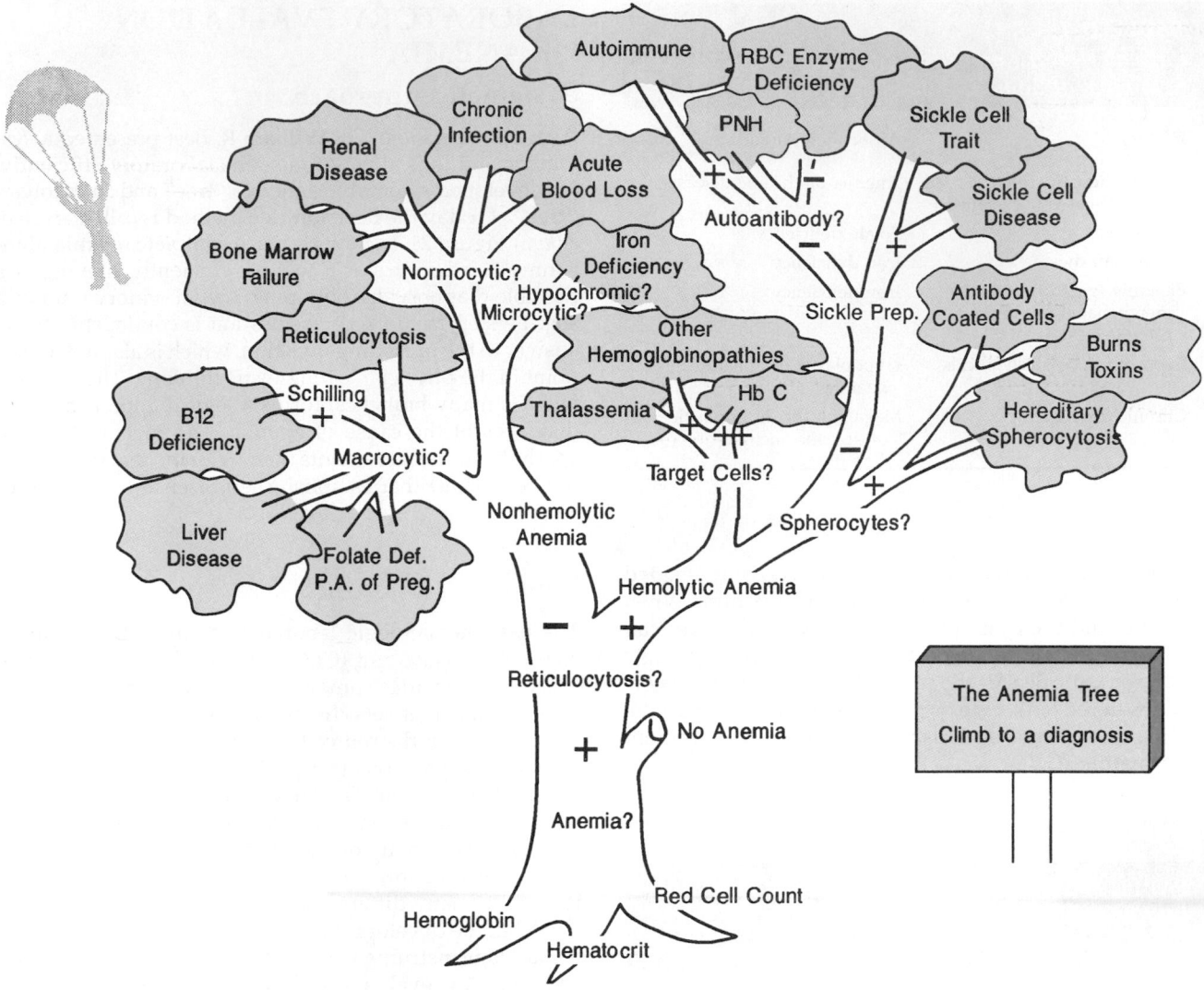

FIGURE 21-1. Following the branches of the anemia tree leads the physician and laboratorian to possible causes of anemia of unknown origin. P. A. of Preg = pernicious anemia of pregnancy.

If a hemolytic process is causing the anemia, increased numbers of reticulocytes should be found in the blood. Various estimates of reticulocyte production, particularly in the face of anemia, are being used with good effect on the diagnostic and therapeutic processes. Examples of such measurements include the absolute reticulocyte count (Chap. 9) and an exciting new parameter called the immature reticulocyte fraction (IRF). The IRF is measured by several flow cytometric reticulocyte counters. It has been described as the "left shifted" reticulocyte count and has been found to be clinically useful in following chemotherapy, erythropoietin therapy, and marrow failure.

The Blood Film Evaluation

At this level of our "tree climbing," the time-honored blood film examination is employed in an effort to discover additional clues that may be helpful. A useful discussion of this sometimes neglected evaluation has recently been published and the interested reader is

encouraged to study this evaluation.[8] Other laboratory tests (*e.g.*, the solubility test for sickling hemoglobin; Chap. 14) may be suggested at this level before the definitive diagnosis is achieved. Each chapter details the peripheral blood film changes associated with the various anemias that are discussed.

The Bone Marrow Examination

A final important hematologic test in the diagnosis of anemia is the bone marrow examination. In the most general sense, any patient with anemia is a candidate for a marrow study. The cause of an unexplained anemia may become evident after a careful study of the bone marrow, but there has been a significant decline in the number of marrow studies that are performed to investigate anemia. Formerly many anemic patients underwent marrow aspiration routinely as part of their diagnostic workup, but it is evident that little additional information is provided by a bone marrow study, for example, in hemolytic anemia. Patients with possible iron deficiency anemia may require an assessment of marrow iron stores; however, the development of peripheral blood assays for serum iron and ferritin allows more efficient estimation of iron stores without bone marrow aspiration or biopsy.

Special studies such as bone marrow biopsy tissue sections or special stains for microorganisms such as those found in histoplasmosis infections may provide specific diagnoses in some cases.

EPILOGUE

Viewers of Figure 21-1 may wonder just why the man is descending in a parachute. As I remember it, Dr. Best, at the end of a presentation, asked whether anyone had wondered why the parachutist was included. He explained that it certainly was possible for the parachutist to land on the proper branch (*i.e.,* the correct diagnosis) but that his chances of hitting that exact branch were not very good. Consequently, he proposed that the use of the logical approach, climbing from the ground up, constitutes a more efficient way of arriving at the correct diagnosis.

References

1. Bessman JD, Gilmer PR, Gardner FH: Improved classification of anemia by MCV and RDW. Am J Clin Pathol 80:332, 1983
2. Best WR: Differential diagnosis of hemolytic anemias. In Sunderman FW, Sunderman RW Jr (eds): Hemoglobin—Its Precursors and Metabolites, p 307. Philadelphia, JB Lippincott, 1964
3. Dacie JW, Lewis SM: Use of haematological techniques in clinical work. In Dacie JW, Lewis SM: Practical Haematology, 6th ed, p 132. Edinburgh, Churchill Livingstone, 1984
4. de Gruchy GC: General principles in the diagnosis and treatment of anaemia. In de Gruchy GC: Clinical Haematology, 4th ed, p 59. Oxford, Blackwell Scientific, 1978
5. Koepke JA, Bull BS: The intralaboratory control of quality. In Lewis SM, Koepke JA (eds): Hematology Laboratory Management and Practice, p 183. Oxford, Butterworth-Heinemann, 1995
6. Koepke JA, Dotson MA, Shifman MA et al: A flagging system for multichannel hematology analyzers. Blood Cells 11:113, 1985
7. Koepke JA, Koepke JF: Hematologic problems—Anemia. In Koepke JA, Koepke JF: Guide to Clinical Laboratory Diagnosis, 3rd ed, p 148. Norwalk, CT, Appleton and Lange, 1987
8. Shively JA: Interpretive aspects of hematology tests with a focus on the blood film. In Lewis SM, Koepke JA (eds): Hematology Laboratory Management and Practice, p 12. Oxford, Butterworth-Heinemann, 1995
9. van Assendelft OW: Interpretation of the quantitative blood cell count. In Koepke JA (ed): Practical Laboratory Hematology, p 61. New York, Churchill Livingstone, 1991
10. Wheby MS: Using a clinical laboratory in the diagnosis of anemia. Med Clin North Am 50:1689, 1966
11. Wintrobe MM: The erythrocyte in man. Medicine 9:195, 1930
12. Wintrobe MM: The diagnostic and therapeutic approach to hematologic problems. In Lee GR, Bithell TC, Foerster J et al (eds): Wintrobe's Clinical Hematology, 9th ed, p 3. Philadelphia, Lea & Febiger, 1993

PART IV

The Leukocytes

CHAPTER 22

The Phagocytic Leukocytes—Morphology, Kinetics, and Function

Louann W. Lawrence

Objectives

1. List and describe the morphologic characteristics of the five principal types of leukocytes that normally circulate in peripheral blood.
2. List criteria for identification of leukocytes and compare the relative usefulness of each criterion.
3. Describe the origin, kinetics, and function of each of the phagocytic leukocytes.
4. Name, describe, and recognize each of the six stages of neutrophil maturation.
5. Recognize which leukocyte stages are normally found in the storage and/or mitotic pools.
6. Differentiate between marginal and circulating pools of leukocytes.
7. Describe the relationship of the mast cell to the basophil and the macrophage to the monocyte.

INTRODUCTION TO THE LEUKOCYTES

The terms *leukocyte* and *white blood cell* are used synonymously to refer to the colorless nucleated cells that circulate in peripheral blood and function as the body's main line of defense against foreign invaders such as bacteria, viruses, and other foreign antigens. In peripheral blood they are present in much smaller numbers than erythrocytes, and they are transported by way of the peripheral blood to areas where they enter the tissues and perform their functions.

Kinetics

Our knowledge of leukocytes is not as extensive as that of erythrocytes. Leukocytes spend a relatively short time in the peripheral blood. The term *kinetics* refers to the dynamic forces that move cells into and out of different body compartments or tissues. Leukocytes are found in three different compartments in the body: bone marrow,

TABLE 22-1
Leukocyte Classification

GRANULOCYTES	NONGRANULOCYTES
Neutrophils	Monocytes
Eosinophils	Lymphocytes
Basophils	
POLYMORPHONUCLEAR	**MONONUCLEAR**
Neutrophils	Monocytes
Eosinophils	Lymphocytes
Basophils	
PHAGOCYTES	**IMMUNOCYTES**
Neutrophils	Lymphocytes
Eosinophils	
Basophils	
Monocytes	

peripheral blood, and tissues. When we examine and count leukocytes in a peripheral blood sample, we are looking at only a small fraction of the body's total leukocyte population. Blood vessels serve principally as a transport system to get the leukocytes to the tissues where most of their functions are carried out. The kinetics of each leukocyte are discussed in more detail later in this chapter and in Chapter 23.

Classification

Five principal types of leukocytes normally circulate in peripheral blood: neutrophils, eosinophils, basophils, monocytes, and lymphocytes. Several different criteria may be used to classify leukocytes (Table 22-1). According to *granularity*, leukocytes may be classified as granulocytes (neutrophils, eosinophils, basophils) and nongranulocytes (monocytes and lymphocytes). The granulocytes contain distinct granules in their cytoplasm, whereas the nongranulocytes lack prominent granules. This classification is not very satisfactory, because the so-called nongranulocytes do, in fact, contain granules (all monocytes contain small, indistinct granules and certain subtypes of lymphocytes contain large azure granules); however,

TABLE 22-2
Criteria for Leukocyte Identification

1. Cell size
2. Nucleus-cytoplasm ratio
   a. High ratio: Nucleus occupies most of cell area with only a small rim of cytoplasm.
   b. Low ratio: Nucleus is small in relation to volume of cytoplasm.
3. Cytoplasm characteristics
   a. Color of background cytoplasm
   b. Presence or absence of granules
   c. Color and size of granules
4. Nuclear characteristics
   a. Shape
   b. Color
   c. Chromatin pattern
   d. Presence or absence of nucleoli

their granules are not their primary identifying characteristic. Another morphologic classification is based on *nuclear segmentation*. Polymorphonuclear cells (neutrophils, eosinophils, basophils) contain a multilobed or segmented nucleus in their mature form, while mononuclear cells (monocytes and lymphocytes) contain a nucleus that may be variable in shape but is a single mass, not segmented. Again, this is not a very satisfactory classification, because the nuclei of immature polymorphonuclear cells are not segmented and because basophil nuclei do not necessarily segment. The third classification system, which is based on the *function* of the cells, divides them into phagocytes and immunocytes. In this text the latter classification system is used. In this chapter, the phagocytic leukocytes (neutrophils, eosinophils, basophils, monocytes) will be discussed, and in Chapter 23 the immune leukocytes (lymphocytes).

Morphology

The major routine method for studying the morphology of leukocytes is the stained peripheral blood film. The use of a Romanowsky-type stain, such as Wright stain, allows for the classification of leukocytes by their various reactions to the different dyes in the stain. (See Chap. 3 for additional discussion of blood film staining.)

Table 22-2 contains a list of criteria for the identification of leukocytes. A competent morphologist keeps these criteria in mind and uses as many as possible when attempting to identify any leukocyte. The most valuable and reliable criterion, especially for deciding whether a cell is mature or immature, is the nuclear chromatin pattern. Several stages of chromatin maturity have been described. Euchromatin denotes immaturity and is characteristic of blast cells. It appears finely granular and is distributed uniformly, with very few if any tiny aggregates (Fig. 22-1). The amount of heterochromatin increases with maturity. It appears as coarse, granular areas forming medium-sized to large aggregates or clumps that are

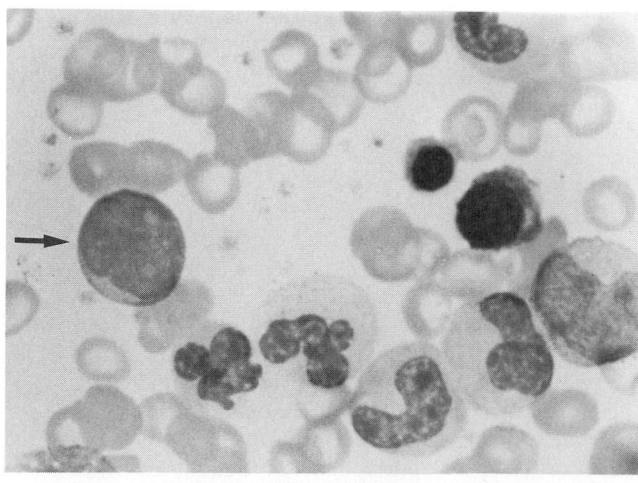

FIGURE 22-1. Differences in chromatin pattern. Compare the appearance of the chromatin pattern in the blast nucleus (*arrow*) to that in the surrounding, more differentiated cells. Note how the chromatin clumping increased between the neutrophil band forms and the segmented form. Note the denseness of the chromatin in the two red cell precursors.

irregularly distributed. Parachromatin, the nonstaining or clear areas between the chromatin clumps, becomes more prominent as cells mature.[25]

The nuclear:cytoplasmic ratio may be used to identify mature cells, but it varies in dividing cells, depending on where the cell happens to be in the mitotic cycle. Because color can vary with each staining system, it is the least reliable criterion for cell identification. Nuclear shape is also a relatively poor criterion, as it is highly susceptible to artifacts and can change considerably in disease states. It is helpful to compare easily identified cells on the same slide with those that are more difficult to identify. One must also keep in mind that cell maturation is an ongoing process and that different stages of cell maturation evolve from one stage to the next rather than in a stepwise process, so that a specific cell may demonstrate characteristics of two maturation stages. A cell may lack one or more of the identification criteria for a particular stage; therefore, the competent morphologist uses as many features as possible to make the best decision.

A brief description of each cell as it appears under light microscopy on Romanowsky-stained films follows.[24] Detailed descriptions of each cell type are presented later in this chapter and in subsequent chapters. The reference ranges listed below are for adults and should be considered as examples only.[19] Reference ranges must be established by each individual laboratory and may vary slightly.

Neutrophil, Segmented

Color Plate 22-1
Synonyms: Seg, polymorphonuclear neutrophil, poly, PMN
Diameter: 10 to 15 μm
Nucleus: Segmented into two to five lobes (some references regard 2–4 lobes as normal); lobes are connected by a threadlike filament that does not contain chromatin. Nuclear chromatin is dark purple and forms densely stained clumps separated by a network of lighter purple bands.
Cytoplasm: Stains light pink with numerous specific or secondary granules that are too small to be resolved individually with the light microscope and give the cytoplasm a grainy appearance. A few purple primary granules may remain visible.
Reference Range:
Relative, 37% to 77%
Absolute, 2.0 to 6.93 $\times$ 10^9/L

Neutrophil, Band

Color Plate 22-2
Synonyms: Nonsegmented neutrophil, neutrophil staff or stab
Diameter: 10 to 15 μm
Nucleus: Elongated, curved, or sausage-shaped with rounded ends and areas of dense clumping at each pole. The beginning of segmentation may be apparent, but the connecting band between lobes is wide enough to reveal two distinct margins surrounding nuclear material. Filaments are not present.
Cytoplasm: Identical to that of segmented neutrophil
Reference Range:
Relative, 0% to 11%
Absolute, 0 to 0.87 $\times$ 10^9/L

Eosinophil

Color Plate 22-3
Synonyms: Eo, acidophil
Diameter: 12 to 16 μm
Nucleus: Dark purple; chromatin pattern similar to neutrophil; usually band-shaped or segmented into only two lobes, occasionally more.
Cytoplasm: Filled with large, spherical, refractive granules of uniform size that stain bright orange-pink. The granules are usually evenly distributed but rarely overlie the nucleus.
Reference Range:
Relative, 1% to 7%
Absolute, 0.05 to 0.67 $\times$ 10^9/L

Basophil

Color Plate 22-4
Synonym: Baso
Diameter: 10 to 14 μm
Nucleus: Light purple staining; may be round, indented, band-shaped, or lobulated. Often difficult to see because of overlying granules. Chromatin pattern is smudged and indistinct.
Cytoplasm: Characterized by densely stained, dark violet to purple-black granules that are variable in size and unevenly distributed. Because the granules are water soluble, only vestiges of granules may be found, and sometimes granules are contained within small vacuoles.
Reference Range:
Relative, 0% to 1.6%
Absolute, 0 to 0.20 $\times$ 10^9/L

Monocyte

Color Plates 22-5 and 22-6
Synonyms: Mono, mononuclear phagocyte
Diameter: 12 to 22 μm
Nucleus: Highly variable in shape; may be round, horseshoe-shaped or lobulated, and usually shows some degree of folding or convolutions. Chromatin is light purple and arranged in loose strands or lacy pattern.
Cytoplasm: Abundant (*i.e.*, nuclear:cytoplasmic ratio is low). Dull, pale, faded, gray-blue; containing fine, indistinct granules giving it a ground-glass appearance. Cell outline may be irregular with occasional pseudopods, and occasional vacuoles may be seen.
Reference Range:
Relative, 2% to 10%
Absolute, 0.3 to 0.90 $\times$ 10^9/L

Normal Lymphocyte

Color Plates 22-7 and 22-8
Synonym: Lymph
Diameter: Small, 6 to 8 μm; medium to large, 8 to 15 μm
Nucleus: Deep purple, compact, densely packed clumps or blocks of chromatin with linear areas of parachromatin. Nucleoli may be visible. Shape may be round, oval, or indented.
Cytoplasm: Ranges from sparse in the smaller forms to abundant in the larger forms. Stains pale to bright sky blue. May contain a few prominent reddish (azurophilic) granules. May be indented by surrounding red cells.
Reference Range:
Relative, 10% to 44%
Absolute, 0.6 to 3.44 $\times$ 10^9/L

Variant Lymphocyte

Color Plates 25-1 and 25-2
Synonyms: Reactive, atypical, stimulated lymphocytes (Chap. 25)
Diameter: Highly variable, 10 to 22 μm
Nucleus: May range from extremely dense to pale and immature-looking; nucleoli may be visible; chromatin may be lumpy or blocked with clearer areas of parachromatin.
Cytoplasm: Usually abundant and ranges in staining intensity from deeply basophilic to pale blue; often appears foamy, or even frankly vacuolated.
Reference Range:
Relative, 0% to 7.5%
Absolute, 0 to 0.66 $\times$ 10^9/L

THE NEUTROPHIL

Morphology

The neutrophil is the most common leukocyte in normal peripheral blood. In the mature form it is easily recognized on a Romanowsky-stained blood film by its distinctive segmented nucleus and pinkish purple or pinkish tan granules in the cytoplasm. Six stages in the maturation of this cell have been defined. They are, from least to most mature, myeloblast, promyelocyte, myelocyte, metamyelocyte, band and segmented form. Collectively they are called the granulocytic or neutrophilic maturation series. The term *granulocytic* is often used synonymously with neutrophilic, but technically, granulocytic refers to eosinophils and basophils, as well as neutrophils. Eosinophils and basophils undergo the same maturation stages as neutrophils, but immature forms are rarely seen in the peripheral blood. It is important to be able to recognize the immature forms of the neutrophil because they are seen in peripheral blood in many conditions. In addition, the ability to differentiate these cells in bone marrow specimens is a necessary skill in many laboratories.

MYELOBLAST

The earliest recognizable form that can be identified by light microscopy as a cell that will mature into one of the myeloid cells is the myeloblast (see Color Plate 22-9). This cell has dark to light blue cytoplasm that contains no visible granules. The nucleus is made up of a smooth, delicate, uniformly distributed chromatin pattern sometimes described as lacy. Myeloblasts usually have two or more distinct nucleoli, which disappear as the cell matures. The nucleus occupies most of the cell, leaving only a small rim of cytoplasm. This is referred to as a high nuclear:cytoplasmic ratio. The approximate cell diameter is 15 to 20 μm, depending on what stage in the mitotic cycle it is in. Cells become relatively larger just prior to mitotic division. Myeloblasts make up about 1% to 2% of the cells in normal bone marrow and normally are not seen in peripheral blood.

The French-American-British (FAB) Cooperative Group introduced a modified definition of myeloblasts, which they believe may be more useful clinically in defining some hematologic disease states.[3,21] The cells are sometimes referred to as type I and type II myeloblasts. Type I is identical to the cell described in the previous paragraph, with no granules in the cytoplasm. Type II blasts have a few (up to 20) primary (azurophilic) granules in their cytoplasm. Their other characteristics are similar to those of the type I blasts, except that their nuclear:cytoplasmic ratio tends to be lower and the nucleus remains in a central position. They do not contain numerous cytoplasmic granules as does the promyelocyte, which is described in the next section (see Color Plate 22-10 and Chap. 34 for further descriptions and pictures of these two forms). A few authors also recognize a type III blast which has greater than 20 granules and a centrally located nucleus (*i.e.*, it does not become a promyelocyte until the nucleus becomes eccentric). Slight differences from one morphologist to another in identifying the various maturation stages are inevitable.

Most morphologists are very cautious in differentiating among types of blasts (myeloblasts, monoblasts, lymphoblasts). When using only light microscopy and Romanowsky stains they have such similar characteristics that it is difficult to distinguish among them. In leukemic diseases when blasts are seen in abundance in the peripheral blood and bone marrow, the use of cytochemical stains or immunologic cell markers helps to distinguish from which cell line the blasts arise. (Chaps. 29 and 34.) The best rule when attempting to identify very immature cells on a peripheral blood film stained with Wright or a comparable type of stain is to identify the cell as a blast without attempting to distinguish its cell line. It is best to be aware of the limits of light microscopy and of the availability of more definitive methods of cell identification.

PROMYELOCYTE

The morphologic definition of a promyelocyte (also known as progranulocyte) is difficult. A majority of morphologists in this country will place a cell in the promyelocyte stage at the first appearance of cytoplasmic granules. However, if attempting to classify a leukemia according the FAB criteria, the so-called type II blast should not be classified as a promyelocyte. It was once thought that promyelocytes could mature into any of the three granulocytes (neutrophil, eosinophil, or basophil), hence the term progranulocyte. It is now known that the cell is committed at a much earlier stage, perhaps during the stage that is recognizable as a blast, to becoming either an eosinophil, basophil, or neutrophil.

The promyelocyte is characterized by large, prominent, reddish purple granules in the cytoplasm called primary or azurophilic granules (see Color Plate 22-11). The background cytoplasm remains dark blue to blue, and the nucleus still appears fairly immature with a uniform, evenly distributed chromatin pattern. Nucleoli may or may not be visible. As the cell matures, the nucleus may be displaced off center and the nuclear:cytoplasmic ratio decreases. This cell is still rather large and may sometimes appear larger than the myeloblast, depending on its stage in the mitotic cycle. Promyelocytes make up 2% to 5% of nucleated cells in the bone marrow and normally are not found in the peripheral blood.

Synthesis of primary granules begins and ends during this stage. As the cell continues to divide, primary granules are diluted among daughter cells. These granules, which are rich in the enzyme myeloperoxidase, are present in all stages including the mature segmented neutrophil, but they become less visible with Wright or a comparable stain.

MYELOCYTE

Myelocytes begin to form a second set of granules referred to as secondary or specific granules. The primary granules become less visible as the secondary granules are being formed, thus cells in this stage may have varying amounts of each type of granule. Some investigators have proposed subdividing this stage into early and late, but it is not usually done because the distinction is not clinically relevant. Secondary granules are smaller and not resolved by most light microscopes and are the granules that eventually fill the cell and give it its characteristic pinkish tan color (see Color Plate 22-12). The cytoplasm of the cell begins to lose cytoplasmic RNA (blue color), but a tinge of blue may remain, especially along the edges of the cell. As the pinkish specific granules begin to form in the Golgi region of the cell, a pink arc may be seen, which is sometimes called the "dawn of neutrophilia." The nucleus becomes more condensed and the chromatin pattern clumped; nucleoli usually are no longer visible. The nuclear:cytoplasmic ratio continues to decrease. The cell size ranges from 16 to 24 μm. Myelocytes are the last stage to undergo mitosis. Cells in subsequent stages continue to mature but do not divide. Neutrophilic myelocytes make up approximately 10% to 20% of nucleated marrow cells and normally are not seen in peripheral blood.

The secondary granules contain lysozyme, acid hydrolases, and a variety of other proteins but not peroxidase. The secondary granule contents and their functions are discussed in the section on neutrophil biochemistry.

METAMYELOCYTE

The cell next matures into a metamyelocyte (also called a *juvenile*), and the shape of the nucleus becomes the chief identification criterion. Until this stage the nucleus has remained round or oval, but now it begins to flatten on one side and to constrict or indent (becoming kidney bean or peanut shaped) (see Color Plate 22-13). Nuclear chromatin condenses even more to become coarsely

clumped. The cytoplasm has lost all traces of blue color (RNA) and appears uniformly pink with pinkish purple secondary granules evenly distributed, much as in the cytoplasm of the mature cell. Metamyelocytes make up approximately 15% to 30% of nucleated marrow cells and normally are not found in the peripheral blood. To differentiate this stage from the next more mature stage (the band), the indentation of the nucleus must be less than half the width of the nucleus.

BAND OR STAB CELL

This is the last stage before the mature cell. Bands are normally present in a small percentage in peripheral blood. Probably the greatest source of variation and discrepancy in leukocyte morphology is identification of the band form. Because an increase in bands in peripheral blood can be clinically relevant, it is important to try to standardize criteria for band identification, at least within an institution. Extremes in band definitions range from "a cell is a band unless a filament is seen between segments" (normals range from 12%–18%) to "if it is indented over two thirds of the total width of the band at its widest point, it is no longer a band" (normals range from 0%–5%). In an attempt to standardize band definitions the College of American Pathologists Survey Committee makes the following recommendation: "Any mature cell of the granulocytic series which has a curved, band-shaped nucleus which has *not* developed a threadlike filament, shall be called a band. If any nuclear chromatin is seen in the bridge between the lobes, then the bridge is not a filament and the cell is a band." The committee also recommends, "Any cell in which the nucleus is so twisted that the entire outline of the nucleus is not visible, due to superimposition of one part of the nucleus upon the other parts, shall be classified as a poly (segmented neutrophil)."[7] These criteria have also been adopted by the National Committee for Clinical Laboratory Standards (NCCLS).[24] By these criteria normal values range from 5% to 10%. Most clinical laboratories use these criteria but still may have discrepancies due to individual judgment and personal interpretation of each cell. Laboratories should develop quality control and training programs to keep band criteria standardized among their own personnel to aid in identifying clinically relevant increases in band forms.

SEGMENTED NEUTROPHIL

This cell gets its name from the characteristic shape of the nucleus. (Refer to morphologic description and adult reference range in the introduction section of this chapter.) Children normally have lower relative numbers of segmented neutrophils; however, since their total leukocyte counts tend to be higher than adults, the absolute values are very similar (3.0–4.0 $\times$ 10^9/L).[29]

Kinetics

LIFE SPAN AND POOLS

The life span of the neutrophil is approximately 9 or 10 days from myeloblast to death. The cell spends its life in three main areas of the body, passing from bone marrow to peripheral blood and into the tissues. The movement does not reverse, *i.e.*, neutrophils do not go back into the

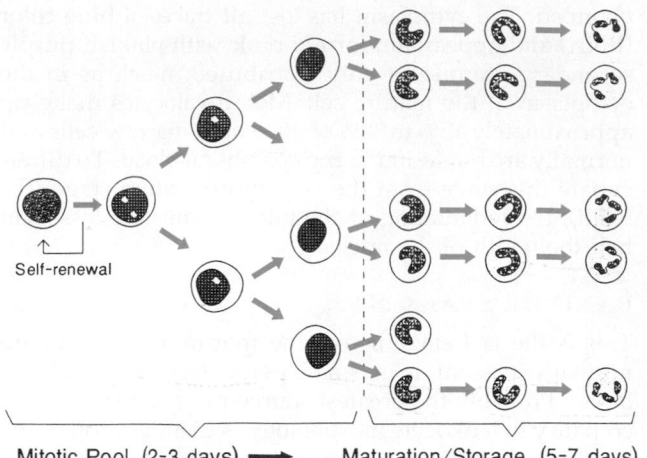

Mitotic Pool (2-3 days) ⟶ Maturation/Storage (5-7 days)

FIGURE 22-2. Bone marrow pools or compartments. Cells capable of division (stem cells, blasts, promyelocytes, and myelocytes) are in the mitotic pool. Nondividing cells (metamyelocytes, bands, and segmented forms) are in the maturation or storage pool.

blood after entering the tissues. In the bone marrow the cells can be pictured as in two separate pools: (1) mitotic and (2) maturation and storage (Fig. 22-2). The mitotic pool contains myeloblasts, promyelocytes, and myelocytes. The maturation and storage pool contains metamyelocytes, bands, and segmented neutrophils. It has been estimated that the cells stay in the mitotic pool for 2 or 3 days and undergo four or five cell divisions. Cells spend 5 to 7 days in the maturation and storage pool, no longer undergoing division but progressively maturing. Under certain reactive or stressful conditions, maturation time may be shortened, divisions may be skipped, and release into the blood may occur prematurely. Appearance of immature neutrophils in the peripheral blood is sometimes referred to as a "shift to the left." During infections, transit time from myelocyte stage to mature cells in the blood may be as short as 48 hours.[1]

Neutrophils move into the peripheral blood, where they remain only 6 to 10 hours before passing into the

tissues, where they perform their principal function and die a short time later. While in the blood they are continuously and rapidly exchanged between two intravascular pools, the circulating and marginated pools (Fig. 22-3). At any one time approximately half of blood neutrophils are not circulating freely but are adhering to vessel walls. These make up the marginated neutrophil pool (MNP). Shifts may occur during stress or exercise or after epinephrine is administered. Such movements from the MNP to the circulating neutrophil pool (CNP) cause transient leukocytosis. This may account for the elevated leukocyte count obtained from a fearful, crying child or an adult in a stressful situation. The value may be normal when it is checked under calmer conditions.[5]

If large numbers of granulocytes are removed experimentally by leukapheresis or by administration of a test dose of endotoxin, mature granulocytes are promptly released into the circulating blood from the marrow neutrophil reserve. This response is similar to the body's response to infection or trauma. In the first 1 or 2 hours the granulocyte count drops then rises by 3.0 to 5.0 × 10⁹ mature cells per liter within about 4 to 5 hours. The initial drop is due to a shift of cells from the CNP to the MNP. The subsequent rise is due to a reversal of this shift as well as to cells being released from the marrow storage pool. The marrow pool is estimated to contain a 4- to 10-day supply of cells. Recent studies suggest that granulocytes are released from the marrow on a first in–first out basis.[1] The more mature cells are released first, probably owing to specific surface receptors that are only contained on mature cells.[18] The higher ratio of band to segmented cells in the marrow as compared to the peripheral blood also supports selective release of segmented cells.[30]

Normally, neutrophils leave the blood and enter the tissues randomly with no relation to how long they have been circulating. They leave by the process of diapedesis, in which they squeeze between junctions in the endothelial cells of vessel walls (see Fig. 22-3). The production rate of neutrophils is an estimated 1.63 × 10⁹ cells per kilogram body weight per day, which enter and leave the blood.[1] This production can increase dramatically in response to inflammatory stimuli.

Little is known about the cells after they move into

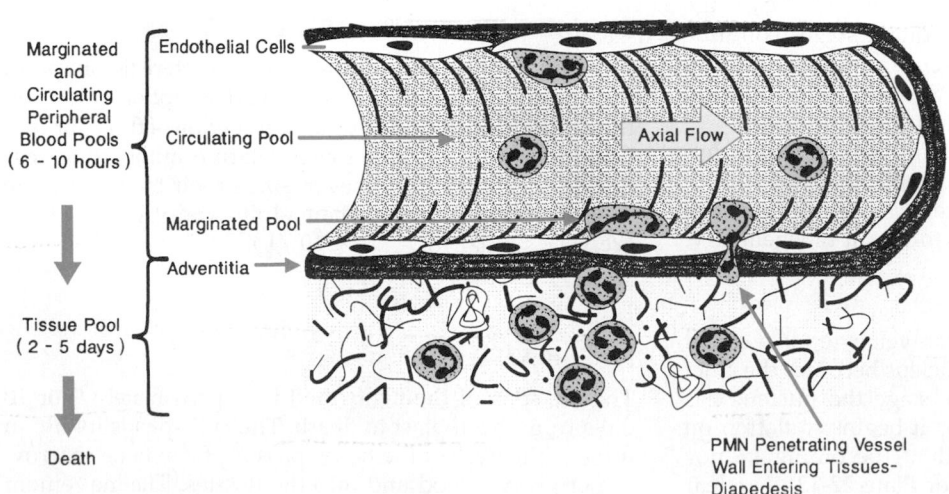

Marginated and Circulating Peripheral Blood Pools (6 - 10 hours)

Endothelial Cells

Circulating Pool

Axial Flow

Marginated Pool

Adventitia

Tissue Pool (2 - 5 days)

Death

PMN Penetrating Vessel Wall Entering Tissues- Diapedesis

FIGURE 22-3. Neutrophil transit from marrow to tissues. The circulating blood has two neutrophil pools: those cells that are circulating (CNP) and those that are adhering to capillary endothelial cells (marginated or MNP).

the tissues. Neutrophils normally migrate into the lung, oral cavity, gastrointestinal tract, liver, and spleen.[1] Their life span is thought to be short because they survive only 2 to 3 days in tissue cultures. If they are not utilized in an area of inflammation or infection they may leave the body by way of secretions in the bronchi or gastrointestinal tract, or in urine. They may die in the tissues, or may be destroyed by other phagocytic cells (monocytes or macrophages).

REGULATORY MECHANISM

Although the details of regulation of maturation of stem cells into mature neutrophils are not clearly understood, hemopoietic growth factors play a major role in this process. These humoral factors are thought to act in a manner similar to erythropoietin on regulation of erythrocyte production. Local control of stem cells by surrounding tissue in the bone marrow (hematopoietic microenvironment) may also play a part in granulocyte regulation. Current evidence suggests that at least four growth factors influence neutrophil maturation and production: granulocyte-monocyte colony-stimulating factor (GM-CSF), granulocyte-colony stimulating factor (G-CSF), interleukin-3 (IL-3), and stem cell factor (*c-kit* ligand or KL).[1] Neutrophils possess specific membrane receptors at various stages of development through which they communicate with these growth factors. GM-CSF influences the production of monocytes and eosinophils also, while G-CSF stimulates only the production of neutrophils. IL-3 and stem cell factor both influence multipotent stem cells early in development and are not specific for neutrophils. G-CSF plays a critical role in regulation of neutrophil production. Studies with animals have shown that administration of antibodies to G-CSF leads to severe neutropenia. Prominent sources of these factors are blood monocytes and macrophages, activated T lymphocytes, endothelial cells, and fibroblasts. As part of the inflammatory response, macrophages and T lymphocytes are activated and release CSFs and other cytokines that cause endothelial and mesenchymal cells to release additional CSFs. Bacterial endotoxins and phagocytosis of bacteria also stimulate increased release of CSFs. These CSFs stimulate marrow production of neutrophils. When the inflammatory stimulus or the microorganisms are contained, the stimulus for CSF production is decreased and neutrophil production returns to normal.

Biochemistry

ENERGY PRODUCTION

The principal biochemical pathway to produce energy in the neutrophil is anaerobic glycolysis (Embden-Meyerhof pathway; Chap. 6). The hexose monophosphate shunt is also active in circulating leukocytes, but it accounts for less than 5% of the glucose consumed. Both pathways are stimulated to increase activity during phagocytosis. This is called a *respiratory* or *metabolic burst* and it plays a role in the killing of microorganisms and detoxification of the cell.[4]

GRANULE CONTENTS

The granules of neutrophils contain enzymes, most of which aid the cell in successfully killing bacteria. The primary or azurophilic granules which first appear in the promyelocyte stage contain myeloperoxidase, lysozyme (muramidase), proteases, and bactericidal cationic proteins. Myeloperoxidase, together with hydrogen peroxide and a halide, aids in killing phagocytosed bacteria. Even though primary granules are not visible in the mature neutrophil, their contents are still present, as evidenced by the positive peroxidase staining of the mature neutrophil. Lysozyme is capable of degrading glycopeptides and hydrolyzing carbohydrates that are constituents of the cell wall of some bacteria. There is evidence of its presence in both primary and secondary granules. Monocytes also contain lysozyme in their granules, in larger quantities than neutrophils.[26]

Secondary granules contain lysozyme, lactoferrin, specific collagenases, plasminogen activator, and vitamin B_{12}-binding proteins, but no peroxidase. Lactoferrin is an iron-binding glycoprotein that competes with bacteria for iron, possibly inhibiting growth. It also may promote neutrophil adherence to endothelial cells.[26]

Alkaline phosphatase is an enzyme in neutrophils that is used as an aid in diagnosis of certain hematologic disorders (Chaps. 29 and 35). It was previously thought to be a component of secondary neutrophilic granules, but more recent studies have determined its location to be in a cytoplasmic organelle that is slightly less dense than the secondary granules. These organelles first appear during the late myelocyte stage, which corresponds with the appearance of alkaline phosphatase in the cell.[2] Although its function *in vivo* is not known for certain, the amount of enzyme activity tends to increase when cellular metabolism increases.

Function

PHAGOCYTOSIS

The overall purpose of the neutrophil is to protect against infection. This function is quite separate from, but interrelated with, the protective function of the other leukocytes. The main mechanism used by the neutrophil is phagocytosis, which is the process of locating, ingesting, and killing bacteria and other foreign invaders. For discussion purposes this process is divided into five steps: motility, recognition, ingestion, degranulation, and killing (Fig. 22-4).

Motility. During locomotion, neutrophils acquire a distinct asymmetric shape that resembles a hand mirror. The "glass" of the mirror is formed by pseudopods and moves in a wavelike motion, or "ruffles," as it moves forward. The "handle" is a narrow tail of cytoplasm that seems to drag behind. The pseudopods that are formed during locomotion are filled with filament networks, which are polymers of actin, a muscle protein. Another muscle protein, myosin, also is present, and it catalyzes hydrolysis of adenosine triphosphate (ATP) to provide energy for the contraction of the actin fibers.[26] Neutrophils increase their glycolytic rate during locomotion and ingestion, in

Chemotaxis:
a. Directed motility   b. Diapedesis   c. Recognition and ingestion

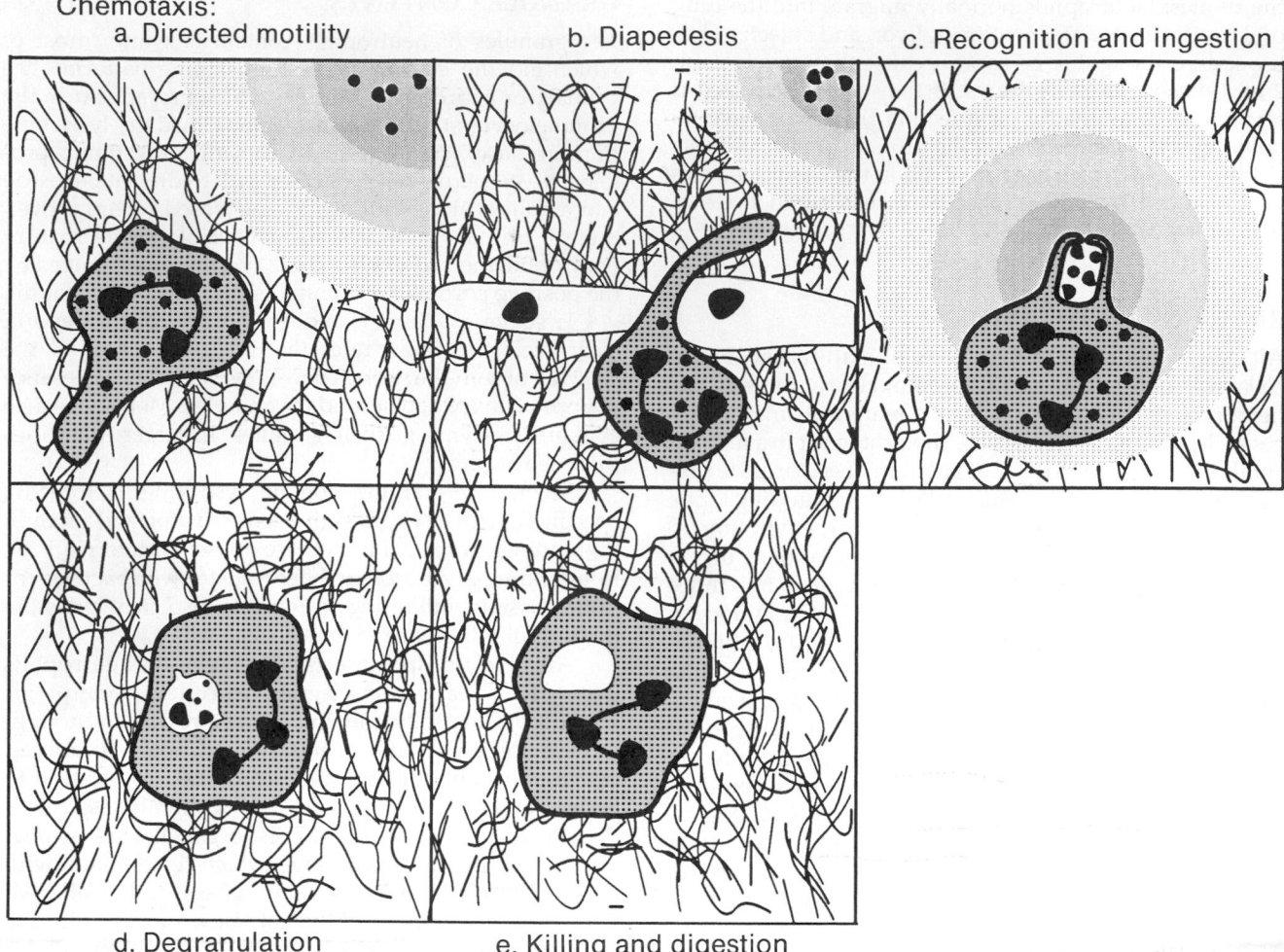

d. Degranulation   e. Killing and digestion

FIGURE 22-4. Phagocytosis is a function of neutrophils and monocytes. The act of phagocytosis includes directed motility, diapedesis, recognition and ingestion, degranulation, and killing and digestion.

order to maintain a supply of ATP to sustain their motion and other activities.

The neutrophil normally moves randomly in a zigzag motion. In order to successfully attack invading microorganisms, the neutrophil is guided or drawn by a process called chemotaxis. In this process, chemical stimuli (chemotactic factors) are generated and released by interactions between tissues and microorganisms or other antigens. Chemotactic factors activate the neutrophil by binding to specific cell surface receptors, causing the neutrophil to roll along the wall of a capillary, adhere to the wall, and eventually squeeze through the endothelial cells (diapedesis) toward the stimulus. Chemotactic factors form a gradient, and the neutrophil moves in the direction of the highest concentration of the chemical. Neutrophils tend to respond faster than monocytes to chemotactic stimuli. The end result is *directed* migration of the neutrophil toward the source of the stimulus.

One of the better known chemotactic factors is a low-molecular weight fragment, C5a, which is derived from the cleavage of proteins of the complement system. The C5a fragment is an anaphylatoxin that causes smooth muscle contraction and is also the most potent of the

chemotactic factors.[26] Factors that are liberated from the bacteria themselves are also known to be chemotactic but are not well defined. One bacterial factor, endotoxin, is known to activate coagulation factor XII (Hageman factor), which initiates the coagulation and fibrinolytic systems. Fibrinopeptide B, plasminogen activator, and kallikrein are then generated from the activation of these systems and are known to be chemotactic factors. Lymphocytes and monocytes may liberate substances that are chemotactic for neutrophils. Other known chemotactic factors are metabolic products of arachidonic acid that are known to exist in inflammatory fluids and are produced by platelets.[26]

Recognition. Once the neutrophil has found its way to the site of invasion it must be able to recognize the offending organism or substance. Some bacteria resist recognition because of a capsule. Antibodies and complement substances that coat the organisms and aid the neutrophil in recognizing what to ingest are referred to as *opsonins*, from a Greek word meaning "to prepare for dining." Opsonins react with specific receptors on the neutrophil membrane, which in turn trigger the act of ingestion.

Some bacteria can be recognized and ingested by neutrophils without any help, but other pathogens (*e.g.*, *Streptococcus*, *Pneumococcus*, and *Meningococcus* organisms) are not ingested until they have been opsonized. The main opsonins are IgG antibodies and byproducts of the same complement-mediated reactions that produce chemotactic factors. Aided by IgM antibody, a large fragment of the third component of complement, C3, binds to the surface of microorganisms and allows the neutrophil to recognize them. A glycoprotein, called fibronectin, found in plasma and the outer membrane of fibroblast and endothelial cells has also been shown to coat particles and enhance their ingestion by binding the particle to the phagocyte.[27]

Ingestion. When a neutrophil comes into physical contact with a foreign particle, its pseudopods flow around the particle or microorganism and fuse together. This completely surrounds the particle in a phagosome. The neutrophil membrane also becomes sticky, in order to firmly adhere to the particle. If a neutrophil is moving randomly and happens to collide with an ingestible particle, it immediately forms a phagosome around the particle, even though no chemotactic factor is present.

Degranulation. Cytoplasmic granules within the neutrophil migrate to the phagosome and fuse with it. This fusion allows the contents of the granule to be released into the phagosome. This complex biochemical process requires increased energy from the neutrophil in the form of ATP, which is supplied by the metabolic burst described previously.

Killing. The neutrophil actively metabolizes oxygen to produce toxic substances for killing ingested foreign particles. An oxidase in the cell membrane is activated during ingestion, and reduced pyridine nucleotide (NADPH) is the source of the reducing power. Two principal toxic metabolites produced are superoxide anion (O_2^-) and hydrogen peroxide (H_2O_2). Superoxide anion is the first reaction product of oxygen, and at acid pH is further reduced to hydrogen peroxide. As glycolysis increases during ingestion, lactic acid is generated, which effectively lowers the pH of the phagosome. The acid environment in the phagosome not only enhances the reduction of superoxide anion to hydrogen peroxide but is in itself bactericidal. Both superoxide and hydrogen peroxide permeate cell membranes and are highly toxic to bacteria (as well as to animal cells). The enzyme myeloperoxidase, which is found in the primary granules of the neutrophil, helps potentiate the killing action of hydrogen peroxide in the presence of ascorbic acid and halides. Lysozyme hydrolyzes the mucopeptide cell wall of a few species of bacteria.

Because the oxygen metabolites are toxic also to the host's cells, they are kept in check by several detoxification mechanisms. First, they are localized in the phagosomes and thus are sealed off from other parts of the cell. An enzyme, superoxide dismutase, rapidly converts any superoxide that escapes into the cell into hydrogen peroxide. Another enzyme, catalase, destroys hydrogen peroxide in the cytoplasm. Reduced glutathione and the hexose monophosphate shunt also act to detoxify hydrogen peroxide and to regenerate NADPH (Fig. 6-7).

A defect in any of the steps described above in the phagocytic process can result in a disease state. Patients with such defects suffer recurrent infections. An example of a defect in locomotion and ingestion is a disorder known as Chédiak-Higashi syndrome (Chap. 26). In this rare congenital disorder the inability of cells to respond to chemotactic gradients renders patients very susceptible to infections.

THE EOSINOPHIL

Eosinophils are formed in the bone marrow from a committed precursor cell, which is morphologically indistinguishable from the myeloblast. They undergo the same maturation stages as the neutrophil in the bone marrow and spend a short time in the blood in transit to the tissues where they perform their functions.

Morphology

The eosinophil can first be distinguished from the neutrophil at the promyelocyte stage. Eosinophilic promyelocytes, myelocytes, and metamyelocytes are difficult to distinguish because the size and numbers of granules tend to mask other morphologic features. Immature eosinophils have a few large blue granules, which are lost by attrition as the cell undergoes subsequent mitotic divisions. As the cell matures, specific granules form and, upon staining with Romanowsky stain, take on a refractive, orange appearance. Because of the low percentage of these cells in the bone marrow and peripheral blood, they are not routinely differentiated into the several maturation stages; rather, they are merely divided into mature and immature forms. In pathologic conditions in which the percentage of eosinophils is greatly increased, it may be clinically relevant to identify the different stages (see Color Plates 22-14 and 22-15). The mature eosinophil is described in the introduction section of this chapter.

Kinetics

The eosinophil goes through its maturation stages in the bone marrow, and cells are stored there several days before being released into the peripheral blood where they circulate with a half-life of about 18 hours before migration into the tissues.[31] They appear to survive longer in the tissues than neutrophils, most likely at least 6 days. While in the tissues, they are found mostly in the skin or on mucosal surfaces of the respiratory and gastrointestinal tracts. Of the body's total number of eosinophils, only approximately 1% are found in the blood. Death and elimination are similar to neutrophils.[32]

Three hemopoietic growth factors, produced primarily by T lymphocytes, have been shown to influence eosinophil development, GM-CSF, IL-3, and interleukin-5 (IL-5). Of these only IL-5 promotes terminal maturation of eosinophils.[32] Studies suggest that IL-5 is the only growth factor specific for eosinophils and may be responsible for causing increases in eosinophils when other cells remain in normal amounts.[31]

Biochemistry

The principal source of energy for eosinophils is glycolysis. They also experience a metabolic burst or increase in glycolysis prior to phagocytosis, as seen in neutrophils. All enzymes of the hexose monophosphate shunt are found in the eosinophil.

The outer, less dense matrix of eosinophil granules contains hydrolytic enzymes, one of which is peroxidase. The peroxidase in eosinophil granules is found in higher concentration and differs biochemically and antigenically from the peroxidase found in neutrophil granules, but the function is similar to the peroxidase in neutrophils. The inner core of the eosinophil granules contains basic protein rich in arginine, lysine, and phospholipids. More than 50% of the protein is made up of major basic protein (MBP), an arginine-rich protein that is cytotoxic to *Schistosoma mansoni*[14] and plays a major role in the ability of the eosinophil to damage this and other parasitic invaders.[6]

When a large number of eosinophils disintegrate in secretions or exudates, Charcot-Leyden crystals may be seen. These hexagonal bipyramidal crystals have been found in nasal mucus of patients with allergic asthma, pleural fluid of patients with pulmonary eosinophilic infiltrates, and stool of patients with parasitic infections. Charcot-Leyden crystals were originally described as aggregates of the crystalloid core of eosinophil granules, but they have since been shown to be composed of lysophospholipase, which is localized in the plasma membrane of eosinophils.[15]

Function

Eosinophils function as phagocytes but appear to move more slowly and to have less intracellular killing ability than neutrophils. They respond to chemotactic factors such as bacterial products and complement components but appear to prefer factors secreted by mast cells and basophils (histamine) and antigen-antibody complexes. It has been proposed that eosinophils are drawn to the site of immediate hypersensitivity reactions by mast cell chemotactic factors and may contribute to the inactivation of mast cell products and local control of the reaction.[6] Conversely, recent evidence suggests that eosinophils play a key role in the pathogenesis of asthma and other pulmonary diseases by damaging infiltrated bronchial tissue and lung parenchyma.[20]

Another important function of eosinophils is their ability to damage the larval stages of parasitic helminths. *Schistosoma mansoni* has been studied most extensively. Eosinophils attach to the parasite, only after opsonization with IgG, IgE,[32] or complement, and extend long projections over the parasite surface. They then degranulate and the contents of their granules break down the parasite. Degradation products of the parasite are then phagocytosed by a different population of eosinophils. Other leukocytes may assist in the phagocytosis process.[14]

THE BASOPHIL

The basophil is the least common of the leukocytes and makes up 0% to 1.6% of total peripheral blood leukocytes and only 0.3% of nucleated blood cells in the marrow.

Basophils are formed in the bone marrow, and their maturation stages parallel those of the neutrophil except that the nucleus does not always segment. Although basophils are derived from the same uncommitted multipotent stem cell as other granulocytes, the basophil clearly has its own committed precursor cell.[28]

Morphology

Because so few basophils are present in both peripheral blood and bone marrow, staging usually is not done, except to differentiate mature from immature basophils.

The mature basophil is described in the introduction section of this chapter. Their large size helps to differentiate basophil granules from neutrophils with dark-staining (toxic) granules. Immature basophils have fewer granules, an immature-looking nucleus, and discernible basophilia in the cytoplasm (see Color Plates 22-16 and 22-4).

Relationship to Mast Cell

Mast cells are cells that resemble basophils and are normally distributed throughout the connective tissues, especially around blood and lymph vessels and peripheral nerves and rarely in the bone marrow. Mast cells are larger than basophils and usually have a small round nucleus and more abundant cytoplasm, which usually makes up about two thirds of the cell. Their granules stain darkly, like those of the basophil, but they are more numerous, more closely packed, and smaller. Usually the granules do not overlie or obscure the nucleus as they do in basophils (see Color Plate 27-2). Mast cells have a long life span and are capable of proliferation in the tissues. They develop from a hematopoietic progenitor cell and migrate to the tissues, where they complete maturation.[12] Their relationship to basophils is still unclear. Although mast cells and basophils share some morphologic characteristics and functional similarities, currently there is no proof that they develop from a common progenitor cell, or that the basophil is a circulating precursor of the mast cell.[9]

Kinetics

Basophils are thought to have a short life span, similar to that of the eosinophil. Exactly what happens to them after they enter the tissues is uncertain. Several hemopoietic growth factors have been shown to influence basophil production, including IL-3, IL-5, and GM-CSF. However, IL-3 is the principal one responsible for basophilic growth and differentiation.[9] Mature basophils are recruited from the circulation to sites of allergic reactions through lymphocyte-derived chemotactic signals reacting with surface receptors on the cells.[16] Increased numbers of basophil progenitor cells have been found in the circulation of atopic (*i.e.*, allergic) persons. Basophil precursor cells may also be stimulated to differentiate into mature cells by a similar response. Basophil progenitor cells may arrive at allergen-stimulated tissue sites where they undergo differentiation. This process may also elicit further bone marrow release of basophil progenitors.[8]

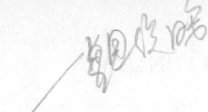

Biochemistry and Function

The cytoplasmic granules of basophils and mast cells synthesize and store histamine and contain other mediators of the inflammatory response. Basophils are thought to be the repositories of virtually all of the histamine in normal human blood. Basophils have previously been reported to contain heparin, but some studies show they contain very little.[11] Basophil granules lack hydrolytic enzymes, although peroxidase activity is present.

Basophils have been reported to ingest sensitized erythrocytes and antigen-antibody complexes and to exert a sluggish motility. Their phagocytic capacity is substantially less than that of neutrophils or eosinophils. By far the more important function of basophils is their role in immediate hypersensitivity reactions. Basophils and mast cells have specific receptors for Ig E, which trigger degranulation when appropriate antigens are present. Clinical manifestations of this immediate hypersensitivity reaction may be some forms of bronchial asthma, urticaria, allergic rhinitis, and anaphylaxis to drugs, insect stings, and other antigens. Basophils, along with mast cells, may aid in host defense against some parasitic infections by undergoing anaphylactic degranulation at infection sites.[17]

Basophils also play a role in lymphocyte-mediated delayed hypersensitivity reactions. T lymphocytes stimulated by antigen or mitogen have been shown to generate substances that activate basophils to release histamine.[28]

THE MONOCYTE

The monocyte is sometimes classified with the lymphocyte because both are mononuclear cells and are morphologically similar. Functionally, however, monocytes more closely resemble the granulocyte, since phagocytosis is one of the main monocytic functions. The monocyte also participates in cellular and humoral immunity in several other ways that will be discussed later in this chapter. The monocyte is often described as part of the *mononuclear phagocyte system*, which includes macrophages found in tissues and body fluids. The term *reticuloendothelial system* was previously used to denote these same cells as well as various other tissue cells, but it is now considered outdated. The macrophage is the tissue cell counterpart of the blood monocyte. Both share phagocytosis as their major function, and kinetic studies indicate that the blood monocyte is the precursor of most, although perhaps not all, macrophages.[10]

Morphology

PROMONOCYTE

The precursor cells of blood monocytes are monoblasts and promonocytes. Both precursor cells are very difficult to identify morphologically. Most morphologists agree that monoblasts are in the marrow but that they are indistinguishable from myeloblasts using light microscopy.[10] Monoblasts have been identified in leukemic states, but these cells are products of a malignancy and do not necessarily resemble normal monoblasts. A promonocyte stained with a Romanowsky stain has the gray-blue cytoplasm characteristic of the mature monocyte and may have an indented or lobulated nucleus. The nuclear chromatin appears immature, with fine, evenly distributed chromatin. Nucleoli may or may not be visible. It is fairly large (12–18 μm) and has a high nuclear:cytoplasmic ratio (see Color Plate 22-17).

MONOCYTE

Although the mature monocyte has a diameter similar to that of the neutrophil in a wet mount (12–15 μm), it often appears slightly larger than the other leukocytes on a peripheral blood film owing to its strong tendency to adhere and spread on glass surfaces. Monocytes are described in the introduction section of this chapter.

Kinetics

LIFE SPAN

Monocytes are formed in the bone marrow from the same progenitor cells that form neutrophils. It is not known at which point in cellular maturation the cell becomes committed to being either a monocyte or a neutrophil. The first recognizable cell in the marrow, the promonocyte, is an actively dividing cell which undergoes at least three divisions as it matures to the monocyte, taking 30 to 48 hours. Monocytes lose their ability to divide and leave the marrow shortly after completing their last division, usually within 24 hours. There is no large marrow reserve pool for monocytes as there is for granulocytes. Monocytes stay in the peripheral blood for about 70 hours where they are divided into circulating and marginated pools, and then move into the tissues, probably never to return to the blood.[22] Once in the tissues, monocytes differentiate into macrophages and may remain in the tissue several months, possibly longer. Although most macrophages are derived from blood monocytes, macrophages in the tissues are capable of cell division and may be largely self-sustaining.[13] During inflammatory conditions, the number of monocytes entering and leaving the circulation is increased and their transit time is shortened (see Color Plate 22-18).[22]

REGULATORY MECHANISM

Monocyte production is regulated by a group of hemopoietic growth factors, as described earlier in this chapter for other cell types. The factors that have been related to monocyte production and regulation are GM-CSF, IL-3, monocyte colony-stimulating factor (M-CSF) and interleukin-6 (IL-6).[13] Although many tissues of the body produce these factors, cells of the monocyte-macrophage system are important sources, as are T lymphocytes, which are responding to mitogen or antigen. Other substances released by macrophages, such as prostaglandins, are thought to inhibit monocyte production, thereby creating a balance.

Biochemistry

Monocytes depend on aerobic glycolysis for their energy and phagocytosis. They have only a small amount of stored glycogen, so they must depend on externally supplied substrates. Most macrophages depend on anaerobic glycolysis; the exception is the alveolar macrophage, located in the lung, which relies heavily on aerobic glycolysis.[23]

Mature monocytes contain a variety of lysosomal enzymes, such as acid phosphatase, β-glucuronidase, lysozyme, lipase, peroxidase, and many others. These enzymes are helpful in the wide variety of monocyte functions. Monocytes are not as rich in peroxidase as the neutrophil, and the macrophage contains no peroxidase at all. Lysozyme is released continuously by monocytes and macrophages rather than during degranulation only, as in granulocytes. It functions mainly as a bacteriolytic enzyme, but it may have an enhancement effect on phagocytosis and a potential antineoplastic effect. Cytochemically, monocytes give a positive reaction for nonspecific esterases (NSE) that are inhibited by sodium fluoride. The nonspecific esterase stain is often used to differentiate monocytes from cells of the granulocyte series in which NSE is not inhibited by sodium fluoride (Chap. 29).[13]

Surface receptors allow monocytes and macrophages to attach to and ingest immunoglobulin-coated particles. Monocytes and macrophages have receptors for IgG, IgA, IgE, and complement C3.[23]

Function

PHAGOCYTOSIS

The cells of the monocyte-macrophage system participate in phagocytosis in a manner similar, but not identical, to that described in the section on neutrophils. The neutrophil is generally thought to be the more efficient phagocyte, except when the particle to be engulfed is large in relation to the cell, in which case the monocyte is more efficient. Monocyte motility is slow compared to that of neutrophils. Studies show that neutrophils arrive at the scene of tissue damage first and monocytes tend to come along later to ingest cellular debris. Macrophages are influenced by a migration inhibition factor released by T lymphocytes which causes them to remain at the site of infection. Chemotactic factors that attract monocytes include antigen-antibody complexes, complement components, kallikrein, factors released by activated T lymphocytes, and substances produced by bacteria.

The killing potency of macrophages is greatly enhanced when the cells are "activated." Activation refers to the process of enhancing motility, metabolism, enzyme activity, and killing capacity. Activation may result from the cell coming in direct contact with microorganisms or their byproducts, or from soluble substances, called lymphokines, released by sensitized T lymphocytes and lymphocytes called natural killer cells. Morphologically, activated macrophages are larger and have more granules; biochemically, metabolism of glucose increases by way of the hexose monophosphate shunt. Activated macrophages release greater amounts of enzymes, complement components, chemotactic factors for neutrophils, interferon, and pyrogen. They utilize the same oxygen metabolites (superoxide anion and hydrogen peroxide) as the neutrophil to kill foreign organisms. Microorganisms such as *Mycobacterium, Listeria, Salmonella, Brucella,* and certain fungi and protozoa that are known to parasitize macrophages and replicate within them may be inhibited or destroyed when the macrophages become activated. Activated macrophages secrete interleukin-8 (IL-8), a potent chemotactic factor which attracts neutrophils.[23]

OTHER FUNCTIONS

In addition to phagocytosis, mononuclear phagocytes also play a role in cellular and humoral immunity in close association with T lymphocytes. Mononuclear cells phagocytize and process (degrade and chemically modify) antigens and present them to T lymphocytes. The T lymphocytes in turn respond by secreting lymphokines, which activate resting macrophages. After killing the microorganism, the activated macrophages liberate substances (prostaglandins) that suppress or turn off the T-cell reaction.

Macrophages release a soluble factor, interleukin 1, which stimulates T lymphocytes. This factor promotes replication of T lymphocytes that are responding to an antigen.[13] Mononuclear phagocytes also are known to secrete various substances that regulate the inflammatory response, numerous components of the complement system, and endogenous pyrogen, which causes fever by its effect on the hypothalamus. They also produce interferon, which may participate in conferring protection against viral infections. Macrophages produce transcobalamin II, the primary transport factor for vitamin B_{12} (Chap. 12). Monocytes and macrophages secrete substances such as plasminogen activator, plasmin inhibitor, platelet activation factor, and a tissue thromboplastin-like procoagulant, and thereby participate in the coagulation cascade and in fibrinolysis. The cells of the monocyte-macrophage system also secrete G-CSF and GM-CSF, which promote the proliferation of myeloid stem cells into the neutrophil and monocyte cell lines.

CHAPTER SUMMARY

The phagocytic leukocytes are significant as the body's main line of defense against infection. By recognizing them morphologically on a stained blood film, their presence and concentration in the peripheral blood may be evaluated. It must be noted, however, that this is a very incomplete picture because of the short time they spend in the vascular space. Recognizing the immature forms of these cells provides indicators of disease and marrow stress. The limitations of light microscopy when trying to identify immature cells must not be overlooked.

A discussion of the process of phagocytosis and its relationship to other functions of these cells has been presented. The interrelationship of all the cells and their functions is necessary for them to operate with maximum efficiency to keep the body free of foreign invaders.

Case Study 22-1

A 17-year-old boy was brought to the emergency room following an automobile accident, with a suspected broken leg. A CBC was ordered immediately and his white blood cell count was 8.5×10^9/L. One hour later additional tests were ordered and another CBC was performed. This time the white blood cell count was 14.0×10^9/L. Other CBC parameters remained fairly stable. Laboratory error and patient misidentification were ruled out as causes of the increased white blood cell count in the second sample. What is a possible explanation for this rapid change in white blood cell count?

Case Study 22-2

A new clinical laboratory scientist in the hematology laboratory is consistently getting a lower percentage of band neutrophils when performing differential counts. What is a possible explanation? What should the supervisor do to correct the situation?

Review Questions

22-1. The correct order for the neutrophil's maturation stages is

  A. myelocyte, myeloblast, metamyelocyte, promyelocyte, band, segmented.
  B. promyelocyte, myelocyte, myeloblast, metamyelocyte, segmented, band.
  C. myeloblast, promyelocyte, myelocyte, metamyelocyte, band, segmented.
  D. myeloblast, promyelocyte, metamyelocyte, myelocyte, band, segmented.

22-2. When distinguishing between mature and immature leukocytes, the most reliable morphologic characteristic is

  A. cell size.
  B. nuclear chromatin pattern.
  C. cytoplasmic color.
  D. nuclear shape.

22-3. The best technique to follow when identifying leukocytes is to

  A. use as many morphologic criteria as possible.
  B. use cell size as the most important criterion.
  C. rely heavily on color.
  D. use nuclear-cytoplasmic ratio exclusively for identification of immature cells.

22-4. A gray-blue cytoplasm with a "ground-glass" appearance is found most frequently in the

  A. myeloblast.
  B. lymphocyte.
  C. basophil.
  D. monocyte.

22-5. The stages of granulocytes normally found in the mitotic pool are

  A. myeloblast, myelocyte, metamyelocyte, and promyelocyte.
  B. metamyelocyte, band, segmented, and myeloblast.
  C. myeloblast, promyelocyte, and myelocyte.
  D. promyelocyte, myelocyte, and metamyelocyte.

22-6. Basophils share functional and morphologic characteristics with

  A. mast cells.
  B. monocytes.
  C. macrophages.
  D. myelocytes.

22-7. The most immature stage of neutrophil maturation which is no longer capable of mitosis is the

  A. promyelocyte.
  B. myelocyte.
  C. metamyelocyte
  D. band.

References

1. Babior BM, Golde DW: Production, distribution, and fate of neutrophils. In Beutler E, Lichtman MA, Coller BS, Kipps TJ (eds): Williams Hematology, 5th ed. New York, McGraw-Hill, 1995
2. Bainton DF: Neutrophilic leukocyte granules: From structure to function. Adv Exp Med Biol 336:17, 1993
3. Bennett JM, Catovsky D, Daniel MT et al: Proposals for the classification of the myelodysplastic syndromes. Br J Haematol 151:189, 1982
4. Beutler E: Metabolism of neutrophils. In Beutler E, Lichtman MA, Coller BS, Kipps TJ (eds): Williams Hematology, 5th ed. New York, McGraw-Hill, 1995
5. Boggs DR, Winkelstein A: White Cell Manual, 4th ed. Philadelphia, FA Davis, 1983
6. Butterworth AE, David JR: Eosinophil function. N Engl J Med 304:154, 1981
7. College of American Pathologists: Identification of Blood and Bone Marrow Cells, Quality Evaluation Program. Skokie, IL, CAP, 1972
8. Denburg JA, Telizyn S, Belda A et al: Increased numbers of circulating basophil progenitors in atopic patients. J Allergy Clin Immunol 76:466, 1985
9. Denburg JA: Basophil and mast cell lineages in vitro and in vivo. Blood 79:846, 1992
10. Douglas SD, Ho W: Morphology of monocytes and macrophages. In Beutler E, Lichtman MA, Coller BS et al (eds) Williams Hematology, 5th ed. New York, McGraw-Hill, 1995
11. Galli SJ, Dvorak HF: Basophils and mast cells. Structure, function and role in hypersensitivity. In Gupta S, Good RA (eds): Cellular, Molecular, and Clinical Aspects of Allergic Disorders. New York, Plenum, 1979
12. Galli SJ, Dvorak AM: Production, biochemistry and function of basophils and mast cells. In Beutler E, Lichtman MA, Coller BS, Kipps TJ (eds): Williams Hematology, 5th ed. New York, McGraw-Hill, 1995
13. Ganz T, Lehrer RI: Production, distribution, and fate of monocytes and macrophages. In Beutler E, Lichtman MA, Coller BS, Kipps TJ (eds): Williams Hematology, 5th ed. New York, McGraw-Hill, 1995
14. Glauert AM, Butterworth AE, Sturrock RF et al: The mechanism of antibody-dependent, eosinophil-mediated damage to schistosomula of Schistosoma mansoni in vitro: A study by phase-contrast and electron microscopy. J Cell Sci 34:187, 1978
15. Gleich GJ, Loegering BS, Adolphson CR: Eosinophils and bronchial inflammation. Chest 87(Suppl):10S, 1985
16. Goetzl EJ, Foster DW, Payan DG: A basophil-activating factor from human T lymphocytes. Immunology 53:227, 1984
17. Huntley JF: Mast cells and basophils: A review of their heterogeneity and function. J Comp Pathol 107:349, 1992
18. Jagels MA, Hugli TE: Mechanisms and mediators of neutrophilic leukocytosis. Immunopharmacology 28:3, 1994
19. Koepke JA, Dotson MA, Shifman MA: A critical evaluation of the manual/visual differential counting method. Blood Cells 11:173, 1986
20. Kroegl C, Virchow JC, Luttmann W, Walker C, Warner JA: Pulmonary immune cells in health and disease: the eosinophil leukocyte (Part 1). Eur Respir J 7:519, 1994
21. Kouides PK, Bennett JM: Morphology and classification of myelodysplastic syndromes. Hematol Oncol Clin North Am 6:485, 1992
22. Langermans JAM, Hazenbos WLW, Van Furth R: Antimicrobial functions of mononuclear phagocytes. J Immunol Methods. 174:185, 1994
23. Lehrer RI, Ganz T: Biochemistry and function of monocytes and macrophages. In Beutler E, Lichtman MA, Coller BS,

Kipps TJ (eds): Williams Hematology, 5th ed. New York, McGraw-Hill, 1995

24. National Committee for Clinical Laboratory Standards: Reference leukocyte differential count (proportional) and evaluation of instrument methods. Approved Standard, NCCLS document H20-A, vol 12, no 1. Villanova, PA, NCCLS, 1992

25. Shafer J: White Blood Cell Morphology. Workshop Manual, ASMT Region III. Orlando, FL, 1975

26. Smolen JE, Boxer LA: Functions of neutrophils. In Beutler E, Lichtman MA, Coller BS, Kipps TJ (eds): Williams Hematology, 5th ed. New York, McGraw-Hill, 1995

27. Stossel TP: Leukocytes II. Phagocytosis and its disorders. In Beck WS (eds): Hematology, 4th ed. Cambridge, MA, MIT Press, 1985

28. Valent P: The phenotype of human eosinophils, basophils, and mast cells. J Allergy Clin Immunol 94:1177, 1994

29. Van Assendelft OW: Reference values for the total differential leukocyte count. Blood Cells 11:79, 1985

30. Van Furth R, Raeburn JA, VanZweet TL: Characteristics of human mononuclear phagocytes. Blood 54:498, 1979

31. Wardlow AJ: Eosinophils in the 1990s: New perspectives on their role in health and disease. Postgrad Med J 70:536, 1994

32. Wardlow AJ, Kay AB: Eosinophils: production, biochemistry, and function. In Beutler E, Lichtman MA, Coller BS, Kipps TJ (eds): Williams Hematology, 5th ed. New York, McGraw-Hill, 1995

CHAPTER 23

Immune Leukocytes— Morphology, Kinetics, and Function

F. Sue Allison

Objectives

1. Identify three distinguishing physiologic characteristics of lymphocytes.
2. Compare and contrast the morphology of lymphocytes, large granular lymphocytes, microblasts, rubricytes, and plasma cells using light and electron microscopy.
3. Explain the hierarchy of lymphoid cell development.
4. Discuss the migration and recirculation of lymphocytes.
5. Classify each stage of lymphoid cell development relative to major surface markers.
6. Discuss the functions of lymphocytes.

Lymphocytes play a major role in maintenance of health and in the response to and recovery from disease. Variations in quality or quantity of lymphocytes provide diagnostic data and are indicators of the response to therapy. Accurate evaluation of lymphocytes depends on knowledge about their formation, migration, differentiation, and function.

PHYSIOLOGIC CHARACTERISTICS OF LYMPHOCYTES

Three physiologic characteristics of lymphocytes that help distinguish them from other normal blood cells have been outlined by Müller-Hermelink and are discussed below.[31]

Lymphocytes Are Not Obligate End Cells

An obligate end cell is a mature cell that is committed to perform one or more functions and die. Granulopoiesis produces end cells (neutrophils) that are no longer capable of proliferation and therefore vanish after the fulfillment of their function. Lymphopoiesis differs in that primary lymphoid organs (*i.e.*, bone marrow and thymus) generate incompletely differentiated cells capable of both proliferation and the production of end cells that perform a function and die (*e.g.*, plasma cells).

Lymphocytes Are a Heterogeneous Group of Cells

Some lymphocyte precursors migrate to the thymus where they are induced through hormone-like substances to become T cells, which are primarily responsible for cell-mediated immunity. Other precursors develop into B cells, which fulfill the function of humoral immunity (antibody production). Another group of lymphocytes, natural killer (NK) cells, are capable of lysing a variety of target cells. Some lymphocytes do not develop along either the T- or B-cell pathway. Differences in maturation, cell markers, and responses to mitogenic stimulation exemplify the heterogeneity of these cells even though they may appear identical on examination with routine stains and light microscopy.

Lymphocytes Are Predestined to Migrate

Lymphocytes generally spend several hours to days in tissue, then migrate back and forth between the peripheral blood and the lymphatic tissue. This migration between blood, lymphatics, and tissue is referred to as *recirculation*. Although other blood cells also migrate, they tend to go in one direction only (*i.e.*, they do not return to the blood). Both T and B cells are normal inhabitants of marrow and both freely migrate to and from body tissues.[46]

CHARACTERIZATION OF LYMPHOCYTES AND PLASMA CELLS

Romanowsky-Stained Films: Light Microscopy

Lymphocytes are divided arbitrarily by size into categories of small (diameter 7–10 μm) and large (diameter 11–25 μm) cells. Small lymphocytes have a large nuclear:cytoplasmic ratio with relatively scant cytoplasm. Large lymphocytes contain more abundant cytoplasm. The nucleus is round or oval (occasionally kidney-shaped) and is composed predominantly of dense blocks of heterochromatin with central and peripheral areas of condensation. Areas of parachromatin are unstained or lightly stained and indistinct (see Color Plate 23-1). Lymphocytes are usually mononuclear; however, one or two binucleated lymphocytes per 10,000 may be observed.[4] The nucleolus may not be obvious when stained by ordinary techniques, especially in small lymphocytes. The scant amount of blue cytoplasm in a small lymphocyte is usually devoid of granules; however, medium-sized to larger cells with more cytoplasm may demonstrate azurophilic (red-violet) granules that are usually prominent (0.3–0.6 μm).

Large granular lymphocytes (LGL) are characterized by a nuclear diameter that is significantly larger than that of the small lymphocyte. The cytoplasm is light-blue, frequently unevenly stained, and abundant. The nuclear:cytoplasmic ratio is decreased. Granules located next to the Golgi complex are large and a red-violet color (see Color Plate 23-2).[19]

Transformed lymphocytes are morphologically altered cells that reflect lymphocyte reaction to antigen. Their morphology is described in detail in Chapter 25.

Plasma cells are round or oval mononuclear cells, 10 to 28 μm in diameter, with smooth or irregular margins (see Color Plate 23-3). The eccentrically located nucleus is composed of blocks of heterochromatin resembling a tortoise shell.[4] Abundant nongranular cytoplasm usually appears deep blue because of the numerous ribosomes (RNA). The area immediately next to the nucleus containing the Golgi complex is unstained (perinuclear chromophobic area or area of Höf). The periphery of the cytoplasm has a "layered look," which is explained by the presence of flattened parallel sacs of rough endoplasmic reticulum (RER). The cytoplasm may contain round, discrete globules that are unstained, pale blue, or occasionally red. These globules contain immunoglobulin (Ig) and are called Russell bodies. When they fill the cytoplasm, the cells may appear to contain a cluster of grapes and are referred to as morula, grape, or Mott cells (see Fig. 39-4).

Problems in Identification of Lymphocytes

Mononuclear cells with blue, nongranular cytoplasm frequently are difficult to identify for novices. Generally, close observation of nuclear chromatin structure, amount of cytoplasm, and comparison with other cells on the same blood film are helpful.

DISTINGUISHING LYMPHOCYTES FROM BLAST CELLS

Common features of blast cells (particularly microblasts) and lymphocytes are similar size, a round purple nucleus which may contain nucleoli, and scant blue cytoplasm. The nuclear chromatin of the blast cell reveals fine, delicate strands that have a stippled or sievelike appearance (predominance of euchromatin) and that stain evenly and lightly (pink-purple). In contrast, the lymphocyte nucleus contains dense, clumped, or coarse blocks of heterochromatin that stains dark purple, with sharp demarcations of unstained or lightly stained parachromatin (compare Color Plates 22-7 and 22-9).

DISTINGUISHING LYMPHOCYTES FROM MONOCYTES

Large lymphocytes and monocytes may be confused unless the chromatin pattern is examined carefully. Whereas lymphocyte heterochromatin is in the form of blocks, the monocyte heterochromatin appears linear, lacy, stringy, or ropy and frequently has "brainlike" convolutions. The overall staining intensity of the monocyte nucleus is usually less than that of the lymphocyte. Nuclear shape may be helpful: the lymphocyte nucleus is round, ovoid, or kidney-shaped; that of the monocyte is often folded or U-shaped. Finally, the character of the cytoplasm is characteristic: lymphocyte cytoplasm is clear blue, whereas the monocyte contains extremely small azure granules in a blue-gray cytoplasm that gives it an opaque or ground-glass appearance (compare Color Plates 22-5 with 23-1).

DISTINGUISHING LYMPHOCYTES FROM RUBRICYTES

Lymphocytes and rubricytes may be of similar size and both contain dense blocks of nuclear chromatin. The nuclear parachromatin of the lymphocyte tends to stain light purple with deep purple heterochromatin, giving the appearance of crushed velvet. Parachromatin in the rubricyte is colorless, and the chromatin is in small dense spherical clumps, giving a checkerboard appearance.

Generally, the cytoplasm of the lymphocyte tends to be clear blue, whereas the rubricyte may have a mingling of blue (RNA) and pink (hemoglobin), giving the cytoplasm an overall "muddy" or gray appearance (see Color Plate 6-7).

Electron Microscopy

LYMPHOCYTES

Transmission electron microscopy of lymphocytes enables visualization of detailed nuclear structure and cytoplasmic organelles (Fig. 23-1). The nucleus has a double membrane containing nuclear pores. A large nucleolus is usually seen and frequently is surrounded by blocks of chromatin. The Golgi complex is small, and mitochondria are small and sparse. There is very little rough endoplasmic reticulum. Large granular lymphocytes contain cytoplasmic granules of different sizes located near the Golgi complex that are usually bound by unit membranes. Many vesicles are seen in the area immediately next to the Golgi complex.

PLASMA CELLS

The plasma cell nucleus contains blocks of heterochromatin with remnants of a nucleolus. The cytoplasm is laden with RER, which surrounds the nucleus (see Fig. 23-2 and Color Plate 23-3). The Golgi complex is large and pushes into the nucleus. Large, elongated mitochondria are present in the cytoplasm, usually around the Golgi complex. Sparse lysosomes may be observed.

Cytochemistry

Cytochemical reactivity routinely used to evaluate lymphocytes consists primarily of stains to differentiate acute lymphoblastic leukemia from acute nonlymphoblastic leukemia. The various reactions are described in the chapter devoted to cytochemistry (Chap. 29).

Cell Markers

A greater understanding relative to pathophysiology, treatment, and prevention of disease has been facilitated through the discovery of cell markers by the use of monoclonal antibodies (MAbs). The lymphocyte, with its unique subsets, has served as the prototype for these techniques.

A simple system for classifying leukocyte differentiation antigens was needed. Therefore, an internationally recognized system of nomenclature, *cluster designation (CD)*, was established for groups of two or more MAbs that recognize a similar epitope (antigenic determinant) on normal and neoplastic cells and cell lines. A summary of some of the most frequently used CDs and the primary subpopulations of targeted lymphocytes appears in Table 23-1.[3,37]

LYMPHOPOIESIS

Sites of Formation

Lymphocyte-producing tissue consists of the *primary lymphoid organs (PLO)*, which include the bone marrow and thymus, and *secondary lymphoid tissue (SLT)*, which includes the lymph nodes, spleen, tonsils, and Peyer's patches (lymph nodules in the submucosa of the small bowel), as well as numerous foci of subendothelial and subepithelial lymphocytes, monocytes, and macrophages. The PLO supply the SLT with partially differentiated lym-

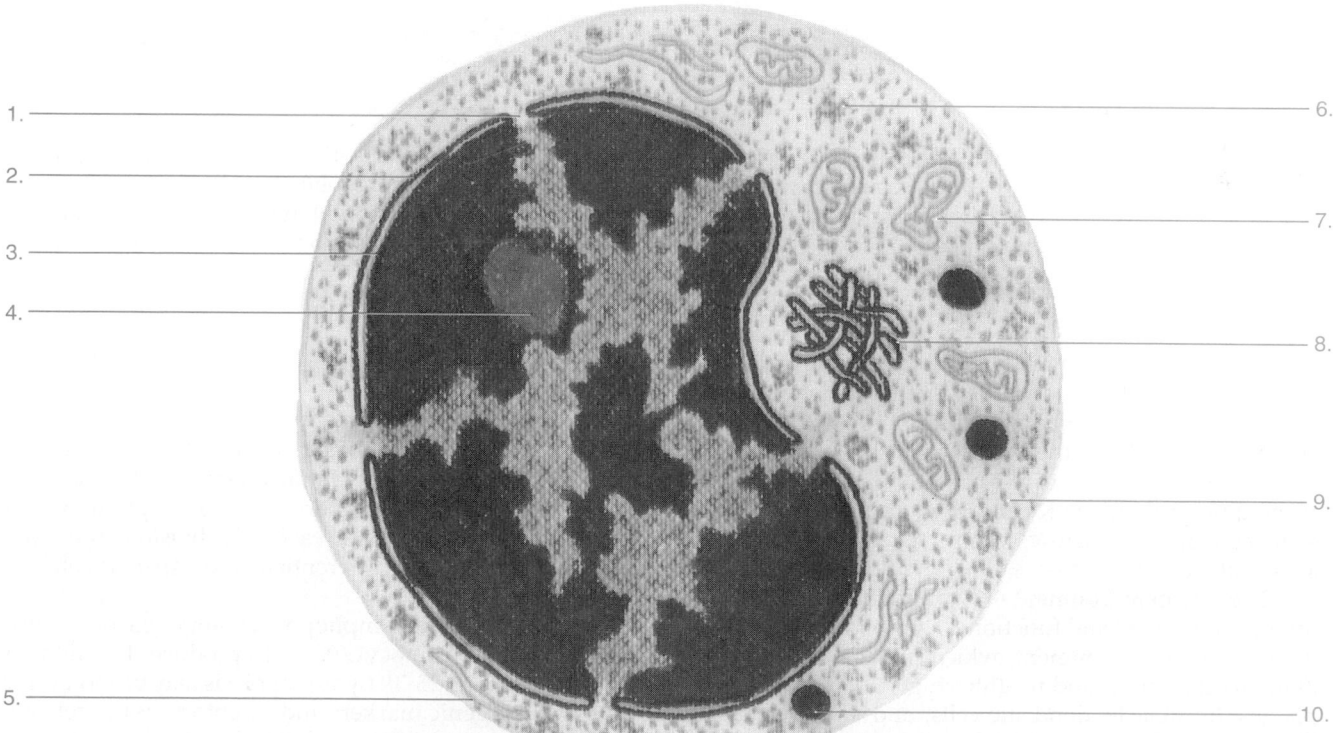

FIGURE 23-1. A drawing of the electron microscopic appearance of a normal mature lymphocyte: (1) nuclear pore; (2) the nuclear envelope; (3) perinuclear chromatin; (4) nucleolus; (5) rough endoplasmic reticulum; (6) aggregate of glycogen; (7) mitochondrion; (8) Golgi complex; (9) polyribosome; (10) azurophilic granule. (Courtesy of Thomas F. Dutcher, MD.)

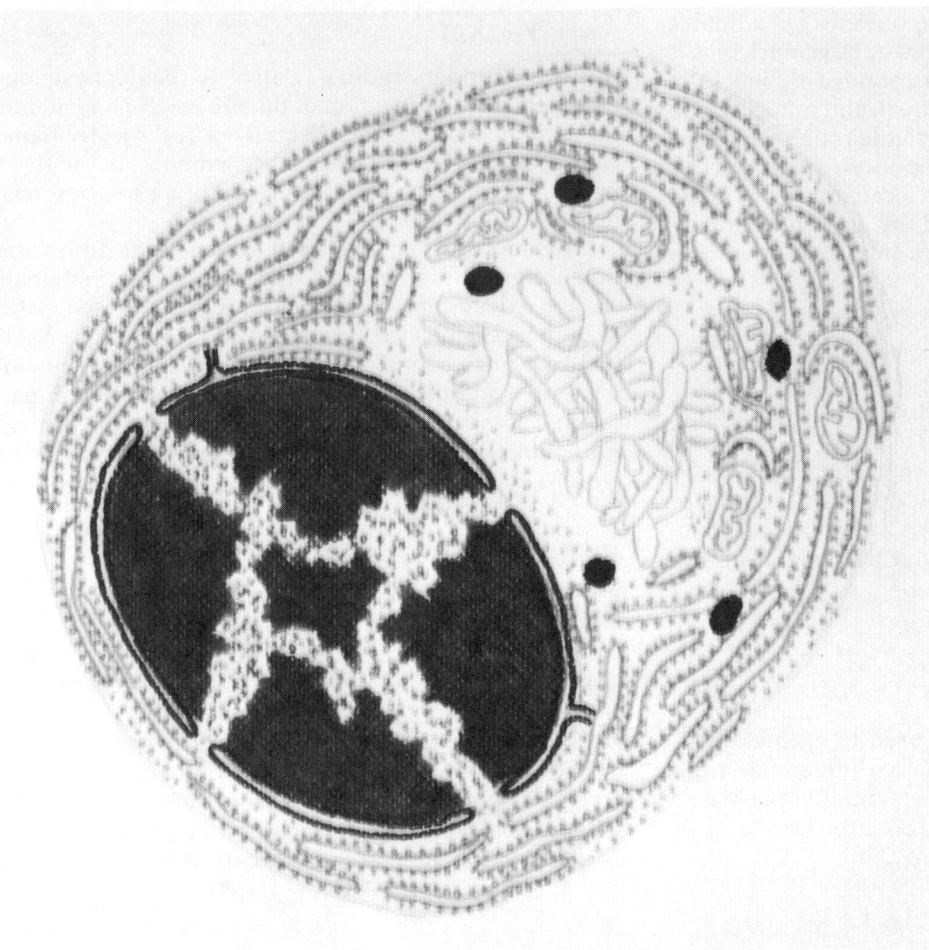

FIGURE 23-2. Drawing of the electron microscopic appearance of a normal plasma cell. (Courtesy of Thomas F. Dutcher, MD.)

phocytes. Lymphopoiesis in the PLO is continuous and antigen independent (*i.e.*, it requires no antigenic stimulation). In the SLT, lymphocytes become immunocompetent in response to antigen stimulation.

Immunocompetent cells develop along defined pathways of lymphoid differentiation which are determined, at least in part, by the microenvironment encountered by progenitor cells. The marrow supplies the thymus with a multipotential thymocytic progenitor (pro/pre–T cell) that requires the thymic microenvironment to differentiate into a T cell.[48] On the other hand, the marrow's own microenvironment appears to be responsible in part for B-cell differentiation. NK cells originate from a totipotent stem cell in the marrow, where the majority of these cells mature.[37]

The microenvironment of lymphoid cells is critical to their development and function. A lymphoid cell interacts with its microenvironment, which includes extracellular matrix components and neighboring cells such as macrophages, fibroblasts, dendritic cells, and endothelial cells (EC). Soluble factors, which are produced by cells in the microenvironment as well as by certain blood cells, interact with cell-surface receptors on lymphoid cells and with one another to promote proliferation and differentiation of the lymphoid cells. These factors are referred to as *cytokines* or *interleukins (IL)*.[33] Cell-adhesion molecules

(CAMs) serve as ligands or coreceptors for many surface proteins and facilitate lymphocyte adhesion to other cells or structures. The ability of lymphocytes to adhere to other cells and structures enables them to migrate, home, and recirculate.[26]

Bone Marrow Lymphopoiesis

The hierarchy of lymphoid cell development begins with the totipotent hematopoietic stem cell.[7–10,34] Totipotent stem cells dwell primarily in the marrow and are capable of self-replication. A proportion of their progeny lose some totipotentiality with each cell division until they become committed to differentiate into a specific cell type (see Fig. 5-5).

The committed lymphopoietic stem cell or colony-forming unit–lymphocyte (CFU-L) produces functionally diverse cells (Fig. 23-3). Lymphopoiesis may be monitored by using antigenic markers and receptors on the cell surface, by cytochemistry, and by detection of gene rearrangement which normally occurs during lymphocyte maturation. The CFU-L is characterized by the presence of HLA-DR, the terminal deoxynucleotidyl transferase (TdT) nuclear enzyme, the stem cell antigen (CD34),[37] and c-kit (also known as stem cell factor; Fig. 23-4).[24,37]

TABLE 23-1
Recommended Cluster Designation Nomenclature

Cluster Designation (CD)	Primary Subpopulation
B CELL	
CD10	Early pre–B, stage I thymocytes
CD19	Pre–B, B cells
CD20	Most B cells, ~1/2 of pre–B cells
CD21	Majority of blood B cells; mantle zone and primary follicle B cells
CD22	Most B cells, ~1/2 of pre–B cells
CD23	B cell activation antigen
CD37	B cells
CD40	B cells
CD72	Pan–B cells
CD73	B cells, T subset
CD74	B cells, macrophages
CDw75	Mature B cells, T subset
CD76	Mature B cells, T subset, PMNs
CDw78	Pan–B cells, macrophage subset
T CELL	
CD1	T cells, Langerhans cells
CD2R	Activated T cells
CD4	T cells, (helper/inducer)
CD7	T cells and thymocytes
CD8	T cells, (suppressor/cytotoxic)
CD27	T and plasma cells
CD28	CD8 cytotoxic T cells
CD38	Lymphoid progenitors, germinal center B and plasma cells, proliferating T cells
CD45RA	B cells, naive T cells, NK cells, monocytes
CD45RO	Memory T cells, myeloid cells
NK CELL	
CD2	T cells, most NK cells
CD3	Activated T cells
CD7	Most T cells and thymocytes
CD11b	Monocytes, T cells
CD16	NK cells, some T cells, monocytes (weak)
CD56	NK cell, some T cells
CD57	NK cell, some T cells

PMN = polymorphonuclear neutrophils; NK = natural killer.

B CELLS

Differentiation along the B-cell pathway may proceed in the bone marrow; however, the precursor cell may also migrate to a peripheral organ such as the spleen, where it acquires the markers of a B cell.[43,45] The earliest recognizable B cell in humans is the pro–B (*progenitor*) cell, which is characterized by receptors such as CD19 and TdT but contains no immunoglobulin.[20] Differentiation of the pro–B to pre–B (*precursor*) cell requires immunoglobulin gene rearrangement (Fig. 23-4) and is dependent on a variety of substances, including IL-7, which initiates Ig-heavy chain (IgHC) expression. Immunoglobulin synthesis can be upregulated (caused to be increased) by *c-kit* (stem cell factor).[5]

The initial pre–B cell is a large, rapidly dividing cell with a convoluted nucleus and is followed by a small pre–B cell that appears a few days later and divides slowly.[11] Large and small pre–B cells are present in the marrow throughout life. Small pre–B cells may be seen in blood from newborn infants as well as in patients with aplastic anemia, after marrow transplantation, and in lymph nodes following local antigenic stimulation. They are mononuclear cells, 10 to 20 μm in diameter, and contain a large nucleus with strikingly homogeneous nuclear chromatin without visible nucleoli.[30] The nucleus may be cleft. When cytoplasm is visible, it is medium to deep blue, extremely scant, and devoid of granules, inclusions, and vacuoles (see Color Plate 23-4). The term *hematogone* has been used to describe this cell.[28,30] Other authors have supported the view that these cells are pre–B cells.[8,12]

Pre–B cells retain the HLA-DR antigen, CD19, and other surface markers, and a few test positive for TdT.[7,11] Stages of pre–B cell differentiation have been identified, but they are beyond the scope of this chapter.

The common denominator in the differentiation of all B cells is the rearrangement of immunoglobulin genes. Germline Ig genes are organized in discrete segments that must be rearranged in order to be functionally transcribed. These are the variable (V), diversity (D), and joining (J) gene segments. When successful VDJ$_H$ rearrangements occur, the production of μ-heavy chains (HC) in pre–B cells is evident.

Immature B cells, the next stage of differentiation, are characterized by the absence of CD10 and TdT, the first appearance of surface membrane Ig (sIg), and intracytoplasmic HCs of IgM type. B cell–specific antigens (*e.g.*, CD20, CD22, and CD40) appear. CD19, the marker that is retained from the pro–B cell stage until differentiation into the plasma cell, continues to be demonstrable.[37]

Mature B cells are those that demonstrate sIg. Shortly after the appearance of sIg molecules, light chains (LC) are synthesized, joined with HC, and inserted into the plasma membrane. LC synthesis begins with an individual cell synthesizing either lambda (λ) or kappa (κ) chains, but not both. Only mature B cells that bind antigen with their unique combination of Ig-HC and -LC can be activated and multiply (Fig. 23-4).[53]

Mature B cells migrate to secondary lymphoid tissue where the antigen-dependent phase of development occurs as a specific antigen is encountered. In humans, approximately 10% of cells of B lineage are precursors that are active in regeneration, whereas greater than 90% are resting mature B cells.[42]

NATURAL KILLER CELLS

The bone marrow presently appears to be the primary developmental site for natural killer (NK) cells and there is evidence that differentiation of these cells can occur in the thymus (Fig. 23-3).[48] NK cells represent a morphologically homogeneous population of large granular lympho-

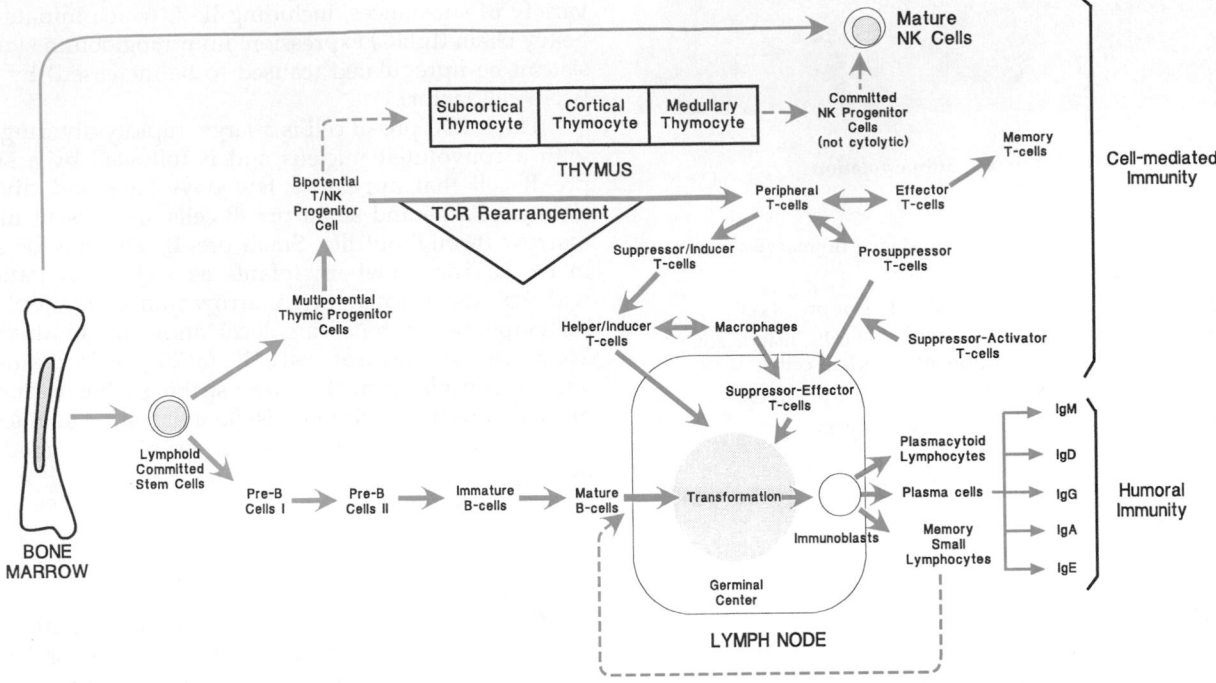

FIGURE 23-3. Diagram of the immune system. (Modified from Callihan TR, Holbert JM Jr, Berard CW: Neoplasms of terminal B-cell differentiation: The morphologic basis of functional diversity. In Sommers SC, Rosen PP [eds]: Malignant Lymphomas, a Pathology Annual Monograph, p 172. Norwalk, CT, Appleton-Century-Crofts, 1983; and Spits H, Lanier LL, and Phillips JH: Development of human T and natural killer cells. Blood 85:2657, 1995.)

cytes, the majority of which are characterized by the presence of CD2, CD11b, CD16, and CD56 antigens and are nonadherent and nonphagocytic.[41,52] The most aggressive NK cells express CD16 and CD56, and they are controlled by the IL-2 cytokine.

Thymic Lymphopoiesis

The prothymocyte (pro–T cell) also originates from the CFU-L in the marrow. It is characterized by the presence of antigens such as c-kit, pan–T cell antigens CD2 and CD7, HLA-DR, and cytoplasmic CD3, the hallmark of the T cell lineage (Fig. 23-4).[37] The pro–T cell migrates to the thymus to develop through interaction with a variety of stromal cells in the thymic microenvironment (e.g., dendritic epithelial cells, macrophages, interdigitating dendritic cells) and with other developing T cells.[48] Thymic hormones (i.e., the thymosins) also play a crucial role in the differentiation of T cells.[35] The thymus, a small gland that lies behind the sternum, is composed of a framework of epithelial cells. After infancy it slowly atrophies, essentially disappearing by adulthood.

Internally, the thymus is composed of a spongy network of endothelial cells organized into a medulla (central region) and cortex (peripheral region) enclosed within a capsule (Fig. 23-5). The cortical region is distinguished by the presence of large lymphocytes that are dividing rapidly in the absence of antigen. Under the influence of the thymus, these cells undergo changes in surface antigens and become immunocompetent subpopulations of T lymphocytes as they migrate toward the medulla.

The three discrete stages of human intrathymic differentiation have been defined as early (subcapsular), com-

mon (cortical), and mature (medullary) thymocytes, based on their reactivity with monoclonal antibodies (Table 23-2).[48] As the developing cells travel from the subcapsular region across the cortex into the central medulla, they undergo proliferation, T cell–receptor (TCR) gene rearrangement, major histocompatability complex (MHC) restriction (see later), and molecular and functional maturation.[40]

The definitive marker for T cells is the T cell antigen receptor (TCR) signaling complex (TCR/CD3). TCRs are disulfide-linked cell surface heterodimers, either $\alpha\beta$ or $\gamma\delta$. T cells in the secondary lymphoid tissue (SLT) and blood generally demonstrate $\alpha\beta$ heterodimers, whereas epithelial tissues contain a predominance of TCR $\gamma\delta$ cells.[16,54] TCR-β gene rearrangement is essential for progression from an early triple negative thymocyte (CD3−, CD4−, CD8−) to the double positive stage (CD4+, CD8+; Table 23-2).[48] When successful rearrangement of TCR-β occurs, CD3 is expressed in conjunction with TCR.[48] As the T cell develops within the thymus, CD3/TCR, CD4, and CD8 surface markers are acquired in the cortex. Two subsets of lymphocytes eventually develop: those exhibiting CD4 on their surface (helper cells) and those having CD8 on their surface (suppressor or cytotoxic cells).[35] At the same time self-reactive and defective cells are destroyed. Only 5% of thymocytes leave the thymus,[40] and most of these migrate to SLT.

An important part of T cell development in the thymus is major histocompatibility complex (MHC) restriction. The MHC is a cluster of genes located on the short arm of chromosome 6. These genes code for antigenic proteins or molecules on cell surfaces. T cells are programmed to recognize antigen only when it is linked to

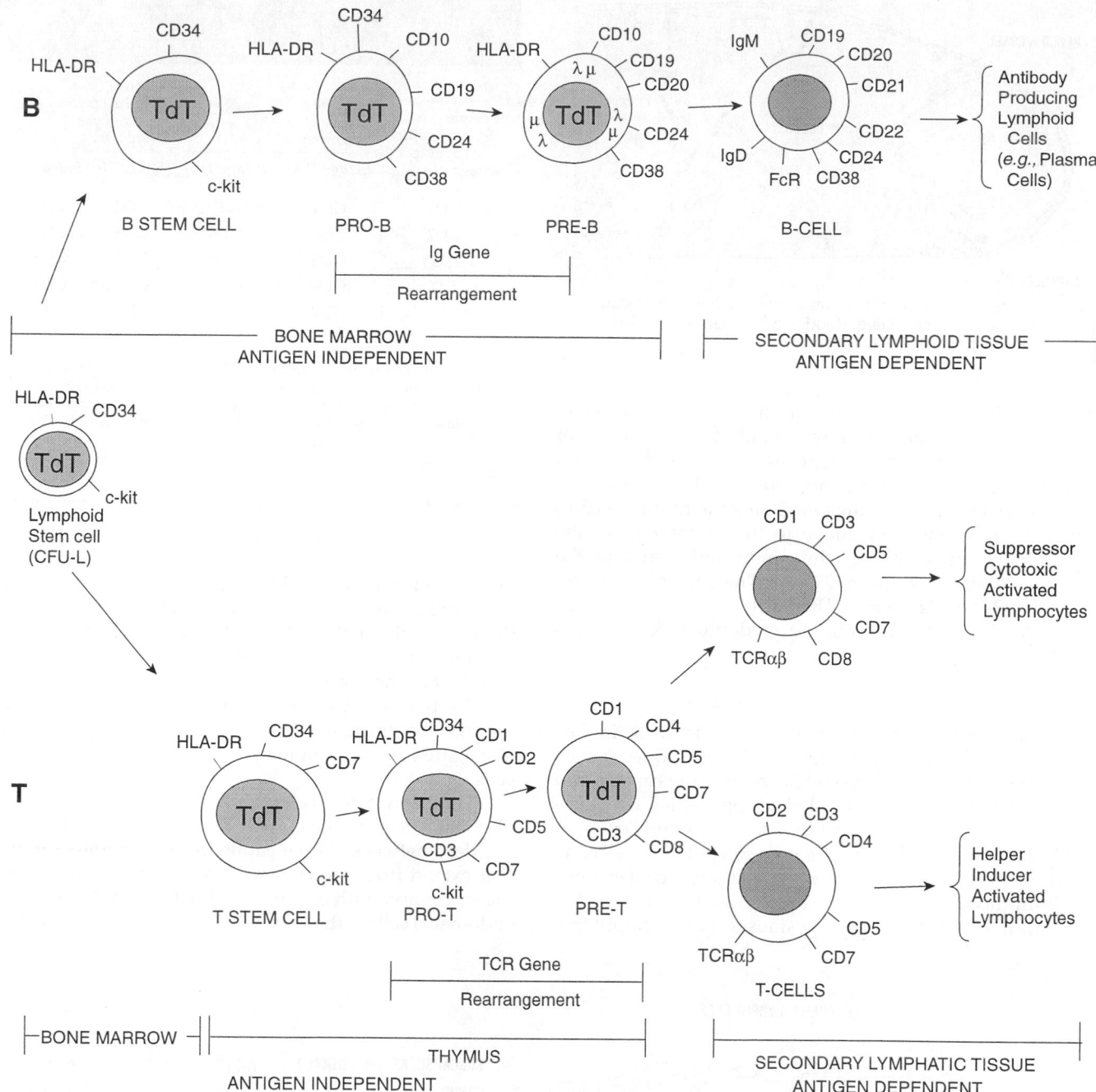

FIGURE 23-4. Pattern of surface antigen expression during maturation of T and B lymphocytes.

certain MHC molecules on a target cell surface. This is known as MHC restriction. For example, helper T cells (T_H or CD4 lymphocytes) have a class II MHC restriction, meaning that T_H can only recognize antigens complexed with class II surface molecules. Conversely, cytotoxic lymphocytes (CD8) are class I MHC restricted.

Secondary Lymphoid Tissue Lymphopoiesis

B and T cells home to clearly defined areas, a process called *ecotaxis*. The principal areas of dynamic lymphopoiesis are the germinal centers inside lymphoid follicles

in the spleen, lymph nodes, Peyer's patches, and other mucosal associated lymphoid tissue. Newly formed small lymphocytes are released by the secondary lymphoid tissue into the blood late in the course of an antibody response.

SPLEEN

The spleen is composed of red pulp (primarily erythrocytes), white pulp (primarily leukocytes), and a marginal zone (Fig. 6-8). Major components of each include vessels, reticular cells, and free cells within a reticular meshwork.

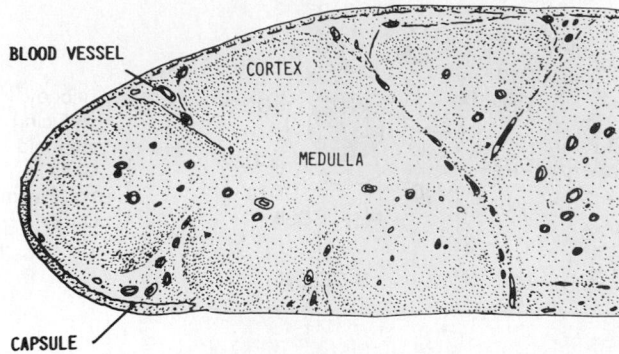

FIGURE 23-5. Diagram of thymus showing lobules composed of medullary and cortical tissue. (Modified from Burnet M: The thymus gland. Sci Am 207:53, 1962.)

TABLE 23-2
Stages of Intrathymic Differentiation

Early (Subcapsular) Thymocyte (Stage I)	Common (Cortical) Thymocyte		Mature (Medullary) Thymocyte (Stage III)	
	(Stage IIA)	*(Stage IIB)*	*Subset 1*	*Subset 2*
CD1	CD1	CD3$^{+/-}$	CD2	CD2
CD2	CD2	CD4	CD3	CD3
CD38	CD3	CD8	CD4	CD5
TdT	CD4		CD5	CD8
	CD7		CD7	CD38
			CD38	

CD = Cluster designation; TdT = terminal deoxynucleotidyl transferase
Modified from Reinherz EL et al: Discrete stages of human intrathymic differentiation: Analysis of normal thymocytes and leukemic lymphoblasts of T-cell lineage. Proc Natl Acad Sci USA 77:1588, 1980; and Lanier LL, Allison JP, Phillps JN: Correlation of cell surface antigen expression on human thymocytes by multicolor flow cytometric analysis: Implications for differentiation. J Immunol 137:2501, 1986.

T cells move from the marginal zone of the white pulp to the periarteriolar lymphoid sheaths (PALS) of the white pulp (T-dependent area). T cells then begin migrating from the spleen and are gone in 5 or 6 hours.

B cells move from the marginal zone to the PALS to mix with T cells, then move to the upper part of the germinal centers of the white pulp and return to the venous sinuses of the red pulp. This process requires approximately 24 hours.[13] These differences in migration patterns and times explain the predominance of B cells in the spleen.

LYMPH NODES

Lymph nodes are enclosed in a capsule with a continuous endothelial lining. The anatomy of lymph nodes is such that afferent lymphatic vessels penetrate the capsule and transport lymphatic fluid called lymph, loaded with antigen, into the node to be filtered. The lymph enters a subcapsular sinus, where it comes in contact with many lymphocytes and macrophages. The subcapsular sinus communicates with cortical and subcortical sinuses that communicate with medullary sinuses, which empty into the efferent lymphatics. The lymph exits through the efferent lymphatics into the thoracic duct, which drains into the venous circulation. Within the capsule, lymph nodes are divided architecturally into the cortex and medulla (Fig. 23-6). The cortex contains primary and secondary follicles that are surrounded by a layer of lymphocytes referred to as the mantle zone. The medulla contains cord-like aggregates of lymphocytes as well as many plasma cells.

The artery entering a lymph node gives rise to arterioles that extend to the cortex. There they split into a rich capillary network. These capillaries empty into venules that extend from the cortex to the medullary cords and finally connect with the vein leaving the lymph node. The endothelial cells in the venule area closest to the capillaries

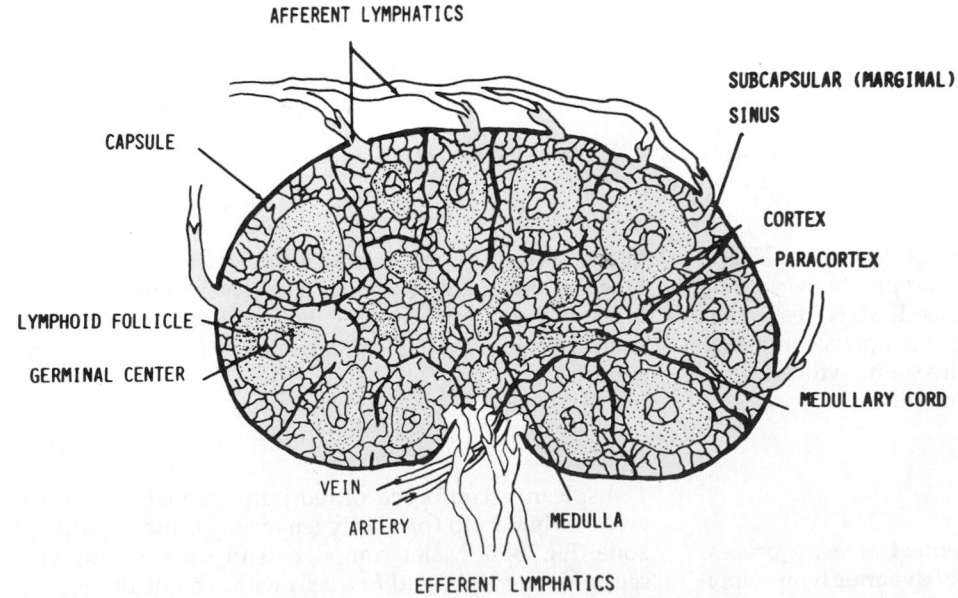

FIGURE 23-6. Diagram of the framework of a lymph node. T cells predominate in the paracortex, B cells in the germinal centers. (Modified from Wintrobe MM, Lee GR, Boggs DR et al: Clinical Hematology, p 277. Philadelphia, Lea & Febiger, 1981.)

(postcapillary venules) have special endothelial cells that allow lymphocytes to migrate from the blood into the lymph node.

Two routes of lymphocyte entry into the lymph node are therefore possible: (1) through afferent lymphatics and (2) from blood through the endothelial lining of postcapillary venules (Fig. 23-7). The T cell journeys to the paracortex between the germinal centers and the medullary cords. These areas of dense accumulations of T cells scattered among interdigitating reticulum cells and epithelioid venules are referred to as *thymus-dependent zones.*

B cells congregate in the germinal centers,[13] move to the medulla, and exit the efferent lymphatics. Thus, germinal centers in the cortex of the lymph node and medullary cords in the deep portion of the lymph node constitute *B cell–dependent zones.*

Lymphoid follicles accomplish T-cell dependent, antigen-induced B cell proliferation and differentiation. Germinal centers appear to be the site of the transformation of the B cell from a small to a large lymphocyte. The transformed B cell leaves the germinal center as an immunoblast and moves toward the medullary cords where it continues to mature into a plasmacytoid lymphocyte and/or plasma cell.

LYMPHATIC AGGREGATES

Dense accumulations of lymphocytes that are not encapsulated are found in loose connective tissue throughout the gastrointestinal, respiratory, and urogenital tracts. Since much of this lymphoid tissue is associated with mucosal surfaces, it is referred to as mucosa-associated lymphoid tissue (MALT).

LYMPHOKINETICS

Lymphokinetics is the process of lymphocyte multiplication, maturation, storage, and migration to tissues, including sites of infection or cell damage.

Mitosis and Multiplication

Radioisotopic labeling of lymphocytes provides information about lymphokinetics and the life span of these cells. The rate at which radioisotope-labeled cells appear in various tissues is used to measure their rate of production and their migration patterns. The marrow has the fastest turnover of lymphocytes; the thymus is second fastest.

Pre–B cells represent approximately 0.6% of all nucleated cells in the marrow and approximately 6% of lymphoid cells.[11] Pre–B cells require 3 to 4 days to develop into B cells. Although many cells die before leaving the marrow, the surviving lymphocytes leave the marrow within 1 to 2 days and home to the spleen.[35]

T cell lymphopoiesis cannot be sustained by stem cells developed within the thymus; it requires a continuous supply of marrow precursors.[35]

Life Span

Defining lymphocyte life span is difficult. There is a high rate of lymphocyte production and turnover in the marrow and thymus. Both short-lived and long-lived populations of peripheral mature lymphocytes exist. Most lymphoid cells have a short life span.[14] Lymphocyte interactions with the environment influence their life span.[14]

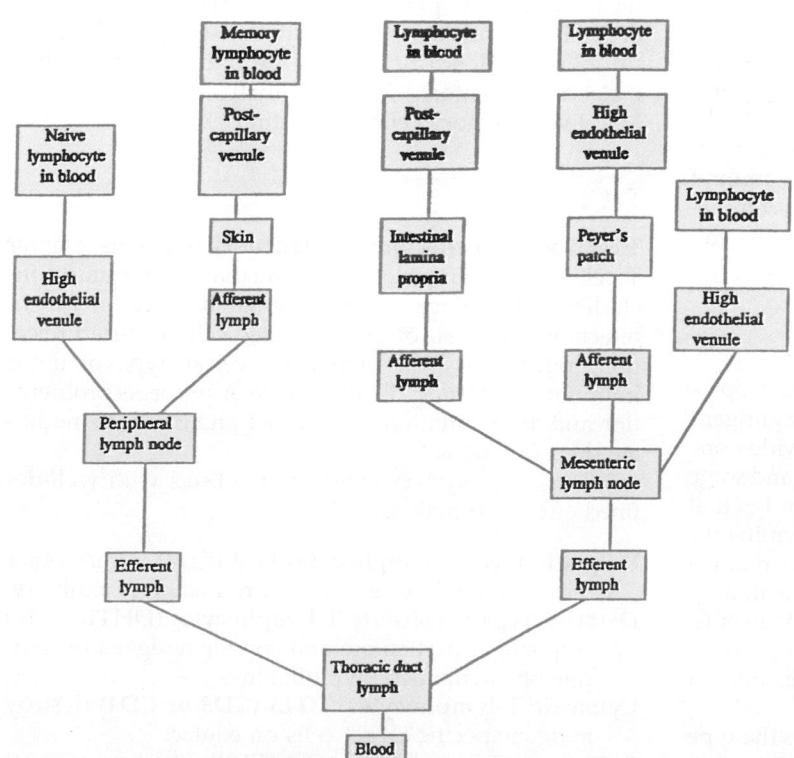

FIGURE 23-7. Lymphocyte recirculation routes. (From Springer TA: Traffic signals for lymphocyte recirculation and leukocyte emigration: The multistep paradigm. Cell 76:307, 1994, with permission.)

Migration of Lymphocytes

The process of migration involves the lymphocyte adhering to, traversing, and then detaching from endothelium.[50] *Trafficking* or *homing* refers to the circulation and migration of cells to specific tissues. For the lymphocyte to move into tissue, interaction with endothelial cells lining blood vessels must occur. Various molecules (*i.e.*, selectins, chemokines, chemoattractant receptors, and Ig superfamily members such as integrin ligands, and integrins) mediate lymphocyte adhesion either to activated endothelial cells or to specialized endothelium in lymphoid organs called high endothelial venules (HEV).[50] The HEV express specific surface proteins (vascular addressins) that selectively bind subsets of circulating lymphocytes with homing receptors.[10]

Lymphocytes interact with normal endothelial cells in a precisely regulated manner and migrate into lymphoid and nonlymphoid tissue; naive T cells (those not yet exposed to antigen) migrate into the lymph nodes, and memory T cells migrate primarily into the nonlymphoid tissue where they were originally stimulated.[46] Naive and memory T lymphocytes enter the lymph node by different routes (see Fig. 23-7).[50] Lymphocytes in search of foreign antigens travel through both nonlymphoid and lymphoid tissues.[50] Once in the tissues, lymphocytes move among other cells in the lymph nodes, skin, spleen, lung, or intestinal mucosa. The time spent in blood or lymph is minimal compared to time spent moving through tissues. Migrating lymphocytes reenter the bloodstream through the thoracic duct, migrate through endothelial cells of postcapillary venules, or enter the lymph nodes through multiple afferent lymphatics and leave by the efferent lymphatics (Fig. 23-7).[50]

FUNCTION

The major function of lymphocytes in the immune system is antigen recognition and the generation of an appropriate immune response. The interaction of T and B cells with one another and with other cell systems (*e.g.*, endothelial and macrophage systems) as well as the amount of antigen, the anatomic site of antigen entry, and complement, all play crucial roles in the outcome of the immune response.

B Cells

B cells differentiate into plasma cells that secrete glycoprotein Igs in response to stimulation by foreign antigens (humoral immunity). The secretion of Igs provides one mechanism of defense against pyogenic bacteria and some viruses. The B cell system produces a variety of Igs that react with an infinite number of antigenic determinants. Synthesis of Igs by plasma cells is essential to the removal and degradation of many foreign substances. The binding of antigen by antibody begins a succession of events, including adherence of immune complex to receptors on leukocytes, complement activation, and neutralization of toxins and viruses.

The physical state of the antigen determines the type of cell interaction that is necessary to activate the resting B cell. For example, soluble antigens require modification by macrophages in addition to factors produced by T cells. Particulate antigens, such as bacteria, cells, and viruses, may be presented directly to lymphocytes or may require partial degradation by macrophages before presentation.

B cells, T cells, and macrophages all produce cytokines, which are biologically active substances that affect other cells. In certain situations, cytokines may substitute for antigen. Several cytokines produced by activated T cells directly regulate growth and maturation of B cells. Examples include B-cell growth factors I (IL-4) and II (IL-5), B-cell differentiation factor (IL-6), IL-2, B-cell stimulatory factor-2, and interferon (IFN)-γ.[35,47]

Mature resting B cells can be activated into the G_1 phase of the cell cycle (see Fig. 5-6) by antigen or by polyclonal B cell activators (PBA), which are substances (*e.g.*, microbial cell constituents) that can activate all B cell clones independent of their antigenic specificity.[35] Once activated, both IgM and IL-4 are required for progression to the S phase (DNA synthesis).[35] In addition to T-cell–derived growth factors for B cells, there is evidence that normal stimulated B cells generate and respond to endogenous B-cell growth factor.[22,32]

Mitogens are substances commonly used to evaluate lymphocyte function because they stimulate lymphocyte transformation and mitosis. They include pokeweed mitogen (PWM), lipopolysaccharide (LPS), *Staphylococcus aureus* Cowan I (SAC), concanavalin-A (con-A), and phytohemagglutinin (PHA). The Epstein-Barr virus (EBV) can also stimulate lymphocytes. Most marginal zone B cells have EBV receptors (CD21)[37] that are T cell independent.[37,51] Early activation of peripheral blood B cells can be identified by activation antigens CD23 and CD77.[35]

The end result of B cell activation is production of memory cells and plasma cells. The generation of B memory cells depends on their affinity for (strength of binding to) follicular dendritic cells in the follicles surrounding the germinal centers.[49] High affinity B cells are exported as long-lived memory cells. Low affinity B cells die *in situ*.[49]

T Cells

T cells perform effector and regulatory functions. *Effector* T cells are responsible for cell-mediated immunity, including defense against intracellular bacterial or fungal infections, cytolysis of virus-infected cells, allograft rejection, graft-versus-host reaction, and certain types of tumor immunity. *Regulatory* T cells induce or suppress proliferation and differentiation of effector T and B cells to moderate their functions.

The T cell system consists of subsets with well-defined effector functions:

Helper/inducer T lymphocytes (T$_H$) (CD4) induce other T cells and help B cells in the production of antibody.
Delayed hypersensitivity T lymphocytes (DHTL or T$_D$) respond to particulate and soluble antigens by producing chemotactic lymphokines.
Cytotoxic T lymphocytes (CTL) (CD8 or CD4) destroy antigen-specific target cells on contact.[35]
Suppressor T lymphocytes (T$_S$) (CD8) actually represent

three cells: an inducer, an effector, and a transducer, a trio that regulates humoral and cell-mediated responses.[35]

HELPER/INDUCER T CELLS

Helper/inducer T cells (T_H) are required by some antigens in order to activate B cells to produce antibodies. T_H can activate B cells either by (1) release of soluble stimulating interleukins, which does not require physical contact between the T_H and B cell or (2) by physical contact, which requires major histocompatibility complex (MHC) identity between the T_H and B cell. T_H cells have the CD4 surface marker (among others) and are MHC class II restricted (*i.e.*, they recognize only target cells with class II molecules on their membrane surface; see Thymic Lymphopoiesis).[37,38]

In response to antigen or mitogen stimulation, the helper/inducer T cell system orchestrates a complex and varied set of functions. These responses can be studied *in vitro* using mitogens that trigger T cell responses like those that occur during activation by specific antigens *in vivo*.

IL-2 (CD25), a T cell–produced growth factor, stimulates the proliferation and differentiation of activated T cells.[37] The production of IL-2 is dependent on IL-1, a cytokine released by macrophages,[35] which stimulates CD4 cells to produce IL-2.[35]

DELAYED HYPERSENSITIVITY T LYMPHOCYTES

In response to appropriate antigen in delayed-type hypersensitivity (DTH) reactions, delayed hypersensitivity T lymphocytes (DHTL) produce chemotactic lymphokines, which either confine or activate macrophages (migration-inhibition factor [MIF] and macrophage-activating factor [MAF]) and may recruit uncommitted lymphocytes. An example of delayed hypersensitivity is allergic contact dermatitis produced by agents such as cosmetics or the plant allergens associated with poison ivy.

MIF has been identified as IL-4, which induces membrane alterations resulting in the clumping and immobilization of cells. MAF has been identified as interferon (IFN)-γ.[35] Although IFN-γ was characterized initially for its antiviral quality, other functions have been attributed to it.[27] These include inhibition of tumor cell growth, enhancement of NK cell activity and antibody-dependent cell-mediated cytolytic (ADCC) activities (see following), alteration of cell membranes to increase antigen expression on several cell lines, and activation of macrophages.[28]

CYTOTOXIC T LYMPHOCYTES

Both CD4 and CD8 subpopulations of lymphocytes contain cytotoxic T lymphocytes (CTL). The characteristics of CTL are summarized in Table 23-3 along with other types of cytotoxic lymphocytes also discussed in this chapter. Note that of the three cell-mediated cytotoxic lymphocytes, CTL are the only ones that must recognize the MHC-coded antigens on the target cell membrane surface. Furthermore, CTL must be induced to perform their cytotoxic function. IL-2 produced by CD4$^+$ T_H cells induces antigen-stimulated CD8$^+$ cells to become cytotoxic. The T cell receptor on CD8$^+$ cells recognizes only MHC class I molecules (*i.e.*, it is MHC class I restricted). CTL also have the ability to recycle to fulfill their function. For example, they can kill a target cell and then proceed to a second cell to continue their cytotoxic activity.

SUPPRESSOR T CELLS

Suppressor T cells (T_S) regulate both cell-mediated and humoral immunity and have the CD8 surface marker (among others).[35] The suppressor function is complex and involves the interaction of at least three types of T cells.

TABLE 23-3
Characteristics of Lymphocytes Involved in Cell-Mediated Cytotoxicity

	Cytotoxic T (CTL) Cell	Natural Killer (NK) Cell	Killer (K) Cell
Lymphocyte class	T cell	non-T, non-B*	non-T, non-B
Cytoplasmic granules†	Few	Several	Several
Characteristic phenotype‡	CD8 or CD4	Expresses many including CD16, CD8, and sometimes CD3, among others	Variable
Surface receptors	α/β or γ/δ	Unknown	Fc receptor
Mechanism of cytotoxicity	Inducible	Natural (nonimmunologic)	Antibody dependent (ADCC)§
MHC restriction‖	Class I (CD8) or Class II (CD4)	None	None

* Although classified as non-T, non-B, NK cells do express some T cell surface markers.
† Cytoplasmic granules contain substances involved in the cytolytic process.
‡ NK and K cells have no unique surface marker.
§ Antibody-dependent cell-mediated cytotoxicity.
‖ MHC (major histocompatibility complex) restriction refers to the ability of cells to recognize target cells only if they have certain MHC-coded molecules (e.g., class I or II) on their surface.

Put simply, the T_S system involves an inducer cell, an effector cell, and a transducer cell that provides communication between the inducer and effector cells. T_S have MHC restrictions that are different from T_H cells and CTL but these are not well understood.[35] Much remains to be learned about the structure and function of T_S.

Large Granular Lymphocytes

Large granular lymphocytes (LGL) are large cells with pale blue cytoplasm, a low nuclear:cytoplasmic ratio, and cytoplasmic azurophilic granules. LGL are cytotoxic but lack clear markers for B or T cells. At least three classes of lymphocytes exhibit LGL morphology, each with distinct activities. These include natural killer (NK) cells, killer (K) cells, and lymphokine-activated killer (LAK) cells (see below). LGL reside primarily in the blood and spleen[2] and have the capacity to exert both natural killing and antibody-dependent killing.[6,15] Two to six percent of the peripheral blood leukocytes or approximately 10% of the peripheral blood lymphocytes are LGL.[35]

The LGL cells represent a defined subset of mononuclear cells based on surface markers and mechanisms of cytotoxicity. The characteristic surface marker for all classes is Fcγ RIII for IgG (CD16).[35] They appear to be more efficient in the production of interferon-γ, colony-stimulating factors, and IL-2 than other lymphocytes.[23]

NATURAL KILLER CELLS

Natural killer (NK) cells (see Table 23-3) appear to participate in many different immunologic functions. These have been summarized as (1) recognition and lysis of certain tumor cells and virus-infected cells without MHC restriction; (2) resistance to certain bacterial, fungal, and parasitic agents; (3) immune regulation; (4) regulation of hematopoiesis; and (5) natural resistance to allogeneic grafts.[41]

NK cells recognize their targets naturally (nonimmunologically); that is, previous sensitization or activation is not required for NK cell activity. Nevertheless, NK cell activity can be enhanced by the cytokine interferon-γ. When exposed to IL-2, proliferation of NK cells occurs without requiring an antigen receptor.[35]

NK cells react spontaneously against a wide variety of syngeneic, allogeneic, and xenogeneic cells. Targets for destruction by NK cells include malignant cells, virus-infected cells, fetal cells, subpopulations of thymus cells, bone marrow cells, and macrophages.[21] NK cells may fulfill an important function early in host defense before the antibody-dependent immune mechanisms have been mobilized.[55] The spleen and blood contain the majority of mature NK cells that exhibit maximum NK function.[1,2]

KILLER CELLS

K cells, like NK cells and CTL, are cytotoxic lymphocytes (Table 23-3). However, there is a major difference in the cytotoxicity mechanism of the three cell types. K cells do not react specifically with cell membrane antigens of their target cell, but they effect binding and cytotoxicity by way of antibodies that are already bound to antigens in the cell membrane of target cells. This mechanism is referred to as antibody-dependent cell-mediated cytolysis (ADCC). K cells display high affinity for IgG Fc receptors (FcR). K cell activity has been demonstrated in virus infections, tumors, and autoimmune diseases.[31]

LYMPHOKINE-ACTIVATED KILLER CELLS

Lymphokine-activated killer (LAK) cells represent a subset of cytolytic cells that are activated directly by IL-2.[18] LAK cells do not express some NK surface antigens and thus are phenotypically different from NK cells.[17] Differences among these cells are observed generally in the kinetics of activation, target cell specificity, stimuli responsible for activation, and the phenotype of the precursor. Another characteristic that distinguishes LAK cells from NK cells is their ability to mediate the lysis of fresh tumor target cells that are resistant to NK cell lysis.[35]

Cytokines

In addition to the cytokines discussed previously and the specific and nonspecific helper/inducer and cytolytic/suppressor factors, activated B and T lymphocytes secrete a variety of other cytokines. These cytokines are proteins that function principally to moderate effector cell number and function. Cytokines have been divided into families which include, the interferons, tumor necrosis factor (TNF)–related molecules, Ig superfamily members, chemokines, and hematopoietins (*e.g.*, granulocyte–macrophage colony-stimulating factor [GM-CSF]).[36,44] The cytokine *tumor necrosis factor* is a type of cytotoxin that is produced mainly by both macrophages and activated T lymphocytes and has tumoricidal activity against a range of tumor cells *in vitro*.[29]

CHAPTER SUMMARY

From their origin in marrow to differentiation in the thymus or secondary lymphoid tissue (SLT), lymphoid cells may become programmed for immediate action or may circulate "immortally" in anticipation of a summons to action. These characteristics make the lymphocyte a cell with remarkable capabilities. It differs from other defensive cells such as granulocytes in that it may have a life span of several years or may die *in situ* within hours or days without participating in the war on foreign antigens.

The three major populations of lymphocytes include B cells, T cells, and large granular lymphocytes that are generally considered non-T, non-B cells. Effective immunocompetence is dependent on the heterogeneity, quantitative balance, and interaction of these populations of lymphocytes with one another and with other cells in their microenvironment.

It is essential for the clinical laboratorian to be able to morphologically identify small lymphocytes, large (granular or nongranular) lymphocytes, transformed lymphocytes, and plasma cells in blood and bone marrow. Identification of lymphoid cell cytochemistry and cell markers is vitally important to the evaluation and differentiation of the numerous lymphocyte subpopulations, which are vital in the diagnosis and treatment of many lymphoproliferative disorders.

Case Study 23-1

A 14-year-old female was seen by her physician because of fever, sore throat, and swollen lymph nodes in her neck for 3 days. Laboratory data included the following: WBC 13.0 × 10⁹/L; RBC 4.27 × 10¹²/L; Hb 12 g/dL; Hct 0.36 L/L; MCV 84 fL; MCH 27.8 pg; MCHC 32.9 g/dL; PLT 315 × 10⁹/L. The differential (200 cell count) was neutrophils segmented 15%; eosinophils 2%; monocytes 5%; lymphocytes 59%*; and transformed (variant) lymphocytes 19%.†

1. What two cells are most likely to be confused with small lymphocytes?
2. State the evidence, pro and con, that the cells classified as lymphocytes were correctly identified.
3. The 19% of cells classified as transformed lymphocytes have CD2, CD3, CD7, and CD8 surface markers. What does this mean?

Case Study 23-2

The bone marrow of a 2-year-old female was being evaluated to determine remission of acute lymphoblastic leukemia following bone marrow transplantation. Fifteen percent of 1000 cells scanned on coverslip preparations of Romanowsky-stained marrow were mononuclear cells approximately 10 μm in diameter with a 2:1 nuclear:cytoplasmic ratio, homogeneous chromatin without visible nucleoli, and scant to nonvisible blue, nongranular cytoplasm. Several of these cells had a nuclear cleft. These cells were absent from the peripheral blood film.

The following results were obtained from the immunophenotype of the bone marrow cells: CD2⁻, cytoplasmic CD3⁻, CD7⁻, CD10⁺, CD19⁺, CD20⁻, CD22⁻, CD34⁻, TdT⁺, *c-kit*⁻. The cells were reported as blast cells of the B lineage, characteristic of the CFU-L.

1. Based on the hierarchy of lymphoid cell development relative to morphology and immunophenotype characteristics, discuss the accuracy of the final report and its interpretation.
2. State the most likely cause for the presence of these cells in this patient's bone marrow.

Review Questions

23-1. A characteristic that distinguishes lymphocytes from other normal blood cells is

   A. migration to and from the peripheral circulation.
   B. homogeneous maturation of subsets.
   C. heterogeneous microscopic morphology.
   D. development of end cells destined to die.

23-2. On a Romanowsky-stained peripheral blood film, a cell was observed to have a diameter of 7 μm, an oval nucleus with fine, delicate chromatin strands, and a predominance of euchromatin. It had scant, blue, nongranular cytoplasm. The cell should be classified as a

   A. monocyte.
   B. lymphocyte.
   C. microblast.
   D. rubricyte.

---

* Cells approximately 8.5 μm in diameter; large nuclear:cytoplasmic ratio; dense blocks of central and peripheral heterochromatin; parachromatin tends to stain light purple, giving a "crushed velvet" appearance; blue, nongranular cytoplasm.

† Cells approximately 20 μm in diameter with a round nucleus. Minimal marginal nuclear clumping and a tendency for the central chromatin to be linearly arranged with visible nucleoli; large amount of evenly blue-stained cytoplasm, frequently with a "foamy" appearance; variation in morphology from cell to cell.

23-3. Natural killer cells are

   A. dependent on antibody for cytotoxicity.
   B. non-T, non-B cells.
   C. B lymphocytes.
   D. MHC restricted.

23-4. A major function of CD4⁺ lymphocytes is to

   A. cytolyze virus-infected cells.
   B. produce IL-2.
   C. produce immunoglobulin.
   D. phagocytize pyogenic microbes.

For the following questions, choose from these answers:
   A. 1 and 3 are correct
   B. 2 and 4 are correct
   C. 1, 2, and 3 are correct
   D. Only 4 is correct
   E. All are correct

23-5. Molecules that mediate migration of lymphocytes include

   1. selectins.
   2. Ig superfamily members.
   3. integrins.
   4. chemokines.

23-6. Pre–B cells are characterized by

   1. the presence of sIg.
   2. possessing the TCR/CD3 complex.
   3. the presence of CD4 antigen.
   4. originating in the bone marrow.

23-7. Cytotoxic T cells (CTL) are characterized by

   1. CD8 or CD4 surface markers.
   2. major histocompatibility complex restriction.
   3. a few cytoplasmic granules.
   4. destroying antigen-specific targets on contact.

References

1. Abo T, Cooper MD, Balch CM: Characterization of HNK-1⁺ (Leu-7) human lymphocytes 1. Two distinct phenotypes of human NK cells with different cytotoxic capability. J Immunol 129:1752, 1982
2. Abo T, Miller CA, Gartland GL et al: Differentiation stages of human natural killer cells in lymphoid tissues from fetal to adult life. J Exp Med 157:273, 1983
3. Bernard A, Boumsell L: The clusters of differentiation (CD) defined by the first international workshop on human leukocyte differentiation antigens. Hum Immunol 11:1, 1984
4. Bessis M (Brecher G, trans): Blood Smears Reinterpreted. Berlin, Springer International, 1977
5. Billips LG, Petitte D, Dorshkind K et al: Differential roles of stromal cells, interleukin-7, and kit-ligand in the regulation of B lymphopoiesis. Blood 79(5):1185, 1992
6. Bradley TP, Bonavida B: Mechanism of cell mediated cytotoxicity at the single cell level. IV. Natural killing and antibody-dependent cellular cytotoxicity can be mediated by the same human effector cell as determined by the two-target conjugate assay. J Immunol 129:2260, 1982
7. Burrows PD, Cooper MD: B-cell development in man. Curr Opin Immunol 5:201, 1993
8. Caldwell CW, Poje E, Helikson MA: B-cell precursors in normal pediatric bone marrow. Am J Clin Pathol 195:816, 1991
9. Callihan TR, Holbert JM Jr, Berard CW: Neoplasms of terminal B-cell differentiation: The morphologic basis of functional

diversity. In Sommers SC, Rosen PP (eds): Malignant Lymphomas, p 169. Norwalk, CT, Appleton-Century-Crofts, 1983

10. Carlos TM, Harland JM: Leukocyte-endothelial adhesion molecules. Blood 84:2068, 1994
11. Cooper MD, Lawton AR: Pre-B cells: Normal morphologic and biologic characteristics and abnormal development in certain immunodeficiencies and malignancies. In Pernis B, Vogel HJ (eds): P&S Biomedical Sciences Symposia, Cells of Immunoglobulin Synthesis, p 411. New York, Academic Press, 1979
12. Davis RE, Longacre TA, Cornblett J: Hematogones in the bone marrow of adults. Am J Clin Pathol 102:202, 1994
13. Ford WL: Lymphocyte migration and immune responses. Prog Allerg 19:1, 1975
14. Freitas AA, Rocha BBL: Lymphocyte lifespans: Homeostasis, selection and competition. Immunol Today 14(1):25, 1993
15. Gastl G, Niederwieser D, Marth C et al: Human large granular lymphocytes and their relationship to natural killer cell activity in various disease states. Blood 64:288, 1984.
16. Godfrey DI, Kennedy J, Mombaerts P et al: Onset of TCR-B gene rearrangement and role of TCR-B expression during CD3⁻, CD4⁻, CD8⁻ thymocyte differentiation. J Immunol 152:4783, 1994
17. Grimm EA, Ramsey KM, Mazumder A et al: Lymphokine-activated killer cell phenomenon. II. Precursor phenotype is serologically distinct from peripheral T lymphocytes, memory cytotoxic thymus-derived lymphocytes and natural killer cells. J Exp Med 157:884, 1983
18. Grimm EA, Robb RJ, Roth JA et al: Lymphokine-activated killer cell phenomenon. III. Evidence that IL-2 is sufficient for direct activation of peripheral blood lymphocytes into lymphokine-activated killer cells. J Exp Med 158:1356, 1983
19. Grossi CE, Cadoni A, Zicca A et al: Large granular lymphocytes in human peripheral blood: Ultrastructural and cytochemical characterization of the granules. Blood 59:277, 1982
20. Hagman J, Grosschedl R: Regulation of gene expression at early stages of B-cell differentiation. Curr Opin Immunol 6:222, 1994
21. Herberman RB, Ortaldo JR: Natural killer cells: Their role in defenses against disease. Science 214:24, 1981
22. Jurgensen CH, Ambrus JL, Fauci AS: Production of B-cell growth factor by normal human B cells. J Immunol 136:4542, 1986
23. Kasahara T, Djeu JY, Dougherty SF et al: Capacity of human large granular lymphocytes (LGL) to produce multiple lymphokines: Interleukin 2, interferon, and colony stimulating factor. J Immunol 131:2379, 1983
24. Keller G: Haematopoietic stem cells. Curr Opin Immunol 4:133, 1992
25. Lanier LL, Allison JP, Phillips JN: Correlation of cell surface antigen expression on human thymocytes by multicolor flow cytometric analysis: Implications for differentiation. J Immunol 137:2501, 1986
26. Law C-L, Clark EA: Cell-cell interactions that regulate the development of B-lineage cells. Curr Opin Immunol 6:238, 1994
27. Lee SH, Aggarwal BB, Rinderknecht E et al: The synergistic antiproliferative effect of gamma interferon and human lymphotoxin. J Immunol 133:1083, 1984
28. McKenna RW, Bloomfield CD, Brunning RD: Nodular lymphoma: Bone marrow and blood manifestations. Cancer 36:428, 1975
29. Meager A: Cytokines, p 144. Englewood Cliffs, Prentice-Hall, 1991
30. Muehleck SD, McKenna RW, Gale PF et al: Terminal deoxynucleotidyl transferase (TdT)-positive cells in bone marrow in the absence of hematologic malignancy. Am J Clin Pathol 79:277, 1983

31. Müller-Hermelink HK, Lennert K: The cytologic, histologic and functional basis for a modern classification of lymphoma. In Lennert K (ed) (Frederick DD, Soehring M, trans): Malignant Lymphomas Other than Hodgkin's Disease, pp 3, 17. New York, Springer-Verlag, 1979
32. Muraguchi A, Nishimoto H, Kawamura N et al: B cell-derived BCGF functions as autocrine growth factor(s) in normal and transformed B lymphocytes. J Immunol 137:179, 1986
33. Ogawa M: Differentiation and proliferation of hematopoietic stem cells. Blood 81:2844, 1993
34. Palacios R, Samaridis J: Bone marrow clones representing an intermediate stage of development between hematopoietic stem cells and pro-T lymphocyte or pro-B-lymphocyte progenitors. Blood 81:1222, 1993
35. Paraskevas F, Foerster J: The lymphocytes. In Lee GR, Bithell TC, Foerster J et al (eds): Wintrobe's Clinical Hematology, 9th ed, p 354. Philadelphia, Lea & Febiger, 1993
36. Paul WE, Seder RA: Lymphocyte responses and cytokines. Cell 76:241, 1994
37. Pirruccello SJ, Johnson DR: Reagents for flow cytometry: Monoclonal antibodies and hematopoietic cell antigens. In Keren DF, Hanson CA, Hurtubise PE (eds): Flow Cytometry & Clinical Diagnosis, p 56. Chicago, ASCP Press, 1994
38. Poppema S, Bhan AK, Reinherz EL et al: Distribution of T cell subsets in human lymph nodes. J Exp Med 153:30, 1981
39. Reinherz EL, Kung PC, Goldstein G et al: Discrete stages of human intrathymic differentiation: Analysis of normal thymocytes and leukemic lymphoblasts of T-cell lineage. Proc Natl Acad Sci USA 77:1588, 1980
40. Ritter MA, Boyd RL: Development in the thymus: It takes two to tango. Immunol Today 14(9):462, 1993
41. Ritz J, Schmidt RE, Michon J et al: Characterization of functional surface structures on human natural killer cells. Adv Immunol 42:181, 1988
42. Rolink A, Melchers F: Generation and regeneration of cells of the B-lymphocyte lineage. Curr Opin Immunol 5:207, 1993
43. Rosenberg N, Kincade PW: B-lineage differentiation in normal and transformed cells and the microenvironment that supports it. Curr Opin Immunol 6:203, 1994
44. Rothstein G: Origin and development of the blood and blood forming tissues. In Lee GR, Bithell TC, Foerster J et al (eds): Wintrobe's Clinical Hematology, 9th ed. p 41. Philadelphia, Lea & Febiger, 1993
45. Ryser JH, Vassalli P: Mouse bone marrow lymphocytes and their differentiation. J Immunol 113:719, 1974
46. Shimizu Y, Newman W, Tanaka Y et al: Lymphocyte interactions with endothelial cells. Immunol Today 13(3):106, 1992
47. Sidman CL, Marshall JD, Shultz LD et al: Gamma interferon is one of several direct B cell-maturing lymphokines. Nature 309:801, 1984
48. Spits H, Lanier LL, Phillips JH: Development of human T and natural killer cells. Blood 85:2654, 1995
49. Sprent J: T and B memory cells. Cell 76:315, 1994
50. Springer TA: Traffic signals for lymphocyte recirculation and leukocyte emigration: The multistep paradigm. Cell 76:301, 1994
51. Thorley-Lawson DA, Mann KP: Early events in Epstein-Barr virus infection provide a model for B-cell activation. J Exp Med 162:45, 1985
52. Timonen T, Ortlando JB, Herberman RB: Characteristics of human large granular lymphocytes and relationship to natural killer and K cells. J Exp Med 153:569, 1981
53. van Noesel CJM, van Lier RAW: Architecture of the human B-cell antigen receptors. Blood 82:363, 1993
54. Weissman IL: Developmental switches in the immune system. Cell 76:207, 1994
55. Yang J, Zucker-Franklin D: Modulation of natural killer (NK) cells by autologous neutrophils and monocytes. Cell Immunol 86:171, 1984

CHAPTER 24

Laboratory Evaluation of Leukocytes

Joan C. Terrell

Objectives

1. Describe the manual cell counting procedure, including appropriate specimen diluents, specimen dilution using the Thoma and Unopette system, dimensions of various hemocytometers, cell enumeration, and calculation of cells/L.
2. Describe steps in the manual differential procedure, including slide identification, low power scanning, platelet and WBC estimation, oil immersion cell enumeration and observation, and reporting criteria.
3. Recognize sources of error in manual cell counting and leukocyte differential counts.
4. Describe quality control monitoring procedures for manual cell counting and leukocyte differential counts.
5. Calculate total leukocyte count correction when nucleated red blood cells are present on the peripheral blood film.
6. Calculate indirect absolute cell values and recall both relative and absolute reference ranges.
7. Recall factors affecting WBC reference ranges.
8. Identify special considerations when evaluating blood films, including patient age, specimen age, and effects of anticoagulants on a blood film.

This chapter emphasizes the procedures for manual counting and differentiation of leukocytes. Manual cell counts and differentiation were originally the only means of enumerating and classifying cellular elements in blood and body fluids. To a large extent the laboratory evalua-tion of leukocytes, erythrocytes, and platelets has now been automated (Chaps. 41 and 42). Leukocyte identification and classification is referred to as the *leukocyte differential count*.

If automated leukocyte evaluation is available, why must laboratory scientists learn manual techniques for evaluating them? There are several reasons.

For every automated method there should be a back-up method, and in some laboratories that method is the manual one. Not all samples can be evaluated by auto-mated methods for one reason or another. For example, when a leukocyte count is extremely low or high, it may be necessary to perform a manual count because of loss of instrument linearity (capability to count cells accu-rately) at the extreme ends of the spectrum. Other samples that may require manual cell counting include those with abnormal proteins, clumped platelets, or antibody ele-ments in the plasma that interfere with an instrument in its ability to count leukocytes.

Extremely abnormal leukocytes, such as those seen in leukemia, may not, in some cases, be accurately differ-entiated by automated methods, although today some methods are proving to be very accurate in identifying abnormal cells. For laboratories with automated leukocyte differential capabilities, the decision to perform manual differential counts on certain specimens is in the hands of each individual laboratory. The fact remains that there will be specimens that require a manual differential count for some time to come.

MANUAL LEUKOCYTE COUNTS

Manual cell counts are performed with the aid of an apparatus called a hemocytometer (Fig. 24-1). The areas of the hemocytometer generally used for counting leuko-cytes as well as erythrocytes and platelets (Chap. 56) are indicated in Figure 24-2. In practice, erythrocytes no longer are counted manually on the hemocytometer be-cause this is a very inaccurate and imprecise method. Today, erythrocyte counts are performed on single-chan-nel or multichannel instruments. The formulas presented for calculating total cellular elements in the procedures that follow may be applied to any cellular element. In today's automated laboratories manual counting is used principally for cells in abnormal specimens and in cere-brospinal fluid (CSF) and other body fluids (Chap. 30).

Manual Leukocyte Counts

PRINCIPLE. A suitably diluted specimen is loaded onto a hemocytometer and the cellular elements are identified and counted microscopically and reported as number of cells per liter (cells/L).

SPECIMEN REQUIREMENTS. Whole blood anticoagulated with EDTA is preferred, although heparin or ammonium potassium oxalate may be used if an EDTA specimen is not available. Specimens must not have any clots. Specimens diluted prior to their receipt in the laboratory must be labeled with the name of the diluent and the ratio of specimen to diluent.

REAGENTS AND EQUIPMENT

1. Hemocytometer (Levy counting chamber with improved Neubauer ruling; Fig. 24-1). The two ruled areas on either side of the hemocytometer each have an area of 9 mm². These areas are divided into a counting grid that enables the microscopist to accurately count cellular elements (Fig. 24-2). The depth of the chamber between coverslip and ruled area is 0.1 mm (Fig. 24-1). Hemocytometers must meet the National Bureau of Standards (NBS) specifications, as indicated by the NBS initials on the chamber.
2. Coverslip, optically flat, designed for hemocytometers
3. Thoma diluting pipette or Unopette
4. Pipette suction apparatus (Clay Adams)
5. Diluents for leukocyte counting. These must be capable of lysing erythrocytes without destroying leukocytes. One of the following diluents may be used:
   Acetic acid, 2% (v/v). Combine 2 mL glacial acetic acid with distilled water to 100 mL in a volumetric flask. Always add acid slowly to water to avoid splashing the acid.
   Hydrochloric acid (HCl), 1% (v/v). Combine 1 mL concentrated HCl with distilled water to 100 mL in a volumetric flask.
   Türk's solution. Combine 3 mL glacial acetic acid, 1 mL aqueous gentian violet (1% w/v), and 96 mL distilled water. Türk's solution enhances leukocyte nuclear definition.
6. Diluents for platelet counting. These must preserve platelet integrity while inhibiting their aggregation (Chap. 56).
7. Diluents for CSF and other body fluids. See Chapter 30 for special handling of fluids. Cells in body fluids are counted without dilution in some cases.

GENERAL PROCEDURE FOR SPECIMEN PREPARATION. *Note:* Protective gloves should be worn whenever handling the specimen, pipettes, or counting chambers, or anything with which the specimen may come into contact.

1. Place a dampened gauze square in the bottom of a Petri dish with two halves of a wooden stick placed on gauze to serve as a stand for the hemocytometer.
2. Place whole blood on rotator for at least 1 to 2 minutes, or hand invert at least 60 times.[4] (Complete but gentle inversion is required to mix blood but avoid hemolysis.) Other body fluids must also be suitably mixed to ensure specimen homogeneity. Specimen samples for manual counts must be diluted immediately after the specimen is mixed.
3. Choose appropriate dilution for anticipated cell count (Table 24-1). Dilutions ranging from 1 part in 10 (1:10) to 1 part in 1000 (1:1000) may be made using Thoma pipettes (Fig. 24-3). A 1:10 or 1:20 dilution is commonly made with the WBC pipette and a 1:100 or 1:200 dilution with the RBC pipette.
4. Attach mechanical pipette suction device to WBC pipette.
5. To make a 1:20 dilution, draw a sample of whole blood specimen to exactly the 0.5 mark (Fig. 24-3) on pipette stem. If blood is drawn just slightly above this mark, use a nonabsorbent material (*e.g.*, Parafilm) to remove excess blood and ensure blood is exactly at the 0.5 mark in pipette. If blood is

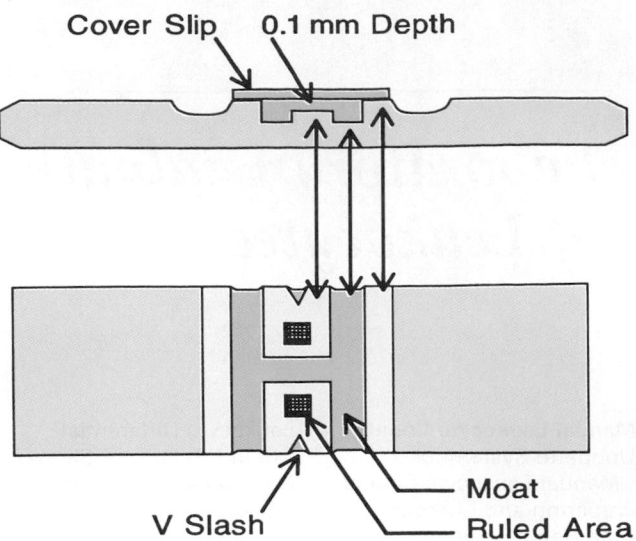

FIGURE 24-1. The Neubauer hemocytometer.

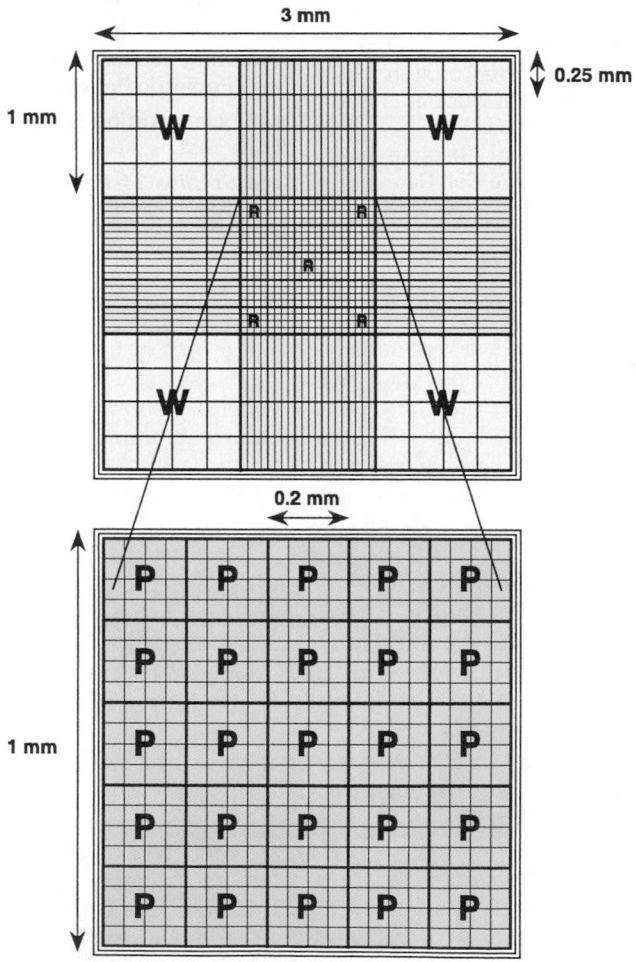

FIGURE 24-2. The ruled area of the Neubauer hemocytometer. There are nine large (1 mm) squares. Each of the four corner 1-mm squares is subdivided into 16 smaller squares and is marked **W** to indicate use for counting leukocytes. The center 1-mm square is subdivided into 25 smaller squares, each 0.04 mm². The squares marked **R** were used for counting erythrocytes when they were historically counted manually. The higher magnification of this center square (*below*) illustrates all 25 0.04-mm² squares marked **P** where platelets are counted.

TABLE 24-1
Recommended Dilutions for Manual WBC Count Specimen Preparation Based on Anticipated WBC Count

Anticipated WBC Count ($\times 10^9$/L)	Recommended Dilution	Type of Thoma Pipette
0.1–3.0	1:10	WBC
3.1–30.0	1:20	WBC
>30.0	1:100	RBC
≥100.0	1:200	RBC

drawn too far above the 0.5 mark, the procedure should be repeated using a new pipette, since excess blood sticking to the pipette wall will cause an inaccurate dilution.

6. Tilt pipette so that stem is slightly above horizontal and wipe stem carefully with slightly dampened gauze, moving from pipette bulb toward tip. *Caution:* Do not allow capillary attraction to draw fluid from tip onto gauze. Gauze or any absorbent cloth tends to absorb the liquid portion of blood, causing an erroneous increase in cell counts.

7. Gently rotating pipette between forefinger and thumb, draw diluent steadily into pipette exactly to the 11 mark (Fig. 24-3). This results in a 1:20 dilution of blood to diluent in the pipette bulb.

8. Immediately cover tip of pipette with gloved middle finger and carefully remove suction device. To avoid handling of specimen, the pipette should be placed on a mechanical pipette shaker and shaken for approximately 3 minutes. If this device is not available, place gloved thumb and middle finger over open tips and vigorously rotate pipette back and forth perpendicular to the axis of the pipette, moving only the wrist, for 30 to 45 seconds. This ensures even dispersion of lysed erythrocytes (see Sources of Error section).

9. Repeat this procedure with a second pipette to obtain two dilutions of the same specimen.

CALCULATION OF DILUTION. When using a WBC pipette, divide by 10 the value on stem to which the blood sample is drawn to obtain sample dilution (see example below).

When using an RBC pipette, divide by 100 the value on stem to which the blood sample is drawn to obtain sample dilution. In each case the denominator (*i.e.*, 10 or 100) represents 1 unit less than the dilution mark above the bulb on the pipette (*e.g.*, for the WBC pipette, 11 − 1 = 10) (see Fig. 24-3). One part is subtracted to account for one part of diluent that remains in

the pipette stem, which is not part of the mixture of sample and diluent in the pipette bulb.

For example, using a WBC pipette, if blood is drawn to the 0.5 mark and diluent to the 11 mark, the resulting dilution is $0.5 \div 10$ or 1:20. If blood is drawn to the 1 mark and diluent to the 11 mark, the dilution is 1:10. The same principle applies to calculating dilutions in the RBC pipette.

SOURCES OF ERROR
1. Failure to adequately mix blood specimen at least 1 minute on the rotator, or 60 inversions by hand, just prior to taking a sample for counting renders cell counts inaccurate.
2. Failure to immediately mix blood and diluent in Thoma pipette produces clumps of erythrocyte stroma, which entrap leukocytes and make accurate counting impossible.
3. Using diluent contaminated with blood causes erroneous results.
4. Bubbles in Thoma pipette cause an inaccurate dilution.
5. Drawing blood too far past the appropriate dilution mark and then drawing it out causes an inaccurate dilution, because some of the blood may stick to pipette walls.

Unopette System for Manual Leukocyte Counts

The Unopette system (Becton Dickinson, Rutherford, NJ[3]) provides a series of reservoirs containing premeasured diluent and pipettes that automatically measure the appropriate amount of sample required for diluting blood specimens in preparation for manual counting. Various reservoirs are available with appropriate diluting fluids for leukocyte, platelet, and eosinophil counts. Reservoirs are also available for performing dilutions to obtain a complete blood count from a skin puncture specimen or to measure erythrocyte osmotic fragility. The standard Unopette reservoir used for leukocyte counts contains 0.475 mL of a 3% aqueous solution of glacial acetic acid.

The same techniques are used for Unopettes, no matter what laboratory procedure is to be performed. The manufacturer's instructions must be followed carefully to ensure accurate results.

Preparing and Charging the Hemocytometer

Whether using a Thoma pipette or Unopette, the hemocytometer (Levy counting chamber with improved Neu-

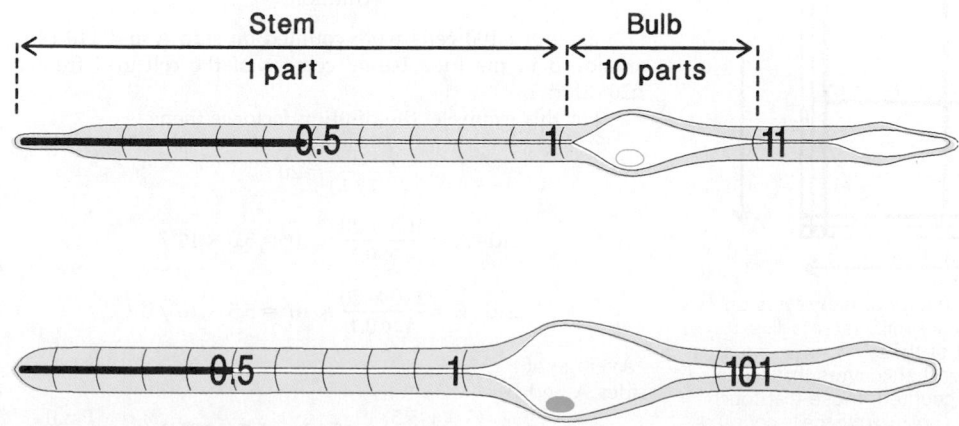

FIGURE 24-3. Thoma pipettes used to dilute specimens for cell counts. Upper pipette is used to make 1:10 or 1:20 dilutions. Lower pipette is used to make 1:100 or 1:200 dilutions for elevated leukocyte counts; this pipette was historically used for manual erythrocyte counts, which are no longer performed.

bauer ruling) is used to count the cells and must be scrupulously cleaned prior to use.

1. Just before using, always clean the hemocytometer and coverslip with distilled water, and then with absolute methanol, and dry thoroughly using only microscope lens paper to avoid leaving lint particles or scratches on cell counting grid area or coverslip. *Caution:* Do not use gauze for drying. It can scratch the grid surface. *Caution:* Carefully dry moat areas and do not allow fingers to touch any surface contacted by diluted specimen.
2. Place special coverslip on hemocytometer so that it partially covers both V slashes or V-shaped channels (Fig. 24-1). (Never use disposable slide coverslips, since they bend and thus reduce the counting volume.)
3. Ensure that the mixture in diluting pipette or Unopette is well mixed.
4. Charge from Thoma diluting pipette (or follow instructions for charging on package insert from Unopette).
   a. Allow approximately one fourth of mixture in bulb to flow onto a waste cloth. Discard cloth in biohazardous waste.
   b. Firmly place a *dry* gloved finger over *dry* end of pipette to stop sample flow and place pipette tip on one of the hemocytometer V slashes at approximately a 30-degree angle. *Caution: Do not disturb coverslip.*
   c. Slowly release finger to allow mixture from bulb to flow evenly and completely under coverslip and over surface of ruled area. Be sure to fill area completely, but do not overfill or underfill.
   d. Use second dilution prepared in separate pipette to fill opposite side of hemocytometer and repeat loading procedure. Place hemocytometer in Petri dish and cover; allow to stand for approximately 5 minutes to allow cells to settle.

Microscopic Cell Counting Procedure

The cells included in the microscopic count of each square on the hemocytometer counting chamber are determined as illustrated in Figure 24-4. All cells touching any one

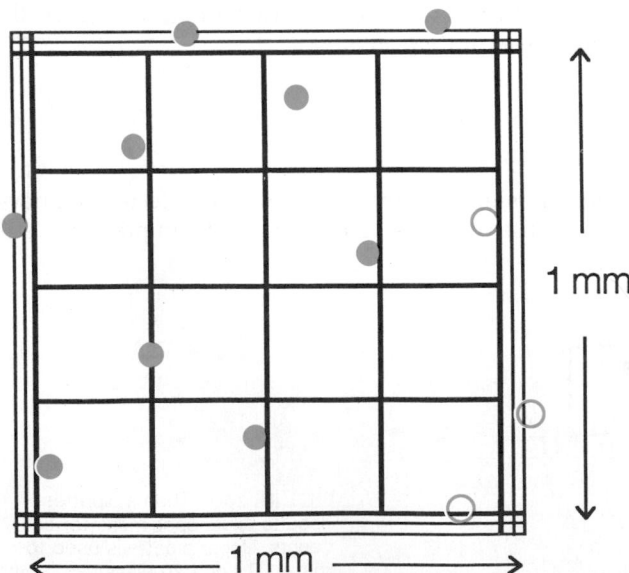

FIGURE 24-4. Rules for microscopic counting of leukocytes on the Neubauer hemocytometer. One square millimeter is illustrated. Leukocytes are counted in eight of these 1-mm squares, four on each side of the hemocytometer. Leukocytes that touch the top or left triple boundary lines are counted; those that touch the bottom or right boundaries are not. (*Solid circle,* cells counted; *open circle,* cells not counted.)

of the triple lines at the top or left of the square being evaluated are counted. All cells touching any one of the triple lines at the bottom or to the right are excluded from the count. This convention is used to count any cellular element in any square of the hemocytometer. Standard areas of the counting chamber used for counting leukocytes, erythrocytes, and platelets are illustrated in Figure 24-2. Standard counting areas for these elements exist in modern laboratory practice, the actual areas counted vary widely. Professional laboratorians must be prepared to adapt the use of the hemocytometer to the specimen being examined.

Microscopic Cell Counting

PROCEDURE

1. Rotate the low-power objective of the microscope into viewing position. *Caution:* This step is important to avoid damaging the hemocytometer and microscope objective lenses.
2. Carefully place hemocytometer on microscope stage. Move X/Y motion control knobs so that center of one hemocytometer counting area is directly under objective.
3. To assist in focusing, move low-power objective as close as possible to hemocytometer, using coarse adjustment knob. Do not force knob.
4. While looking into oculars, turn coarse adjustment knob so that hemocytometer and low-power objective begin moving farther apart until grid lines come into focus. Leukocyte nuclei appear as slightly iridescent but not refractile objects. The cells should look like small dark or black dots. If necessary, adjust the light intensity, lower the condenser, or partially close the iris diaphragm to obtain an optimal field of view.
5. Using X/Y motion control knob, move hemocytomer so that top left square of counting area is in center of field of view. This is where leukocyte count is begun.
6. Begin counting cells in upper left 1 × 1-mm square of ruled area.
7. For a standard leukocyte count, identify and count the cells over the four 1-mm-square corners of each side of the hemocytometer (areas marked W in Fig. 24-2).
8. Calculate the number of leukocytes per liter for each side of the hemocytometer. Average the results and report this number.

CALCULATIONS

Cells ($\times 10^9$/L) =

$$\frac{\text{Total cells counted} \times \text{Specimen dilution factor}}{\text{mm}^2 \text{ counted} \times 0.1 \text{ mm}} \times 10^6$$

(*Note:* 0.1 mm is the depth of fluid in chamber.) To calculate any dilution factor, set up this equation:

$$\frac{1}{\text{dilution}}$$

Example: 100 cells were counted on side A and 110 cells on side B in the four 1-mm^2 corners of the cell grid from a 1:20 dilution.

For this example, the dilution factor is then:

$$\frac{1}{1/20} = 20$$

$$\text{Side A} = \frac{100 \times 20}{4 \times 0.1} \times 10^6 = 5.0 \times 10^9/\text{L}$$

$$\text{Side B} = \frac{110 \times 20}{4 \times 0.1} \times 10^6 = 5.5 \times 10^9/\text{L}$$

Average of sides A and B =

$$\frac{(5.0 + 5.5)}{2} \times 10^9/\text{L} = 5.3 \times 10^9/\text{L} = \frac{\text{Final}}{\text{WBC count}}$$

TABLE 24-2
Current SI Units Conversion from Former Reporting Units for Leukocytes (WBC), Erythrocytes (RBC), and Platelets (PLT)*

Cell Type	Former Reporting Units	Current Reporting Units	Former Example	Current Example
WBC	$\times 10^3/mm^3$	$\times 10^9/L$	$8.0 \times 10^3/mm^3$	$8.0 \times 10^9/L$
RBC	$\times 10^6/mm^3$	$\times 10^{12}/L$	$4.5 \times 10^6/mm^3$	$4.5 \times 10^{12}/L$
PLT	$\times 10^3/mm^3$	$\times 10^9/L$	$350 \times 10^3/mm^3$	$350 \times 10^9/L$

* The examples in the Former column are equivalent to those in the Current column.

In the past, cell counts for blood and body fluids were reported in cells per cubic millimeter (mm^3). This was subsequently changed to cells per microliter (μL; $1\ mm^3 = 1\ \mu L$). It is now recommended that laboratories report these counts in SI units (Chap. 9; see Table 9-6), in which counts are reported as cells/L, as in the formula above. By SI convention, cell counts are reported as illustrated in Table 24-2.

QUALITY CONTROL. Quality control in manual counting is primarily a function of the technical expertise of the laboratorian. A quality control program for manual counts should monitor the following items:

1. Specimens must be checked individually for clots. Clotted specimens are unsuitable for counting any cellular element.
2. Diluting with either Thoma pipettes or Unopettes must be done with scrupulous attention to technique. Only Thoma pipettes that meet NBS specifications should be used. Such pipettes have an indication on the stem of the accuracy of pipette measurement (*i.e.*, $\pm$ 0.5%). Pipettes with cracked or chipped tips should be discarded in a waste container designated for broken glass or sharp objects.
3. Only hemocytometers that meet NBS specifications should be used.
4. Levels of reservoir diluent in Unopettes should be checked visually to ensure that the volume appears correct. The reservoirs can be used only prior to their expiration date (check storage container for lot number and expiration date). Pipettes with expired reservoirs are useful for practice.

Cells must be evenly distributed over the hemocytometer surface. For a standard leukocyte count within the reference range, there should be no more than a 15-cell difference between the highest and lowest total number of cells found among the eight 1-mm-square corner squares counted.[17] Total cells counted on each side of the counting chamber should agree within 10% of each other.[4] Counts that do not meet this standard should not be reported. Rather, the procedure should be repeated carefully using an acceptable, well-mixed specimen.

Even with a skilled laboratorian and meticulous attention to detail, manual counting has a high percentage of imprecision and error that cannot be avoided. This error is attributed to the small number of cells counted; the uncontrollable variation in cell distribution when the sample is loaded on the hemocytometer; the error in graduations of the pipette and hemocytometer; and various operator errors in the dilution process or loading process. For leukocyte counts using a 1:20 dilution, the 95% confidence limits are approximately 15%. For example, given a manual leukocyte count of $5.0 \times 10^9/L$ performed using a 1:20 dilution, the 95% confidence limits for the count are approximately $5.0 \pm 0.8 \times 10^9/L$.

LEUKOCYTE REFERENCE RANGES. Each laboratory should determine its own population reference range (Chap. 44).

In 1952 the normal adult leukocyte reference range reported in one study was 4.5 to $11.0 \times 10^9/L$, based on manually counted samples.[2] Current published reference ranges are based on automated, electronically, or optically counted samples.

Because leukocyte counts are age dependent, a single meaningful reference range cannot be established. Table 24-3 defines total leukocyte reference ranges as a function of age. These ranges were derived with automated cell counters. Other studies of absolute leukocyte reference ranges for adults have been published.[8,24] Many other factors cause variations in individual leukocyte counts, including time of day,[2,24] stress,[18] and exercise.[1] Black subjects usually have lower reference ranges based on lower absolute neutrophil values,[5,14,31] although in one study of American blacks, a decreased neutrophil count was not evident.[8]

With more sophisticated automated instruments and greater care in selecting normal sample populations, according to some investigators, the upper limit of the adult reference range may be lower than that based on manual counts.[27]

MANUAL DIFFERENTIAL CELL COUNTS

Performing differential cell counts is an art form. Skill is acquired only through practice based on a solid background of technical knowledge. The steps required to perform a complete differential are discussed in detail here.

PRINCIPLE. A blood film review is first performed on an appropriately prepared and stained blood film, which involves a systematic microscopic scan to estimate leukocyte count, identify morphologic erythrocyte abnormalities, and estimate platelet number. Finally leukocytes are classifed into group types.

SPECIMEN REQUIREMENTS. Whole unclotted blood is required for preparing the peripheral blood film. Fresh peripheral blood from a skin puncture is the specimen of choice for a manual differential count, but if anticoagulated blood must be used, K_3EDTA or K_2EDTA (1.5 ± 0.15 mg/mL) is recommended. EDTA is preferred, because it prevents formation of artifacts and acceptably preserves blood for up to 4 hours.[23] Blood samples should be kept at room temperature. Use of an anticoagulant introduces certain morphologic changes in the leukocytes, which become increasingly exaggerated with storage time. Examples of these changes include vacuoles in the cytoplasm of granulocytes and karyorrhexis (nuclear disintegration) (Chap. 3). When final evaluations of blood films are made, the amount of time the cells were allowed to interact with EDTA before the films were prepared and stained should be taken into consideration.

REAGENTS AND EQUIPMENT. The reagents and equipment for both manual and automated preparation and staining of

TABLE 24-3
*Leukocyte Values in Humans**

Age	Total Leukocytes ($\times 10^9$/L)	Neutrophils			Eosinophils	Basophils	Lymphocytes	Monocytes
		Total	Band	Segmented				
12 hr	13.0–38.0	6.0–28.0 68%	2.33† 10.2%	13.2 58%	0.02–0.95 2.0%	0–0.5 0.4%	2.0–11.0 31%	0.40–3.6 5.3%
1 wk	5.0–12.0	1.5–10.0 45%	0.83 6.8%	4.7 39%	0.07–1.10 4.1%	0–0.25 0.4%	2.0–17.0 41%	0.30–2.7 4.8%
12 mo	6.0–17.5	1.5–8.5 31%	0.35 3.1%	3.2 28%	0.05–0.70 2.6%	0–0.2 0.4%	4.0–10.5 61%	0.05–1.1 4.8%
6 yr	5.0–14.5	1.5–8.0 51%	0–1.0 3.0%	1.5–7.0 48%	0–0.65 2.7%	0–0.2 0.6%	1.5–7.0 42%	0.0–0.8 4.7%
14 yr	4.5–13.0	1.8–8.0 56%	0–1.0 3.0%	1.8–7.0 53%	0–0.50 2.5%	0–0.2 0.5%	1.2–5.8 37%	0.0–0.8 4.7%
21 yr	4.5–11.0	1.8–7.7 59%	0–0.7 3.0%	1.8–7.0 56%	0–0.45 2.7%	0–0.2 0.5%	1.0–4.8 34%	0.0–0.8 4.0%

* Values listed first for each age are absolute counts ($\times 10^9$/L); values listed second, as percentages, are relative counts.
† Band count at 12 hours includes a small percentage of myelocytes.
(From Altman PL, Dittmer DS: Blood and Other Body Fluids, p 125. Bethesda, MD, Federation of American Societies for Experimental Biology, 1961, with permission.)

peripheral blood films for manual differential counts are discussed in Chapter 3. Blood films should be stained within one hour of preparation.

    MICROSCOPE PREPARATION. Too often the microscope is taken for granted. Like other instruments, it requires daily performance checks. The Koehler illumination procedure (Chap. 4) should be performed prior to each session with the microscope, particularly when performing differential counts, to ensure the best resolution and clarity in viewing hematopoietic cells.

PROCEDURE

I. **Check slide identification.** Check blood film identification to ensure that film and automated count report identification match.

II. **Perform patient specimen orientation.** To become familiar with the patient specimen, carefully review the automated count report, noting the number of leukocytes and platelets, the number and size (MCV) of erythrocytes, the hemoglobin concentration (MCHC) of erythrocytes, and the RDW, if measured. During the differential process, the above information is compared to the actual findings on the blood film. Any extreme discrepancy (*e.g.*, a reference range platelet count on the automated report but only a rare platelet on the blood film) should be investigated immediately and resolved before the differential count is reported.

III. **Perform low-power scan to review blood film adequacy.**

  A. **Check feather edge (Fig. 24-5) for fibrin threads.** Fibrin threads may be present even in films made from specimens that do not contain gross clots. Fibrin threads tend to entrap larger leukocytes and are accompanied by platelet clumping. Neither a differential count nor a platelet estimate should be attempted on blood films that exhibit fibrin threads.

  B. **Examine film edges for excess leukocytes.** The edges of even the best-prepared blood films have accumulations of granulocytes and monocytes, but in films that are spread too thin, most of the large cells are pushed to the film edges, leaving relatively more lymphocytes in the center. Blood film edges should contain less than two to four times more leukocytes per field than the number present in the body of the film.[23,30]

  C. **Verify acceptable number of leukocytes.** In a total leuko-

cyte count of no less than 4.0×10^9/L, the acceptable working area should contain at least 300 leukocytes.[23] This may be quickly ascertained by someone experienced in scanning blood films.

  D. **Verify stain quality.** The stain should clearly distinguish between dark purple nuclear material and bright red-orange erythrocytes (Chap. 3).

  E. **Examine erythrocyte distribution patterns and shapes.** Erythrocytes normally repel one another. In the examination area of a well-prepared blood film, the erythrocytes should be distributed evenly and singly (or just slightly overlapping) in at least a lateral strip along the thinner end of the blood film. The cells should not be distorted. This strip should be the diameter of one low-power field. In the presence of abnormal serum globulins the erythro-

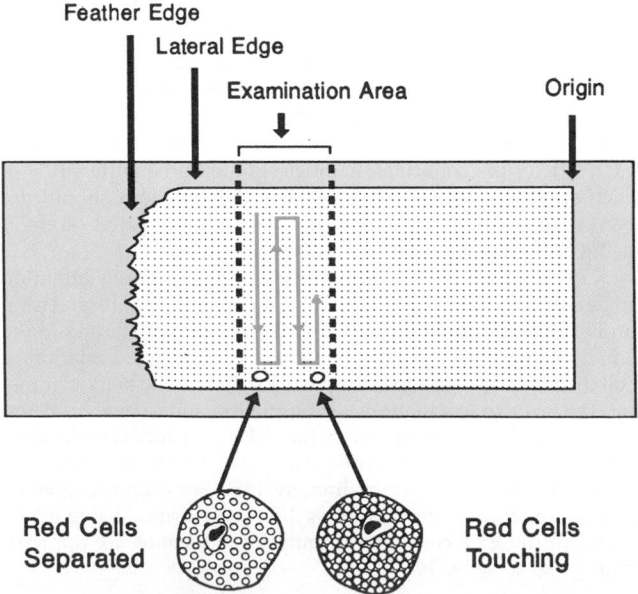

FIGURE 24-5. Illustration of a properly made push-wedge peripheral blood film showing the "battlement" pattern for leukocyte differential procedure.

cytes may assume rouleaux formations (Chap. 8). In the presence of certain antibodies to RBC surface antigens (*e.g.*, cold agglutinins), erythrocyte clumping or agglutination may be seen. The presence of either rouleaux or agglutination should be indicated on the differential report (Chap. 8).

The presence of certain abnormal erythrocyte shapes can be readily detected under low-power scan (*e.g.*, target cells, sickle cells, spherocytes). The many types of anisocytosis and poikilocytosis that should be indicated on the differential report are discussed in Chapter 8.

IV. **Perform oil-immersion examination of the blood film.**

A. **Prepare blood film with oil.** Evenly spread a thin layer of nondrying type B immersion oil over the blood film in the examination area toward the feather edge. Use oil sparingly and never substitute other types of lubricants for immersion oil, because substitutes may damage optical lense mounting.

B. **Calculate ratio of electronic platelet count to platelets per oil-immersion field.** Before platelet estimates can be performed, the laboratory must calculate the ratio of the electronic platelet count to the number of platelets per oil-immersion (or high-power) field of view. This must be done once for every microscope brand in the laboratory that is used for platelet estimates because of the slight differences in the field of view among microscope brands. Once this ratio is calculated, it may be used to determine an estimation factor for platelet estimates that may be used until there are major repairs or changes to the instrument used to obtain the electronic platelet counts or until a new microscope is used for the estimates. Any major changes of this nature warrant a close check of the current ratio, and possibly recalculation of the ratio, particularly when new equipment is introduced. The procedure for calculation of this ratio and estimation factor is as follows:

1. Perform electronic platelet counts on 30 consecutive fresh patient blood samples. Make sure the platelet count is in control.
2. Prepare and stain one peripheral blood film for each sample.
3. For each film, under oil-immersion microscopy, find an area where 50% of the red cells are overlapping in doublets or triplets. Then count the number of platelets in 10 consecutive fields.
4. Divide by 10 the total number of platelets found to obtain the average number per single oil-immersion field.
5. Divide the electronic platelet count by the average number of platelets per oil field.
6. Add the numbers obtained in step 5 and divide by 30 (the number of observations in this analysis) to obtain the average ratio of the platelet count–to–platelets per oil-immersion field.
7. Round the number calculated in step 6 to the nearest whole number to obtain an estimation factor, the number of peripheral blood platelets represented by one platelet in an oil-immersion field. Table 24-4 provides an example of this calculation. Each laboratory should perform this calculation using its own microscope and electronic equipment.

C. **Estimate platelet count.** Once the platelet estimation factor is calculated (step 7 above), the laboratory scientist may simply calculate the average number of platelets per oil-immersion field on all subsequent specimens and multiply this number by the estimation factor to obtain the platelet estimate. For example, in the hypothetical laboratory data represented in Table 24-4, if the average number of platelets found for any given sample on oil-immersion

fields is 17, the platelet estimate calculation would be $17 \times 15 \times 10^9/L = 255 \times 10^9/L$.

The following guidelines are provided to facilitate platelet estimates:

1. The approximate reference range for platelets is 140 to $440 \times 10^9/L$.
2. There are approximately 10 to 40 red cells per platelet in normal peripheral blood. Thus, an oil-immersion field ($1000\times$ magnification) containing 100 red cells should have 3 to 10 platelets, whereas a field with 200 red cells should have 5 to 20 platelets.
3. As with leukocyte estimates, platelet estimates in the presence of abnormal hematocrit values tend to be biased. A somewhat more sophisticated method for estimating platelet counts makes use of the Miller disk (see Fig. 9-7), which has also been used for reticulocyte counts. This method assumes that the ratio of platelets to red cells should be the same as the ratio of these two cell types in the blood sample. If this ratio is not similar to the one found by the hematology analyzer, the analyzer may have generated an erroneous platelet count. Although this method is more tedious than the method described here, it yields more reliable information.[19]
4. Accurate estimates are possible only when there are no platelet clumps, or at most, rare clumps of two to three platelets. Larger or more numerous platelet clumps cause inaccurate estimates. If clumps are noted, the original blood specimen should be reexamined for clots. If clots are not found, platelet clumping in the presence of EDTA should be suspected and noted on the specimen report.
5. Platelet estimate reports and leukocyte differential count reports should also indicate the presence of large or morphologically abnormal platelets. Because of their size they could be counted by automated counting instruments as erythrocytes or even lymphocytes, resulting in an inaccurate platelet total.
6. If different brands of microscopes are used in the same laboratory, they may have different field-of-view diameters, so a correction factor is required to calculate all counts performed on the microscope with the larger (or smaller) field of view to ensure consistency in reporting (Chap.4). Otherwise, the estimation factor should be calculated for each microscope brand used in any given laboratory (Table 24-4) and used appropriately for platelet estimates.

D. **Estimate leukocyte count.** Total leukocyte counts can be estimated roughly under either high-power scan ($400\times$) or oil-immersion microscopy ($1000\times$). The same procedure described in Table 24-4 for platelets can be applied to determining a leukocyte count estimation factor. Leukocyte count estimates should always be a part of the blood film review to verify the automated leukocyte count. Many laboratories report the estimated blood film leukocyte count only as low, normal, or high. In general, this is the best practice, since it is difficult to estimate the leukocyte count very accurately. Experience is the biggest factor in being able to perform leukocyte estimates accurately and consistently.

An accurate estimate depends on an acceptable anticoagulated specimen free from clots, a well-prepared blood film, a well-trained laboratory scientist, and development and use of an estimation factor appropriate for the microscope in use. An estimation factor must be determined for each microscope brand used in the laboratory. If there are any questions about the accuracy of an automated leukocyte count when it is compared to the estimate, the specimen identification should be rechecked,

TABLE 24-4
*Calculation of the Platelet Count Estimation Factor**

Sample Number	Electronic Platelet Count ($\times 10^9$/L)	Average No. Platelets Per Oil-Immersion Field (Based on 10 Fields)	Electronic Platelet Count Divided by Average No. Platelets per Oil-Immersion Field
1	252	17.1	14.737
2	301	24.1	12.490
3	282	18.6	15.161
4	60	4.0	15.000
5	257	16.8	15.298
6	388	26.1	14.866
7	290	18.9	15.344
8	246	15.9	15.472
9	450	29.1	15.464
10	56	4.1	13.659
11	10	0.8	12.500
12	312	19.3	16.166
13	252	16.2	15.556
14	90	5.8	15.517
15	136	8.6	15.814
16	298	21.0	14.190
17	362	22.9	15.808
18	95	5.8	16.379
19	280	18.3	15.301
20	157	12.0	13.083
21	240	15.5	15.484
22	200	12.8	15.625
23	15	1.5	10.000
24	281	18.9	14.868
25	195	13.5	14.444
26	198	13.1	15.115
27	71	4.4	16.136
28	262	18.1	14.475
29	328	21.3	15.399
30	188	12.9	14.574
		Total:	443.925

$$\frac{SUM}{n} = \frac{443.925}{30} = 14.798 \approx 15.0$$

Therefore: 1 platelet per oil field $\approx 15.0 \times 10^9$/L

* Due to slight differences in the field of view, this must be done for each microscope brand (e.g., Nikon, American Optical, Olympus) used in the laboratory, to obtain accurate peripheral film platelet estimates. This table presents sample platelet estimate data from a hospital laboratory showing platelet counts obtained from a Coulter Model S Plus IV and manual platelet counts obtained from peripheral blood films under oil immersion microscopy using the laboratory's own microscope brand. The ratio of platelet count to platelets per oil-immersion field was calculated and the average of these ratios was taken to determine the actual number of peripheral blood platelets represented by one platelet on an oil-immersion field.

the automated count should be repeated, and a new blood film should be prepared and evaluated. A manual count may also be performed if necessary.

Estimates should never be attempted without a knowledge of the hematocrit value of the specimen from which the film was made. As the hematocrit increases, the leukocyte estimate tends to be falsely decreased; as the hematocrit decreases, the leukocyte estimate tends to be falsely increased. Leukocytes should be evenly distributed over the examination area. Leukocyte clumping or the presence of endothelial or epithelial cells should be included in the comments of the differential count report.

E. **Perform differential leukocyte count.**
1. Classify at least 100 leukocytes. Larger numbers (200–400) yield more precise results. Leukocyte differentiation involves the counting and morphologic classification of 100 leukocytes reviewed while using a specific search pattern in the appropriate examination area of a blood film. The "battlement" track method is used to count leukocytes (see Fig. 24-5).[23] Another recommended method is the "lengthwise" or "longitudinal" pattern in which cells are counted in consecutive fields in strips or rows from the tail end straight back toward the thick end of the film.[23] Again, leukocytes should only be differentiated in areas where erythrocytes are distributed evenly and singly (or just slightly overlapping), making leukocytes more easily identifiable. As many strips as necessary are counted until the desired number of leukocytes is counted. Each intact leukocyte must be classified, including distorted cells that can be clearly identified (e.g., fragile eosinophils). Skipping cells that look unfamiliar skews the results and is inaccurate and unacceptable practice. They should be classified as unidentified cells. Chapters 22 and 23 present a

detailed description of the appearance of mature and immature leukocytes.

2. Report results of the 100 cells classified as a percentage. These results are considered *relative* cell counts. For example, if 60 neutrophils were found among 100 leukocytes counted, this would be reported as 60% neutrophils. When manual differential counters are used, the technologist must verify that the sum of the percentages equals 100%.

3. Keep a separate count of nucleated red blood cells (NRBCs). NRBCs are counted separately while classifying the 100 leukocytes. They should be reported as the number per 100 leukocytes counted. If more than 5 NRBCs are found per 100 leukocytes, the automated leukocyte count must be corrected because NRBCs, being as large as small leukocytes, erroneously elevate the automated leukocyte count. The calculation for correction of the leukocyte count when NRBCs are present is discussed below in the section on Calculations.

4. Note and report abnormal leukocyte morphology. Leukocytes may appear abnormal or demonstrate inclusions, which must be noted on the differential count report. For example, toxic granulation in neutrophils is an indication of infection or chemical toxicity. The many abnormal morphologic features that may occur are reviewed in Chapters 25 and 26.

5. Identify and grade abnormal erythrocyte morphology (Chap. 8). Erythrocyte morphology is observed first under low-power scan for major abnormalities. It should also be observed during leukocyte differentiation and, finally, as a separate evaluation under oil immersion microscopy. Although abnormalities of erythrocyte shape and size may be observed under low power, erythrocyte inclusions such as malaria, basophilic stippling, Howell-Jolly bodies, and others can be visualized with certainty only by using oil-immersion microscopy (Chap. 8).

6. Identify and report in the differential comments any miscellaneous nonleukocyte abnormal cells, such as endothelial cells or NRBCs, that are found during the differential. Such cells are not included in the 100-cell leukocyte differential count. Table 24-5 provides a description of well known miscellaneous cells and the normal and abnormal conditions under which they are found.

QUALITY CONTROL FOR DIFFERENTIAL CELL COUNTS. As for manual cell counts, quality control for differentials is basically a function of the expertise, alertness, and attention to detail of the laboratory scientist; however, when differentials are performed in an institution by a group of laboratory scientists, the following steps should be taken to ensure uniform reporting within the group:

1. Agree on the definition of all terms used (*e.g.*, band or stab neutrophil, variant or atypical lymphocyte, Downey cell, Türk cell).

2. Establish 95% confidence limits within the group for differential performance and reporting (Table 24-6). This should be done on a cell-by-cell basis. Whenever available, a cell count from a properly calibrated automated instrument that counts large numbers of cells should be used as the true value. For example, if five laboratory scientists each perform a 100-cell differential on the same blood film, and the true number of peripheral blood lymphocytes according to the instrument count is 8%, then the reported value of each laboratory scientist, according to Table 24-6, should be between 3% and 16% lymphocytes. This ensures that all personnel are reporting differential results within the 95% confidence limits. The auto-

mated three-part differential count, which includes granulocytes, lymphocytes, and monocytes, can be used as the mean or observed value *a* in Table 24-6, to establish confidence limits for manual differentials. Note in Table 24-6 that, as more cells are differentiated, the confidence interval range becomes tighter (*i.e.*, the differential count becomes more accurate).

3. Regularly circulate unfamiliar slides among the group members and compare results with established confidence limits.

4. Establish a required level of accuracy that new laboratory personnel must achieve before being cleared to report differential count results.

5. Establish a list of abnormalities, which, if observed on the differential study, must be reviewed by the supervisor or clinical pathologist before results are reported (*e.g.*, presence of blasts or any unclassified cells).

Calculations for Correction of Leukocyte Count in the Presence of Nucleated Erythrocytes

When more than five nucleated red blood cells are found during a 100-leukocyte differential count, correction of the automated leukocyte count is necessary. The correction calculation is as follows:

$$\frac{WBC \times 10^9/L \times 100}{NRBC \text{ per } 100 \text{ leukocytes} + 100} = \text{corrected WBC count}$$

For example, given a WBC count of $24.0 \times 10^9/L$ and an NRBC count of 20/100 WBC,

$$\frac{24.0 \times 10^9/L \times 100}{20 + 100} = 20.0 \times 10^9/L,$$
$$= \text{Corrected WBC count}$$

Calculation of Absolute and Relative Cell Counts

Performance of the routine leukocyte differential count yields results in terms of relative cell counts (*i.e.*, the percentage of total leukocytes represented by a specific cell type). Table 24-7 provides examples of how to convert relative cell counts to "indirect" absolute cell counts. The formula follows:

$$\text{Indirect relative cell count} \times \frac{\text{Total WBC count}}{\text{count}} = \frac{\text{Absolute}}{\text{cell count}}$$

The percentage of each cell group observed on the differential is used in this formula to obtain the indirect absolute cell count for each cell type. The results should be compared to the established laboratory reference range. Table 24-3 provides a sample reference range chart for absolute leukocyte counts at various ages.

This calculation is referred to as the indirect absolute cell count because it is only an estimate of the actual number of cells per liter of any given cell type. The direct absolute cell count requires actually counting each cell type, either manually or by automated methods.

Absolute cell counts provide much more accurate assessments of the actual number of each cell type in the peripheral blood. As automated counting of specific cell types becomes more universal, absolute values are becoming the standard reporting format. Note in Table 24-7 two

TABLE 24-5
Miscellaneous Cells that May Be Found During the Peripheral Blood
*Film Differential Count**

Cell Type	Description	Normal Conditions Under Which Cells are Found	Abnormal Conditions Under Which Cells are Found
Smudge cells	Nuclear remnants of lymphocytes; formed during blood film preparation. Appearance is similar to a thumbprint. Chromatin is structureless.	A few may be found normally.	Disease characterized by abnormal proliferation of lymphocytes (*e.g.*, chronic lymphocytic leukemia)
Basket cells	Nuclear remnants of granulocytic cells with netlike chromatin pattern; formed during blood film preparation.	A few may be found normally.	Some leukemias
Necrotic cells	Granulocytic cells with pyknotic nuclei and no filaments between segments	None	Prolonged exposure to EDTA; chemotherapy (rarely)
Phagocytic cells	Neutrophil that has engulfed foreign substance (*e.g.*, bacteria, fungus)	None	Overwhelming septicemia, bacterial and fungal infections, erythrophagocytosis in which neutrophil engulfs RBC
Endothelial cells	These large cells (20–30 μm), which line the veins, often have a stretched, ovoid appearance. They have a single nucleus with dense chromatin and no nucleoli. Cytoplasm is abundant and appears translucent. Cells may appear in sheets. Usually found at feather edge; distinctive appearance when compared to blood cells.	Found occasionally in blood obtained by venipuncture or capillary puncture	This cell is considered a contaminant. It must not be confused with clumps of malignant cells.
Megakaryocyte fragments	Medium to large, nude nuclei that stain dark purple.	Newborns	Aberrant platelet production, myelofibrosis, essential thrombocythemia, extreme hypoxia
Nucleated red blood cells (NRBCs)	Varies according to cell maturity (Chap. 6). Usually no attempt is made to classify the maturity of NRBCs; they are only counted, and the number per 100 WBC is reported.	Newborns	NRBCs may be found in many abnormal conditions (*e.g.*, hemolysis, leukemia, myeloproliferative disorders, and others)

* These cells are not counted as part of the 100 leukocytes but should be mentioned in the comments when they are observed.

different specimens with the same "normal" differential count results. One has a leukocyte count of 8.0×10^9/L, which is within the adult reference range, and the other has a leukocyte count of 2.0×10^9/L, which is below the reference range. Calculation of the absolute neutrophil and lymphocyte counts reveals that, although the differential results appear normal for both, the specimen with the 2.0×10^9/L leukocyte count indicates an absolute decrease in neutrophils and lymphocytes in the peripheral blood.

Leukocyte Differential Count Reference Ranges

Table 24-3 provides a relative mean leukocyte number for each normal leukocyte type for subjects ranging in age from newborn through adult. Ranges are shown for absolute counts. Table 24-8 provides a sample reference

range for the leukocyte differential count in terms of relative numbers based on data from 507 healthy adults.[32] Each laboratory should develop its own reference range for the differential count to include gender and age reference ranges. Relative cell counts should always be considered in terms of the total leukocyte count (*i.e.*, converted to an absolute count) for proper interpretation of the results, as just discussed.

Comments and Sources of Error

Although morphologic evaluation of a stained blood film is one of the most important hematologic procedures, the manual differentiation of leukocytes is an inaccurate and unreproducible method that is subject to errors that cannot be totally eliminated, including sampling errors, uncontrollable errors in cell distribution on the blood film, and human inconsistency in cell interpretation.

TABLE 24-6
Confidence Limits* for Percentages of Specific Cell Types Identified by Manual Differential Counts

a (Observed Percentage of Specific Cell Type)	n (Total Cells Counted in Differential)			
	100	200	500	1000
0	0 4	0 2	0 1	0 1
1	0 6	0 4	0 3	0 2
2	0 8	0 6	0 4	1 4
3	0 9	1 7	1 5	2 5
4	1 10	1 8	2 7	2 6
5	1 12	2 10	3 8	3 7
6	2 13	3 11	4 9	4 8
7	2 14	3 12	4 10	5 9
8	3 16	4 13	5 11	6 10
9	4 17	5 14	6 12	7 11
10	4 18	6 16	7 13	8 13
15	8 24	10 21	11 19	12 18
20	12 30	14 27	16 24	17 23
25	16 35	19 32	21 30	22 28
30	21 40	23 37	26 35	27 33
35	25 46	28 43	30 40	32 39
40	30 51	33 48	35 45	36 44
45	35 56	38 53	40 50	41 49
50	39 61	42 58	45 55	46 54

* Confidence coefficient, 95%.

Example: If 6% monocytes were identified in a 100-cell differential (n = 100), there is a confidence coefficient of 95% that the true value is between 2% and 13% and a 5% chance that it is not.

For a over 50, obtain confidence limits by reading limits for 100 − a in the table and subtracting them from 100.

Example: The 95% confidence limits for 75% neutrophils counted in a sample where 100 cells were counted (n = 100) are between 65% and 84%.

From Rumke CL: Variability of results in differential counts on blood smears. Triangle, Sandoz Journal of Medical Science 4:156, 1960. Copyright Sandoz Ltd, Basle, Switzerland, with permission.

TABLE 24-8
Total Leukocyte Count and Relative Leukocyte Count Reference Ranges for Adults*

Total leukocytes	$4.1–10.9 \times 10^9$/L
Neutrophils	47.0–79.5%
Lymphocytes	12.5–40.0%
Monocytes	2.0–11.0%
Eosinophils	0.0–7.5%
Basophils	0.0–2.0%

* Counts are based on analysis of blood from 507 healthy adults. Although not shown in this table, bands may also normally be seen in the peripheral blood (approximately 0.0 to 6.0%). These ranges will vary; therefore, each laboratory must determine its own reference ranges. Other chapters in this text list slightly different reference ranges for these cell types to emphasize the variance that normally exists in studies of different individuals from institution to institution.

From Zacharski LR, Elveback LR, Linman JW: Leukocyte counts in healthy adults. Am J Clin Pathol 56:148, 1971, with permission.

Certain cell types, particularly monocytes, eosinophils, and basophils, may be distributed in a nonrandom manner on a blood film. High percentages of these cell types, especially if in a limited area of the film, should be rechecked before the numbers are reported.

Differential counts on leukocyte numbers in excess of 35.0×10^9/L can be performed on 200 cells to improve precision. As the leukocyte total rises, the total number of leukocytes counted should increase proportionally to ensure sampling from a sufficiently large portion of the examination area.

As leukocyte totals drop below 2.0×10^9/L, some laboratories may perform differential counts on fewer than 100 cells; however, this is not recommended because when fewer cells are counted, the imprecision of the differential increases tremendously (see Table 24-6). It is recommended that if less than 100 cells can be found, a

TABLE 24-7
Example of Conversion of Relative Cell Counts Obtained from Two Sample Leukocyte Differentials to Indirect Absolute Cell Counts*

	Relative Cell Count (%)	×	Total Leukocyte Count ($\times 10^9$/L)	=	Absolute Cell Count ($\times 10^9$/L)	Adult Reference Range ($\times 10^9$/L)
PATIENT A SAMPLE: "NORMAL" DIFFERENTIAL WITH LEUKOCYTE COUNT IN REFERENCE RANGE						
Neutrophils	75%		8.0		6.0	1.8–7.7
Lymphocytes	18%		8.0		1.4	1.0–4.8
Monocytes	6%		8.0		0.5	0.0–0.8
Eosinophils	1%		8.0		0.1	0.0–0.45
PATIENT B SAMPLE: "NORMAL" DIFFERENTIAL WITH LEUKOCYTE COUNT BELOW REFERENCE RANGE						
Neutrophils	75%		2.0		1.5	1.8–7.7
Lymphocytes	18%		2.0		0.4	1.0–4.8
Monocytes	6%		2.0		0.1	0.0–0.8
Eosinophils	1%		2.0		0.02	0.0–0.45

* Both relative and absolute counts must be compared to laboratory reference ranges. Absolute counts provide a more accurate assessment of the types of leukocytes present in the peripheral blood as shown by comparison of the "normal" differential in a sample with a leukocyte count within the reference range to the exact same "normal" differential from a patient with a leukocyte count below the reference range. Note that comparison of the absolute values to the reference ranges shows that the neutrophils and lymphocytes are within the reference range for patient A but they are both below the reference range for patient B.

buffy coat preparation should be made in which leukocytes are concentrated before being spread on a glass slide (Chap. 3). The stained smear is then observed for abnormal cells; a differential is not possible on the buffy coat preparation. Such preparations have two drawbacks, including a preparation method that causes morphologic changes in the leukocytes and uneven distribution of cell types, and the procedure itself which is time consuming. Counting fewer than 100 cells on a blood film is unacceptable.

A note of the *actual* number of cells counted *must* be included in the differential report if more than 100 or fewer than 100 cells are counted; however, the differential should be converted to 100% for reporting purposes unless the laboratory manager directs otherwise.

Because of their life-threatening implications, certain blood film findings may have to be reported immediately to the attending physician: schistocytes, which may indicate a hemolytic condition; blast forms (if never or not recently reported in the patient); neutrophilic phagocytosis of microorganisms indicating the presence of systemic infection; sickle cells; and erythrocytic microorganisms, among others. Laboratory policies and procedures should clearly indicate which findings demand immediate reporting to the physician after confirmation by a supervisor or clinical pathologist.

ABSOLUTE EOSINOPHIL COUNTING PROCEDURE

Occasionally, an absolute eosinophil count is still requested for diagnostic purposes, because it may be more accurate and clinically meaningful to determine the absolute number of eosinophils in a volume of blood than to determine the relative number from the differential count. Decreased eosinophil numbers (eosinopenia) are associated with hyperadrenalism (Cushing's disease). Increased eosinophil numbers (eosinophilia) occur with allergic reactions, parasitic infestations, brucellosis, and certain leukemias.

Absolute eosinophil counts may be direct or indirect. Calculation of the indirect count was discussed earlier and generally is used simply to verify the direct absolute count. It is recommended that an automated method (*e.g.,* a five-part differential instrument; Chap. 42) be used, if at all possible, to obtain absolute eosinophil counts.

Absolute Eosinophil Counts

PRINCIPLE. Using a suitably diluted specimen and appropriate stain, eosinophils can be identified and counted microscopically after a specimen is loaded on a hemocytometer. Phloxine in the stain causes eosinophils to appear red under light microscopy. Leukocytes, except the eosinophils, are lysed by sodium carbonate and water. Erythrocytes are lysed by propylene glycol in the diluting fluid. Heparin, if present in the diluting fluid, inhibits leukocyte clumping. Sodium carbonate also enhances eosinophil granule staining. The count is reported in terms of cells per liter.[28]

SPECIMEN. Whole blood anticoagulated with EDTA or heparin may be used. Skin puncture blood samples are also acceptable.

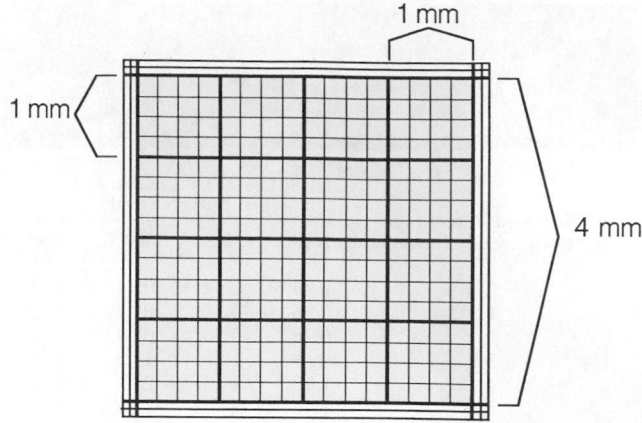

FIGURE 24-6. One ruled area of a Fuchs-Rosenthal hemocytometer. This special hemocytometer has two such counting areas, each with 16 1-mm-square areas for increased accuracy of eosinophil and basophil counting. Chamber depth is 0.2 mm, so that total volume is 6.4 mm³ (0.2 mm × 16 mm² × 2 counting areas).

REAGENTS. A prepared kit is available that uses the Unopette system for absolute eosinophil counts. The reservoir contains phloxine B solution in propylene glycol and distilled water. A 25-μL capillary pipette is used to aspirate the blood sample and make a 1:32 dilution in the reservoir. Alternatively, stains including Pilot's solution or Randolph's stain, may be prepared by the laboratory as described elsewhere.[28]

EQUIPMENT
Thoma WBC diluting pipette (or eosinophil Unopette reservoir and 25-μL pipette).

A special hemocytometer with a larger counting volume than that of the Neubauer, for eosinophil counts. Either the Fuchs-Rosenthal or Speirs-Levy hemocytometer is acceptable.

Fuchs-Rosenthal hemocytometer (Fig. 24-6). This hemocytometer has two ruled areas each consisting of one 4 × 4-mm square. The hemocytometer's depth is 0.2 mm. Total volume in each ruled area is therefore 16 mm² × 0.2 mm, or 3.2 mm³. Total volume that may be counted on the chamber is 2 × 3.2 mm³, or 6.4 mm³.

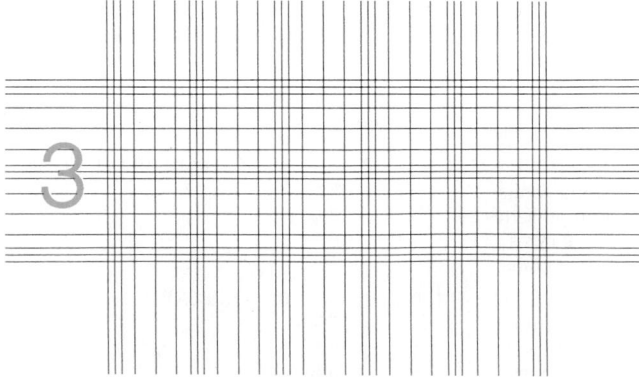

FIGURE 24-7. One counting area of a Speirs-Levy hemocytometer. This special hemocytometer has four such counting areas, each with ten 1-mm squares arranged in two horizontal rows of five. Eosinophils or basophils may be counted using this chamber. Chamber depth is 0.2 mm, so that total volume is 8 mm³ (0.2 mm × 10 mm² × 4 counting areas). An identification number engraved on the left side of each counting area and visible under the microscope facilitates orderly counting.

Speirs-Levy hemocytometer (Fig. 24-7). This hemocytometer has four counting areas, each consisting of ten 1×1-mm squares in two horizontal rows of five squares. Hemocytometer depth is 0.2 mm. Total volume of each counting area is 10×1 mm$^2 \times 0.2$ mm, or 2.0 mm^3. Total volume that may be counted on the chamber is 4×2.0 mm^3, or 8 mm^3. Either two or all four counting areas may be counted during the procedure.

For procedure and calculations for absolute eosinophil counts, see Randolph,[28] the first edition of this textbook, or the eosinophil Unopette System (Becton Dickinson, Rutherford, NJ[3]) package insert. Calculations are similar to those described earlier for manual leukocyte counts.

ABSOLUTE BASOPHIL COUNTING PROCEDURE

Direct absolute basophil counts occasionally are requested for diagnostic purposes, because the indirect absolute count derived from the differential count is not very reliable (the differential reference range for basophils being 0 to 2%). This count may be used to confirm *basophilia*, or an increase in the basophil count. It also may indicate *basopenia*, a decrease in the basophil count. Basophilia is associated with chronic myelogenous leukemia, polycythemia vera, myelofibrosis, myxedema, colitis, and sometimes chronic hemolytic anemia. Basopenia often occurs with allergic reactions. Refer to Cooper[6] for details on this seldom performed procedure, which calls for Cooper and Cruickshank stain and counting stained basophils on a Fuchs-Rosenthal or Speirs-Levy hemocytometer.

CONSIDERATIONS IN EVALUATING LEUKOCYTES FROM PEDIATRIC PATIENTS

Pediatric reference ranges for leukocytes and the morphologic appearance of children's leukocytes deserve special consideration because they are different from those of adults. A number of textbooks are available on the subject of normal and abnormal pediatric hematology.[16,22,26]

The reference range of newborns' total leukocyte count is higher than at any other time of life (see Table 24-3). Although it declines significantly within 1 week, the high side of the reference range remains above that of adults into the teenage years.

One of the most striking features on the blood film of a newborn is the normal presence of nucleated red blood cells. There may be as many as 24 per 100 leukocytes differentiated, but normally they are seen only during the first few days of life.

Immature leukocytes are also typical on the newborn's blood film. Usually there is a shift to the left (Chap. 25), which reflects the finding of immature granulocytes, including metamyelocytes, myelocytes, and occasionally, a promyelocyte.[15] These immature cells generally disappear within the first few days of life.

Table 24-3 presents the leukocyte reference ranges in terms of absolute and relative numbers for various age groups. Note that 12 hours after birth, the absolute neutro-

phil and monocyte counts can be higher than at any other age. Within 2 weeks, however, the neutrophil count may drop to within normal adult ranges.[25] Monocytes are increased during the first year of life but are normal thereafter.[29] Eosinophil counts may be higher during the first year of life than at any other time, but also decline gradually with age.[7] No significance has been detected in the relationship of basophil counts and age.[29]

Note also that the absolute lymphocyte count at birth may be higher than that of adolescents and adults. Seven days after birth, the count may actually be higher than it was at birth, and this elevation may persist into the first year of life. The count begins to decline gradually with increasing age, although even teenagers may normally have a higher absolute lymphocyte count than adults.

Of particular interest in the pediatric differential count is evaluation of the lymphocytes, which can be baffling. There may be many variations in the appearance, size, and color of lymphocytes, which are caused by disease states in both adults and children. But in pediatric patients, the problem of identifying lymphocytes is compounded because the *normal* morphology of children's lymphocytes differs from that of adults. One reason for this is the fact that significant numbers of pre–B and pre–T lymphocytes circulate in the peripheral blood of infants as compared to adults (Chap. 23 and Color Plate 27-14). Institutions where performance of pediatric differential counts is required should consult textbooks of pediatric hematology for guidance in establishing the criteria for differentiating between normal and abnormal lymphocytes.

A few megakaryocyte fragments may also be found on the newborn's peripheral blood film (see Table 24-5).

ANTINUCLEAR ANTIBODY (ANA) TEST

Autoantibodies called antinuclear antibodies (ANA) directed against a variety of intracellular nuclear proteins are a classic finding in the sera from patients with systemic rheumatic diseases, including systemic lupus erythematosus (SLE), an autoimmune disease.[10] More than 25 autoantibodies to specific nuclear antigens have been identified. Sera from patients with SLE typically contain at least 3 of these autoantibodies.[21] Although ANA testing is sensitive, it is not specific for SLE; an abnormal ANA may indicate other disorders as well.

The immunofluorescent ANA test is now used in many laboratories to assist in the diagnosis of systemic rheumatic disease, including SLE.[13,17] The use of mitotically active (actively dividing) human epithelioid cells and genetic modification techniques have increased both the sensitivity and diagnostic usefulness of current immunofluorescent ANA tests.[10] Positive results show fluorescence which requires the use of a fluorescent microscope.

An indirect immunoenzyme antibody technique (which also uses mitotically active human epithelioid cells) is also available for ANA testing, in which positive results yield a color reaction that is visible by light microscopy.[11,12] Regardless of methodology, use of reference sera available from the Centers for Disease Control and Prevention (CDC) is strongly recommended for quality control.[21] Sera giving equivocal results should be tested using the ELISA (enzyme-linked immunoabsorbent assay) methodology for identification of specific antibodies.[20]

CHAPTER SUMMARY

Today the performance of manual leukocyte counts has been virtually replaced by automated counting techniques, but because instruments are not infallible, laboratory scientists are obligated to learn the art and science of manual leukocyte counting. In addition, manual leukocyte differential counts are increasingly being replaced by automation, but there will always be abnormal specimens that require a manual blood film review.

The Neubauer hemocytometer, Thoma pipette or Unopette, and microscope are the key pieces of equipment used in manual leukocyte counting. Hemocytometers and Thoma pipettes must meet NBS specifications. The proper specimen dilution must be selected based on the approximate expected result (see Table 24-1). It is important to know the dimensions (length, width, depth) of the Neubauer chamber in order to correctly quantitate leukocytes (see Figs. 24-1 and 24-2). The formula for any cell count is as follows:

$$\text{Cells} \times 10^9/\text{L} = \frac{\text{Cells counted} \times \text{Dilution factor}}{\text{mm}^2 \text{ counted} \times \text{Depth}} \times 10^6$$

The dilution factor is calculated as 1 divided by the dilution. Leukocyte reference ranges are shown in Table 24-3.

The differential count procedure includes leukocyte, erythrocyte and platelet evaluation. The leukocyte differential is reported in terms of the relative number or percentage of each leukocyte category on the peripheral blood film. This relative number can be converted to the absolute number of cells per liter of blood, which is a more valuable and accurate assessment of cell quantities (see Table 24-7).

Manual eosinophil and basophil counts provide absolute cell count results that may be useful in certain diagnostic situations. The Fuchs-Rosenthal (see Fig. 24-6) or Speirs-Levy (see Fig. 24-7) hemocytometers should be used for these counts.

Case Study 24-1

During the monthly quality control check of laboratorians' differential performance accuracy and agreement, the following results were collected for a selected specimen for lymphocytes based on a manual 100-cell differential count. The same specimen was analyzed on an instrument that provides automated differentials based on examination of 10,000 leukocytes; this value is considered the "truth."

Automated	Tech 1	Tech 2	Tech 3	Tech 4	Tech 5
10%	7%	14%	2%	17%	10%

1. Do all laboratorians' results fall within the 95% confidence interval for a 100-cell differential count, assuming that the automated result of 10% is the most reliable value? Explain.

Case Study 24-2

The differential count on a newborn (>12 hrs old) with a total leukocyte count of 30.0 × 10⁹/L was segmented neutrophils 70%, band forms 10%, lymphocytes 5%, monocytes 15%; nucleated RBCs 8 per 100 WBCs; smudge cells 10; and megakaryocyte fragments 6.

1. Identify any findings, including relative and absolute cell counts, that are abnormal or outside of the reference range for a newborn.
2. Does the automated WBC count require correction? If so, what is the corrected value?
3. What values and information should be included in the final differential report?

Review Questions

24-1. The most commonly used hemocytometer is the

A. Becton Dickinson.
B. Fuchs-Rosenthal.
C. Levy with improved Neubauer rulings.
D. Speirs-Levy.

24-2. The range of possible dilutions using Thoma pipettes is

A. 1:10 to 1:200.
B. 1:10 to 1:1000.
C. 1:20 to 1:100.
D. 1:20 to 1:1000.

24-3. If nucleated red blood cells are seen during a leukocyte differential count they are

A. counted and reported as a percentage of the 100-cell differential.
B. counted and reported but not included as a percentage of the 100-cell differential.
C. not significant and therefore not counted.
D. counted but only reported if there are more than 5 per 100 WBCs.

24-4. If fibrin threads are observed during the low-power scan of the thin edge of a stained blood film, the technologist should

A. do the differential only on the central portion of the blood film.
B. not attempt platelet estimate but proceed with WBC differentiation.
C. not proceed further with the differential.
D. proceed with the differential noting presence of fibrin on report.

24-5. A student was given a specimen with an automated WBC count of 10 × 10⁹/L and asked to count the WBC manually. Given the inherent error of manual counting, which of the following ranges are in the 95% confidence limits which the student should achieve?

A. 9.0–10.0 × 10⁹/L
B. 8.0–12.0 × 10⁹/L
C. 8.5–11.5 × 10⁹/L
D. 8.8–11.2 × 10⁹/L

24-6. If a manual leukocyte count is anticipated to be less than 3.0 × 10⁹/L, the recommended dilution is

A. 1:200
B. 1:100
C. 1:20
D. 1:10

Exercises

24-1. Two hundred fifty leukocytes were counted on a hemocytometer in the four WBC squares (each 1 × 1 mm) on side A and 265 were counted in the same areas on side B. A WBC pipette was used to dilute the patient's blood (0.5 part blood and diluent drawn to the 11 mark). What is the final leukocyte count?

24-2. An automated leukocyte count was flagged as erroneous because it was above the linear range. After observing the peripheral blood film, it was determined that there was an average of 70 leukocytes per oil-immersion field. The calculated estimation factor for the microscope in use was 1 WBC = 1.5×10^9/L peripheral blood leukocytes.

A. What is the approximate leukocyte count based on the peripheral blood findings and estimation factor?
B. What manual dilution should be made for counting on the hemocytometer? What type of pipette should be used?
C. Given this dilution and 170 cells counted in the four usual WBC (1×1 mm) squares on side A and 184 counted in the same areas on side B, what is the final leukocyte count?

24-3. A differential count revealed 20 nucleated red blood cells per 100 leukocytes in a sample with 20.0×10^9/L leukocytes. Is a leukocyte count correction needed? If so, what is the corrected count?

24-4. Calculate leukocytes ($\times 10^9$/L) for the following values:

Dilution of Blood	Number of Squares	Area of Each Square	Depth of Chamber	Total Cells Counted
A. 1:10	4	1 mm^2	0.1 mm	194
B. 1:20	4	1 mm^2	0.1 mm	383
C. 1:10	8	1 mm^2	0.1 mm	273
D. 1:200	8	1 mm^2	0.1 mm	207
E. 1:32	40	1 mm^2	0.2 mm	50 (eosinophils)

24-5. A differential count showed 8 eosinophils in 100 leukocytes. Given a leukocyte count of 8.4×10^9/L, what is the indirect absolute number of eosinophils per liter? Show calculations. Is this result within the usual reference range?

References

1. Ahlborg B, Ahlborg G: Exercise leukocytosis with and without beta-adrenergic blockade. Acta Med Scand 187:241, 1970
2. Albritton EC: Standard Values in Blood. Philadelphia, WB Saunders, 1952
3. Becton Dickinson and Company: Laboratory Procedures Using the Unopette Brand System, 8th ed. Becton Dickinson, Rutherford, NJ, 1977
4. Brown BA: Routine hematology procedures, pp 94, 119; and Special hematology procedures, pp 197–199. In Brown BA (ed): Hematology: Principles and Procedures, 6th ed. Philadelphia, Lea & Febiger, 1993
5. Caramihai E, Karayalcin G, Aballi AJ et al: Leukocyte count differences in healthy white and black children 1 to 5 years of age. J Pediatr 86:252, 1975
6. Cooper JR, Cruickshank CN: Improved method for direct counting of basophil leukocytes. J Clin Pathol 19:402, 1966
7. Cunningham AS: Eosinophil counts–Age and sex differences. J Pediatr 87:426, 1975
8. England JM, Bain BJ: Total and differential leukocyte count. Br J Haematol 33:1, 1976; Br Med J 1:306, 1975
9. Fairbanks VF, Fahey JL, Beutler E: Clinical Disorders of Iron Metabolism, 2nd ed, p 178. New York, Grune & Stratton, 1971
10. Fritzler MJ, Miller BJ: Detection of autoantibodies to SS-A/Ro by indirect immunofluorescence using a transfected and overexpressed human 60 kD Ro autoantigen in HEp-2 Cells. J Clin Lab Analysis 9:218, 1995
11. Fritzler MJ, Wall W, Gohill J et al: The detection of autoantibodies on HEp-2 cells using an indirect immunoperoxidase kit (Colorzyme). Diag Immunol 4:217, 1986
12. Immuno Concepts: Colorzyme ANA Test System: An indirect enzyme antibody test for the semi-quantitative detection of antinuclear antibody in human serum; to be used as an aid in the detection of systemic rheumatic disease (package insert). Sacramento, CA, Immuno Concepts, 1989
13. Immuno Concepts: Fluorescent ANA Test System: An indirect fluorescent antibody test for the semi-quantitative detection of antinuclear antibody in human serum; to be used as an aid in the detection of systemic rheumatic disease (package insert). Sacramento, CA, Immuno Concepts, 1988
14. Karayalcin G, Rosner F, Sawitsky A: Pseudo-neutropenia in Negroes. A normal phenomenon. NY State J Med 72:1815, 1972
15. Kato K: Leukocytes in infancy and childhood. A statistical analysis of 1,081 total and differential counts from birth to fifteen years. J Pediatr 7:7, 1935
16. Lanzkowsky P: Manual of Pediatric Hematology and Oncology, 2nd ed. New York, Churchill Livingstone, 1995
17. Miale JB: Appendix–methods. In Miale JB (ed): Laboratory Medicine Hematology, p 913. St Louis, CV Mosby, 1982
18. Milhorat AT, Small SM, Diethelm O: Leukocytosis during various emotional states. Arch Neurol Psychiatr 47:779, 1942
19. Mogodam L: Application of the Miller disc for the estimation and quality control of the platelet count. Lab Med 11:131, 1980
20. Nakamura RM, Bylund DJ: Contemporary concepts for the clinical and laboratory evaluation of systemic lupus erythematosus and "lupus-like" syndromes. J Clin Lab Analysis 8:347, 1994
21. Nakamura RM, Bylund DJ, Tan EM: Current status of available standards for quality improvement of assays for detection of autoantibodies to nuclear and intracellular antigens. J Clin Lab Analysis 8:360, 1994
22. Nathan DG, Oski FA: Hematology of Infancy and Childhood, 4th ed. Philadelphia, WB Saunders, 1993
23. National Committee for Clinical Laboratory Standards: Leukocyte Differential Count (Proportional) and Evaluation of Instrumental Methods; Approved Standard H20-A, vol 12, no 1. Villanova, PA, NCCLS, 1992
24. Orfanakis NG, Ostlund RE, Bishop CR et al: Normal blood leukocyte concentration values. Am J Clin Pathol 53:647, 1970
25. Osgood EE, Baker RL, Brownlee IE et al: Total, differential and absolute leukocyte counts and sedimentation rates of healthy children four to seven years of age. Am J Dis Child 58:61, 1939
26. Oski FA, Naiman JL (ed): Hematologic Problems in the Newborn, 3rd ed. Philadelphia, WB Saunders, 1982
27. Patrick CW, Keller RH: The New Morphology: Combining Traditional Cytomorphology with Automated Differential Information, Cytogenetics and Molecular Probes, Monoclonal Antibodies and Immunophenotyping, Laser Flow Cytometry and Cell Sorting. Workshop Manual, Annual Meeting, New Orleans, 1986. Washington, DC, American Society for Medical Technology, 1986
28. Randolph TG: Differentiation and enumeration of eosinophils in the counting chamber with a glycol stain: A valuable technique in appraising ACTH dosage. J Lab Clin Med 34:1696, 1949
29. Rothstein G: Origin and development of the blood and blood forming tissues. In Lee GR, Bithell TC, Foerster J et al (eds): Wintrobe's Clinical Hematology, 9th ed, p 41. Philadelphia, Lea & Febiger, 1993
30. Stiene-Martin EA: Causes for poor leukocyte distribution in manual spreader-slide blood films. Am J Med Technol 46:624, 1980
31. van Assendelft OW et al: The differential distribution of leukocytes. In Koepke JA (ed): Differential Leukocyte Counting, p 11. Skokie, IL, College of American Pathologists, 1979
32. Zacharski LR, Elveback LR, Linman JW: Leukocyte counts in healthy adults. Am J Clin Pathol 56:148, 1971

PART V

Leukocyte Abnormalities (Nonmalignant)

CHAPTER 25

Nonmalignant, Reactive Disorders of Leukocytes

E. Anne Stiene-Martin
Virginia Haight

Objectives

1. Define leukocytosis, leukopenia and pancytopenia.
2. Describe various reactive morphologic alterations that occur in circulating leukocytes.
3. List the common nonmalignant causes for quantitative increases and decreases in granulocytes, monocytes, and lymphocytes and state the term used to refer to each (*e.g.*, neutrophilia).

4. Define leukemoid reactions and describe the morphologic differences between reactive and malignant alterations in leukocytes.
5. Describe and differentiate type I, II and III lymphocytes.

Leukocytes function to protect the body against invasion by foreign organisms or antigens. In so doing they undergo visible changes (reactive or toxic changes) that are evaluated microscopically in the clinical laboratory. These changes are the most common type of leukocyte abnormality seen in the clinical hematology laboratory and may be subdivided into quantitative variations (alterations in numbers) and qualitative variations (morphologic alterations). This chapter will discuss the common causes of quantitative changes and will describe the more frequently encountered morphologic alterations. The discussion on reactive lymphocytes will address specific disease entities that are accompanied by reactive lymphocytes such as infectious mononucleosis. Such alterations must be distinguished from those seen in neoplastic leukocytes as well as those resulting from genetic abnormalities. Ways of making these distinctions will be described.

To discuss quantitative abnormalities in leukocytes, it is necessary to define reference ranges for total leukocytes as well as for each cell type. These may vary among laboratories because of differences in cell counting proce-

TABLE 25-1
Definitions of Increased and Decreased Numbers of Leukocytes According to Cell Type

Cell Type	Term	Cell Count (× 10⁹/L)
Neutrophils	Neutrophilia	>8.0
	Neutropenia	<1.75
	Agranulocytosis	<0.5
Eosinophils	Eosinophilia	>0.7
	Eosinopenia	<0.05
Basophils	Basophilia	>0.3
	Basopenia	<0.005
Monocytes	Monocytosis	>1.0
	Monocytopenia	<0.03
Lymphocytes	Lymphocytosis	>4.5 (adult)
		>9.0 (infant)
	Lymphopenia	<0.9

dures, instrumentation, methods used to establish reference values, and in patient populations. The lower level for total leukocytes in adults is usually somewhere between 3.0 and 4.0 × 10⁹/L, and the high, between 10.0 and 11.0 × 10⁹/L.[81] Pediatric values are significantly different. One source reports reference ranges for children to be 4.5 to 13.5 and for infants 6.0 to 17.5 × 10⁹/L.[42] *Leukocytosis* (defined in adults as leukocyte counts greater than 11.0 × 10⁹/L) may be caused by an increase in one or more of the cell types that normally circulate in peripheral blood or by the presence of abnormal cell types. Conversely, *leukopenia* is defined as a total leukocyte count of less than 3.0 × 10⁹/L and is due to a decrease in neutrophils (neutropenia or granulocytopenia), lymphocytes (lymphopenia), or all cell types (pancytopenia). Eosinophils, basophils, and monocytes are normally present in such low numbers that individual decreases do not produce leukopenia. Table 25-1 defines the criteria used in this chapter to identify increases or decreases in specific cell types.

NEUTROPHILS

Quantitative Abnormalities

In determining whether an absolute increase or decrease in neutrophils exists, the age and ethnicity of the subject must be taken into account.[81] Children tend to have higher neutrophil counts than adults; blacks tend to have lower counts than Caucasians.[72,81] When calculating the absolute value of circulating neutrophils (the product of the total leukocyte count and the percentage of neutrophils), all stages of neutrophil maturation, *excluding* blasts and progranulocytes, are included.

NEUTROPHILIA

Three major causes of neutrophilia are infection, inflammation, and malignancy. Reactive neutrophilias may be either acute (transient) or chronic and frequently are accompanied by increased numbers of immature forms (neutrophilic left shift). Table 25-2 lists common reactive causes of neutrophilia and is subdivided into those involving pathology and those that are physiologic.

Bacterial infections, especially those caused by cocci, may produce striking neutrophilia. Not all bacteria cause neutrophilia; some in fact suppress neutrophil production, resulting in a neutropenia to be described below. The degree of neutrophilia produced by infections depends on virulence of the organism as well as the age and health (resistance) of the patient. Children tend to develop more profound neutrophilia than adults. Conversely elderly persons, as well as those who have nutritional deficits or who are immunocompromised for whatever reason, may produce only moderate responses or none at all when challenged with the same infection.

Neutrophilia associated with inflammatory responses to tissue injury or destruction occurs in a wide variety of situations (see Table 25-2). The basic mechanism for neutrophilia in these cases is release of substances by dead or dying cells that act as chemotactic agents, or stimulators of marrow cell release or production.

Inflammatory responses may also occur in the presence of neoplasms, especially those that are growing fast or are producing substances that induce marrow output of neutrophils.[68] Metabolic disorders such as diabetes, renal dysfunction, or liver disease may produce circulating toxic substances (related to ketoacidosis, uremia, azotemia) and stimulate a neutrophilic response. Acute hemorrhage, especially when internal, stimulates neutrophilia,[27] presumably as a result of a combination of factors including cell destruction and promotion of neutrophil release. Regardless of whether the neutrophilia is associated with infection or inflammation, the underlying cause of increased marrow production and release is related to

TABLE 25-2
Causes of Reactive Neutrophilia

PATHOLOGIC

Infections (localized or generalized)
    Pyogenic bacteria
    Certain viruses
    Actinomyces fungi
    Some spirochetal and rickettsial organisms

Inflammatory responses to tissue destruction
    Serosal
    Visceral
    Blood cell destruction
    Posttraumatic (surgical, accidental)
    Thermal injury
    Chemicals/drugs/venoms
    Parasitic invasions

Other inflammatory responses
    Neoplastic growth
    Metabolic disorders
    Acute hemorrhage

Drugs
    Corticosteroids
    Lithium

PHYSIOLOGIC

Response to therapy

Pseudoneutrophilia caused by physical or emotional stimuli

the elaboration of cytokines (substances produced by one cell that affect another cell) such as prostaglandins, epinephrine, tumor necrosis factor, and platelet activating factor.[2]

Adrenocorticosteroids can also cause neutropenia. It may be related to inhibition of neutrophil migration.[7] Lithium, a common antidepressant drug, appears to cause neutrophilia through direct stimulation of hematopoiesis.[9] Likewise, the use of recombinant hematopoietic growth factors such as rhG-CSF and rhGM-CSF is believed to cause both increased cell production as well as enhanced release from marrow stores.[34,71]

Physiologic neutrophilia is usually caused by a shift of marginated cells to the circulating pool, a condition sometimes referred to as pseudoneutrophilia. (See Chap. 22 for a discussion of marginal and circulating pools of leukocytes.) This neutrophilia is generally transient, lasting only a few hours, is mediated by the release of catecholamines[52] and is not characterized by any significant increase in immature forms.

NEUTROPENIA

Neutropenia is the most common cause of leukopenia. The term *agranulocytosis* is used to designate extreme neutropenia ($<0.3 \times 10^9$/L). Neutropenia usually renders the patient vulnerable to infection; however, the relationship between neutrophil count and the number of neutrophils delivered to the tissues is not consistent, which may explain why some persons with neutropenia do not experience more infections.[83] Table 25-3 lists the major causes of neutropenia.

Decreased production of neutrophils may be inherited or acquired. Inherited forms are rare and include a variety of poorly understood syndromes. They include defective stem cell development and disorders of cellular development or function that result secondarily in decreased circulating numbers.

TABLE 25-3
Causes of Neutropenia

DECREASED NEUTROPHIL PRODUCTION

Inherited stem cell disorders

Acquired stem cell disorders
    Chemical toxicity (*e.g.*, benzene)
    Marrow replacement
    Nutritional deficiencies
    Cytotoxic drugs

INCREASED NEUTROPHIL DESTRUCTION

Infections
    Overwhelming
    Certain bacteria
    Viral

Immune reactions
    Isoimmune
    Autoimmune
    Drug-induced

Sequestration

Pseudoneutropenia

Malignant myeloproliferative disorders

Acquired forms of decreased neutrophil production are common. Destruction or injury to stem cell compartments results in hypoplastic or aplastic marrow with concomitant decreases in all cell types. Agents capable of causing moderate to severe marrow suppression include ionizing radiation, chemicals such as benzene, and a wide variety of cytotoxic drugs used in combating malignancy. Marrow replacement by tumor, fibrous tissue, or hematopoietic malignancy may also result in pancytopenia. In some cases neutropenia may be a preleukemic manifestation.[45] Vitamin B_{12} or folate deficiency causes ineffective hematopoiesis leading to decreases in all cell types.

The second category of neutropenic states includes those caused by increased neutrophil destruction due to infections, immune mechanisms, or hypersensitivity states. Any infection that overwhelms the marrow's capacity to produce adequate numbers of neutrophils will result in neutrophils being consumed or recruited to the tissues faster than they are released by the marrow. This type of neutropenia is seen most frequently in debilitated patients who have little or no marrow reserves, elderly persons, and infants.

Typhoid, paratyphoid, and brucellosis are bacterial infections commonly associated with leukopenia and neutropenia. Viral infections characterized by neutropenia include measles, yellow fever, infectious hepatitis, infectious mononucleosis, and rubella.[56] The neutropenia of viral infections is often noted in the early stages of the disease.

Neonatal isoimmune neutropenia results from transplacental transfer of maternal IgG antibodies directed against fetal neutrophils.[44] Acquired autoimmune neutropenia has been described and is analogous to autoimmune hemolytic anemia or immune thrombocytopenic purpura, but not as common.[10] Antineutrophil antibodies have also been described in collagen vascular diseases (lupus erythematosus, Felty's syndrome)[8] and following transfusion of blood products.

Drug hypersensitivity can result in agranulocytosis.[35] The list of drugs believed to cause this disorder is extensive and growing. The first drug to be implicated, in the late 1920s, was amidopyrine. Since then, with the ongoing introduction of new drugs such as cephalosporin, reports of agranulocytosis invariably followed. Drug-induced agranulocytosis affects women more frequently than men (2.5:1) and is more often seen in middle age than in young adults. The underlying disorder may be a genetic tdefect that prevents proper metabolism of the drug. Removal of the offending drug generally results in prompt recovery.

A third mechanism of neutropenia is sequestration or trapping. Splenic enlargement, regardless of cause, may lead to neutropenia, which is usually relatively mild. Neutrophils may also be sequestered in pulmonary vasculature after chemotactic stimuli or during hemodialysis.[16]

Finally, patients may have a decreased number of circulating neutrophils because of a shift from the circulating pool of neutrophils to the marginal pool. This may be referred to as *pseudoneutropenia* because the total blood granulocyte pool is not decreased. It may occur during hypersensitivity reactions or viral infections, and after hypothermia.[74]

Qualitative Abnormalities

Morphologic alterations in neutrophils in response to stress, infection, or inflammation often are called *toxic changes*. These changes (Table 25-4) include the presence of increased numbers of immature forms (left shift) and morphologic evidence of maturation abnormalities (*e.g.*, ring-shaped band forms), alterations in functional activity, or degenerative changes.

A *neutrophilic left shift* is defined as the presence of increased numbers of circulating nonsegmented or immature neutrophils. Release of marrow stores results in greater numbers of circulating neutrophilic band forms and metamyelocytes. Continued marrow stimulus is accompanied by increased marrow production of neutrophils and the presence of neutrophilic myelocytes in the circulation. Small numbers of promyelocytes and blast forms may be found in peripheral blood from individuals with severe or overwhelming infections. (See Chap. 22 for morphologic description of immature neutrophils.) The importance of recognizing and reporting the various stages of neutrophil development in peripheral blood is underscored by the fact that a change in the ratio of nonsegmented to segmented neutrophils appears to be one of the best indicators of the severity of infection.[14]

The presence of a neutrophilic left shift and circulating nucleated red cells is referred to as a *leukoerythroblastic reaction*. Synonyms include leukoerythroblastic anemia and leukoerythroblastosis. The reaction may be mild or severe and may be present in a wide variety of conditions that have as a common feature, stress or damage to marrow and development of extramedullary hematopoiesis. The conditions most commonly associated with striking and sustained leukoerythroblastic reactions are those involving the presence of a space-occupying lesion in the marrow (myelophthisis) such as metastatic tumor, fibrosis, lymphoma, or leukemia. Mild and transitory leukoerythroblastic reactions may be a minor component of several conditions, including hemolytic anemia, severe infections, cardiac failure, uremia, and megaloblastic anemia.[15] Although it is a nonspecific reaction, leuko-erythroblastosis provides important evidence of underlying disease or stress to the hematopoietic compartment.

Morphologic evidence of neutrophil activation, degeneration or alterations in function can be subdivided into two categories of abnormalities: cytoplasmic and nuclear.

CYTOPLASM

Cytoplasmic alterations in toxic neutrophils are those most frequently cited in the literature. They include toxic granulation, Döhle bodies, cytoplasmic vacuoles, degranulation, pseudopodia, and swelling.

Toxic granules are believed to be altered primary granules.[51] Primary granules, although present in neutrophils under normal circumstances, are not prominent with ordinary Romanowsky stains (*e.g.*, Wright stain). Neutrophil stimulation by foreign organisms or antigens may cause alterations in these granules, resulting in different staining characteristics.[49] Toxic granules are described as being larger than secondary granules and dark blue-black in color after staining. Much has been written about the significance and prognostic value of quantitating toxic granulation. Generally it can be said that the greater the proportion of affected neutrophils, the graver the prognosis.[43] It is important to differentiate between true toxic granulation, artifactual granules caused by poor staining technique, and the abnormal metachromatic granules seen in some genetic disorders of mucopolysaccharide metabolism (Chap. 26). True toxic granules may be distinguished by their tendency to cluster within the cell and by the fact that not all neutrophils will be equally affected (Fig. 25-1). Dark granules caused by both overstaining and Alder-Reilly bodies (Chap. 26) generally are distributed throughout the cell, and all cells tend to be affected equally.

Döhle bodies (see Color Plate 25-1) are cytoplasmic inclusions consisting of ribosomal RNA arrayed in parallel rows.[6] They are found in segmented and band neutrophils. With Romanowsky stains they appear as pale blue, round or elongated bodies between 1 and 5 μm in diame-

---

TABLE 25-4
Toxic Neutrophil Morphology

Circulating immature forms
    Mild: Increased band and metamyelocyte forms
    Moderate: Circulating myelocytes and occasional promyelocytes
    Marked: Circulating blast forms

Morphologic abnormalities
    Cytoplasmic
        Toxic granules
        Döhle bodies
        Vacuolation
        Degranulation
        Pseudopods
        Swelling
    Nuclear
        Pyknotic and/or necrotic
        Hypersegmentation
        Nuclear projections
        Ring forms

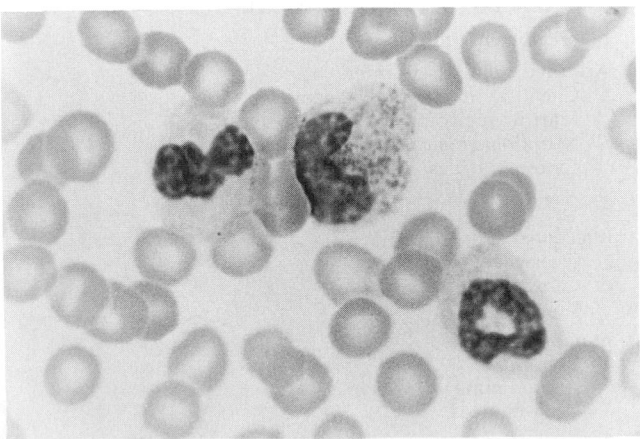

FIGURE 25-1. Toxic granulation. Note that the center neutrophil contains toxic granules whereas the other two do not. This suggests that the granulation is not artifact. In addition, the neutrophil to the lower right contains a ringed nucleus.

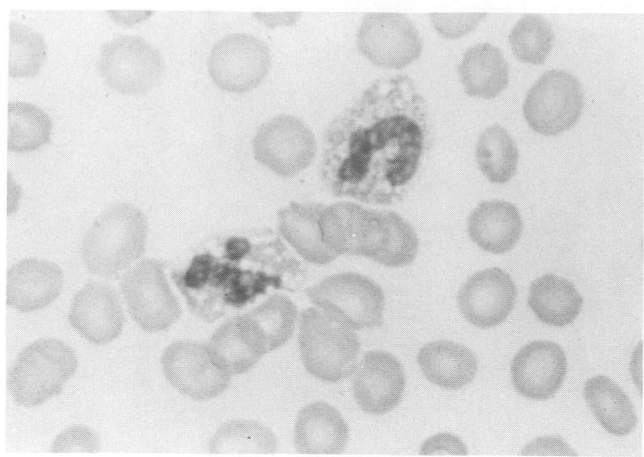

FIGURE 25-2. Autophagocytic vacuoles. Note their small size and distribution throughout the cell.

ter that are usually located in close apposition to cell membranes. It should be noted that the anticoagulant EDTA affects the staining characteristics of Döhle bodies so that they may be more gray than blue and may even disappear in blood that is stored in EDTA. Döhle bodies are relatively nonspecific in that they are associated with a wide range of conditions, including pregnancy.[1] They are transient in that they are seen most often during the first 1 to 3 days after an insult (*e.g.*, infection, burn, surgery), after which they tend to disappear. What causes them to form is not known.

It is important to differentiate between the transient Döhle body seen after infection or tissue damage and the larger spindle-shaped inclusion seen in the May-Hegglin anomaly (Chap. 26). Light microscopic differentiation can usually be made based on size (May-Hegglin bodies often are greater than 5 μm in diameter), the cell types affected (May-Hegglin inclusions are found in all types of granulocytes), and the fact that May-Hegglin bodies are not transient.[13]

Cytoplasmic vacuolation is caused by phagocytosis, either of self (autophagocytosis) or of extracellular material. Autophagocytosis may be caused by drugs such as sulfon-

amides and chloroquine,[65] by prolonged storage of cells, or by degranulation on exposure to certain toxins or high doses of radiation.[38] Generally, autophagocytic vacuoles tend to be small in size (1–2 μm) and evenly distributed throughout the cytoplasm (Fig. 25-2). Phagocytic vacuolation due to ingestion is seen commonly in septic processes caused either by bacteria or fungi. Phagocytic vacuoles can be quite large (up to 7 or 8 μm), are not evenly distributed, and often are outlined by visible toxic granules (Fig. 25-3).

Numerous studies have correlated the presence of vacuolated neutrophils with bacteremia.[50] Vacuoles as well as toxic granulation are indicative of neutrophils with decreased bactericidal properties.[75] Consequently, assuming a fresh specimen, the presence of vacuolation in more than 10% of neutrophils can be very significant.[50] Vacuolation and toxic granulation have been reported in patients receiving neutrophil production–stimulating growth factors[12] and in patients receiving growth factors.[71]

True vacuolation must be distinguished from that due to excessive delay between blood collection and blood film preparation. Vacuolation due to delay tends to be autophagocytic (*i.e.*, small, evenly distributed vacuoles) and the vacuoles are reported to stain yellow rather than red with neutral red.[6]

Cytoplasmic degranulation is a normal function of neutrophils that have been activated or injured.[23] Primary granules are emptied into the phagosome, whereas secondary granules are secreted into the extracellular environment.[27] Degranulation often is accompanied by disruption of cellular membranes during the process of making the blood film.

Cytoplasmic pseudopodia are rare alterations in toxic neutrophils. They are granule-free protrusions of cytoplasm that give the neutrophil an ameboid character (Fig. 25-4). They may be indicative of sluggish or depressed neutrophil locomotion known to be caused by a variety of bacterial and therapeutic agents.[26] They are seen most frequently in association with cytotoxic agents. Prolonged specimen storage in EDTA may cause artifactual pseudopodia, which must be distinguished from toxic cytoplasmic pseudopodia.

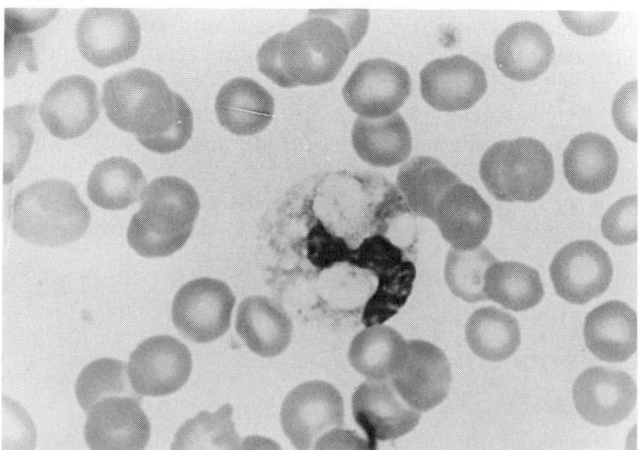

FIGURE 25-3. Phagocytic vacuoles. Compared to autophagocytic vacuoles, these are considerably larger and few in number.

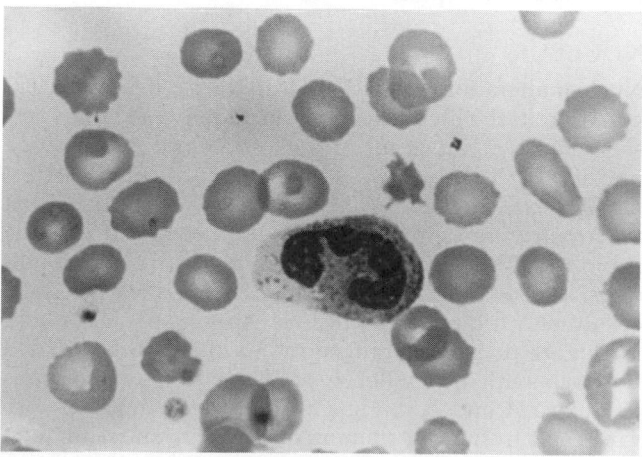

FIGURE 25-4. Granule-free cytoplasmic pseudopod. This may reflect either aberrant cell locomotion or prolonged delay in anticoagulant.

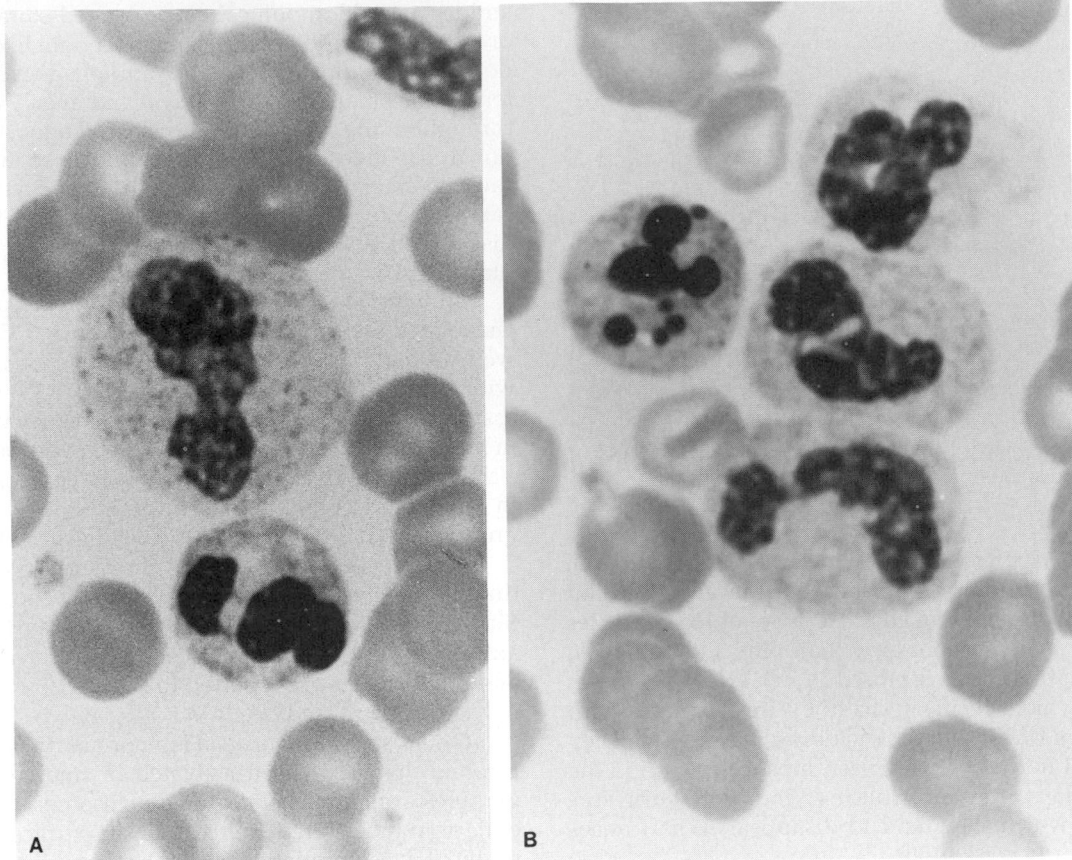

FIGURE 25-5. **(A)** The two neutrophils in this field are exhibiting anisocytosis or variation in size. In addition, the lower neutrophil contains a pyknotic nucleus. **(B)** Necrotic (dead) neutrophil on the left. Compare the nuclear structure of this cell to the three viable neutrophils at right.

Cytoplasmic swelling may be caused by actual osmotic swelling of the cytoplasm[60] or by increased adhesiveness to the glass slide by stimulated neutrophils. Regardless of cause, the result is perceptible variation in neutrophil size within a population or neutrophilic anisocytosis (Fig. 25-5A). A swollen or edematous neutrophil, sometimes referred to as a *macropolycyte*, must be distinguished from the large hypersegmented neutrophils resulting from vitamin B_{12} or folate deficiency. Giant neutrophils have also been reported in patients with AIDS.[22]

NUCLEUS

Nuclear alterations in toxic neutrophils have received less attention in the literature. They include pyknosis, hypersegmentation, nuclear projections, and ring-shaped nuclei.

Pyknotic nuclei are shrunken and dense nuclei that apparently are dehydrated.[65] They may be in cells just about to die and are seen most frequently in septic conditions. They should be distinguished from dead (necrotic) cells that are rarely seen in fresh specimens and whose nuclei are dense and broken into two or more rounded portions with no evidence of filamentous connections (compare A and B in Fig. 25-5). Nuclear pyknosis also can result from poor staining or preparation techniques, but that can be detected since most cells are equally affected. Unfortunately, there is some confusion in the literature because some authors describe necrotic cells as being pyknotic.

Hypersegmented nuclei are commonly seen in long-term chronic infections. The neutrophils may be either large or normal size. There may be more than one cause.[61] More recently there have been reports of macropolycytes with hypersegmented nuclei in response to recombinant G-CSF.[12] In some cases, hypersegmented neutrophils may reflect borderline folate deficiency; in others, it may reflect a degenerative process.

Toxic nuclear projections are hairlike projections seen most frequently in band forms. The projections usually are only on the inner side of the band form, the side that faces the centriole (Fig. 25-6).[6] Toxic nuclear projections have been reported in patients with metastatic carcinoma or after irradiation.

Ringed nuclei (see Fig. 25-1) are seen in both toxic states and malignant myeloproliferative states.[41] Small numbers of neutrophils with ringlike nuclei may be seen early in infections, when leukocytosis is prominent and band forms are increased to levels of 30% or more.

EOSINOPHILS
Quantitative Abnormalities
EOSINOPHILIA

Eosinophilia may be inherited, malignant, or reactive. Hereditary eosinophilia has been reported in a few families as an autosomal-dominant trait.[57] Eosinophilia usually is benign, and the major concern is to differentiate inher-

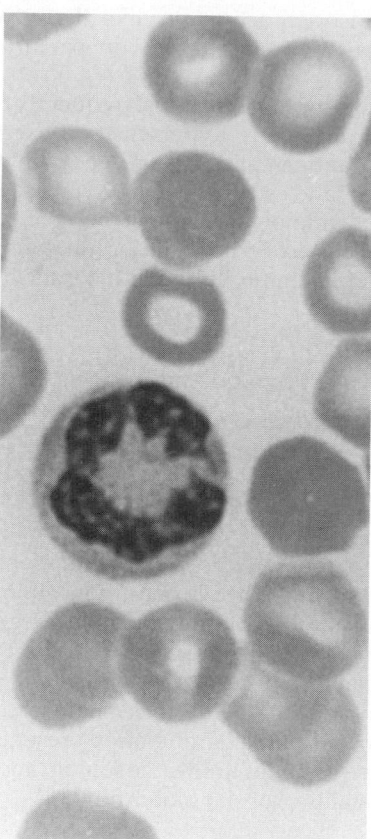

FIGURE 25-6. Toxic nuclear projections. Note the hairlike projections on the inner side of the nucleus.

TABLE 25-5
Changes in Eosinophil Number

Eosinophilia
  Infestation by tissue-invading parasites
  Allergic reactions
    Respiratory (asthma, hay fever)
    Skin disorders (psoriasis, eczema)
  Hypersensitivity disorders
    Loeffler's syndrome
    Pulmonary infiltrates with eosinophilia (PIE)
    Tropical eosinophilia
  Malignancies of myeloid cells
  Certain infections (*e.g.*, scarlet fever)
  Miscellaneous disorders
    Familial
    Post-irradiation
    Certain poisons
    Periarteritis nodosa
Eosinopenia
  Decreased production
  Acute bacterial infection
  ACTH administration

at levels above $1.5 \times 10^9/L$. The underlying cause may be parasitic, allergic, neoplastic (eosinophilic leukemia), or idiopathic (unknown). Persistent hypereosinophilia is cause for concern, since there tends to be eosinophil infiltration into all tissues with resulting tissue damage and organ dysfunction such as cardiomyopathy. Consequently, the hypereosinophilic syndrome is generally monitored carefully, and therapy to suppress eosinophils such as antihistamines, cytotoxic drugs, or leukopheresis may be instituted.

EOSINOPENIA

Eosinopenia is difficult to detect using manual differentials and total leukocyte counts, since zero percent eosinophils is frequently considered to be within the reference range based on a 100-leukocyte differential count. The various automated five-part differential systems are capable of detecting eosinopenia. It may result from production abnormalities similar to those listed previously for neutropenia. In addition, eosinopenia is a characteristic finding in most acute bacterial infections. Reappearance of eosinophils in the peripheral blood generally is a sign of recovery from the infection. The mechanism for the eosinopenia of acute infections is not known. It may be a combination of factors, including sequestration, margination, and chemotaxis.[3]

Eosinopenia is also a well known outcome of ACTH administration if adrenal function is normal. Glucocorticoids, prostaglandins, and epinephrine will depress eosinophil levels.[84] The mechanism of these eosinopenias is felt to be a combination of increased margination and decreased marrow release.

Qualitative Abnormalities

Circulating immature eosinophils (left shift) are extremely rare in reactive conditions, even in the face of markedly increased eosinophils. Morphologic evidence of stimulation and activity includes degranulation, vacuolation, and hypersegmentation.

ited eosinophilia from reactive forms to be described below.

Reactive eosinophilia is most frequently associated with two categories of disorders (Table 25-5): parasitic invasion of tissue and allergic or hypersensitivity disorders. In addition, an eosinophilic response may be seen in collagen-vascular diseases, neoplastic disorders, and some immune deficiency states.[82]

Eosinophilia is associated with parasites that invade and cause tissue destruction, but it is not characteristic of protozoal infections. Eosinophils have unique capabilities for suppressing virtually all helminthic organisms (trematodes, nematodes, and cestodes). There is a significant positive correlation between eosinophil count and parasite death.[17] Eosinophil attraction to parasites appears to be T lymphocyte–directed and antibody dependent.[11] Parasite killing is mediated through eosinophil degranulation,[53] release of crystalloid major basic protein and cationic proteins, and peroxidation.

The role of the eosinophil in allergic reactions involves modulation of the inflammatory response resulting from basophil or mast cell degranulation. Immediate hypersensitivity reactions produce a wide variety of products that influence eosinophil traffic (Chap. 22). Activation of the immune system and basophil or mast cell degranulation may very well be the underlying mechanism for a wide variety of eosinophilia-producing conditions.

The term *hypereosinophilic syndrome* denotes a condition in which there is persistent and extreme eosinophilia

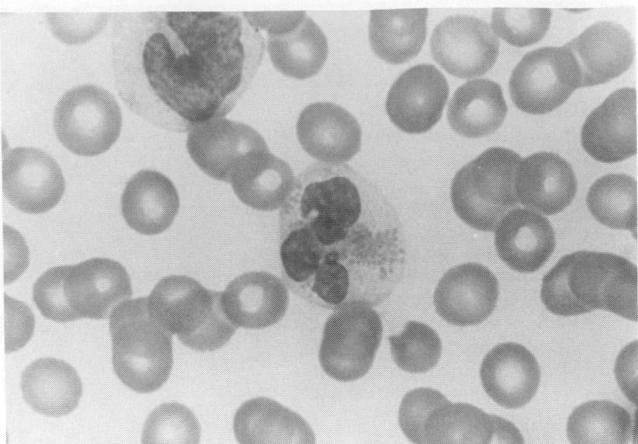

FIGURE 25-7. Reactive eosinophil exhibiting degranulation and three nuclear lobes (hypersegmentation).

Degranulation is probably the most prominent reactive eosinophil alteration. The result is a cell with a few scattered eosinophil granules in pale blue to colorless cytoplasm (Fig. 25-7). The act of degranulation renders the cytoplasmic membrane somewhat vulnerable to the making of a blood film. Thus, eosinophilias frequently are characterized by increased numbers of broken or disrupted eosinophils on the blood film. Eosinophil degranulation should be reported only if the specimen is fresh, as eosinophils are prone to degranulate in stored blood. It should be noted that eosinophils with decreased granules may also be seen in malignant myeloproliferative disorders. These usually can be differentiated from reactive eosinophils by the accompanying blood picture (*i.e.*, other evidence of malignancy).

Vacuolation of eosinophils is seen occasionally. The vacuoles tend to be quite small and their significance is unknown.

Hypersegmentation is the only relatively common nuclear alteration in reactive eosinophils. Since normal eosinophils have only two nuclear lobes, eosinophil hypersegmentation is defined as three or more lobes or a mean greater than 2.5 lobes. The causes of eosinophilic hypersegmentation are probably similar to those described previously for neutrophils.

BASOPHILS
Quantitative Abnormalities

The normal number of circulating basophils is so low that reference values have been difficult to obtain, owing to the fact that 1000-cell differential counts would be necessary to calculate reliable absolute values.[29] Differential counters that are capable of identifying basophils within populations of 10,000 leukocytes or more provide a means of defining the lower normal limits for basophils (0.005–0.010 × 10⁹/L).

BASOPHILIA

Basophilia is present in many of the disorders that cause eosinophilia. This is not surprising in view of the evidence that eosinophils and basophils may share a common stem cell.[20] Also basophil activation, like that of eosinophils, appears to be controlled at least in part by T lymphocytes.[30]

Reactive basophilias are most frequently cited in association with immediate hypersensitivity reaction, long-term foreign antigen stimulation,[73] hypothyroidism, ulcerative colitis, and estrogen therapy.[79] There is a transient basophilia of unknown origin in newborn infants and following exercise.[54] Striking basophilia is often seen in the malignant myeloproliferative disorders (Chap. 35).

BASOPENIA

Basopenias have been described during acute infections, stress, hyperthyroidism, and increased levels of glucocorticoids.[79]

Qualitative Abnormalities

There is little to nothing in the literature about basophil morphology during reactive conditions. Immature forms do not circulate in reactive basophilia. Degranulation is the single morphologic alteration that may be detected. Degranulation may be seen after ingestion of a fatty meal[73] or as a consequence of antigen-related stimulation.[66,79] Evaluation of basophil degranulation presents some problems, as these granules are water soluble and may be lost during the staining of the blood film.

MONOCYTES
Quantitative Abnormalities

If reference ranges for monocytes are based on Romanowsky-stained morphology, the lower limits are 0.03 to 0.09 × 10⁹/L and upper limits are 0.85 to 1.0 × 10⁹/L. If, on the other hand, monocytes are identified using enzymatic[39] or surface markers, the upper limit of normal may be significantly higher (*e.g.*, 1.8 × 10⁹/L). It should be noted at this point that calculation of absolute values from a manual differential count should be based on at least a 200-cell differential count, because of the tendency of these cells to cluster along the edges of spreader-slide blood films.

MONOCYTOSIS

Owing to the fact that monocytes and neutrophils share a common stem cell (CFU-GM), it is not surprising to note that many of the conditions listed as causes of neutrophilia are also accompanied by absolute monocytosis. The monocytosis is usually inconspicuous in the presence of the more noticeable neutrophil response. For example, 6% monocytes in 25 × 10⁹/L leukocytes represents an absolute monocytosis which might be overlooked.

Monocytosis may be reactive or malignant. Inherited forms have not been described. The monocytosis seen in malignant myeloproliferative disorders is discussed in Chapters 33 through 35. Causes of reactive monocytosis are listed in Table 25-6.

Although a wide variety of acute bacterial infections have been reported to be accompanied by monocytosis, three in particular are cited most consistently: tuberculo-

TABLE 25-6
Causes of Reactive Monocytosis

Bacterial infection
    Tuberculosis
    Subacute bacterial endocarditis (SBE)
    Syphilis

Inflammatory responses
    Surgical trauma
    Tumors
    Collagen vascular disease
    Gastrointestinal disease

Recovery from neutropenia (relative)

Myeloproliferative disorders

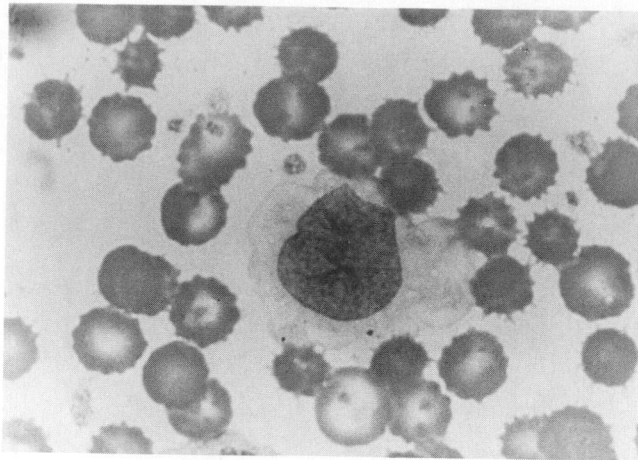

FIGURE 25-8. An immature-appearing monocyte reflecting a type of reactive monocytic "left shift."

sis, subacute bacterial endocarditis (SBE), and syphilis. Tuberculosis is thought to elicit increased monocytes because of their role in the cellular response to the bacillus (granuloma formation).[32] Monocytosis in such cases is believed to reflect active disease. Some of the monocytes in patients with SBE may mature in the peripheral blood, resulting in circulating histiocytes or macrophages. This is considered to be highly significant and is discussed below under qualitative changes. The spirochetes of syphilis cause widespread interstitial inflammation and invasion of lymphatic and vascular systems. In these patients, monocytosis may be a response to inflammation or be related to the cells' role in the immune system.

Monocytosis may also be seen in inflammatory reactions to tissue destruction such as surgical trauma or tumors.[33]

There is little or no marrow storage of monocytes; therefore, they are released into the circulation before neutrophils are. Because of this, relative monocytosis frequently heralds recovery from agranulocytosis or marrow hypoplasia.

MONOCYTOPENIA

Monocytopenia may be seen following administration of glucocorticoids[78] or during overwhelming infections that also cause neutropenia.

Qualitative Abnormalities

Reactive morphology in monocytes includes the presence of immature monocytes in the circulation (a type of monocytic left shift; Fig. 25-8) and monocyte transformation into macrophages.[80] Morphologic changes associated with transformation into macrophages include increases in cytoplasmic volume and spreading ability (cell diameters sometimes approach 50 μm), increased numbers of dense granules representing both primary and secondary lysosomes, and increased evidence of both phagocytic and pinocytic activity (cytoplasmic vacuolation, intracellular debris, and highly irregular cytoplasmic borders). In addition, the nuclear chromatin pattern may become reticular (netlike) with visible nucleoli.

The finding of macrophages (Fig. 25-9) in the peripheral blood of patients suffering from septic processes such as SBE has been described in the literature over several

years. In our experience, these cells may make their appearance in the peripheral blood long before blood cultures are positive, making their identification very important. They will most often be found in the edges of the blood film, owing to their large size.

A final monocyte alteration that might be considered a reactive change is an alteration in the nucleus to a long, thin, bandlike shape that frequently appears highly contorted (Fig. 25-10). Explanations for this finding are not found in the literature; however, they are seen frequently in the same preparations as hypersegmented neutrophils and may also reflect incipient folate deficiency.

LYMPHOCYTES

Terminology

Various terms have been used to describe the lymphocytes seen in nonmalignant reactive disorders: variant lymphocytes, reactive lymphocytes, atypical lymphocytes, virocytes, stress lymphocytes, Downey cells, transformed lymphocytes, transitional lymphocytes, and glandular fever cells, among others.

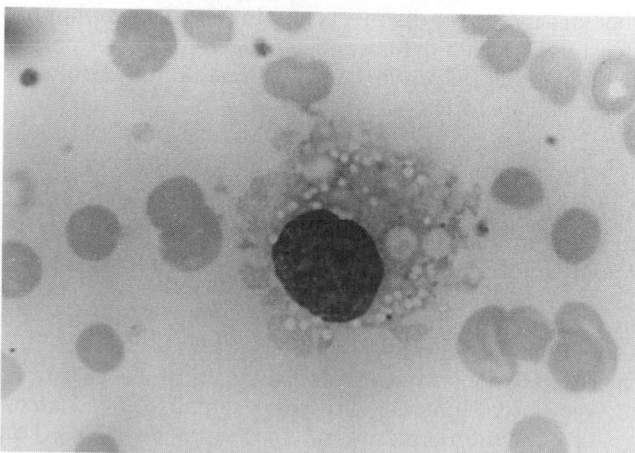

FIGURE 25-9. A circulating macrophage that was found in the feathered edge (tail) of a blood film taken from a patient who was septic.

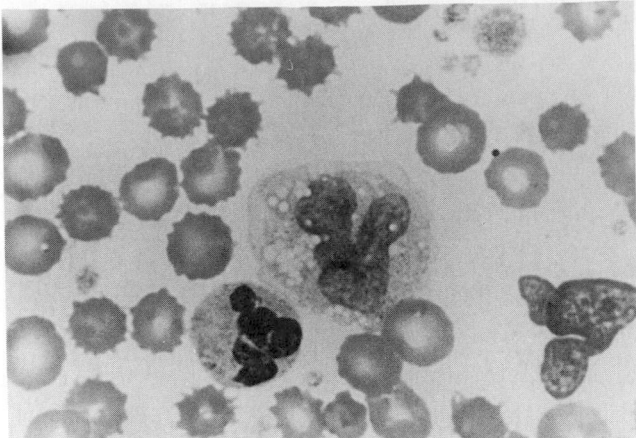

FIGURE 25-10. A toxic monocyte containing a highly contorted nucleus that may be reflecting incipient folate deficiency.

TABLE 25-7
Causes of Lymphocytosis with and without Variant Morphology

Absolute lymphocytosis with variant lymphocytes
    Infectious mononucleosis
    Acute viral hepatitis
    Cytomegalovirus infections
Relative lymphocytosis with variant lymphocytes
    Toxoplasmosis
    Viral-related disorders
        Measles
        Mumps
        Chickenpox
        Rubella
        Viral pneumonia
    Immune disorders
        Drug reactions
        Serum sickness
        Idiopathic thrombocytopenia
        Autoimmune hemolytic anemia
    Nonviral infections
        Tuberculosis
        Syphilis
        Malaria
        Typhus
        Brucellosis
        Rickettsia
        Diphtheria
Absolute lymphocytosis with normal lymphocytes
    Acute infectious lymphocytosis
    Bordetella pertussis infection
Relative lymphocytosis with normal lymphocytes
    Neutropenia

While *virocytes* is an adequate term to describe reactive lymphocytes in most patients who have a known viral infection, there are other causes of altered lymphocytes in which no virus is implicated. Because such lymphocytes are normal cells reacting to a stimulus, whether it be viral or other, the designation *reactive lymphocytes* has gained considerable popularity in several institutions. A less definitive but quite popular term is *atypical lymphocytes*. The National Committee for Clinical Laboratory Standards has proposed *variant lymphocytes* as the term of choice. Table 25-7 lists the conditions in which variant (reactive) lymphocytes are found in peripheral blood.

Morphology of Variant Lymphocytes

The most important feature of variant lymphocyte morphology is the recognition of its benign nature. The pertinent fact is that these lymphocytes are normal cells that have been altered as the result of a normal response to stimulus.

Downey and McKinlay,[21] who provided the classic description of the reactive lymphocyte, found enough variation in its structure to classify variant (reactive) lymphocytes into three distinct types. In reactive lymphoproliferative disorders, these cells are seen in the peripheral blood in either one or various combinations of the following three categories.

TYPE I

Also called plasmacytoid lymphocyte and Türk's irritation cell, type 1 cells are differentiated cells that are functionally immunocompetent and probably of B-cell origin.

Size: 9 to 20 μm in diameter
Shape: Oval or round
Nucleus: Heavy strands or dense blocks of chromatin irregularly clumped with sharp, small, defined areas of parachromatin; nuclear shape may be indented or oval. Nuclear membrane is distinct.
Cytoplasm: Basophilia varies, but usually the cytoplasm is moderately basophilic. It may be vacuolated, with darker areas of basophilia at the periphery. It may also have a foamy appearance and may contain azurophilic granules (see Color Plate 25-2).

TYPE II

These cells are sometimes referred to as the infectious mononucleosis (IM) cell because they predominate in IM.

Size: 15 to 25 μm in diameter
Shape: Irregular or scalloped
Nucleus: The chromatin strands are not as condensed as those of type I. Masses of chromatin are interspersed throughout. Nuclear shape is round or oval and is rarely lobulated. Nuclear banding frequently is seen in EDTA specimens. Nucleoli usually are not visible.
Cytoplasm: Abundant and often indented by surrounding structures. Nucleus:cytoplasm ratio is 1:2 to 1:4. The cytoplasm has few vacuoles and usually is pale, except for basophilia at the periphery of the cytoplasm and radiating from the nucleus. Azure granules may or may not be present. This cell often has been described as resembling a fried egg or a flared skirt (see Color Plate 25-3).

TYPE III

Transformed lymphocytes or reticular lymphocytes are cells in an intermediate stage of transformation, the process through which the resting small lymphocyte under-

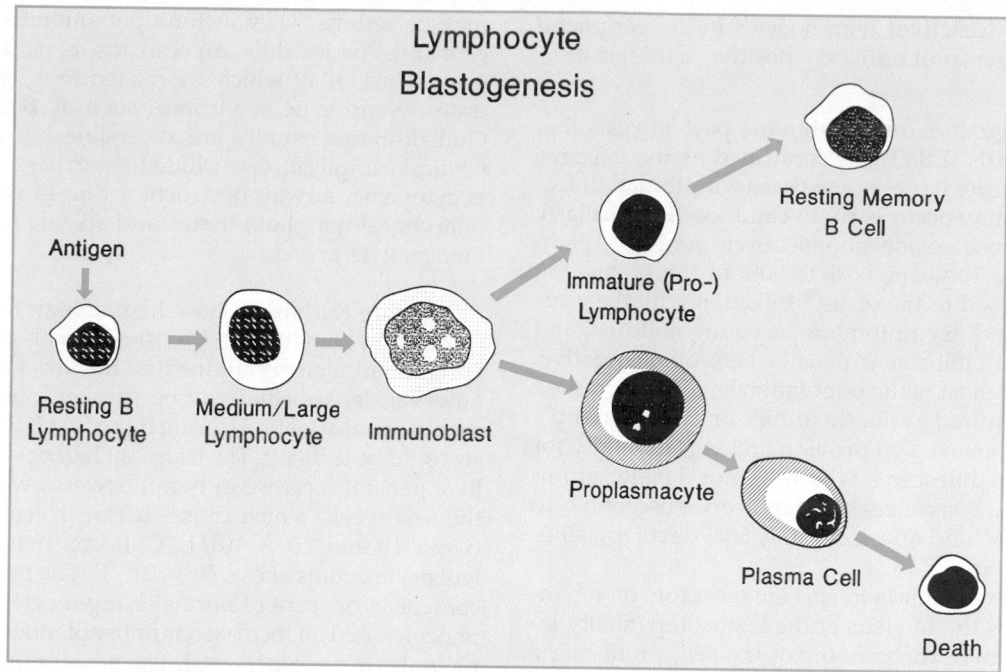

FIGURE 25-11. Diagram of morphologic changes associated with lymphocyte transformation in response to antigen stimulation. The B-cell line is used as an example.

goes blast transformation and ultimately becomes a fully immunocompetent T lymphocyte or plasma cell.

Size: 12 to 35 μm in diameter
Shape: Round or irregular
Nucleus: Finely reticulated nuclear chromatin (immature). Chromatin strands are finely dispersed with loose, indistinct clumping and poorly defined parachromatin. Nucleoli are usually highly visible and elongated or irregular in shape.
Cytoplasm: Abundant and may or may not be basophilic. A clear perinuclear area (see Color Plate 25-4) may be seen.

Note that chromatin structure (quantity and distribution) and parachromatin features are of paramount importance in distinguishing these cells from monocytes. One major precaution should be noted here: Variant (reactive) lymphocytes are particularly vulnerable to effects of delay in blood film preparation and storage in anticoagulant (EDTA). Therefore, fresh specimens (*i.e.*, blood films made within 30 minutes of collection) are an absolute necessity. Prolonged exposure to EDTA can lead to bizarre morphology that mimics that seen in malignancy, such as clefted nuclei, mitotic forms, necrotic (dead) cells, and numerous broken cells.

Lymphocyte Transformation

The lymphocyte morphology described above reflects the cumulative events following antigenic stimulation in which the stimulated lymphocyte undergoes structural and biochemical changes, transforming the small lymphocyte to the blastlike cell, a process called *blastogenesis* (Fig. 25-11 and Color Plate 25-5). Transformation can be induced *in vitro* by specific and nonspecific antigens. The most commonly used are phytohemagglutinin (PHA) for T-cell stimulation and pokeweed mitogen (PWM) for both T- and B-cell stimulation leading to mitosis. Cultures using PHA show nuclear changes in 4 hours and RNA production within 8 hours; at the end of 72 hours most cells are transformed and in mitosis.

When lymphocyte transformation is studied with the transmission electron microscope, the nucleus becomes larger and clearer and the cytoplasm contains an enlarged Golgi apparatus, which increases rapidly and occupies a significant space in the cell's center. Ribosomes increase in number, and mitochondria increase in volume. The endoplasmic reticulum develops slightly if it is a T cell and considerably if it is a B cell. Azurophilic granules increase in number and nucleoli become elongated and enlarged.

Scanning electron microscopy reveals a pronounced shape change from round to "hand mirror" shape—an indication of increased motility. A uropod (viscous posterior portion of the cytoplasm) becomes very prominent. The uropod region contains the Golgi complex, where proteins are accumulated.

Absolute Lymphocytosis with Variant Lymphocyte Morphology

INFECTIOUS MONONUCLEOSIS

Definition. *Infectious mononucleosis (IM)* is a clinically acute contagious viral disease that affects primarily young adults and teenagers. It is not often seen before 10 or after 40 years of age. When it does affect adults 40 years or older, it is generally more severe. The disease is self-limited and benign, but serious complications can occur which occasionally may be fatal. The disease is characterized by variant (reactive) lymphocytes in the peripheral blood and a heterophil antibody-positive serologic test.

Pathophysiology. It is only within the past 30 years that Epstein-Barr virus (EBV) was confirmed as the infective agent in IM. Studies have shown that asymptomatic infection with EBV may occur early in childhood, particularly in children whose socioeconomic environment is poor, and that by age 10 years, 60% to 90% of the population have been exposed to the virus.[24] Infection with the virus is often mild and asymptomatic in young children, and sera from these children is usually heterophil negative. By age 40 years, most of the population have been exposed to and have acquired antibody to EBV antigen. Anti-EBV antibodies are believed to provide lifelong immunity for most persons. Adolescents who have not developed immunity (who are seronegative) are very susceptible to infection by EBV, and approximately 50% develop a clinically acute disease.

EBV selectively binds to specific receptors on B lymphocytes, enters the nucleus at the histocompatibility locus, and takes over the genome of the cell, producing a virally altered cell surface. During the first week of the disease these B cells proliferate, producing infected clones of B cells. Normal immunoglobulin-secreting B cells also increase with the aid of T helper cells and in response to the infected B cells. Such a polyclonal B-cell response results in hypergammaglobulinemia.

The antibody response in turn activates T lymphocytes, inducing blastogenesis. Blastogenic T cell response is shown to increase with time, and during transformation, T lymphocytes acquire cytotoxic potential. The increased number of circulating reactive lymphocytes directly reflects this T-cell proliferation. During the second week of the disease, T-helper cell activity increases until finally T-suppressor cells become activated and shut down T-helper activity. The balance that is achieved between helper and suppressor cells invokes the immunoregulatory mechanism, returning the immune response to normal.[40]

Persons with immune disorders of impaired T-cell function are not able to control proliferation of infected B cells; the result is long-lasting complications in which B-cell lymphomas may develop. Likewise, individuals who are immunosuppressed for purposes of organ transplant may express a post-transplant lymphoproliferative disorder caused by EBV infection.[58]

Clinical Features. The incubation period of IM is about 11 days. Onset is usually accompanied by low-grade fever, which may then elevate to levels as high as 106°F. Fever, sore throat, and cervical lymphadenopathy are the presenting symptoms in more than 80% of cases. Splenomegaly is found in about 50% of cases and hepatomegaly in approximately 10%. Occasionally the patient may present at the prodromal stage (incubation period), when the only manifestation is nonspecific malaise and fatigue and no hematologic or secondary changes are evident, making the diagnosis difficult. This prodromal stage may last 4 to 5 days, and the disease lasts for 1 to 3 weeks.

Complications are rare, but when they occur they may be serious. They include pneumonitis, meningoencephalitis, pericarditis, myocarditis, hepatitis, and laryngeal edema, all of which are related to lymphocytic infiltrates. Neurologic syndromes such as Bell's palsy and Guillain-Barré usually are reversible but can be fatal.[4] Clinical complications include hemorrhage due to thrombocytopenia, airway obstruction due to enlargement of pharyngeal lymphoid tissue, and splenic rupture if splenomegaly is present.[31]

Laboratory Features. Classic hematologic findings are absolute lymphocytosis ($>5 \times 10^9$/L), with more than 20% variant lymphocytes. In the first few days after infection, however, leukopenia may be present. Should a patient seek medical attention during these first few days, diagnosis could be difficult. The transient leukopenia is followed by a general increase in lymphocytes toward the end of the first week, which causes a rise in leukocytes to between 10 and 20×10^9/L. Children may present with leukocyte counts above 50×10^9/L. The peripheral blood contains a mixture of normal lymphocytes, variant lymphocytes, and an increased number of monocytes. Eosinophils also may be increased. The proportion of the various cell types changes as the disease progresses. All three types of variant lymphocytes may be found, although type II predominates. Cells vary greatly in size and shape, in nuclear chromatin pattern (coarse to fine nuclear clumping), and in cytoplasmic features such as vacuolation (foamy appearance) or smooth homogeneous cytoplasm. These lymphocytes usually appear 4 to 5 days after onset of the disease and persist for upwards of 30 days. Since variant or reactive lymphocytes are found in a variety of other illnesses, the percentage may help to distinguish IM from other diseases. Forty percent or more is strongly suggestive of IM. Occasionally when clinical findings suggest IM, hematologic or serologic findings fail to confirm the diagnosis. In such instances cytomegalovirus (CMV) infection or toxoplasmosis should be suspected.

Examination of bone marrow usually is not indicated, but occasionally it may be necessary to rule out leukemia. It is usually normal but may be hypercellular, with hyperplasia of the erythroid, myeloid, and megakaryocytic lines. Variant lymphocytes may be present, but the overall number of lymphocytes usually is not increased. Cells resembling the Reed-Sternberg cell of Hodgkin's disease may be seen (Fig. 38-1).[67]

The classic serologic finding is the presence of the so-called heterophil antibody. When it was discovered that the sera of patients with IM caused agglutination of sheep red cells, the antibody was called a heterophil antibody, meaning that it reacted with antigens that were not responsible for its production. Earlier, in 1911, Forssman had described a nonspecific antigen, the Forssman antigen, in the tissues of various animals, including the guinea pig. Antibodies to this antigen are present in the sera of normal persons in low titers (1:56). IM heterophil antibody *is not* absorbed or is only slightly absorbed by Forssman antigen but *is* absorbed by beef erythrocytes. Therefore, the presence of the heterophil antibody that is not absorbed by Forssman antigen is the *sine qua non* (*i.e.,* diagnostic) of IM.

Two types of serologic tests for IM are available: the classic test described above and an antibody test specific for EBV. The classic test has been largely replaced by rapid tests (slide or tube), (*e.g.* the Monospot test), available from several manufacturers.[46] All such tests should be interpreted in conjunction with clinical and hematologic findings. Thus, if lymphocyte morphology resembles that in IM and results of the heterophil test are negative, other viral diseases should be considered. Occasionally, the heterophil test is negative early in the course of the disease. If hematologic and clinical findings support the diagnosis of IM, the serologic test should be repeated in 2 to 7 days. For heterophil-negative or unusual cases, EBV-specific antibodies can be assayed by immunofluorescence techniques. Immunofluorescent antibody tests are mandatory for diagnosis of IM if other criteria have not been met. During the course of the disease, patients may develop a variety of EBV antibodies, which differ in reactivity and specificity.[37] These include the heterophil group, which are IgM antibodies. Also included are IgI and IgM antibodies to viral capsid antigen (VCA), diffuse (D) component of early antigen (EA) complex, and IgI antibodies to EBNA (nuclear associated antigen).

If hepatitis is suspected as a complication of IM, alkaline phosphatase, lactate dehydrogenase (LD), alanine aminotransferase (ALT), and aldolase values are elevated. Uric acid levels may be increased.

CYTOMEGALOVIRUS INFECTION

Definition and Clinical Features. A disease caused by cytomegalovirus (CMV) closely resembles IM. CMV is the most common agent causing fetal infection. Clinical symptoms differ from those of IM inasmuch as patients do not have tonsillitis or enlarged lymph nodes. One of the most distinguishing features is that patients generally do not complain of a sore throat. Lethargy is unusual, and most CMV infections appear to be subclinical. Fever and splenomegaly are common in middle-aged adults. Hepatomegaly may be found in 50% of patients, as compared to only 10% in IM patients. At onset of illness, malaise, fever, and chills are common. A rash may be present. Symptoms may persist for a longer period (3 weeks) than in IM. The incubation period is 35 to 40 days for adults and 20 to 25 days for children. CMV occurs commonly in adults, whereas IM is unusual after age 35. An increased incidence of CMV has been noted in homosexual men, and CMV has been implicated as a possible agent of Kaposi's sarcoma. CMV in newborns may cause cytomegalic inclusion disease, hepatosplenomegaly, jaundice, cataracts, and mental retardation. It is thought that the disease is transmitted to the child perinatally from virus in cervical secretions, or possibly by blood transfusion. The risk of CMV viremia in bone marrow transplant patients is high.[47]

Pathophysiology. CMV is a cell-associated herpes virus similar to EBV. The virus is found in urine, oral and cervical secretions, and semen, as well as in leukocytes. Since CMV resides in cervical secretions and semen, transmission in adults is primarily venereal. CMV was first recognized in 1962, when open heart surgery patients developed a severe febrile illness with skin rash, splenomegaly, and marked lymphocytosis that resembled IM. More than half of all adults possess antibodies to CMV.

Laboratory Findings. Lymphocytosis with variant or reactive lymphocytes similar to those seen in IM is always present. In contrast to infectious mononucleosis, T cells are not increased in CMV. The leukocyte count rarely exceeds $15 \times 10^9/L$; however, higher counts have been reported. A normochromic, normocytic anemia often occurs and results of the direct antiglobulin test (DAT) may be positive. Platelet number may be decreased and may be low enough to produce petechiae.

IgM and IgG antibodies to CMV antigen can be demonstrated. Complement-fixing antibody with a fourfold rise in the antibody titer is considered diagnostic. IgM antibody to CMV has also been found in patients with IM. IgM cytolytic antibody to CMV-infected cells is seen in patients with primary CMV infection. Results of heterophil antibody tests are negative, and there is no increase in EBV titers. Occasionally, other laboratory abnormalities occur, including cold agglutinins, antinuclear antibodies, and cryoglobulins.

CMV infection is probably most commonly acquired from transfusion of large amounts of fresh blood.[5] CMV is found in the leukocytes of some transfused blood. Infection of the patient is either due to direct transmission of CMV from donor blood or to activation of latent infection in the recipient. Symptoms appear 3 weeks to 3 months after transfusion. Seroconversion (finding CMV antibodies in the patient's serum) increases with the quantity of blood transfused (*i.e.*, 6%–10% with 1–5 units of blood and up to 40%–60% with 10–15 units of blood).

Absolute Lymphocytosis with Normal Lymphocyte Morphology

ACUTE INFECTIOUS LYMPHOCYTOSIS

Acute infectious lymphocytosis is a benign and self-limited disorder usually found in children between the ages of 1 and 10 years, and occasionally up to 14 years of age. The causative agent may be viral or nonviral; however, an enterovirus–coxsackie A subgroup has been isolated in stool specimens of 21% of patients and may be responsible for the extreme lymphocytosis seen in this disease. The fact that the disease occurs in clusters and outbreaks is suggestive of a contagious agent. The incubation period appears to be between 12 and 20 days. The disease may last from 3 to 5 weeks to as long as 2 months.

Generally, patients with infectious lymphocytosis are asymptomatic. If symptoms do occur, they usually are fever, upper respiratory infection, diarrhea, and abdominal pain. No organomegaly is noted.

The one striking laboratory finding is an extreme leukocytosis that may exceed $100 \times 10^9/L$, although most patients exhibit leukocytes from 40 to $50 \times 10^9/L$. The leukocytosis is the result of marked T-lymphocyte proliferation. The morphology is that of small resting lymphocytes, uniform in size and structure with scant cytoplasm. Variant or reactive morphology is conspicuously absent. Bone marrow examination reveals a slight increase in small lymphocytes. Serology is negative for the heterophil antibody.

BORDETELLA PERTUSSIS INFECTION

Bordetella pertussis is another infection in which 70% to 90% of leukocytes on the peripheral blood film are normal-looking lymphocytes. The increase in small lymphocytes may be due to redistribution from tissue pools to circulating pools caused by a lymphocyte-promoting factor (LPF). Studies in mice indicate that LPF attaches to lymphocytes and blocks their movement from blood to lymph nodes, thus increasing the number of circulating lymphocytes and decreasing lymphocytes in the lymph nodes. Leukocyte counts range from 15 to 50 × 10⁹/L. The leukocytosis and lymphocytosis are more pronounced than in any other febrile illness except IM.

Relative Lymphocytosis with Variant Lymphocyte Morphology

TOXOPLASMOSIS

A lymphadenopathic variety of *Toxoplasma* (*Toxoplasma gondii*) infection is similar in clinical presentation to IM, causing fever and enlarged lymph nodes; however, the result of the heterophil antibody test is negative. Up to 10% of seronegative IM cases may be toxoplasmosis. The clinical symptoms ultimately help to differentiate between IM and toxoplasmosis. In IM, lymphatic involvement is often confined to posterior cervical lymph nodes, whereas there tends to be generalized involvement of lymphatic tissue in toxoplasmosis. Splenomegaly and sore throats are less common in toxoplasmosis.

Laboratory features usually are benign, with normal hematologic parameters, the exception being a relative increase in lymphocytes and the presence of reactive lymphocytes. Rarely is absolute lymphocytosis seen. Morphology of the variant lymphocytes is variable; some may have scant amounts of cytoplasm, making them resemble the lymphoblasts of acute leukemia. Cells of the IM type (type II) are not often seen. Current tests for confirmation are indirect fluorescent antibody and indirect hemagglutination techniques.

MISCELLANEOUS DISORDERS

Lymphopenia and neutropenia develop soon after the onset of measles, mumps, chickenpox, hepatitis, and roseola, followed within a few days by a relative lymphocytosis. There is always a pleomorphic blood picture, and variant lymphocytes are a dominant finding. As recovery occurs and the blood picture normalizes, small lymphocytes increase and some of the large lymphocytes become plasmacytoid (type I). Immune responses, recent immunizations, hypersensitivity reactions, and autoimmune diseases all produce the same type of lymphoid reactions. The absolute number of lymphocytes does not increase, but an increase in mitotic forms and increased DNA synthesis are noted. Occasionally, immature lymphocytes (type III) may be seen. The immature appearance of these lymphoid cells may cause confusion with malignant lymphoproliferative disorders.

Ten percent of patients with thyrotoxicosis have neutropenia and relative lymphocytosis. The blood changes are probably due to a disturbance of adrenocortical function.

Lymphopenia

A decrease in the number of circulating lymphocytes could be due to decreased production, alterations in lymphocyte traffic, or lymphocyte destruction.

Lymphopenia due to alterations in lymphocyte traffic has been documented in a wide variety of conditions. Heavy exertion causes a significant increase in epinephrine which, in turn, is believed to cause decreases in the number of circulating lymphocytes.[59] Steroid therapy inhibits lymphocyte migration into lymph nodes thereby disrupting lymphocyte recirculation. This may be due to steroid effects on the lymphocyte's ability to adhere.[69] Morphine administration results in a 30% decrease in circulating lymphocytes. It has been suggested that the opioid affects both lymphocyte recirculation by stimulating the release of adrenal hormones as well as decreasing lymphocyte proliferation.[25] Recently, it has been shown that the lymphopenia seen in patients with acute appendicitis is caused by the selective recruitment of memory T lymphocytes by the inflamed appendix.[76] Lymphocyte depletion related to destruction or premature death has been reported in HIV-1 infection, systemic lupus erythematosus,[62] after intensive chemotherapy treatment for cancer,[48] and after exposure to epoxy resins[19] or nitrogen dioxide.[70]

LEUKEMOID REACTIONS

Distinguishing Between Reactive and Malignant Morphology

Leukemoid reactions are reactive leukocytoses that resemble the blood findings seen in leukemia. Some investigators have defined a leukemoid reaction as one in which the total leukocyte count is greater than 50 × 10⁹/L or blast forms are found in the blood. It may be either myeloid or lymphoid.

Neutrophilic leukemoid reactions (NLR) may present with excessively high leukocyte counts and a severe left shift, including occasional blast forms, and thus they resemble the blood picture of chronic myeloid leukemia (CML). They have been reported in patients with tuberculosis, metastatic tumor, and, in the experience of the authors, they may accompany deep or occult abscesses. Differentiation between NLR and CML usually can be made on the basis of both morphology and cytochemistry. Morphologically, CML involves all granulocytes, so increased numbers of eosinophils, basophils with immature forms, or both are a hallmark of CML. NLR, on the other hand, generally involves only neutrophils, with eosinophil and basophil numbers being normal or *decreased*. The neutrophil alkaline phosphatase value may be used to differentiate the two entities cytochemically. It tends to be increased in a neutrophilic reaction and decreased in CML. It suffices to say that the presence of circulating blast forms does not necessarily indicate leukemia and should be investigated further.

Lymphocytic leukemoid reaction (LLR) refers to any condition in which the lymphocytic leukocytosis is so marked that it gives the impression of possible leukemia. Infectious mononucleosis in children may present with leukocyte counts in excess of $50 \times 10^9/L$, which may lead to an impression of acute lymphocytic leukemia. Likewise, patients with infectious lymphocytosis may have a peripheral blood picture that is reminiscent of chronic lymphocytic leukemia. Children who are critically ill with *Bordetella pertussis* infection may have a leukemoid response, with a leukocyte count above $50 \times 10^9/L$.

Since both reactive and malignant lymphocytosis may exhibit immature-looking cells, to distinguish between the two entities requires skill and experience. The major morphologic differentiation lies in the heterogeneity of variant lymphocytes (polymorphism). This means that within a single specimen both large cells and small cells; basophilic and pale cells; and cells with immature chromatin and cells with densely clumped chromatin are observed. Malignancies, on the other hand, usually are clonal, and all abnormal cells appear very similar to one another.

CHAPTER SUMMARY

This chapter has addressed the reactions of leukocytes to infection, stress, or trauma including changes in numbers as well as appearance. Cytoplasmic and nuclear alterations in granulocytes and monocytes as well as three major types of variant (reactive) lymphocyte morphology have been described in detail. Disorders that commonly result in reactive lymphocyte abnormalities have been discussed, with emphasis on infectious mononucleosis (IM). The importance of differentiating between reactive morphology and artifact as well as distinguishing between reactive and malignant morphology has been stressed.

Case Study 25-1

The patient was a 34-year-old white male complaining of severe headache and drowsiness. History was negative except for severe sinusitis with accompanying fever 3 weeks prior to admission. The patient did not have a fever on admission. Laboratory data included the following: The leukocyte count was markedly increased at $106 \times 10^9/L$, whereas the red cell parameters were relatively normal: RBC $4.60 \times 10^{12}/L$; Hb 14.8 g/dL; Hct 0.45 L/L; MCV 98 fL; MCH 32 pg; MCHC 33 g/dL; the platelet count was also in the normal range at $226 \times 10^9/L$. The leukocyte differential was based on 300 cells with the following results: blasts, 2%; promyelocytes, 5%; neutrophil (N) myelocytes, 7%; N. metamyelocytes, 14%; N. band forms, 11%; N. segmented forms 52%; lymphocytes, 6%; monocytes, 3%; eosinophils, 0%; basophils, 0%; and 2 nucleated red blood cell per 100 leukocytes. Sixty percent of neutrophils from myelocyte to segmented stage contain toxic granulation; 5% contain Döhle bodies.

1. What is the evidence, pro and con, for a diagnosis of chronic myeloid leukemia?
2. Is the toxic granulation most likely true or artifactual? Why?
3. Is the monocyte number increased or normal in absolute numbers?
4. The patient's neutrophil alkaline phosphatase value was 316 (normal, 65–165). What does this mean?

Case Study 25-2

A 45-year-old woman was shaking with chills and fever that began after she inhaled toxic fumes. Two days later, she noticed a rash over her back and trunk. She was admitted to the hospital suffering from generalized body soreness, coughing, malaise, and fever. Her admission laboratory findings were: WBC $5.9 \times 10^9/L$; Hb 11.6 g/dL; PLT $30 \times 10^9/L$ and a leukocyte differential revealed neutrophils (N) segmented forms 24% and toxic; N band forms, 72%; lymphocytes, 2%; monocytes, 2%. On day 2, the patient's Hb had fallen to 7.7 g/dL and her platelets had decreased to $13.0 \times 10^9/L$. Consequently, the patient was transfused with 2 units of packed red cells and several units of platelets.

The patient's condition began to stabilize on the fourth day. Her Hb was 10.0 g/dL and her PLT was $120 \times 10^9/L$. The neutrophils no longer looked toxic and there was no evidence of phagocytosis. However, on a follow-up leukocyte differential performed in the outpatient laboratory on day 24, a marked reactive lymphocytosis was noted, which persisted for 2 weeks. Her leukocyte count and differential were: WBC $14.0 \times 10^9/L$; neutrophils, seg. 20%; neutrophils, band 10%; lymphocytes, 60% (variant); monocytes, 10%.

1. Judging from the clinical information and admission laboratory findings, what is the most likely cause of the thrombocytopenia and the left shift of the neutrophils?
2. Considering the patient's clinical history and treatment, what is the most likely cause of the reactive lymphocytosis?
3. What is the absolute lymphocyte count on day 24?
4. What laboratory tests are needed to confirm the diagnosis?

Review Questions

25-1. A neutrophilia can be caused by

A. infection that overwhelms bone marrow production capacity.
B. splenomegaly.
C. typhoid infection.
D. metabolic disorder.

25-2. The term that refers to the presence of ribosomal RNA remnants in the cytoplasm of toxic neutrophils is

A. left-shift.
B. Döhle body.
C. leukoerythroblastic reaction.
D. toxic granulation.

25-3. A toxic monocytosis should alert the technologist to examine the blood film for circulating

A. macrophages.
B. megakaryocytes.
C. tumor cells.
D. plasma cells.

25-4. A patient whose circulating eosinophils exceed $2.0 \times 10^9/L$ over an extended period of time may be vulnerable to

A. parasites.
B. bacterial infection.
C. organ dysfunction.
D. viral disorders.

25-5. If a patient has infectious mononucleosis, one would expect to see significant numbers of variant lymphocytes that resemble

A. immunoblasts.
B. plasma cells with foamy cytoplasm.

C. large lymphocytes with scalloped edges.
D. small lymphocytes with azure granules.

25-6. A reactive lymphocytosis (lymphocytic leukemoid reaction) usually can be distinguished from a malignant lymphocytosis because reactive lymphocyte populations are more likely to have

A. immature appearing cells.
B. clonal morphology.
C. pleomorphic morphology.
D. all of the above

References

1. Abernathy MR: Döhle bodies associated with uncomplicated pregnancy. Blood 27:380, 1966
2. Altenburg SP, Bozza PT, Martins MA et al: Adrenergic modulation of the blood neutrophilia induced by platelet activating factor in rats. Eur J Pharmacol 256:45, 1994
3. Bass DA, Gonwa TA, Szejda P et al: Eosinopenia of acute infection: Production of eosinopenia by chemotactic factors of acute inflammation. J Clin Invest 65:1265, 1980
4. Bailey RE: Diagnosis and treatment of infectious mononucleosis. Am Fam Physician 49:879, 1994
5. Baumgartner J, Glauser MP, Burgo-Black AL et al: Severe cytomegalovirus infection in multiply transfused, splenectomized trauma patients. Lancet 2:63, 1982
6. Bessis M: Living Blood Cells and Their Ultrastructure. Berlin, Springer-Verlag, 1973
7. Bishop CR, Rothstein CR, Ashenbrucker HE et al: Leukokinetic studies. XIII. A non steady-state kinetic evaluation of the mechanism of cortisone-induced granulocytosis. J Clin Invest 50:1678, 1971
8. Bishop CR: The neutropenias of Felty's syndrome. Am J Hematol 2:203, 1977
9. Boggs DR, Jouce RA: The hematopoietic effects of lithium. Semin Hematol 20:129, 1983
10. Boxer LA, Greenberg MS, Boxer GJ et al: Autoimmune neutropenia. N Engl J Med 293:748, 1975
11. Butterworth AE: The eosinophil and its role in immunity to helminth infection. Curr Top Microbiol Immunol 77:127, 1977
12. Campbell LJ, Maker DW, Tay DLM et al: Marrow proliferation and appearance of giant neutrophils in response to recombinant human granulocyte colony stimulating factor (rhG-CSF). Br J Haematol 80:298, 1992
13. Cawley JC, Hayhoe FGS: The inclusions of the May-Hegglin anomaly and Döhle bodies of infection. Br J Haematol 22:491, 1972
14. Christensen RD, Bradley PP, Rothstein G: The leukocyte left shift in clinical and experimental neonatal sepsis. J Pediatr 98:101, 1981
15. Clifford GO: The clinical significance of leukoerythroblastic anemia. Med Clin North Am 50:779, 1966
16. Craddock PR, Fehr J, Brigham KL et al: Complement and leukocyte-mediated pulmonary dysfunction in hemodialysis. N Engl J Med 296:769, 1977
17. David JR, Vadas MA, Butterworth AE et al: Enhanced helminthotoxic capacity of eosinophils from patients with eosinophilia. N Engl J Med 303:1147, 1980
18. Davidsohn I et al: The differential test for infectious mononucleosis. J Lab Clin Med 45:561, 1955
19. Demers PA, Schade WJ, Demers RY: Lymphocytopenia and occupational exposures among pattern and model makers. Scand J Work Environ Health 20:107, 1994
20. Denburg JA, Telizyn S, Messner H et al: Heterogeneity of human peripheral blood eosinophil-type colonies: Evidence for a common basophil-eosinophil progenitor. Blood 66:312, 1985
21. Downey H, McKinlay C: Acute lymphadenosis compared with acute lymphatic leukemia. Arch Intern Med 32:82, 1923
22. d'Onofrio G, Mancini S, Tamburrini E et al: Giant neutrophils with increased peroxidase activity. Another evidence of dysgranulopoiesis in AIDS. Am J Clin Path 87:584, 1987
23. Falloon J, Gallen JI: Neutrophil granules in health and disease. J Allerg Clin Immunol 77:653, 1986
24. Fleisher G, Paradise J: Atypical lymphocytosis in children. Ann Emerg Med 10:424, 1981
25. Flores LR, Wahl SM, Bayer BM: Mechanisms of morphine-induced immunosuppression: Effect of acute morphine administration on lymphoycte trafficking. J Pharmacol Exp Ther 272:1246, 1995
26. Forsgren A, Schmeling D: Effect of antibiotics on chemotaxis of human leukocytes. Antimicrob Agents Chemother 11:580, 1977
27. Gallen JI: Neutrophil specific granules: A fuse that ignites the inflammatory response. Clin Res 32:320, 1984
28. Gerber P, Hamre D, Moy RA et al: Infectious mononucleosis: Complement-fixing antibodies to herpes-like virus associated with Burkitt lymphoma. Science 161:173, 1969
29. Gilbert HS, Ornstein L: Basophil counting with a new staining method using Alcian blue. Blood 46:279, 1975
30. Goetzl EJ, Foster DW, Payan DG: A basophil-activating factor from human T lymphocytes. Immunology 53:227, 1984
31. Gordon MK, Rietveld JA, Frizelli FA: The management of splenic rupture in infectious mononucleosis. Aust N Z J Surg 65:247, 1995
32. Groopman JE, Golde DW: The histiocytic disorders: A pathophysiologic analysis. Ann Intern Med 94:95, 1981
33. Grzelak I, Olszewski WL, Engeset A: Influence of operative trauma on circulating blood monocytes: Analysis using monoclonal antibodies. Eur Surg Res 16:105, 1984
34. Hansen PB, Knudsen LM, Johnsen HE et al: Stimulation tests for the bone marrow neutrophil pool in malignancies. Leuk Lymphoma 16:237, 1995
35. Hartl W: Drug allergic agranulocytosis (Schultz's disease). Semin Hematol 2:313, 1965
36. Henle G, Henle W, Diehl V: Relation of Burkitt's tumor-associated herpes-type virus to infectious mononucleosis. Proc Natl Acad Sci USA 59:94, 1968
37. Hewetson JF, Rocchi G, Henle W et al: Neutralizing antibodies to Epstein-Barr virus in health populations and patients with infectious mononucleosis. J Infect Dis 128:283, 1973
38. Holley TR, vanEpps DE, Harvey RL et al: Effect of high doses of radiation on human neutrophil chemotaxis, phagocytosis and morphology. Am J Pathol 75:61, 1974
39. Horowitz DA, Allison AC, Ward P: Identification of human mononuclear leukocyte populations by esterase staining. Clin Exp Immunol 30:289, 1977
40. Klein E, Ernberg I, Masucci MG et al: T-cell response to B cells and Epstein-Barr virus antigens in infectious mononucleosis. Cancer Res 41:4210, 1981
41. Knecht H, Eichhorn P, Streuli RA: Granulocytes with ring-shaped nuclei in severe alcoholism. Acta Haematol 73:184, 1985
42. Koepke JA, Koepke JF: Guide to Clinical Laboratory Diagnosis, 3rd ed. Norwalk, CT, Appleton & Lange, 1987
43. Kugel MA, Rosenthal N: Pathological changes in polymorphonuclear leukocytes during progress of infection. Am J Med Sci 183:657, 1932
44. Lalezari P, Nussbaum G, Gelman S et al: Neonatal neutropenia due to maternal isoimmunization. Blood 15:236, 1960
45. Lensink DB, Barton A, Appelbaum FR et al: Cyclic neutropenia as a premalignant manifestation of acute lymphoblastic leukemia. Am J Hematol 22:9, 1986
46. Linderholm M, Bowman J, Juto P et al: Comparative evalua-

tion of nine kits for rapid diagnosis of infectious mononucleosis and Epstein-Barr virus-specific serology. J Clin Microbiol 32:259, 1994

47. Ljungman P, Aschan J, Azinge JN et al: Cytomegalovirus viremia and specific T-helper cell responses as predictors of disease after allogeneic marrow transplantation. Br J Haematol 83:118, 1993

48. Mackall CL, Fleisher TA, Brown MR et al: Lymphocyte depletion during treatment with intensive chemotherapy for cancer. Blood 84:2221, 1994

49. Mackie PH, Mistry DK, Wozniak JT et al: Neutrophil cytochemistry in bacterial infection. J Clin Pathol 32:26, 1979

50. Malcolm ID, Flegel KM, Katz M: Vacuolation of the neutrophil in bacteremia. Arch Intern Med 139:675, 1979

51. McCall CE, Katayama I, Cotran RS et al: Lysosomal and ultrastructural changes in human "toxic" neutrophils during bacterial infection. J Exp Med 129:267, 1969

52. McCarthy DA, Macdonald I, Grant M et al: Studies on the immediate and delayed leucocytosis elicited by brief (30 min) strenuous exercise. Eur J Appl Physiol 64:513, 1992

53. McLaren DJ: The role of eosinophils in tropical disease. Semin Hematol 19:100, 1982

54. Morgan DJR, Moodley PI, Elliott EV et al: Histamine, neutrophil chemotactic factor and circulating basophil levels following exercise in asthmatic and control subjects. Clin Allerg 12(Suppl):29, 1982

55. Moses HL, Glade PR, Kasel JA et al: Infectious mononucleosis: Detection of herpes-like virus and reticular aggregates of small cytoplasmic particles in continuous lymphoid cell lines derived from peripheral blood. Proc Natl Acad Sci USA 60:489, 1968

56. Nagaraju M, Weitzman S, Baumann G: Viral hepatitis and agranulocytosis. Am J Digest Dis 18:247, 1973

57. Naiman JL, Oski FA, Allen FH et al: Hereditary eosinophilia. Report of a family and review of the literature. Am J Hum Genet 16:195, 1964

58. Nalesnik MA, Starzl TE: Epstein-Barr virus, infectious mononucleosis and post transplant lymphoproliferative disorders. Transplant Sci 4:61, 1994

59. Nieman DC, Henson DA, Johnson R et al: Effects of brief, heavy exertion on circulating lymphocyte subpopulations and proliferative response. Med Sci Sports Exerc 24:1339, 1992

60. O'Flaherty JT, Kreutzer DL, Ward PA: Neutrophil aggregation and swelling induced by chemotactic agents. J Immunol 119:232, 1977

61. Oria J, Yoneda S: Variation of the form and structure of the nucleus in various types of plurisegmented neutrophils. In Damashek W, Taylor FHL (eds): George R Minot Symposium in Hematology. New York, Grune & Stratton, 1949

62. Osman C, Swaak AJ: Lymphocytotoxic antibodies in SLE: A review of the literature. Clin Rheumatol 13:21, 1994

63. Paul JR, Bunnell W: The presence of heterophile antibodies in infectious mononucleosis. Am J Med Sci 183:90, 1932

64. Pfeiffer E: Drusenfieber. Yahrb Kinderheilk 29:257, 1889

65. Ponder E, Ponder RV: The cytology of the polymorphonuclear leukocyte in toxic conditions. J Lab Clin Med 28:316, 1942

66. Pruzansky JJ, Ts'ao C, Krajewski DV et al: Quantification of ultrastructural variations in enriched blood basophils: Correlation of morphological changes and antigen-induced histamine release. Immunology 47:41, 1982

67. Reynolds DJ, Banks PM, Gulley ML: New characterization of infectious mononucleosis and a phenotypic comparison with Hodgkin's disease. Am J Pathol 146:379, 1995

68. Robinson WA: Granulocytosis in neoplasia. Ann NY Acad Sci 230:212, 1974

69. Sackstein R, Borenstein M: The effects of corticosterids on lymphocyte recirculation in humans: Analysis of the mechanism of impaired lymphocyte migration to lymph nodes following methylprednisolone administration. J Investig Med 43:68, 1995

70. Sandstrom T, Leden MC, Thomasson L et al: Reductions in lymphocyte subpopulations after repeated exposure to 1.5 ppm nitrogen dioxide. J Ind Med 49:850, 1992

71. Schmitz LL, McClure JS, Litz CE et al: Morphologic and quantitative changes in blood and marrow cells following growth therapy. Am J Clin Pathol 101:67, 1994

72. Shaper AG, Lewis PP: Genetic neutropenia in people of African origin. Lancet 2:1021, 1971

73. Shelley WB, Jiuhlin L: Degranulation of the basophil in man induced by dietary lipemia. Am J Med Sci 242:221, 1961

74. Shenaq SA, Yawn DH, Saleem A et al: Effect of profound hypothermia on leukocytes and platelets. Ann Clin Lab Sci 16:130, 1986

75. Solberg CO, Hellum KB: Neutrophil granulocyte function in bacterial infections. Lancet 2:727, 1972

76. Soo KS, Michie CA, Baker SR et al: Selective recruitment of lymphocyte subsets to inflamed appendix. Clin Exp Immunol 100:133, 1995

77. Sprunt T, Evans F: Mononuclear leucocytosis in reaction to acute infections. Johns Hopkins Hosp Bull 31:357, 1920

78. Thompson J, VanFurth R: The effect of glucocorticoids on the proliferation and kinetics of promonocytes and monocytes of the bone marrow. J Exp Med 137:10, 1973

79. Thonnard-Neumann E: The influence of hormones on the basophilic leukocytes. Acta Haematol 25:261, 1961

80. Tomkins E: The monocytes. Ann NY Acad Sci 59:832, 1955

81. van Assendelft OW: Reference values for the total and differential leukocyte count. Blood Cells 11:77, 1985

82. Weller PF, Goetzl EJ: The human eosinophil. Am J Pathol 100:793, 1980

83. Wright DG, Meierovics AI, Foxley JM: Assessing the delivery of neutrophils to tissues in neutropenia. Blood 67:1023, 1986

84. Zucker-Franklin D: Eosinopenia and eosinophilia. In Williams WJ et al (eds): Hematology, 4th ed. New York, McGraw-Hill, 1990

CHAPTER 26

Nonmalignant Hereditary Disorders of Leukocytes

Angela Foley

Objectives

1. Identify and describe the inherited nuclear and cytoplasmic abnormalities seen in granulocytes, the monocyte–macrophage system, and the immune leukocytes.
2. Compare and contrast the inherited morphologic and/or functional abnormalities of granulocytes, monocyte–macrophage system, and immune leukocytes and include genetics, pathophysiology, and clinical and laboratory findings.

Inherited anomalies involving leukocytes may be associated with morphologic and/or functional aberrations in one or more of the circulating leukocyte populations. These disorders must be correctly identified and not confused with some of the more common reactive or malignant diseases which may express similar hematologic abnormalities. Although most of these disorders are relatively rare, this chapter presents those that are most relevant to the practice of the clinical laboratory scientist.

INHERITED ABNORMALITIES OF GRANULOCYTE MORPHOLOGY

Nuclear Abnormalities

PELGER-HUËT ANOMALY

Pelger-Huët anomaly results in hyposegmentation of the granulocyte nucleus with increased density and coarseness of chromatin. There are two forms of the anomaly: "true," which is inherited, and "pseudo," which is ac-

quired. True Pelger-Huët anomaly is inherited as an autosomal dominant trait, and its distribution is worldwide. The cells appear to be both cytochemically and functionally normal.

Typically, in the heterozygous condition, the neutrophil nucleus either consists of two symmetric, rounded lobes connected by a fine filament, or it fails to segment and thus resembles a peanut or dumbbell. The bilobed nuclei are commonly described as appearing like pince-nez spectacles (Fig. 26-1). Segmentation beyond two lobes is uncommon. In the rare homozygote, the nuclei remain round. Careful examination of the chromatin, which is coarse and densely clumped, indicates that these cells are fully mature.

The acquired or "pseudo" Pelger-Huët form is commonly associated with myeloproliferative disorders (Chaps. 34 and 35), myelodysplastic syndromes (Chap. 33), some infections, and drug therapy. In the acquired form, a number of the cells contain round nuclei such as those seen in the homozygotic form of Pelger-Huët anomaly. In addition, the cytoplasm of cells in the acquired form frequently is hypogranular. The distinction between the two forms is based on morphologic evidence of diseases associated with the acquired form and on the family history.

It is of practical importance to recognize the Pelger-Huët anomaly so that it is not confused with a neutrophilic left shift. A differential on a patient with Pelger-Huët anomaly might be reported by the unwary as containing numerous myelocytes, metamyelocytes, and bands, when in actuality, all of the granulocytes are fully mature. These cells should be reported as mature neutrophils or placed in a separate category with a comment that they are Pelger-Huët cells. Careful observation of the nuclear shape and texture should facilitate the distinction.

HEREDITARY NEUTROPHIL HYPERSEGMENTATION

This is an autosomal dominant trait in which peripheral blood neutrophils are noticeably hypersegmented, with a mean of four lobes. Normally, segmented neutrophils seldom have more than five lobes, and a mean lobe count is usually slightly less than three. This condition, which is rare, is not associated with disease. It is important to be aware that hypersegmentation is not necessarily attributable to vitamin B_{12} or folic acid deficiency (Chap. 12).

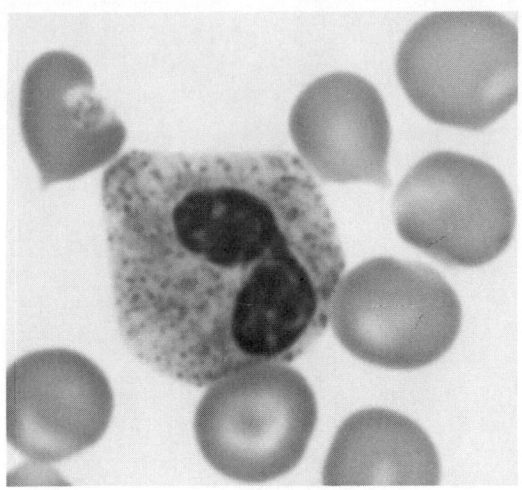

FIGURE 26-1. Pelger-Huët neutrophil showing typical nuclear shape (pince-nez or dumbbell). (original magnification ×1000)

Cytoplasmic Abnormalities

MAY-HEGGLIN ANOMALY

May-Hegglin anomaly is a rare syndrome characterized by leukopenia, variable thrombocytopenia, giant platelets, and gray-blue staining inclusions in the cytoplasm of the granulocytes and monocytes (see Color Plate 26-1). Inheritance is autosomal and dominant. Most persons with this anomaly do not experience clinical symptoms; however, approximately one-third of affected people develop hemorrhagic problems of variable severity.

The inclusions of May Hegglin are similar in appearance and composition to Döhle bodies, but they are larger, more spindle shaped, and are found in all leukocytes.[4] The large platelets may be hypogranular and platelet counts are most commonly in the 40 to 80 × 10⁹/L range. Bleeding times may be prolonged and clot retraction abnormal (Chap. 56). The degree of abnormality seems to be proportional to the extent of thrombocytopenia, which may be more accurately reflected by total platelet mass than platelet number.[18] Electron microscopy studies suggest that abnormal microtubule organization may play a role in the defective platelet formation in this disorder.[12] Platelet aggregation studies are normal (Chap. 56).

ALDER-REILLY ANOMALY

Alder-Reilly anomaly is inherited as an autosomal recessive trait and is characterized by the presence of abnormally large azurophilic and basophilic granules resembling severe toxic granulation in the cytoplasm of granulocytes seen on Wright stained peripheral blood (see Color Plate 26-2). These inclusions do not appear to affect function and are referred to as Alder-Reilly bodies. They are not seen consistently in the peripheral blood of patients exhibiting incomplete expression of the anomaly but can be found on careful examination of bone marrow macrophages and lymphocytes. When the anomaly is completely expressed, all of the granulocytes, some of the lymphocytes, and monocytes in both the bone marrow and the peripheral blood are affected. In addition, the granules of basophils and eosinophils are so bizarre that

they can be differentiated only by their peroxidase reaction, eosinophils being positive and basophils negative.[23] Leukocyte alkaline phosphatase is generally normal.

This anomaly may be seen in association with a group of storage diseases in which protein–carbohydrate complexes called mucopolysaccharides accumulate in the cytoplasm of tissue and blood cells. These storage abnormalities will be discussed later in this chapter.

INHERITED ABNORMALITIES OF GRANULOCYTE FUNCTION

For proper function, phagocytes must be able to move randomly as well as directionally along a chemotactic gradient. Once they have arrived, they must be able to recognize and ingest the offending agent. Subsequently, they must be able to release their granule contents into the phagosome and undergo a respiratory burst to complete the destruction of the ingested antigen (see Fig. 22-4). Defects in any of these abilities related to motility and killing may result in disease.

Defective Motility

Hyperimmunoglobulin E, lazy leukocyte syndrome, and leukocyte adhesion deficiency are examples of diseases associated with defective motility of phagocytes.

HYPERIMMUNOGLOBULIN E

Hyperimmunoglobulin E or Job's syndrome is an uncommon condition characterized by defects in neutrophil and monocyte chemotaxis and marked elevations in the level of circulating IgE.[26] The molecular basis for this syndrome remains unknown, but occurrence in successive generations suggests an autosomal dominant mode of inheritance.[15,20] The cells respond very slowly to chemotactic agents. As a result, bacteria have more time to multiply in the tissues before they are attacked. Like the biblical Job, the patients suffer from persistent boils and recurrent "cold" staphylococcal abscesses. (These abscesses are described as cold because the usual signs of inflammation [heat and redness] are absent.) The mechanism for the poor phagocyte response is unknown. However, it has been proposed that the increased level of IgE is the result of insufficient suppressor T-cell function.[14] Evidence also suggests that a chemotactic inhibitor released by mononuclear cells may be responsible for the increased susceptibility to bacterial infections.[14]

LAZY LEUKOCYTE SYNDROME

Lazy leukocyte syndrome is a rare condition in which, as its name suggests, both random and directed movement of the cells are defective.[22] The mode of inheritance is unknown. Bone marrow reserves of granulocytes are normal, but release of cells from the marrow to the peripheral blood is poor.[19] As a result, neutropenia is a consistent finding. The cells fail to respond to inflammatory stimuli but otherwise appear to have normal phagocytic and bactericidal activity. The clinical features include low-grade fever and recurrent infections involving the gums, mouth, and ears. Surprisingly, some patients have only mild clinical signs.

Normal neutrophils contain actin filaments that are closely associated with the cell's ability to form pseudopods and move. Ultrastructural and biochemical studies suggest that the cells in lazy leukocyte syndrome contain defective actin filaments.[3]

LEUKOCYTE ADHESION DEFICIENCY

Leukocyte adhesion deficiency is a rare autosomal recessive disorder characterized by recurrent skin and soft tissue infections, neutrophilia, impaired pus formation, and poor wound healing. Affected individuals have a deficiency or total lack of three leukocyte surface glycoproteins designated CD11/18 complex. This family of glycoproteins has also been referred to as the $\beta2$ integrins and are essential for normal leukocyte motility and transendothelial migration.[1] In addition, they serve as major receptors for the C3b opsonic complement component and are necessary for phagocytosis and respiratory burst activation.[7] Neutrophils from individuals with this disorder generally fail to migrate to inflammatory sites and those that do are unable to recognize opsonized microorganisms. Affected individuals have persistent neutrophilia ranging from 15 to $60 \times 10^9/L$, which may exceed $100 \times 10^9/L$ during infections.

Defective Killing

The inability to kill microorganisms may be secondary to a failure of granule release, as in the Chédiak-Higashi syndrome, or inability to ingest the organism, as is seen in congenital deficiency of the complement component C3. In addition, defects in oxidative metabolism, as in chronic granulomatous disease of childhood, and myeloperoxidase deficiency, will affect the bactericidal capacity of phagocytes.

CHÉDIAK-HIGASHI SYNDROME

Chédiak-Higashi syndrome is a genetic disorder first recognized because of the presence of giant cytoplasmic granules in the phagocytes and lymphocytes (Fig. 26-2 and Color Plate 26-3). The syndrome affects at least six species: humans, mink, cattle, mice, cats, and killer whales. It is inherited as an autosomal recessive trait and is manifested in all species in much the same way. It has been extensively studied because of the availability of animal models and because two animal models, *i.e.*, cattle and mink, are of economic importance. Affected individuals display partial albinism, are more susceptible to a variety of common infectious agents, and have hemorrhagic tendencies. In later or accelerated stages of the disease, hepatosplenomegaly, liver failure, lymphadenopathy with lymphoma-like morphology, and neuropathy may develop. Death usually results from overwhelming infection.

Partial albinism is the result of a relative pigmentary dilution. Melanocytes are responsible for skin pigmentation. In Chédiak-Higashi syndrome, there is abnormal

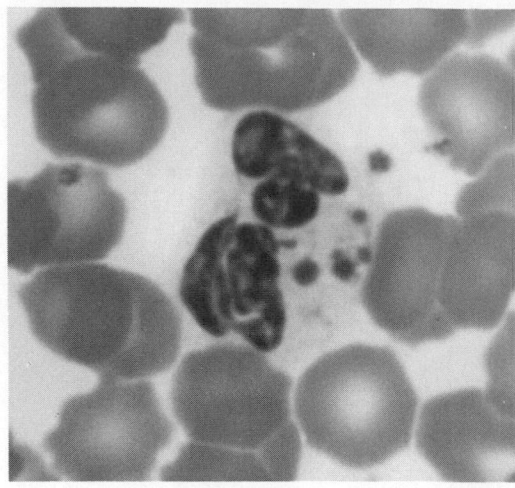

FIGURE 26-2. Chédiak-Higashi syndrome. Neutrophil exhibits characteristic giant lysosomes. Source of this blood film was an Aleutian mink. (original magnification ×1000)

packaging of melanosomes into large melanin-containing structures, which, being fewer in number and more widely scattered, absorb less light. Thus, the skin, hair, and eyes of affected individuals appear lighter than normal. The patient often is described as having silvery hair and pale skin and suffers from photophobia.

Recurrent infections, most commonly with staphylococci and other gram-positive organisms, can be attributed to abnormal phagocyte function.[29] While ingestion of bacteria and oxygen metabolism is normal, neutrophils and other phagocytes are unable to release their granule content and exhibit delayed killing. Cytolytic function of natural killer cells and cytotoxic T lymphocytes is also defective.[2] Recent studies suggest that the basic defect in Chédiak-Higashi lies in a membrane fusion protein which is crucial for the secretion of the lysosomal compartment of various hematopoietic cells.[2]

The most striking laboratory feature is the presence of the large, abnormal cytoplasmic granules in granulocytes, monocytes, and lymphocytes. These can be readily observed on Wright-stained blood films and accentuated with peroxidase stain. Routine coagulation studies are normal except for the bleeding time, which is prolonged. Platelet aggregation studies are abnormal regardless of the aggregating agent used because of the abnormal release of granule contents, with a decreased availability of ADP and serotonin. Anemia, leukopenia, and thombocytopenia frequently develop with time.

CONGENITAL C3 DEFICIENCY

Congenital deficiency of the complement component C3 is rare and is inherited as an autosomal recessive trait. Heterozygous carriers have approximately half the normal C3 activity (adequate for disease resistance). Homozygotes or compound heterozygotes suffer from repeated severe infections with encapsulated bacteria, which, because of the failure of opsonization (coating) by C3b, are poorly recognized and inefficiently phagocytosed.[13]

CHRONIC GRANULOMATOUS DISEASE

Chronic granulomatous disease (CGD) is a rare condition, usually detected in childhood, in which phagocytes ingest but cannot kill catalase-positive organisms because of the lack of an appropriate respiratory burst (Chap. 22). It is caused by mutations in one of several genes encoding for respiratory burst oxidase proteins that are either components of cytochrome b or located in the cytosol of the resting phagocyte. There are two modes of inheritance for CGD. In some families the gene is clearly sex-linked, whereas in others the condition is transmitted as an autosomal recessive trait with the defective gene being located on chromosome 16.[6]

In CGD, catalase-positive organisms survive and multiply in the phagosome because they neutralize their own hydrogen peroxide. Catalase-negative organisms, which are unable to neutralize their peroxide, are destroyed in a normal fashion in CGD because they generate enough peroxide for the phagocyte's microbicidal system to function. From this standpoint, they might be considered "suicide" organisms.

In CGD there is a drastic decrease in oxygen uptake and a decrease in the generation of a series of oxygen metabolites that are necessary for microbial killing. The deficient metabolites include hydrogen peroxide (H_2O_2) and superoxide (O_2^-), hydroxyl radical, and singlet oxygen. The last metabolite, which has the same chemical formula as atmospheric oxygen, has a distorted electron cloud around the two oxygen nuclei and is highly unstable. Its decay to the ground state is associated with emission of light, called *chemiluminescence*.

There are two approaches to the evaluation of the respiratory burst (*i.e.*, chemiluminescence and NBT reduction). Chemiluminescense, which is the emission of low-level light pulses by stimulated cells, can be measured in luminometers.[28] Light pulses result from the oxidation of other molecules by the singlet oxygen produced in the burst. Normally, resting cells do not emit light, and activated cells do. In CGD, neither resting nor stimulated cells emit light. The respiratory burst can also be evaluated by nitroblue tetrazolium (NBT) reduction in the phagocyte. When NBT, a yellow water-soluble dye, is reduced, it is converted to an insoluble blue formazan. Normal activated phagocytes ingest and reduce NBT to a blue-black intracytoplasmic precipitate using the O_2^- they generate in the respiratory burst. Because burst activity is necessary for this reduction, patients with conditions in which the burst is lacking are unable to reduce NBT.

The clinical features of CGD are variable. In mild cases, they may first appear in adolescence or adulthood. They include chronic pyogenic infections, lymphadenopathy, and hepatosplenomegaly. Healing is often accompanied by granuloma formation (*i.e.*, accumulations in the skin and other tissues of masses of macrophages and giant cells). Recurrent pneumonia is common and often is the cause of death.

MYELOPEROXIDASE DEFICIENCY

Myeloperoxidase (MPO) deficiency is a relatively common disorder inherited in an autosomal recessive fashion. Its incidence has become apparent with the development of differential cell counters that use myeloperoxidase activity for cell identification.[21] It is a benign condition in which patients are rarely troubled by infections. Without MPO, bacterial killing is slowed but complete.

INHERITED DISORDERS OF THE MONOCYTE–MACROPHAGE SYSTEM

Monocytes and macrophages are responsible for ingestion and disposal of foreign substances, unwanted biosynthetic products of cells, and their breakdown products, including lipids, carbohydrates, proteins, and nucleotides. There are several mechanisms associated with the abnormal accumulation of a specific substance that causes a macrophage to become overloaded resulting in macrophage storage disease. These mechanisms may be summarized as (1) an abnormal increase in catabolism causing true overload in cellular breakdown products that overwhelms the normal enzyme systems, as may be seen, for example, in myeloproliferative disorders and hemolytic anemias; (2) the lack of an enzyme necessary to metabolize the substances; and (3) indigestibility of ingested particles. This section will cover those inherited storage diseases that are a result of the lack of single enzymes necessary for the degradation or catabolism of various lipids or carbohydrates.

Mucopolysaccharidoses

Mucopolysaccharidoses (MPS) are a group of closely related syndromes resulting from genetically determined deficiencies of specific enzymes involved in the degradation of mucopolysaccharides. Mucopolysaccharides are carbohydrates that contain hexosamine and are found in mucus among other things. The mucopolysaccharidoses include Hurler (MPS I), Hunter (MPS II), Sanfilippo (MPS III), Morquio or Morquio-Ullrich (IV), Maroteaux-Lamy (MPS VI), and Sly (glucuronidase deficiency [MPS VII]) syndromes. In all but one form, the mode of inheritance is autosomal recessive; Hunter disease, the exception, is transmitted as a sex-linked recessive trait. Hurler and Hunter syndromes were given the name "gargoylism" because of characteristic facial and skeletal abnormalities. These disorders differ in severity and expression, depending on the extent of the enzyme deficiency and the particular tissues in which the abnormal product accumulates. The affected enzymes normally cleave terminal sugars from polysaccharide chains attached to a core protein. When there is a block in the removal of this terminal sugar, degradation of the rest of the polysaccharide is halted. These chains therefore accumulate within the lysosomes of cells in various tissues and organs, including leukocytes. Cells in affected tissues are swollen and have apparent ballooning and clearing of their cytoplasm. Electron microscopy shows the cleared areas to be full of minute vacuoles that contain mucopolysaccharides.[16] In peripheral blood and bone marrow, there is variable expression of the abnormalities consisting of metachromatic granules in leukocytes and histiocytes (as described under Alder-Reilly anomaly). It should be noted that these granules are sometimes referred to as "Alder-Reilly bodies" or as "Reilly bodies." Because they are metachromatic, they will stain purple with toluidine blue.

Lipid Storage Diseases

Lipid storage diseases are genetically determined disorders in which the macrophages of one or more tissues become overloaded with lipid. These diseases result from the lack of a functional enzyme required for breakdown of lipids that have been ingested by phagocytes. Expression of the disease depends on the particular enzyme that is depressed or missing. Transmission is autosomal recessive, and, except for Gaucher disease type II, the highest incidence is seen in Ashkenazic (northern European) Jews, possibly reflecting an inbred population. This chapter will present only those disorders in which lipid storage in macrophages accounts for the major clinical manifestations, namely Gaucher and Niemann-Pick disease.

GAUCHER DISEASE

Gaucher disease is the most common of the lipidoses. It is characterized by the lack of the enzyme beta-glucosidase, with the resultant macrophage accumulation of glucocerebrosides in the spleen, liver, and bone marrow. Three types of Gaucher disease have been identified that differ in age of onset and severity.

Type I, the most common form, is called the "adult" form of the disease, although the symptoms usually begin in childhood or early adulthood. Accumulation of lipid-laden macrophages in the spleen causes pronounced splenomegaly (Color Plate 26-4). Overloaded liver macrophages interfere with the circulation of blood through the sinusoids, and liver function tends to deteriorate. The accumulation of Gaucher cells in the marrow causes bone lesions, and bone pain is probably the most troublesome clinical problem from the patient's standpoint. The central nervous system is not affected. Some patients, depending on the age when the disease first appears, have normal life spans. Death may occur because of liver disease, bleeding, or sepsis.

Type II, the infantile or cerebral form of Gaucher disease, is much more severe because of central nervous system involvement. Neurologic deterioration progresses rapidly, and death usually occurs within the first few years of life.

Type III, the juvenile form of Gaucher disease, first becomes apparent in early childhood. The central nervous system is only occasionally involved. Hepatosplenomegaly and bone involvement develop rapidly, and the life expectancy is short.

Regardless of the type, leukopenia, thrombocytopenia, and various degrees of anemia are common and related to the extent of splenomegaly. The anemia is normochromic and normocytic. Masses of Gaucher cells may be found in the bone marrow, spleen, liver, and other affected tissues. The Gaucher cell is a large macrophage with a small, usually eccentrically placed, nucleus. Its cytoplasm is distended by glucocerebrosides, which give it a characteristic crinkled appearance like crumpled tissue paper (Fig. 26-3). These cells are strongly periodic acid–Schiff (PAS) positive. The measurement of beta-glucosidase in leukocytes or fibroblasts is helpful in identifying homozygotes and heterozygotes for the purpose of genetic counseling. Because activity in the heterozygous state overlaps with the normal range, DNA analysis may be necessary for definitive diagnosis. Prenatal diagnosis can be made by measuring beta-glucosidase activity or examining DNA in cultured amniocentesis cells. Characteristically, serum acid phosphatase is markedly elevated in all forms of Gaucher disease and is helpful in confirming the diagnosis.

"Pseudo"-Gaucher cells may be seen in a variety of disorders including chronic myelocytic leukemia, Hodgkin disease, multiple myeloma, rheumatoid arthritis, and AIDS. These patients possess a normal enzyme system which is unable to process the excess lipid burden presented by increased cell turnover.

NIEMANN-PICK DISEASE

Niemann-Pick is a clinically and biochemically heterogeneous disorder in which there is abnormal accumulation of sphingomyelin and cholesterol in mononuclear phagocytic cells and some parenchymal cells throughout the body. The disorder is generally divided into five categories, designated A through E. This chapter will discuss only types A (neuropathic) and B (non-neuropathic), because they account for the vast majority of reported cases. In both types there is deficient activity of the lysosomal hydrolase, acid sphingomyelinase. Type A appears in infancy and is characterized by failure to thrive, marked hepatosplenomegaly, neurologic deterioration, and death by age 3 years. Type B, the adult form, occurs much less frequently and also appears in infancy. Patients have hepatosplenomegaly but no neurologic involvement. They experience a milder disease course and often survive into adulthood.

In both forms of the disease, the bone marrow contains numerous macrophages whose cytoplasm is swollen by many small, uniform lipid droplets. Such macrophages are often described as "foam" cells (Fig. 26-4). Peripheral

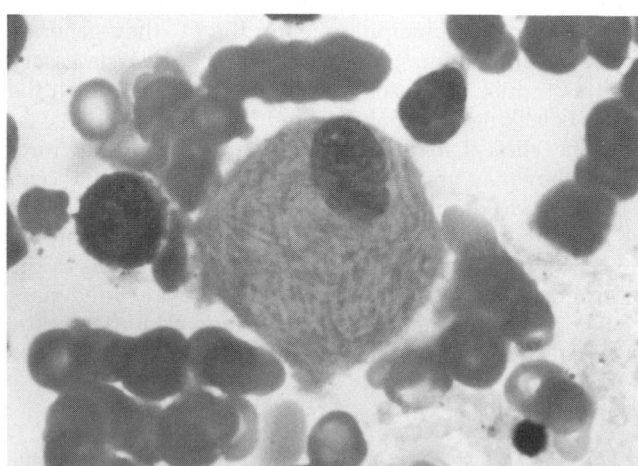

FIGURE 26-3. Gaucher cell. Note striations in cytoplasm of this abnormal macrophage. (original magnification ×1000)

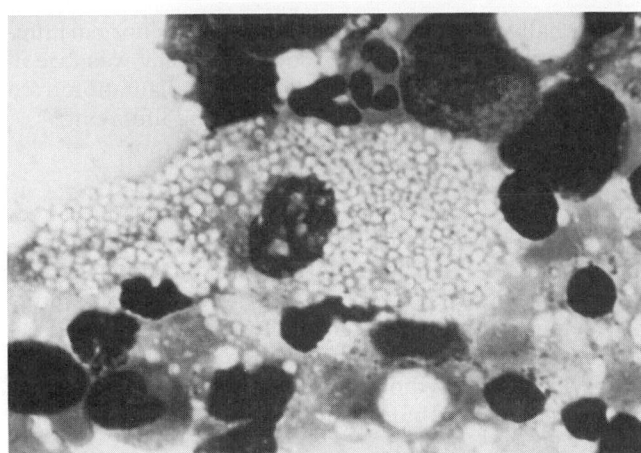

FIGURE 26-4. Niemann-Pick cell. Note lipid droplets in cytoplasm. (original magnification ×1000)

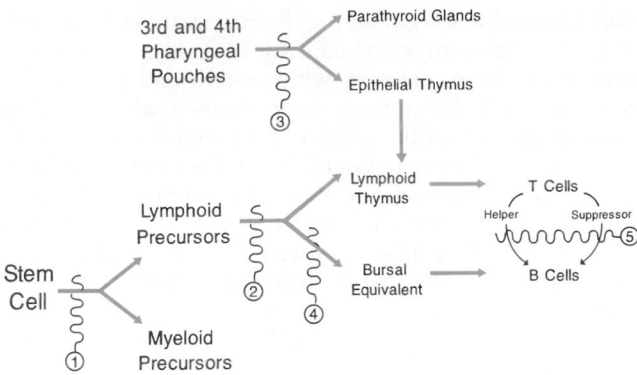

FIGURE 26-5. Ontogeny of immunocompetent cells. Numbered points indicate where development of these cells might be interrupted in pathologic conditions: (1) decrease in all cells—aplasia; (2) combined immunodeficiency; (3) defective T-cell production and cellular immunity; (4) defective B-cell production and antibody production; (5) defective communication between T and B cells or abnormal ratios of T to B cells.

blood monocytes and lymphocytes may also contain cytoplasmic vacuoles revealed by electron microscopy to be lipid-filled lysosomes.

Precise diagnosis and differentiation from similar lipidoses can be accomplished by identification of sphingomyelin in biopsies of tissues containing the affected cells or by establishing a deficiency of the enzyme sphingomyelinase. Antenatal diagnosis can be made using leukocytes or cultured fibroblasts from amniotic fluid.

Sea-blue histiocytes are macrophages that contain a substance which stains blue with Romanowsky-type stains. They lack diagnostic specificity and have been observed in the marrow of patients with a variety of disorders including chronic erythemic myelosis, chronic myelocytic leukemia, Hodgkin disease, hyperlipemic states, multiple myeloma, sickle cell disease, Niemann-Pick disease, and others.[17] Sea-blue histiocyte syndrome, once thought to be a separate disease entity, is now accepted to be the adult form of Neimann-Pick disease (type B).[27]

INHERITED DISORDERS OF IMMUNE LEUKOCYTES

Serious disease is associated with failure of lymphoid development in the bone marrow and thymus and with failure of the thymus itself to develop. Figure 26-5 summarizes the ontogeny of immunocompetent cells, the potential points of interruption, and the effects of interruption at each point. See Chapter 23 for a detailed discussion of lymphopoiesis. Immunologic deficiencies can be classified as B-cell deficiencies, T-cell deficiencies, and combined T- and B-cell deficiencies.

B-Cell Deficiencies

Assessment of B-cell function is based both on the level of serum immunoglobulins and on the ability of the patient to produce immunoglobulins against protein and polysaccharide antigens (*i.e.*, tetanus toxin and pneumococcal polysaccharide vaccines). A history of successful immunization against toxoids such as diphtheria or per-

tussis is evidence of a previous normal humoral response. Circulating numbers of B cells can be measured utilizing immunofluorescence, monoclonal antibodies, and flow cytometry (Chap. 43). Sex-linked agammaglobulinemia and common variable immunoglobulinemia are examples of B-cell deficiencies.

SEX-LINKED (BRUTON) AGAMMAGLOBULINEMIA

Sex-linked agammaglobulinemia is transmitted by the mother to her male children. It becomes obvious when the infant is about 6 months of age and has essentially lost the protection of maternal IgG that crossed the placenta during intrauterine life. At this time, the child contracts a series of bacterial infections involving the usual childhood pathogens but fails to develop immunity against them. All classes of immunoglobulins are either absent or extremely low. Peripheral blood lymphocytes are normal in number although they tend to be exclusively T cells. There is an absence of B cells in the blood, bone marrow, and secondary lymphoid tissues. It is clear that the T-cell system is functioning normally, because these children develop lasting immunity to most viral infections. Therapy includes the use of antibiotics and passive immunization with pooled human gamma globulin.

COMMON VARIABLE IMMUNOGLOBULINEMIA (CVI)

CVI is a heterogeneous group of disorders characterized by hypogammaglobulinemia, recurrent bacterial infections, and various immunologic abnormalities including increased incidence of autoimmune disease and malignant lymphoproliferative disorders. B cells of affected individuals are unable to differentiate into mature antibody producing plasma cells. This inability may be the result of a number of different molecular aberrations including intrinsic B-cell defects, T- and/or B-cell activation defects, and/or defective T-cell lymphokine production or surface molecule expression.[9] Patients with CVI have normal numbers of circulating B cells but decreased levels of immunoglobulins, specifically IgG. They also fail to respond to immunization with protein and polysaccharide antigens. In contrast to patients with sex-linked agammaglobulinemia, men and women are equally affected and, in most patients, onset does not occur until the second or third decade of life. Although the pathogenesis of CVI remains unclear, recent studies indicate that susceptibility may in some cases be determined by a gene or genes near the major histocompatibility class III region.[25]

T-Cell Deficiencies

T-cell deficiencies arise either from failure of development of the thymus or from a blockage of the stem cell destined to develop in the thymus.

There are a number of approaches to the laboratory evaluation of T-cell status. The first is study of hypersensitivity through skin testing with agents that induce a delayed hypersensitivity response in most normal adults. A history of normal recovery from viral infections supports the existence of normal cell-mediated immunity. Also, the numbers of circulating T cells can be measured using flow cytometry or sheep cell rosette techniques. DiGeorge syndrome is a classic example of pure T-cell deficiency.

DiGEORGE SYNDROME (CONGENITAL THYMIC APLASIA)

This is a congenital anomaly characterized by defective development of the thymus and parathyroid glands. This abnormality results from an abnormal development of the third and fourth pharyngeal pouches resulting in thymic hypoplasia, hypoparathyroidism and immunodeficiency. Affected infants display tetany (intermittent, sudden spasms usually involving the extremities) secondary to a lack of parathyroid hormone and subsequent hypocalcemia. Other characteristics of this syndrome include congenital heart defects and facial dysplasia. Those infants who survive the neonatal period are susceptible to repeated viral, fungal, and bacterial infections. The defect involves a deletion of the chromosome 22q11 region. Although most cases lack hereditary predisposition, some familial cases have been reported.[8] Transplantation of fetal thymus tissue into affected children has been successful in populating thymus-dependent areas with lymphocytes and restoring T-cell function.

Combined B- and T-Cell Deficiencies

SEVERE COMBINED IMMUNODEFICIENCY DISEASE (SCID)

SCID is characterized by a rapid succession of serious infections beginning in early infancy with death occurring usually before the age of 2 years. The disorder may be transmitted in an autosomal or sex-linked recessive fashion which accounts for the 3:1 ratio of males to females affected with the disorder.[24] Affected infants exhibit profound lack of T cells in the blood and lymphoid tissue. B cells may be normal or decreased in number but are functionally impaired, even when present in normal numbers. Until recently, survival beyond infancy was rare in afflicted individuals. Bone marrow transplantation from histocompatible donors has proven to be lifesaving.

WISKOTT-ALDRICH SYNDROME

In this disease, both T- and B-cell function is impaired. The disorder is characterized by eczema, thrombocytopenia, and recurrent bacterial and viral infections. Inheritance is sex-linked recessive with affected boys rarely surviving beyond adolescence. There is an increased occurrence of lymphoreticular malignancies in those affected individuals who do survive past childhood.[5] Serum IgM levels are low, but IgG and IgA levels may be normal or increased.

ATAXIA TELANGIECTASIA

Ataxia telangiectasia is a rare condition in which there is ataxia (progressive loss of muscular coordination) associated with telangiectasia (dilation of small blood vessels). It is transmitted as an autosomal recessive disease with the defective gene or genes being linked to the chromosome 11q22-23 region.[10] Virtually all patients have a dysplastic or hypoplastic thymus with a minimal T-cell population and defective cellular immunity. IgG levels are normal, however about 80% of patients lack both serum and secretory IgA. Death usually occurs in the second or third decade of life secondary to chronic respiratory infection or lymphoreticular malignancy.

CHAPTER SUMMARY

Genetically determined abnormalities of leukocytes may affect morphology, function, or both and may involve any cell line. All the abnormalities addressed in this chapter are relatively rare compared with reactive or malignant alterations. Because of this, there is always the concern that those disorders characterized by morphologic abnormalities might be mistaken for more common acquired morphologic abnormalities or vice versa. Table 26-1 lists those hereditary morphologic abnormalities that might be confused with acquired abnormalities and gives some possible distinctions.

Case Study 26-1

The following profile was generated on a 20-year-old male patient admitted to the hospital for elective surgery: WBC 6.2 × 10⁹/L; RBC 5.1 × 10¹²/L; Hb 15.6 g/dL; Hct 0.48 L/L; MCV 94.1 fL; MCH 30.6 pg; MCHC 32.5 g/dL; PLT 255 × 10⁹/L. The automated differential indicated an abnormal WBC population. On performing a manual differential, the laboratorian noted that the majority of neutrophils were band forms or bilobed with a "pince-nez" appearance. The chromatin appeared coarse and densely clumped.
1. What is the most likely cause of the differential findings?
2. How should these cells be reported?
3. Why is it important that these cells be correctly identified?

Case Study 26-2

A 5-year-old girl was admitted to the hospital for evaluation of recurrent infections, bleeding problems, and marked hepatosplenomegaly. She had been previously identified as having

TABLE 26-1
Hereditary vs Acquired Morphologic Abnormalities

Inherited Form	Acquired Form	Distinctions	
Pelger-Huët (PH)	Neutrophilic left shift (NLS)	PH	Characteristic dumbbell shape; chromatin dense and clumped
		NLS	Chromatin in immature neutrophils is not dense; less clumping
	Pseudo–Pelger-Huët (PPH)	PPH	Presence of several round nuclei; hypogranularity and other evidence of malignancy
Hypersegmentation (HS)	B_{12} or folate deficiency (B/F)	HS	Does not respond to therapy; is not transient
		B/F	Oval macrocytes
May-Hegglin (MH)	Döhle bodies (DB)	MH	Larger inclusions (>1 μm); present in all granulocytes and monocytes; accompanied by giant platelets
		DB	Smaller inclusions (1 μm or less) only in neutrophils
Alder-Reilly (AR)	Toxic granules (TG)	AR	All cells are affected; granules evenly dispersed in cells; granules not peroxidase positive
		TG	Granules clustered in neutrophils; not all cells affected; granules are strongly peroxidase positive
Chédiak-Higashi (CH)	Neutrophils with ingested organisms (IG)	CH	Patient history of lifelong infections; physical appearance (partial albinism); all cell types may have abnormal granules; granules are golden brown
		IG	Only phagocytes contain material; ingested organisms stain purple; other evidence of toxicity

Chédiak-Higashi syndrome and displayed subtle signs of partial albinism. Important laboratory findings: Hb 6.0 g/dL; PLT 81 × 10^9/L; WBC 5.9 × 10^9/L; reticulocytes 7%; differential is 30% neutrophils, 3% monocytes, 67% lymphocytes. Many cells contained abnormal granules pathognomonic for Chédiak-Higashi syndrome. Bone marrow aspirates and biopsy showed widespread lymphohistiocytic infiltration characteristic of the accelerated (lymphomalike) phase of the syndrome. The abnormal blood chemistry findings were: total bilirubin 2.0 mg/dL; markedly elevated AST and ALT; prothrombin time 15 seconds (control 12 seconds); and markedly decreased IgG.

Her infection responded well to antibiotic therapy. Her anemia and thrombocytopenia were treated with packed RBCs and PLTs. Prednisone and vincristine were given to reduce the hepatosplenomegaly. However, these measures were of only transient help, and she required repeated therapy periodically until her death 1 year later.

1. What is the most likely cause of the anemia and thrombocytopenia?
2. What factors contributed to her bleeding problem?
3. What laboratory results reflected progressive liver failure?

Review Questions

26-1. Nuclear hyposegmentation with normal neutrophil function is associated with

    A. Alder-Reilly anomaly.
    B. Chédiak-Higashi anomaly.
    C. May-Hegglin anomaly.
    D. Pelger-Huët anomaly.

26-2. The defect in Chédiak-Higashi anomaly involves a(n)

    A. mucopolysaccharide metabolic defect.
    B. membrane fusion protein defect.
    C. opsonization defect.
    D. respiratory burst defect.

26-3. Gaucher disease is characterized by a deficiency of the enzyme

    A. β-galactosidase.
    B. β-glucosidase.
    C. hexoseaminadase A.
    D. sphingomyelinase.

26-4. In chronic granulomatous disease there is

    A. abnormal phagocytosis with normal superoxide production.
    B. normal phagocytosis with abnormal nitroblue tetrazolium (NBT) reduction.
    C. normal phagocytosis with decreased myeloperoxidase production.
    D. abnormal phagocytosis with normal chemiluminescence.

26-5. Laboratory features of sex-linked (Bruton's) agammaglobulinemia include

    A. normal immunoglobulin levels and decreased numbers of circulating T cells.
    B. decreased immunoglobulin levels and normal numbers of circulating lymphocytes which are exclusively T cells.
    C. decreased immunoglobulin levels and decreased numbers of circulating B and T cells.
    D. normal immunoglobulin levels and decreased numbers of circulating B cells.

References

1. Arnout MA: Leukocyte adhesion molecule deficiency: Its structural basis, pathophysiology and implications for modulating the inflammatory response. Immunology Rev 114:145, 1990
2. Baetz K, Isaaz S, Griffiths G: Loss of cytotoxic T lymphocyte

function in Chédiak-Higashi syndrome arises from a secretory defect that prevents lytic granule exocytosis. J Immunol 154:6122, 1995

3. Boxer LA, Hedley-White ET, Stossel TP: Neutrophil actin dysfunction and abnormal neutrophil behavior. N Engl J Med 291:1093, 1974

4. Cawley JJ, Hayhoe FGJ: The inclusions of the May-Hegglin anomaly and Döhle bodies of infection: An ultrastructural comparison. Br J Haematol 22:491, 1972

5. Cotelingam JD, Witebsky FG, Hsu SM et al: Malignant lymphoma in patients with the Wiskott Aldrich syndrome. Cancer Invest 3:515, 1985

6. Curnutte JT: Chronic granulomatous disease: The solving of a clinical riddle at the molecular level. Clin Immunol Immunopathol 67:52, 1993

7. Dinauer MC: Leukocyte function and non-malignant leukocyte disorders. Curr Opin Ped 5:80, 1992

8. Driscoll DA, Budarf ML, Emmanuel BS: A genetic etiology for DiGeorge syndrome: Consistent deletions and microdeletions of 22qll. Am J Hum Genet 50:924, 1993

9. Farrington M, Grosmaire LS, Nonyaama S et al: CD40 ligand expression is defective in a subset of patients with common variable immunodeficiency. Proc Natl Acad Sci USA 91(3):1099, 1994

10. Gatti RA, Berkel I, Boder E et al: Localization of an ataxia telangectasia gene to chromosome 11q22-23. Nature 336:577, 1988

11. George JN: Thrombocytopenia due to diminished or defective platelet function. In Williams WJ, Beutler E, Lichtman MA et al (eds): Hematology, 5th ed. New York, McGraw-Hill, 1995

12. Greinacher A, Meuller-Eckhardt C: Hereditary types of thrombocytopenia with giant platelets and inclusion bodies in the leukocytes. Blut 60:53, 1990

13. Katz Y, Wetsel RA, Schlesinger M et al: Compound heterozygous complement C3 deficiency. Immunology 84(1):5, 1995

14. Leung DYM, Geha RS: Clinical and immunologic aspects of the hyperimmunoglobulin E syndrome. Hematol Oncol Clin North Am 2:81, 1988

15. Lindenbaum C, Chatwani A, Dyerr R: Hyperimmunoglobulinemia E and pregnancy: A case report. Am J Obstet Gynecol 157:1273, 1987

16. Loeb H, Jonniaux G, Resibois A et al: Biochemical and ultrastructural studies in Hurler's syndrome. J Pediatr 73:860, 1968

17. Long RG, Lake BD, Pettit JE et al: Adult Niemann-Pick disease: Its relationship to the syndrome of the sea-blue histiocyte. Am J Med 62:627, 1977

18. McDunn S, Hartz W, Ts'Ao C et al: Coronary thrombosis in a patient with May-Hegglin anomaly. Am J Clin Path 95(5):715, 1991

19. Miller ME, Oski FA, Harris MB: Lazy leukocyte syndrome: A new disorder of neutrophil function. Lancet 1:665, 1971

20. Nielsen H, Valerius NH, Schaffalitzky OB: Selective defect of phagocyte responsiveness to N-f-Met-Leu-Phe in a familial syndrome of recurrent cold abscesses. J Infect Dis 153:1184, 1986

21. Parry M, Root RK, Metcalf JA et al: Myeloperoxidase deficiency: Prevalence and clinical significance. Ann Intern Med 95:293, 1981

22. Patrone F, Dallegri F, Rebora A et al: Lazy leukocyte syndrome. Blut 39:265, 1979

23. Rampini VS, Adank W: Hamatologische Befunde bei Patienten mit Gargoylismus und heterozygoten Gerntrgern. Helv Pediatr Acta 19:101, 1964

24. Rosen FS: Immunodeficiency diseases. In Williams WJ, Beutler E, Lichtman MA et al (eds): Hematology, 5th ed. New York, McGraw-Hill, 1995

25. Schaffer FM, Palermos J, Zhu ZB et al: Individuals with IgA deficiency and common variable immunoglobulinemia share polymorphisms of major histocompatibility complex class III. Proc Natl Acad Sci USA 91(3):1099, 1994

26. Schopfer K, Baerlocher K, Price P et al: Staphylococcal IgE antibodies, hyperimmunoglobulinemia E, and *Staphylococcus aureus* infections. N Engl J Med 300:835, 1979

27. Strigaris K, Kokkinis K, Liberopoulos S et al: Liver lesion on CT and ultrasonography in adult Niemann-Pick disease related to sea-blue histiocyte syndrome—A case report. Hepato-Gastroenterol 40:240, 1993

28. Whitehead TP, Kricka LJ, Carter TJN et al: Analytical luminescence: Its potential in the clinical laboratory. Clin Chem 25:1521, 1979

29. Wolff SM, Dale DC, Clark RA et al: The Chédiak-Higashi syndrome: Studies of host defenses. Ann Intern Med 76:293, 1972

PART VI

Special Hematologic Evaluations

CHAPTER 27

Preparation and Evaluation of Bone Marrow

Karen G. Lofsness
Ella M. Spanjers

Collection of Marrow Specimens

Processing of Specimens
Aspirate
Clotted Specimens
Material for Sectioning

Staining of Specimens
Routine Staining
Evaluation of Stain Quality
Special Stains
Staining Sectioned
  Material

Normal Marrow Cells
Macrophages

Mast Cells
Osteoblasts
Osteoclasts

Evaluation of Marrow Preparations
Cellularity and
  Composition of Sections
Low-Power Scan of Films
  and Imprints

Marrow Differential

Preparation of the Final Report

6. Given a well-prepared H&E-stained trephine section at a magnification of 100×, recognize normocellular, hypercellular, and hypocellular marrow.
7. Summarize the procedure for performing a bone marrow differential. Given the results of a marrow differential in percentages, calculate the M:E ratio.

The collection, processing, and examination of bone marrow is one of the more complex procedures done in the clinical laboratory and one of the most difficult to perform properly. It is a technique that requires a great deal of skill and expertise, and it is not learned quickly. In order to obtain the maximum amount of information from the bone marrow sample, all steps must be executed carefully, from beginning to end.

The basic procedure described in this chapter is one that has been used effectively by our laboratory for many years.[21] It has been modified and updated as better equipment has become available and the demand for new diagnostic tests has multiplied. Figure 27-1 illustrates, in flowchart format, our protocol for collecting, processing, and evaluating bone marrow samples. The portions of the procedure that are primarily the responsibility of the hematology laboratory are described in detail here.

Approximately 1800 bone marrow collections are performed by our laboratory each year. For almost all patients, the site of choice is the posterior iliac crest. Both a trephine biopsy and aspirated marrow are obtained in nearly all cases. There are probably as many methods of processing bone marrow specimens as there are laboratories collecting them. The procedure described in this

Objectives

1. Briefly explain the process of collecting a bone marrow specimen.
2. Differentiate between a bone marrow aspirate and a trephine biopsy.
3. Describe the four layers observed in a normal bone marrow specimen after centrifugation.
4. Discuss the source, preparation, and purpose of each of the following bone marrow specimens: direct film, concentrated film, "crush" preparation, particle section, trephine section, and imprint.
5. Given a well-prepared Wright-Giemsa–stained bone marrow aspirate film at a magnification of 1000×, recognize the following cells: macrophage, mast cell, osteoblast, and osteoclast.

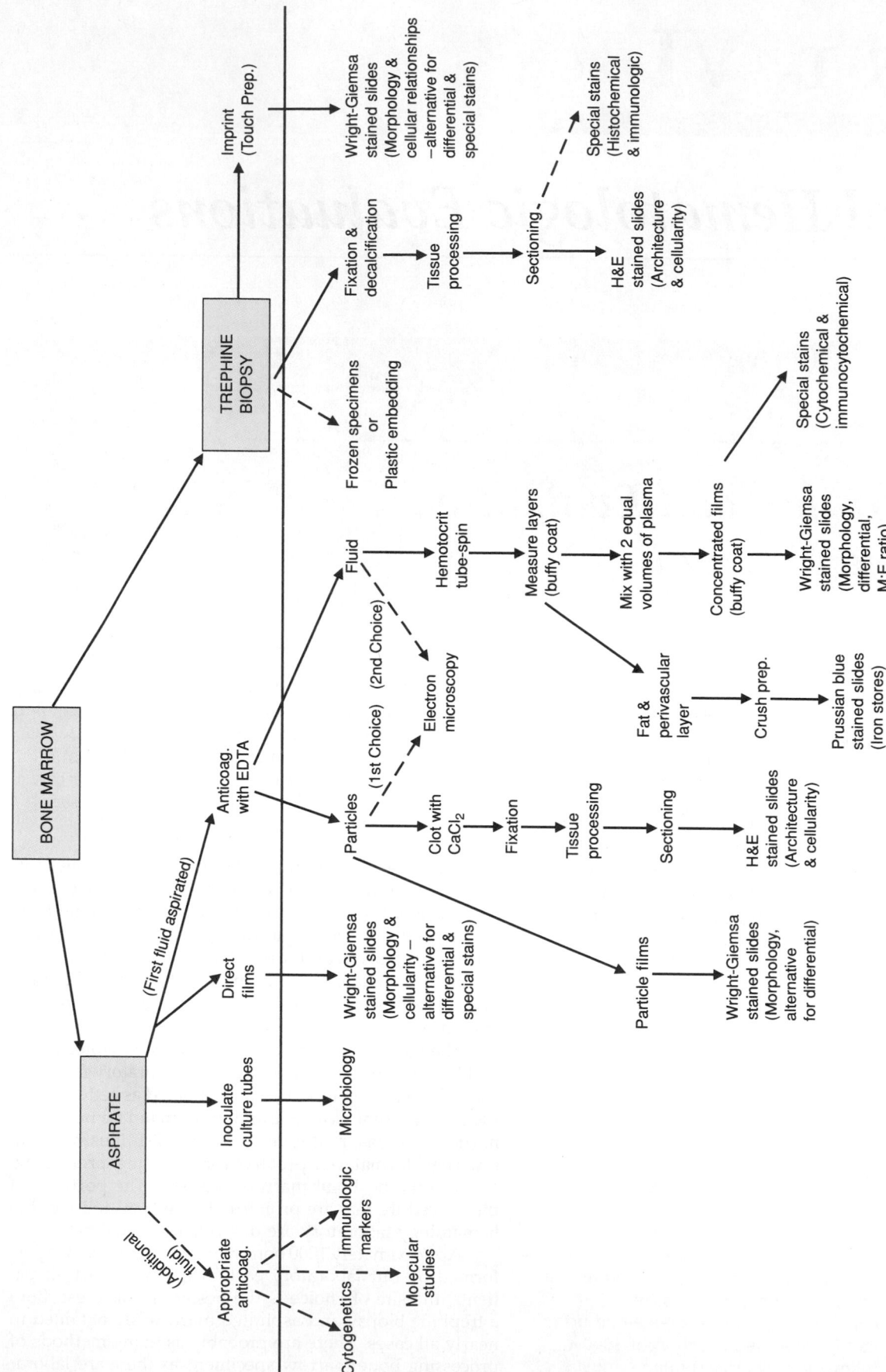

FIGURE 27-1. Flowchart of protocol described in this chapter for collecting, processing, and evaluating bone marrow samples. Procedures above solid horizontal line take place at bedside; those below line are performed in laboratory. *Solid arrows* = routinely performed procedures; *broken arrows* = optional tests.

chapter is recommended because it is flexible, there is a high yield of acceptable marrow samples, and almost every portion of the marrow obtained is utilized in some way. The various preparations complement each other and, when interpreted correctly, provide a great deal of information about the hematologic status of the patient.[5]

COLLECTION OF MARROW SPECIMENS

A medical technologist or medical laboratory assistant trained in preparing bone marrow specimens assists the person performing the bone marrow procedure. The assistant often has to act as a supportive influence, depending on the reaction of the patient to the procedure. Although a physician has usually described the test to the patient and obtained permission to perform it, the assistant may have to review the technique briefly. While assisting in the technical part of the bone marrow procedure and preparing the specimens, the assistant must be alert for any problems that might arise concerning the patient.

Necessary Supplies

Before the procedure is started, the assistant should clear a working area and have all supplies readily at hand. Disposable sterile bone marrow trays are commercially available, but additional supplies usually are necessary for obtaining the extra specimens that have become a part of the routine procedure in many hospitals and clinics. Trays designed by the laboratory can be set up and sterilized by the central supply area, and some of the supplies can be washed, resterilized, and reused. The following equipment is recommended for inclusion in this tray:

Aspiration needle (*e.g.*, University of Illinois sternal needle)
Trephine biopsy needle (*e.g.*, Jamshidi needle) (*Note:* Disposable needles are now recommended for all patients, and they cannot be sterilized with the tray. They may be distributed as a separate item with the tray.)
Two or more 30- to 35-mL syringes (glass or plastic) for aspiration
One small syringe (and accompanying needles) for local anesthetic
Sponges, forceps, medicine cups (for cleaning the area)
Towels for drapes
Gauze squares (4 × 4 inch)
Lancet (for small incision)
Sterile gloves, solutions for cleaning the area, a local anesthetic, and tape for a pressure bandage can be obtained separately.

The supplies necessary for the bone marrow preparation by the assistant at the bedside can be carried in an inexpensive plastic carrying tray:

Alcohol swabs
Lancets (for capillary puncture)
Surgical blades (size 22)
2 × 2-inch gauze squares
Glass slides
Spreader device
Small battery-operated fan
Vials (17 × 80 mm) containing anticoagulant (EDTA) or commercially prepared EDTA tubes
Vials of freshly prepared fixative. (*Note:* Due to environmental concerns, fixatives that contain zinc chloride, rather than mercury, should now be used.)
Marking pencil

Additional supplies may include extra 30- to 35-mL syringes, extra aspiration and biopsy needles, heparin, saline, and various microbiologic culture tubes.

BLOOD FILMS

Whenever possible, capillary puncture blood films should be prepared before the bone marrow is obtained, because stress to the patient can alter peripheral counts. A spreader device, such as that illustrated in Figure 27-2, should be used for all films. Twelve to fifteen blood films are made to ensure sufficient material for special stains as well as Wright-Giemsa staining. Ideally, anticoagulated blood is avoided for studying morphology because of the resulting changes in cell structure. Exceptions may be made in cases in which a capillary puncture could be harmful to the patient.

All films should be dried as quickly as possible to avoid drying artifact. A small fan may be used to dry films prepared at the bedside. This will enable the assistant to continue more quickly with the other steps of the procedure. For safety reasons, ''waving'' the slides to dry them is no longer recommended.

An alternative method for preparing films of blood and bone marrow is the coverslip technique. It provides even cellular distribution but requires more training to produce acceptable specimens. Coverslips are difficult to handle and process for both routine and special staining. Descriptions of the coverslip technique can be found in several references,[10,12,23] and it is described in Chapter 3.

TREPHINE BIOPSY

The trephine biopsy is a solid core of bone and marrow tissue obtained using a specialized needle with a cutting edge. This biopsy should be obtained before the aspiration to avoid any disruption of marrow architecture at the site.[5] The trephine specimen is placed on gauze (which helps absorb excess blood), and immediately imprinted by touching the slide to the specimen. This avoids damaging the specimen with forceps and lessens the possibility of contamination. Several imprints from the same specimen should be made on at least two slides.

Bilateral trephine biopsies are frequently performed (on both the left and right posterior iliac crests), and more than one biopsy may be obtained from the same side. Each specimen should be imprinted separately and the slides labeled so that imprints from the same bone can be identified. This is important for counting purposes, special stains, and estimating cellularity. Occasionally, imprints are the only material available for morphologic and cytochemical study.

After imprinting, the biopsies are put into vials of fixative. The biopsies from the right side should be fixed and processed separately from those from the left side, although all specimens from the same side can be processed together.

ASPIRATION

The aspiration of bone marrow follows immediately after the biopsy and usually is done on only one side. A 30- to 35-mL syringe is used to aspirate 1 to 3 mL of marrow. After the aspiration, the syringe should be kept horizontal with back pressure to avoid accidentally expressing the specimen until it is transferred to the vial described in the next paragraph. Speed in working with the aspirate is important, because the presence of megakaryocytes and the release of thromboplastin from tissue damage result in a shortened clotting time.

The aspirate is immediately transferred to a 2-dram (10 mL) glass vial containing powdered disodium EDTA (1 mg/mL of marrow) and mixed gently. The inside surface of the vial should be such that megakaryocytes and platelets do not adhere to it (*e.g.*, plastic). The amount of EDTA can be estimated after an

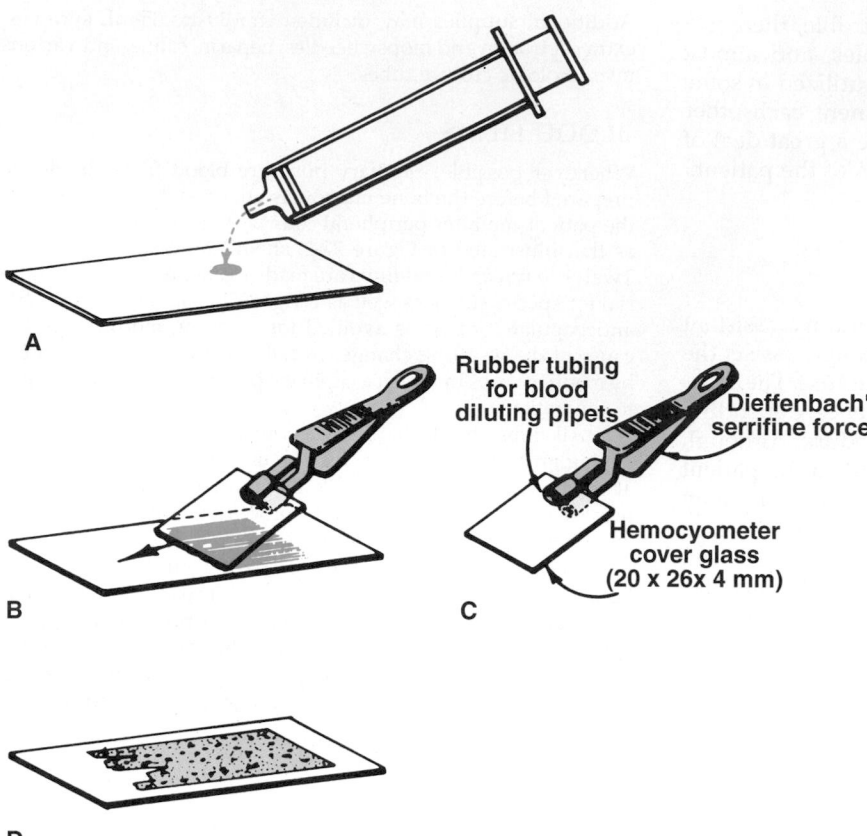

FIGURE 27-2. Spreading technique used to prepare peripheral blood films and for direct and buffy coat preparations of marrow. Spreader device (**C**) consists of hemocytometer coverglass held by clamp forceps (Dieffenbach's serrefine) with rubber tubing on ends to lessen coverglass breakage. Small drop of blood or marrow is expressed onto clean glass slide (**A**). Marrow is quickly spread (**B**) and dried immediately. This technique produces thin, uniform film slightly narrower than the slide (**D**). (From Brynes RK, McKenna RW, Sundberg RD: Bone marrow aspiration and trephine biopsy: An approach to a thorough study. Am J Clin Pathol 70:753–759, 1978, with permission.)

initial weighing to visualize 1 mg. The amount used can vary somewhat without causing significant morphologic changes or clotting of the specimen. Preparing two vials, one for less than 1 mL of bone marrow and one for up to 3 mL, will help prevent problems. Commercially prepared dry disodium EDTA tubes can be used, but the smaller diameter of these tubes makes it more difficult to transfer the marrow. The larger vial surface area also provides faster and more thorough mixing with the anticoagulant and results in inhibition of specimen clotting. Because the trephine biopsy is performed first, disruption of the area may initiate coagulation and cause clotting of the aspirate, even with speed and correct technique.

DIRECT FILMS

The small amount of marrow remaining in the syringe is sufficient for making direct films at the bedside. A drop of the marrow is expressed onto each of five or six slides and then distributed with a spreader device (see Fig. 27-2). If one large drop can be expressed onto a slide, the spreader can be dipped into the drop and then spread across individual slides. If the amount of marrow aspirated is insufficient for an anticoagulated specimen, as many films as possible should be made from the marrow in the syringe. This will provide slides for special stains, as well as Wright-Giemsa staining.

Occasionally, when a "dry tap" (the inability to aspirate marrow into the syringe) occurs, a small amount of marrow may be present in the aspiration needle. This marrow can be obtained for direct films if the top opening of the needle is covered with a gloved index finger while it is being removed from the patient and a stylet is pushed into the needle as it is held over a slide.

If fluid cannot be aspirated for an anticoagulated specimen or for direct films, small pieces of an unfixed trephine specimen

(after imprinting) can be cut off with a surgical blade and the freshly cut surface imprinted on a slide. One or more of these cut pieces also can be crushed between two slides. The slides are pulled apart while in a parallel position while applying gentle pressure. These preparations often provide representative material for morphologic interpretation when the trephine biopsy does not imprint well, in addition to providing extra material for special stains. This procedure is done in the laboratory, and the specimen should be taken there on a gauze square slightly moistened with saline.

SPECIAL PROCEDURES

Trephine biopsies for special preparations such as frozen sections, plastic embedding, or electron microscopy are usually obtained by cutting off, with a surgical blade, a representative piece of the biopsy after it has been imprinted. Biopsies for immunophenotyping must not come in contact with saline, and a separate piece should be cut off and put on dry gauze. The remaining portion of the specimen is immediately transferred to freshly prepared fixative at the bedside, and the special preparation is taken to the laboratory on saline-moistened gauze for processing according to the procedure(s) requested.

Electron microscopy preparations are most satisfactory when made from particles of marrow. However, the buffy coat is more often available, and a technique has been described for processing it from a portion of the marrow aspirated for morphologic study.[15] Trephine specimens processed for electron microscopy are acceptable but are more difficult to section.

Bone marrow aspirates for special laboratory procedures are obtained *after* the specimen for morphologic study, because subsequent aspirations usually are more diluted with sinusoidal blood. The specimens for cytogenetic or immunologic studies are aspirated into individual 30- to 35-mL syringes that have been heparinized at the bedside with 0.5 mL of heparin (1000 USP U/mL) per 3 mL of marrow and capped to prevent loss of the fluid. Specimens for molecular studies are collected in commercially prepared evacuated ACD (acid citrate dextrose) tubes. Specimens for culture are drawn in a separate sterile syringe and transferred under aseptic conditions to the appropriate culture tubes.

SAFETY PRECAUTIONS

All blood and bone marrow specimens should be considered potentially infectious and are to be handled using universal blood and body fluid precautions.[6] Gloves should always be worn when collecting or handling blood or bone marrow samples. Persons collecting bone marrow may wish to use additional barrier precautions, which include wearing a gown and mask as well as the gloves.

If a disposable tray has not been used, the entire marrow tray should be sterilized before being cleaned for reuse. Disposable trephine and aspiration needles are recommended for all patients. Any nondisposable laboratory supplies that have been exposed to blood or bone marrow during collection or processing of the specimen should be soaked for at least 1 hour in a solution of 1% sodium hypochlorite (bleach) or another recommended disinfectant before cleaning.

The further processing of blood and bone marrow specimens in the hematology laboratory should also be carried out using universal blood and body substance precautions. Gloves must be worn, and working behind a clear protective shield is recommended. Although a small fan may be used to dry films prepared in an individual patient's room, blood or bone marrow films prepared in the open laboratory area should not be dried with electric fans or by waving the slides in the air. In the laboratory, satisfactory drying of films can be accomplished by using a fan in a vented hood.

PROCESSING OF SPECIMENS

Aspirate

The bone marrow aspirate is a suspension of blood, fat, and solid units or particles of developing hematopoietic cells. The aspirate should be processed in the laboratory as soon as possible, preferably within 1 hour. Artifact caused by time delay will vary with different specimens.

The aspirate is gently mixed and poured into a disposable Petri dish. The fluid marrow is removed from around the particles with a 9-inch disposable Pasteur pipette and is transferred to one or more disposable Wintrobe hematocrit tubes. During this procedure, the fluid should be kept mixed by agitation with the tip of the Pasteur pipette to prevent uneven cellular distribution if more than one tube is filled. At the same time, gently tipping the Petri dish back and forth will aid in mixing and help to flow the fluid away from the particles, because it is important to retain them for films and section material. Even though particles are not always obtained in sufficient numbers for sectioning, films should still be made from any particles present.

Particle preparations are made by gently squashing a particle between two slides and then pulling the slides apart while in a parallel position. Several particle films should be prepared. After the excess fluid is removed from the remaining particles, they are aggregated and clotted together by gently adding drops of 0.015 M $CaCl_2$ around the outside of the aggregate to prevent dispersing the particles. When they can be collected as a clot with a dissecting needle, the particles are transferred to freshly prepared fixative. Occasionally no solid clot is obtained, and the

particles are then aspirated into a Pasteur pipette and expressed gently into the fixative.

The Wintrobe tube containing the fluid specimen of marrow is covered and centrifuged for 8 to 10 minutes at 850 × g (approximately 2800 rpm) in a tabletop centrifuge with a horizontal head. Normally, four main layers are present after centrifugation (see Fig. 27-8A). Reading from top to bottom, the layers and their reference ranges[5] are:

	Iliac	Sternum
Fat and perivascular cells	1%–3%	1%–3%
Plasma	No reference range	
Buffy coat (myeloid and erythroid nucleated cells)	3%–5%	5%–8%
Erythrocytes	No reference range	

The plasma and erythrocyte layers have no expected range, because they can vary widely depending on the amount of marrow dilution with sinusoidal blood. The total amount of fluid aspirated can be estimated from the Wintrobe tubes, because they hold approximately 1 mL. If less than 1 mL but more than 0.3 mL of marrow is present in the tube, the layer percentages can be calculated quite accurately.

Particles present in the centrifuged marrow will be found in either the fat layer or the buffy coat layer, depending on whether fat is present in the specimen. Usually, the presence of particles will not alter the volume of the layers significantly. Particles may also appear as a separate layer directly below the fat and then can be recorded independently.

The fat and perivascular layer is distinct and can be measured easily. However, the buffy coat may show several layers, and care must be taken to include the entire layer of nucleated cells. Erythroblasts usually layer just above the erythrocytes, and their respective colors may differ only slightly.

With a clean Pasteur pipette, "crush" preparations are made from the fat and perivascular layer using the method described for particle preparations. This layer is rich in macrophages and is used to demonstrate storage iron in the marrow by staining with the Prussian blue reaction. The more perivascular material present, the greater the reliability of the storage iron estimation.

The excess plasma is removed, leaving a volume equal to more than one but less than two times the buffy coat layer. Using a clean pipette (to avoid contamination with fat), the remaining plasma and the buffy coat layer are transferred to a paraffin-lined 10 × 35-mm disposable tissue culture dish or watchglass to make the concentrated preparations. The fluid is gently and thoroughly mixed with a glass stirring rod or the cleaned end of a Wintrobe tube and remixed after every four to five slides to prevent uneven distribution of cells. To ensure sufficient material for special stains, 20 to 25 films are prepared using the spreader device shown in Figure 27-2. If the buffy coat layer is small and more than one Wintrobe tube is available from the same aspirate, the buffy coat layers can be combined to obtain more preparations.

Clotted Specimens

Bone marrow aspirates containing fibrinous material or small clots are processed using the previously described techniques, but an attempt is made to avoid this material in the fluid to be centrifuged. Some of the megakaryocytes may be lost, but the other cellular distribution remains fairly reliable. If particles are not available, the clots should be processed for sectioning.

Solidly clotted marrow specimens or those containing large clots can be processed to obtain preparations for morphologic study and special stains, although the cellular distribution is unreliable. The clot is mashed to obtain fluid for centrifuging and processing by using a flat surface or cutting through it repeatedly with a Pasteur pipette. Particles are sometimes released with this procedure, and they can be spread and processed as described previously. If no particles are available, pieces of the clot should be processed for sectioning. Clotting of the specimen should be noted in the final report.

Material for Sectioning

Trephine biopsies and particle aggregates are processed for sectioning either mechanically or by hand. The biopsies and particles are prepared similarly, with the exception that trephine specimens must first be decalcified.

The paraffin block is sectioned at 3 μm, and cut at least half way through the specimen or until only a small amount of tissue is retained in the block. Serial sections from various areas of the ribboned material are mounted on albumin-coated slides and labeled separately, so that any specified area can be remounted if special stains are indicated.

The paraffin ribbons should be stored for a time to ensure they are available until all special stain requests have been completed. Special studies are often done in retrospect, and sections stored for 6 months or longer can still be mounted satisfactorily.

STAINING OF SPECIMENS

Routine Staining

All films should be well dried before they are stained; drying fixes the cells and helps prevent poor staining. A Romanowsky stain containing both Wright and Giemsa stains is preferred, because Giemsa increases the staining intensity of the azurophilic granules. However, an excess of Giemsa stain can cause difficulty in distinguishing between the neutrophilic and monocytic series because of the amount and intensity of reddish granulation produced.

Slides from each type of bone marrow preparation are stained for morphologic study. If sufficient material is available, it is recommended that the following be stained with Wright-Giemsa stain:

Three peripheral blood films (preferably capillary puncture specimens)
Two direct marrow films
Four or five buffy coat preparations
One particle preparation
One trephine imprint (from each biopsy)

One buffy coat film of marrow is also stained for iron to check for the presence of sideroblasts.[7] The crush preparation of the fat and perivascular layer is stained for storage iron by a Prussian blue method; if this specimen is not available, the buffy coat preparation should be examined for iron-containing macrophages.

Evaluation of Stain Quality

The quality of the Wright-Giemsa stain should be assessed microscopically under oil by noting both the color and the contrast of cellular structures. Examination of the granulation in leukocytes is particularly important. Even the smaller granules, such as those in the neutrophil precursors, monocytes, and platelets, should appear sharp and distinct.

If the stain is not dark enough or the contrast in colors is not well defined, the slide usually can be improved by restaining. If the quality is still not acceptable, the staining solutions may

be old or contaminated. They should be checked before attempting to stain fresh material.

Precipitated stain interferes with evaluating cell morphology and is not acceptable. If precipitate is present, it can sometimes be dissolved by rinsing the slide quickly in absolute methanol and immediately washing with water.

Special Stains

If possible, unfixed slides from each type of preparation are retained for special stains. The various cytochemical and immunocytochemical stains require different fixation methods, and the reactions may be decreased or completely inhibited if the wrong fixative is used. For example, absolute methanol decreases or completely inhibits the myeloperoxidase reaction.

Some of the special staining reactions are preserved longer if the films are desiccated. Storing some of the preparations in a desiccator is recommended if the type of special stain needed is not immediately apparent.

The more commonly performed cytochemical stains (Chap. 29) for bone marrow films include periodic acid–Schiff (PAS), myeloperoxidase, Sudan black, chloroacetate esterase, nonspecific esterase, and tartrate-resistant acid phosphatase (TRAP). Immunocytochemical stains, such as TdT (terminal deoxynucleotidyl transferase), are becoming more popular as better procedures are developed and their diagnostic value becomes more apparent.

Staining Sectioned Material

Prior to staining, sections are fixed to the slides by heating in an oven at 58° to 62°C for 30 to 40 minutes and cooling to room temperature. Routine hydration of the sections is then carried out, and tissues fixed with solutions containing mercury are treated with an iodine and sodium thiosulfate solution to remove residual mercury.

The hematoxylin and eosin (H&E) stain is performed routinely on all sectioned material. Optimum staining times will vary depending on the fixative used and the type of specimen (trephine or particle section); there is even variation between specimens of the same type. Particle sections need less staining time than trephine specimens.

After staining with hematoxylin, individual sections should be examined microscopically to evaluate the intensity of the stain. Sections can be restained before continuing if they appear too light, or decolorized with a recommended acid solution if they appear too dark.

The sections are counterstained in an alcoholic eosin solution and after transfer to the first xylene solution are checked microscopically for color contrast. Excess eosin, which can mask cellular detail, is removed by reversing the staining steps back through the various concentrations of alcohol. If the eosin color appears too light, the procedure is reversed back to the eosin step, the sections restained, and then carried through the stages of alcohol to xylene.

The preparation stained with H&E should appear crisp, with prominent nuclear detail, reddish eosinophil granules, and pale pink megakaryocyte cytoplasm.

Iron stains should be done routinely on the particle sections only, because trephine biopsies lose some stainable iron in the decalcification process and cannot be used for an accurate estimation of storage iron. The enzyme stains are unsatisfactory on decalcified tissue, but other special stains such as PAS, reticulin, acid-fast, fungal, and many immunohistochemical stains can be done as requested, usually in specified areas of the sectioned material.

NORMAL MARROW CELLS

In addition to the developing hematopoietic cells described elsewhere in this text, several other cell types are present in normal marrow. Although macrophages, mast cells, osteoblasts, and osteoclasts are not seen frequently, it is important to be able to identify them because they may be confused with other cells, both normal and pathologic.

Macrophages

The most mature cell in the mononuclear phagocyte system is the macrophage or histiocyte (see Color Plate 27-1). Macrophages are the progeny of the blood monocytes and perform essential phagocytic and immunologic functions. They are widely dispersed throughout the tissues of the body, and their morphology differs somewhat with their location.

In the bone marrow, macrophages are relatively large cells, with a diameter as much as 30 μm or more. On film preparations (Fig. 27-3) they are spreading, irregularly shaped cells, and pseudopods are often seen. The nucleus is usually oval, indented, or elongated. The chromatin, which stains lilac to light reddish purple with Romanowsky stains, is spongy or reticular in pattern. One or more nucleoli are often visible. The abundant cytoplasm is usually light gray to blue, although it sometimes has a pinkish tinge. The azurophilic granules vary in both number and size. In addition to the granules, cytoplasmic vacuoles are often seen and may be prominent. Other evidence of phagocytosis, such as engulfed erythrocytes, leukocytes, platelets, microorganisms, pigments, or other debris, may be present.

Macrophages stain positively with nonspecific (alpha-naphthyl acetate or alpha-naphthyl butyrate) esterase. They show negative to weakly positive activity with myeloperoxidase and chloroacetate esterase. Prussian blue stains may be used to demonstrate the increased storage iron that accumulates in macrophages in such conditions as sideroblastic anemia, excessive blood transfusions, and the anemia of chronic disease.

Because they are larger cells, macrophages tend to be pulled to the sides and feather edges of film preparations and should be searched for there. In normal marrow, macrophages comprise less than 1% of the nucleated cells. Their numbers are increased in disorders characterized by rapid cellular turnover, such as the hemolytic anemias, idiopathic thrombocytopenic purpura, and solid tumors.[22] Morphologically abnormal macrophages are seen in storage disorders such as Gaucher disease, in which a specific enzyme deficiency causes the accumulation of partially degraded lipid material in the macrophages, resulting in the characteristic cells (see Fig. 26-3).[11,22]

Mast Cells

The origin of mast cells (also called tissue basophils) is uncertain, but they are widely distributed in the body. Tissue mast cells participate in inflammatory and hypersensitivity reactions, during which they release their granule contents outside the cell, causing localized edema and inactivation of toxic agents.[4]

On Romanowsky-stained bone marrow films, mast cells are from 12 to 25 μm in diameter (Fig. 27-4 and Color Plate 27-2). They are usually rounded or oval, although they occasionally appear elongated or spindle shaped. The nucleus is round or oval and centrally located. It stains a uniform medium purple, but its structure is usually obscured by the intense cytoplasmic granulation. The background cytoplasm is colorless to slightly pink, and it is packed with densely staining dark purple to blue-black uniform spherical granules. Mast cells often stain so darkly that they are not easily recognized, and they may be mistaken for artifacts or cellular debris.

Mast cell granules contain both histamine and heparin, and they stain metachromatically with toluidine blue. Mast cells also stain positively with chloroacetate esterase.

Although mast cells superficially resemble basophils and may even share an ancestor, they are not the same cells. Mast cells are usually larger than basophils, and the granulation is more intense. In contrast to the irregular size and shape of basophil granules, the granules of mast cells are uniform and spherical. Mast cell granules are not water soluble.[22] The granules of both cell types contain histamine and heparin, and both stain metachromatically. However, mast cell and basophil granules differ ultrastructurally and in other chemical constituents.

Mast cells are rarely seen in normal bone marrow. They may be increased in refractory anemias, chronic

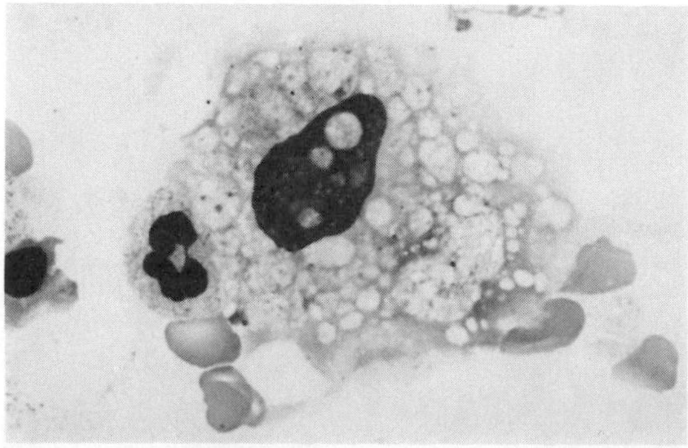

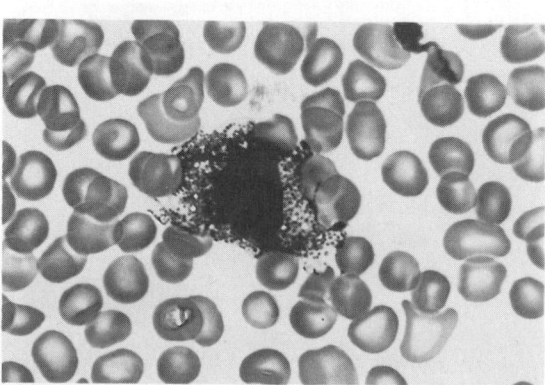

FIGURE 27-3. Macrophage. Abundant cytoplasm with prominent vacuoles, some of which overlie nucleus. (original magnification ×1000)

FIGURE 27-4. Mast cell. Nuclear structure obscured by dense, uniform granulation. (original magnification ×1000)

renal failure, some lymphoproliferative disorders (*e.g.*, Waldenström macroglobulinemia), and systemic mastocytosis (an accumulation of mast cells in the tissues).[22]

Osteoblasts

Osteoblasts are specialized cells that synthesize new bone matrix. Although they are seen occasionally on films of aspirated bone marrow, osteoblasts are actually related to the marrow stromal network and are not part of the hematopoietic system.[22]

On film preparations, osteoblasts appear as oval, elongated cells approximately 30 μm in length (Fig. 27-5 and Color Plate 27-3). The nucleus is round to oval, relatively small, and eccentrically located. It sometimes appears to be partially extruded from the cell, and the cytoplasm streams out behind the nucleus, giving the cell a "waterbug" or "comet" appearance. The chromatin is coarsely reticular, and one or more distinct nucleoli usually are seen. The basophilic cytoplasm is abundant, and the cytoplasmic border appears frayed or indistinct. There is often a rounded lighter-staining area (corresponding to the Golgi apparatus) within the cytoplasm at some distance from the nucleus. The texture of the cytoplasm is not smooth; it may have a grainy, fibrillar, or even slightly bubbly appearance. However, granules usually are not seen.

Morphologically, osteoblasts may be confused with plasma cells, as they both tend to have eccentric nuclei and basophilic cytoplasm (compare Color Plates 23-3 and 27-3). However, osteoblasts are larger than plasma cells, and the pale-staining area in the cytoplasm is separated from the nucleus. In plasma cells, this lighter area is perinuclear.

Osteoblasts often appear in clusters or aggregates and may be mistaken for tumor cells. They are seen occasionally in marrow films from infants and children but are rare in adult marrow except when active bone formation or repair is occurring, as in Paget disease, metastatic tumor, or at the site of a recent biopsy.[9]

Osteoclasts

Osteoclasts are large multinucleated cells that are involved in bone demineralization and resorption. It is

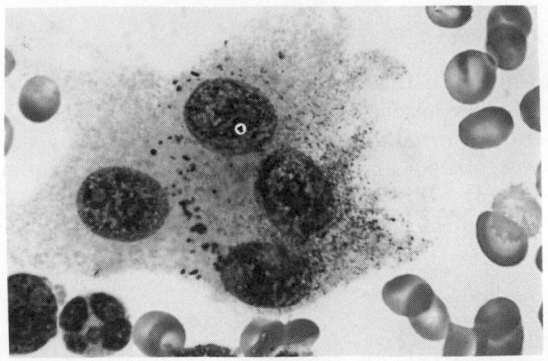

FIGURE 27-6. Osteoclast. Separate nuclei, granular cytoplasm with larger inclusions. (original magnification ×1000)

likely that they are formed from the fusion of circulating monocytes and macrophages.[22]

The most distinctive characteristic of osteoclasts on a bone marrow film is their impressive size, which can reach 100 μm or greater (Fig. 27-6 and Color Plates 27-4 and 27-5). These giant cells are irregularly shaped and have an indistinct ruffled cytoplasmic border. Osteoclasts contain a variable number of discrete nuclei, which are not connected to one another and may be scattered throughout the cell. The nuclei are round or oval and similar in size. They have a fine reticular chromatin pattern, and at least one prominent nucleolus usually is seen in each nucleus. The cytoplasm ranges from cloudy light blue to light pink. It is filled with azurophilic granules, which are irregular in both size and distribution within the cell. Larger purple-pink cytoplasmic inclusions are sometimes seen.

Because of their similar size and appearance, osteoclasts may be misidentified as megakaryocytes, and examination of the nuclear structure is the best way to distinguish them. In the osteoclast, each nucleus is separate; they are not attached to one another. Megakaryocyte nuclei are multilobulated; the segments are connected and may appear superimposed on one another (Fig. 27-7 and Color Plate 27-6). Nucleoli, if visible in megakaryocytes, are small and inconspicuous. In addition, cytoplasmic granulation in megakaryocytes is much more uniform.

Like osteoblasts, osteoclasts are more common in the marrow of infants and children and are rarely seen in

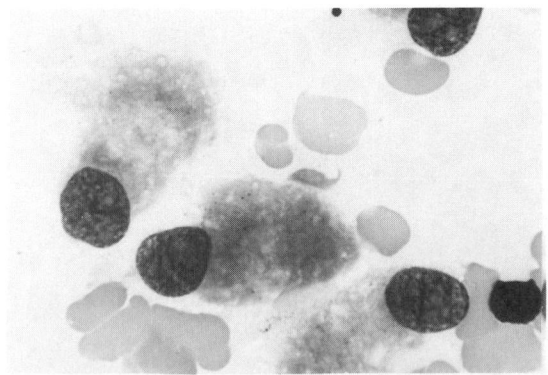

FIGURE 27-5. Osteoblasts. Nucleus partially extruded, with cytoplasm streaming behind. Lighter cytoplasmic area separated from nucleus. (original magnification ×1000)

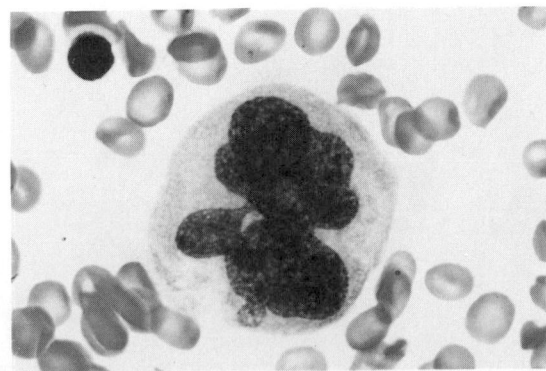

FIGURE 27-7. Megakaryocyte. Multilobulated nucleus, uniform cytoplasmic granulation. (original magnification ×1000)

normal adult marrow. Osteoclasts are increased when bone remodeling or destruction is taking place, as in osteolytic bone disease. They may also be found associated with metastatic tumors[23] or at the site of recent marrow biopsy.[9] Color Plates 27-7 and 27-8 are drawings of large cells found in bone marrow. Color Plates 27-9 through 27-13 show a variety of abnormal cells that may be confused with megakaryocytes.

EVALUATION OF MARROW PREPARATIONS

Prior to the microscopic examination of any bone marrow slides, the peripheral blood films obtained at the time of marrow collection should be evaluated. Erythrocyte, platelet, and leukocyte morphology are assessed, and except in cases of extreme leukopenia, a 300-cell differential (100 cells on each of three slides) should be performed.

Cellularity and Composition of Sections

Because of the time involved in processing bone marrow sections, blood and marrow films will have been examined by the time the sections have been processed and stained. For continuity in interpreting bone marrow preparations, the person examining the films should also evaluate the architecture, cellularity, and morphology of the stained section material.

The ratio of marrow fat to hematopoietic elements is normally about 1:2 in adults. Iliac marrow may be slightly less cellular than sternal marrow. The amount of marrow fat generally increases with the age of the patient.[22] Less fat is seen on films than on sections, because the aspirated marrow is somewhat diluted by sinusoidal blood. Al-

though some biopsies show areas of variable cellularity, the overall cellularity of the specimen should be judged as normal, increased, or decreased. The relative cellularity of typical normocellular, hypercellular, and hypocellular marrows, comparing the buffy coat layer, the trephine sections, and the direct films of each, are shown in Figures 27-8 through 27-10.

Using low-power magnification, each section on each slide is evaluated for the following: cellularity, cellular distribution (compare to film preparations), megakaryocytes, abnormal aggregates or infiltrates (*e.g.*, tumor nodules or granulomata), fibrosis (confirm with reticulin stain), and abnormal intracellular and extracellular material.

Some findings may need further examination under oil magnification. Special stains of specific areas may subsequently be requested.

Low-Power Scan of Films and Imprints

All bone marrow slides that have been Wright-Giemsa stained (direct, buffy coat, and particle preparations and trephine imprints) should first be examined under low power (100× to 200× total magnification). The entire slide is scanned for irregular cellular distribution and large or abnormal cells or aggregates. On film preparations, particular attention should be directed to the sides and feather edges, as larger cells and clusters of cells tend to accumulate there.

Although megakaryocyte numbers are best estimated from trephine sectioned material,[8] film preparations should also be examined, keeping in mind that any clotting will decrease the number of megakaryocytes. The feather edge of the concentrated (buffy coat) preparation is the best area in which to evaluate megakaryocyte num-

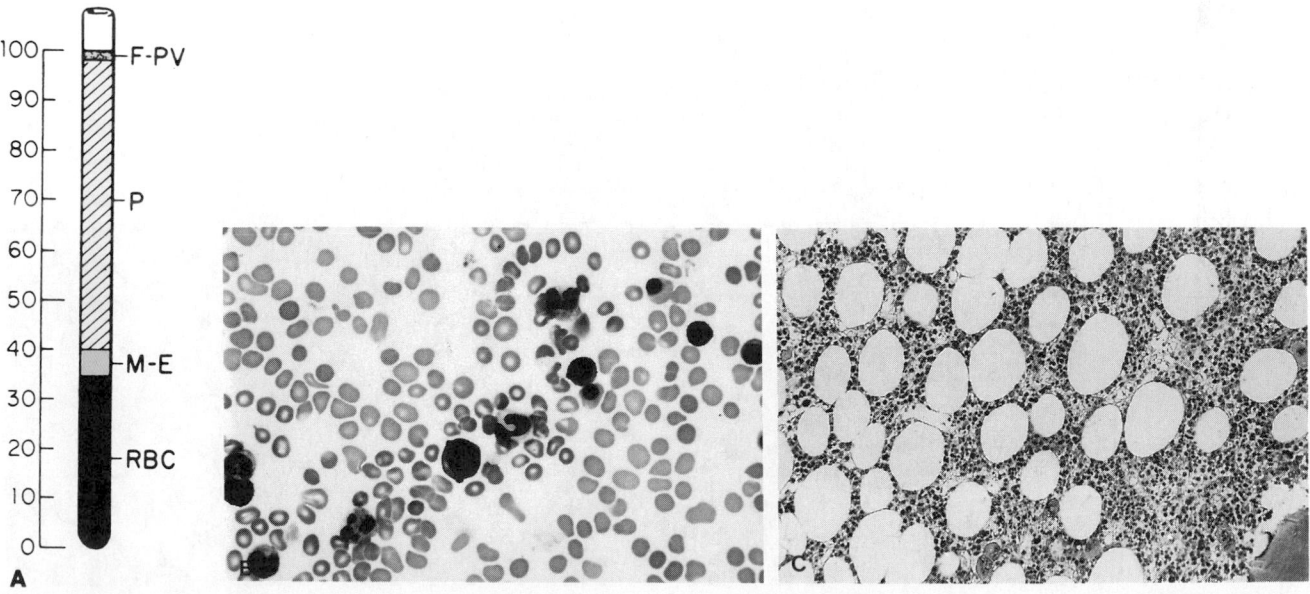

FIGURE 27-8. Normocellular bone marrow (marrow transplant donor). Wintrobe tube (**A**) shows normal fat and perivascular layer (2%) and normal myeloid–erythroid (buffy coat) layer (5%). Direct film (**B**) at 400× original magnification and trephine biopsy section (**C**) at 100× original magnification are both normocellular. (Part *A* from Brynes RK, McKenna RW, Sundberg RD: Bone marrow aspiration and trephine biopsy: An approach to a thorough study. Am J Clin Pathol 70:753–759, 1978, with permission.)

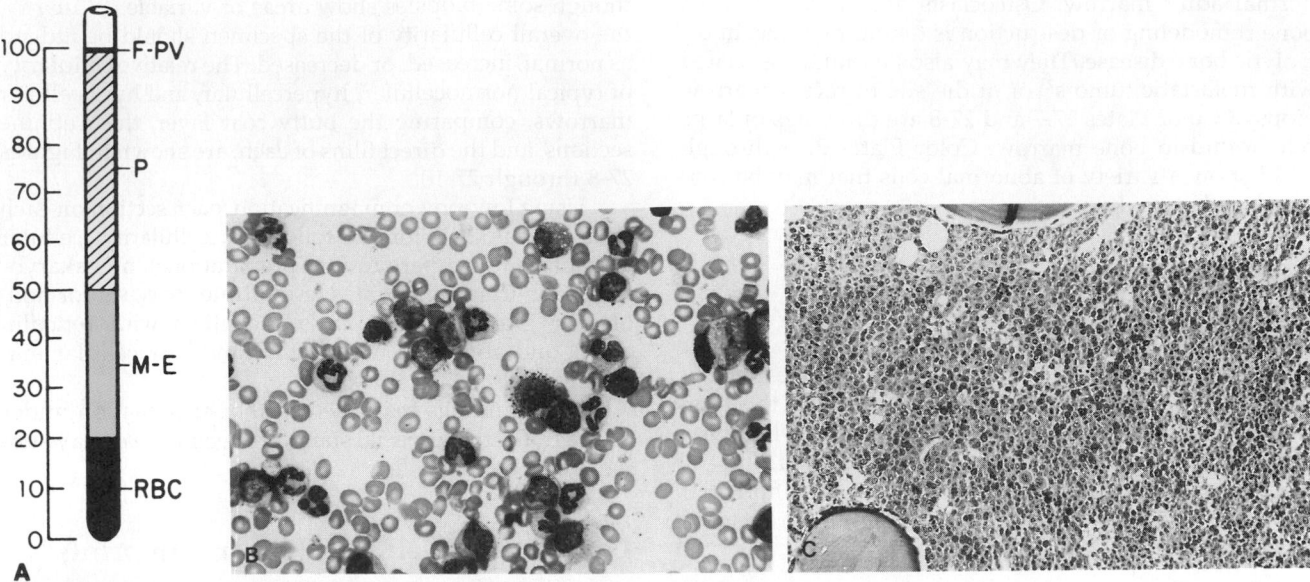

FIGURE 27-9. Hypercellular bone marrow (chronic myelogenous leukemia). Wintrobe tube (**A**) shows decreased fat and perivascular layer (trace) and markedly increased myeloid–erythroid (buffy coat) layer (30%). Direct film (**B**) at 400× and trephine biopsy section (**C**) at 100× are both markedly hypercellular. (Part *A* from Brynes RK, McKenna RW, Sundberg RD: Bone marrow aspiration and trephine biopsy: An approach to a thorough study. Am J Clin Pathol 70:753–759, 1978, with permission.)

bers and morphology. Normally, clumps of from 2 to 6 megakaryocytes should be seen frequently along the feather edge, as well as scattered individually throughout the slide. In cases of peripheral blood thrombocytopenia, megakaryocyte numbers and maturation should be evaluated thoroughly.

Other large or unexpected cells that may be detected during the low-power scan include macrophages, mast cells, osteoblasts, and osteoclasts. Higher-power magnification should be used to confirm any unusual findings.

Tumor cells usually, but not always, occur in clumps or sheets (see Color Plates 27-10 and 27-11) in the marrow and sometimes will not be present on every preparation. When metastatic tumor is suspected, the entire set of stained slides (from both the trephine biopsy and the

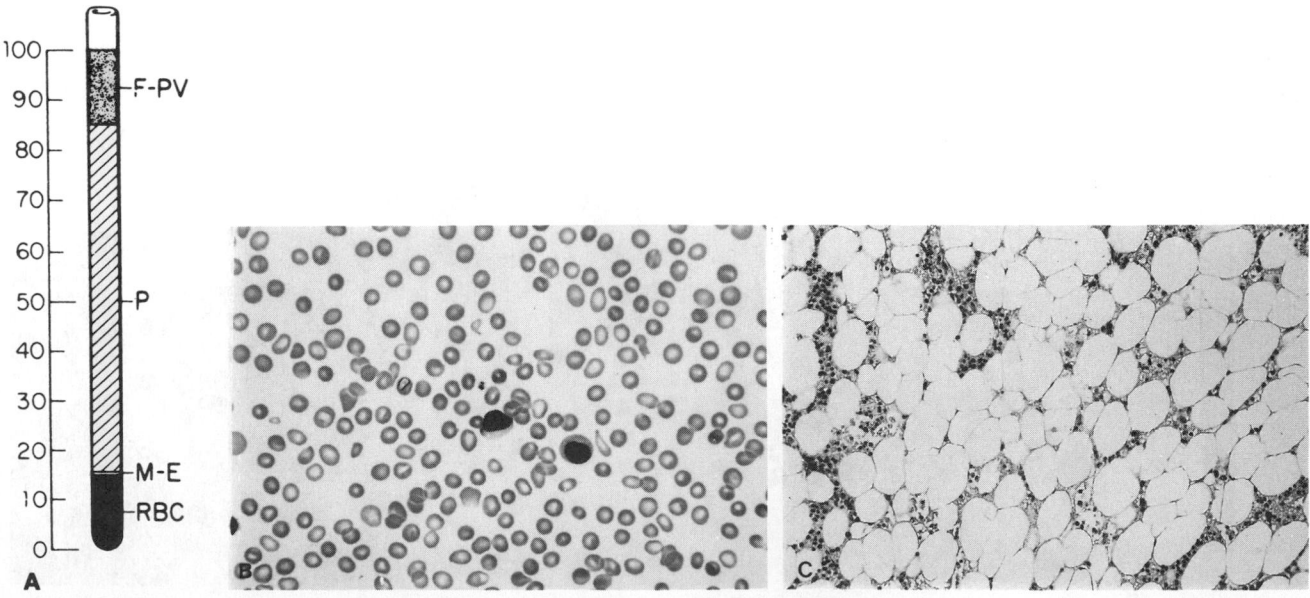

FIGURE 27-10. Hypocellular bone marrow (aplastic anemia). Wintrobe tube shows markedly increased fat and perivascular layer (15%) and decreased myeloid–erythroid (buffy coat) layer (trace). Direct film (**B**) at 400× and trephine biopsy section (**C**) at 100× are both markedly hypocellular. (Part *A* from Brynes RK, McKenna RW, Sundberg RD: Bone marrow aspiration and trephine biopsy: An approach to a thorough study. Am J Clin Pathol 70:753–759, 1978, with permission.)

aspirate) must be examined completely before the marrow can be reported as being negative for tumor cells.

The last step in the low-power scan is the selection of the best slides and the optimal area for the differential count.

MARROW DIFFERENTIAL

After the low-power microscopic examination is completed, the marrow differential is performed. The concentrated (buffy coat) specimen is preferable because it is a relatively uniform preparation, most of the fat and particles having been removed by centrifugation. A large number of randomly distributed cells can be examined rapidly,[5] which is particularly advantageous with hypocellular marrows. However, the direct film, particle preparation, or touch imprint of the trephine biopsy also can be used for the differential count. These preparations have the advantage of being unaltered by anticoagulant.

PROCEDURE

A thin well-stained area of the slide in which the cells are evenly distributed and cellular damage is minimal should be selected and the differential performed using an oil-immersion lens and 1000× total magnification. Consecutive fields are examined, and all cells are identified. In addition to tallying the cell types, any morphologic abnormalities such as variations in cell size or structure, nuclear or cytoplasmic inclusions, mitotic figures, abnormal lobulation, or multinucleation should be recorded.

Unlike the peripheral blood differential, which includes only leukocytes in the total percentage, it is customary to include all nucleated hematopoietic cells in a bone marrow differential. However, because they are large cells and are not evenly distributed on the slide, megakaryocytes and macrophages are often reported as appearing increased, decreased, or normal in number rather than being included in the differential total.

It is recommended that at least 500, and preferably 1000, cells be counted for a marrow differential. This is best accomplished by counting 500 cells on each of two slides, which not only lessens the variability attributable to uneven cellular distribution, but also allows the examiner more opportunity to discover morphologic abnormalities. In cases of extremely hypocellular marrow or if only direct films can be obtained, fewer cells can be counted. However, the practice of routinely counting only 100 or 200 cells for marrow differentials should be discouraged, because the statistical variability is too great for this method to provide valid results.[17]

REFERENCE RANGES

Although several "normal" marrow differential ranges can be found in the literature,[8,10,14,18,19,20,23] the variables involved in this procedure make it difficult to compare these studies or to adapt their data for use in one's own laboratory. The following factors can influence the determination of a reference range:

Number of subjects studied
Their age, sex, and state of health: Were they randomly selected and truly "normal"?
Method used to collect and process the marrow
Amount of dilution with sinusoidal blood
Type of specimen used for counting: direct, concentrate, particle smear, or imprint
Counting procedure used
Number of cells counted

Criteria used for cell identification and classification
Number of observers and their expertise

Because of these variables, each laboratory should establish its own reference range, if possible, or at least compare a published range with known normals before adapting it.

The values used for adult bone marrow differentials on concentrated preparations in the authors' laboratory are shown (as an example) in Table 27-1. These ranges have been modified over the years and are considered guidelines rather than absolute limits between normal and abnormal. Our routine method of classifying and recording marrow differentials diverges somewhat from that in most published studies. Instead of subdividing cell lines into individual stages of maturity (*i.e.*, neutrophil myelocyte, basophilic normoblast), we combine most cell lines and report them as a group (*i.e.*, eosinophils and precursors). We have found this method to be advantageous for several reasons: it is faster; there is less variation in cell classification among individual observers; and the report is easier to interpret. When a significant increase or decrease in any specific stage of maturation is seen, it is always noted in the morphologic report. Type I and type II myeloblasts and promyelocytes are tabulated separately, because their percentages are important in the diagnosis and classification of the acute leukemias and the myelodysplastic syndromes according to the French-American-British (FAB) criteria.[1-3]

Pediatric bone marrow differential ranges are subject to the same variables listed previously. Most studies agree that the expected values in children differ somewhat from those of adults. In one study of normal infants, it was found that the number of marrow lymphocytes increases during the first month of life, and they remain the predominant leukocyte in the bone marrow at least through the 18th month. There is a corresponding decrease in both the granulocyte and the erythroblast populations.[16] Some of the small "lymphocytes" seen in the marrow of infants appear quite immature, with a fine, smooth chromatin pattern and relatively little cytoplasm. These cells might well represent hematopoietic stem cells or progenitor cells (Color Plate 27-14).

MYELOID:ERYTHROID (M:E) RATIO

The relative proportions of the two principal bone marrow cell lines (myeloid and erythroid) can be expressed numerically as the M:E ratio. One method of determining this ratio compares the relative number of developing granulocytes (neutrophils,

---

TABLE 27-1
Guidelines for Adult Bone Marrow Differentials in Concentrated Smears, 1000-Cell Counts

Cell Type	Range (%)
Erythroblasts	18–24
Myeloblasts, type I	0–1
Myeloblasts, type II	0–2
Promyelocytes	1–4
Neutrophils and precursors	53–63
Monocytes and precursors	0–2
Eosinophils and precursors	1–3
Basophils and precursors	0–1
Lymphocytes	8–12
Plasma cells	0–2

eosinophils, and basophils) with the relative number of erythrocyte precursors. For example, the M:E ratio for the following differential would be 60% myeloid to 15% erythroid, or 4:1:

Neutrophils and precursors	50%
Eosinophils and precursors	8%
Basophils and precursors	2%
Lymphocytes	20%
Monocytes	5%
Erythroblasts	15%

The expected marrow M:E ratio in adults ranges from 2:1 to 4:1. It may be somewhat higher in infants.[9,23]

Some authors exclude eosinophils and basophils and include only the neutrophils and their precursors in the myeloid component of the M:E ratio,[23] whereas others prefer a "WBC to nucleated RBC" ratio, including the lymphocytes, monocytes, and plasma cells with the granulocytes.[8] Which cell lines to include and whether to express this ratio in reverse as an "E:M ratio" seems to be a matter of personal preference.

PREPARATION OF THE FINAL REPORT

The bone marrow report should describe all the significant findings, both positive and negative, in a concise and understandable format. The person preparing the final report should have examined all the different marrow preparations and reviewed the pertinent clinical information.

General information on the collection procedure, such as the anatomic site used, whether the biopsy was unilateral or bilateral, and whether any difficulty was encountered in obtaining marrow should be included. The approximate volume of marrow aspirated is recorded, along with the relative volumes (in percent) of the specific layers after centrifugation.

The differential report should state the preparation used for counting, the number of cells counted, and the relative percentages of each cell line, both normal and abnormal. Any irregularities in maturation or morphology are reported. The appearance of an abnormal or malignant population of cells, such as leukemic blasts, should be described in detail.

Megakaryocyte and macrophage numbers are reported as increased, decreased, or within normal limits. Any abnormal morphologic features in these cell lines should be described. If mast cells, osteoblasts, or osteoclasts are seen, their appearance should be noted.

The results (both positive and negative) of all routine and special staining procedures are reported.

The cellularity of the marrow, as evaluated on the trephine sections, is reported as normocellular, hypercellular, or hypocellular. Any abnormalities of marrow architecture should be described, including the presence of any focal lesions (e.g., tumor nodules or granulomas). An estimate of megakaryocyte numbers from the sections is recorded also.

The differential from the peripheral blood films taken at the time of marrow collection is included in the bone marrow report. Abnormalities of erythrocyte, platelet, and leukocyte morphology should be described.

The report concludes with a summary of the significant findings, integrating data from all marrow and blood preparations examined. On followup marrow studies, comments comparing previous reports should be included. By interpreting these bone marrow findings in light of known clinical information and the results of other laboratory tests, the examiner arrives at a final impression (which may include or exclude a definite diagnosis). Confirmatory tests may be suggested or helpful references cited.

The final bone marrow report is the means by which the results of this complex study are communicated to the clinician. A variety of sample report forms for recording bone marrow studies have been published,[8,14,19,20] and computerized systems have been described.[13,24] It is the responsibility of each laboratory to consider the needs of the institution it serves and devise a bone marrow evaluation and reporting system that will provide the greatest benefit to clinicians and patients.

CHAPTER SUMMARY

The preparation and evaluation of bone marrow is an extremely important laboratory test and yet is difficult to perform properly. This chapter describes a step-by-step procedure that generates several types of marrow preparations, including a direct marrow film, a buffy coat preparation of nucleated marrow cells, a "crush" preparation of fat and perivascular cells and sections that may consist of clotted marrow, concentrated marrow particles, or bone core specimens. The differences between marrow aspirate and trephine biopsies are discussed. Routine and special stains for marrow films as well as staining procedures for sectioned materials are described. Cells that are normally found in the marrow but not usually seen in peripheral blood films, including macrophages, mast cells, osteoblasts, and osteoclasts, are described. Finally, a method for evaluating marrow preparations is discussed, including evaluation of cellularity, bone marrow differential, and preparation of the final report.

Review Questions

27-1. All of the following bone marrow collection procedures take place at the patient's bedside EXCEPT

    A. imprinting trephine sections.
    B. preparing particle films.
    C. inoculating culture tubes.
    D. preparing direct films.

27-2. The bone marrow trephine biopsy is

    A. anticoagulated with EDTA.
    B. stained for iron.
    C. often obtained from both iliac crests.
    D. performed after the aspirate is collected.

27-3. After centrifugation of a normal bone marrow aspirate, the uppermost layer in the Wintrobe hematocrit tube consists of

    A. myeloid–erythroid cells.
    B. nucleated red blood cells.
    C. fat and perivascular cells.
    D. osteoblasts and osteoclasts.

27-4. The bone marrow specimen that is preferable for staining by the Prussian blue method to evaluate iron stores is the

A. "crush" preparation.
B. trephine biopsy section.
C. direct marrow film.
D. trephine biopsy imprint.

27-5. On a Wright-Giemsa–stained bone marrow aspirate film at 1000 × magnification, a cell that is 80μ in diameter with multiple separate nuclei, abundant granular cytoplasm, and large purple-pink inclusions is most likely a

A. macrophage.
B. mast cell.
C. osteoblast.
D. osteoclast.

27-6. An H&E-stained bone marrow trephine section that shows a significantly increased amount of fat would be described as

A. hypocellular.
B. normocellular.
C. hypercellular.
D. a poor specimen.

27-7. The results of a bone marrow differential are: 40% neutrophils and precursors; 20% lymphocytes; 20% monocytes; and 20% red cell precursors. The M:E ratio for this patient is

A. 1:2.
B. 2:1.
C. 3:1.
D. 4:1.

References

1. Bennett JM, Catovsky D, Daniel MT et al: Proposals for the classification of the acute leukaemias. Br J Haematol 33:451, 1976
2. Bennett JM, Catovsky D, Daniel MT et al: Proposals for the classification of the myelodysplastic syndromes. Br J Haematol 51:189, 1982
3. Bennett JM, Catovsky D, Daniel MT et al: Proposed revised criteria for the classification of acute myeloid leukemia. Ann Intern Med 92:620, 1985
4. Bessis M: Blood Smears Reinterpreted. Berlin, Springer-Verlag, 1976
5. Brynes RK, McKenna RW, Sundberg RD: Bone marrow aspiration and trephine biopsy: An approach to a thorough study. Am J Clin Pathol 70:753, 1978
6. Centers for Disease Control: Recommendations for prevention of HIV transmission in health care settings. MMWR 36(Suppl 2):1S, 1987
7. Dacie JV, Lewis SM: Practical Haematology, 4th ed. New York, Grune & Stratton, 1968
8. Diggs LW, Bell A: Bone marrow. In Schmidt RM (ed): CRC Handbook in Clinical Laboratory Science, vol 2, section 1. Boca Raton, FL, CRC Press, 1980
9. Henry JB: Clinical Diagnosis and Management by Laboratory Methods, 18th ed. Philadelphia, WB Saunders, 1991
10. Kass L: Bone Marrow Interpretation. Philadelphia, JB Lippincott, 1979
11. Kitchens CS: Clinical observations of human bone marrow macrophages. Medicine 56:503, 1977
12. Koepke JA: Examination of the bone marrow. In Koepke JA (ed): Laboratory Hematology. New York, Churchill Livingstone, 1984
13. Martin PJ, Johnson-Taylor R: A simple questionnaire for use in computerizing bone marrow aspirate reports. Med Lab Sci 41:295, 1984
14. Miale JB: Laboratory Medicine, 6th ed. St Louis, CV Mosby, 1982
15. Parkin JL, Brunning RD: Unusual configurations of endoplasmic reticulum in cells of acute promyelocytic leukemia. J Natl Cancer Inst 61:341, 1978
16. Rosse C, Kraemer MJ, Dillon TL et al: Bone marrow cell populations of normal infants: The predominance of lymphocytes. J Lab Clin Med 89:1225, 1977
17. Rumke CL: The statistically expected variability in differential leukocyte counting. In Koepke JA (ed): Differential Leukocyte Counting. Skokie, IL, College of American Pathologists, 1977
18. Rywlin AM: Histopathology of the Bone Marrow. Boston, Little, Brown & Co., 1976
19. Schleicher EM: Bone Marrow Morphology and Mechanics of Biopsy. Springfield, IL, Charles C Thomas, 1973
20. Silver RT: Morphology of the Blood and Marrow in Clinical Practice. New York, Grune & Stratton, 1981
21. Sundberg RD: Aspiration biopsy of bone marrow. Bull U Minn Hosp 21:471, 1950
22. Trubowitz S, Davis S: The Human Bone Marrow: Anatomy, Physiology, and Pathophysiology. Boca Raton, FL, CRC Press, 1982
23. Wintrobe MM, Lee GR, Boggs DR et al: Clinical Hematology, 8th ed. Philadelphia, Lea & Febiger, 1981
24. Youness E, Drewinko B: A computer-based reporting system for bone marrow evaluation. Am J Clin Pathol 69:333, 1978

CHAPTER 28

Hematopoietic Stem Cells for Transplantation

Lynne H. Lyons
Gary Van Zant

Objectives

1. Compare autografts and allografts with respect to definition and hematopoietic sources and list advantages and disadvantages for each.
2. Identify and explain the principle of at least three graft manipulations and state whether it is usually performed on bone marrow, peripheral blood or both.
3. List at least four laboratory assays that evaluate a graft. For each describe the principle and the specific information it provides.

Bone marrow or stem cell transplantation can be performed to replace genetically defective cells or to rescue a patient after attempting to eradicate a tumor using aggressive chemo- or radiotherapy, which also ablates the bone marrow including stem and progenitor cells as a side effect (Table 28-1). Bone marrow transplantation is a procedure that involves a graft of hematopoietic cells that is infused to repopulate a patient's marrow. The graft must contain pluripotent stem cells and hematopoietic progenitors that produce mature blood cells (Chap. 5). Until recently, bone marrow has been used exclusively as a source of these cells; however, peripheral blood cells from patients or normal donors who have been treated to mobilize their blood cell progenitors into the circulation are now being used increasingly. Grafts may be autologous (from the same individual) or from a carefully selected (allogeneic) donor.[1,2]

Before receiving the graft, the patient is conditioned with ablative high-dose chemotherapy or total body irradiation, or both, and in some cases the graft is manipulated before infusion to purge tumor cells or to select particular hematopoietic populations. During the recovery phase, as with the ablative phase, the patient is isolated for infection prophylaxis and requires continuous laboratory monitoring and blood component support. It is usually assumed that engraftment occurs when the absolute neutrophil count is higher than 0.5×10^9/L on three consecutive days. Marrow repopulation occurs in stages, with platelets usually being the slowest blood cell lineage to reach normal levels. The entire process usually takes 10 to 60 days depending on the patient's disease and often on the amount of prior chemotherapy received.

ALLOGENEIC TRANSPLANTATION OF MARROW

In searching for a donor, siblings then parents and close relatives are the first choice. If a donor cannot be identified in this pool, the National Marrow Donor Program can search its registry for a matched unrelated donor.

A potential donor's leukocytes are typed for human leukocyte antigens (HLA). Because these antigens regulate immune interaction, the laboratory must verify donor–recipient compatibility and identify the best possible match. A six-antigen match is the standard for a histocompatible donor, for whom the HLA-A, -B and -DR loci are identical on both chromosomes. Donor–recipient mismatches of these three antigens are principally responsible for causing graft-versus-host disease (GVHD). Most individuals are heterozygous, with two different alleles at each locus (*i.e.*, one from each parent), thus accounting for the six crucial antigens. Mononuclear cells from histocompatible donors are infused into an allogeneic recipient without further processing. The entire quantity of donor marrow collected, including erythrocytes, is usually given if there is no major or minor ABO incompatibility.[6]

If no histocompatible donor is found, a haploidentical relative with a five of six antigen match is considered. Successful transplantation diminishes with mismatched antigens, but a graft from a one-antigen mismatched sibling is usually better than a graft from a matched, unrelated donor because of the many mismatches in minor histocompatibility antigens that have a cumulative effect. A transplant center can rely exclusively on treating the ensuing GVHD or the graft can be depleted of T lymphocytes before infusion to minimize GVHD. There is an inverse relation between GVHD and graft rejection as long as the GVHD remains low grade (*i.e.*, a low-grade GVHD generally decreases the severity of graft rejection). Note, however, that depletion and not elimination is rec-

TABLE 28-1
Common Disorders for Transplantation

Malignant	Nonmalignant
Leukemias	Aplastic anemias
Multiple myeloma	Thalassemias
Lymphomas	Immunodeficiencies
Solid tumors	Metabolic anomalies

ommended because residual T lymphocytes are beneficial for the graft-versus-leukemia (GVL) effect described in the next section.[7]

AUTOLOGOUS TRANSPLANTATION

An autologous transplant is most feasible in solid tumor disease with no metastasis to the bone marrow. However, successful transplants are possible in hematopoietic malignancies, such as chronic myelogenous leukemia, if the patient can be harvested during a period when tumor cells with the Philadelphia chromosome are absent.[15] In other cases of bone marrow disease, there are techniques to purge the autologous graft of tumor cells before infusion.

Obtaining a graft by leukapheresis is the least invasive technique. The patient is treated with a chemotherapeutic drug, such as cyclophosphamide or granulocyte colony-stimulating factor (G-CSF), a cytokine that mobilizes stem and progenitor cells from marrow into the circulation.[10] The patient's peripheral blood mononuclear leukocytes which are enriched with stem cells can then be collected on successive days until the desired number of stem and progenitor cells which are Cluster of Differentiation (CD) 34$^+$ is obtained, usually in two to three leukaphereses. If the patient has been heavily pretreated or does not mobilize stem cells well, bone marrow may be harvested to maximize the yield.

A search for donors and extensive workups are avoided with autologous transplantation. The major advantages of an autologous graft include earlier engraftment and the absence of GVHD. On the other hand, GVHD is closely associated with the so-called graft-versus-leukemia/tumor (GVL) effect which provides an immunologic advantage against residual malignant cells that the body may harbor.[9] Without GVL benefit, the physician must rely more on the ablative therapy to eradicate all tumor cells.

GRAFT CRYOPRESERVATION

Autologous harvests of peripheral blood or bone marrow are cryopreserved (stored at very low temperatures) until transplant. Occasionally cryopreservation of an allogeneic graft is required when scheduling constraints exist between the donor's availability and the recipient's treatment regimen. The major objective of freezing the cells is to maintain cell viability until the graft is needed.

Osmotic changes that occur during the freezing process must be gradual enough to prevent the cells from losing too much water as the solute concentration of the suspending medium increases when ice crystals form. Therefore, cryoprotectants add a membrane permeable solute to help control both intracellular dehydration and the amount of external crystallization during the slow freezing process.[14]

There are two methods of freezing. The controlled-rate method uses a programmable, liquid nitrogen-cooled chamber to gradually reduce the temperature of the graft until heat of fusion (just prior to freezing), which is the critical transition phase during which injury from crystallization could occur. Thereafter, temperature reduction proceeds at a faster rate to near −80°C after which the cells are transferred to a liquid nitrogen freezer (−196°C) where good cell viability can be maintained for several years.

An alternative method is mechanical or "dump" freezing for which cells in cryoprotectant are placed in a −80°C freezer. The principle is essentially the same as the controlled-rate method in that the temperature of the cells falls to −80°C at a rate comparable with the former method. For longer storage these cells can be maintained in liquid nitrogen.

GRAFT ENGINEERING

Graft engineering is a part of the larger discipline of biomedical engineering and is a term that reflects the cellular manipulations carried out by a modern clinical laboratory in support of a bone marrow transplant program.[3] The cellular manipulations may be broken down into two main areas: manipulations for allogeneic transplants and those for autologous transplants. The needs for each are distinct.

Allogeneic Transplants

Even closely matched donor–recipient combinations carry a probability of the recipient developing GVHD, a life-threatening posttransplant complication. The probability of developing GVHD and the subsequent disease severity increases with the extent of HLA mismatch.[7] Because T lymphocytes in the graft are primarily, but probably not solely, responsible for causing GVHD, their removal is the main goal of engineering a proper allograft. T cells may be removed by two general methods—a negative cellular selection to selectively remove T cells (T-cell depletion), or a positive cellular selection for non-T cells (CD34 selection). Each gives a graft depleted of T cells, but is otherwise quite different.

T-CELL DEPLETION

Selective removal of T cells (negative selection) has been achieved by several methods, usually sharing a common immunologic theme, because the cell surface antigens (or surface markers) of these cells are well known.[12] Chief among them are CD3, CD5, CD4, CD8 and the T-cell receptors (TCR), TCRα/β and TCRδ/γ. Cytolytic T-cell–specific monoclonal antibodies and complement arguably offer the most direct means of T-cell removal. In practice, the success of the method is dependent on the antibody used and, predictably, the expertise of the technical personnel, usually clinical laboratory scientists. Typically, a 1.0- to 3.0-log depletion is achieved by this method, which means that between 10% and 0.1% of the T cells remain.

Other widely used immunologic-based methods include antibodies coupled to magnetic beads (immunomagnetic beads) that selectively confine the cells to which they are attached to a magnetic field, allowing the unlabeled, nonmagnetic, cells to be collected separately; and panning (as in panning for gold) where the antibodies are attached to the growth surface of a tissue culture dish or flask and the T cells remain adherent when the other cells are gently removed. In this use of the analogy, the "gold nuggets" (T cells) are discarded. The graft, after T-cell depletion by negative selection, largely resembles, both qualitatively and quantitatively, the graft before manipulation except for the depleted T-cell population. Morphologically identifiable precursor cells of the various blood cell lineages are still present, as are the blast cells and primitive progenitors.

CD34 SELECTION

Selection of cells positive for the CD34 antigen enriches the stem and progenitor cells in a graft. This method excludes T cells that lack the CD34 cell surface antigen.[11] The product of this method is a graft consisting largely of stem and progenitor cells—the purity of which depends on how well the selection method is performed. A clean separation is important because the level of tumor cell depletion is directly related to stem cell purity. Morphologically, a CD34+-selected graft is composed largely of undifferentiated blast cells (see Color Plate 28-1).

Because harvest of an allograft from a donor can usually be scheduled to coincide with the completion of a patient's ablative therapy, the graft is typically infused immediately at completion of any manipulative procedures, including T-cell depletion. Thus the graft usually need not be cryopreserved.

Complicating the subject of T-cell depletion is the issue of a GVL effect.[5] The chances of relapse are generally less with allografts than autografts and a major reason for this is the heightened immune surveillance that occurs in response to allogeneic cells. Presumably such an immune response is responsible for eliminating residual tumor cells in the patient. The GVL effect is introduced here because it is believed that T cells in the graft are at least partially responsible. Total T-cell depletion, although reducing the possibility of GVHD, may also eliminate the beneficial GVL effect. Thus T-cell depletion becomes a balance of desirable and undesirable outcomes. It is now generally believed that too stringent a T-cell depletion is undesirable, and sufficient T cells should remain in the allograft to stimulate a GVL effect while at the same time not causing high-grade GVHD. Alternatively, T cells may be given to the patient after transplant to stimulate a cellular immune response. The effectiveness of such post-transplant buffy coat infusions is being evaluated in clinical trials.

Autologous Transplants

Autografting has a separate set of problems, not the least of which is the significant possibility of harvesting tumor cells along with marrow or blood. Such cells may cause tumor relapse after the transplant. Therefore, the role of engineering an autograft takes the form of purging tumor cells from it after removal from the patient and before reinfusion.[8] The same strategies of negative or positive cellular selection described above may be used in purging. Negative selection (removal) of carcinogenic cells requires the exploitation of some unique property of the tumor cell as compared with normal hematopoietic cells. There are several possibilities, some quite specific and others not.

PURGING TUMOR CELLS

Among the more specific strategies is an immune-based approach using antibodies. For example, breast cancer cells are usually epithelial in origin, and thus antibodies directed against epithelial cells in general, although not specific for breast carcinoma, have efficacy in purging because epithelial cells are not normally found in marrow or blood. Removal of them by any of the immuno-based methods discussed in the preceding section applies here (i.e., cytolytic monoclonal antibodies, immunomagnetic methods, or panning). Tumors of other tissues may require a more specific approach because they may have overlapping sets of antigens with hematopoietic cells. A further complication is that tumor cells are by nature aberrant cells and may have an altered pattern of cell surface antigens—some that are appropriate for that tissue may be absent, or inappropriate ones may be expressed. It is impractical to raise new antibodies specific for every patient's cancer.

A less specific means of negative selection takes advantage of the fact that tumor cells tend to be rapidly dividing and, therefore, are subject to being killed by cell cycle-specific drugs, such as 4-hydroperoxycyclophosphamide (4-HC), the active form of cyclophosphamide.[8] Hematopoietic progenitors, but not most stem cells, are also rapidly dividing and are killed along with tumor cells when an autograft is purged using 4-HC. When the surviving, but partially depleted stem cell population is transplanted, slow engraftment times are common. Patients, therefore, are dependent on frequent platelet and red cell infusions and are subject to a prolonged period of neutropenia and danger of infection. Nonetheless, there is evidence showing that this type of pharmacologic purging, although toxic to many blood-forming cells in the graft, is more toxic to tumor cells and leads to a clinically important reduction of cells capable of causing relapse, while at the same time preserving enough stem cells to engraft. Several clinical studies are presently investigating ways to selectively make hematopoietic cells resistant to cycle-active cytotoxic drugs. These include (1) selectively and reversibly producing nonreplicating hematopoietic cells or (2) making them capable, through gene therapy, of pumping out the cytotoxic drugs before they can harm the hematopoietic cells.

As with T-cell depletion of an allograft, positive selection of CD34$^+$ cells results in depletion of contaminating tumor cells in the autograft. Because of the availability of several commercial CD34$^+$ cell selection devices for clinical studies, this method of purging is currently popular and has the added benefit of resulting in a significant volume reduction of the graft, thereby simplifying cryopreservation and storage.

Ex Vivo Numerical Expansion

Increasing the number of stem and progenitor cells in a graft after it has been removed from the donor is a technique that holds great promise (at least conceptually) for the processing laboratory and ultimately the patient.[4] It has several attractive possibilities that meet existing needs for the manipulation of both allografts and autografts. For the former, it offers the possibility of culturing cells in the presence of specific growth factors or pharmacologic agents to optimize the numbers and types of immune cells to foster a GVL effect, while at the same time minimizing the induction or severity of GVHD.

In the same context, blood cells harvested from the umbilical cords of newborn infants contain populations of stem cells with two unique attributes: (1) they are capable of extensive and prolonged proliferation in culture; and (2) they lack many of the HLA antigens characteristic of stem cells from adult marrow or blood. The latter attribute raises the possibility of creating a universal donor bank of stem cells from cord blood collections. A significant problem with this approach is that the number of cells obtained from an umbilicus is not sufficient to engraft an adult. However, their extensive capacity for proliferation raises the possibility of generating an adult-sized graft through expansion in culture. Early feasibility studies along these lines are underway at several research centers.

Numerical expansion of stem cells in autografts offers two significant advantages over current methods.[17] First, the size of the harvest, whether it be marrow or blood, need not be very large, thus minimizing the chances of collecting metastatic tumor cells. Recent studies have suggested that, with an expansion step, enough stem cells for engraftment could be generated from a 100- to 200-mL collection of blood from a cytokine-stem/progenitor-cell–mobilized adult patient. Standard procedures now require two to four leukaphereses in which two to five blood volumes are processed each session. Second, the usual 1- to 2-week culture period required for stem and progenitor cell expansion offers an opportunity to purge the graft. There is evidence that at least some leukemia cells do not survive under culture conditions in which normal stem and progenitor cells proliferate. In addition, active purging methods may be used in conjunction with the expansion step to augment any passive purging obtained in culture. For example, tumor-specific monoclonal antibodies, vaccines or cytolytic cells could be added during culture.

Last, expansion of the stem cells that have been spared after an *ex vivo* purge of tumor cells with a chemotherapeutic agent such as 4-HC may facilitate the regeneration of the stem cell compartment, thereby reducing the length of time required for engraftment and, consequently, the patient's susceptibility to infection and dependence on transfusions.

LABORATORY ASSESSMENT

The laboratory is responsible for characterizing the graft before and after manipulation, with checkpoints along the way. Such data provide quality control and quality assurance for the product infused into the patient.

There are several parameters that must be determined to characterize the quality of the graft. Total leukocyte and differential counts must be performed; viability measurements using dye exclusion to verify a healthy cell population; and sterility tests for bacterial and fungal microbes are done to avoid transmission of infection.

Phenotypic characterization of the cell surface antigen repertoire involves labeling a sample of the graft with fluorescent-labeled monoclonal antibodies and analyzing it with a fluorescence-activated cell sorter (FACS; Chap 43). This flow cytometric technique can categorize and quantitate cells of interest (*e.g.*, stem cells and T cells). FACS analysis before and after manipulation provides timely information of depletion or enrichment of particular cell populations.

A limiting dilution assay (LDA) functionally demonstrates T-cell depletion. As its name suggests, samples taken before and after depletion are serially diluted to produce two sets of cultures with decreasing cell numbers. Replicates of each dilution are cultured in multiwell plates and scored for growth. The cell dilutions at which replicate cultures foster growth and no growth provide information from which the frequency of T cells (or other progenitors) can be calculated by using Poisson statistics, and the log of depletion can be determined. Progenitor cell assays permit the growth of colony-forming unit–granulocyte, erythrocyte, monocyte, megakaryocyte (CFU-GEMM), CFU-GM (granulocyte, monocyte) and burst-forming unit–erythrocyte (BFU-E) colonies using a specialized media with defined cytokines (Chap. 5). These colonies are counted and their numbers used to measure the progenitors in the graft.[13] Both of these assays require culturing for 14 days before assessments can be made.

FUTURE DEVELOPMENT

This field is in its infancy and will undergo significant growth over the next several years. High-dose chemotherapy requiring stem cell support has become an important treatment for an increasing number of cancers and myelodysplastic disorders, and the list will continue to grow. The possibilities for innovative manipulation of hematopoietic grafts to customize them for specific transplant and disease settings are as diverse as our imaginations. In the allogeneic setting, new ways of depleting T cells responsible for GVHD, while at the same time fostering GVL, will be developed. Research will establish which immune cells are responsible for the two effects and readily available cell separation methods will soon follow to allow the engineering of grafts tailored to enhance GVL while preventing GVHD.

In the autologous setting, myriad purging methods will be developed—driven by the advent of new technology and specific needs. Advances in cell separation technologies will permit large-scale and rapid isolation of cell populations, either enriched for stem and progenitor cells or depleted of tumor cells. New technologies for the accurate and rapid determination of tumor cell contamination will make quality control of grafts much easier.

Automated bioreactors for the culture of marrow and blood will be available for use in the laboratory to produce custom grafts to fit specific needs. Unwanted cell populations may be depleted, whereas beneficial populations may be expanded through the selective application of growth factors, antibodies or nutrients during the culture period.

Lastly, culture methods will make possible the combination of genetic engineering with graft engineering. Genetically altered grafts will produce cures of certain genetic diseases; for example, some of the lysosomal storage diseases and the thalassemias. In addition, it may be possible to endow stem cells, through genetic engineering, with much greater resistance to chemotherapeutic drugs, thus permitting further escalation of doses to selectively kill cancer cells.

CHAPTER SUMMARY

Bone marrow, peripheral blood, and even umbilical cord blood grafts can rescue patients who have received ablative therapy for certain malignant and nonmalignant diseases. When transplanting a T-cell–depleted allogeneic graft, the risk of graft rejection must be weighed against the benefit of low-grade GVHD

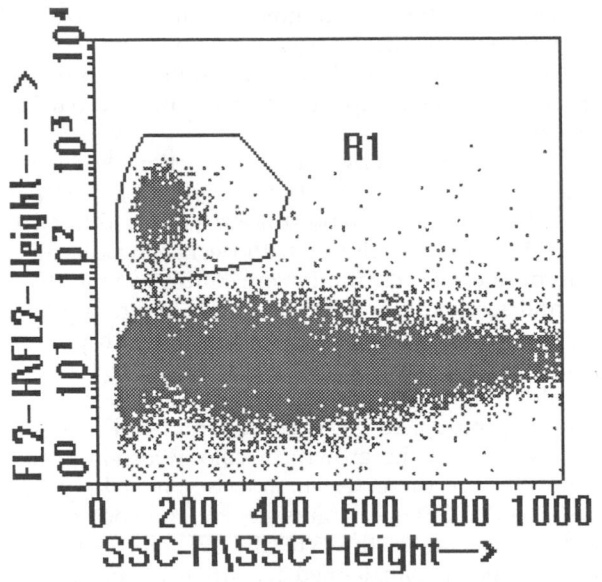
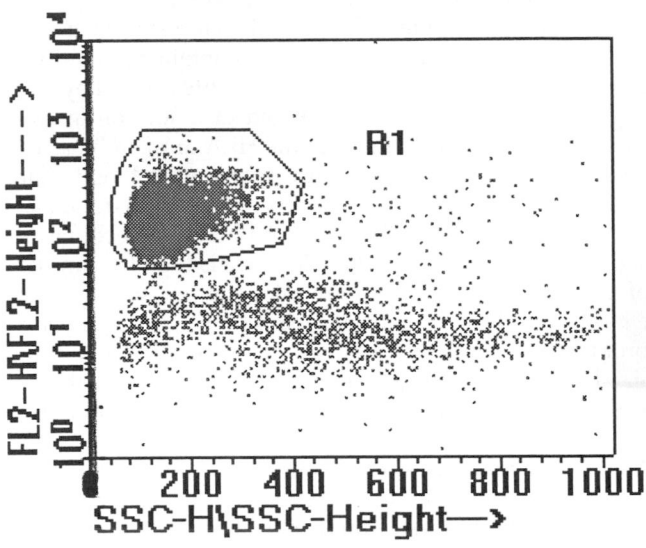
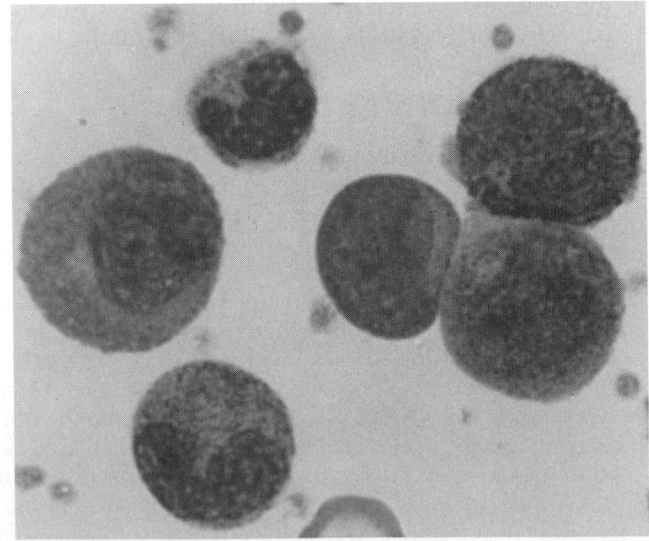
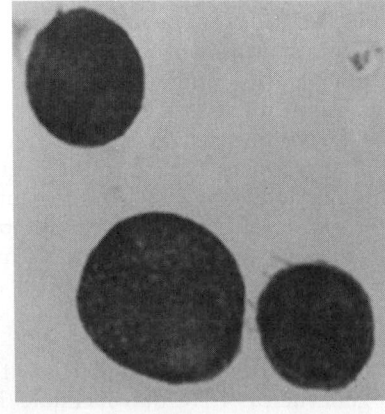

FIGURE 28-1. **(A)** FACS analysis of the leukapheresis starting sample with cell morphology. **(B)** FACS analysis of the eluate product and CD34⁺ cell morphology. Note increase in CD34 cells (circled area).

and the desirable GVL effect. Therefore, obtaining the desired log depletion of T cells with monoclonal antibody is extremely important. These factors are absent with cryopreserved autologous grafts; however, the possibility of reinfusing tumor cells is of concern. Several methods to purge grafts of T cells and tumor cells have been outlined as well as methods to purify the graft by selecting CD34$^+$ cells rendering a reduced cell volume for cryopreservation and subsequent infusion. Culturing stem cells from an autologous graft or cord blood offers solutions to problems encountered in transplantation.

Before and after manipulation, the laboratory must define, as much as possible, the quality of the graft. This involves documenting that the desired outcome occurred and that the remaining stem and progenitor cells are viable and in sufficient numbers for successful engraftment.

Finally, new monoclonal antibodies, chemotherapeutics and separation techniques are imminent. Sensitive and specific purging methods, and cell expansion systems sometimes coupled with genetic engineering will provide better cure rates and target more diseases. Graft engineering is at the exciting interface between basic research and clinical application and, because it makes use of evolving technology, new procedures to benefit patients are continuously being developed. The future will include manipulations not yet fully appreciated, but will surely include those applying advances in molecular biology, including gene therapy.

Case Study 28-1

A 48-year-old man with non-Hodgkin lymphoma and marrow involvement qualified for an autologous transplant. He was given cyclophosphamide, and 2 days later daily G-CSF therapy was begun. His daily leukocyte counts, beginning day 6 of stem cell mobilization therapy were: day **6**, 2.5×10^9/L; day **7**, 0.1×10^9/L; day **8**, 0.2×10^9/L; day **9**, 4.5×10^9/L; day **10**, 7.0×10^9/L; day **11**, 10.0×10^9/L; day **12**, 19.0×10^9/L; and day **13**, 33.5×10^9/L. The patient was leukapheresed and 48.2×10^9 cells were treated with biotinylated anti-CD34 and passed through an avidin column. The following fractions were assayed for CD34$^+$ cells and the percentage positive results are indicated for each: leukapheresis (169 mL), 6.1%; after antibody, 6.3%; unadsorbed, 1.5%; and eluate (69.6 mL), 92.8%.

Figure 28-1 morphologically contrasts the starting sample and final product. After high-dose cytotoxic therapy and radiation the patient was infused with his cryopreserved graft. On the 9th day following the transplant (+9), the patient had an absolute neutrophil count of 0.52×10^9/L. Counts on days +10 and +11 were 0.58 and 0.64×10^9/L, respectively.

1. Given the expected WBC response, what was the optimum time to leukapherese and why?
2. Explain the expected CD34 (stem cell) yield for each fraction. Do these data meet the expectation?
3. When did the patient engraft? Explain why this could occur so rapidly.
4. What advantage would this graft have over an unmanipulated one? Consider the risk of relapse.

Case Study 28-2

A 20-year-old man with acute myelogenous leukemia (AML) was transplanted with bone marrow harvested from his father. The allograft was fractionated with a Ficoll gradient to obtain a mononuclear fraction and was treated with cytolytic anti-T–lymphocyte monoclonal antibody and complement. Below are the laboratory data evaluating the graft:

Marrow Sample	Cells Viable (%)	FACS CD3$^+$, CD5$^+$ and TCR$^+_{\alpha\beta}$(%)	LDA Proliferation Frequency
Untreated	96	26.2	1/37
Treated	>99	<0.1	1/13,032
		LOG DEPLETION	
		>2.4	2.54

Marrow Sample	Stem Cell Culture Colonies Per 10^9 Nucleated Cells		
	CFU-GEMM	*BFU-E*	*CFU-GM*
Untreated	3	112	284
Treated	3	62	491

1. Why was a T-cell depletion performed?
2. Did this manipulation affect the progenitor cells?
3. (a) Flow cytometry and the LDA are different methods with different principles. What are they? (b) Was the graft sufficiently depleted? (c) Do the results correlate?
4. What might be the consequences to a patient if T cells are ineffectively depleted? If too large a depletion is achieved?

Review Questions

28-1. A metastatic breast cancer patient who did not respond to chemotherapeutic treatment is mobilized with G-CSF and scheduled for an autologous harvest and transplant. This is the best approach because

A. metastatic bone marrow involvement would not interfere.
B. there is too little time for cord blood manipulation, the source of choice because HLA antigens are absent.
C. there is obviously no histocompatible sibling donor.
D. autologous peripheral blood is the least invasive stem cell source, with a faster engraftment rate.

28-2. Allogeneic grafts are

A. never cryopreserved.
B. histocompatible if two of three antigens are matched.
C. sometimes T-cell depleted.
D. bone marrow grafts that require tumor cell purging.

28-3. An autologous graft from a patient with bone marrow involvement is best processed by

A. positive selection of CD34$^+$ cells followed by a purge for residual tumor cells.
B. adding cord blood rich in CD34$^+$ cells.
C. T-cell depletion with monoclonal antibody and cytolysis.
D. immediate controlled-rate cryopreservation.

28-4. Specific monoclonal antibodies are used in graft engineering for

A. positive selection of T cells.
B. purging unwanted cells from autografts.
C. use after cytolytic purges.
D. enhancing *ex vivo* expansion of stem/progenitor cells.

28-5. Which statement is FALSE?

A. An assay to show enrichment of stem and progenitor cells before and after processing is the limiting dilution assay.
B. CD34$^+$ cells are enriched by T-cell depletion.
C. *Ex vivo* cytolic drugs must be adjusted to kill tumor but not stem or progenitor cells.
D. A graft sample is cultured to show that viable stem and progenitor cells were infused.

References

1. Amos TAS, Gordon MY: Sources of human hematopoietic stem cells for transplantation—a review. Cell Transplant 4:547, 1995
2. Armitage JO: Bone marrow transplantation. N Engl J Med 330:827, 1994
3. Bronzino JD: Introduction. In The Biomedical Engineering Handbook, p iii. Boca Raton, CRC Press, 1995
4. Brugger W, Heimfeld S, Berenson RJ et al: Reconstitution of hematopoiesis after high-dose chemotherapy by autologous progenitor cells generated ex vivo. N Engl J Med 333:283, 1995
5. Champlin R: Optimizing the composition of bone marrow for allogeneic transplantation. J Hematother 4:53, 1995
6. de Magalhaes-Silverman M, Donnenberg AD, Pincus SM et al: Bone marrow transplantation: A review. Cell Transplant 2:75, 1993
7. Gale RP: Graft-versus-host disease. Immunol Rev 88:193, 1985
8. Gee A: Purging of peripheral blood stem cell grafts. Stem Cells 13(suppl 3):52, 1995
9. Horowitz MM, Gale RP, Sondel PM, et al: Graft-versus-leukemia reactions after bone marrow transplantation. Blood 75:555, 1990
10. Kessinger A, Armitage JO, Landmark JD: Autologous peripheral hematopoietic stem cell transplantation restores hematopoietic function following marrow ablative therapy. Blood 71:723, 1988
11. Krause DS, Fackler MJ, Civin CI et al: CD34: Structure, biology and clinical utility. Blood 87:1, 1996
12. Martin PJ, Hansen JA: Quantitative assays for detection of residual T cells in T-depleted human marrow. Blood 65:1134, 1985
13. Messner HA: Assessment and characterization of hemopoietic stem cells. Stem Cells 13(suppl 3):13, 1995
14. Rowley SD: Hematopoietic stem cell cryopreservation: A review of current techniques. J Hematother 1:233, 1992
15. Savage DC, Goldman JM: Approaches to the treatment of chronic myelogenous leukemia. Int J Hematol 60:1, 1994
16. Stiff PJ, Koester AR, Weidner MK et al: Autologous bone marrow transplantation using unfractionated cells cryopreserved in dimethylsulfoxide and hydroxyethyl starch without controlled-rate freezing. Blood 70:974, 1987
17. Van Zant G, Rummel SA, Koller MR et al: Expansion in bioreactors of human progenitor populations from cord blood and mobilized peripheral blood. Blood Cells 20:482, 1994

Suggested Readings

Armitage JO, Antman KH (eds): High-Dose Cancer Therapy, 2nd ed. Baltimore, Williams & Wilkins, 1995

Forman SJ, Blume KG, Thomas ED (eds): Bone Marrow Transplantation. Oxford, Blackwell Scientific Publications, 1994

Gee A (ed): Bone Marrow Processing and Purging. Boca Raton, FL, CRC Press, 1991

Stamatoyannopoulos G, Nienhuis AW, Majerus PW, Varmus H (eds): The Molecular Basis of Blood Diseases. Philadelphia, WB Saunders, 1994

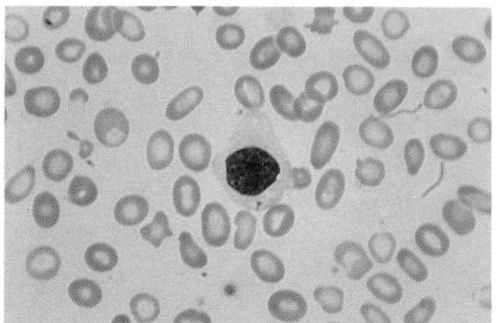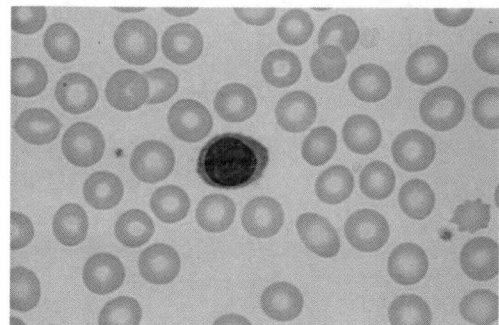

PLATE 23-1. Large and small lymphocytes. The nucleated cell in (**A**) is a large lymphocyte with abundant, clear, almost colorless cytoplasm. The nucleated cell in (**B**) is a small resting lymphocyte. Compared with the larger lymphocyte, this cell has a higher nuclear:cytoplasmic ratio and a denser chromatin pattern. (1000×)

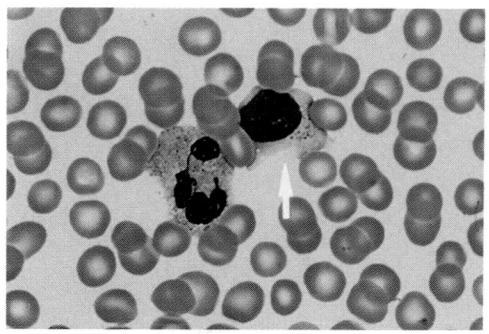

PLATE 23-2. Large granular lymphocyte. The *arrow* is pointing to a medium-to-large lymphocyte with large pinkish granules in its cytoplasm. The other cell is a segmented neutrophil. (1000×)

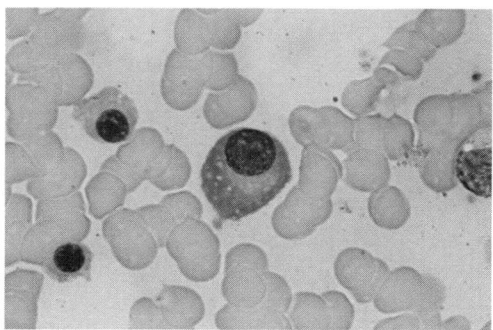

PLATE 23-3. Normal bone marrow plasma cell and two rubricytes. The perinuclear chromophobic area in the cytoplasm is striking in the deeply basophilic cytoplasm. (*Courtesy Ann Bell, M.A.*)

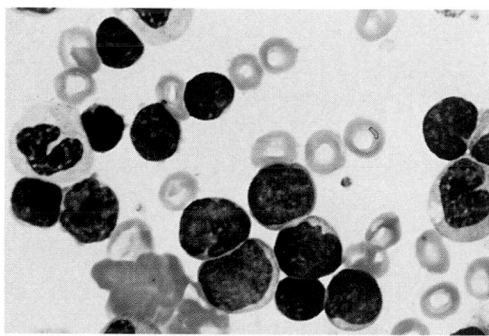

PLATE 23-4. Hematogones in bone marrow stained with Wright-Giemsa. Strikingly homogeneous nuclear chromatin without visible nucleoli and with extremely scant, blue, agranular cytoplasm are observed. Nuclear cleavages appear in a few of the cells. (*Courtesy Richard D. Brunning, M.D.*) See Color Plate 27-14 for a lymphocyte found in newborn infants that has also been referred to as a *hematogone*.

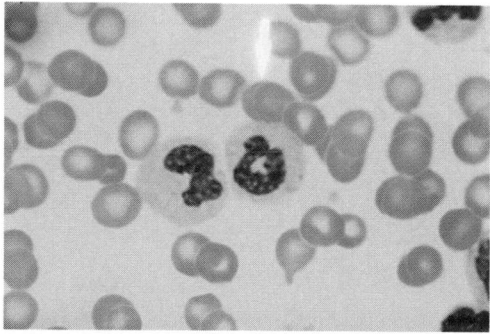

PLATE 25-1. Döhle body. The neutrophil in the center of the field (*arrow*) contains a Döhle body just inside the plasma membrane. The color of Döhle bodies varies from blue to gray, depending on the type of specimen. (1000×)

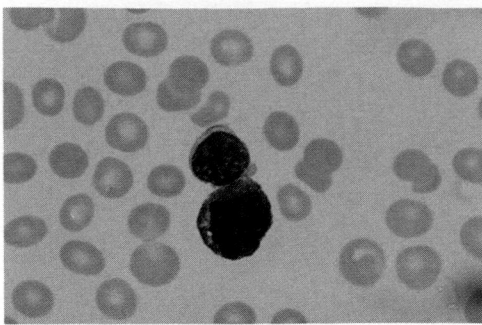

PLATE 25-2. Reactive lymphocyte, type I. The smaller cell is a small normal lymphocyte. The larger cell is a type I variant lymphocyte, also known as a *plasmacytoid lymphocyte* or a *Türk irritation cell*. Note the extremely blue cytoplasm. (1000×)

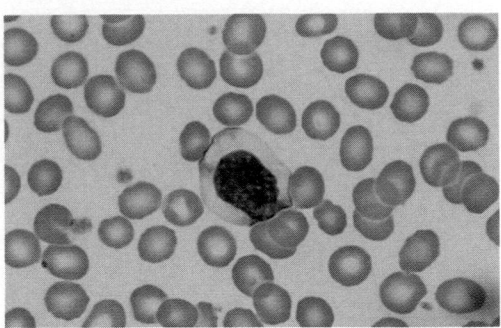

PLATE 25-3. Reactive lymphocyte, type II. Note the abundant clear cytoplasm with radiating basophilia, which gives it a flared skirt or fried egg appearance. Also note the nuclear banding. (1000×)

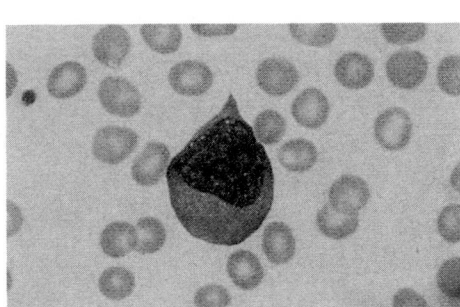
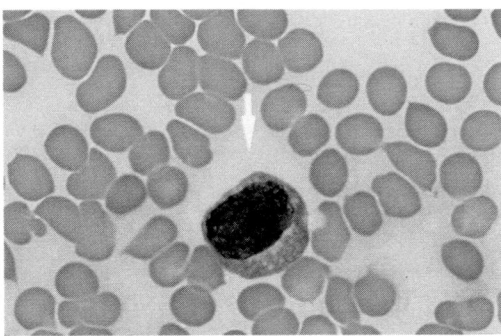

PLATE 25-4. Two examples of type III variant lymphocytes. Note the visible nucleoli in both. The cytoplasm in (**A**) is quite basophilic, indicating that this is probably a B-cell blast. Type III variant lymphocytes also may have clear or pale cytoplasm, such as seen in (**B**). Color Plate 25-5 contains a third example of a type III variant lymphocyte.

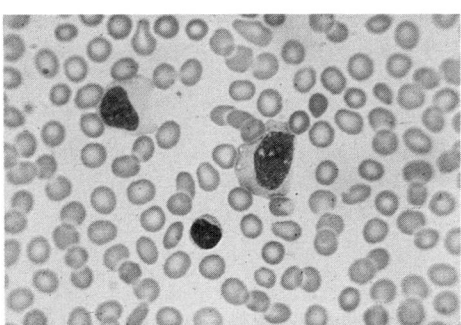

PLATE 25-5. Blastogenesis. These three cells represent three phases of blastogenesis. The lowest cell is a small resting lymphocyte. When this cell is stimulated by antigen, it swells in size (both nucleus and cytoplasm) and eventually becomes a large lymphocyte (upper left). The process of transformation continues until the cell becomes a blast capable of division (the type III lymphocyte on the right). (400×)

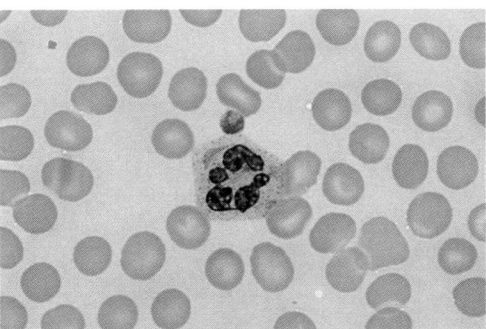

PLATE 26-1. Neutrophil from patient with May-Hegglin anomaly. Note large spindle-shaped basophilic inclusion in the cytoplasm (upper left). (1000×)

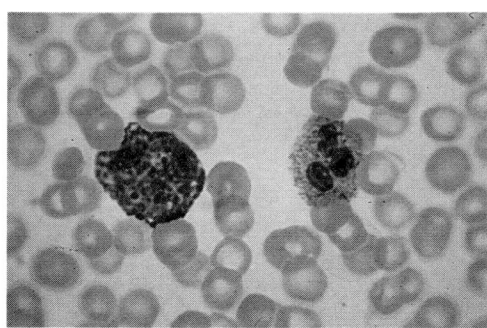

PLATE 26-2. Alder-Reilly syndrome. *(Left)* A normal basophil. *(Right)* Neutrophil with large azurophilic granules ("Alder-Reilly bodies"). *(From American Society of Hematology Slide Bank, 1977, used with permission.)*

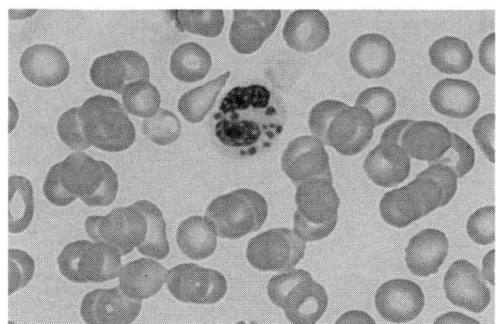

PLATE 26-3. Chédiak-Higashi. The segmented neutrophil contains several large greyish granules (giant lysosomes) that are characteristic of this disorder. (1000×)

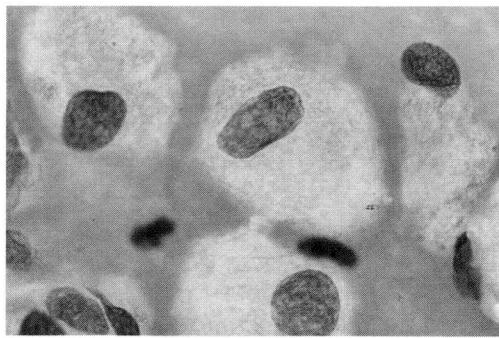

PLATE 26-4. Imprint of splenic tissue from a patient with Gaucher disease. Four typical macrophages can be seen. Note the faint striations in the cytoplasm of the macrophages that are characteristic of this disorder. These cells are strongly PAS positive. (1000×)

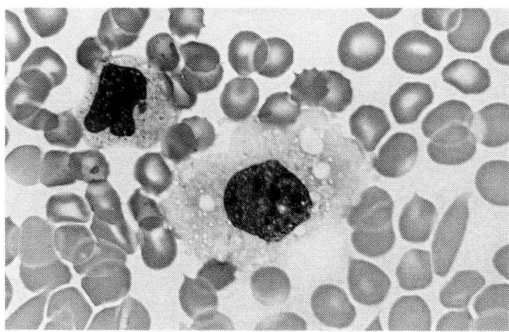

PLATE 27-1. Macrophage. Note the abundant, vacuolated cytoplasm. The other cell is a band-form neutrophil. See Color Plate 22-18 for another example of a macrophage. (1000×) *(Courtesy of Karen Lofsness.)*

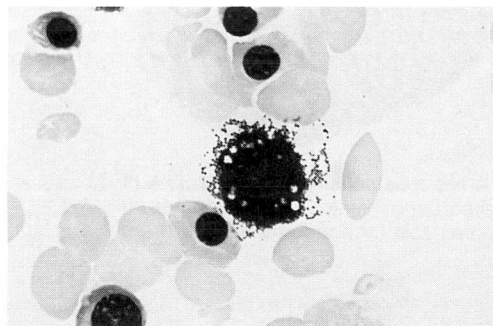

PLATE 27-2. Tissue mast cell. This cell's nucleus is rarely seen because it is masked by the large number of metachromatic (purple-black) granules of identical size. In this case, the cell's plasma membrane has been disrupted in the making of the marrow film, and several granules have been pushed out of the cell. (1000×) *(Courtesy of Karen Lofsness.)*

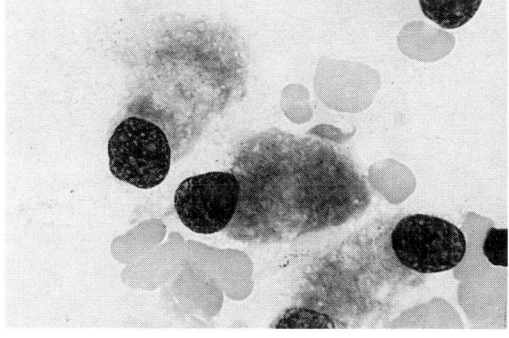

PLATE 27-3. Osteoblasts. Note how the nucleus is so eccentric that it appears to be outside of the cell in some cases. These cells have been described as looking like water bugs. See Color Plate 27-8 for a drawing of this cell. (1000×) *(Courtesy of Karen Lofsness.)*

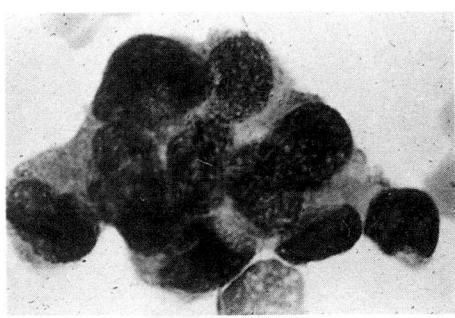

PLATE 27-10. Tumor cells. Nuclei have a variable color and chromatin clumping. Nucleoli are common and cells are variable in size and shape and the cytoplasmic borders may be difficult to distinguish as the cells tend to clump. Cytoplasm color is variable.

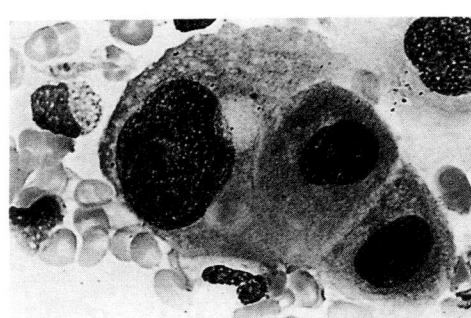

PLATE 27-11. Tumor cells. Nuclei have variable color and chromatin clumping and nucleoli are common. The cells are variable in size and shape and the cytoplasmic borders may be difficult to distinguish. The cells tend to clump and the cytoplasmic color is variable.

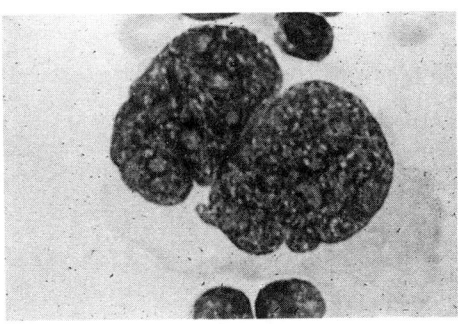

PLATE 27-12. Reed-Sternberg Cell. Nuclear lobes are often mirror images. The nucleoli are more prominent than those of a megakaryoblast. Cytoplasmic color is variable. See also Color Plate 55-14.

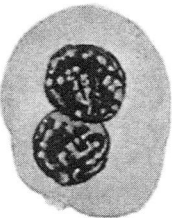

PLATE 27-13. Multinucleated red cell precursor. The cytoplasm is polychromatophilic or pink and it is nongranular. The nuclear chromatin is clumped. This cell is smaller than a megakaryocyte.* See also Color Plate 55-12.

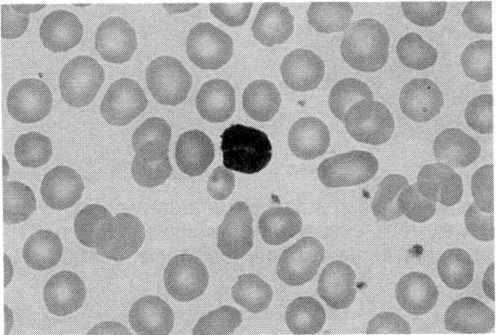

PLATE 27-14. Lymphocyte from a newborn baby. Note the scanty cytoplasm and the clefted (grooved) nucleus. This is believed to represent a pre-B cell that has not been stimulated by antigen. This cell is sometimes referred to as a *hematogone* (see Color Plate 23-4). This cell is very similar morphologically to the maligant lymphoblast seen in acute lymphoblastic leukemia (see Color Plate 36-2). Care must be taken not to misidentify these cells as their malignant counterparts. (1000×)

* From Diggs LW, Sturm D, Bell A: The Morphology of Human Blood Cells, 5th ed. Abbott Park, IL, Abbott Laboratories, 1985, with permission

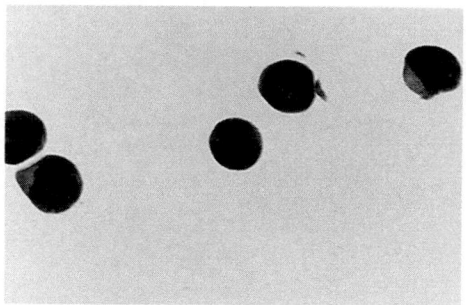

PLATE 28-1. Wright stain morphology of CD34+ stem cells that have been selected and purified for transplantation.

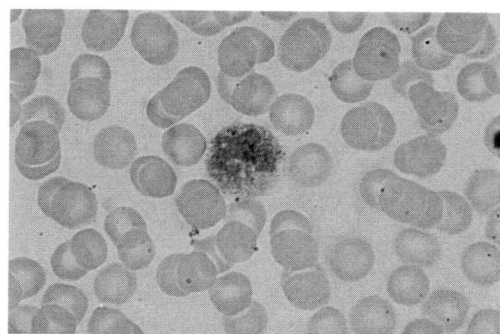

PLATE 29-1. Leukocyte alkaline phosphatase. A segmented neutrophil stained for alkaline phosphatase. This cell might be scored as 2+ or 3+ depending on the laboratory. Due to the subjectivity in scoring, it is imperative that each laboratory establish its own reference range. (1000×)

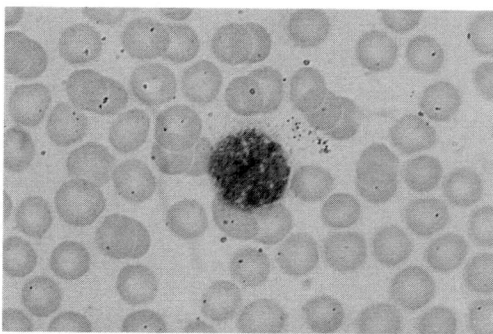

PLATE 29-2. Leukocyte alkaline phosphatase (LAP). A segmented neutrophil stained for alkaline phosphatase. This cell was scored as 4+ but others might score it as 3+. See also Color Plate 35-5 for an LAP with another (red) azo dye. Compare it with Color Plate 29-1. (1000×)

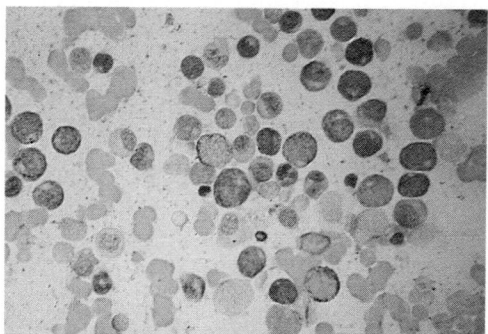

PLATE 29-3. Naphthyl AS-D chloroacetate (specific) esterase-positive neutrophilic cells.

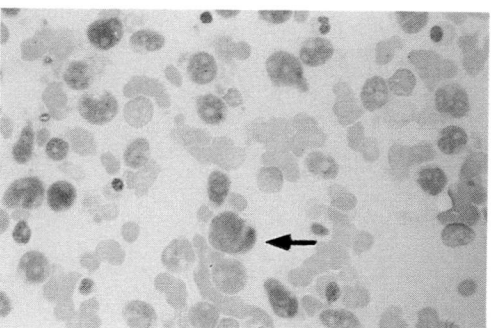

PLATE 29-4. Alpha naphthyl (nonspecific) esterase-positive blast (see *arrow*). See also Color Plate 33-3 for an example of a dual esterase stain showing both specific and nonspecific staining in the same field.

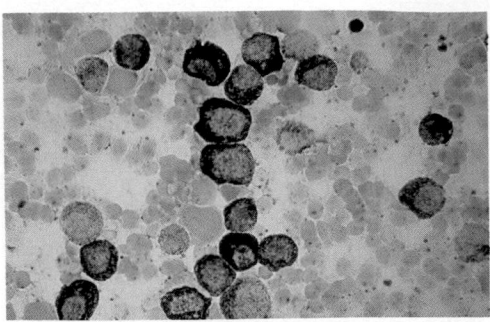

PLATE 29-5. Myeloperoxidase-positive blasts with negative lymphocytes in the field.

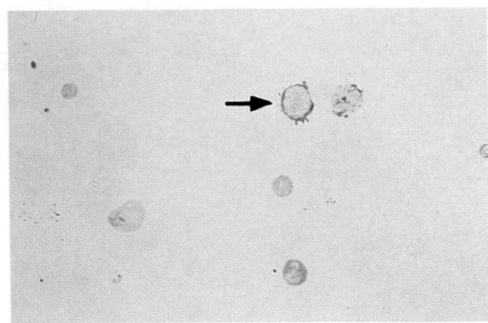

PLATE 29-6. PAS positivity in erythroid precursor in a patient with FAB M6 leukemia (see *arrow*).

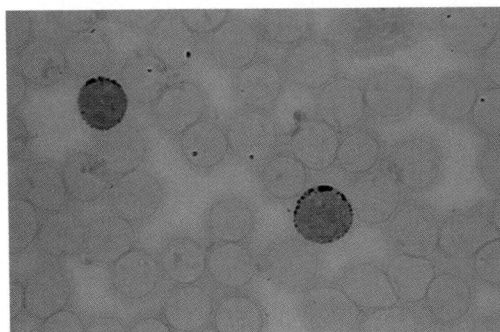

PLATE 29-7. PAS positivity in two lymphoblasts from a patient with L1 ALL. Note the coarse, granular (chunky) appearance of reaction.

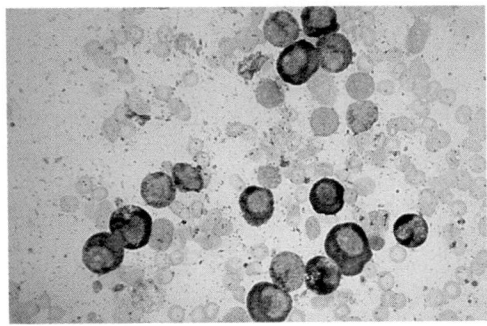

PLATE 29-8. Sudan black B–positive blasts with negative lymphocytes in the field.

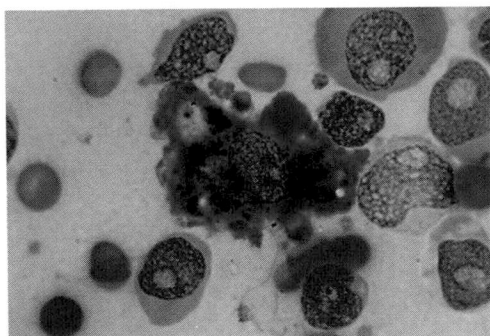

PLATE 29-9. Prussian blue positive macrophage. The green color in the cytoplasm indicates the presence of ferric (Fe^{3+}) iron stores. The intensity of the green color reflects the concentration of iron stores. This particular macrophage is "loaded." (1000×) (*Courtesy of Jean Shafer.*)

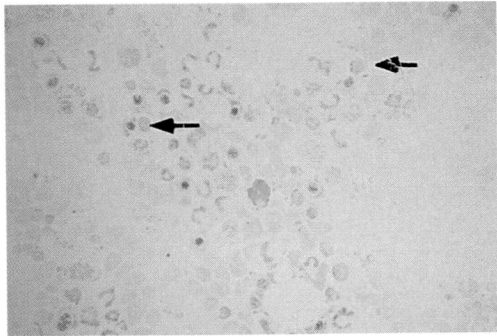

PLATE 29-10. Positive iron stain with ringed sideroblasts noted by *arrows*.

CHAPTER 29

Cytochemistry

Barbara J. Helbert
Edward S. Rappaport

Objectives

1. Evaluate the need to provide cytochemical procedures in an individual laboratory.
2. Describe the principles of the cytochemical procedures discussed in this chapter.
3. Discuss the common usages for each of the cytochemical procedures.
4. Correlate cytochemical results to disease processes.
5. Identify sources of error in the performance of each cytochemical procedure discussed in this chapter.
6. Discuss the mechanics of immunocytochemistry and some of its uses.
7. Discuss the advantages and disadvantages of cytochemistry when compared to other methods of cell identification, such as molecular probes and flow cytometry.

HISTORY OF CYTOCHEMISTRY

Since Anton van Leeuwenhoek first used lenses in the 1600s to magnify bacteria, protozoa, and blood cells, scientists have been searching for specific methods to aid in cellular identification. The work of Ehrlich and others provided the first staining methods later modified to the Romanowsky-Giemsa combinations currently in use for morphologic identification of blood cells using the light microscope. These stained films of blood or bone marrow often require more art than science in cellular identification. The quality of the films and stain is variable and dependent on the skill of the laboratorian. Even if good films are made and stained properly, much depends on experience of the morphologist for cell classification.

Histochemistry or cytochemistry, defined as the application of chemical processes to cells and tissues to reveal their chemical composition, has been in existence since the early 1800s. *Histochemistry* usually refers to staining performed on cut sections of tissue whereas *cytochemistry* is performed on films of cells. The usefulness of cytochemistry includes identification of: (1) malignant cell types on the basis of cytoplasmic or nuclear chemistry; (2) cellular constituents that are present in abnormal form or amount; (3) lack of cellular constituents; and (4) cells exhibiting functional abnormalities. In general, cytochemical stains are done on both peripheral blood and bone marrow films where most cells are intact. Procedures in histochemistry designed for use with cut sections of tissue are frequently adapted to stain intact cells. The primary value of cytochemical stains is to help identify the lineage of malignant cells present in a patient with leukemia.[1]

FACTORS TO CONSIDER BEFORE INITIATING CYTOCHEMICAL STAINS

Many factors must be considered when a laboratory initiates the performance of special staining procedures:

1. **Testing volume should be adequate.** The laboratory should look at numbers of bone marrow examinations performed per year. If the number is low (*e.g.,* less than 50), special stains would be ordered infrequently because only a portion of bone marrow examinations would require staining. In such cases, the laboratory should seriously consider the use of a commercial or reference laboratory to perform the occasional cytochemical procedure.
2. **Cost of testing.** Most procedures are available in kit form for staining. These kits are expensive, and in many cases kit components cannot be purchased separately to replenish only selected reagents. Making buffers or counterstains from chemical components is equally costly and requires an inventory of chemicals. Such an inventory may include hazardous chemicals, which present other problems for the laboratory with regard to storage and federal, state, and local regulations.
3. **Consistent laboratorian technique.** If stains are performed infrequently, techniques may suffer. It is often said that staining is an art, and repetition will improve technique. If a laboratorian is uncertain of procedural steps or performs them incorrectly, improper results may occur, requiring repeat staining or giving incorrect diagnostic information. This adds to the cost of the stains and more importantly, may lead to improper

care of the patient. In addition, even if the staining technique is beyond reproach and an excellent stained product is generated, if it is not examined within a reasonable time, changes may occur in the stain that can affect the interpretation (*e.g.*, fading or interaction with light).

4. **Carcinogenic activity of staining components.** Many of the substrates used for cytochemical staining procedures are documented carcinogens. Kit directions should be specifically followed for these components. For the protection of the laboratorian, a hood should be available for staining components that come in powder form and must be diluted for test performance. Masks, gloves, and other protective equipment that is standard in the laboratory should be required when performing these staining procedures.

5. **Expiration of stain components.** If stains are performed infrequently, the kit components may expire, rendering them unusable. The laboratory is required to institute a regular expiration date check on kit components to ensure that expiration has not occurred even if the kits are not being used.

6. **Diagnostic relevance of staining procedures.** As immunology and molecular biology procedures are developed, cytochemical staining procedures play a smaller role in the diagnostic process. Immunologic methods using flow cytometry (Chap. 43) are providing specific antigenic identification of cells which is being used to develop treatment protocols and follow patient course in many of the leukemias, especially those found in children. Immunocytochemical methods using the microscope will be described briefly in this chapter. Molecular biology (Chap. 31) seeks to identify genetic changes on a single gene to find the source of the leukemic process or to identify a single circulating leukemic cell. These two disciplines are most likely the future foundation of cell identification, treatment protocols, and monitoring of patient response to therapy.

PROCEDURAL SUMMARIES

There are many common components to the staining procedures discussed in this chapter. They are as follows:

1. Before staining can begin, an adequate bone marrow or peripheral blood film must be made. Peripheral blood films can only be used when the malignant cells are circulating, otherwise a bone marrow specimen is necessary.
2. Films that are too thick or too thin may cause problems with fixation. Inadequately fixed films will wash off the slides or wrinkle during the staining process, very often at the end of the procedure after much time and effort has been expended.
3. Concentration methods such as buffy coat preparations (Chap. 3) or cell separation using Ficoll medium can be used for cytochemical staining when low numbers of abnormal cells are present. Cytocentrifuge preparations (Chap. 30) or touch prints from the bone marrow biopsy are further sources of material for staining.
4. If possible, all films should be allowed to dry a minimum of 4 hours and no more than 48 hours at room temperature before staining begins. The use of heat to dry the films may cause problems in staining and should be used with caution.
5. Equipment such as Coplin jars, graduated cylinders, beakers,

forceps, funnels, pipettes, coverslips, filter paper, mounting media, and a microscope should be available for all procedures. These materials must be kept clean if used more than one time for staining. Use of disposables is recommended when available.
6. Recently some of the cytochemical staining procedures have been adapted for use with a 500-watt microwave oven; the oven decreases the time necessary for stain performance.[17] These microwave techniques are in extensive use for cut sections of tissue.
7. Most of the staining substrate mixtures are sensitive to pH, heat, and light. Changes in one or more of these factors may be responsible for false-negative or false-positive results in many cases.
8. Kit or procedure manual directions must be followed explicitly for consistent results.

ENZYMATIC TECHNIQUES

Phosphatases

Acid and alkaline phosphatases are a group of isoenzymes capable of liberating phosphate from many monophosphate esters.

ACID PHOSPHATASE

Acid phosphatase is located in lysosomes and is present in all hematopoietic cells.[8] Focal staining of T lymphocytes is seen and can be used in the preliminary identification of T-cell subsets of acute lymphocytic leukemia (ALL). The staining procedure requires a fixation with either cold methanol-acetone or room temperature citrate-acetone. Slides should be allowed to air-dry thoroughly after fixation. The staining substrate is naphthol AS-BI phosphate and N,N-dimethylformamide with an azo dye such as fast garnet GBC in an acetate buffer. The slides are incubated for 45 to 60 minutes. During the staining process, phosphate is released from naphthol AS-BI by acid phosphatase enzymatic hydrolysis. The naphthol may then couple with the azo dye to form an insoluble precipitate, which is deposited at the site of activity. Films are counterstained with Mayer's hematoxylin solution for 3 to 4 minutes, followed by a tap water wash. A normal blood film should be used as a control, since acid phosphatase is present in all cell lines. A positive reaction is indicated by the presence of dark red granules if fast garnet was used as the azo dye. An intense positive reaction is seen in platelets and plasma cells. Moderate activity is seen in monocytes. Weak, mostly granular reactivity is seen in neutrophils of all maturation stages. Lymphocytes and erythroblasts will show little activity. The blasts in approximately 90% of T-cell ALL will show discrete positive granules.

Stained slides should be mounted with a solvent-based mounting media to avoid fading of the positive color. Most procedures suggest avoiding exposure to light and heat while performing this stain. The incubation mixture can be placed in a closed cabinet after slides have been added or the Coplin jar can be wrapped in aluminum foil to effectively block all light from the reaction mixture. Enzyme activity is stable for about 2 weeks in unfixed films and longer if the films are fixed, allowed to air-dry, and stored at $-20°C$.

TARTRATE-RESISTANT ACID PHOSPHATASE (TRAP)

Acid phosphatase (AcP) activity in normal cells is inhibited by the addition of L(+)-tartaric acid to the staining substrate. This inhibition of activity does not occur in the abnormal cells of hairy cell leukemia because of the presence of AcP isoenzyme 5 in these cells.[8] The addition of a tartrate solution to the phosphatase incubation mixture can therefore be used for identification of hairy cells. The procedure is the same as described above, with the addition of tartrate solution to the staining substrate. Hairy cells will remain positive in the substrate whereas activity will be absent in other lymphocytes. Acid phosphatase and tartrate-resistant acid phosphatase can be added simultaneously if necessary for cell identification. Positive TRAP is characteristic, but not pathonomonic of hairy cells.

ALKALINE PHOSPHATASE

Alkaline phosphatase (AlkP) is present in the cytoplasm of neutrophils and is referred to as leukocyte alkaline phosphatase (LAP) or neutrophil alkaline phosphatase (NAP). Eosinophils are rarely positive and basophils are generally negative. All other leukocytes are usually negative.[13] EDTA should be avoided as a specimen anticoagulant because enzyme activity may be inhibited. Films from capillary puncture or from the venipuncture needle without anticoagulant should be used.

The principle of the stain is identical to the acid phosphatase reaction, except that the reaction is performed at an alkaline pH. The staining procedure involves fixation of a peripheral blood film with citrate-formaldehyde-acetone fixative at room temperature. Slides are rinsed and immersed in the staining solution consisting of naphthol AS-BI phosphate, N,N-dimethylformamide, and fast blue BB or fast red violet LB for 15 to 20 minutes. Rinsed slides are counterstained with neutral red solution if using fast blue, and Gill No. 3 hematoxylin if using fast red violet. A positive reaction is indicated by the presence of blue-black precipitate at sites of enzyme activity if using fast blue and a red precipitate if using fast red violet. The stained films should be coverslipped with an aqueous mounting medium to avoid fading. Blood from a woman in the third trimester of pregnancy makes an excellent positive control because the LAP is normally increased during late pregnancy. Lymphocytes on the blood film can serve as a negative control. Slides can be made, fixed, and air-dried for 30 to 60 minutes before storing at −20°C; enzyme stability lasting up to 1 year.[13]

A method of scoring individual neutrophils has been developed and used to evaluate LAP activity. Presence of positive staining is graded in 100 mature neutrophils and bands by rating each from 0 to 4 on the basis of quantity and intensity of staining. Only neutrophils should be scored, so it is important to be able to recognize all cell types when using the counterstaining procedure. Table 29-1 describes the rating system. When 100 neutrophils are scored, the number of neutrophils rated in each category is multiplied by the rating. These values are totaled to obtain the final score. Reference totals range from 13 to 160; however, due to the subjectivity inherent

TABLE 29-1
Criteria for Scoring Leukocyte Alkaline Phosphatase (LAP) Reaction Product in Neutrophils

Score	Amount of Precipitated Dye
0	No granules in the cytoplasm
1	Few (could be counted), small granules occupying <50% of the cytoplasm
2	Moderate stained granules occupying 50%–80% of cytoplasm
3	Strongly stained granules occupying 80%–100% of cytoplasm and beginning to coalesce
4	Strongly-stained granules packed into the cytoplasm. The nucleus is the only cell component that remains visible.

in this scoring system (each laboratorian may rate the individual cells differently based on his or her interpretation of the scoring system), each laboratory should establish its own reference range. Experience in scoring will eliminate some of these differences, but it may still be necessary to have more than one technologist score the slides from a single sample for consistency. Color Plates 29-1 and 29-2 show 2+ and 4+ cells, respectively.

In addition to third-trimester pregnant women, scores are elevated in polycythemia rubra vera, any leukemoid reaction responding to infection or stress, myelofibrosis, and in the presence of tumor metastasis. Scores are decreased in viral infections, chronic myelogenous leukemia (CML), and paroxysmal nocturnal hemoglobinuria (PNH). A small number of individuals have inherited hypophosphatemia, which results in low LAP scores.

The hematologic value of the LAP score is to distinguish early CML from infection or polycythemia vera. In addition, the LAP is proposed as a means of distinguishing between malignant and benign paraproteinemias,[15] as a predictor of the metastatic state of breast and colorectal cancer,[19] and as a prognostic test for lung cancer.[18]

Esterases

Esterases are enzymes capable of hydrolyzing aliphatic and aromatic esters at acid or neutral pH.[7] The biochemistry of these enzymes is complex and multiple isoenzymes exist which are cell specific. Table 29-2 shows the isoenzyme numbers and cellular locations.

TABLE 29-2
Cellular Location of Esterase Isoenzymes

Esterase Isoenzyme No.	Cellular Location
1, 2, 7, 8, 9	Mast cells, neutrophils
3, 4, 5, 6	Monocytes, megakaryocytes, plasma cells

Those isoenzymes designated 1, 2, 7, 8, and 9 are commonly referred to as "specific" esterases found in neutrophils and mast cells, while 3, 4, 5, and 6 are known as "nonspecific" and are found in monocytes, megakaryocytes, and plasma cells. The principle of esterase staining is very much like the phosphatase stains. In the presence of an esterase, the ester will be released from an alpha-naphthol or naphthyl ester substrate, and the resulting alpha-naphthol is freed to bind with an azo dye.

Staining techniques for both the specific and nonspecific esterases are quite similar except for differences in substrates. Films are fixed in a citrate-acetone-formaldehyde solution for 30 seconds and then washed with running deionized water. Fixed films are then incubated in a buffered staining solution—naphthol AS-D chloroacetate-ester/fast red violet LB (specific) or alpha-naphthyl acetate-ester/fast blue BB (nonspecific). Timing will vary according to substrate. They are then rinsed in running water. Gill No. 3 or Mayer's hematoxylin may be used to counterstain for 2 to 3 minutes. The slides are then rinsed and dried. These procedures can be performed on the same film by incubation with the alpha-naphthyl acetate solution first, and then the naphthol AS-D chloroacetate solution followed by the counterstain procedure. Combining the two stains is usually a matter of personal preference but could be of use when diagnostic material is limited. The presence of enzyme activity is noted by red granulation for the specific (chloroacetate) esterase stain (see Color Plate 29-3) and brown to dark brown for the nonspecific (alpha-naphthyl) esterase stain (see Color Plate 29-4).

A film of normal bone marrow aspirate can be used as a control, because neutrophils and mast cells will stain positive with chloroacetate while monocytes, megakaryocytes, basophils, and plasma cells will be positive with alpha-naphthyl acetate. Auer rods are strongly chloroacetate-positive in cases of acute myelocytic leukemia. Some focal positivity with the specific procedure occurs in the cytoplasm of T lymphocytes.[6] The alpha-naphthyl acetate (nonspecific) esterase stain will show weak positivity for erythroid precursors, which may prove confusing when evaluating immature cells. Sodium fluoride solution can be added to the incubation mixture, which will inactivate the monocyte esterase isoenzyme to resolve the question of lineage. A second substrate, alpha-naphthyl butyrate, can be used as a substitute for alpha-naphthyl acetate ester and is slightly more specific for the monocyte esterase. The procedure would be the same as for the alpha-naphthyl acetate.

Peroxidases

Peroxidases are enzymes that rapidly catalyze the oxidation of substrates including phenols in the presence of hydrogen peroxide. The enzyme is present in the primary granules of neutrophils and is absent in lymphocytes and erythroid lines in all stages of development. Eosinophils will be strongly positive and monocytes may show a weak reaction.[4] Benzidine has been used in the past as the color indicator (it turns blue-green upon oxidation). However, because of its strong carcinogenic properties, use of benzidine is under strict regulation. Consequently, benzidine is impractical to store and use because it presents an unnecessary carcinogenic exposure to laboratory employees. Methods currently employ the diaminobenzidine salt (DAB) as the substrate.

Films are fixed in cold formalin/acetone or gluteraldehyde/acetone fixative. The staining substrate is a diaminobenzidine solution with fresh 1% hydrogen peroxide added just before slide incubation. Slides are counterstained in Gill No. 3 hematoxylin.

A positive reaction is indicated by the presence of gray-black granulation in the cytoplasm of the cells (see Color Plate 29-5). Eosinophils will stain red-brown. Patients with myelodysplastic syndromes may exhibit variable reactions with this stain depending on cellular maturation.[2] Patients have been identified with hereditary myeloperoxidase deficiency in whom all neutrophils and monocytes show negative staining. In these cases, the eosinophils are unaffected and contain stainable peroxidase. A normal peripheral blood film can be used as a control for the staining procedure (neutrophils will be positive and lymphocytes will be negative).

Problems with this stain can often be traced to:

1. **Use of weak hydrogen peroxide.** It is important that this component be fresh when used.
2. **Fixation.** Peroxidase is sensitive to methanol and formaldehyde.
3. **Freshness of the specimen.** Films should be fresh when stained, because peroxidase deteriorates when slides are stored longer than 2 weeks.

Recently, a chemiluminescence assay for the demonstration of intracellular myeloperoxidase has been reported that appears to be highly sensitive in that it was able to detect undifferentiated myeloid leukemia (M0) blasts.[3]

NONENZYMATIC TECHNIQUES

Carbohydrates

Leukocytes contain glycogen as a primary carbohydrate storage component. Glycogen can be converted to glucose when needed by the cells. Glycogen is present in all neutrophils and their precursors, increasing in concentration from diffuse (1+) to concentrated granules as the neutrophils mature. Basophils, monocytes, and megakaryocytes contain varying amounts of glycogen, but normal lymphocytes and erythroid precursors do not.[20]

The periodic acid–Schiff (PAS) reaction is used to ascertain whether glycogen is present in cells. It is a two-step reaction: (1) periodic acid is used to form aldehyde groups from glycogen and (2) the Schiff reagent (a colorless solution composed of leukofuchsin) reacts with the aldehyde groups, creating a bright reddish pink color.

Films are fixed with formalin/ethanol and then washed in running tap water. Slides are kept in the periodic acid for 15 to 20 minutes before being washed and placed in the Schiff reagent for 15 to 20 minutes. The counterstain is Gill No. 3 hematoxylin. Normal peripheral blood films can be used for control, because neutrophils should be bright pink.

The diagnostic usefulness of this stain applies to three types of patients: (1) cases of FAB (French-American-British) M6 erythroleukemia (Chap. 34), in which the erythroid precursors show granular PAS positivity in early forms with later forms diffusely positive (see Color Plate 29-6);[1] (2) those with Gaucher disease, in whom Gaucher cells can be distinguished from Niemann-Pick cells by their strong PAS positivity; and (3) most (80%) of acute lymphatic leukemia (ALL) cases exhibit some lymphoblasts containing "chunky" granular PAS positivity (Color Plate 29-7). There is conflicting evidence of the prognostic significance of the PAS reaction in these patients.[9]

Problems with this stain include (1) background staining if the slides are not rinsed thoroughly in running tap water; (2) false-negative results caused by outdated periodic acid or Schiff reagent (if the Schiff reagent is not crystal clear, it should be discarded); and (3) the colorless Schiff reagent that will stain anything it touches a bright pink. This includes laboratorians and their clothing.

Lipids

A wide variety of substances in cells fall into the category of lipids. Simple, compound, and derived lipids can be found in cell membranes and within cellular organelles. Lipids are often associated with proteins and are referred to as lipoproteins. Neutrophils contain lipids in both primary and secondary granules. Lipids also occur in monocytic lysosomal granules but are rarely seen in lymphocytes. Sudan black B (SBB) stains many of these lipids by an uncertain mechanism, possibly a combination of chemical reaction and selective absorption.[14] The SBB reaction gives similar results to the peroxidase reaction (*i.e.*, positive in granulocytes and monocytes and negative in lymphocytes), but it is much more stable and can be performed on a specimen after several months. Furthermore, the reagents are not carcinogenic, which is an advantage to the laboratory in terms of storage and personnel safety. On the other hand, the peroxidase stain is faster and somewhat more sensitive. Each laboratory must select which stain to perform. There is usually no reason to perform both.

Films are fixed with buffered formalin/acetone for 30 to 60 seconds and then washed in running water. They are then placed in the staining solution consisting of Sudan black B in a phenol phosphate buffer for 30 to 60 minutes. Slides are washed in 70% ethanol for 2 to 3 minutes and then in distilled water for the same time before counterstaining in hematoxylin (Harris) or nuclear fast red. A normal blood film can be used for a control, because neutrophils will be strongly positive containing a brown-black precipitate (see Color Plate 29-8) and lymphocytes should be negative. Neutrophil precursors should be slightly positive at the blast stage, increasing as they mature. The blasts of acute granulocytic leukemia are often strongly SBB positive due to cytoplasmic–nuclear asynchrony associated with malignant cells. Aüer rods are intensely positive. Problems occur when the pH varies from neutral. False-negative results may occur due to overfixation. In addition, SBB may stain nonspecific cellular lipid and be falsely positive.

Iron

Iron is an important component of the human red blood cell. Its presence in the hemoglobin of the red blood cell ensures that oxygen can be carried by the cell to the tissues of the body. When hemoglobin is broken down, the released iron is stored by macrophages in the bone marrow in the form of hemosiderin or ferritin until it is reused by the body. It is important in many disorders to determine the amount and location of iron stores in the bone marrow. This is easily quantitated by Perl's Prussian blue reaction in which ferric ions (Fe^{3+}) react with acidic potassium ferrocyanide ions to form ferric ferrocyanide, which appears as a blue-green precipitate.[12]

Films are fixed in methanol for 1 to 2 minutes then air-dried. Slides are then placed in the staining solution consisting of equal parts 2% potassium ferrocyanide in distilled water and 2% HCl for 60 minutes. The stain solution can be placed in a 37°C water bath or incubator to decrease staining time to 15 to 20 minutes. Slides are rinsed with distilled water and then counterstained with nuclear fast red. Control films from a patient with increased iron stores can be made and held for several months. This stain is technically simple but problems of overstaining occur if tap water is used for the rinse steps (rust in the water is stained by the reaction). False-negative results can occur if the HCl is omitted or if potassium ferricyanide is used by mistake.

Blue-green precipitate in macrophages is indicative of the presence of iron (see Color Plate 29-9) and is evaluated as absent, decreased, normal, or increased (some laboratories use a scale of 0–4+). Iron granules should also be seen in a fraction of the red cell precursors (referred to as *sideroblasts*). Absence of sideroblasts in the face of normal or increased stores is associated with the anemia of chronic disease (iron block; Chap. 13). Impaired iron utilization by red cell precursors, which occurs in a number of conditions including dysmyelopoietic syndromes, will produce iron deposits in mitochondria, which form a ring around the nucleus of the red cell precursors (see Color Plate 29-10). These "ringed sideroblasts" are important in the diagnosis of the dysmyelopoietic syndrome known as refractory anemia with ringed sideroblasts[2] (Chap. 33). In addition, ringed sideroblasts have been noted in post-transplant marrows as part of a transient dyserythropoiesis seen in a large percentage (87%) of patients after bone marrow transplantation.[10]

IMMUNOCYTOCHEMISTRY

Immunocytochemistry may be defined as the identification of the immunologic phenotype of a given cell population through the use of specific monoclonal or polyclonal antibodies against selected cell antigens. Various specimens may be used including cell suspensions, paraffin or cryostat sections, films, imprints, or cytocentrifuge preparations. A slide-based technique is advantageous because it allows for counting of designated cell populations and because a permanent slide can be filed for future review. Slide-based immunocytochemistry has also been cost effective because no expensive equipment is required. However, as the price of flow cytometers continues to decrease, the labor-intensive aspect of slide-based immunocytochemistry will shift the balance of cost effectiveness toward the use of flow cytometry as the method of choice for quantifying cell populations (Chap. 43). Regardless of whether the cells are counted manually with a microscope or automatically with a flow cytometer, the principle is the same. A primary antibody against the cell antigen is applied to the specimen. This is followed by a secondary antibody against the Fc portion of the primary antibody. The secondary antibody carries a tag of some type that can be visualized. The tag may be an enzyme, which will form a colored precipitate in the presence of its substrate (*e.g.*, peroxidase or alkaline phosphatase), or it may be a fluorescent tag.

Hematologic uses of immunocytochemistry include (1) identification of terminal deoxynucleotidyl transferase (TdT) enzyme;[21] (2) identification of megakaryocytic precursors that cannot be adequately identified with Wright-Giemsa stains for the diagnosis of acute megakaryocytic leukemia (M7 AML);[22] (3) identification of the phenotype of the neoplastic cell in acute leukemias (lymphoid *vs* myeloid and subtypes);[11] (4) increased accuracy in the evaluation of CSF specimens from patients with possible malignancy involving the CNS.[16]

THE FUTURE OF CYTOCHEMISTRY

The use of cytochemical stains to separate lymphoblastic from myeloblastic disorders remains a part of the diagnostic process when a patient presents to the physician with acute leukemia. However, the development of more specific immunologic procedures (Chap. 43) has caused these stains to become less important.[5] Many new treatment protocols depend more on immunologic markers than peroxidase positivity when patients are first evaluated for leukemia. This trend is especially noticeable in children in whom the presence or absence of immunologic markers will help to determine treatment protocols and predict patient outcome. Molecular biology is also taking a role in diagnostic procedures with leukemia patients (Chap. 31) that will further erode the need for a battery of cytochemical stains. In a climate of increasing pressure on the laboratory to provide relevant, cost-effective testing with best utilization of laboratorian time, cytochemical stains may become a luxury that most laboratories cannot afford.

CHAPTER SUMMARY

Cytochemistry has been an integral part of the diagnostic process in the identification of cell lineage in patients with leukemic and other bone marrow disorders. The procedures are not complicated but do require attention to detail and strict adherence to directions either from a procedure manual or kit. Practice will improve technique and provide consistent results, and it is important to have sufficient testing volume to provide this repetition. Problems with procedures will be recognized when proper positive and negative control material is provided and thoroughly evaluated with the staining results. No single cytochemical stain result should be used for a diagnostic decision. The methods in use and being developed in immunology, molecular biology, and immunocytochemistry take cell identification to a

new level and most probably represent the future of the diagnostic process. Will the cytochemical stains be eliminated? The answer to this question is not completely clear, but the primary goal of the laboratory is to provide the physician with all the necessary information to diagnose, treat, and monitor the patients. Cytochemistry still has a place in that mission.

Case Study 29-1

A 78-year-old man had been diagnosed with refractory anemia several years previous to this physician visit. Packed-cell transfusion had been necessary with no further therapy. The patient went to the physician complaining of increasing infections, fever, and weakness. CBC revealed an anemia and the presence of a nucleated red blood cell on differential analysis. The bone marrow aspirate was found to show erythroid hyperplasia with bizarre RBC precursors and the presence of blasts of unknown origin. The cytochemical staining pattern of the blasts showed them to be peroxidase negative, Sudan black B negative, and PAS positive.
1. What is implied when a cell is said to be PAS positive?
2. What is the most likely diagnosis in this case?

Case Study 29-2

An elderly male complained of weight loss and anorexia. A CBC revealed anemia, thrombocytopenia, and the presence of numerous blasts. After cytochemical stains the blasts were reported to be peroxidase negative, Sudan black B negative, naphthol AS-D chloroacetate esterase negative, alpha-naphthyl acetate esterase positive.
1. In the cytochemical staining pattern in this case, only one stain is positive. What is another name given to this stain?
2. What cell line is usually positive with this stain?
3. What is another substrate that has similar results?
4. What is the most likely diagnosis in this case?

Review Questions

29-1. The following results were obtained from a patient with an elevated leukocyte count when the peripheral blood film was stained for leukocyte alkaline phosphatase and neutrophils were scored as follows: 6 cells–0; 25 cells–1+; 25 cells–2+; 30 cells–3+; 14 cells–4+.

After calculating the total LAP score, it is evident that this patient most likely has

A. chronic myelogenous leukemia.
B. acute lymphatic leukemia.
C. a leukemoid reaction.
D. paroxysmal nocturnal hemoglobinuria (PNH).

29-2. Hairy cells can be identified when performing the acid phosphatase stain by adding _____ to the incubation mixture.

A. formalin
B. tartrate
C. diaminobenzidine
D. naphthol AS-BI chloroacetate

29-3. Schiff reagent is used to stain

A. lipids.
B. iron.
C. nuclear material.
D. carbohydrates.

29-4. A laboratorian was asked to perform a cytochemical staining battery on bone marrow aspirate films from a patient who was suspected of having leukemia. After Sudan black B staining, the stains showed wrinkling of the film. The control slide showed the proper cellular reaction. The peroxidase stain was set up and, prior to the counterstaining step, the bone marrow aspirate film and control slide blood film washed off their slides. The problems could both be a result of

    A. incorrectly performed fixation steps.
    B. use of improper anticoagulant to make the films.
    C. incorrect pH of the incubation mixture.
    D. use of contaminated water to rinse the slides.

References

1. Bennett JM, Catovsky D, Daniel MT et al: Proposals for the classification of the acute leukaemias. Br J Haematol 33:451,1976

2. Bennett JM, Catovsky D, Daniel MT et al: Proposals for the classification of the myelodysplastic syndromes. Br J Haematol 50:189, 1982

3. daFonseca LM, Brunetti IL, Rego EM et al: Characterization of myeloid or lymphoid acute leukemia by a chemiluminescence assay. Comparison with immunocytochemistry using an antimyeloperoxidase antibody. Acta Haematol 90:19, 1993

4. Hayhoe FGJ, Quaglino D: Haematological Cytochemistry. Edinburg, London, New York, Churchill Livingstone, 1980

5. Klobusicka M: Possibilities and limitations of cytochemical methods in diagnosis of acute leukemia. Micron 25:317, 1994

6. Knowles DM II, Halper JP, Machin GA et al: Acid alpha naphthyl acetate esterase activity in human neoplastic lymphoid cells. Usefulness as a T cell marker. Am J Pathol 96:257, 1979

7. Li CY, Yam KW, Yam LT: Esterases in human leukocytes. J Histochem Cytochem 21:1, 1973

8. Li CY, Yam LT, Yam KW: Acid phosphatase isoenzyme in human leukocytes in normal and pathologic conditions. J Histochem Cytochem 18:473, 1970

9. Lilleyman JS, Britton JA, Anderson LM et al: Periodic acid Schiff reaction in childhood lymphoblastic leukaemia. The Medical Research Council Working Party on Childhood Leukaemia. J Clin Pathol 47:689, 1994

10. Macon WR, Tham KT, Greer JP et al: Ringed sideroblasts: A frequent observation after bone marrow transplantation. Mod Pathol 8:782, 1995

11. Nagal K, Sohda H, Kuriyama K et al: Usefulness of immunocytochemistry for phenotypical analysis of acute leukemia, improved fixation procedure and comparative study with flow cytometry. Leuk Lymphoma 16:319, 1995

12. Preece A: Gomori's iron reaction. A Manual for Histologic Technicians, 3rd ed, p 244. Boston, Little, Brown and Co., 1972

13. Rutenberg AM, Rosales CI, Bennett JM: An improved histochemical method for the demonstration of leukocyte alkaline phosphatase activity: Clinical application. J Lab Clin Med 65:698, 1965

14. Sheehan HL, Storey GW: An improved method of staining leukocyte granules with Sudan black B. J Pathol Bacteriol 59:336, 1947

15. Stasi R, Bruno A, Venditti A et al: Leukocyte alkaline phosphatase score in plasma cell dyscrasias: Correlation with disease severity and circulating levels of granulocyte colony stimulating factor. Leuk Lymphoma 17:479, 1995

16. Tani E, Costa I, Svedmyr E et al: Diagnosis of lymphoma, leukemia, and metastatic tumor involvement of the cerebrospinal fluid by cytology and immunocytochemistry. Diagn Cytopathol 12:14, 1995

17. Valle S: Special stains in the microwave oven. J Histotechnol 9:237, 1986

18. Walach N, Gur Y: Leukocyte alkaline phosphatase and carcinoembryonic antigen in lung cancer patients. Oncology 50:279, 1993

19. Walach N, Gur Y: Leukocyte alkaline phosphatase as a probable predictor of the metastatic state in breast and colon cancer patients. Oncology 52:12, 1995

20. Wislocki GB, Rheingold JJ, Dempsey EW: The occurrence of the periodic acid-Schiff reaction in various normal cells of blood and connective tissue. Blood 4:562, 1949

21. Witzig TE, Phyliky RL, Li CY et al: T-cell chronic lymphocytic leukemia with a helper/inducer membrane phenotype. A distinct clinicopathologic subtype with a poor prognosis. Am J Hematol 21:139, 1986

22. Zucker-Franklin D, Greaves MF, Grossi CE et al: Atlas of Blood Cells, Function and Pathology. Philadelphia, Lea and Febiger, 1981

CHAPTER 30

Laboratory Evaluation of Body Fluids

Joy Jarvis Gall

Objectives

1. State four general conditions detected and monitored by laboratory analysis of body fluids.
2. State the primary differences in appearance and in *general* composition between cerebrospinal fluid (CSF) and serous fluid; between serous fluid and synovial fluid.
3. State the reference ranges for erythrocyte and leukocyte counts in CSF, and the types of cells normally present.
4. Contrast the predominant cell types seen in CSF in the different phases of bacterial meningitis and viral meningitis.
5. State four features of CSF that can differentiate traumatic tap from true hemorrhage and describe the cell types consistent with marrow contamination.
6. Describe the hematologic examination of body fluids, to include macroscopic observation, procedure for hemocytometer erythrocyte and leukocyte counts, preparation and examination of cytocentrifuge preparations, and reporting results.
7. State ten sources of error in performing cell counts and differentials, and one remedy for each.
8. Define an effusion. State at least three criteria for classifying an effusion as a transudate or an exudate, and the clinical significance of each classification.

The evaluation of body fluids is often treated as an afterthought by clinical laboratory texts and educational programs. Consequently, the attitude of students and veteran laboratorians alike toward body fluids is frequently one of apprehension, and even avoidance. Armed with knowledge and a bit of experience, the laboratorian can accomplish the processing and examination of body fluids with the same confidence, skill, and accuracy as if performing routine CBC and differentials.

Generally, the purpose of laboratory analysis of body fluids, regardless of type, is to detect and monitor one of four conditions: *infection, hemorrhage, malignancy,* or *inflammation.* These will be discussed in detail in this chapter.

Body fluids are quite diverse, with extreme variation in physical properties, cell count, and cell types. Each sample must be treated individually. A comprehensive treatment of body fluids is beyond the scope of this text. However, every laboratory engaging in body fluid examination should have books devoted exclusively to this topic on hand for reference.[9,18]

The body fluids to be discussed can be divided into three types: cerebrospinal fluid, serous fluid, and synovial fluid.

CEREBROSPINAL FLUID

General Considerations

Three membranes, or meninges, cover the brain and spinal cord (Fig 30-1). These membranes, from outside inward, are the *dura mater,* a thick fibrous material containing several dural venous sinuses, just beneath the cranium; the *arachnoid mater* or membrane, which is complex, weblike, and contains the surface cerebral blood vessels; and the *pia mater,* delicate and directly in contact with the brain. Cerebral spinal fluid (CSF) is located in the *subarachnoid space,* or under the arachnoid membrane, in the thin space between the arachnoid membrane and pia mater. The capillaries of the pia mater form the choroid plexus (see Color Plate 30-1) that project into the ventricular system of the brain. Most CSF is formed in these choroid plexus, and circulates over the brain and around the spinal cord. Resorption into the venous circulation occurs by the villi in the arachnoid membrane, which extend into the dural sinuses and form an interface

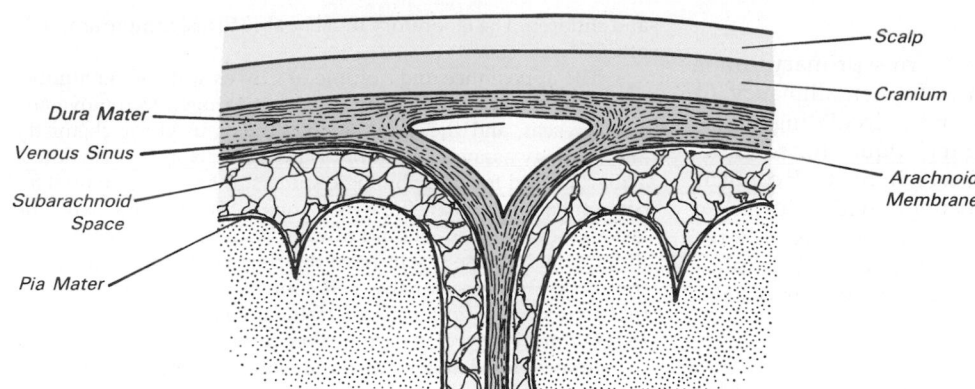

FIGURE 30-1. Outer subarachnoid system of CNS.

between CSF and blood.[1] There is a constant turnover of CSF, at a rate of about 20 mL per hour. Total volume of CSF is 90 to 150 mL in adults, 60 to 100 mL in children, and 10 to 60 mL in neonates and infants.

The function of CSF is to cushion and protect the brain and spinal cord from sudden changes in pressure and provide a site for metabolic exchange of nutrients and waste. Unlike most tissues, the brain and spinal cord do not communicate directly with blood for this exchange. Rather, CSF acts as a buffer between blood and central nervous system tissues.

The blood–brain barrier determines the rate of passage of plasma constituents from blood to CSF and brain. Some substances diffuse freely, some are regulated within narrow limits, and some are blocked completely.

The anatomic components of the blood–brain barrier are the choroid plexus epithelium and the endothelium of all the capillaries in contact with the CSF. The choroid plexus epithelium capillaries are enclosed by specialized ependyma. The capillary endothelial cells differ from those in other tissues in that tight junctions are present between adjacent cells. Thus, a physical barrier is formed. Constituents which diffuse freely between plasma and CSF, such as glucose, urea, and creatinine, require hours to equilibrate. Large molecules, such as many proteins and drugs, diffuse very slowly or not at all, and do not enter CSF from blood. CSF normally contains less than 1% of the total protein present in plasma. In addition to diffusion, active transport and secretion also occur. Together these mechanisms accomplish the regulation of passage of substances between blood and CSF. Concentration of most constituents in CSF varies from that in blood.

Abnormalities of CSF

INFECTIONS

Analysis of CSF is the primary diagnostic tool for infections of the meninges, or *meningitis*, for which it is highly sensitive and specific. Meningitis can be bacterial, viral, treponemal (tertiary syphilis), tuberculous (as in tuberculosis), fungal (*e.g.,* histoplasmosis or cryptococcus), and rarely, amebic. CSF is useful but is somewhat less sensitive in detecting other central nervous system (CNS) infections, such as encephalitis, brain abscess, and paraspinal abscess.

The most important application of CSF evaluation is the diagnosis of acute bacterial meningitis and its differentiation from aseptic (viral) meningitis. Bacterial meningitis is rapidly fatal if untreated but usually responds completely to early, appropriate antibiotic treatment. A delay of mere hours in treatment may result in permanent neurologic impairment (*e.g.,* sensorial deafness). If suspicion is strong, empirical antibiotic treatment may be instituted immediately based in part on cell count and differential results, and prior to availability of culture results. Viral meningitis, however, is less serious, usually self-limiting, and requires only supportive treatment. Immunocompromised patients, including those with acquired immunodeficiency syndrome (AIDS), are susceptible to a variety of opportunistic infections.

HEMORRHAGE

Subarachnoid hemorrhage (SAH), or bleeding into the subarachnoid space where CSF circulates, is confirmed with 100% sensitivity by detection of blood in CSF. Specificity, however, is only 80%, owing to introduction of blood into CSF by traumatic tap in as many as 20% of patients.[15] Although computed tomography (CT) scan has only moderate sensitivity for detection of SAH, a positive CT scan with a clear patient history can obviate the need for CSF examination.

SAH has many causes, one of which is cerebral aneurysm. Ruptured cerebral aneurysm occurs in 28,000 people per year in North America, and is associated with death or permanent disability in two-thirds of patients. Rupture is commonly preceded by a minor hemorrhage hours, days, or weeks before. This minor leak is most always heralded by a moderate to severe, unremitting headache of sudden onset and unusual location. Various other symptoms such as nausea and vomiting may accompany it. This event is often misdiagnosed as migraine, neuralgia, or even gastroenteritis. If this minor leak is diagnosed, surgery can be performed to repair the aneurysm with excellent results. In one study, CT scan was negative in 55% of patients with a minor leak. CSF examination, when performed, was always positive.[14] Sensitivity of CSF examination for detecting other types of intracranial hemorrhage ranges from 25% to 50%.[15]

MALIGNANCY

Malignancy in CNS may take three forms: primary tumor of the CNS, secondary metastasis from malignancy in other tissues, or seeding of the CSF by circulating leukemia or lymphoma cells. Imaging techniques for solid tumors or the finding of malignant cells in the CSF confirm suspected CNS malignancy in patients with neurologic symptoms. Periodic examination of CSF is frequently requested for patients with certain leukemias and lymphomas because of their great propensity for invasion of CSF.

DEMYELINATING DISORDERS

Demyelinating disorders include multiple sclerosis (MS) and Guillain-Barré syndrome (infectious polyneuritis). CSF in patients with MS may contain normal protein levels but elevated levels of IgG. Polyacrylamide gel electrophoresis with isoelectric focusing of gamma globulin may be used in the diagnosis.[2,9] Guillain-Barré syndrome is typically associated with a very high CSF protein (e.g., 200 mg/dL).[15] Myelin basic protein, a component of myelin nerve sheath, is released into CSF during demyelinating diseases, as well as other inflammatory conditions. Plasma cells may be seen in both MS and Guillain-Barré.

Sample Collection and Handling

CSF may be obtained by cisternal puncture, lateral cervical (neck) puncture, ventricular cannulas (shunts), or lumbar puncture (LP). All but LP usually require the expertise of a neurosurgeon.[15]

LP is the most commonly performed method for collection of CSF. The most common complication of LP is headache, with reported incidence of 10% to 35%, which can persist for several days. It is caused by decreased pressure and residual CSF leakage after the tap.[4]

Traumatic tap is the inadvertent puncture of local blood vessels before reaching the subarachnoid space, contaminating the CSF with peripheral blood. The first CSF collected ranges from pink to red, corresponding to slightly to grossly bloody. Once the subarachnoid space is reached, subsequent fluid contains less blood and gradually clears as collection proceeds. Blood from a traumatic tap lessens from tube 1 to tube 3 or 4. Depending on the skill of the person performing the tap, trauma should be minimal, and fluid should be crystal clear by the last tube. Normal CSF is clear and colorless, resembling water. Peripheral blood contamination invalidates many CSF determinations, or makes their interpretation extremely difficult. Grossly bloody taps may contain clots.

Bone marrow contamination of the sample can take place if the needle penetrates vertebral marrow. Nucleated red blood cells (NRBC) in all stages and immature leukocytes in the sample can be evidence of bone marrow contamination. Peripheral blood contamination may present this picture as well, if NRBC and a left shift are present in the peripheral blood, as is often the case with neonates. In leukemic patients with circulating blasts, care must be taken to avoid confusion of marrow or blood contamination of CSF with CNS involvement from leukemia.

SAMPLE HANDLING

Technique. CSF is collected in 3 or 4 sterile tubes numbered sequentially in order of collection and labeled. Anticoagulant is not required because CSF contains negligible fibrinogen and does not clot. Although 1 to 4 mL may be placed in each tube, frequently the volumes are much less, especially from infants and children. The laboratory must be able to test minute amounts of CSF.

The appearance and volume of CSF as well as the number of each tube are recorded. Tube 1 is centrifuged to remove any cells present, and the supernatant fluid is used for chemistry and serology assays. The color of this supernatant is also noted. Tube 2 is used for microbiologic studies. It has less potential for contamination by skin flora than tube 1. Tube 3 or 4, with the last aliquot obtained, should always be used for cell count and differential because it will have the least contamination from a traumatic tap. Occasionally, cell counts may be ordered on all tubes to aid in distinguishing a traumatic tap from hemorrhage. Excess fluid is saved in case further tests are indicated.

Immediate delivery to the laboratory and prompt processing and analysis of the CSF are essential for two reasons. First, the serious nature of illness involving the CNS requires swift action. Second, even slight delay adversely affects some CSF determinations, particularly glucose and cell counts which deteriorate quickly. CSF is hypotonic (specific gravity is 1.007). It also has a very low concentration of proteins and lipids. These factors contribute to rapid cell destruction. For example, the initial neutrophil count decreases by 32% in 1 hour and by 50% in 2 hours post collection. Significant reduction in lymphocytes and monocytes is not seen until after 3 hours.[19] Lysis of erythrocytes in CSF begins 1 hour after SAH or introduction into CSF by traumatic tap. If delay is unavoidable, tubes for chemistry and cell counts should be refrigerated. Tubes for culture should *not* be refrigerated, however, due to loss of some fastidious organisms.

For most cases of bacterial meningitis, a delay would not confuse the interpretation of laboratory data. However, there are some situations, such as the differentiation of early bacterial meningitis from aseptic (viral) meningitis in which prompt cell counts may be critical.

Laboratory Tests

ROUTINE TESTS

There is general agreement that a cell count with a cell concentrate differential and protein and glucose levels should be performed on all CSF.[10]

Cell Count with Differential. The cell count with differential is a sensitive and often specific indicator of disease. Presence of RBC, in the absence of traumatic tap, indicates hemorrhage. The degree of increase and the presence or absence of certain leukocyte types are consistent with different disease entities. Malignant cells and microorganisms may be detected during the cell differential examination.

Protein Level. Protein elevation (>45 mg/dL) in CSF is a sensitive but nonspecific finding in the majority of diseases affecting CSF. Four mechanisms are responsible for protein elevation in CSF during a disease process: (1) increased permeability of the blood–brain barrier; (2) decreased removal of protein molecules at the arachnoid villi; (3) mechanical obstruction to circulation of CSF; and (4) increased synthesis of immunoglobulin by lymphocytes and plasma cells within the CNS.

Falsely elevated CSF protein results from traumatic tap. Note that neonates normally have relatively high CSF protein (150 mg/dL) owing to an immature blood–brain barrier.

Glucose Level. Decreased glucose (<40 mg/dL) has long been highly associated with acute or chronic bacterial, tuberculous, fungal, amebic, or parasitic meningitis. It is useful as a screen for these infections, and favors their diagnosis over viral meningitis. However, a low glucose level can be an insensitive and nonspecific indicator of such infections. Glucose can be normal in 45% of patients with bacterial meningitis.[7,15] Conversely, it can be decreased in 25% of viral meningitis cases.[12]

Three mechanisms are involved in decreasing CSF glucose: impaired glucose transport; increased glycolytic activity of the CNS; and glucose utilization by WBCs, microorganisms, or malignant cells. CSF glucose should *always* be interpreted in conjunction with a simultaneous blood glucose level. Hypoglycemia (low blood glucose) decreases CSF levels even in the absence of CNS disease. Conversely, recently elevated blood glucose will increase CSF glucose, falsely raising the CSF level to normal in the presence of disease. A traumatic tap will also obscure the true CSF glucose level.

ADDITIONAL TESTS

It has been recommended that if the CSF pressure, cell counts with a cell concentrate differential, and protein are normal, no further testing is necessary. Immunocompromised patients, suspected bacterial meningitis in children, and suspected MS are exceptions to this recommendation. If these guidelines are followed, an estimated 48% of additional tests could be eliminated.[7]

The outcome of routine screening tests and clinical history determine which additional tests are indicated. Such tests are numerous, some are highly specialized, and some are just emerging from research to clinical application. Table 30-1 lists many in current use.

TABLE 30-1
Additional Tests Performed on CSF

Tests	Application/Comments
MICROBIOLOGY	
Gram stain	Preliminary classification of bacteria
Acid-fast stains, cultures	Tuberculosis
India ink, nigrosin stain	Cryptococcus
Bacterial cultures	Both CSF and blood
Viral cultures	Limited value; moderate sensitivity; feces, urine, saliva, or throat cultures sometimes more sensitive for systemic virus invading CSF; slow turnaround time
Fungal cultures	Limited value; may require large volume of CSF
Antibiotic sensitivities	
Limulus amoebocyte lysate for endotoxin assay	Positive in gram-negative infections
Wet mount, immunofluorescent methods, electron microscopy	Amoebic meningoencephalitis due to *Naegleria fowleri*
SEROLOGY	
Countercurrent immunoelectrophoresis	Bacterial and fungal antigens; faster than culture
Latex agglutination	
Enzyme-linked immunosorbent assay (ELISA)	
Serum viral antibody titer increase	Most sensitive, but impractical owing to large numbers of potential viruses
FTA-ABS (fluorescent treponemal antibody with absorption)	With positive serum FTA (fluorescent treponemal antibody) in syphilis patients
VDRL	
Fibrin derivative D-dimer by latex agglutination	Differentiate subarachnoid hemorrhage (SAH; present) from traumatic tap (absent)
CYTOLOGY AND IMMUNOPATHOLOGY	
Stains, monoclonal antibodies for immunophenotypic studies, tumor markers	Malignant cell identification
MOLECULAR GENETICS	
Polymerase chain reaction	Detects small numbers of malignant cells using minimal volume of CSF
CHEMISTRY	
Protein electrophoresis	Gamma globulin (IgG) increase
Beta-2 transferrin	Present only in CSF, not serum, tears, nasal secretions, etc.; confirm CSF leakage from nose, ears, or eyes after head injury
Beta-2 microglobulin	CNS leukemia, lymphoma
Myelin basic protein	Demyelinating disorders, trauma
C-reactive protein	Meningitis
Lactate dehydrogenase	Bacterial *vs* viral meningitis; SAH, stroke, malignancy
Creatine kinase	Prognosis after brain damage
Lactate	Meningitis

Hematologic Examination

Hematologic examination includes macroscopic observations, erythrocyte (RBC) and leukocyte (WBC) counts (usually by hemocytometer), and examination of cells which have been concentrated on a glass slide and stained with Wright stain.

Procedures presented are examples only and offer general guidelines gleaned from the many methodologies in use. Each laboratory must review the literature and establish its procedures according to its personnel, equipment, and patient population.

MACROSCOPIC OBSERVATIONS

Procedure

1. Record appearance, which includes both *color* and *clarity*. CSF should be colorless. If not colorless, (slightly xanthochromic [faintly pink or yellow], xanthochromic, slightly bloody, or bloody), the sample may be centrifuged to remove intact cells and the color of the supernatant is recorded. Clarity may be clear, slightly cloudy (turbid), cloudy, or bloody. Note any other inclusions, such as clots or bits of tissue. Consistency is normally that of water. Record it only in rare cases of increased viscosity from capsular polysaccharides of *Cryptococcus*.
2. Record tube number. Ideally, tube 3 or 4 is used for hematology. However, more than one tube may be submitted for cell counts, in an attempt to distinguish SAH from traumatic tap. Note type of container.
3. Record volume.

Sources of Error. Normal CSF is clear and colorless. Xanthochromia generally results from RBC lysis, release of hemoglobin into the CSF, and subsequent conversion of hemoglobin to bilirubin. The term *xanthochromia* is used when reporting orange or yellow color of CSF because it implies an abnormal yellow. Conversely, *yellow* is used in reference to serous and joint fluids since it is their normal color.

An elapse of 1 hour or more after collection before examining CSF will allow RBCs introduced during traumatic tap to lyse, thus producing xanthochromia not originally present. This may give a false impression of SAH.

Solutions containing iodine used to disinfect the skin prior to LP are amber in color, and are sometimes dried on the exterior of the transparent plastic CSF tube. This may go unnoticed, and the clear CSF is erroneously viewed through the iodine as xanthochromic.

Due to the difficulty of CSF recollection, cell counts and differential may be performed on samples with small clots; however, a comment that clots were present and adversely affect accuracy must be included. A completely clotted sample should not be counted but may be resuspended so that a film can be made, stained and examined for specific cell types or abnormalities.

Comments and Clinical Significance. Turbidity becomes perceptible if the WBC count exceeds 200×10^6/L; the RBC count exceeds 400×10^6/L; microorganisms, lipids, or radiographic contrast media are present; or if protein is increased. Lipids result from fat embolism or fat aspirated during LP. Pink or red color becomes noticeable as the RBC count rises from SAH or traumatic tap.

Infrequent causes of xanthochromic CSF include (1) bilirubin secondary to elevated serum direct bilirubin and jaundice with a normal blood–brain barrier (BBB); (2) high total bilirubin as in neonates with an immature BBB; (3) elevated CSF protein (>150 mg/dL); (4) hypercarotenemia due to the yellow pigment

beta-carotene from increased intake of yellow vegetables in food faddism; and (5) melanin pigment produced by meningeal malignant melanoma.

Clotting is absent with SAH. However, clots may form in bloody CSF from traumatic tap. Clots may also be present with extreme protein elevation as in Froin's syndrome (subarachnoid block), or in suppurative (pus-producing) or tuberculous meningitis.

COUNTING CELLS IN CSF

General Considerations. Reference ranges for blood cells in CSF are found in Table 30-2. Cell counts in most CSF samples are well below the lower limits of accuracy and background count of electronic cell counters. As previously mentioned, even a slightly cloudy specimen has WBC and RBC counts in the range of 200 to 400 cells $\times$ 10^6/L. Typical electronic counters may have a lower limit below which cell counts are not accurate (*e.g.*, 200×10^6/L for WBC and $20,000 \times 10^6$/L for RBC). Therefore, manual counting of undiluted CSF using a hemocytometer is usually required. Cloudy or bloody samples may require dilution prior to manual count. Purulent or grossly bloody CSF may be counted electronically, with certain precautions.

Laboratorians accustomed to manual WBC and platelet counts by hemocytometer on whole blood are often uncomfortable with CSF counts for a number of reasons. First, counts vary widely from zero to thousands. For this reason, there is no predetermined dilution to use. Second, the area counted for CSF must be adjusted depending on the number of cells present. Generally, the fewer the cells, the more area is counted. Third, RBC in CSF are not lysed and must be distinguished from WBC. Finally, CSF may contain unfamiliar cells such as lining cells, histiocytes, and malignant cells not seen in whole blood. Hence, more *judgment* must be exercised when counting CSF cells.

It is advisable to first examine undiluted CSF using the hemocytometer to assess the situation. Ascertain whether cells are countable. RBC or WBC may predominate, with great disparity in the numbers of each. If cells are packed in a single layer or overlapping, dilution will

TABLE 30-2 *Reference Ranges for WBCs and RBCs in CSF*		
	WBC	
Patient Age (Years)	*SI Units (/L)*	*Conventional Units (/μL)*
<1	$0–30 \times 10^6$	0–30
1–4	$0–20 \times 10^6$	0–20
5–puberty	$0–10 \times 10^6$	0–10
Adult	$0–5 \times 10^6$	0–5
	RBC	
	SI Units (/L)	*Conventional Units (/μL)*
All ages	0×10^6	0

be necessary. The lowest dilution to use for each cell type to render it reasonably easy to count is determined through experience. If the estimated count of RBC or WBC is within the range of the electronic cell counter, automated counts may be feasible.

Accurate dilutions of small volumes can be prepared with automatic pipettes found in most laboratories. The Unopette system (Becton Dickinson, Rutherford, NJ) of disposable reservoirs filled with various premeasured diluents and accompanying pipettes may be appropriate in some cases.

There are two ways to report cell counts in CSF. One is to report the RBC count and the total nucleated cell count. Nucleated cells include WBC, ependymal cells, histiocytes, malignant cells, and NRBC. This method has the advantage of being easier, since discrimination between nucleated cell types is not required. However, it offers less useful information to the clinician, who is interested primarily in the exact WBC count and secondarily in the presence of other cell types.

The preferred method is to report both the WBC and RBC counts. This necessitates recognition and omission of non-leukocytes. Later, non-leukocytes may be identified and semiquantitated on the differential examination. Discrimination between leukocytes and non-leukocytes may prove difficult on some specimens. In these cases, all nucleated cells on the chamber may be counted and the count corrected for all non-leukocytes based on the WBC differential. Other cells are enumerated separately per 100 WBC. Correction is calculated in a similar manner to the correction of a whole blood WBC count for NRBC (Chap. 24). Regardless of whether WBC or total nucleated cells are reported by the laboratory, the report should be clearly stated, and consistency should be maintained.

Procedure for Manual RBC Count

1. Thoroughly mix the sample.
2. Insert a plain microhematocrit capillary tube into the appropriate CSF sample and fill about three-fourths full, or using an adjustable automatic pipette, withdraw 11 μL of mixed sample.
3. Transfer the undiluted CSF to one side of a Neubauer hemocytometer with coverslip in place by touching the tip of the capillary tube to the edge of the coverslip or by expelling the measured sample from the pipette. Rotate the chamber, and fill the other side. Verify that fluid is properly mounted (*i.e.*, the chamber should be completely filled with no micro- or macro-flooding). Cells will settle in about 1 minute.
4. Scan both sides on low power (10× objective). Observe for even distribution of cells. Determine whether dilution of RBCs is needed.
5. If distribution is poor, reload. If dilution is needed, prepare the desired dilution using isotonic saline and reload.
6. Refer to the Neubauer hemocytometer (Fig. 24-2). Determine the area to be counted. Guidelines for choosing the area to count are:[9]
   a. If less than 200 cells are present in all 9 squares (roughly <20 cells per square), count all 9 squares. Area counted is 9 mm².
   b. If more than 200 cells are present in all 9 squares, count the four corner squares. Area counted is 4 mm².
   c. If more than 200 cells are present in 1 square, count five of the squares *within the center square* for an area of 0.2 mm².
7. Count RBC in the appropriate area using high power (40×).

It is a good idea to count WBC separately as well, for comparison to the WBC count to be performed later.

8. Count the same number of squares on the other side. Cell counts on the two sides should agree within 10% of the lower count. Greater differences require a repeat of steps 1 through 8.[9]
9. Calculate the number of RBC per microliter (μL) or per liter (L) in the CSF (Chap. 24). It should be noted that frequently there is no dilution of CSF. For example, using undiluted CSF, if 4 WBC are counted in nine squares of a Neubauer chamber, the calculation would be

$$\text{Total WBC} / \mu\text{L} = \frac{4 \times 10}{9} = 4 \quad \text{or} \quad \frac{4}{0.9} = 4$$

Sources of Error in Manual RBC Counts. Normal RBC appear round with translucent, smooth centers, and are equal to or smaller than WBC in size. They may have a faint grayish or greenish cast. However, they can vary considerably in size and appearance. They may be shrunken or swollen. When *crenated*, the projections give a more textured look, causing confusion with small WBCs such as lymphocytes. *Ghost cells* are RBC membranes from which hemoglobin has laked (leaked). They are barely visible and difficult to count. Presence of ghost cells will falsely lower the RBC count, and a comment to this effect should be reported.

WBC are the size of RBC or larger, round, and colorless. Their texture is grainy, resembling frosted glass. The nucleus may or may not be discernible. Lining cells, macrophages, and many malignant cells are larger than WBC and have round nuclei. They may be clumped. Histiocytes often contain large vacuoles or debris.

Incorrect cell identification is common with inexperience. Crenated RBC and lymphocytes have a subtle difference in texture that is indistinguishable to the novice. Counting WBC as RBC or vice versa produces falsely high values. A combination of errors usually occurs. Counting WBC separately while performing the RBC count is helpful in revealing these errors. This count is used to cross-check the later count done on stained WBC, and they should be similar. If not, error in the RBC count is likely.

As with any manual cell count, proper technique is crucial to accurate results. Incomplete mixing, micro-flooding (resulting in lifting of the coverslip and an inaccurate count), macro-flooding (overflow into the moat resulting in a falsely decreased count), poor cell distribution, or calculation error will invalidate results. Calculation errors are all too common. To state the obvious, it is imperative that the dilution used, if any, and the area counted be remembered and used properly in the calculation. For example, if 1/5th of the middle square is counted, 5 mm² is sometimes erroneously used instead of 0.2 mm² for area counted. Actually, *5/25 of one mm²* was counted, not 5 mm².

Elapse of 1 hour or more between LP and cell counts produces falsely low counts because of cell lysis. Counting too slowly allows evaporation and receding of the fluid in the chamber and falsely increases the count. Too much light renders unstained cells invisible, and counts of zero may be erroneously reported. The contrast should be increased by lowering the condenser, partially closing the diaphragm, and decreasing the light intensity.

Yeast forms, if not budding, can be easily mistaken for RBCs. Yeast is somewhat more refractile. Yeast may also be seen after RBC lysis on the chamber for WBC count, and on the stained slide.

Differentiating Subarachnoid Hemorrhage (SAH) from Traumatic Tap. Normally there are no RBC in pure CSF. If present, they originate from SAH or from peripheral blood contamination during collection. The clinician attempts to determine the cause of RBC in CSF by correlating patient history and examination, CT scan, and CSF hematologic findings.

Presence of xanthochromia (if noted within 1 hour of collection), an approximately consistent RBC count in all tubes, positive D-dimer,[13] and macrophages containing RBC, hemosiderin, or hematoidin seen on the stained slide are all strong evidence of hemorrhage. Conversely, absence of xanthochromia, decreasing RBC numbers in sequentially collected tubes, negative D-dimer, lack of erythrophagia, and clotting are more consistent with traumatic tap. Declining RBC count in serial tubes is not specific; counts may be divergent in either case. RBC crenation is *not* a distinguishing characteristic.

A study compared xanthochromia and RBC count in sequential tubes to D-dimer for differentiation of traumatic LP from SAH. Only D-dimer *clearly* differentiated between the two, with 100% sensitivity and specificity.[13]

It must be remembered that SAH and traumatic tap are not mutually exclusive; they can be concurrent.

Procedure for Manual Leukocyte Count. This method makes use of a solution of powdered crystal violet dissolved in concentrated glacial acetic acid (add stain to acetic acid until a deep purple color is achieved) in sufficient quantity to produce purple staining of WBC nuclei in CSF. Undiluted glacial acetic acid alone is often used to lyse RBC and to improve visibility of WBC. It is strong enough to be effective in a very minute quantity, resulting in negligible dilution of the CSF. Addition of crystal violet stain further enhances nuclear detail.

1. Coat the inside of a plain microhematocrit capillary tube with crystal violet–acetic acid solution. Tap the end of the tube several times on absorbent pad to drain excess stain. Set aside.
2. Insert a *clean* capillary tube into well-mixed CSF and fill about three-fourths full. *To avoid contaminating the CSF, do not place the stain-coated tube directly into the CSF.*
3. Transfer the CSF from the plain tube to the coated tube by placing the tubes end-to-end and allowing the CSF to flow into the coated tube.
4. Mix the fluid with the stain by holding the tube horizontally and slowly tilting it back and forth while rolling it between the fingers, being careful not to spill. Expel the first couple of drops onto an absorbent pad before mounting it on the chamber. (These first drops can be mostly stain. The column of CSF pushes some of the stain coating forward as it enters the coated tube.)
5. Properly load both sides of a Neubauer chamber. Wait about 3 minutes for RBC to lyse, WBC to stain, and settling.
6. Scan both sides on low power. Observe for even distribution of WBC. Determine if dilution is needed (see General Considerations).
7. Decide what area is to be counted using the guidelines previously presented. Count the WBCs in the appropriate area using high power. They will have a purple nucleus and transparent cytoplasm.
8. Count the same number of squares on the other side. If agreement is poor, repeat the procedure. Calculate the WBC count (Chap. 24).

Sources of Error. Counting other nucleated cells as WBCs causes a positive error. Staining makes cell identification easier. Lining cells, histiocytes, and most malignant cells are larger with a round nucleus and abundant cytoplasm. Macrophages may contain vacuoles or debris. RBC may be resistant to lysis in neonates or when rbc are high. These may be counted as WBC.

NRBC are sometimes present. They most resemble lymphocytes, but with a smoother nuclear texture and more clear cytoplasm. They should be omitted from the count unless identification is too difficult. In such cases, they are included and the WBC count is corrected after counting the number of NRBC per 100 WBC on the CSF differential (Chap. 24).

Yeast forms will stain, if not heavily encapsulated, as a solid purple round, oval, or budding form. Bacteria will stain as well. Stained debris and yeast can be mistaken for WBC. If both distinct nucleus and cytoplasm are not visible, or if the material is refractile, it is not a cell. WBC counts are also subject to poor technique and calculation error.

The count should be compared with the unstained WBC tallied during the RBC count. A significant difference indicates error in the count or calculations. Because stained WBC are relatively easy to count, the error often is in the unstained count, making the RBC count suspect as well. The discrepancy must be resolved.

As with all laboratory testing, one should always question whether the results *make sense.* For example, a WBC count of zero is unlikely if several thousand RBC are present. In one instance a student gave a cursory glance for stained WBC and saw none, although 12,000 RBC/μL were present. Her supervisor noticed the inconsistency and reexamined the chamber. The WBC were very pale. New stain solution with insufficient crystal violet had been prepared. The stain was adjusted, and the count repeated. Many WBC were indeed present.

If a traumatic tap is likely, the ratio of WBC to RBC in the patient's PB may be compared with that in the CSF. If these ratios are approximately equal, the WBC are most likely due to PB contamination. If the ratio is higher in CSF, increased WBC are probably present in the CSF, indicating CNS disease. This correction is only approximate and is quite prone to error. The clinician usually makes this determination.

Electronic Cell Counts and Sources of Error. Most manufacturers of automated cell counters do not recommend them for body fluid counts. Their indiscriminate use will produce invalid counts and obstruct or damage the instrument. However, most laboratories do use them under specific conditions. Success can be achieved in carefully selected situations with certain precautions. The undiluted sample should always be previewed on the chamber and RBC and WBC counts estimated to verify that one or both are within the range of accuracy of the instrument. Often, for example, RBC are countable on the instrument, but WBC require a manual count, or *vice versa.* Also, the sample should be observed for nucleated cells other than WBC. Most instruments count these as leukocytes and mathematical correction based on the CSF WBC differential may be necessary. Finally, the presence of other interfering materials such as yeast, crystals (especially in joint fluids), or cell clumps should be noted, because they may invalidate automated counts and occlude flow cells or apertures, making dilution and manual count preferable. If a fluid is viscous, hyaluronidase must be added before counting.[9]

CONCENTRATING CELLS FOR WBC DIFFERENTIAL IN CSF

Formerly, a WBC differential was performed directly from the hemocytometer. Cells were classified as mononuclear or polymorphonuclear in an attempt to differentiate lymphocytes and monocytes from neutrophils. This was accomplished with great difficulty and considerable inaccuracy. Furthermore, the mononuclear category included immature neutrophils, blasts, lymphoma cells, tumor cells, lining cells, NRBC, and pyknotic neutrophils. Additionally, only a relatively small number of cells were available for classification, and no permanent slide was retained. The only advantage was that no special equipment was required. This method is now obsolete and unacceptable, except in rare instances in which an additional three drops of CSF are unavailable for concentration. Stained preparations of concentrated nucleated cells must be examined on all CSF samples including those with normal WBC counts.

Centrifugation, sedimentation, and filtration have all been used in an attempt to concentrate cells in CSF. Each suffers from several disadvantages, which include (1) use of 3 to 5 mL of CSF; (2) variable and incomplete cell recovery; (3)much cellular distortion and damage; (4) relatively long time required; (5) high level of skill required; and (6) the necessity for wet fixation of cells. Wet fixation is unsuitable for Wright-Giemsa staining, which requires air-dried slides fixed in methanol.

Today cytocentrifugation is the concentration method of choice. This method has many advantages. It uses relatively little sample, is fast, requires little skill, and provides good cell recovery with minimal distortion. Several slides can be spun simultaneously. Preparations are suitable for a variety of stains. The one disadvantage is the requirement for the special centrifuge and accompanying chambers (Fig. 30-2).

Procedure

1. One to 10 drops of CSF are placed in the cup of the cytocentrifuge chamber. Two drops of 22% albumin are added to increase yield and reduce cell distortion. The chamber is spun at low speed (200–1000 rpm) in a specialized centrifuge for 5 to 10 minutes. The fluid passes through the tube in the chamber toward a glass slide (Fig. 30-2). Cells are deposited on the

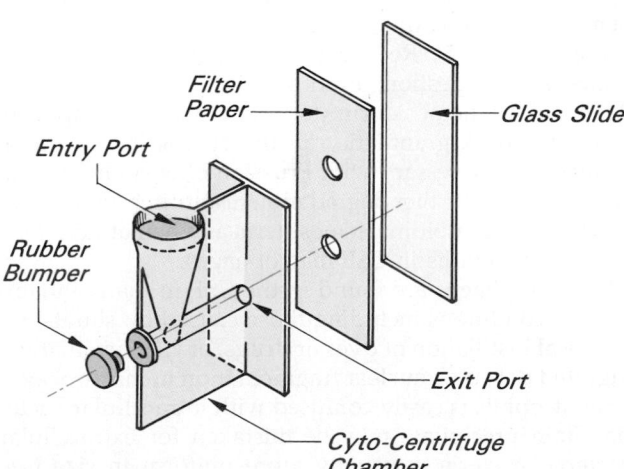

FIGURE 30-2. Cytocentrifuge technique for CSF concentration. Rubber bumper creates closed system between entry port where CSF is introduced and glass slide. This figure shows one of twelve chambers available in cytocentrifuge. The CSF and any cells contained therein leave chamber through exit port; excess fluid is absorbed by filter paper, and concentrated cells are deposited on glass slide. (Courtesy of Shandon, Inc., Publication No. CYTI, Pittsburgh, PA, December, 1976.)

slide in a concentrated button about 6 mm in diameter. Excess fluid is absorbed by filter paper surrounding the cell button. Slides are removed and air dried, ready for fixation and staining.

2. Wright-Giemsa stain is used for the routine examination and WBC differential. Additional slides can be prepared for microbiology stains, cytochemistries, and immunocytologic stains.

3. The entire cell button is scanned using low power (10×), paying particular attention to the edges. The examiner should be alert for any unusually large, unfamiliar, or suspicious cells or clumps of molded cells. Malignant cells can be rare and often are located on the edges. If suspicious cells are found, the slide should be referred to a pathologist for review and any unstained slides saved for possible additional testing.

4. Using an oil objective (50× or 100×), a WBC differential is performed in the same manner as on a peripheral blood film. If fewer than 100 WBC are present, all cells should be counted. This is the *relative differential*, expressed as a percentage of each WBC type.

5. If an *absolute differential* is to be reported, the percentage of each WBC type is multiplied by the total WBC count. The sum of the individual cell counts should equal the total WBC count.

6. The absolute differential is sometimes converted to total mononuclear WBC and total polymorphonuclear WBC for reporting. Mononuclear includes lymphocytes and monocytes. Polymorphonuclear includes all neutrophil stages, eosinophils, and basophils. Eosinophils are enumerated separately if present in significant numbers, typically more than 10%.[12] In addition to reporting these categories, any immature or abnormal cells must be reported separately.

7. Normal lining cells and histiocytes are usually not included in the differential. Their exact numbers are not clinically significant. They may be mentioned and semiquantitated as few, moderate, or many.

8. Any additional findings are also reported. These might include microorganisms, such as bacteria, yeast forms, or amoebae; reactive lymphocytes; histiocytes containing erythrocytes, hemosiderin, or hematoidin; NRBC; and pyknotic cells.

References Ranges for Leukocyte Differential in CSF. Lymphocytes and monocytes are the normal cellular components of CSF. Lymphocytes (70%) predominate in adults, and monocytes and macrophages (80%) predominate in neonates and young children.[9,17]

Before the use of cell concentrates for differential, any neutrophils were considered pathognomonic. However on cytocentrifuge preparations of normal CSF, a small number may be seen (up to about 8%)[9] and probably originate from minute peripheral blood contamination during LP. Their significance should be evaluated relative to the total number of cells present as well as the clinical picture and other laboratory findings.

A few lining cells and macrophages are normal. Ependymal cells and choroid plexus cells may rarely be seen in children, especially those with hydrocephalus and ventricular shunts.

Morphologic Evaluation

NORMAL CELLS

Most hematopoietic cells in CSF appear the same as they do in peripheral blood. Some artifacts from cytocentrifugation do occur, with lymphocytes particularly affected. The nuclear chromatin is more finely textured and the nucleolus more apparent, giving a false impression of immaturity. Nuclear shape is often irregular. Lymphocytes of infants, which normally tend to look somewhat immature on the peripheral film, can look similar to the lymphoblasts seen in acute lymphoblastic leukemia (ALL) after cytocentrifugation, especially on the edges of the button. Patient age and history should be considered when identifying these cells.[16]

A rare reactive lymphocyte may be seen. These are medium to large with abundant, deeply basophilic cytoplasm. Monocytes can sometimes be difficult to differentiate from macrophages—this is not surprising since macrophages are usually derived from monocytes. Both are relatively pale-staining cells with abundant pale-gray cytoplasm, which often contains vacuoles and finely textured chromatin. The monocyte nucleus can be ovoid, horse-shoe shaped, or lobular. Macrophages tend to be larger, and nuclear shape is round to oval.

Choroid plexus cells and ependymal cells are small, mature cells with low nuclear:cytoplasmic (N:C) ratio (see Color Plate 30-1). The nucleus is about the size of a red cell. They may be seen in clusters.

REACTIVE CELLS AND ORGANISMS

A *reactive lymphocytosis* (see Color Plate 30-2) features a broad spectrum of lymphocytes exhibiting various degrees of stimulation, from small resting cells to medium to large ones with varying amounts of deep blue cytoplasm and nucleoli. This diversity helps to differentiate a reactive population from the monotonous (clonal) picture in malignant conditions such as leukemia or lymphoma.

Increased CSF lymphocytes predominate in viral meningitis and occasionally in *early* bacterial meningitis (15%).[9] Lymphocytosis is common in acute bacterial meningitis when the CSF leukocyte count is 1000×10^6/L or less.[9] Lymphocytosis also occurs in *Listeria monocytogenes* meningitis; tuberculous, syphilitic, and fungal meningitis; partially treated bacterial meningitis; degenerative disorders such as multiple sclerosis and Guillain-Barré syndrome; and other inflammatory conditions. Lymphocytes can also be involved in a mixed-cell reaction.

Monocytes increase in CSF with other cells as part of a mixed-cell reaction in most infections and diseases. They usually do not predominate.

Neutrophils are subject to cytocentrifuge artifact. The nuclear segments are fanned out around the periphery of the cell. They deteriorate quickly in CSF, and *pyknotic* (degenerated) neutrophils (see Color Plate 30-3) are often seen. Nuclear lobes lose their chromatin pattern and become dense, dark-staining spheres. When the nucleus becomes a single mass, these necrotic neutrophils are frequently mistaken for NRBC. The difference lies in the cytoplasm which more closely matches the pinkish, finely granular look of neutrophils rather than the smooth appearance of NRBC cytoplasm.

Neutrophils commonly enter CSF from peripheral blood (PB) contamination during collection, and this must always be considered. Likewise, immature neutrophils frequently result from PB contamination in a patient with a left shift, or from bone marrow (BM) contamination (see Color Plate 30-4). In the latter, various stages of NRBC are present, and blasts may be seen. BM contamination is most common in infants and young children but occurs in adults as well. This picture should not be confused with leukemic cells in CSF. In addition to marrow, another common source of NRBC in CSF is peripheral blood contamination in infants who have circulating NRBC.

It is suggested that an eosinophilia of 10% or more is probably clinically significant and should be reported.[12] The most common cause of CSF eosinophilia is an allergic reaction to foreign material in the CNS. The culprit is usually a shunt, implanted to drain CSF into the peritoneal cavity or the venous system to control hydrocephalus in children.[9,21] Eosinophilia is often mild, but has been reported to be as high as 78%.[21] This is a local reaction and is not accompanied by a concomitant PB eosinophilia. A common cause of eosinophilia in some settings is invasion of the CNS by parasites like *Toxocara cati*, *Taenia solium*, cysticercosis, *Angiostrongylus cantonensis* (Southeast Asia), larva migrans, and others.

Basophils and mast cells can be seen in small numbers in various conditions. Their significance is unclear, but they may accompany eosinophilia.

Plasma cells frequently accompany reactive lymphs in CSF. They are seen in acute viral infections; subacute or chronic inflammatory processes such as tuberculosis, syphilis, sarcoidosis, and subacute sclerosing panencephalitis; multiple sclerosis; and Guillain-Barré syndrome.

Primitive cell clusters (PCCs) of probable germinal matrix origin mature to neuronal cells. They can be seen in CSF of premature infants suffering intraventricular hemorrhage or in infants with hydrocephalus. These immature blastlike cells are molded into clusters. They must be distinguished from normal choroid plexus cells and ependymal cells, from malignant CNS cells, and from lymphoblasts. Choroid plexus and ependymal cells cluster like PCCs, but have a lower nuclear-to-cytoplasmic ratio and a more mature nucleus. Malignant cells cluster as well but are larger. Lymphoblasts are nearly identical to PCCs, but they do not mold (conform) to one another. Age and history aid in the differential identification.[3]

Macrophages (with ingested RBCs, hemosiderin, or hematoidin [hematin]) are seen after hemorrhage (see Color Plate 30-5). Red cells are ingested within a few hours. After digestion, a red cell-sized vacuole appears. After 2 days, hemosiderin (form of stored iron) appears as coarse, dark granulation in the cytoplasm. It can be confirmed if necessary with Prussian blue stain for iron. After 2 weeks, further degradation results in bright amber crystals of hematoidin. Hemosiderin and hematoidin may persist for months in CSF macrophages.

Macrophages are found in the CSF in many inflammatory conditions including those caused by shunts, intrathecal instillation of dyes or drugs, or CNS irradiation. Ingested debris or nuclear fragmentation in macrophages or neutrophils is easily confused with intracellular bacteria. Stain precipitate may be mistaken for extracellular bacteria. Bacteria is usually more uniform in size (see Color Plate 30-6), and clustering, such as pairs, tetrads, or chains, can often be found. A Gram stain should be performed for confirmation.

Yeast and other fungal organisms are often unsuspected, but may be detected on cytocentrifuge preparations. Yeast may be oval or budding, and they may be encapsulated, and stain dense, dark purple. Other fungi can appear as pale blue bodies with an adjacent clearing within an oval structure.

Amoebae must be differentiated from macrophages. They have sky blue cytoplasm and a distinct, finely granular, violet nucleus.[9]

MALIGNANT CELLS

Solid Tumor Cells (Carcinoma). Tumors can originate in the CNS or metastasize from other sites. Common metastatic tumors, in order of frequency, originate in the lung, breast, kidney, and gastrointestinal tract. Melanoma and choriocarcinoma may also metastasize to the CNS.[9] Table 30-3 presents general characteristics of malignant cells. Mesothelial cells are not found in CSF. Any cell resembling mesothelial cells in CSF is highly suspicious for malignancy. Suspicious cells should be referred to a pathologist.

Hematopoietic Malignancies. Patients rarely present with CNS involvement by leukemia or lymphoma at the time of diagnosis. Rather, the malignant cells appear in the CSF during apparent remission induced by chemotherapy, which does not cross the blood–brain barrier to CSF. Therefore, treatment protocol requires periodic monitoring of CSF for leukemic or lymphoma cells.

Acute lymphoblastic leukemia (ALL) commonly invades the CNS. Lymphoblasts are seen on cytocentrifuge concentrates even when the CSF leukocyte count is normal (0 to 5×10^6/L). This can signify CNS relapse, subsequent marrow relapse and dictate the need for intensified systemic therapy and intrathecal therapy.[16] Although lymphoblasts have characteristic morphology (see Color Plate 30-7), they may be confused with normal lymphocytes exhibiting cytocentrifuge artifact, normal lymphocytes in neonates, or PCCs of germinal matrix origin.

Acute myelocytic leukemia (AML) invades the CNS less commonly. Of the AMLs, monocytic and acute progranulocytic leukemias are most likely to feature CNS involvement.

Cells of diffuse non-Hodgkin lymphoma in the CSF vary greatly depending on the type of lymphoma. Cells range from small, cleaved lymphoid cells to large and highly undifferentiated (blastlike) cells. Cells may exhibit molding. Any uniform or monotonous picture of lymphoid cells should raise suspicion of malignancy. Immunophenotypic analysis can be useful to distinguish reactive lymphocytosis from lymphomas.

In cases of multiple myeloma, immature and abnormal plasma cells may be present in CSF.

Whenever leukemia or lymphoma cells are seen in CSF, peripheral blood contamination with circulating blasts or bone marrow contamination must be ruled out.

SEROUS FLUID

Physiology of Serous Fluid

Serous (serum-containing) fluid includes pleural, pericardial, and peritoneal fluids, which are normally present in small amounts between two mesothelium-lined membranes that cover the lungs, heart, and abdominal organs, respectively. Serous fluid functions to reduce friction between the membranes thus facilitating movement of the organs within. The membranes are called serous membranes. One lines the organ itself within the cavity, and the other lines the cavity wall. Normally there is very little space between these two membranes; however, fluid accumulates in abnormal conditions.

Unlike CSF, serous fluid is an ultrafiltrate of plasma which is continuously produced and reabsorbed. Formation and resorption are controlled by capillary hydrostatic pressure, plasma oncotic (osmotic) pressure, capillary permeability, and lymphatic resorption. Systemic or local diseases that influence these factors can result in abnormal accumulation of serous fluid, called an *effusion*. When an effusion is present, it is removed therapeutically to relieve pressure exerted by the fluid on the organs and for laboratory evaluation.

Sample Collection and Handling

Collection is by aseptic needle aspiration. Complications are rare. Aspiration of pleural fluid is called *thoracentesis*. Aspiration of pericardial fluid is referred to as *pericardiocentesis*, and that of peritoneal (ascitic) fluid is *paracentesis*. As with CSF, traumatic tap can occur, causing contamination with peripheral blood. Blood is nonhomogeneous, and clears as aspiration proceeds. The fluid can be distributed into tubes as follows: (1) EDTA for gross appearance, cell counts, cell differential and morphology; (2) heparin for chemistry assays; (3) sterile heparin for microbiology; (4) heparin for cytology; and (5) a tube without anticoagulant to detect clotting. Blood for serum chemistries should be drawn simultaneously for comparison.

TABLE 30-3
Distinguishing Between Benign Mesothelial Cells and Malignant Cells

Benign	Malignant
Characteristic in size	Often large, giant
Cell clusters in flat sheets	Three-dimensional clumps; tumor balls
Cells touch, not molded	Molding
Distinct cell borders within cell groups	Indistinct cell borders in clumped cells
Cannibalism very rare	Cannibalism (cells within cells) common
Orderly, uniform appearance	Disorderly, bizarre
Round or oval nucleus	Irregular nuclear shape
If multinucleated, even number of uniform nuclei	If multinucleated, dissimilarity of nuclei
No nuclear molding	Nuclear molding
Nucleoli small or moderate	Nucleoli prominent, multiple, or irregular
Normal mitosis	Abnormal mitosis
Even chromatin pattern	Varied chromatin pattern within a cell
Low nuclear:cytoplasmic ratio	High nuclear:cytoplasmic ratio
Cytoplasmic membrane smooth, ruffled, or scalloped	Cytoplasmic tags
Artifactual nuclear clefts	Deep nuclear clefts

Laboratory Tests

IDENTIFICATION OF EFFUSIONS AS TRANSUDATES OR EXUDATES

It is diagnostically helpful to determine whether an effusion is a transudate or an exudate through laboratory evaluation.

A *transudate* is an ultrafiltrate of plasma which results from filtration of blood serum across a physically intact vascular wall. Its accumulation usually results from alteration of capillary hydrostatic pressure or plasma oncotic pressure by a systemic disease such as congestive heart failure, alcoholic liver cirrhosis, or hypoproteinemia associated with nephrotic syndrome. Once identified as a transudate, further testing of the effusion is not usually needed.

An *exudate* accumulates actively in association with vascular wall damage or decreased lymphatic resorption caused by local infection, hemorrhage, malignancy, or inflammation. Infections include tuberculosis, pneumonia, and peritonitis. Malignant proliferation damages vessel walls and obstructs lymphatic ducts. It is a major cause of exudates and is the most common cause of hemorrhage into serous fluid. Other causes of hemorrhage are pulmonary infarction and trauma. Inflammation may be associated with rheumatoid disease or systemic lupus erythematosus.

Table 30-4 summarizes tests for identification of effusions as transudates or exudates. No one test is sufficient, and there is some overlap of values. Therefore a constellation of test results is evaluated.

ADDITIONAL TESTS

The exudate may be submitted for gram and acid-fast staining; aerobic, acid-fast, anaerobic, and fungal cultures; cytology and tumor markers; pH; and enzymes such as lipase, amylase for pancreatic disease, or alkaline phosphatase for small intestine injury.

Hematologic Examination

Macroscopic observation, erythrocyte and leukocyte counts, and preparation and examination of Wright-stained cytocentrifuge preparations are essentially the same as for CSF. The following additions or exceptions are noted.

Because pale yellow is the color of normal serous fluid, the term *xanthochromic* is not used, because it implies hemoglobin degradation after hemorrhage. Even if Hb degradation did occur, it cannot be interpreted in the presence of the underlying yellow color.

A milky white or lipemic fluid is referred to as chylous or pseudochylous. *Chylous* fluids contain lipids leaked from lymphatic ducts secondary to trauma or malignancy. *Pseudochylous* fluids contain cholesterol crystals and cellular debris and are seen in tuberculosis and rheumatoid arthritis.

Green peritoneal fluid may contain bile from perforation of the gallbladder or intestine, or from cholecystitis or pancreatitis.

The acetic acid/crystal violet solution for manual WBC counts cannot be used on fluids with high protein content. Acetic acid causes protein to precipitate, causing trapping and clumping of WBC. Both RBC and WBC can be counted in undiluted, unstained fluid as described for CSF RBC counts. If dilution is necessary, isotonic saline can be used. One percent ammonium oxalate with or without methylene blue added can be used for WBC counts.

Fluids with high protein content and increased viscosity may require reduction or elimination of albumin used in the cytocentrifuge preparation.

TABLE 30-4
Identification of Effusions as Transudates or Exudates

Test/Observation	Transudate	Exudate
Color	Pale yellow	Pale yellow, yellow, or red
Clarity	Clear	Clear, cloudy, or turbid
Total protein*	<30 g/L, or <50% of serum level	>30 g/L or >50% of serum level
Specific gravity	<1.015	>1.015
WBC count	$<300 \times 10^6$/L	$>500 \times 10^6$/L
Fibrinogen	Absent; does not clot	Present; may clot
Glucose	Varies with serum level	<Serum level with some infections or high cell counts
Lactate dehydrogenase (LD)*	<200 U/L, or <60% of serum level	>200 U/L, or >60% of serum level due to cellular debris
RBC count	Low (absence of traumatic tap)	$>100,000 \times 10^6$/L if hemorrhage from malignancy, trauma, or pulmonary infarction
Cholesterol (pleural)*	<60 mg/dL	>60 mg/dL
Bilirubin (pleural)*	<60% of serum level	>60% of serum level
Serum-ascites albumin concentration gradient (*i.e.*, serum albumin minus ascites fluid albumin)*	1.1–2.1 g/dL	0.2–1.0 g/dL

* *Most reliable.*
Data from Kjeldsberg C, Knight J: *Body Fluids*, 3rd ed. Chicago, American Society of Clinical Pathologists, 1993; and Ringsrud K, Linne J: *Urinalysis and Body Fluids: A Color Text and Atlas*. St. Louis, Mosby, 1995.

Morphologic Evaluation

Neutrophils predominate in most bacterial infections and inflammatory processes.

Lymphocytes, reactive (or variant) lymphocytes, and a few plasma cells predominate in tuberculosis, viral infections, and malignancy. Plasma cells may be seen in pleural fluids from patients with rheumatoid arthritis.

Eosinophilia (greater than 10%) is characteristic of pneumothorax, hypersensitivity syndromes, and parasitic infections.

Monocytes and macrophages are present in normal, reactive, and malignant fluids.

Mature RBC are present in most effusions. They are greatly increased in malignancy, trauma, and infarction. Malignancy is the most common cause of bloody effusions.

Mesothelial cells of the serous membranes desquamate into most serous fluid. They are *not* found in CSF. They are 12 to 30 μm in diameter and occur singly, in sheets, or rarely in three-dimensional clusters (see Color Plate 30-8). The abundant cytoplasm is gray to deep blue with perinuclear pallor and may contain small vacuoles. Sometimes the cell resembles a "fried egg." Nuclei may be single or multiple and are smooth, round, and dark purple with uniformly distributed, stippled chromatin and 1 to 3 round nucleoli. Mesothelial cells are capable of becoming macrophages. Reactive mesothelial cells may contain large vacuoles and exhibit phagocytosis. They may undergo a morphologic transformation demonstrated by loss of basophilia and development of foamy vacuolization, thus becoming indistinguishable from macrophages. Intermediate forms are seen.

Mesothelial cells have no clinical significance, although they are characteristically absent in tuberculous effusions. The primary concern is to become familiar with them (see Color Plate 30-9), recognize them as normal, and avoid confusion with malignant cells. Table 30-3 compares distinguishing features of mesothelial cells and malignant cells. Samples containing cells suspicious for tumor (carcinoma) are referred to cytology for identification.

The detection of malignant cells is one of the most important reasons for examination of fluids (see Color Plate 30-10). Lung cancer is the leading cause of malignant pleural and pericardial effusions, followed by breast cancer. Mesothelioma, ovarian and gastrointestinal carcinoma, and malignant melanoma also frequently produce effusions. Mesothelioma is characterized by viscous or gelatinous fluid, resembling synovial fluid. Lymphoma is associated with chylous effusion.

SYNOVIAL FLUID

Physiology

Synovial fluid (SF), or joint fluid, is colorless to pale yellow and clear with a consistency similar to that of raw egg white.[6] It is an ultrafiltrate of plasma. It differs from serous fluid in that it contains hyaluronate (hyaluronic acid), a high molecular weight mucopolysaccharide polymer; and lubricin,[9] a specialized protein. These are secreted by the

TABLE 30-5 *Classification of Joint Diseases*	
I. Noninflammatory (often degenerative)	Osteoarthritis Traumatic arthritis Neuroarthropathy
II. Inflammatory (often immunological)	Rheumatoid arthritis Systemic lupus erythematosus Reiter's disease Rheumatic fever Scleroderma Erythema multiforme (allergic)
III. Septic	Bacterial, tuberculous, fungal
IV. Crystal-induced	Gout, pseudogout, apatite gout
V. Hemorrhagic	Traumatic injury Hemophilia Anticoagulation Malignancy (infrequent)

Data from Kjeldsberg C, Knight J: *Body Fluids*, 3rd ed. Chicago, American Society of Clinical Pathologists, 1993; and Ringsrud K, Linne J: *Urinalysis and Body Fluids: A Color Text and Atlas.* St. Louis, Mosby, 1995.

synovial membrane which lines the interior of the joint cavity. The hyaluronate-protein complex imparts stickiness and high viscosity to synovial fluid and enhances its function as a joint lubricant. Synovial fluid also transports nutrients to the joint cartilage.

Effusions develop with joint disease or joint trauma. Symptoms may include pain, swelling, and reduced mobility. Joint diseases are classified in five categories (Table 30-5) and more than one condition can coexist. Reference ranges for each category may be found in texts devoted to body fluids.[11]

Sample Collection and Handling

Sterile needle aspiration of synovial fluid (*arthrocentesis*) is performed for collection and therapeutically to relieve symptoms. Complications are rare. Traumatic tap may occur.

Although normal synovial fluid does not clot, diseased fluid may. Therefore, anticoagulant is required. Three tubes are collected: (1) liquid EDTA for cell count, differential, and crystal examination; (2) sterile sodium heparin for microbiology; and (3) a plain tube to observe for clotting and for chemistries. Powdered EDTA, lithium heparin, and oxalate are contraindicated because they can confuse the crystal analysis. Blood is collected simultaneously for comparative serum levels.

Cell count and leukocyte differential should be performed within 1 hour to avoid deterioration of neutrophils. Chemistries should be assayed promptly or the specimen refrigerated. If complement is to be assayed, it must be done within 2 to 3 hours or the specimen frozen at $-70°C$ since complement is especially heat labile.

Hematologic Examination

MACROSCOPIC OBSERVATIONS

Cloudiness or turbidity is proportional to cell count and number of crystals. Lipemic SF may contain cholesterol crystals. Black or gray discoloration may be seen in prosthetic arthroplasty. As with serous fluid, xanthochromia is difficult to interpret.

In addition to color and clarity, viscosity is noted. Viscosity is high in normal synovial fluid. When poured, normal and noninflammatory fluids form a string 4 to 5 cm long. If the string breaks before reaching 3 cm, viscosity is reduced. Low viscosity indicates joint inflammation. Enzymes in inflammatory synovial fluid depolymerize hyaluronate.

COUNTING CELLS AND CYTOCENTRIFUGE PREPARATIONS

Unless inflammation has sufficiently reduced its viscosity, synovial fluid can be impossible to work with. Its tendency to form strings can cause it to snap out of a pipette and back into the container. Pretreatment with hyaluronidase (1 drop of 0.05% buffered hyaluronidase to 1 mL of synovial fluid; incubate at room temperature for 4 minutes)[9] may be necessary to permit proper mixing and accurate counts.

As with CSF and serous fluid, manual cell counting of undiluted synovial fluid is the method of choice. However, acetic acid cannot be used in stains or diluents because it precipitates hyaluronate, causing cell clumping. Methylene blue (0.1%) enhances WBC. If dilution is required, isotonic saline or hyaluronidase diluent are used. Diluents that lyse red cells in bloody fluid for WBC counts are hypotonic saline, 1% ammonium oxalate with or without methylene blue, and absolute basophil diluent.[9] *Note:* Oxalate in diluent can crystallize, giving a false impression of crystals in synovial fluid. Cells may need 30 minutes to settle on the hemocytometer before counting because of viscosity.

Albumin is omitted in cytocentrifuge preparations because synovial fluid and some serous fluids already contain adequate protein. Excess protein causes WBC to appear as compact, dark-staining spheres, and neutrophils to resemble lymphocytes. If synovial fluid is highly viscous and the leukocyte count is high, a slide-on-slide pull-apart technique (Chap. 3) may produce acceptable slides.

CRYSTAL EXAMINATION

It is imperative that all unknown synovial fluid be examined for crystals. Crystals found in synovial fluid include monosodium urate (MSU), calcium pyrophosphate dihydrate (CPPD), cholesterol, steroids, hydroxyapatite and other basic calcium phosphates, calcium oxalate, and artifacts.

A polarizing lens permits passage of light vibrating in only one direction or plane, blocking the rest. If a second polarizing lens is parallel to the first, the polarized light passes on through it. If one of the lenses is turned perpendicular to the other, all light is blocked. This is referred to as *maximum extinction*. When applied to microscopy, the field becomes completely dark.

Some crystals, when placed between crossed polarizing lenses, are capable of rotating the plane of polarized light, enabling it to pass through the second polarizing lens. The crystal is therefore visible as bright and white in the dark field. Such crystals are commonly said to "polarize," and are properly referred to as "optically active."

Another property of certain crystals is birefringence. *Birefringence* is double refraction, or the bending of light into two components that emerge from the crystal as two parallel rays of polarized light, one vibrating parallel to the optic axis and one at right angles to it. These two rays travel at different speeds and have a different index of refraction. Birefringence has either a positive or negative sign.

Polarized light is used primarily to detect MSU, which is diagnostic of urate gout and CPPD crystals present in pseudogout and associated with degenerative arthritis. Both are birefringent, but with opposite signs. Strength of birefringence also differs: MSU exhibits strong birefringence whereas CPPD is weakly birefringent.

Many artifacts and debris can confuse crystal analysis. The reader is referred to texts devoted to body fluid analysis for detailed descriptions of these crystals as well as artifacts.

Morphologic Evaluation

Leukocyte and macrophage morphology is like that previously described in CSF and serous fluids. *Synovial lining cells* in synovial fluid resemble mesothelial cells seen in serous fluid. They have no clinical significance. In contrast to CSF and serous fluid, malignant cells only rarely invade synovial fluid.

Neutrophils exceeding 80% correlate strongly with septic arthritis. They may have intracellular bacteria or crystals. *Ragocytes* or *RA cells* are neutrophils with dark purple inclusions consisting of IgG, IgM, complement, rheumatoid factor, and immune complexes. They are seen in rheumatoid arthritis and other inflammatory synovial fluid.

Macrophages may contain clumps of apatite crystals which appear as dark purple inclusions with alizarin red. They may also contain hemosiderin or hematoidin after bleeding into the joint.

Cartilage cells are typically seen in osteoarthritis, and may also be present due to trauma.

MISCELLANEOUS FLUIDS

Peritoneal Lavage

One purpose of peritoneal lavage is to diagnose internal bleeding due to blunt trauma to the abdomen. One liter of isotonic solution is infused into the peritoneal cavity and recovered. If blood is not visible, a sample is sent to the laboratory for cell counts. If positive, surgical repair may be indicated. Sample reference ranges for positive lavage are RBC more than 100,000/μL and WBC more than 500/μL.[12]

Bronchoalveolar Lavage

The purpose of bronchoalveolar lavage (BAL) is to sample the lower respiratory tract for cell count and differential, cytology, chemistries, or culture. A bronchoscope is used to instill saline into the alveolar spaces and aspirate it for laboratory evaluation.[5,8]

Alveolar macrophages may contain more coarse granulation than other macrophages, especially if the patient smokes. Unlike macrophages in other fluids, they are sometimes included in the differential.

Bronchial lining cells have a unique appearance. They are rectangular or columnar with an extremely eccentric nucleus and one ciliated end. They may be viewed as a contaminant, implying that bronchial rather than alveolar cells have been sampled.[5,18] Unlike other lining cells, their percentage may be included in the differential, since their relative number reflects the quality of the sample obtained.

One application of BAL is the identification of opportunistic infections such as *Pneumocystis carinii* or *Aspergillus* species in immunocompromised patients. *Pneumocystis* pneumonitis is strongly suggested by a decrease in alveolar macrophages, an increase in neutrophils, the presence of plasma cells and immunoblasts, and basophilic foamy or honeycomb acellular areas.[5] Silver stain for cysts confirms the diagnosis.

Eosinophils in Urine Sediment and Nasal Discharge

Cytocentrifuge preparations of urine sediment and smears of nasal discharge are stained and examined for eosinophils. Eosinophils are associated with allergic rhinitis and allergic interstitial nephritis due to hypersensitivity to drugs such as penicillin.

Wright, Diff-Quik®, or Papanicolaou stain may be used. Hansel secretion stain (methylene blue and eosin-Y in methanol; Lide Laboratories, Inc., St. Louis, MO 63034) is also excellent for demonstrating eosinophils.[8]

A major source of error is mistaking neutrophils for eosinophils. Unlike whole blood, which varies little in consistency and pH, urine and nasal discharge are highly variable. Achieving proper staining can be difficult when using pH-dependent stains, such as Wright stain. A common consequence is that neutrophils can appear very red as compared to their usual appearance in blood or other body fluids. Therefore, lobularity and granule size and refractility must be used as criteria for identification. It is helpful to remember that if all the cells look the same, they are likely to be neutrophils. If eosinophils are present, even in high percentages, some neutrophils are usually present as well. Eosinophils are quite striking and blatantly obvious when compared to the neutrophils.

CHAPTER SUMMARY

Body fluids are tested to diagnose and monitor four general conditions: infection, hemorrhage, malignancy, and inflammation. WBC and RBC counts and leukocyte differentials are performed on most samples. Careful examination of a Wright-stained slide prepared by cytocentrifugation should always be included for leukocyte differential and to detect microorganisms and malignant cells. The most important conditions diagnosed by CSF examination are bacterial meningitis and subarachnoid hemorrhage (SAH). Leukemia, lymphoma, and carcinoma are also detected in CSF. Acute lymphoid leukemia (ALL) is the leukemia which most commonly invades CSF.

Serous fluid exists in small amounts between membranes which line potential cavities housing organs. Effusions are increased amounts of fluid which accumulate in these cavities due to abnormal conditions and are designated as transudates or exudates based on their etiology and laboratory values. Transudates result from a systemic disease such as congestive heart failure. Exudates result from local disease, and further testing is indicated to determine the cause. Familiarity with normal mesothelial cells must be acquired to allow differentiation from malignant cells.

Synovial fluid is present in small amounts in joints for lubrication. Its high viscosity causes technical difficulties in counting and cytocentrifuge slide preparation. In addition to cell counts and differential, examination for crystals is essential. Peritoneal and bronchoalveolar lavages may also be submitted for cell counts and differential. Neutrophils tend to stain red in urine sediment and nasal smears, and are commonly mistaken for eosinophils.

Case Study 30-1

A 9-month-old girl was admitted to the hospital with bruising. A CBC and differential revealed the following: WBC 283 × 10^9/L; Hb 6.3 g/dL; Hct 0.19 L/L; platelets 4 × 10^9/L; and 93% blasts. Bone marrow examination, positive TdT, and cell marker studies resulted in a diagnosis of acute lymphocytic leukemia. A CSF cell count and differential was WBC 2 × 10^6/L; RBC 5180 × 10^6/L; leukocyte differential: blasts 80%, lymphocytes 14%, and monocytes 6%.

1. What is the reference range for CSF cell counts for a 9-month-old child? Is the CSF cell count abnormal in this case?
2. Do the blasts in the CSF indicate active CNS invasion by leukemia? What calculation can be useful to determine this? What additional information is needed?
3. Does acute lymphocytic leukemia (ALL) commonly invade the CNS?

Case Study 30-2

A 31-year-old man was admitted to the hospital with pneumonia, skin rash, and genital herpes. He was diagnosed with acquired immunodeficiency syndrome (AIDS), *Pneumocystis carinii* pneumonia (PCP) detected by bronchoalveolar lavage, and disseminated cryptococcus infection with positive blood culture. A CSF cell count was 0 RBCs and 0 WBCs.

1. Does the normal cell count rule out CNS infection?
2. Since the count is normal, is examination of a cytocentrifuge preparation necessary or likely to be helpful in the diagnosis?
3. Will the yeast organisms stain with Wright stain? What would they look like?
4. What other tests performed on CSF can assist in the diagnosis of fungal meningitis?

Review Questions

30-1. While performing an RBC count on undiluted, unstained CSF, 200 RBC and 6 WBC were counted in 9 mm². While performing the WBC count on the same CSF, undiluted and stained with acetic acid/crystal violet stain, 190 WBC were seen in 9 mm². Based on the above information, one can conclude that

  A. the RBC count on the unstained CSF and the WBC count on the stained CSF should be reported.
  B. RBC were mistaken for WBC on the stained count.
  C. WBC were mistaken for RBC on the unstained count.
  D. the CSF should be recollected.

30-2. A 6-month-old baby was brought to the ER because of fever. CBC and differential results were: WBC 15 × 10^9/L, Hct 0.35 L/L, platelets 250 × 10^9/L; segmented neutrophils 15%, bands 10%, lymphocytes 65%, monocytes 10%. A lumbar puncture was performed to rule out meningitis. CSF counts were WBC 250 × 10^6/L, RBC 50 × 10^6/L. The cytocentrifuge preparation revealed NRBC in all stages, and all stages of neutrophil precursors including blasts. This picture is most consistent with

A. peripheral blood contamination from traumatic tap.
B. invasion of the CNS by acute myelocytic leukemia.
C. fulminating bacterial meningitis.
D. bone marrow contamination.

30-3. In distinguishing subarachnoid hemorrhage (SAH) from traumatic tap, SAH is associated with

A. a positive D-dimer.
B. decreasing red cell number in sequentially drawn tubes.
C. absence of xanthochromia.
D. small clots in tube no. 1.

30-4. Which statement is NOT true of bacterial meningitis?

A. Neutrophils always predominate in CSF in all phases of the illness.
B. CSF glucose is often decreased.
C. Lymphocytes can predominate in CSF in the early stages.
D. CSF protein is often increased.

30-5. Serous fluid differs from synovial fluid in that serous fluid

A. is not an ultrafiltrate of plasma.
B. is highly viscous.
C. has the consistency of raw egg white.
D. lacks hyaluronate.

30-6. An exudate is most likely to exhibit

A. specific gravity <1.015.
B. WBC count >500×10^6/L.
C. total protein <30 g/L.
D. a close association with a systemic condition such as congestive heart failure.

References

1. Adams R, Victor M: Principles of Neurology, 5th ed, pp 11–16. New York, McGraw-Hill, 1993
2. Bentz J: Laboratory investigation of multiple sclerosis. Lab Med 26(6):393, 1995
3. Fischer J, Davey D, Gulley M et al: Blastlike cells in cerebro-spinal fluid of neonates possible germinal matrix origin. Am J Clin Pathol 91:255, 1989
4. Fishman R: Lumbar puncture and CSF examination. In Rowland L (ed): Merritt's Textbook of Neurology, 9th ed, pp 93–97. Philadelphia, Williams & Wilkins, 1995
5. Fleury J, Escudier E, Pocholle M et al: Cell population obtained by bronchoalveolar lavage in *Pneumocystis carinii* pneumonitis. Acta Cytol 29(5):721, 1985
6. Glasser L: Reading the signs in synovia. Diagn Med 3(6):35, 1980
7. Hayward R, Shapiro M, Oye R: Laboratory testing on cerebrospinal fluid: A reappraisal. Lancet 1:1, 1987
8. Henry J (ed): Clinical Diagnosis and Management by Laboratory Methods, 18th ed. Philadelphia, WB Saunders, 1991
9. Kjeldsberg C, Knight J: Body Fluids, 3rd ed. Chicago, American Society of Clinical Pathologists, 1993
10. Knight J: The laboratory examination of cerebrospinal fluid. Medical Laboratory Products, Feb, 1988
11. Knight J: The laboratory examination of synovial fluid. Medical Laboratory Products, Aug, 1987
12. Krieg A, Kjeldsberg C: Cerebrospinal fluid and other body fluids. In Henry J (ed): Clinical Diagnosis and Management by Laboratory Methods, 18th ed. Philadelphia, WB Saunders, 1991
13. Lang D, Berberian L, Lee S et al: Rapid differentiation of subarachnoid hemorrhage from traumatic lumbar puncture using the D-dimer assay. Am J Clin Pathol 93:403, 1990
14. Leblanc R: The minor leak preceding subarachnoid hemorrhage. J Neurosurg 66:35, 1987
15. Marton K, Gean A: The spinal tap: A new look at an old test. Ann Intern Med 104:840, 1986
16. Odom L, Wilson H, Cullen J et al: Significance of blasts in low-cell-count cerebrospinal fluid specimens from children with acute lymphoblastic leukemia. Cancer 66:1748, 1990
17. Pappu L, Purohit D, Levkoff A et al: CSF cytology in the neonate. Am J Dis Child 136:297, 1982
18. Ringsrud K, Linne J: Urinalysis and Body Fluids: A Color Text and Atlas. St. Louis, Mosby, 1995
19. Steele R, Marmer D, O'Brien M et al: Leukocyte survival in cerebrospinal fluid. J Clin Microbiol 23:965, 1986
20. Talstad I: Electronic counting of spinal fluid cells. Am J Clin Pathol 81:506, 1984
21. Tzvetanova E, Tzekov C: Cerebrospinal fluid of children with shunts implanted for the treatment of internal hydrocephalus. Acta Cytol 30:277, 1986

CHAPTER 31

Molecular Testing in Hematology

Jennifer K. Morrow

Objectives

1. List four features of human genomic DNA that directly affect the specificity of molecular testing.
2. List and compare the three major types of molecular test formats.
3. List three uses of molecular information in hematologic diseases and give examples.

Over the past decade, laboratory methods developed initially as research tools for molecular biology have begun to find their way into the clinical laboratory. The tremendous potential of these techniques to analyze disease at the genetic/molecular level was quickly recognized and much effort has been invested in adapting them to the clinical setting. Although molecular testing is useful in virtually every area of medicine, hematopathology has particularly benefited from its use. It is important for all clinical laboratorians to be familiar with the terminology and types of procedures in use and to be aware of appropriate clinical uses.

BASIC PRINCIPLES OF MOLECULAR BIOLOGY

Structure and Features of DNA

The basic functions and structure of DNA are described in Chapter 5 but features crucial to the understanding of molecular testing will be emphasized in this section. These are the following:

1. A single strand of DNA is made up of a chain of phosphorylated deoxyribose sugars, each attached to a purine (adenine [A], guanine [G]) or pyrimidine (cytosine [C], thymine [T]) base forming nucleotides. The sugars are hooked together between the hydroxyl group of the 3' carbon on one end and the phosphate group on the 5' carbon of the next one. Therefore, every strand will have a free 5' phosphate on one end and a free 3' hydroxyl on the other. This imparts a structural direction or *polarity* on each strand.

2. The two strands of the DNA double helix run in opposite directions; the beginning 3' carbon of one strand is across from a free 5' carbon on the opposing strand. Thus, they are said to be *antiparallel*.

3. Each strand consists of a *linear sequence* of the four nucleotide bases (A, T, G, and C) that are so arranged that they come in close contact with the nucleotide bases on the opposing strand.

4. Interstrand pairing of complementary bases (G:C and A:T) is by *hydrogen bonding* (two hydrogen bonds between A and T and three between G and C).

5. DNA synthesis (*in vivo* and *in vitro*) is unidirectional, proceeding from 5' to 3' end with growth of the new strand only at the 3' end.

6. Genomes of different organisms are unique and distinguishable one from another. The human genome consists of double-stranded DNA molecules organized into chromosomes within cell nuclei.

Hybridization

Almost every molecular assay depends on the concept of *hybridization*, which refers to the interaction between two complementary nucleotide sequences (Fig. 31-1). It is worthwhile to note that these interactions can take place between DNA or RNA molecules. Hybridization reactions often involve a relatively small piece of nucleotide base sequence, which is used to search for its complementary sequence in a complex milieu of nucleotide base sequences—there are three billion base pairs for human genomic DNA. These short detector sequences of nucleotides are called either *probes* or *primers* depending on the procedure in which they are used. A common analogy is that a probe is equivalent to a magnet that can pull a needle out of a haystack.

Hybridization reactions depend on unwinding and separating the two strands of a DNA helix. This is referred to as *denaturation of DNA* and can be accomplished in several ways, the simplest being heating. In the presence of complementary base sequences (the entire strand or shorter pieces), hydrogen bonds can reform or hybridize (*i.e.*, hybridization). Hybridization allows very high specificity, which is desirable in clinical testing.

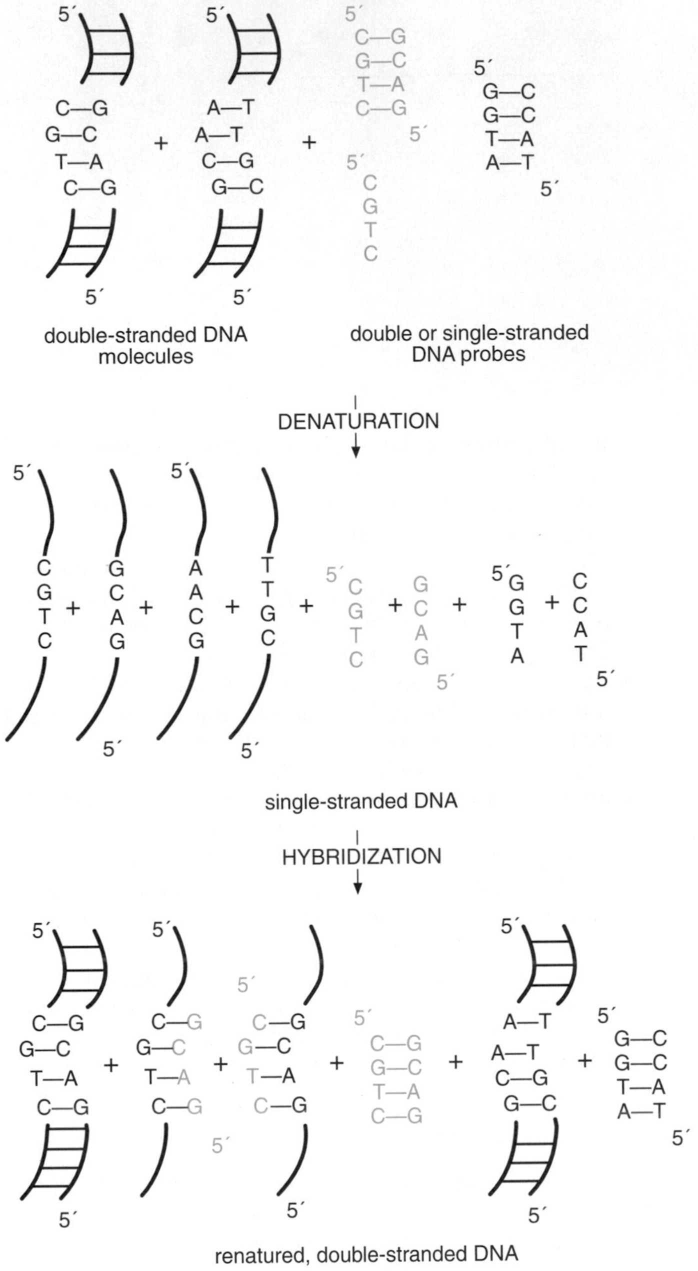

FIGURE 31-1. Hybridization of complementary DNA sequences. Following denaturation (by thermal or chemical means), the DNA becomes single-stranded. Under the appropriate conditions, hydrogen bonds form between complementary bases of the DNA sample and the DNA probe to remake double-stranded molecules. The sizes of probes and base sequences shown are for illustrative purposes only. The probes complementary to one of the double-stranded DNA molecules are shown in color. Note that both double- and single-stranded DNA probes may be used.

MOLECULAR TESTING

Due to the large size and complexity of the human genome, it was previously difficult, if not impossible, to study selected small parts. The discovery and development of a number of molecular tools have enabled research and clinical laboratory scientists to study and characterize a disease process at its most fundamental level; that is, the genetic difference that is associated with or causative of that condition. These tools include:

- A variety of microbial enzymes that are capable of
  — cutting DNA strands at specific locations (restriction endonucleases)
  — synthesizing new DNA strands (polymerases)
  — connecting DNA pieces (ligases)

- Microbial vectors into which foreign DNA can be cloned, characterized, and sequenced (recombinant DNA technology; used to introduce foreign DNA into host cells)
- Substrates that bind nucleic acids (used for nucleic acid separation, purification, and detection)

Technical training, quality control, and quality assurance programs are crucial for all clinical testing but especially for molecular testing,[12,13,18,25–27,52] since there is no standardization of test procedures at the present time. Proficiency test surveys (administered by the College of American Pathologists) for a few molecular tests are now available. As of this writing, the Association for Molecular Pathology is spearheading efforts to establish guidelines and certification for laboratories performing molecular testing.

Method Guidelines

Since the analyte is nucleic acid (DNA or RNA), the specimen must contain nucleated cells, thereby excluding mature red blood cells as a source. Most commonly the specimen is peripheral blood, but bone marrow or tissue biopsy may be required. For some procedures, paraffin-embedded fixed tissue is a convenient and adequate source. Specimen requirements are specific for each particular test. A variety of methods is available for the removal and purification of nucleic acids from cells. The choice of the target nucleic acid is mostly determined by the nature of the molecular event being tested, but still it is necessary to be aware of an important difference between DNA and RNA. Whereas DNA is very stable, RNA is very labile. Thus, working with RNA requires many additional precautions with specimen collection, processing, and analysis because of its inherent susceptibility to degradation.

The choice of method(s) to use for a particular test depends on a number of factors:

1. The type of molecular change to be identified (*e.g.*, a change involving one or a few bases in contrast to one in which larger chromosomal regions are affected)
2. The number and variety of the molecular changes for a particular condition (whether or not there is a single unique change in all cases, such as seen in sickle cell anemia)
3. The clinical question being asked
4. The experience and capabilities of the laboratory
5. Practical issues such as cost, turnaround time, and test sensitivity

Molecular testing procedures are numerous and varied in format but can be grouped into three general categories: probe, amplification, or sequence based. Listed in Table 31-1 are well established methods as well as some newer ones. Each category, with examples, will be discussed separately. Readers are referred to review articles that further discuss many of these methods.[11,29]

Probe Analysis

All probe-based assays depend on the use of a *known* nucleic acid sequence, or probe, to detect (by hybridization) its complementary sequence in an unknown sample (Fig. 31-2). The probe is usually tagged with a discernible marker in order to demonstrate that hybridization has occurred. *In situ* hybridization (ISH) is performed on cells immobilized on microscope slides and results are interpreted at the intracellular location of the target sequence. A few positive cells can easily be detected in a negative background when conditions are optimal but this can be difficult to achieve. The use of fluorescent labeled probes (FISH) has enhanced basic ISH to allow the analysis of metaphase and interphase chromosomes.

Originally, hybridization assays were carried out in solution, a method that is unsuited for many applications. Thus, the discovery of materials that could serve as a solid support greatly facilitated the use of hybridization as an analytic tool. Commonly, these are membranes onto which nucleic acids are transferred (blotted) and then probed. The *dot/slot blot* is a procedure in which specimens (often cell lysates) are filtered or spotted onto a membrane in an array such that each specimen is contained within a small circular (dot) or oblong (slot) area. This method is procedurally simple and can easily test multiple samples. Interpretation of weak reactions, however, can be problematic. Two frequently used modifications of the dot/slot blot technique are (1) allele specific hybridization in which replicate blots are analyzed separately with probes representing normal or mutant sequences; and (2) reverse dot blot in which the probes (instead of the target) are bound to the membrane allowing the analysis of one specimen with many different probes.

Although ISH and dot/slot blot analyses reflect the presence or absence of a target sequence, they yield no other information about it. In conjunction with the discovery of restriction endonucleases, a technique involving their use was invented by Dr. E.M. Southern. This provided a significant advance in our ability to analyze the structure and organization of genes. Complex DNA molecules could be cut by enzymes into small fragments, separated by gel electrophoresis, transferred to a membrane, and probed for specific sequences. Long the dependable workhorse of molecular laboratories, Southern blotting gives results reflecting the sequence, size, and chromosomal or gene location of the hybridized fragment(s). However, because it is composed of many steps and manipulations, it requires a high level of training and a number of quality control measures. In a similar procedure known as a *Northern* (a play on Dr. Southern's name) *blot*, RNA is electrophoresed and probed. This method, however, is used more often to study gene expression rather than as a diagnostic procedure.

Amplification Analysis

Amplification-based techniques arose mainly out of the need for better test sensitivity, particularly when a specimen is very small or of poor quality or when the target nucleic acid is present in very low amounts or degraded. In general, they are simpler to perform and yield faster and more sensitive results than most blotting methods.

Although these techniques differ significantly in their principles of operation, they are similar in that they all result in an increased ability to detect the target sequence. This may be accomplished by three different means: (1) synthesizing copies of the target such as the *polymerase chain reaction (PCR)* or *nucleic acid sequence-based amplification (NASBA)*; (2) using target sequence probes that increase their numbers only when the target sequence is present such as the *ligase chain reaction (LCR)* and *Qβ replicase (QBR)*; and (3) using secondary enzymes and coupled substrates in a manner similar to immunoassays to enhance the detection signal, such as *branched DNA (bDNA)*. Some of these methods may prove to be most useful in infectious disease testing. An example of each type is diagrammed in Fig. 31-3.

The first and most widely used amplification method, PCR, will be discussed in this chapter. Conceptually sim-

TABLE 31-1
Molecular Testing Methods

Type	Ref.	Advantages	Disadvantages
PROBE BASED			
In situ hybridization (ISH)	5, 46, 50	Gives intracellular localization of target sequence Cell morphology remains intact Cell type is identifiable	Poor discrimination of subtle sequence differences Nonspecific background interpretation Tedious
Dot/slot blot	37, 42	Relatively fast Easily performed Gives a yes or no answer Easily quantitated Many samples can be tested at once Does not require DNA purification	No size determination Susceptible to nonspecific probe binding Controls are crucial because it gives a yes or no answer
Southern blot	48	Gives a size determination Gives a chromosomal location Very reproducible	Labor intensive Complex, multistep procedure Requires purified high m.w. DNA Long time until results obtained Difficult to automate
Northern blot	49	Gives mRNA size information Can quantitate mRNA expression	Technical difficulties of working with RNA Not very useful clinically
AMPLIFICATION BASED			
Polymerase chain reaction (PCR)	39, 41	High sensitivity Fast to perform and get results Can perform using DNA that is degraded or not purified Requires a very small quantity of specimen Semiautomatable with thermal cycler	Sensitive to contamination Requires some template sequence information Difficult to perform for quantitation purposes
Nucleic acid sequence-based amplification (NASBA)	31	High sensitivity Isothermal reactions Useful for detection of RNA templates	Requires three enzymes The difficulties of working with RNA
Ligase chain reaction (LCR)	2	High sensitivity Good single base change discrimination	Must know entire target sequence Limited by the number of target molecules present False positives may result from nonspecific primers
Qβ replicase (QBR)	28	Ribosomal RNA target present in multiple copies per cell Isothermal reactions High sensitivity in short time Automated	The difficulties of working with RNA Must confirm positive results Less sensitive than PCR Background amplification
Branched DNA	51	Good quantitative assay Less prone to product contamination	Less sensitive than enzymatic amplifications Nonspecific background
SEQUENCE BASED			
Restriction enzyme digestion	38	A known sequence difference is usually identifiable Easily performed and interpreted	Requires a known sequence difference between normal and mutant alleles
Single-stranded confirmation polymorphism analysis (SSCP)	45	Can discriminate between small sequence differences Can screen a large region of DNA	Further analysis is needed to characterize the differences
Denaturing gradient gel electrophoresis (DGGE)	14	Good single base change discrimination	Complex electrophoretic technique
Direct DNA sequencing	43, 47	Gives ultimate information on genetic differences or similarities Good for distinguishing polymorphism	Unless automated, is technically complex and error prone Automated instruments are expensive
Genosensor technology	4	Miniaturized DNA sequencing Rapid and economical Multiprobe information Microchip format	In early stages of development

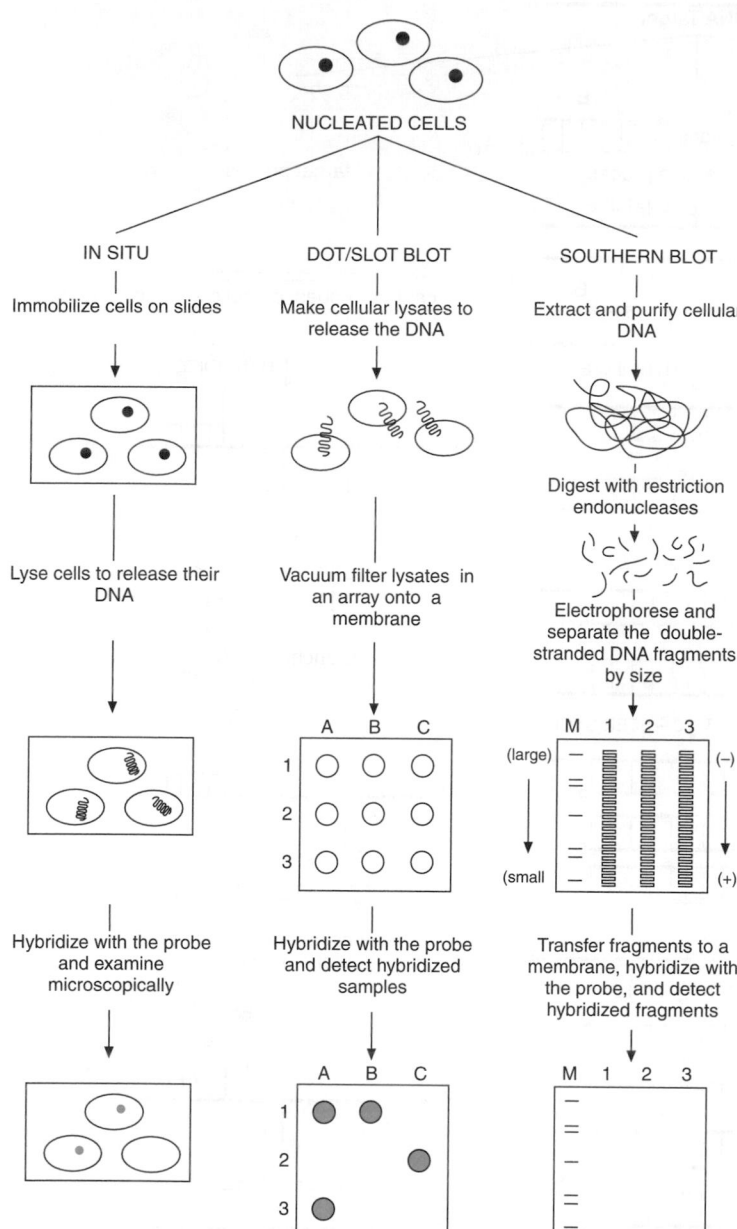

FIGURE 31-2. Probe methods. All three types shown require the use of a DNA target and a DNA probe tagged with a marker (isotopic or nonisotopic) that allows the detection of hybridized DNA molecules. The bottom drawings represent the visual results for each method. Red indicates a positive hybridization between the probe and its complementary target sequence. The interpretation of these results are as follows. **In situ:** Two of the three cells examined contain the sequence probed for. **Dot/slot blot:** Of the nine different specimens analyzed, only four (1A, 1B, 2C and 3A) are positive for the sequence of interest. **Southern blot:** The sizes of the DNA fragments from three individuals (1, 2, and 3) are compared to known size markers (M). The pattern of hybridization reveals that 1 and 2 share a fragment of similar size and that 3 is different from both.

ple, the basic method consists of repetitive cycles of three reactions, each carried out at different temperatures. The specificity is imparted with the use of oligonucleotide primers matching opposite DNA strands on either end of the region of interest, which hybridize to their complementary target sequences. The bound primers serve to initiate bidirectional synthesis of the targeted DNA sequence by a unique DNA polymerase capable of functioning at and not destroyed by the high temperatures necessary to denature DNA. Each PCR cycle results in the doubling of the number of target molecules, and after 30 cycles at least one million copies can be made. An analogy is that we now have a haystack full of needles (targets). A common method variation is *reverse transcriptase PCR (RT-PCR)*, in which RNA is isolated and a DNA copy made before proceeding to the PCR step. The RT-PCR technique is particularly useful for analyzing chromosomal translocations.

The PCR products can be analyzed in a variety of ways, but most simply by gel electrophoresis for size determination. The main consideration for clinical use of PCR is the prevention of contamination of future PCRs with the products of past analyses, which could result in false-positive values. There are a number of physical and chemical ways in which to accomplish this.

Sequence Analysis

Taking advantage of the sequence of bases in a nucleic acid is the ultimate way in which to evaluate molecular differences or similarities. *Restriction enzymes* make double-stranded cuts in DNA at sites unique to each enzyme that are very specific (*i.e.*, at a particular sequence of bases). Consequently, when DNA from different origins are subjected to a specific restriction enzyme, they will be cut at different locations and result in different sized

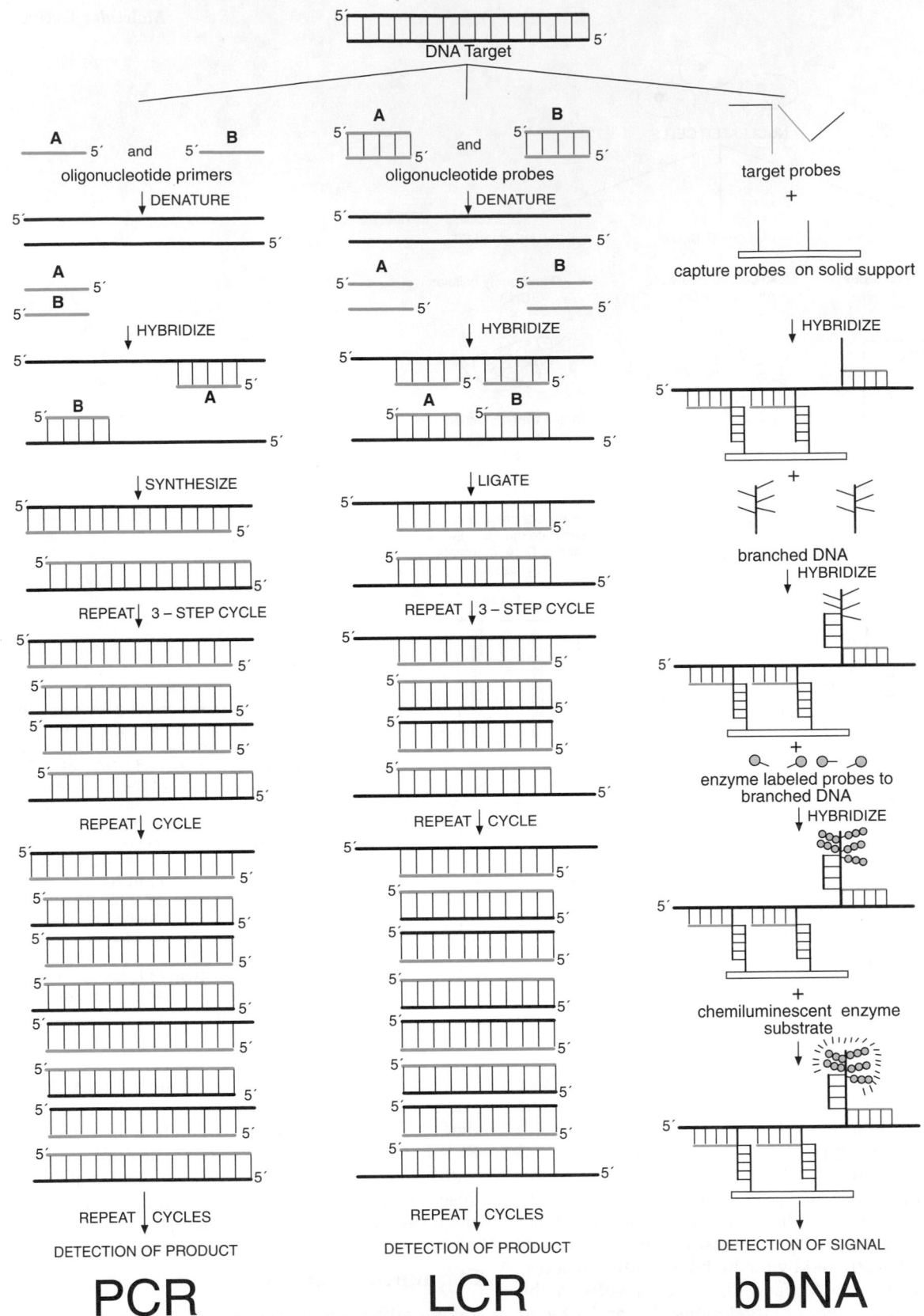

FIGURE 31-3. Amplification-based methods. Diagrams show the basic steps of the three different types of amplification using DNA as the targeted template. Either the target sequence (polymerase chain reaction [PCR]), probe sequence (ligase chain reaction [LCR]), or signal (branched DNA [bDNA]) is amplified by the mechanisms shown. Shown in red are primers and newly synthesized sequences for PCR, probes and newly ligated sequences for LCR, and probes for the target and bDNA sequences for the bDNA method. The hashed lines ||||| represent areas of double-stranded base pairing.

fragments. The DNA fragments can then be separated by gel electrophoresis. If the DNAs are different, the electrophoresis will show different patterns of fragments. Some newer polyacrylamide gel electrophoretic techniques such as *single-stranded conformation polymorphism (SSCP)* or *denaturing gradient gel electrophoresis (DGGE)* analysis have the resolving power to discriminate between the gel migration of DNAs, which are different *by only one base.*

The definitive way to compare nucleic acid sequences is by *direct sequencing of DNA,* in which the actual base sequence is determined. This can be done manually or by machine but neither method is readily adaptable in most clinical laboratories. An exciting future technology is the use of computer chips containing arrays of nucleotide sequence recognition elements. This format potentially could greatly enhance the speed and reduce the cost of DNA sequencing and of mutation detection and thus make it cost effective for most clinical laboratories.

SUMMARY

In summary, although each method is distinct, many actual clinical tests involve combinations of methods and modifications of the basic method. For instance, it is common to perform an amplification followed by a hybridization in order to confirm the identity of the amplification product and to increase the sensitivity of the assay. Many of these formats are not easily incorporated into the traditional clinical laboratory setting because of their complexity, labor intensity, and the high costs of reagents and instruments. Molecular testing will become more widespread with advances in automation, development of test kits, and cost reductions.

HEMATOLOGIC APPLICATIONS

Hematology has long been a beneficiary of the use of molecular methods for the identification of genes and genetic changes associated with specific diseases. Table 31-2 gives the best known hematologic molecular markers, their clinical correlates, and the analytical methods most often used to detect them. The types of genetic changes range from those occurring on a single chromosome (most inherited erythrocyte and hemostasis disorders) to those involving the interchange of DNA between chromosomes (most of the leukocyte disorders). Two examples illustrating hematologic analyses are shown in Figure 31-4.

Erythrocytes

The globin gene was one of the earliest genes to be fully characterized and its mutations correlated with a spectrum of disorders. Although there exist good diagnostic tests for most erythrocyte disorders, the high specificity of molecular detection is particularly useful for prenatal and carrier testing. Technically, it is much easier to test for a disease like sickle cell anemia in which all cases result from the same single nucleotide base substitution. Testing is much more complex for the thalassemias owing to the large number of different mutations that cause many variants of the disease.

Leukocytes

The identification of the molecular changes in leukocytes that accompany the development of leukemias and lymphomas is proving valuable in diagnosis, staging, prognosis, monitoring of residual disease, and evaluation of therapies. The vast majority of these changes are chromosomal translocations, in which pieces of chromosomes are physically interchanged. Identification of these chromosomal abnormalities by molecular methods is much faster than the traditional cytogenetic methods, which may take up to two weeks. When a chromosomal rearrangement moves the regulatory region of an actively transcribed gene adjacent to a gene normally involved in cell proliferation or differentiation, the result may lead to neoplastic transformation. Such is the case for many of the hematopoietic malignancies in which there are rearrangements involving regulatory regions of the genes of the immune system.

Molecular markers associated with specific leukemias and lymphomas are useful in a variety of ways. They may assist in diagnosis and classification and may also be predictive of therapeutic response. For example, the chromosomal translocations t(8;21) in M2 acute myeloid leukemia (AML), t(15;17) in M3 AML, and inv(16) in M4 AML (Chap. 34) are thought to be markers of cells that respond well to therapy. Others seem to be more indicative of a bad prognosis, perhaps due to faster disease progression or resistance to treatment. These include t(4;11) (except in very young children), t(9;22) (the Philadelphia chromosome), and t(1;19) in cases of acute lymphoblastic leukemia (ALL, Chap. 36). The specific location on a chromosome where a break and translocation occurs may differ between patients. More clinical studies are needed to determine whether they also differ in predicting prognosis.

The rearrangements within genes of the immune system that occur during normal differentiation of B and T lymphocytes are good lineage markers when they are detectable in clonal expansions of cells that contain the same gene rearrangement (Fig. 31-4, *top*). Rearrangements also are unique markers for a given patient's malignancy that help in determining whether subsequent malignancies are recurrences of the original or of different cell origin. Additional molecular alterations such as mutations in the p53 tumor suppressor gene often precede or accompany disease progression, but their clinical utility awaits further study.

The high sensitivity of molecular methods makes them the preferred way to assess minimal residual disease and to detect early relapse. In fact, some of the amplification techniques are able to detect one abnormal cell in a mixture of a million normal cells. However, there seem to be differences between diseases and the significance of low levels of abnormal cells. For several categories of acute leukemia (*e.g.,* M2 and M4 AML), it is common for a PCR detectable level of leukemic cells to persist even during clinical remission. For others, PCR negativity might be a goal of therapy, and a return to PCR positivity may signal relapse (Fig. 31-4, *bottom*).

There are a number of pathogens which are directly or indirectly associated with hematologic conditions for

TABLE 31-2
Molecular Markers of Hematologic Disorders

Disorder	Marker	Ref.	Method	Cases Characterized
ERYTHROCYTES				
Sickle cell anemia	Single base substitution in the 6th codon of the β-globin gene	40	PCR, ASO, SB or combinations	All cases
α-Thalassemias	Usually deletions in the α-globin gene; point mutations less common	3	PCR, REA	Heterogeneous disease with many different genetic changes
β-Thalassemias	Usually point mutations in the β-globin gene	15	PCR, ASO, REA, SEQ, or combinations	Heterogeneous disease with many different genetic changes
LEUKOCYTES				
Acute Myeloblastic Leukemia (AML)	t(8;21)	19	RT-PCR	18% to 40% of M2 cases
	t(15;17)	17	RT-PCR	70% to 100% of M3 cases
	inv (16)	21	RT-PCR	30% of M4 cases
	11q23 abnormalities	7	RT-PCR	75% of infantile cases
Chronic Myeloid Leukemia (CML)	t(9;22) (Philadelphia chromosome)	32	RT-PCR	90% to 95% of cases
Acute Lymphoblastic Leukemia (ALL)	t(1;19)	8, 9	RT-PCR	Precursor B-cell lineage
	11q23 abnormalities	7, 8	SB, RT-PCR	75% of infantile cases (B cell)
	t(4;11)	8, 9	RT-PCR	60% of infantile cases (B cell)
	t(9;22)	8, 9	RT-PCR	25% to 33% of adult cases (B cell)
	t(1;14)	8	PCR	T-cell lineage
	T-cell receptor gene rearrangements	9, 20	SB, PCR	Majority of T-cell cases
Lymphoma	t(11;14)	44	PCR, SB	50% to 60% of mantle cell
	t(14;18)	22	PCR, SB	85% to 95% of follicular
	t(8;14)	34	RT-PCR	75% to 80% of Burkitt's
	3q27 abnormalities	33	SB	27% to 45% of diffuse large cell
	Ig heavy chain gene rearrangements	20	PCR, SB	95% of B-cell lineage
	T-cell receptor gene rearrangements	20	SB, PCR	95% of T-cell lineage
	p53	23, 36	PCR, SB, SSCP, SEQ	Mycosis fungoides Progression indicator
HEMOSTASIS				
Hemophilia A	Substitutions, deletions, insertions, or rearrangements within the factor VIII gene	35	REA, PCR, SSCP, SB	Heterogeneous spectrum of genetic changes; hundreds of known mutations
Hemophilia B	Usually point mutations in the factor IX gene; others are deletions or insertions	16	REA, PCR/SEQ	33% of all cases due to one point mutation; hundreds of other known mutations
Factor V defect	Single base substitution in codon 506 of the factor V (Leiden) gene	30	PCR/REA	Most inherited cases of high risk for deep vein thrombosis

PCR = polymerase chain reaction; ASO = allele specific hybridization; SB = Southern blot; REA = restriction enzyme analysis; SEQ = sequencing; RT-PCR = reverse transcriptase PCR; SSCP = single strand conformation polymorphism.

which molecular detection is increasingly useful. This is particularly true for organisms difficult or slow to grow in culture. Molecular methods allow for their rapid identification as well as their detection at low levels of infectivity. These include Epstein-Barr virus (Burkitt's lymphoma), human immunodeficiency virus (HIV; immunodeficiency disorders), human T-cell lymphotrophic virus (HTLV-I adult T-cell leukemia), and parvovirus B19 (life-threatening transient aplastic crisis in sickle cell anemia patients). The reader is referred to the literature for a review of this information.[10]

Hemostasis

The identification of a causal molecular defect in hemophilia A or B is complicated by a large number of different possible mutations. Thus, molecular analysis is best used for prenatal and carrier testing in families with previously diagnosed cases. A recent discovery was that there are single-base substitutions in the coagulation factor V (Leiden) gene that result in mutant factor V proteins that function abnormally in the coagulation pathway. Several studies have found that one particular mutation in the

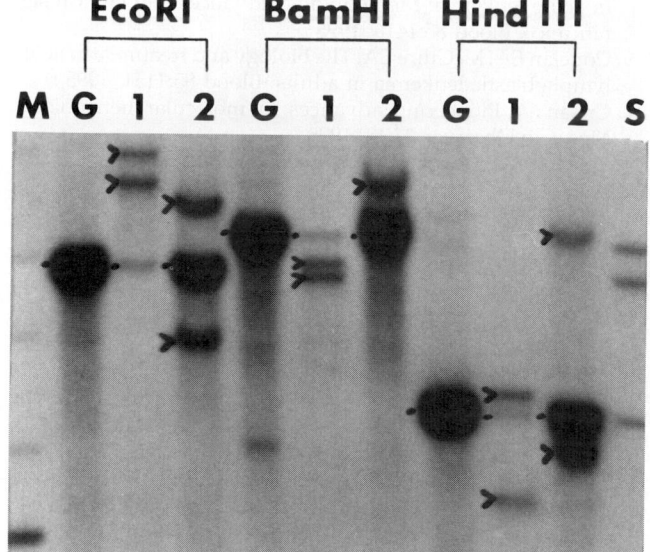

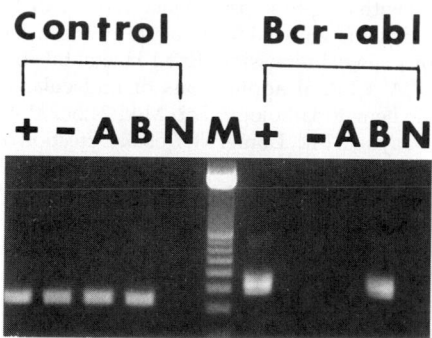

FIGURE 31-4. Molecular analyses using Southern blotting for B-cell gene rearrangement (*top*) and PCR/gel electrophoresis for the t(9;22) (*i.e.*, Philadelphia chromosome *bcr-abl*) translocation (*bottom*).

Top, DNAs from lymph nodes of patients 1 and 2 were digested with the enzymes EcoRI, Bam HI, and Hind III, the fragments electrophoresed, and the blot probed (radioactively) for the immunoglobulin kappa light chain gene. The pattern of hybridizing fragments was compared to that of germline (G) DNA and the sizes to markers (M). Those marked with ● are unrearranged (same as G) and those with > represent clonal rearrangements. The sensitivity control (S) shows that a population of clonal cells of 5% is easily detectable.

Bottom, RNAs from cells known to be positive (+) or negative (−) for *bcr-abl* and a CML patient's post–bone marrow transplant (BMT) bone marrow at day 100 (A) and day 180 (B) were amplified by RT-PCR for a control gene (present in all cells) and for the *bcr-abl* translocation (present only in affected cells). The PCR products were electrophoresed in agarose and visualized with the UV fluorescent dye ethidium bromide. All samples except a control reaction with no DNA (N, negative) were positive for the control gene as expected. When tested for the *bcr-abl* transcript, the positive cells made a 300-base pair product (sized by markers [M]) whereas nothing was amplified in the negative cells. The results for the patient's specimens were negative at day 100 post–BMT with a return to PCR positivity at day 180 post–BMT.

factor V gene may be the most common genetic indicator of susceptibility to venous thrombosis.[30]

Although in-depth discussion is beyond the scope of this chapter, it is worth mentioning that not only have nucleic acids become analytes in the clinical laboratory but they are also being investigated as therapeutic agents through the use of recombinant DNA techniques. In theory, defective genes could be repaired, replaced, or neutralized using normal (nondefective) genes or gene sequences.[1,6,24]

CHAPTER SUMMARY

Structural and functional characteristics of nucleic acids are the basis for a variety of research techniques now entering the realm of clinical laboratory medicine. Using these highly specific and sensitive methods, it is now possible to identify and characterize genetic alterations that correlate with clinical conditions. Because this is such a new and different area of clinical testing which uses methods and terminology foreign to most clinical laboratorians, it is important that today's clinical laboratory scientist understand the underlying scientific principles and become familiar with the different types of molecular techniques.

These techniques were reviewed and comments made on their features and limitations. Examples were given to show how molecular analysis has dramatically affected and enhanced the study of hematologic diseases. These genetic tools allow for more accurate disease diagnosis, prognosis, and therapy evaluation.

In order for molecular testing to be more widely performed, it will be necessary to simplify test formats with diagnostic kit development and to develop automated procedures. Although costs are likely to decrease (with procedural changes and increased commercial competition), the higher costs of molecular testing should be offset by the invaluable information they provide—information that can lead to faster implementation of appropriate treatments. Thus, in the long run, the result is more effective and cost efficient for patient care.

Case Study 31-1

An 18-year-old male visited his physician reporting symptoms of fatigue, pallor, and moderate weight loss. Physical examination revealed hepatosplenomegaly. Laboratory examination of peripheral blood showed a marked elevation in total WBC accompanied by a significantly low hematocrit and platelet count. The bone marrow was packed with blasts. Flow cytometry yielded the following profile: CD2+, CD3+, CD7+, CD19−, CD22−, TdT+, and CALLA−. To support and confirm these results, gene rearrangement studies were performed. They detected a clonal population of cells with rearrangements in the T-cell receptor β genes but not the immunoglobulin heavy- or light-chain genes. Karyotyping was reported as normal. The patient was initially diagnosed as having acute lymphoblastic leukemia (ALL) and treated with chemotherapy. He then underwent a bone marrow transplant, but he relapsed 2 years later.

1. What is the lineage of the malignant cells? Why?
2. How can the gene rearrangement results be used to monitor this patient's disease and therapeutic response?
3. What other molecular marker is sometimes found with this disease that indicates a poor prognosis?

Case Study 31-2

A 25-year-old female was pregnant with her first child. Although she and her husband both had positive family histories for sickle cell anemia, neither had been evaluated for carrier status. They decided to seek genetic counseling and testing.

1. What is the nature of the sickle cell anemia mutation? Is it easier or more difficult to test for than the thalassemias and why?
2. For this pregnancy, is it necessary or preferred to perform molecular testing on the parents as well as the fetus? Why? What would be the implications for future pregnancies?

Review Questions

31-1. Molecular testing

    A. can take advantage of the structural polarity of individual DNA strands.

    B. cannot be used to distinguish human DNA from mouse DNA.

    C. is often based on nonspecific interactions between complementary nucleotide bases.

    D. cannot detect small differences in the linear base sequence of DNA from different origins.

31-2. The most accurate statement about molecular test procedures is that

    A. mature erythrocytes provide a good specimen source.

    B. it is not possible to determine the linear sequence of bases in a piece of DNA.

    C. a probe is a piece of nucleic acid used to search and select for its complementary target sequence.

    D. amplification based assays were developed to improve test specificity.

31-3. Molecular evaluation of hematologic conditions

    A. has prognostic but no diagnostic value.

    B. can identify genetic abnormalities that may affect treatment decisions.

    C. is simple when there are multiple variants of the causative genetic defect.

    D. cannot be used to identify immune system gene rearrangement in B and T lymphocytes.

References

1. Askari FK, McDonnell WM: Antisense-oligonucleotide therapy. New Engl J Med 334:316, 1996
2. Barany F: Genetic disease detection and DNA amplification using cloned thermostable ligase. Proc Natl Acad Sci USA 88:189, 1991
3. Baysal E, Huisman THJ: Detection of common deletional α-thalassemia-2 determinants by PCR. Am J Hematol 46:208, 1994
4. Beattie KL, Beattie WG, Meng L et al: Advances in genosensor research. Clin Chem 41:700, 1995
5. Bhatt B, Burns J, Flannery D et al: Direct visualization of single copy genes on banded metaphase chromosomes by nonisotopic in situ hybridization. Nucleic Acids Res 16:3951, 1988
6. Blau HM, Springer ML: Gene therapy—A novel form of drug delivery. New Engl J Med 334:316, 1995
7. Bower M, Parry P, Carter M et al: Prevalence and clinical correlations of MLL gene rearrangements in AML-M4/5. Blood 84:3776, 1994
8. Campana P, Pui C-H: Detection of minimal residual disease in acute leukemia: Methodologic advances and clinical significance. Blood 85:1416, 1995
9. Copelan EA, McGuire EA: The biology and treatment of acute lymphoblastic leukemia in adults. Blood 85:1151, 1995
10. Crisan D: Pioneering advances in molecular hematology. Med Lab Observer 27:48, 1995
11. Dowton SB, Slaugh RA: Diagnosis of human heritable diseases—Laboratory approaches and outcomes. Clin Chem 41:785, 1995
12. Farkas DH: Launching a DNA lab. Med Lab Observer 27(5):42, 1995
13. Farkas DH: QA initiatives for the DNA lab. Med Lab Observer 27(6):44, 1995
14. Fodde R, Losekoot M: Mutation detection by denaturing gradient gel electrophoresis (DGGE). Hum Mutat 3:83, 1994
15. Galanello R, Barella S, Ideo A et al: Genotype of subjects with borderline hemoglobin A2 levels: Implications for β-thalassemia carrier screening. Am J Hematol 46:79, 1994
16. Giannelli F, Green PM, High KA et al: Haemophilia B: Database of point mutations and short additions and deletions—second edition. Nucleic Acids Res 19(Suppl):2193, 1991
17. Grignani F, Fagioli M, Alcalay M et al: Acute promyelocytic leukemia: From genetics to treatment. Blood 83:10, 1994
18. Grody WW: Proficiency testing in diagnostic molecular pathology. Diag Molec Pathol 3:221, 1994
19. Guerrasio A, Rosso C, Martinelli G: Polyclonal haemopoieses associated with long-term persistence of the AML1-ETO transcript in patients with FAB M2 acute myeloid leukemia in continuous clinical remission. Brit J Haematol 90:364, 1995
20. Hanson CA: Clinical applications of molecular biology in diagnostic hematopathology. Lab Med 24:562, 1993
21. Hebert J, Cayuela J-M, Daniel M-T et al: Detection of minimal residual disease in acute myelomonocytic leukemia with abnormal marrow eosinophils by nested polymerase chain reaction with allele specific amplification. Blood 84:2291, 1994
22. Horsman DE, Gascoyne RD, Coupland RW et al: Comparison of cytogenetic analysis, Southern analysis, and the polymerase chain reaction for the detection of t(14;18) in follicular lymphoma. Am J Clin Pathol 103:472, 1995
23. Imamura J, Miyoshi I, Koeffler HP: p53 in hematologic malignancies. Blood 84:2412, 1994
24. Kirkland MA, O'Brien SG, Goldman JM: Antisense therapeutics in haematological malignancies. Brit J Haematol 87:447, 1994
25. Klosinski DD, Matta N, Hunter S: Workforce adaptations and the future of molecular pathology. Lab Med 23:747, 1992
26. Klosinski DD, Hunter SV, Farkas DH: Operational requirements of a molecular pathology laboratory. Clin Lab News 20(8):10, 1994
27. Klosinski DD: Is a career in molecular pathology for you? Med Lab Observer 27(7):38, 1995
28. Kramer FR, Lizardi PM: Replicatable RNA reporters. Nature 339:401, 1989
29. Landegren U, Kaiser R, Caskey CT et al: DNA diagnostics—Molecular techniques and automation. Science 242:229, 1988
30. Liu X-Y, Nelson D, Grant C et al: Molecular detection of a common mutation in coagulation factor V causing thrombosis via hereditary resistance to activated protein C. Diag Molec Pathol 4:191, 1995
31. Malek L, Darasch S, Davey C et al: Application of NASBA™ isothermal nucleic acid amplification method to the diagnosis of HIV-1 (abstract). Clin Chem 38:458, 1992
32. McClure JS, Litz CE: Chronic myelogenous leukemia: Molecular diagnostic considerations. Hum Pathol 25:594, 1994
33. Nakamura Y, Miki T, Kawamata N et al: Biallelic DNA rearrangements and deletions within the bcl-6 gene in B-cell non-Hodgkin's lymphoma. Brit J Haematol 90:404, 1995
34. Offit K, Chaganti RSK: Chromosomal aberrations in non-

Hodgkin's lymphoma: Biologic and clinical correlations. Hematol Oncol Clin North Am 5:853, 1991

35. Pienemen WC, Deutz-Terlouw PP, Reitsma PH et al: Screening for mutations in haemophilia A patients by multiplex PCR-SSCP, Southern blotting and RNA analysis: The detection of a genetic abnormality in the factor VIII gene in 30 out of 35 patients. Br J Haematol 90:442, 1995

36. Prokocimer M, Rotter V: Structure and function of p53 in normal cells and their aberrations in cancer cells: Projection on the hematologic cell lineages. Blood 84:2391, 1994

37. Rabin D, Dattagupta N: A simple DNA diagnostic method for human genetic disorders. Hum Genet 75:120, 1987

38. Ross DW: Restriction enzymes. Arch Pathol Lab Med 114:906, 1990

39. Saiki RK, Scharf S, Faloona F et al: Enzymatic amplification of β-globin genomic sequences and restriction site analysis for diagnosis of sickle cell anemia. Science 230:1350, 1985

40. Saiki RK, Chang C-A, Levenson CH et al: Diagnosis of sickle cell anemia and β-thalassemia with enzymatically amplified DNA and nonradioactive allele-specific oligonucleotide probes. New Engl J Med 319:537, 1988

41. Saiki RK, Gelfand DH, Stoffel S et al: Primer-directed enzymatic amplification of DNA with a thermostabile DNA polymerase. Science 239:487, 1988

42. Saiki RK, Walsh PS, Levenson CH et al: Genetic analysis of amplified DNA with immobilized sequence-specific oligonucleotide probes. Proc Natl Acad Sci USA 86:6230, 1989

43. Sanger F: Determination of nucleotide sequences in DNA. Science 214:1205, 1987

44. Segal GH, Masih AS, Fox AC et al: CD-5 expressing B-cell non-Hodgkin's lymphomas with *bcl*-1 gene rearrangement have a relatively homogenous immunophenotype and are associated with an overall poor prognosis. Blood 85:1570, 1995

45. Sekiya T: Detection of mutant sequences by single-strand conformation polymorphism analysis. Mutat Res 288:79, 1993

46. Singer RH, Lawrence JB, Villnave C: Optimization of *in situ* hybridization using isotopic and non-isotopic detection methods. Biotechniques 4:230, 1986

47. Smith LM, Sanders JZ, Kaiser RJ et al: Fluorescence detection in automated DNA sequence analysis. Nature 321:674, 1986

48. Southern EM: Detection of specific sequences among DNA fragments separated by gel electrophoresis. J Mol Biol 98:503, 1978

49. Thomas PS: Hybridization of denatured RNA and small DNA fragments transferred to nitrocellulose. Proc Natl Acad Sci USA 77:5201, 1980

50. Trask B: Fluorescence *in situ* hybridization: Application in cytogenetics and gene mapping. Trends Genet 1:149, 1991

51. Urdea MS, Fultz T, Anderson TJ et al: Branched amplification multimers for the sensitive, direct detection of human hepatitis viruses. Nucleic Acids Symp Ser 24:197, 1991

52. Walker RH: Molecular pathology programs of the College of American Pathologists. Lab Med 25:654, 1994

Suggested Readings

Bernstam VA: Gene Level Diagnostics in Clinical Practice. Boca Raton, FL, CRC Press, 1992

Farkas DH: Molecular Biology and Pathology. A Guidebook for Quality Control. San Diego, Academic Press, 1993

Farkas DH: DNA Technology. Clinics in Laboratory Medicine. Philadelphia, WB Saunders, 1996

Heim RA, Silverman LM: Molecular Pathology: Approaches to Diagnosing Human Disease in the Clinical Laboratory. Durham, NC, Carolina Academic Press, 1994

Ross DW: Introduction to Molecular Medicine. New York, Springer-Verlag, 1992

Stamatoyannopoulos G, Nienhuis AW, Majerus PW et al: The Molecular Basis of Blood Diseases. Philadelphia, WB Saunders, 1994

Watson JD, Hopkins NH, Roberts JW et al: Molecular Biology of the Gene. Menlo Park, CA, Benjamin/Cummings Publishing, 1987

PART VII

Malignant Myeloproliferative Disorders

CHAPTER 32

Introduction to the Hematopoietic Malignancies

E. Anne Stiene-Martin

Objectives

1. Describe the events that can lead to a malignancy.
2. Discuss the morphologic evidence of malignancy.
3. Discuss the various means for classifying hematopoietic malignancies.

Three terms will be used interchangeably within the chapters that compose this unit. They are malignant, cancerous and neoplastic. The term *malignant* simply means deadly or capable of producing death. *Cancerous* is a term used to describe an invasive growth that spreads destructively. *Neoplastic* refers to a growth of abnormal tissue such as a tumor, and may be either benign or malignant.

A malignant neoplastic cell is one in which DNA has undergone mutations leading to a transformed cell capable of proliferation that does not respond to normal control mechanisms.[3] Two types of genes may be mutated: proto-oncogenes and tumor suppressor genes. Proto-oncogenes are normal genes that govern some aspect of cell growth and proliferation. They include genes responsible for development of growth factors, growth factor receptors, transducing proteins (*e.g.*, G proteins) and nuclear proteins involved in proliferation (*e.g.*, cyclins).[1] Mutation of a proto-oncogene may result in the generation of an

oncogene which, in turn, is responsible for the synthesis of an abnormal protein that causes aberrant and unregulated growth and proliferation of that cell. Tumor suppressor genes are normal genes that inhibit or regulate the cell cycle. The loss of these genes through mutation results in a cell that is incapable of controlling its own growth. In some instances, more than one mutational event must take place before a cell becomes fully neoplastic.

Genetic mutations leading to malignancy can occur through various mechanisms: (1) a structural mutation that the cell is unable to repair (*e.g.*, a change, deletion or insertion of one or more DNA nucleotides); (2) translocation of segments of genetic material between chromosomes [*e.g.*, t(9;22) found in chronic myelogenous leukemia]; (3) amplification or repeated duplication of a gene segment; and (4) insertion of viral DNA into the genome. In some cases, the appearance of a mutated clone of cells (*i.e.*, a malignancy) can be related to a precipitating cause such as exposure to a chemical (*e.g.*, benzene), ionizing radiation or alkylating agents such as those used in chemotherapy. Likewise, a few malignancies can be traced to a viral infection of cells.[2,4] At other times the malignancy is idiopathic (*i.e.*, there is no known triggering factor).

Regardless of cause, the outcome is a cell that undergoes unregulated proliferation resulting in a clone of identical, proliferating cells. The rate of proliferation is not necessarily faster than normal cells. In fact, the rate of proliferation may be slower than normal. One or more years may elapse between the first appearance of a malignant cell and symptoms of a tumor or neoplasm.

For a time, normal and malignant cells exist side by side in the bone marrow. Eventually, however, the malignant cells will fill the available space, and normal cells will be either inhibited or crowded to the point at which they cannot survive. These events are frequently manifested in the peripheral blood by decreases in red cells (anemia) and platelets (thrombocytopenia). The malignant cells may or may not circulate in the peripheral blood. If they do, the leukocyte count may be normal or increased; if they do not, there usually is a leukopenia. If not treated, the patient usually succumbs to infection secondary to the severe granulocytopenia or bleeding secondary to the lack of platelets.

Sometimes, whether a cell or group of cells is malignant can be determined by their appearance (morphology). Table 32-1 lists various types of morphologic evidence of malignancy. Such evidence of abnormal growth, development or proliferation is indicated by using the prefix "dys" before the term denoting growth and development (poiesis). For example, if one were to find giant, multinucleated red cell precursors, the term *dyserythropoiesis* might be used. Likewise, one might use the term *dysmegakaryocytopoiesis* if abnormally small or vacuolated megakaryocytes were seen.

If abnormal cells are present in both the bone marrow and the peripheral blood, the term *leukemia* is used. If the abnormal cells are confined to the bone marrow and do not circulate, the term *aleukemic leukemia* is used. Another possibility is neoplastic growth of cells confined to lymphatic tissue (such as lymph nodes), resulting in solid lymphatic tumors. The term *lymphoma* is appropriate in these cases, the suffix "oma" meaning "tumor." If the lymphoma spreads to the bone marrow and peripheral blood, the term *leukemic lymphoma* is sometimes used.

TABLE 32-1
Morphologic Evidence of Malignancy

NUCLEAR

Shape abnormalities (clefting, contortions)

Multinuclearity

Megaloblastoid (nonresponsive to vitamin B_{12} or folate)

Hyposegmentation (pseudo–Pelger-Huët) or hypersegmentation

Giant or prominent nucleoli

Increased mitotic figures

CYTOPLASMIC

Abnormal granules (*e.g.*, Auer rod)

Mixed granulation (*e.g.*, basophil and eosinophil)

Decreased granulation

Increased fragility (cytoplasmic fragmentation)

OVERALL

Abnormal size (gigantism or dwarfism)

Tendency to cluster or clump

Clonal morphology (all abnormal cells appear similar)

Classification of the leukemias can be achieved in several ways. First, they can be classified according to the stem cell line involved (myeloid or lymphoid). The myeloid leukemias are those involving granulocytes, monocytes, erythrocytes or megakaryocytes. Other terms that might be used to describe the myeloid leukemias are *myeloproliferative disorders* or *nonlymphocytic* leukemias. The latter term is used most frequently in reference to the acute nonlymphocytic or myeloproliferative leukemias (ANLL), also called acute myeloblastic leukemias (AML). Thus, "ANLL" and "AML" are used interchangeably. The lymphoid malignancies are those involving B or T lymphocytes and may be either leukemias or lymphomas.

The advent of flow cytometry and the availability of monoclonal antibodies that are specific for cell surface markers that identify myeloid and lymphoid cells has caused some blurring of the distinction between leukemias of these two cell lines. The terms mixed, hybrid, bilineal, biclonal and biphenotypic have emerged recently to describe a small percentage (5%–10%) of leukemias having markers for both myeloid and lymphoid cell lines within the same population or even on the same cell.

Leukemias may also be classified as acute and chronic forms. These adjectives originally referred to the expected life span of the patient. That is, patients with acute leukemia had a life span measured in days, weeks, or months, whereas patients with chronic leukemia might survive for 1 to 2 years. The advent of chemotherapy has drastically altered the life expectancy in these diseases such that today, patients with "acute leukemia" may achieve a remission with therapy and live 5 to 15 years or longer. The terms *acute* and *chronic* have been retained, however, to denote the number of primitive (blast) cells in the peripheral blood or bone marrow. Leukemias are generally considered acute if more than 30% blast forms are found in the peripheral blood or more than 50% blasts are found in the bone marrow. Conversely, if a patient has less than 10% blasts in the peripheral blood, the leukemia is more likely to be considered chronic, depending on other findings. This leaves a gray area (10%–30% blasts), which is categorized as subacute, chronic, or chronic in transformation to acute, depending on other hematologic findings and the clinical history.

As discussed in the following chapters, the acute leukemias have been further subdivided according to morphologic criteria by a group of representatives from France, America and Britain (FAB classification). The acute myeloblastic or nonlymphocytic leukemias (AML or ANLL) have been subdivided into eight classifications (M0 to M7), whereas the acute lymphoblastic leukemias (ALL) have been subdivided into three classifications (L1 to L3). These will be described in great detail in Chapter 34 (AML) and Chapter 36 (ALL).

The chronic leukemias have not been similarly subclassified. The chronic myeloproliferative disorders include chronic granulocytic (myelocytic) leukemia (CGL or CML), polycythemia vera (PV), agnogenic myeloid metaplasia with myelofibrosis (AMM), and primary (essential) thrombocythemia (ET). These will be discussed in Chapter 35. The chronic lymphoproliferative leukemias include chronic lymphocytic leukemia (CLL), prolymphocytic leukemia (PLL), and hairy cell leukemia (HCL), which will be addressed in Chapter 37.

The solid tumors of lymphatic tissue (lymphomas) will be classified and discussed in Chapter 38, whereas Chapter 39 addresses a unique lymphoid malignancy that cannot be classified as either a leukemia or a lymphoma in the strictest sense: the plasma cell dyscrasias.

The concept of "preleukemia," in which there is morphologic evidence that leukemia might occur later, has interested investigators for a number of years. At present, the only definable syndromes that might be preleukemic are proliferative disorders of myeloid cells; lymphatic preleukemia is rare and poorly defined. The terms *myelodysplastic* or *dysmyelopoietic* syndromes are commonly used to refer to these disorders. These have also been subclassified by the FAB group and will be discussed in Chapter 33.

Review Questions

32-1. A proto-oncogene is a normal gene that governs some aspect of cellular

A. death.
B. proliferation.
C. secretion.
D. all of the above.

32-2. Leukemias generally are considered acute if more than _____% blasts are found in the peripheral blood.

A. 10
B. 20
C. 30
D. 40

32-3. Morphologic evidence of malignancy includes which of the following: (1) abnormal size; (2) abnormal inclusions such as Döhle bodies; (3) multinuclearity; (4) a wide variation in the appearance of the abnormal cells?

A. 1 and 3 are correct.
B. 2 and 4 are correct.
C. 1, 2 and 3 are correct.
D. 4 only is correct.
E. All are correct.

References

1. Drucker BJ: Oncogenes, growth factors and signal transduction. N Engl J Med 321:1383, 1989
2. Manzari V, Gismondi A, Barillari G et al: HTLV V: A new human retrovirus in a TAC-negative T-cell lymphoma/leukemia. Science 238:1581, 1987
3. Pollock R, Chen S, Powess S et al: Transformation mechanisms at the cellular level. Adv Viral Oncol 4:3, 1984
4. Wyke J: Principles of viral leukemogenesis. Semin Hematol 23:189, 1986

CHAPTER 33

The Dysmyelopoietic Disorders

Robert V. Pierre

Objectives

1. Distinguish the dysmyelopoietic syndromes (DMPS) from chronic myeloproliferative disorders and acute nonlymphocytic leukemia.
2. List the five FAB classifications of DMPS and significant laboratory features of each.
3. List several chromosomal abnormalities associated with DMPS.
4. List the laboratory tests most useful in the diagnosis of DMPS and explain why they are useful.
5. Briefly discuss the treatment and prognosis for patients with DMPS.

DEFINITION OF DYSMYELOPOIETIC SYNDROMES AND RELATION TO OTHER CLONAL MYELOPROLIFERATIVE DISORDERS

The dysmyelopoietic syndromes (DMPS) belong to a group of disorders called clonal myeloproliferative disorders that occur most often in elderly persons. In such disorders, an abnormal group or clone of cells arises from an abnormal myeloid stem cell in the bone marrow. Recall that the myeloid stem cell is the precursor from which all erythrocytes and leukocytes (except lymphocytes) come (see Fig. 5-5). There are three major groups of clonal myeloproliferative disorders including the DMPS (discussed in this chapter), the chronic myeloproliferative disorders (CMPD; Chap. 35), and the acute nonlymphocytic leukemias (ANLL; Chap. 34). It is helpful to understand the relation among these three groups.

The disease process in the DMPS (also called myelodysplastic syndromes) involves the production of myeloid cells that demonstrate *dysplasia*. Dysplasia in cells is demonstrated in many ways including abnormalities in size, shape, maturation, organization, or combinations thereof. The DMPS differ from CMPD in that the DMPS generally have no overproduction of a cell line. The DMPS are more often characterized by peripheral blood cytopenias secondary to either an absolute decrease in precursor cells in the marrow or ineffective cell production. There is disagreement about whether the DMPS are truly leukemic, or whether they represent qualitative stem cell abnormalities. The term preleukemia or preleukemic syndrome has been used by many authors as a synonym for DMPS because they have a great potential for transformation to acute leukemia. The DMPS have a clinical course that is shorter than the CMPD but usually longer than that of the ANLL.

DMPS and CMPD are alike in some aspects. In both disorders, the abnormal pluripotential stem cell line coexists in the marrow with the normal stem cell lines. Also the abnormal cells of both DMPS and CMPD have the potential to differentiate into mature although abnormal-appearing end-stage cells. However, the CMPD are different in that the abnormal stem cell also has the potential to differentiate along a single cell line or along more than one cell line simultaneously. Examples are the production of predominantly granulocytes in chronic granulocytic leukemia (CGL), predominantly erythrocytes in polycythemia vera (PV), and predominantly platelets in essential thrombocythemia (ET). An example of the abnormal production of multiple cell lines is agnogenic myeloid metaplasia (AMM). All of these disorders are clonal in nature.[11]

Although CGL is a malignant process, the other CMPD—PV, ET and AMM—are usually viewed as nonmalignant until the later stages of the disorders when they undergo transformation to acute leukemia. The reasons for this view are that cell maturation remains normal until the transformation, there is little cellular dysplasia, and patients generally have relatively long survival times.

The acute nonlymphocytic leukemias (ANLL), also called acute myeloid leukemias, differ from the DMPS and CMPD in that of the three diseases, the blood cells in ANLL show the least (very little) maturation, the most cell dysplasia, and patients with ANLL generally have the shortest survival times.

HISTORY OF DISEASE

Hamilton-Patterson should probably receive credit for the first description of DMPS in 1949.[15] Block and coworkers introduced the term preleukemia in 1953.[4] In 1972, the first specific clinicopathologic entity of DMPS was described as "refractory anemia with excess myeloblasts."[9] Also in 1972, "chronic myelomonocytic leukemia" was described.[38] Although these disorders may have an increase in marrow blasts, the number of blasts is not sufficient (generally less than 30%) to make a diagnosis of acute leukemia. Other terms have been used for disorders that overlap in their features with the DMPS and some forms of ANLL. They include "refractory dysmyelopoietic anemia,"[26] "subacute myeloid leukemia,"[7] and "smoldering acute leukemia."[25] The French–American–British (FAB) group[3] introduced their classification system for the DMPS in 1973, and it is shown in Table 33-1. The DMPS tend to occur more frequently in males than in females, similar to the male preponderance that occurs in overt ANLL.[36] These syndromes are found most frequently in patients older than 50 years of age.[23] The incidence rises markedly in persons 70 to 90 years of age, but DMPS may occur in any aged group, including young

children. The DMPS appear to be more common than overt ANLL.[23]

The cause or causes of DMPS are unknown, except that some cases may be secondary to X-ray therapy, chemotherapy with alkylating agents, or work or hobby exposure to toxic chemicals. Cases without a known history of such exposure are referred to as primary DMPS. Cases with an exposure history are referred to as secondary DMPS. DMPS are not known to be hereditary.

PATHOPHYSIOLOGY

The pathophysiology of DMPS is poorly understood. DMPS represents the growth of an abnormal clone of cells in the marrow, similar to the process in ANLL. Experimental studies[5] have shown that leukemic cells can suppress the growth of normal cells, either by production of a humoral substance or perhaps by recruitment of T lymphocytes that secrete cytokines (substances produced by cells that have effects on other cells). If the suppression affects the normal pluripotential stem cell lines of the marrow, marrow hypoplasia and pancytopenia result. If the suppression affects only the committed stem cell lines, selective marrow hypoplasia with isolated cytopenias in the peripheral blood may occur. This mechanism may explain the cases of DMPS associated with marrow hypoplasia and singular peripheral blood cytopenias. In many cases of DMPS, cytopenias are associated with a cellular to hypercellular bone marrow; this suggests the existence of a mechanism of premature death of bone marrow cells.[24]

Abnormal DMPS stem cell lines have the ability to differentiate to mature end-stage cells that are abnormal in appearance and function.[2,31] The combination of dyserythropoiesis (abnormal maturation of erythrocytes) with ineffective erythropoiesis accounts for the presence of anemia with mature but oval, macrocytic erythrocytes. The presence of neutropenia with morphologically and functionally abnormal mature forms such as "pseudo"–Pelger-Huët forms (see Fig. 26-1) or degranulated neutrophils accounts for the frequent infections and fever seen in patients with DMPS. The suppression of megakaryocytopoiesis or dysplasia of megakaryocytes (dysmegakaryocytopoiesis) accounts for the thrombocytopenia and abnormal-appearing platelets, which frequently have abnormal function as well, resulting in patient bleeding problems.

CLINICAL PRESENTATION

The classic triad of symptoms in patients with DMPS is fatigue, fever and bleeding. Many patients, particularly those with early stages of DMPS, are asymptomatic and are discovered on routine checkups or in the course of investigating other disorders. Physical examination is usually unremarkable, but pallor may be present secondary to anemia, fever may be present because of infection and there may be petechiae or ecchymoses secondary to thrombocytopenia. The spleen may be slightly enlarged, particularly in chronic myelomonocytic leukemia, but there is usually no lymphadenopathy.

TABLE 33-1
FAB Classification of the Dysmyelopoietic Syndromes (DMPS)

Disorder	Abbreviation
Refractory anemia or refractory cytopenia	RA/RC
Refractory anemia with ringed sideroblasts	RARS
Refractory anemia with excess blasts	RAEB
Chronic myelomonocytic leukemia	CMML
Refractory anemia with excess blasts in transformation	RAEBIT

PERIPHERAL BLOOD AND BONE MARROW ABNORMALITIES

Erythropoiesis

Erythropoiesis in the bone marrow shows quantitative abnormalities that range from red cell aplasia (severe decrease in erythropoiesis) to extreme erythroid hyperplasia. The hallmark of DMPS is dyserythropoiesis which is characterized by the abnormal maturation of red cells that is referred to as "megaloblastoid." *Megaloblastoid* is used to signify the resemblance of nucleated red blood cells (NRBCs) in DMPS to the NRBCs that exhibit megaloblastic maturation in vitamin B_{12} deficiency. However megaloblastoid red cells differ in that they have an open nuclear chromatin pattern that is more coarse than that of megaloblastic maturation and makes parachromatin more prominent (see Color Plates 33-1 and 12-5). Also the chromatin may be attached to the nuclear membrane in large clumps. (Chapter 12 outlines more details on the differences between megaloblastic and megaloblastoid morphology.) The NRBC nucleus may be irregular in shape, from simple indentation to complex cloverleaf forms. Multinuclearity and giant NRBC forms may be seen. There may be asynchronous nuclear–cytoplasmic maturation and a left shift in NRBC maturation, with an increase in the number of rubriblasts.

Hemoglobinization of the cytoplasm of NRBCs may be normal or impaired. Impaired hemoglobinization is associated with a microcytic, hypochromic or dimorphic (normochromic and hypochromic) picture in the peripheral blood. Any of the following may also be seen in the peripheral blood: poikilocytes including ovalocytes and teardrops (dacryocytes) among others, NRBCs, basophilic stippling, Howell-Jolly bodies, siderocytes and sideroblasts.

The bone marrow demonstrates increased stainable iron and may reveal pathologic ringed sideroblasts. Pathologic ringed sideroblasts are NRBCs containing iron-filled mitochondria that form a ring around the nucleus. There must be five or more iron granules in a given NRBC, and the granules must occupy at least 30% of the circumference of the nucleus (see Color Plates 33-2 and 13-2).

Granulopoiesis

Granulopoiesis shows quantitative changes, ranging from decreased granulopoiesis to marked granulocytic hyperplasia. Dysgranulopoiesis is manifested by a left shift in granulocytic maturation, with an increase in myeloblasts (see Color Plate 33-4). There may be nuclear abnormalities such as hyposegmentation (pseudo–Pelger-Huët forms) or hypersegmentation of neutrophils. The cells may also show asynchronous nuclear–cytoplasmic maturation, pseudonucleoli secondary to cytoplasmic intrusion into the nucleus and nuclear blebs. Granule abnormalities are common; there may be hypogranulation of the neutrophils or coarse abnormal granules, the pseudo–Chédiak-Higashi abnormality. Rarely, eosinophils and basophils also show hypogranulation. Auer rods may occasionally be found.

Occasionally, it is difficult to differentiate neutrophilic bands from monocytes owing to hypogranulation. There are atypical neutrophils with monocytoid features; this is particularly true in chronic myelomonocytic leukemia. There may also be cells that have the cytochemical features of both neutrophils and monocytes. This is not surprising because the neutrophil and monocyte are both thought to be derived from a common committed stem cell.

The French–American–British (FAB) group[3] has introduced a classification for blasts to assist in the diagnosis of DMPS. The blasts are classified as Types I, II and III on Romanowsky-stained peripheral blood films. A Type I blast has a centrally located nucleus, a fine nuclear chromatin pattern, a prominent nucleolus, and *no granules* in the cytoplasm (see Fig. 34-1 and Color Plate 33-6). A Type II blast has a centrally located nucleus but a slightly more mature nuclear chromatin pattern and a lower nuclear/cytoplasmic ratio. The cytoplasm contains fewer than 20 granules (see Fig. 34-2 and Color Plate 33-7). The Type III blast has more than 20 granules in the cytoplasm. Types II and III blasts have also been referred to as "abnormal progranulocytes (promyelocytes)." The combined total of Types I, II and III blasts is used to calculate the percentage of blasts and classify a disorder as DMPS (Table 33-2) or ANLL. The Type III blast is not synonymous with the abnormal progranulocyte of ANLL type M3 (Chap. 34).

Megakaryocytopoiesis

Megakaryocytes may show quantitative abnormalities ranging from near absence to hyperplasia. Dysplasia of megakaryocytes is a common feature in DMPS. The most frequent abnormality is a maturational arrest, with the majority of megakaryocytes being small to medium-sized cells, with single or bilobed nuclei, whereas normal megakaryocytes usually have four to eight nuclear lobes (see Fig. 55-3). The cytoplasm may show vacuolization and hypogranulation. Micro- or dwarf megakaryocytes may also be found. In rare cases, there are giant megakaryocytes with hypersegmentation of the nucleus (with more than the usual number of separate small individual nuclei); these are so-called osteoblastic megakaryocytes.

The peripheral blood platelets may be decreased, normal, or rarely, increased. They may be hypogranular or have abnormally large granules that appear fused. Micromegakaryocytes or megakaryoblasts may sometimes be found in the peripheral blood (see Color Plate 34-7). Abnormalities of the dense tubular system or open canalicular system (see Fig. 55-6) may give the platelets a Swiss cheese appearance.

SPECIFIC CLINICOPATHOLOGIC FORMS OF DYSMYELOPOIETIC SYNDROMES

When the FAB group created a classification of the DMPS or myelodysplastic syndromes, they did not describe these disorders, but created diagnostic criteria for each of the entities.[3] The five entities are shown in Table 33-1. Table 33-2 summarizes the principal diagnostic criteria.

TABLE 33-2
Laboratory Findings in the FAB Classification of the Dysmyelopoietic Syndromes

	RA/RC	RARS	RAEB	CMML	RAEBIT
Leukocyte count	N to ↓	N to ↓	N to ↓	↑	N to ↓
Platelet count	N to sl ↓	N to sl ↓	N to ↓	N to ↓	N to ↓
Monocytes					
Marrow	—	—	—	At least 20%	—
Blood	—	—	—	>1 × 10⁹/L	—
Blasts in peripheral blood (%)	<1	<1	<5	<5	>5
Blasts in bone marrow (%)	<5	<5	5–20	0–20	20–30
Dyserythropoiesis	+++	++	+/−	+/−	+/−
Dysgranulopoiesis	−	+/−	++	++	+/−
Dysmegakaryocytopoiesis	−	+/−	+/−	+/−	+/−
Siderocytes/sideroblasts	+	+	+/−	−	+/−
Ringed sideroblasts (%)	+/−	>15	+/−	−	+/−

Key: N, normal; ↓, decreased; sl ↓, slightly decreased; +++, moderate to marked; ++, moderate; +, slight; +/−, slight or none.

Refractory Anemia

The principal feature of refractory anemia (RA) is dyserythropoiesis (see Color Plate 33-1), which is manifested by megaloblastoid maturation of erythrocytic precursors and an anemia characterized by oval macrocytes. The patient may be mildly to severely anemic. The mean cell volume (MCV) and the red cell distribution width (RDW) usually are elevated. A dimorphic red cell picture may occasionally be observed owing to impaired hemoglobinization of NRBCs. Dysplastic NRBCs, sideroblasts, and siderocytes may be found in the peripheral blood. The FAB group emphasizes that a decrease in the absolute reticulocyte count (Chap. 9) is characteristic; however, in our experience, the relative reticulocyte count (percentage) is often elevated, and prominent polychromatophilia may be seen on the blood film.

Neither dysgranulopoiesis nor dysmegakaryocytopoiesis are features of RA. The total leukocyte count is normal or low as is the total platelet count (Table 33-2). An elevated leukocyte count suggests an infection or misdiagnosis. The FAB group stipulates that less than 1% of Types I, II and III blasts be present in the peripheral blood and less than 5% in the bone marrow.

Bone marrow cellularity is most often normal or increased. However, marrow hypocellularity does not exclude the diagnosis. Erythrocytic hyperplasia is present with abnormal (megaloblastoid) maturation. The maturation abnormalities may be subtle and can easily be missed or misidentified as megaloblastic. No giant or bizzare multinucleated erythrocytic precursors are seen. Pathologic sideroblasts may be seen in small numbers. Bone marrow iron is normal or increased. Bone marrow fibrosis is not a feature of RA.

Refractory Cytopenia

The FAB group suggested that disorders characterized by peripheral neutropenia or thrombocytopenia without an increase in blasts be called refractory cytopenia (RC). However in my experience, most cases of peripheral neutropenia or thrombocytopenia with hyperplasia of the corresponding precursors in the bone marrow and with maturational arrest are immune- or drug-related phenomena and *not* DMPS. In the past 24 years, we have observed only three patients whose disease could be classified as RC. Two had a chronic idiopathic thrombocytopenic purpura-like picture, and the third had a chronic immune neutropenia-like picture. The conditions of all three evolved into ANLL.

Refractory Anemia With Ringed Sideroblasts

Refractory anemia with ringed sideroblasts (RARS), also called idiopathic acquired sideroblastic anemia (IASA), is similar to RA; however, the absolute requirement for diagnosis of RARS is the presence of pathologic ringed sideroblasts in the bone marrow (see Color Plates 33-2 and 13-2) and impaired hemoglobinization of erythroid precursors with megaloblastoid maturation. Ringed sideroblasts must account for 15% or more of all nucleated red cells in the marrow. Types I, II and III blasts must be less than 1% in the peripheral blood and less than 5% in the bone marrow. The peripheral blood picture is usually that of a dimorphic anemia, with a combination of hypochromic microcytes and oval macrocytes. Sideroblasts and siderocytes may be present in the peripheral blood.

The FAB group specifies that granulopoiesis and mega-karyocytopoiesis should show minimal quantitative and qualitative changes.

Another type of sideroblastic anemia, called primary sideroblastic anemia, is not a DMPS. It may occur in elderly adults as do the DMPS. The peripheral blood and bone marrow findings are identical with those of RARS except that these patients do not have evidence of dys-granulopoiesis or dysmegakaryocytopoiesis. These patients do not appear to have a leukemic transformation potential.

Refractory Anemia With Excess Blasts

Refractory anemia with excess blasts (RAEB) may display any of the erythroid changes of RA or RARS, but must also have dysgranulopoiesis and peripheral cytopenias of two cell lines. The dysgranulopoiesis is more pronounced than in RARS. Between 5% and 20% of Types I, II and III blasts must be present in the marrow. Up to 5% blasts may be observed on the peripheral blood film. There must be progression of granulocytic precursors to mature forms. Dysmegakaryocytopoiesis may be present with mononuclear or bilobed megakaryocytes in the bone marrow. Large, dysplastic platelets and thrombocytopenia may be noted on the peripheral blood film.

Either RA or RARS may pass through progressive stages of the FAB classification, including RAEB, before transforming into leukemia. The FAB classification is a hierarchic classification in that the number of blasts takes precedence over other features in determining the classification. In cases of RA with marked erythrocytic hyperplasia and dysplasia, an increase in bone marrow blasts to 5% or more causes the condition to be classified as RAEB; likewise, when bone marrow blasts increase to 5% or more in RARS, the classification becomes RAEB, in spite of prominent sideroblasts. Although RAEB is considered a DMPS, when a child or young adult presents with the morphologic picture of RAEB, the disease will be rapidly progressive and should be classified and treated as an ANLL type M2 (Chap. 34).

Chronic Myelomonocytic Leukemia

Chronic myelomonocytic leukemia (CMML) has been included in the FAB DMPS classification. The term originally suggested by Zittoun and coworkers[38] has caused some confusion and may be an illogical one. The FAB group does not believe that the DMPS are early stages of leukemia or even necessarily preleukemic, yet the word leukemia is used in the name for CMML. The term chronic myelomonocytic syndrome might be more appropriate.

Although CMML may exhibit any of the dyspoietic features of erythropoiesis, granulopoiesis and megakaryocytopoiesis described in RA, RARS or RAEB, it has several distinctive features and, in fact, is more frequently confused with chronic myeloproliferative disorders (Chap. 35) than with acute leukemia (Chap. 34) or other forms of DMPS. The FAB criteria state that there must be between 0% and 20% blasts in the marrow and less than 5% blasts in the peripheral blood. The distinguishing feature of CMML is a prominent monocytic component in the bone marrow; at least 20% of the marrow cells are monocytic (normal for adults is 0% to 2%), and there are more than 1×10^9 monocytes per liter in the peripheral blood (normal for adults is 0.0 to $0.8 \times 10^9/L$). The monocytes of the peripheral blood and the monocytic component of the marrow may be difficult to recognize because of the dysplasia of the neutrophils and monocytes. It is strongly recommended that a combined (dual) esterase stain (combination α-naphthyl butyrate–chloroacetate esterase stain; Chap. 29) be used for both the peripheral blood film and the bone marrow aspirate if CMML is suspected.[37] The advantage of this stain is that it permits the differentiation of monocytic and neutrophilic components on a single peripheral blood or bone marrow specimen (see Color Plate 33-3).

The total leukocyte count in all of the other DMPS is usually normal or low, but in CMML it is most often elevated and may exceed $100 \times 10^9/L$. The marrow shows striking granulocytic hyperplasia with progression to mature forms. The mature neutrophils in CMML often appear hypogranular.

Interestingly, the FAB group did not recognize that a transition stage of CMML might exist between CMML and overt acute leukemia. We have seen patients with CMML with an increase in their marrow blasts to more than 20% before transformation to ANLL. The condition in such a situation might be referred to as "CMML in transformation."

There is a syndrome that occurs in infants or young children that resembles the CMML seen in adults; however, it often has a more aggressive clinical course. This disorder characteristically has a deletion of chromosome 7 and may have other chromosomal abnormalities. It is referred to as the "myelomonocytic syndrome of infants" or "monosomy 7 syndrome."[6]

Refractory Anemia With Excess Blasts in Transformation

Patients with refractory anemia with excess blasts in transformation (RAEBIT) present with cytopenias and symptoms of brief duration, and their hematologic picture does not fit the definitions of RA, RARS, RAEB or CMML or any of the FAB acute leukemia categories. The FAB criteria for RAEBIT are (1) 5% or more blasts in the peripheral blood and (2) from 20% to 30% blasts in the bone marrow (see Color Plate 33-4). Auer rods may or may not be present. The diagnostic problem with RAEBIT is that it is difficult to differentiate from ANLL type M2 which is characterized by more than 30% blasts in the bone marrow and a high incidence of Auer rods. The clinical course of RAEBIT, particularly in young patients, is that of acute leukemia.[29]

DYSMYELOPOIETIC DISORDERS NOT INCLUDED IN THE FAB CLASSIFICATION

There are a variety of dysmyelopoietic syndromes not included in the FAB classification. Some have been well characterized and others are less well defined (Table 33-3).

Refractory cytopenia not meeting criteria for RA, RARS, RAEB or CMML

Secondary or therapy related disorders

Postleukemic disorders

Single-cell–line aplasias

Paroxysmal nocturnal hemoglobinuria (PNH)

RARS with isodicentric X abnormality

Dysmegakaryocytopoiesis
    With the 5q⁻ chromosome abnormality
    Without the 5q⁻ chromosome abnormality

Acute myelodysplasia with myelofibrosis

Secondary or Therapy-Related Syndromes

The secondary syndromes are an important group of DMPS. Secondary DMPS usually occur following the use of alkylating-type chemotherapeutic agents either alone or in combination with radiation therapy in the treatment of solid malignant tumors such as lymphomas or breast cancer. Radiation alone produces a lower incidence of secondary DMPS and ANLL. The onset of DMPS is usually 2 to 3 years following treatment, but it may be as short as 2 months. Secondary DMPS or acute leukemia following the use of certain drugs used for cancer treatment may occur in even less than 2 months; however, the DMPS phase may be so short before transformation to acute leukemia that it goes unnoticed.

Secondary DMPS often begins as a refractory macrocytic anemia or sideroblastic anemia. It differs from primary DMPS in that it nearly always has pancytopenia with dysplasia in all marrow cell lines and frequently has a hypocellular marrow with an increase in fibrosis. Cytogenetic studies are particularly helpful in secondary DMPS because a very high percentage of cases caused by radiation or alkylating drug exposure have abnormalities of chromosomes 5 and 7. Cases secondary to use of the drugs that cause rapid onset of DMPS have abnormalities of 11q23 and 21q22.

Postleukemic Syndromes

Foucar and associates have described postleukemic DMPS.[12] They observed patients in whom DMPS had progressed to overt ANLL and after therapy, reverted to their pretherapy DMPS status rather than to a normal marrow or persistence of ANLL. We have observed patients who have attained a remission of their ANLL in the form of a DMPS, rather than a complete remission.

Single Cell Aplasias

Single cell aplasias are disorders in which a single cell-line is initially affected. A well-known single cell aplasia is pure red cell aplasia (Chap. 11) that is usually caused by either immune disorders of the bone marrow, viral infection (particularly parvovirus B19), or marrow injury by drugs such as chloramphenicol. Although most of

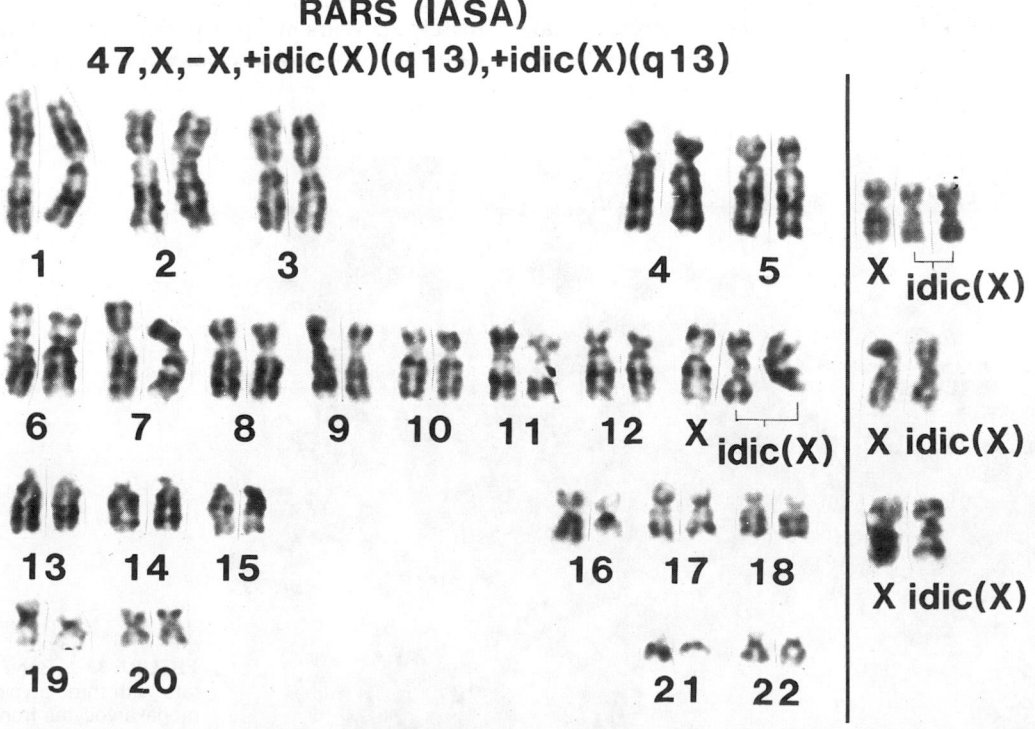

RARS (IASA)
47,X,–X,+idic(X)(q13),+idic(X)(q13)

FIGURE 33-1. GTG-banded 47,X,−X,2idic (X) (q13) karyotype from a patient with refractory anemia with ringed sideroblasts (RARS; *left*) and 2idic (X) (q13) chromosome from three different metaphases (*right*).

these cases are not DMPS, some do represent DMPS because they transform to ANLL. We have followed seven cases of pure red cell aplasia over 18 years and observed one transformation to ANLL.

We have also seen one case of another single-cell aplasia that evolved to an ANLL. The diagnosis was amegakaryocytic thrombocytopenic purpura, a disorder in which there is a deficiency of platelets in the peripheral blood and their precursors in the bone marrow. This disorder might be similar in etiology to a pure red cell aplasia.

Refractory Anemia With Ringed Sideroblasts and Isodicentric X Abnormality

We have observed a group of female patients with RARS and an acquired isodicentric X chromosomal abnormality (Fig. 33-1)[8] in whom the disorder rapidly transformed to ANLL. It is not known whether the breakpoints of this gene rearrangement are at or near the gene that causes the rare inherited (X-linked recessive) form of sideroblastic anemia (Chap. 13).

Refractory Macrocytic Anemia With Megakaryocytic Abnormalities (5q⁻ Syndrome)

The 5q⁻ syndrome should be included among the DMPS because, frequently, the condition goes on to ANLL.[35] The disorder is both a cytogenetic and a clinicopathologic entity. The patient must possess an isolated deletion between bands q15 and q31 of the long arm of chromosome 5, thus the name 5q⁻. There is a striking female preponderance in the disorder. The peripheral blood picture is that of a refractory anemia, with oval macrocytes and normal or increased platelets. The bone marrow is normocellular or hypercellular, with megaloblastoid erythrocytic hyperplasia. The feature that distinguishes this disorder from refractory anemia is the numerous small or medium-sized mononuclear or bilobed megakaryocytes in the bone marrow, which frequently have vacuolated cytoplasm (Fig. 33-2). The type of megakaryocyte found in this disorder is not unique to the 5q⁻ syndrome. They may also be found in RAEB (see that section earlier in this chapter). The combination of a refractory macrocytic anemia, the 5q⁻ chromosome abnormality and atypical megakaryocytes is required for the diagnosis.

Dyspoietic Megakaryocytic Hyperplasia Without 5q⁻ Chromosomal Abnormality

This disorder has been referred to as hyperfibrotic myelodysplasia or myelodysplasia with myelofibrosis. The disorder is characterized by marked megakaryocytic hyperplasia and dysplasia (Fig. 33-3); there may or may not be myelofibrosis present. It differs from acute megakaryocytic leukemia (ANLL type M7; Chap. 34) by having less than 30% blasts. Dyspoiesis of both erythrocytes and granulocytes is also observed. In another variant with megakaryocytic dyspoiesis, the megakaryocytes are large and appear hypermature or hypersegmented. The individual nuclei of the megakaryocyte are separated and distinct (Fig. 33-4).

SURVIVAL AND PROGRESSION TO ACUTE LEUKEMIA

The median survival of patients with DMPS was approximately 2.5 years in a prospective study done at the Mayo Clinic.[23] Tricot and associates found a median survival of

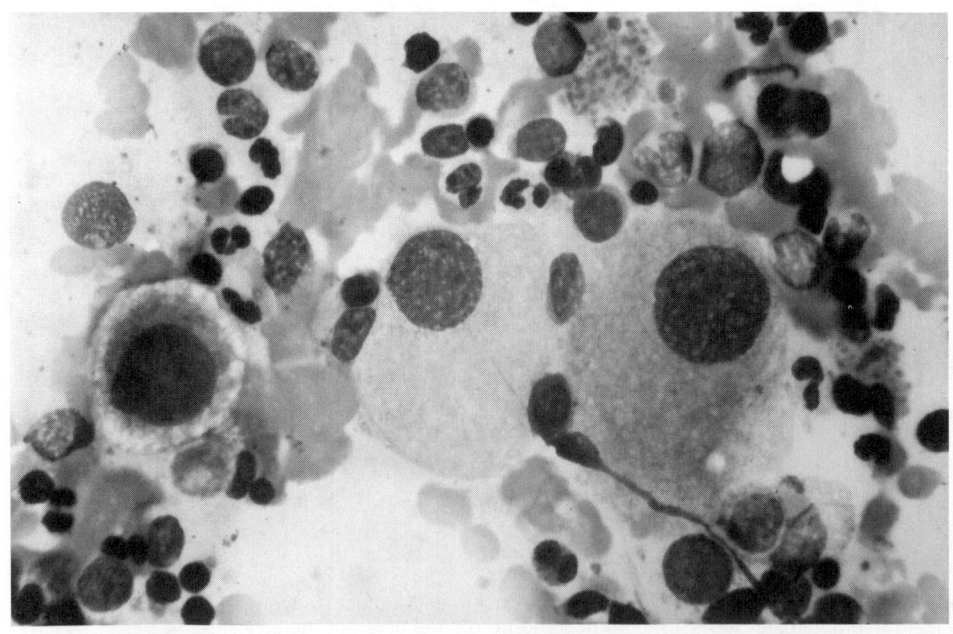

FIGURE 33-2. Bone marrow aspirate with three atypical mononuclear megakaryocytes from a patient with the 5q⁻ syndrome. One cell shows cytoplasmic vacuolization.

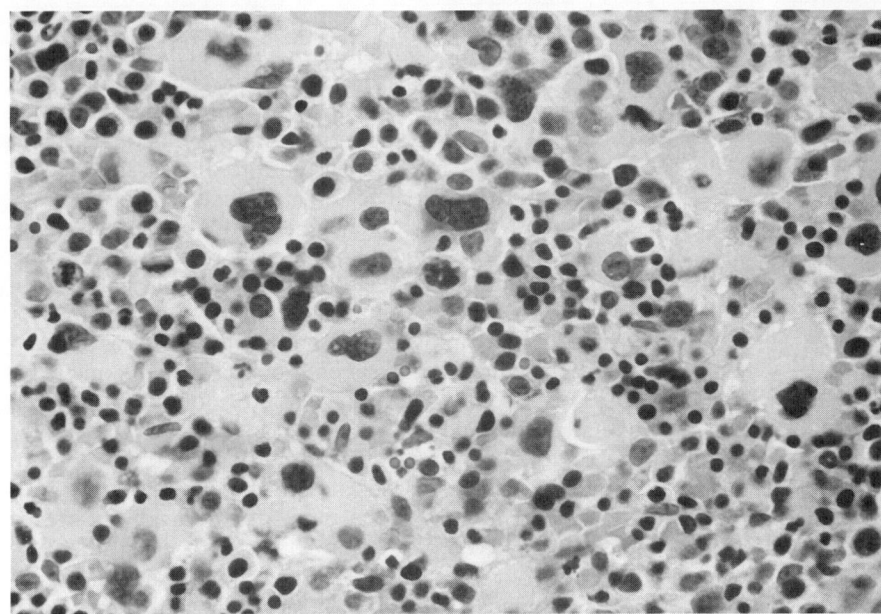

FIGURE 33-3. Bone marrow biopsy section from a patient with a dysmyelopoietic syndrome characterized by striking megakaryocytic dyspoiesis (H & E stain), without the 5q⁻ chromosomal abnormality.

18.5 months for patients with less than 5% marrow blasts and of only 7 months in patients with more than than 5% marrow blasts.[34]

It is apparent that patients with DMPS can die with or without developing acute leukemia, usually from complications of their anemia, neutropenia or thrombocytopenia. Examination of a number of large series of patients with DMPS shows that only approximately 25% of patients go on to overt ANLL (Table 33-4).

LABORATORY TESTS MOST USEFUL IN THE DIAGNOSIS OF DMPS

The diagnosis of DMPS is made from the clinical information, complete blood count, blood film examination, and bone marrow aspirate and biopsy examination. The diagnosis of RAEB, CMML and RAEBIT can be made with

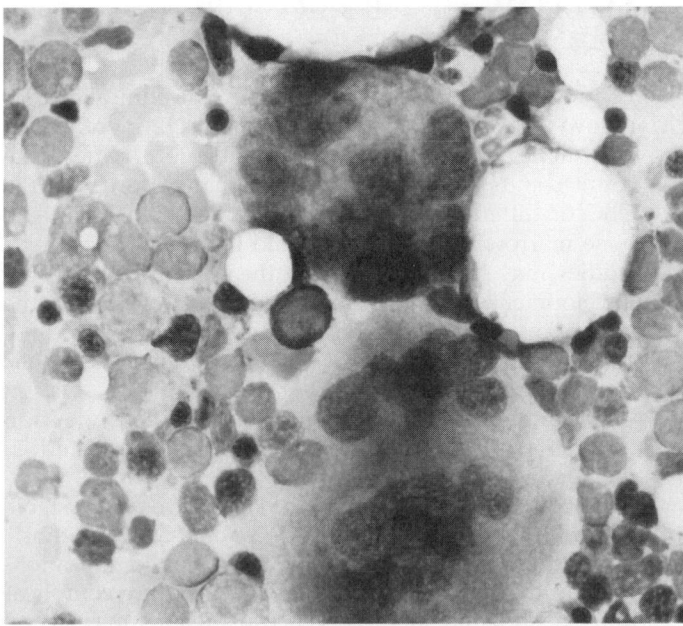

FIGURE 33-4. Bone marrow aspirate from a patient with a dysmyelopoietic syndrome characterized by megakaryocytic dyspoiesis without the 5q⁻ chromosomal abnormality. The majority of megakaryocytes resembled large, hypersegmented forms seen in this photomicrograph.

TABLE 33-4
Frequency of Transformation of DMPS to Acute Nonlymphocytic Leukemia (ANLL)

Series	Number of Patients	Percent (%) with Transformation
Second IWCL[30]	244	21
Weber et al[36]	151	23
Rosenthal and Moloney[26]	117	24
Todd and Pierre[32]	326	22
Juneja et al*[18]	34	18

* Cases of RAEB only.

great accuracy by these standard hematologic examinations and should present no problem to the experienced morphologist. Refractory anemia (RA) or refractory cytopenias (RC) pose a much more serious diagnostic problem, because they are mimicked by a variety of disorders. In a prospective 16-year study of 325 patients with suspected DMPS, 31 patients had spontaneous resolution of their hematologic abnormalities and an additional 15 patients had their condition evolve into typical agnogenic myeloid metaplasia (AMM; Chap. 35).[32] Even in retrospect, these 46 patients (14% of the total) could not be distinguished from those whose condition eventually evolved into acute leukemia. All the patients whose conditions resolved or transformed into AMM were initially said to have RA. No cases of RAEB, CMML or RAEBIT were seen to resolve or transform into other chronic myeloproliferative disorders.

Because morphology alone is not adequate for identification of cases of suspected RA or RARS, additional laboratory tests are mandatory. Serum vitamin B_{12} and folate levels, which should be normal in the DMPS, should always be measured, because early megaloblastic and megaloblastoid maturation can be indistinguishable. Serum iron and ferritin levels and iron stains on the bone marrow aspirate and biopsy should be performed. If pathologic ringed sideroblasts are noted, they should be quantitated by determining their percentage among all nucleated red cells. A reticulin stain should be performed on the marrow to determine whether myelofibrosis is present. A peroxidase and a combined esterase stain should be done on both the peripheral blood and the bone marrow aspirate. The peroxidase stain is used to determine whether acquired peroxidase deficiency is present, and it may make Auer rods visible that are not seen on the Romanowsky stain. The combined esterase stain permits more accurate assessment of the percentage of monocytic cells in the peripheral blood and bone marrow.

The demonstration of a clonal chromosomal abnormality by cytogenetic studies may be helpful in establishing the diagnosis of DMPS in problem cases of RA, RC and RARS. The types of chromosomal changes observed in 40% to 60% of DMPS patients are similar to those observed in ANLL.[20] Secondary or therapy-related DMPS has the same chromosomal abnormalities as secondary ANLL. Secondary DMPS and ANLL have a high frequency of chromosomal abnormalities and abnormalities involving chromosomes 5 and 7.[21] Cytogenetic studies are necessary to classify the 5q⁻ syndrome, the isodicentric X form of RARS and the monosomy 7 syndrome seen in infants, and they may be necessary to distinguish CMML from chronic granulocytic leukemia. In addition, the presence or absence of cytogenetic abnormalities gives prognostic information about both the survival and likelihood of progression to acute leukemia.[19] Major karyotypic abnormalities such as combined $-7,5q^-$ abnormalities or marked hyperdiploidy or hypodiploidy (having more or less than two full sets of homologous chromosomes, respectively) confer a greater possibility of transformation to acute leukemia.

In atypical cases, particularly those who have pathologic ringed sideroblasts, muscle weakness and neurologic abnormalities, toxic exposure to lead or arsenic should be ruled out by serum, urine or tissue studies. We have seen several cases of lead or arsenic toxicity referred to us as suspected DMPS or subacute leukemia (Color Plate 33-5).

In vitro culture for marrow stem cells, particularly for the CFU-GM, may be valuable for establishing the diagnosis of DMPS. However, these studies are mainly research tools and are not widely available for routine use.[14]

Flow cytometric analysis of bone marrow cells (Chap. 43) has been used to determine the fractions of cells in the S and G_2 phases (see Fig. 5-6). Patients who have a higher fraction of cells in these phases have a more stable course.[22] These studies correlate with other studies that show that reduction of proliferative activity correlates with a poor prognosis. Flow cytometry has also been used to measure cellular DNA content and to identify aneuploidy (an abnormal number of chromosomes), both of which are diagnostically helpful.

FOLLOW-UP OBSERVATIONS AND TREATMENT

For patients who appear to have a stable clinical course, follow-up examinations are made at 6- to 12-month intervals. Repeat complete blood cell (CBC) and differential count results are sufficient. If any changes occur in the CBC or differential or in the patient's clinical status, a bone marrow examination should be done. Cytogenetic studies may show a change in the karyotype, with the development of a new abnormality or a change in the karyotype signifying clonal evolution. Evidence of a clonal change is suggestive of an imminent leukemic transformation.

Treatment of patients with DMPS is dependent on two factors: (1) the clinical severity of the process and (2) the age of the patient.

Because patients with DMPS may have a long stable course, it is useful to observe the patient after diagnosis to determine stability. If the patient remains complication-free, no therapy is recommended. If there are complications, such as anemia, red cell transfusions may be required. Neutropenia and thrombocytopenia are of greater concern because long-term leukocyte or platelet transfusion therapy is not feasible. Steroid therapy has been successful in some patients.

A form of therapy based on the principle that leukemic and preleukemic cells can be induced to differentiate by "cell maturation agents," has received extensive evaluation. For example, human leukemic blasts can be induced to differentiate into mature neutrophils by exposure to drugs such as cytarabine (cytosine arabinoside; ara-C),[17,33] *cis*-retinoic acid,[31] or humoral factors that regulate granulopoiesis.[28] Trials of *cis*-retinoic acid and ara-C in low dosage have induced complete remission in some patients and improvement in others, although most patients do not show significant improvement.[11,13,20,31,33]

The more recent introduction of several therapeutic agents including recombinant human erythropoietin (r-HuEPO) and thrombopoietin, CFU-G (stem cells committed to granulocyte production), CFU-GM (stem cells committed to granulocyte and monocyte production; Chap. 5) has made management of these patients somewhat easier. Administration of these agents may decrease the need for transfusion, decrease bleeding manifestations and reduce infections. However, the long-term use of these agents is cost-prohibitive.

Age is an important factor in the selection of therapeutic approach. In young children or young adults whose cytopenias are severe enough to warrant therapy, the disease should be treated as an acute leukemia. In young patients, aggressive antileukemic therapy has proved successful because it induces complete remissions with sustained survival. However, only a small number of DMPS cases occur in young patients. Bone marrow transplantation has been successful in long-term remission of DMPS, and represents the only potentially curative form of therapy currently available.[1] Bone marrow transplantation is limited to patients younger than than 50 years of age, and the disease-free survival at 5 years can range from 35% to 45%.[16]

CHAPTER SUMMARY

The dysmyelopoietic syndromes (DMPS) are clonal proliferative disorders of the bone marrow. Clonal disorders are conditions derived from an abnormality in a single bone marrow precursor cell that leads to an abnormal clone or group of cells.

The DMPS include five major groups according to a number of laboratory observations (*e.g.*, the bone marrow and peripheral blood blast percentage; see Tables 33-1 and 33-2). They are often associated with peripheral blood cytopenias caused either by an absolute decrease in precursor cells or ineffective cell production.

The DMPS are characterized by dysplasia of bone marrow precursor cells and of cells in the peripheral blood. Dysplasia can be demonstrated by abnormalities in size, shape, maturation or organization of cells. Nuclear–cytoplasmic asynchrony and a left shift may be found in both erythrocyte and leukocyte maturation. The bone marrow in any of the major DMPS (except CMML) may reveal pathologic ringed sideroblasts that demonstrate iron-filled mitochondria that form a ring around the nucleus.

The hallmark of DMPS is dyserythropoiesis that is characterized by the abnormal maturation of red cells, referred to as megaloblastoid (resembling megaloblastic). However, megaloblastoid red cells have an open nuclear chromatin pattern that is more coarse than that of megaloblastic maturation with more prominent parachromatin (Chap. 12). The NRBC nucleus may be irregular in shape with multinuclearity. Giant NRBCs may be found.

In DMPS, the peripheral blood may reveal any of the following erythrocyte abnormalities: poikilocytes (*e.g.*, ovalocytes and teardrops), NRBCs, basophilic stippling, Howell-Jolly bodies, siderocytes and sideroblasts.

Granulocytes in DMPS may occasionally show abnormalities such as pseudo–Pelger-Huët forms or hypersegmentation, hypogranulation or coarse granulation, and occasionally Auer rods.

The most frequent abnormality of megakaryocytes is maturation arrest, leading to small to medium-sized cells with single or bilobed nuclei. Peripheral blood platelets may be decreased, normal or, rarely, increased. They may be hypogranular or have abnormally large granules.

The median survival for DMPS patients is 2.5 years before succumbing either to complications of their anemia, neutropenia, or thrombocytopenia or converting to a rapidly fatal acute leukemia.

Case Study 33-1*

A 77-year-old man was admitted to the hospital for excision of a basal cell carcinoma in the nose. His admission CBC revealed a severe macrocytic anemia (Hb, 5.4 g/dL; MCV, 114 fL) and leukopenia (2.9 × 10⁹/L), but platelets were normal. Blood film examination showed a shift to the left with bands, metamyelocytes and myelocytes present (a subsequent blood film revealed 1% blasts). The red cells were dimorphic with macrocytic, normochromic and macrocytic, hypochromic cells exhibiting moderate poikilocytosis. Dacryocytes and oval macrocytes were frequent and occasional NRBC were found.

A bone marrow examination revealed 75% cellularity, a decreased myeloid:erythroid ratio and erythroid hyperplasia. Erythroid precursors were megaloblastoid in appearance. Megakaryocytes were increased in number, and some had single round nuclei. An iron stain showed numerous (25%) ringed sideroblasts.

1. What laboratory findings indicate the presence of a dysmyelopoietic syndrome?
2. State the most likely FAB DMPS classification for this patient's laboratory data and the two findings that are particularly characteristic of this subgroup.

Review Questions

33-1. The DMPS characterized by the greatest number of blasts in the peripheral blood and bone marrow is

A. refractory anemia with excess blasts (RAEB).
B. refractory anemia with excess blasts in transformation (RAEBIT).
C. refractory anemia with ringed sideroblasts (RARS).
D. chronic myelomonocytic leukemia (CMML).

33-2. The percentage of monocytes in the bone marrow indicative of chronic myelomonocytic leukemia (CMML) is

A. more than 5%.
B. 5% to 20%.
C. more than 20%.
D. more than 30%.

* *Modified from Lotspeich-Steininger CA, McKenzie SB: Myelodysplastic syndromes: A review with case studies. J Med Technol 4:5, 1987, with permission.*

33-3. The characteristic laboratory findings in refractory anemia with ringed sideroblasts include _____% marrow ringed sideroblasts and _____% marrow blasts.

   A. more than 15%, less than 5%
   B. more than 15%, less than 1%
   C. more than 20%, less than 5%
   D. more than 5%, 5% to 20%

33-4. In classifying the DMPS, the total percentage of blasts on the peripheral blood film is obtained from combining the percentage of Types

   A. I and II blasts.
   B. I and III blasts.
   C. II and III blasts.
   D. I, II and III blasts.

For the following questions, use the following format to answer:

   A. 1 and 3
   B. 2 and 4
   C. 1, 2 and 3
   D. 4 only
   E. all of the above

33-5. Characteristic abnormalities of erythropoiesis in the DMPS include

   1. megaloblastoid erythroblasts.
   2. cloverleaf-shaped erythroblast nuclei.
   3. asynchronous nuclear/cytoplasmic maturation.
   4. fine nuclear chromatin in erythroblasts with a lack of parachromatin.

33-6. Characteristic abnormalities of granulopoiesis in the DMPS include

   1. a left shift.
   2. hypersegmentation.
   3. pseudo–Pelger-Huët forms.
   4. either hypogranulation or coarse granulation.

33-7. Dysplasia of megakaryocytes in the DMPS may cause morphologic and quantitative abnormalities including

   1. decreased, normal or increased peripheral blood platelets.
   2. hypogranular peripheral blood platelets.
   3. many small megakaryocytes with a single or bilobed nucleus.
   4. many giant megakaryocytes.

33-8. A peripheral blood film or bone marrow from a patient with a DMPS might demonstrate

   1. basophilic stippling and Howell-Jolly bodies.
   2. blasts with granules in the cytoplasm.
   3. Auer rods in blasts.
   4. a cellular or hypercellular bone marrow.

33-9. The best way to identify dysplastic monocytes and distinguish them from neutrophils is to stain the blood or bone marrow film with

   1. reticulin stain.
   2. Wright stain.
   3. peroxidase stain.
   4. combined esterase stain.

References

1. Appelbaum FR, Storb R, Ramberg RE et al: Allogeneic marrow transplantation in the treatment of preleukemia. Ann Intern Med 100:689, 1984

2. Baccarani M, Tura S: Differentiation of myeloid leukaemia cells: New probabilities for therapy. Br J Haematol 42:485, 1979

3. Bennett JM, Catovsky D, Daniel MT et al: Proposals for the classification of the myelodysplastic syndromes. Br J Haematol 51:189, 1982

4. Block M, Jacobson LD, Bethard WF: Preleukemic acute human leukemia. JAMA 152:1018, 1953

5. Broxmeyer HE, Jacobsen N, Kurland J et al: In vitro suppression of normal granulocytic stem cells by inhibitory activity derived from human leukemic cells. J Natl Cancer Inst 60:485, 1978

6. Chessels JM, Sieff CA, Harvey BAN et al: Monosomy 7 in childhood: A preleukaemic state. Br J Haematol 49:129a, 1981

7. Cohen JR, Creger WP, Greenberg PL et al: Subacute myeloid leukemia: A clinical review. Am J Med 66:959, 1979

8. Dewald GW, Pierre RV, Phyliky RL: Three patients with structurally abnormal X chromosomes, each with Xq13 breakpoints and a history of idiopathic acquired sideroblastic anemia. Blood 59:100, 1982

9. Dreyfus B, Rochant H, Sultan C et al: Les anemies refractaires avec exces de myeloblasts dan la moelle. Presse Med 78:359, 1972

10. Fialkow PJ, Jacobson RJ, Singer JW et al: Philadelphia chromosome (Ph[1])-negative chronic myelogenous leukemia (CML): A clonal disease with origin in a multipotent stem cell. Blood 56:70, 1980

11. Flynn P, Miller W, Weisdorf D et al: Treatment of acute promyelocytic leukemia with retinoic acid: Correlation with cell culture studies. Blood 60(Suppl 1):155a, 1982

12. Foucar K, Vaughan WP, Armitage JO et al: Postleukemic dysmyelopoiesis. Am J Hematol 15:321, 1983

13. Gold E, Mertelsmann R, Moore MAS et al: Phase I trial of 13 *cis* retinoic acid in hematologic malignancies. Blood 58(Suppl 1):139a, 1981

14. Greenberg PL, Nichols WC, Schrier SL: Granulopoiesis in acute myeloid leukemia and preleukemia. N Engl J Med 284:1225, 1971

15. Hamilton-Patterson JL: Pre-leukaemic leukaemia. Acta Haemat 2:309, 1949

16. Hoagland H: Myelodysplastic (preleukemia) syndromes: The bone marrow factory failure problem. Mayo Clin Proc 70:673, 1995

17. Housset M, Daniel MT, Degos L: Small doses of Ara-C in the treatment of acute myeloid leukaemia: Differentiation of myeloid leukaemic cell? Br J Haematol 51:125, 1982

18. Juneja SK, Imbert M, Joualt H et al: Haematological features of primary myelodysplastic syndromes (PMDS) at initial presentation: A study of 118 cases. J Clin Pathol 36:1129, 1983

19. Knapp RH, Dewald GW, Pierre RV: Cytogenetic studies in 174 consecutive patients with preleukemic or myelodysplastic syndrome. Mayo Clin Proc 60:507, 1985

20. Koeffler HP: Induction of differentiation of human acute myelogenous leukemia cells: Therapeutic implications. Blood 62:709, 1983

21. LeBeau MM, Albain KS, Larson RA et al: Clinical and cytogenetic correlations in 63 patients with therapy-related myelodysplastic syndromes and acute nonlymphocytic leukemia: Further evidence for characteristic abnormalities of chromosome nos. 5 and 7. J Clin Oncol 4:325, 1986

22. Montecucco C, Ricaardi A, Traversi E et al: Proliferative activity of bone marrow cells in primary dysmyelopoietic (preleukemic) syndromes. Cancer 51:1190, 1983

23. Pierre RV: Preleukemic states. Semin Hematol 11:73, 1974

24. Raza A, Gezer S, Mundle S et al: Apoptosis in bone marrow biopsy samples involving stromal and hematopoietic cells in 50 patients with myelodysplastic syndromes. Blood 86:268, 1995

25. Rheingold J, Kaufman R, Adelson E et al: Smoldering acute leukemia. N Engl J Med 268:812, 1963

26. Rosenthal DS, Moloney WC: Refractory dysmyelopoietic anemia and acute leukemia. Blood 63:314, 1984

27. Saarni MI, Linman JW: Preleukemia: The hematologic syndrome preceding acute leukemia. Am J Med 55:38, 1973

28. Sachs L: Regulatory proteins for growth and differentiation in normal and leukemic hematopoietic cells: Normal differentiation and uncoupling of controls in myeloid leukemia. In Ford RJ, Maizel AL (eds): Mediators in Cell Growth and Differentiation, p 341. New York, Raven Press, 1985

29. Scoazec JY, Imbert M, Crofts M et al: Myelodysplastic syndrome or acute myeloid leukemia? A study of 28 cases presenting with borderline features. Cancer 55:2390, 1985

30. Second International Workshop on Chromosomes in Leukemia: Chromosomes in preleukemia. Cancer Genet Cytogenet 2:108, 1980

31. Swanson GA, Picozzi VJ, Greenberg PL: Effects of retinoic acid and 1,25-$(OH)_2$ vitamin D_3 on hemopoiesis in normals and patients with myelodysplastic states. Blood 62(Suppl 1):155a, 1983

32. Todd WM, Pierre RV: Preleukaemia: A long term prospective study of 325 patients. Scand J Haematol 36(Suppl 45):114, 1986

33. Tricot G, DeBock R, Dekker AW et al: Low dose cytosine arabinoside (ara C) in myelodysplastic syndromes. Br J Haematol 58:231, 1984

34. Tricot G, DeWolf-Peters C, Vlietinck R et al: Bone marrow histology in myelodysplastic syndromes: II. Prognostic value of abnormal localization of immature precursors in MDS. Br J Haematol 58:217, 1984

35. Van Den Berge H, Cassiman JJ, David G et al: Distinctive haematological disorder with deletion of long arm of no. 5 chromosome. Nature 251:437, 1974

36. Weber RFA, Geraedts JPM, Kerkhofs H et al: The preleukaemic syndrome. Acta Med Scand 207:391, 1980

37. Yam LT, Li CY, Crosby WH: Cytochemical identification of the granulocytes and monocytes. Am J Clin Pathol 55:283, 1971

38. Zittoun R, Berndou A, Bilski-Pasquier G et al: Les leucemies myelomonocytaires subaigues: Etude de 27 cas et revue de la literature. Sem Hop Paris 48:1943, 1972

CHAPTER 34

Acute Myeloproliferative Leukemia (Acute Nonlymphocytic Leukemia)

Valerie J. Evans

Objectives

1. List the eight categories of acute nonlymphocytic leukemia based on the FAB classification system and identify the prominent cell type associated with each.
2. Identify the cytochemical and cytogenetic profiles associated with each of the subcategories of acute nonlymphocytic leukemia.
3. Describe the general considerations and techniques utilized for treatment of the acute nonlymphocytic leukemias.

DEFINITION

Acute nonlymphocytic leukemia (ANLL) is a general term applied to all acute leukemias involving cells other than lymphocytes. Another term to define the same group of leukemias is acute myeloid (or myelogenous) leukemia or AML. The two terms will be used interchangeably in this chapter. ANLL or AML is a progressive malignant disease of hematopoietic tissue and is probably a stem cell disorder. It is characterized by a predominance of immature marrow cells that have been blocked at an undifferentiated or partially differentiated stage of maturation with or without involvement of the peripheral blood. Normal myeloid elements are reduced in number, apparently as a result of crowding out by the leukemic cells, and eventually, are replaced if the malignant proliferating clone remains unchecked. If untreated, ANLL has a rapidly fatal course. Death is usually caused by the effects of the resultant pancytopenia (anemia, bleeding and lack of resistance to infection). Acute nonlymphocytic leukemia is principally a disease of adults, but it may occur in any age group. It has a slight predisposition for males.

ETIOLOGY

The cause of ANLL is unclear. It is likely to be a combination or interaction of several factors.[13]

Radiation

Evidence supporting the role of radiation exposure as a factor in the development of leukemia has come from three principal lines of study: (1) radiologists who were occupationally exposed before the establishment of safety standards and practices in clinical radiology; (2) patients treated by radiation for ankylosing spondylitis compared with others with the same disease who were not irradiated; and (3) survivors of the atomic blasts at Hiroshima and Nagasaki. Each of these groups had an increased incidence of leukemia.

Chemicals

Drugs and chemicals that cause bone marrow depression or aplasia are capable of producing leukemia and thus are referred to as *leukemogens*. Some of these are chloramphenicol, phenylbutazone, arsenic-containing compounds, sulfonamides and some insecticides. Certain cytotoxic agents used in the treatment of neoplasms are likewise potentially leukemogenic. These include phenylalanine mustard and cyclophosphamide used to treat multiple myeloma; alkylating agents used to treat several types of cancer, including Hodgkin's disease; and immunosuppressants used to treat immunoinflammatory diseases. Benzene is the only chemical known unequivocally to cause cancer.

Genetics

Chromosomal aberrations, including aneuploidy and breakage, are demonstrated in several diseases associated with an increased incidence of ANLL. These diseases include Down syndrome (trisomy 21), Fanconi's syndrome (excessive chromosomal breakage), Bloom syndrome (marked chromosomal breakage and rearrangement) and D-trisomy. Congenital leukemias are usually nonlymphocytic. Studies of cases of familial leukemia are also highly supportive of the genetic etiology of acute leukemia.

Viruses

There is no conclusive evidence that viruses are causative agents of human leukemia. However, type C RNA viruses are recognized as being the most common class of tumor viruses associated with animal leukemia and lymphoma. These viruses contain an enzyme, reverse transcriptase, which has been detected in human leukemic cells but not in normal blood cells. After invading a host cell, the viral RNA is transcribed in reverse into DNA (*i.e.*, DNA is synthesized from RNA). This is in direct contrast to the normal synthesis of RNA from DNA, thus the name *retrovirus*. The newly synthesized DNA may be incorporated into the host cell's genome next to a normal gene involved in the regulation of cell growth and development (referred to as a *proto-oncogene*).

After insertion of viral DNA, the proto-oncogene may become deregulated or altered, thus forming an *oncogene* which can subsequently cause the transformation of a normal cell to a malignant one. A retrovirus may also incorporate a copy of the oncogenic RNA into its own genome. Thus, in rare circumstances, a retrovirus with a copy of an oncogene in its genome may introduce the activated oncogene into another cell, causing that cell's alteration in some fundamental way and, thus, its transformation into a malignant cell.[29]

CLASSIFICATION

Proper classification of the type of leukemia is necessary for clinicians to make appropriate treatment decisions and extend patient survival. Classification techniques use analysis of many cell features, including morphology, cytochemistry and antigen (or surface marker) analysis by immunochemistry and flow cytometry.

Morphology alone is ineffective in identifying the lineage of all types of leukemia. For example, blast cell morphology, in which the cells are large with primitive nuclei, increased nucleoli and basophilic cytoplasm, may be characteristic of lymphoblasts, myeloblasts or monoblasts. Studies have demonstrated that many cases of acute leukemia have been improperly categorized by morphology alone and have had to be reclassified after cytochemical profiling. Additionally, batteries of special stains may be negative, with no obvious maturation line or intermediate forms being present. These cases are referred to as *undifferentiated leukemias*.

In recent years, ultrastructural studies and cytogenetic and immunologic techniques have been developed to help classify acute leukemia. The study of the ultrastructure of cells by electron microscopy makes it possible to identify specific organelles (*e.g.*, granules that cannot be seen with Romanowsky stains). Specific chromosomal abnormalities are associated with the different subgroups of ANLL and have a prognostic significance.[8] Many monoclonal antibodies have been developed that react

with myeloid cells; these are used in an attempt to subclassify and to predict prognosis.[27] However, immunotyping has not been as helpful in ANLL as it has in the lymphoid leukemias (Chap. 36).[10]

Morphologic Techniques

Categorization of the leukemias classically has been done by assessing the morphology of Romanowsky-stained specimens under light microscopy. This classification is based on the type of normal cell the malignant clone resembles and the stage of maturation of a given cell line. The presence of other abnormal cell types may provide clues to the cell line involved (*e.g.*, pseudo–Pelger-Huët cells would indicate that the affected cell line is granulocytic). The primary distinction to be made when classifying acute leukemias is whether the leukemia is lymphocytic or nonlymphocytic. Romanowsky-stained blasts in acute leukemia reveal certain morphologic characteristics that may be more definitive for one cell type than another. Some of the more important morphologic criteria used to identify blasts are the nuclear:cytoplasmic ratio, the shape of the nuclear outline, the number of nucleoli, and the degree of cytoplasmic maturation. The significance of one specific morphologic abnormality, the Auer rod, is considerable: it defines the leukemia as both acute and nonlymphocytic. Additionally, morphologic criteria for classification of the subtypes of ANLL have been established by French, American and British (FAB) investigators and will be discussed later.

Cytochemical Techniques

Cytochemistry significantly enhances the classification of leukemia. The International Council for Standardization in Haematology (ICSH) has recommended methods for these cytologic procedures.[28] Five enzymes have been standardized: peroxidase, alkaline phosphatase, acid phosphatase, nonspecific esterase, and chloroacetate esterase. Table 34-1 lists the cytochemical findings seen in the different categories of acute nonlymphocytic leukemia, and Chapter 29 describes the various cytochemical procedures.

Immunologic Techniques

The use of monoclonal antibodies to characterize cell lineage in cases of ANLL or AML is now commonly performed.[7] Myeloid cytoplasmic antigens can be detected by immunocytochemical techniques or direct immunofluorescent methods. Flow cytometry permits the detection, quantification, and computed processing of the resultant data. The prognostic significance of surface antigen characterization is most useful in undifferentiated, megakaryocytic and mixed lineage acute leukemia, for which the identification of the myeloid nature of the abnormal cells is not possible by routine morphologic and cytochemical techniques.

In general, the cells seen in the acute nonlymphoid leukemias do not express highly specific immunophenotypes; however, some subsets demonstrate preferential association with some antigens. For example, CD7[+] cells

TABLE 34-1
Cytochemical Findings in ANLL

	Sudan Black B and Peroxidase	Specific Esterase (Naphthol AS-D Chloroacetate)	Nonspecific Esterase		PAS
			α-Naphthyl Acetate	α-Naphthyl Butyrate	
M0	Neg	Neg	Neg	Neg	————
Myelocytic (M1, M2 or M3)	Pos	Pos	Neg	Neg	————
Myelomonocytic, M4	Pos	Pos	Pos	Pos	————
Monocytic, M5	Neg or weak scattered positivity	Neg	Pos	Pos	Pos
Erythroleukemia, M6	————	————	Pos	Neg	Pos
Megakaryocytic, M7	————	————	Pos	Neg	Pos

−, generally not performed, PAS; periodic acid–Schiff reaction.

are associated with CD34 (stem cell) expression and less differentiated morphology (M0 and M1 AML). The myeloid antigens commonly tested for include CD13, CD14, CD15, CD33 and CD41, among others.

Immunologic subtyping may also be of importance in the characterization of mixed lineage leukemias. Cells in these leukemias express antigens at different stages of differentiation and from more than one cell line. Different combinations may occur, *e.g.*, biphenotypic expression in which both myeloid and lymphoid antigens are expressed on the same cells, or bilineage expression in which there are two distinct cell populations, one expressing myeloid antigens and the other lymphoid.

French–American–British System

In 1976, a group of French, American and British investigators proposed a classification for the acute leukemias that would have as its basis Romanowsky-stained films of blood and bone marrow.[2] Known as the FAB classification system, its purpose was to provide a uniform method of subgrouping the different acute leukemias based on a standardized system of nomenclature and morphologic criteria. The criteria for subclassification are based on the morphology of the proliferating cells, principally nuclear morphology, as seen in bone marrow and peripheral blood. Cytochemical distinctions are made where appropriate. Table 34-2 lists some of the chief discriminating factors that may be used to subtype the ANLLs. Use of this standardized system has greatly facilitated the correlation of clinical and laboratory findings and responses to treatment between clinical investigators. It is of value principally in evaluating cases before cytotoxic drug treatment, which may alter morphology.

Specific morphologic criteria are based on two factors: the direction of cell line differentiation and the degree of maturation of the proliferating cells. Eight subclassifications (Table 34-3) of the ANLLs are now recognized. M7, acute megakaryocytic leukemia, was defined almost 10 years after the original classification system was proposed[1,4] and M0, acute myeloid leukemia with minimal differentiation, was only recently defined.[6]

There is a great deal of morphologic heterogeneity and overlap among these subgroups. Counting bone marrow cells to determine the percentage of blasts is neces-sary, because the FAB classification is based on quantitative criteria, in which the total number of blasts is compared with either the total nucleated cells or the total nonerythroid cells in the bone marrow.

Basic to the morphologic criteria of this system is the definition of a blast, of which three types are recognized.[6] Type I blasts show no evidence of cytoplasmic differentiation (Fig. 34-1). Cytoplasmic granules are never present, prominent nucleoli are observed and the chromatin is stippled with no condensation. The nuclear/cytoplasmic (N/C) ratio of the smaller blasts tends to be higher than in larger ones. Type II blasts are similar to Type I but show some evidence of differentiation (Fig. 34-2). A few azurophilic granules may be observed in the cytoplasm, usually fewer than 20. The nucleus is located centrally, and the N/C ratio is low. More than 20 granules in the cytoplasm distinquishes Type III from Type II blasts. These cells exhibit a slightly lower N/C ratio than a Type I blast and have a centrally located nucleus. Cells are classified as promyelocytes, when the following morphologic changes occur: the nucleus becomes eccentric, a well-developed Golgi apparatus is apparent, chromatin has begun to condense, numerous cytoplasmic granules are present that begin to obscure the nucleus, and the N/C ratio diminishes.

M0: ACUTE MYELOBLASTIC LEUKEMIA WITH MINIMAL DIFFERENTIATION

Clinical Presentation. M0 accounts for approximately 5% to 10% of all AMLs. Clinical features are nonspecific and similar to all other AML categories. Many patients present with symptoms of bruising, bleeding or infection. Organomegaly may be seen in some patients. Lymphadenopathy is less commonly observed.

Laboratory Findings. The peripheral blood picture is generally one of pancytopenia. Circulating blasts are seen and blast numbers are variable. Dysplastic maturing granulocytes may be present.

More than 30% blasts are observed in the bone marrow and may compose as much as 90% of the cellular elements. Virtually all of the blasts exhibit Type I morphology, and Auer rods are not found.

Classification of AML M0 cannot be made solely on

TABLE 34-2

Discriminating Factors in the Characterization of FAB Subgroups of ANLL

Subgroup	Clinical Features	Cytochemical Positivity	Cytogenetic Abnormalities	Laboratory Findings
M0	—	Usually none	—	—
M1	—	Sudan black B Peroxidase Naphthol AS-D chloroacetate esterase (low %)	—	—
M2	—	Same as above (higher %)	t(8q$^-$;21q$^+$)	
M3	DIC*	Same as above (close to 100%)	t(15;17)	Prolonged PT and PTT times Low fibrinogen levels Positive fibrin split products test
M4	Tissue infiltrates CNS involvement	Sudan black B Peroxidase Naphthol AS-D chloroacetate esterase α-Naphthyl butyrate and acetate esterase	Chromosome 16 (M4e)	Increased lysozyme
M5	Tissue infiltrates CNS involvement Highest incidence of organ involvement	PAS α-Naphthyl acetate esterase α-Naphthyl butyrate esterase	t(9;11) (M5a)	Increased lysozyme
M6	—	PAS α-Naphthyl acetate esterase α-Naphthyl butyrate esterase	—	Numerous peripheral blood NRBC
M7	Myelofibrosis	Acid phosphatase, PAS	Chromosome 21	Platelet peroxidase

* DIC, disseminated intravascular coagulation; CNS, central nervous system; PAS, periodic acid-Schiff.

TABLE 34-3

Principal Morphologic Criteria in FAB Classification of ANLL

Subgroup	Origin	Cell Types	Nucleus	Cytoplasm
M0	Myelocytic	>30% myeloblasts (Type I)	One or more nucleoli; fine-stippled chromatin	Rare azurophilic granules; rare Auer rod
M1	Myelocytic	>30% myeloblasts (Type I and Type II)	One or more nucleoli; fine-stippled chromatin	Few azurophilic granules; Auer rods
M2	Myelocytic	>30% myeloblasts with >10% granulocytic component	One or more nucleoli; fine-stippled chromatin	Various amounts; numerous azurophilic granules; Auer rods
M3	Myelocytic	Abnormal promyelocytes predominate	Reniform or bilobed shape	Heavy granulation; bundles of Auer rods (fagots)
M4	Myelocytic	>30% blasts >20% granulocytes >20% promonocytes and monocytes	—	—
M5a	Monocytic	Monoblasts predominate, few promonocytes	Lacy chromatin with nucleoli	Basophilic; pseudopods; occasional granules
M5b	Monocytic	Blasts, promonocytes and monocytes Promonocytes predominate in marrow Monocytes predominate in blood	Cerebriform shape with nucleoli	Grayish, ground-glass appearance; fine azurophilic granules
M6	Erythrocytic Myelocytic	>50% erythroid cells in all stages of maturation >30% myeloblasts	Multiple nuclear lobes Multiple nuclei Nuclear fragments Megaloblastic changes	Nuclear:cytoplasmic asynchrony; PAS positivity; gigantism; vacuolization
M7	Megakaryocytic	Megakaryoblasts	Dense chromatin (lymphoid blasts) or fine reticulated chromatin with nucleoli	Scant; blebs and vacuoles; platelet shedding

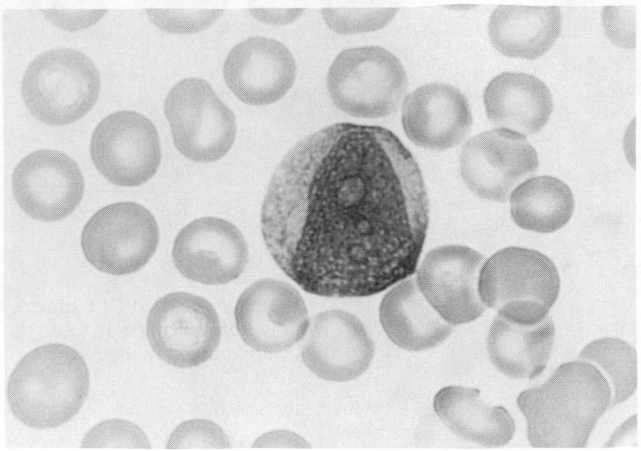

FIGURE 34-1. Type I blast: Blood film from patient with M1 acute myelocytic leukemia without maturation. Note fine nuclear chromatin, prominent nucleoli, and absence of cytoplasmic granules (original magnification ×500; Wright stain).

morphologic or cytochemical grounds. The cytochemical profile of M0 blasts is usually negative, with less than 3% of the blasts demonstrating a positive-staining reaction for myeloperoxidase or Sudan black B. Proof of the myeloid origin of these cells is either (1) by ultrastructural demonstration of peroxidase-positive granules in the endoplasmic reticulum of the blasts or (2) by the reactivity of at least 20% of the blasts for one or more myeloid-related antigens, such as CD13, CD14, CD15, or CD33. The stem cell marker, CD34 may also be positive and may indicate a poor prognosis. The blasts must also demonstrate a negative reaction for lymphoid antigens such as CD10, CD19, CD20, CD22, CD3 and CD5. Terminal deoxynucleotidyl transferase (TdT) positivity may occur in an occasional blast. M0 is usually associated with a poor prognosis because a higher incidence of affected individuals are refractory to chemotherapy compared to those with other types of AML.

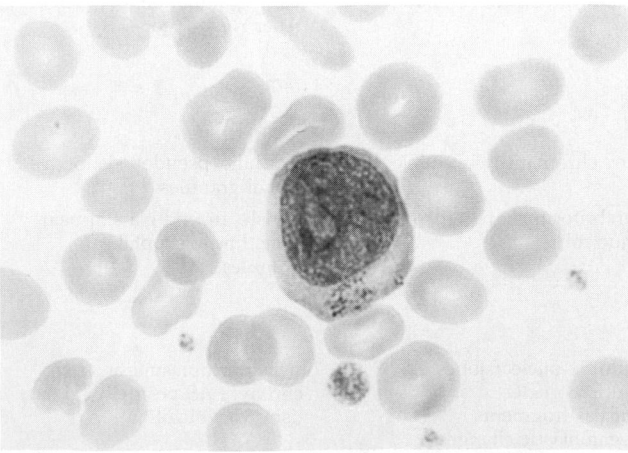

FIGURE 34-2. Type II blast: Blood film from patient with acute myelocytic leukemia without maturation. Note fine nuclear chromatin, prominent nucleoli, and few azurophilic granules in cytoplasm (original magnification ×500; Wright stain).

M1: ACUTE MYELOBLASTIC LEUKEMIA WITHOUT MATURATION

Clinical Presentation. Acute myeloblastic leukemia without maturation is found in all aged groups, with the highest incidence seen in adults. There is no gender predominance. The onset may be sudden or insidious, taking months to years for symptoms to become apparent. Symptoms are related to the degree of cytopenia that develops in the various cell lines and commonly include fever, malaise, fatigue and petechiae (Table 34-4). Organomegaly is variable and may include enlargement of the liver, spleen or lymph nodes; however, most individuals present with little or no organ involvement.

Laboratory Findings. Examination of the peripheral blood reveals that granulocytes, red cells and platelets are reduced in number. The number of circulating blast cells is variable and usually is directly proportional to the total WBC count. In the early stages of M1 AML, the WBC count may be normal or low, with few or no blasts in the peripheral blood, although blasts are increased in the bone marrow. Most patients present with leukocytosis secondary to high numbers of circulating blasts (see Color Plate 34-1).

Nuclear/cytoplasmic maturational asynchrony is a common finding in the malignant cell populations. This may be reflected morphologically (nucleus appears more immature than the cytoplasm) or functionally (*e.g.,* leukemic blasts exhibiting phagocytosis, a property of mature cells).

Characteristically, the bone marrow is hypercellular. Numerous morphologic abnormalities are found in all marrow cell lines, as observed by the presence of dysmyelopoietic neutrophil maturation, dyserythropoiesis and morphologically abnormal megakaryocytes. Table 34-5 lists some of the more common changes (see Chap. 33).

The FAB categorization of M1 leukemia is based on evidence of granulocytic differentiation in the bone marrow. Blast cells may either be type I or a combination of types I and II. Some type II blasts containing at least a few azurophilic granules, Auer rods, or both may be present. Further granulocytic maturation beyond the blast stage is seen in less than 10% of the cells.

The blast count is important, and the total of type I and II blasts must be at least 30% of the nucleated cells in the marrow. If the blast count is less than 30%, the case would be classified as a myelodysplastic syndrome, rather than acute leukemia (Chap. 33).

Cytochemical demonstration of at least 3% Sudan black B- or peroxidase-positive blasts is essential to define the granulocytic nature of M1 acute leukemia. Auer rods will be positive in both reactions. The cytochemical profile for M1 AML also includes positive chloroacetate esterase staining and a negative α-naphthyl acetate esterase reaction. The presence of positivity in leukemic blasts when compared with normal myeloblasts that lack positivity, is a reflection of the asynchrony between cytoplasmic and nuclear maturation characteristic of leukemic cells. CD13, CD14, CD15, CD33 and CD34 myeloid antigens are frequently positive in M1 leukemia. The results of cerebrospinal fluid (CSF) examination usually are neg-

TABLE 34-4
Clinical Features of ANLL

	Signs and Symptoms	Pathophysiology	Supportive Therapy
Anemia	Pallor Lethargy Dyspnea Fatigue Weakness	Bone marrow failure Dyserythropoiesis Decreased RBC survival	Red cell transfusion
Neutropenia	Fever Malaise Infection	Bone marrow failure Dysmyelopoiesis	Granulocyte transfusion Antibiotics Isolation techniques
Thombocytopenia	Hemorrhage Bruising Petechiae Purpura Epistaxis Gingival bleeding Menorrhagia	Bone marrow failure Coagulation defects Qualitative platelet abnormalities	Platelet transfusion
Organ infiltration	Bone tenderness Splenomegaly Hepatomegaly Lymphadenopathy Gum hypertrophy Skin infiltrates Ulceration of the mucous membranes Meningeal syndrome 　　Headache 　　Nausea 　　Vomiting	Extramedullary hematopoiesis Metastatic disease	Radiotherapy

ative because CNS involvement is almost never seen in AML.

M2: ACUTE MYELOBLASTIC LEUKEMIA WITH MATURATION

Clinical Presentation. The presenting symptoms for M2 AML are similar to those of the M1 type. These include manifestations of anemia, infection and a hemorrhagic tendency such as easy bruising, epistaxis, gingival bleeding and petechiae.

Laboratory Findings. The peripheral blood findings commonly include a reduction in the number of normal blood cells and leukocytosis secondary to circulating blast cells (see Color Plate 34-2). The bone marrow is hypercellular with the same morphologic abnormalities in all marrow cell lines that are described in M1. Some cases of M2 demonstrate a marked increase in basophils, eosinophils, or both. The M2 FAB subgroup is distinguished from M1 by the presence of granulocytic cells at or beyond the promyelocytic stage of maturation. In the bone marrow, type I and type II blasts account for more than 30% of the nucleated cells, with 10% or more additional granulocytic cells at various stages of maturation. Less than 20% of the cells are monocytes.

Leukemic alterations in morphology often are observed in peripheral blood, with the presence of pseudo–

TABLE 34-5
Morphologic Abnormalities Associated with ANLL

Dysmyelopoiesis	Dyserythropoiesis	Dysmegakaryocytopoiesis
Nuclear:cytoplasmic asynchrony Leukemic hiatus Nuclear abnormalities Pseudo–Pelger-Huët changes Hypersegmentation Unusual nuclear projections Granule abnormalities 　Increased size and number 　Decreased number or absence 　Auer rods Loss of cellular organelles Irregular cytoplasmic basophilia	Gigantism Multinuclearity Nuclear lobulation Nuclear fragments Pyknosis Megaloblastoid changes Cytoplasmic vacuoles	Giant platelets (megathrombocytes) Hypernuclear and hyponuclear lobulation Micromegakaryocytes Granule abnormalities 　Giant granules 　Abnormal granules

Pelger-Huët and hypogranular neutrophils being most common. Pseudo–Pelger-Huët changes are acquired from the leukemic cell line. The nuclei of these cells may appear rod shaped, dumbbell shaped, or round and nonsegmented. The chromatin may be abnormally condensed. It also is common to see mature neutrophils that appear to be devoid of cytoplasmic granules. Acquired myeloperoxidase deficiency can be demonstrated by cytochemical means. Even neutrophils that have granules may lack myeloperoxidase and may be identified incorrectly as monocytes.

Functional abnormalities may be acquired, with blockages at various stages of maturation. As a result, these cells may exhibit deficiencies in phagocytosis, microbial killing, random locomotion or chemotaxis, or in sequential combinations of these functions.

Cytochemically, M2 blast cells have the same profile as those in M1 except that a larger percentage of the blast forms will be positive for peroxidase or Sudan black B. Serum lysozyme levels and neutrophil alkaline phosphatase also vary among cases of this type and do not contribute diagnostically. Positive reactions with CD13 and CD15 antigens are frequently seen in cases of M2.

Certain cytogenetic abnormalities have a relatively high incidence. A characteristic chromosomal translocation, $t(8q^-;21q^+)$ has been reported in about 10% of cases. This abnormality is associated with low neutrophil alkaline phosphatase levels, a high incidence of cells containing Auer rods, and relatively long survival.

M3: PROMYELOCYTIC LEUKEMIA

Clinical Presentation. The M3 category of AML is found in all age groups (similar to M1 and M2); however, it appears to have a greater propensity for males. The highest male:female ratios occur in the microgranular variant of M3. Clinical symptoms are similar to those of M1 and M2 except that M3 is frequently associated with disseminated intravascular coagulation (DIC; Chap. 52), which is ascribed to the thromboplastinlike activity of the primary granules.

Laboratory Findings. Most cells seen in M3 acute leukemia are abnormal promyelocytes, with heavy granulation filling the cytoplasm and sometimes overlying the nucleus. Indeed, the granules may be so abundant that they obscure the outlines of the nucleus. In contrast, M2 promyelocytes have less granulation, and granules do not obscure the nucleus. Bundles of Auer rods may be seen in the cytoplasm and are referred to as fagots. The nuclei are variable in size and shape, often being reniform (kidney shaped) or bilobed.

The cytochemical profile of M3 leukemia is similar to that of M1 and M2 except that in this disorder, most of the abnormal cells are intensely positive. Many of the hypergranular promyelocytes and the fagot-containing cells are disrupted easily during preparation of bone marrow films, resulting in granules and Auer rods lying free between and on top of cells. This film-making artifact must be distinguished from stain precipitate when interpreting cytochemical stain results (see Color Plate 34-3).

Immunologic studies demonstrate positivity with CD13, CD15, CD11 and CD33 myeloid antigens.

A microgranular variant of acute promyelocytic leukemia is designated M3m.[14,26] Although clinically similar to M3, it is morphologically dissimilar in that the cells appear devoid of granules. In fact, numerous granules are present in these promyelocytes but are below the normal resolution of the light microscope and, therefore, can be detected only by electron microscopy. For this reason, the term "microgranular" is preferable to "hypogranular." By morphologic appearance alone, these cases may appear to resemble a monocytic (M4 or M5) subtype. The blast cells are large, with a deeply notched or folded monocytoid nucleus. The cytoplasm is abundant and may appear to be finely dusted with granules that may lie over the folds of the nucleus. Few cells demonstrate prominent azurophilic granules. Auer rods may be observed. It is important to perform a cytochemical profile on these cases and to demonstrate absence of nonspecific esterase so that these cells are properly distinguished from monocytes (Table 34-1). Sudan black B, peroxidase, and chloroacetate esterase staining should be intensely positive. The prognostic outlook for M3m is worse than that for M3. The condition usually is heralded by initial high blast counts, unlike M3, which is more likely to present with leukopenia.

Cytogenetic studies have revealed a high prevalence (almost 50%) of the chromosomal translocation t(15;17) associated with both the M3 and M3m variants.[20] Chromosomal changes in AML are much less definitive than the Philadelphia (Ph[1]) chromosome found in chronic myelogenous leukemia (CML; Chap. 35). The t(15;17) translocation is a poor prognostic sign. Other translocations have been observed, including t(9;22) and t(8;21).

M4: ACUTE MYELOMONOCYTIC LEUKEMIA

Clinical Presentation. Acute myelomonocytic leukemia (AMMoL) is also known as Naegeli monocytic leukemia. Its clinical presentation is related to symptoms of progressive cytopenia, including fatigue, bleeding diathesis, fever, and organomegaly. Unlike the M1 to M3 types, this subgroup is associated with soft-tissue infiltrates, including gum hypertrophy and infiltration, rectal ulceration, and skin involvement. Meningeal symptoms also are common in M4 leukemia, with headache, nausea, vomiting, blurring of vision, and sometimes intracranial hemorrhage.

Laboratory Findings. Most of the circulating cells in the peripheral blood are blasts and abnormal cells. Some of the highest WBC counts to occur in the AMLs are seen in M4. Both granulocytic and monocytic differentiation is observed in the peripheral blood and bone marrow.

Several morphologic criteria are required for categorization as an M4. In the bone marrow, more than 30% of the nonerythroid cells must be blasts. The sum of myeloblasts, promyelocytes and other maturing granulocytic forms is more than 30%, but less than 80%, of the nonerythroid cells. More than 20% of nonerythroid cells are of monocytic lineage at different stages of maturation. If the monocytic compartment exceeds 80% of the nonerythroid cells, the disease is classified as M5. More than 20% of peripheral blood leukocytes are monocytes or monocytic precursors (see Color Plate 34-4).

Confirmation of the monocytic component of this subgroup requires cytochemistry. The profile includes positive reactions for Sudan black B or peroxidase and both specific and nonspecific esterase. Lysozyme, also known as muramidase, is a low molecular weight enzyme found in neutrophils and monocytes. Monocytes contain larger amounts. Fifty percent of patients with M4 leukemia will excrete large amounts of lysozyme in their urine. Demonstration of serum or urine lysozyme is diagnostically important in M4 for the recognition of the monocytic component of these cells. Levels three times the upper limit of normal are considered significant.

A few cases of M4 AML are characterized by increased marrow eosinophils and classified as M4e. Sometimes, these cells exhibit large basophilic granules mixed with the smaller eosinophilic granules. Nuclei may be single-lobed and unsegmented, similar to pseudo–Pelger–Huët changes. In contrast to normal eosinophils, these cells exhibit distinct chloroacetate esterase and periodic acid–Schiff (PAS) positivity and immunologic positivity with the CD14 myeloid antigen. The M4e variant is associated with a deletion or inversion of the long arm of chromosome 16 and a longer mean survival.

M5: ACUTE MONOCYTIC LEUKEMIA

Clinical Presentation. Acute monocytic leukemia (AMoL), also referred to as Schilling leukemia, is clinically similar to M4; however, the highest incidence of organ involvement is found in this subgroup. Extramedullary tissue masses and CNS involvement are characteristic. The etiology of these symptoms is related to the monocytic component. This leukemia is divided into two categories: M5a, poorly differentiated monocytic leukemia; and M5b, well-differentiated monocytic leukemia. The M5b type differs clinically from M5a in that M5b is associated with a diffuse erythematous skin rash.

Laboratory Findings. Leukocytosis is common. Morphologically, M5a is characterized in both blood and bone marrow by large blast cells with delicate, lacy chromatin (see Color Plate 34-5a). One to three large, prominent vesicular nucleoli are also present. The cytoplasm of these cells is voluminous, and often, one or more pseudopods of basophilic cytoplasm are seen. Azurophilic granulation is rare. Some monocytes are found, along with a small percentage of promonocytes.

The M5b type is characterized by the presence of all stages of monocyte development: monoblasts, promonocytes and monocytes (see Color Plate 34-5b). The percentage of monocytes is usually higher in the peripheral blood than in the bone marrow, where the predominant cell is the promonocyte. Typical promonocytes have cerebriform nuclei with nucleoli. Their cytoplasm is less basophilic than that of monoblasts and has a grayish ground-glass appearance with fine azurophilic granules.

Less than 10% of the nonerythroid cells are granulocytes, and more than 80% are monoblasts, promonocytes

or monocytes. In M5a, more than 80% of the monocytic component are blasts, whereas in M5b, fewer than 80% of the monocytic cells are blasts. A few cells may contain Auer rods, but this finding is much less common than it is in other forms of ANLL. Cytochemically, these cells generally are negative for Sudan black B, peroxidase, and specific esterase, but are strongly positive for nonspecific esterases. Some cells may demonstrate weak scattered Sudan black B or peroxidase activity. The reactivity of these cells for nonspecific esterases will be inhibited by sodium fluoride. CD14 antigen positivity is commonly observed.

Like M4, testing for serum and urine lysozyme reveals very high levels because of the monocytic component of this leukemia. The frequency of DIC is second only to that seen in M3 AML. Cytogenetic abnormalities are relatively nonspecific in M5 leukemia. Rearrangements involving chromosome 11, t(9;11), are the most common.

M6: ACUTE ERYTHROLEUKEMIA

Clinical Presentation. Erythroleukemia was first described by DiGuglielmo in 1917. The term *erythroleukemia* is used when there is a prominent percentage of both neoplastic myeloblasts and erythroblasts. Because of the overlapping morphologic characteristics, it is imperative to distinguish these cases from refractory anemia with excess blasts (RAEB; Chap. 33).

The clinical features of this subgroup are similar to those of the other categories of ANLL.

Laboratory Findings. Peripheral blood findings include a variable leukocyte count, pancytopenia, and most notably, numerous nucleated red blood cells (NRBCs). The presence of NRBCs in the circulation is accompanied by a wide variety of changes in red cell morphology, including anisocytosis, poikilocytosis, macrocytes, oval macrocytes, schistocytes, or mixed populations of hypochromic and normochromic red cells. None of these changes is specific in itself, but together, they are an indication of dyserythropoietic changes in the bone marrow.

The erythrocytic component of an M6 leukemia exceeds 50% of the nucleated cells in the bone marrow. The erythroid cells exhibit various degrees of bizarre morphology, including multiple lobulation of the nucleus with variation in lobe size, multiple nuclei, nuclear fragments, gigantism, vacuolization and megaloblastoid features (see Color Plates 12-5 and 34-6). These findings are referred to as "dyserythropoietic changes." Additionally, more than 30% of the nonerythroid cells in the bone marrow must be type I or type II blasts. These blasts may contain Auer rods. An M6 leukemia frequently progresses to M1, M2, or M4 leukemia.

The red cell precursors in erythroleukemia are cytochemically unusual in that they often demonstrate periodic acid–Schiff (PAS) positivity. This positivity is the result of staining of glycogen and is localized in the cytoplasmic vacuoles of the erythroblasts. As the cells mature, they become richer in glycogen, and the pattern of positivity becomes diffuse rather than localized. Although this reaction is nondiagnostic, it is important to note that most other disorders with megaloblastoid maturation do not demonstrate this pattern of PAS positivity (*i.e.*, a change from granular to diffuse during maturation). The M6 erythroblasts also demonstrate positivity when stained for α-naphthyl acetate esterase and immunologic reactivity with CD33, CA1, anticarbonic anhydrase I, FA6-152 and anti–glycophorin A monoclonal antibodies.

M7: ACUTE MEGAKARYOCYTIC LEUKEMIA

Megakaryoblasts are frequently impossible to recognize by conventional light microscopy techniques. Early reports in the literature describing megakaryocytic leukemia were cases in which there was morphologically recognizable megakaryocytic differentiation. Because ultrastructural staining techniques and surface marker studies have only recently been developed for the recognition of this cell type, M7 was late in being described in the FAB classification system.

Clinical Presentation. The symptoms are similar to those of the other subgroups.

Laboratory Findings. The blast cells of M7 were classified as undifferentiated by previous FAB criteria because of their cytochemical negativity for Sudan black B, peroxidase, and esterase. Blast cells in some cases are small and round with scanty cytoplasm and nuclear chromatin that is dense and heavy, giving the cells a lymphoid appearance. Megakaryocytes in other cases have an undifferentiated appearance, with nuclei that are round with finely reticulated chromatin and one to three prominent nucleoli. There may or may not be granules in the cytoplasm. There is marked heterogeneity in blast cell size, and some of the blasts can be two to three times the size of normal lymphocytes. Some megakaryocytic blasts have cytoplasmic blebs or vacuolization (see Color Plate 34-7). According to the FAB criteria, some cells may appear as small differentiated megakaryocytes (micromegakaryocytes) with platelets shedding from the cytoplasm (see Color Plate 34-7). Others may be seen as naked nuclei with groups of platelets surrounding them. Occasionally, abnormal giant platelets are a prominent finding in the peripheral blood, and platelet counts may be normal or increased. Examination of the bone marrow frequently reveals diffuse reticulin myelofibrosis with aggregates of megakaryocytes localized among sheets of blasts or fibroblasts.[15]

Previously, megakaryoblastic leukemia was frequently not diagnosed. Today, its identification is facilitated by cytochemical and immunologic techniques. Platelet peroxidase (PPO) is an enzyme synthesized early during megakaryocyte maturation.[5] Distinct from myeloperoxidase, PPO is recognized as a specific marker for cells of megakaryocytic origin. Ultrastructural staining for PPO reveals that this enzyme is localized in the nuclear envelope and endoplasmic reticulum, but not in the Golgi apparatus or granules of megakaryocytes. This is unlike myeloperoxidase, which is found in the endoplasmic reticulum, Golgi apparatus and granules of other cell types.

Cytochemical positivity for the α-naphthyl acetate esterase reaction and a negative reaction with α-naphthyl butyrate esterase is unique to megakaryoblasts.[17] Monocytes react positively with both esterase substrates. Acid phosphatase is another cytochemical marker for megakaryoblasts. Diffuse strong positivity is readily seen in the immature stages of this cell line. However, this pattern for acid phosphatase is common in other types of acute leukemia and therefore the acid phosphatase reaction cannot be used as a diagnostic marker for megakaryoblasts. Megakaryocytes are rich in glycogen and will stain intensely with PAS. This reactivity is principally confined to differentiated megakaryocytes, with megakaryoblasts being negative. The strongest PAS reactions will be observed in cells displaying cytoplasmic budding. The associated platelets also are brightly PAS-positive. Finally, some megakaryoblasts may be identified on the basis of their surface glycoproteins IIa and IIIb using immunologic techniques as well as CD41, CD42 and CD61 positivity.

ANLL NOT INCLUDED IN FAB CLASSIFICATION

Several types of ANLL are not included in the FAB classification scheme. These include (1) acute mast cell or acute basophilic leukemias, which are rare disorders in which the cells can be confused with abnormal progranulocytes; (2) hypoplastic acute myeloid leukemia;[21] (3) mixed leukemias, which demonstrate a combination of lymphoid and myeloid characteristics; and (4) secondary leukemias that have evolved from myelodysplastic syndromes. These types are difficult to fit into the FAB classification format.

TREATMENT
General Considerations

The ultimate goal in treating ANLL is to return the bone marrow to its normal state of health and function and to achieve disease-free survival for the patient. Certain factors play an important role in determining how successful therapy will be, specifically the age and pretreatment status. The younger the patient, and the less symptomatic he or she is before treatment, the greater the chance of a significant response. The presence of infection at the time of treatment can reduce the chance of achieving remission by as much as 50%. Although the specific subtype of ANLL is not a significant prognostic factor, patients with M3 disease who have DIC and those with M5 disease with increased likelihood of extramedullary relapse have a somewhat poorer prognosis. Other negative prognostic indicators are an abnormal karyotype at diagnosis and a history of radiation or chemotherapy.

The principal treatment modalities for ANLL are chemotherapy to induce clinical remission, radiation therapy to control leukemic infiltrates, immunotherapy to bolster the patient's immune response to the leukemia, and bone marrow transplantation.

Chemotherapy

The different subtypes of ANLL are treated similarly with the exception of DIC in acute progranulocytic leukemia (M3). Standard treatment programs for ANLL use a combination of drugs with different mechanisms of action and dose-limiting toxicities to achieve the highest remission rates. The two most commonly used cytotoxic agents are cytarabine (cytosine arabinoside; ara-C) and daunorubicin (DNR). When used together, they can produce at least a 65% remission rate.[18] Amsacrine (m-AMSA) is an effective single drug in patients with resistant AML. Table 34-6 lists the mechanisms of action and toxicities of the common chemotherapeutic drugs.

The therapeutic strategy for treating ANLL includes three stages: induction of complete remission (CR), consolidation and maintenance of remission. Complete remission is achieved when bone marrow cellularity returns to normal with less than 5% blasts present. Anything less than a CR is associated with shorter survival and no possibility of a cure. Approximately 20% of patients in whom CR is achieved after first treatment will not relapse.[9] Patients may die from infection or hemorrhage secondary to the effects of chemotherapy before achieving a complete remission. If leukemic infiltrates persist in extramedullary sites (*e.g.*, CNS), even though the bone marrow has returned to normal, complete remission is not achieved. Postremission therapy, consolidation, and intensification using the same chemotherapeutic regimens are given to prevent resurgence of leukemia.

Posttherapeutic susceptibility to infection and bleeding necessitates reverse isolation techniques, intravenous antibiotics and transfusion support until the marrow recovers. Posttreatment peripheral leukocyte counts usually fall to fewer than $0.5 \times 10^9/L$ and may be as low as $0.1 \times 10^9/L$. Platelet values usually will be less than $20 \times 10^9/L$. Characteristically, the leukocyte differential reflects the severe neutropenia and relative lymphocytosis. Residual blast cells may demonstrate morphologic changes attributable to chemotherapy that may make them difficult to recognize. The cytotoxic therapy used in ANLL produces striking megaloblastic changes because of drug interference with DNA synthesis.[12] Additionally, toxic granulation, increased nuclear projections and hyposegmented nuclei may be seen in the neutrophils. Monocytes and lymphocytes demonstrate reactive changes, with lymphocytes appearing to have plasmacytoid features, and monocytes demonstrating increased cytoplasm, increased granules and vacuolization. Red cell morphology is variable. Spherocytes reflect transfused erythrocytes. Polychromasia will increase as red cell production returns to normal in the marrow, and some oval macrocytes may be seen because of the megaloblastoid effect of the antimetabolite therapy. Ineffective erythropoiesis also is evident as coarse basophilic stippling.

Examination of the bone marrow after therapy reveals aplasia with a relative increase in plasma cells, lymphocytes and histiocytes. As the marrow begins to regenerate a few weeks after therapy, an abundance of myeloblasts and promyelocytes is observed that may be confused with a return of leukemia. Red cells in all stages of development may be seen and frequently demonstrate megaloblastoid changes. Myeloid and megakaryocytic morphology is largely normal but may be characterized by megaloblastoid changes.

Treatment of Effects of Cytopenias

The clinical effects of the cytopenias that develop as a consequence of either the crowding out of normal blood cells in the marrow by the leukemic clone or by the reduction of normal numbers of granulocytes, red cells, or platelets as a consequence of chemotherapy, require proper management to prevent early death. Transfusions of packed red cells, platelet concentrates, or, rarely, granulocytes are given. Heparin may be effective in managing bleeding secondary to DIC, antibiotics may be given to attempt prevention of infection, and allopurinol may be necessary to prevent urate nephropathy.[19]

Radiotherapy

Meningeal leukemia occurs in a small percentage of patients with ANLL, particularly those having an M4 or M5 subgroup and presenting with a total leukocyte count higher than $100 \times 10^9/L$. Because systemic chemotherapy cannot cross the blood–brain barrier, radiation or intrathecal chemotherapy is given. Although meningeal leukemia is less frequently associated with ANLL than with ALL, it must be treated effectively to prolong patient survival. The presence of blast cells in the CSF is diagnostic. Treatment usually involves a combination of cranial radiation and intrathecal chemotherapy. Radiotherapy also is given when there is evidence of local tumor masses (chloromas) in other body sites.

TABLE 34-6
Common Chemotherapeutic Agents used in the Treatment of ANLL

Drug	Mode of Action	Toxic Effect
Cytarabine (cytosine arabinoside; ara-C)	Pyrimidine antimetabolite; a cytosine analogue that inhibits DNA synthesis	Myelosuppression; gastrointestinal epithelial injury causing nausea, vomiting, diarrhea and oral mucositis
Daunorubicin (DNR)	Anthracycline antibiotic; binds to DNA and interferes with mitosis and DNA and RNA synthesis	Myelosuppression; alopecia; cardiac toxicity; nausea and vomiting
Amsacrine (m-AMSA)	DNA interaction	Myelosuppression; cardiac toxicity

Immunotherapy

Immunotherapy is a technique in which antibodies are used to treat cancer. It has been used both in an attempt to increase the patient's own immunity to the leukemic cells specifically and to increase the patient's immunity nonspecifically to provide an antileukemic effect.

Using hybridoma technology, monoclonal antibodies can now be produced which have specificity for surface markers on neoplastic cells. Monoclonal antibodies have been used (1) to eliminate leukemic cells *in vitro* from autologous bone marrow preparations for transplant (Chap. 28) and (2) as carriers of strong toxins, although these techniques are still under investigation and also have limitations.

Several agents have been used in immunotherapy, including BCG (a bacterium formerly used to immunize against tuberculosis) and irradiated leukemic cells. The evidence for the efficacy of immunotherapy is inconclusive.[11]

Bone Marrow Transplantation

The mechanism by which marrow transplantation provides an effective defense against leukemia is not well understood. To prepare for transplantation, total-body irradiation of 1000 rad and intensive cyclophosphamide therapy are given to destroy any residual leukemic cells. Candidates for transplantation must be in good clinical condition and in the first clinical remission for the greatest chance of success. Age also is important, with higher survival rates in younger (less than 30 years) patients.

The most serious complication of bone marrow transplantation is graft versus host disease (GVHD), in which the T lymphocytes of the donor marrow destroy the lymphohemopoietic cells of the recipient. See Chapter 28 for a detailed discussion of bone marrow and blood stem cell tranplantation. It is difficult to be assured that all leukemic stem cells have been removed or killed, although polymerase chain reaction technology is showing great promise (Chap. 31).

Differentiation Treatment

One of the newer concepts in the treatment of ANLL is that of manipulating the maturation and differentiation of leukemic cells, rather than killing them.[16,24,25] Leukemic cells are thought to be blocked at an early stage of development and unable to mature to fully functional end cells. Chemically inducing their maturation and differentiation may be an important new modality that might not carry with it the toxic effects of current therapeutic strategies. Differentiation treatments now being studied include retinoic acid, phorbol esters, GM-CSF, G-CSF, and dimethyl sulfoxide (DMSO).

Despite current advances, 25% of patients treated for ANLL will die from complications within the first 12 to 18 months. There is about a 60% long-term survival rate for AML patients who have undergone transplantation during the first clinical remission and approximately a 30% long-term survival rate for those patients who have achieved a second remission.

CHAPTER SUMMARY

Acute nonlymphocytic leukemia (ANLL) is a progressive malignant disease of hematopoietic tissue. Although the etiology of leukemia is unclear, it may be the outcome of the interaction of several factors, including radiation, chemicals, genetics and viruses. This group of leukemias has been identified and subtyped on the basis of cell morphology as seen on Romanowsky-stained films of blood and bone marrow. Techniques such as cytogenetics, cytochemical (see Table 34-4), immunologic and ultrastructural studies are now being employed to aid in diagnosis.

The French–American–British classification scheme is an important method of categorizing acute leukemia that has as its basis standardized nomenclature and morphologic criteria. This system has greatly facilitated the uniform reporting and identification of these leukemias among clinical investigators. By using FAB criteria, the acute nonlymphocytic leukemias can be divided into eight distinct subgroups (see Tables 34-2 and 34-3). These subtypes generally have similar clinical manifestations (see Table 34-3) related primarily to the degree to which the numbers of normal blood cell elements are reduced.

Different subtypes of ANLL are treated similarly. The principal treatment modalities are chemotherapy (see Table 34-6), radiation, immunotherapy and transplantation. Various prognostic factors such as age and pretreatment status are important in determining the rate of therapeutic success. Managing the clinical effects of the profound myelosuppression is necessary after chemotherapy. The prognostic outlook for patients with ANLL is improving.

Case Study 34-1

A 59-year-old white woman was admitted for evaluation of a painful swollen right lower extremity and marked leukocytosis. Physical examination revealed a distended abdomen and splenomegaly 3 to 4 cm below the left costal margin. The entire right lower extremity was markedly swollen with tense edema and the leg was warm and tender to palpitation. There was no lymphadenopathy. Admission laboratory data included: WBC 5.0 × 10^9/L; Hb, 7.4 g/dL; Hct, 0.22 L/L; PLT 19 × 10^9/L; reticulocyte count, 0.1%; leukocyte differential: segmented neutrophils 6%, lymphocytes 16%, monocytes 13%, promonocytes 25%, monoblasts 40%. Red cells were hypochromic and microcytic. Bone marrow aspiration and biopsy were obtained with some difficulty. Sheets of abnormal cells resembling large primitive monocytoid cells with abundant light blue cytoplasm filled the marrow. The nuclei were spongy in appearance, contained one to three vesicular nucleoli, and were consistently irregular in shape. Erythroid and normal myeloid elements were greatly decreased. Serum lysozyme levels were markedly increased.

1. Based on the foregoing description and laboratory results, into which FAB classification would this patient's leukemia most likely fall?
2. What cytochemical determination would most likely be positive in the abnormal cells from this patient's blood and bone marrow?
3. The patient was treated with a course of cytarabine and achieved a remission. A subsequent bone marrow aspiration

revealed red cell precursors with megaloblastoid morphology. What is causing the red cell precursor morphology?

Case Study 34-2

A 63-year-old white male was seen in the emergency room for fever and general malaise. Neither organomegaly nor lymphadenopathy was observed on physical examination. His admission CBC revealed a leukopenia of 2.0×10^9/L, Hb 7.5 g/dL, Hct 0.22 L/L, and PLT 65×10^9/L. The leukocyte differential showed 32% segmented neutrophils, 53% lymphocytes, 8% monocytes, 2% eosinophils and 5% blasts. Red cells were microcytic and normochromic. Bone marrow aspiration revealed a hypercellular marrow filled with sheets of blast cells. These cells were characterized as type I blasts. Aüer rods were not observed. Cytochemically, the blasts were negative for all common myeloid markers including myeloperoxidase and Sudan black B. Surface antigen testing was negative for CD10, CD19 and CD20, but was positive for CD34 and CD7.

1. Based on the above description and laboratory results, into which FAB classification would this patient's leukemia most likely fall?
2. What additional cytochemical profiling could be done to further determine the cell lineage in this case?
3. Is there any prognostic significance associated with the finding of CD34 positivity?

Review Questions

34-1. The total blast cell count in the bone marrow is important when characterizing the acute nonlymphocytic leukemias and must be at least

   A. 40% of the total nucleated cells in the marrow.
   B. 40% of the total white cells in the marrow.
   C. 30% of the total nucleated cells in the marrow.
   D. 30% of the erythroid cells in the marrow.

34-2. The technique(s) used to classify the acute nonlymphocytic leukemias is/are

   A. immunologic.
   B. morphologic.
   C. cytochemical.
   D. all of the above.

34-3. All of the following stains are used to identify the acute nonlymphocytic leukemias EXCEPT

   A. peroxidase.
   B. α-naphthyl butyrate.
   C. naphthol ASD chloroacetate.
   D. TdT.

34-4. Auer rods may be found in all of the following classifications of acute nonlymphocytic leukemia EXCEPT

   A. M0.
   B. M1.
   C. M2.
   D. M3.

34-5. A cytogenetic abnormality is found in almost 50% of patients with which of the following classifications of acute nonlymphocytic leukemia?

   A. M2.
   B. M3.
   C. M5.
   D. M6.

References

1. Bennett JM, Catovsky D, Daniel MT et al: Criteria for the diagnosis of acute leukemia of megakaryocytic lineage (M7). Ann Intern Med 103:460, 1985
2. Bennett JM, Catovsky D, Daniel MT et al: Proposals for the classification of the acute leukaemias: French–American–British Cooperative Group. Br J Haematol 33:451, 1976
3. Bennett JM, Catovsky D, Daniel MT et al: Proposals for the classification of the myelodysplastic syndromes. Br J Haematol 51:189, 1982
4. Bennett JM, Catovsky D, Daniel MT et al: Proposed revised criteria for the classification of acute myeloid leukemia. Ann Intern Med 103:626, 1985
5. Breton-Gorius J, Reyes F, Duhamel G et al: Megakaryoblastic acute leukemia: Identification by the ultrastructural demonstration of platelet peroxidase. Blood 51:45, 1978
6. Catovsky D, Matutes E, Buccheri V et al: A classification of acute leukemia for the 1990s. Ann Hematol 62:16-21, 1991
7. Cheson BD, Cassileth PA, Head DR et al: Report of the National Cancer Institute-Sponsored Workshop on Definitions of Diagnosis and Response in Acute Myeloid Leukemia. J Clin Oncol 8:813-819, 1990
8. Cork A: Chromosomal abnormalities in leukemia. Am J Med Technol 49:703, 1983
9. Coltman CA, Freireich EJ, Savage RA et al: Long term survival of adults with acute leukemia [abstr]. Proc Am Soc Clin Oncol 21:389, 1979
10. Devine SM, Larson RA: Acute leukemia in adults: Recent developments in diagnosis and treatment. CA 44:326-352, 1994
11. Foon KA, Smalley RV, Riggs CW et al: The role of immunotherapy in acute myelogenous leukemia. Arch Intern Med 143:1726, 1983
12. Foucar K, Vaughan WP, Armitage JO et al: Postleukemic dysmyelopoiesis. Am J Hematol 15:321, 1983
13. Fraumeni JF Jr, Miller RW: Epidemiology of human leukemia: Recent observations. J Natl Cancer Inst 38:593, 1967
14. Golomb HM, Rowley JD, Vardiman JW et al: "Microgranular" acute promyelocytic leukemia: A distinct clinical, ultrastructural, and cytogenetic entity. Blood 55:253, 1980
15. Huang MJ, Li CY, Nichols WL et al: Acute leukemia with megakaryocytic differentiation: A study of 12 cases identified immunocytochemically. Blood 64:427, 1984
16. Koeffler P: Induction of differentiation of human acute myelogenous leukemia cells: Therapeutic implications. Blood 62:709, 1983
17. Koike T: Megakaryoblastic leukemia: The characterization and identification of megakaryoblasts. Blood 64:683, 1984
18. Lewis JP, Meyers FJ, Tanaka L: Daunomycin administered by continuous intravenous infusion is effective in the treatment of acute non-lymphocytic leukaemia. Br J Haematol 61:261, 1985
19. Lokich JJ: Managing chemotherapy-induced bone marrow suppression in cancer. Hosp Pract 11(8):61, 1976
20. Misawa S, Lee E, Schiffer CA et al: Association of the translocation (15;17) with malignant proliferation of promyelocytes in acute leukemia and chronic myelogenous leukemia at blastic crisis. Blood 67:270, 1986
21. Needleman SW, Burns CP, Dick FR et al: Hypoplastic acute leukemia. Cancer 48:1410, 1981
22. Reed WP, Newman KA, de Jongh C et al: Prolonged venous access for chemotherapy by means of the Hickman catheter. Cancer 52:185, 1983
23. Robertson MJ, Ritz J: Prognostic significance of the surface antigens expressed by leukemic cells. Leuk Lymphoma 13(Suppl 1):15-22, 1994

24. Ross DW: Leukemic cell maturation. Arch Pathol Lab Med 109:309, 1985
25. Sachs L: Growth, differentiation and the reversal of malignancy. Sci Am 254:40, 1986
26. Savage RA, Hoffman GC, Lucas FV: Morphology and cytochemistry of "microgranular" acute promyelocytic leukemia (FAB M3m). Am J Clin Pathol 75:548, 1981
27. Scott CS, Den Ottolander GJ, Swirsky D et al: Recommended Procedures for the Classification of Leukemias and Lymphoma, vol 2, pp 37–49. Harwood Academic Publishers, 1993
28. Shibata A, Bennett JM, Castoldi GL et al: Recommended methods for cytological procedures in haematology. Clin Lab Haematol 7:55, 1985
29. Weinberg RA: A molecular basis of cancer. Sci Am 249:126, 1983

Recommended Reading

Bloomfield CD (ed): Chronic and Acute Leukemias in Adults. Boston, Martinus Nijhoff, 1985
Goldman JM, Preisler HD (eds): Hematology 1: Leukemias. London, Butterworths, 1984
Thiel E, Thierfelder S (eds): Leukemia: Recent Developments in Diagnosis and Therapy. Berlin, Springer-Verlag, 1984
Wiernik PH, Canellos CP, Kyle RA, Schiffer CA (eds):Neoplastic Diseases of the Blood, vol 1. New York, Churchill Livingstone, 1985

Chronic Myeloproliferative Disorders

Irma T. Pereira

Objectives

1. Discuss the five chronic myeloproliferative disorders relative to (a) their similarities and (b) the labortory findings that best differentiate them.
2. List the diagnostic criteria for polycythemia vera.
3. Describe and discuss the various therapeutic regimens used to treat the chronic myeloproliferative disorders.
4. Describe the Philadelphia chromosome and its significance.

The chronic myeloproliferative disorders (CMPDs) were identified in 1951 by Dameshek[23] as a unified group of independent yet similar conditions that previously had been classified as separate entities. The disorders are polycythemia vera (PV), chronic myelogenous leukemia (CML), agnogenic myeloid metaplasia (AMM), and essential thrombocythemia (ET). Chronic neutrophilic leukemia, a rare disorder, was later added to the group. One could speculate that the CMPDs are all the same disease, each with a slightly different manifestation. The CMPDs could be compared with identical quintuplets: all have the same parent (an abnormal hematopoietic stem cell) and they look alike, but each has its own individuality.

This chapter seeks to explain the integral and sometimes confusing relations of the CMPDs as well as to point out the exceptions to these generalizations. Although classic descriptions will be presented, it must be remembered that the CMPDs can vary dramatically; and coexistence with or transformation to other CMPDs or even lymphoid diseases can take place at any time during their course.

In most patients with CMPD the diagnosis can be readily made from the peripheral blood film. However, additional procedures are usually necessary to confirm the diagnosis or to determine the prognosis.

GENERAL CONSIDERATIONS

CMPDs usually are found in patients in their fifth and sixth decades. The abnormal proliferation of cells associated with the CMPDs is considered to be clonal (*i.e.*, they begin in a single abnormal cell). The abnormality probably arises in a pluripotential stem cell, because usually, more than one line of myeloid cells is involved.

The best evidence of CMPD clonality comes from studies of women who are heterozygous for the glucose-6-phosphate dehydrogenase (G6PD) enzyme, producing both isoenzymes A and B.[36] The gene for G6PD is carried only on the X chromosome, and the female genotype for the G6PD isoenzymes may be homozygous (X^AX^A or X^BX^B) or heterozygous (X^AX^B). According to the Lyon hypothesis (Chap. 5), one X chromosome in each cell is inactivated, and all progeny of that cell retain that inactivation. Therefore, in G6PD-heterozygous women, although each cell makes only one isoenzyme, any tissue, including hematopoietic tissue, will produce a mixture—some cells will produce isoenzyme A and others, isoenzyme B. However, when a hematopoietic neoplastic disease is present in a G6PD-heterozygous woman, all of the patient's malignant hematopoietic cells produce only one isoenzyme. The cells of other tissues continue to be mixed, some producing isoenzyme A and others, isoenzyme B. This finding has led to the conclusion that all the neoplastic cells come from a single cell, and that the CMPDs have a clonal origin.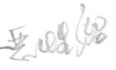

Cells involved in the CMPDs include mature and immature granulocytes, erythrocytes, and platelets. Common features are splenomegaly; mild to marked leukocytosis, thrombocytosis and/or erythrocytosis. Various degrees of marrow fibrosis are considered by some investigators to be a secondary feature resulting from increased numbers of abnormal megakaryocytes and platelets.[16,57,68] See Table 35-1 for the pathogenicity of the CMPDs.

All of the CMPDs have strong interrelations, as demonstrated by the frequent transformations between them (Fig. 35-1). In addition, many CMPDs terminate in acute myelogenous leukemia (AML; blast transformation). A small percentage of cases terminate in acute lymphoblastic leukemia (ALL).

TABLE 35-1
Pathogenicity of Myeloproliferative Diseases

Disorder	Age (yr)	Sex	Ph¹ Chromosome	Main Cell Type Affected	Survival (yr)	Main Cause of Death
CML	>30	M > F	+	Granulocytes	2–5	Blast transformation; hemorrhage; infection
PV	>50	M > F	–	Erythrocytes	~10–15	Thrombosis or hemorrhage, PPMM; blast transformation
AMM	>50	M = F	–	Fibroblasts	~5	Marrow failure; blast transformation; hemorrhage or thrombosis; heart, hepatic, or kidney failure; infection
ET	>50	M = F	–	Platelets	~1–5	Hemorrhage or thrombosis; blast transformation
CNL	?*	?*	–	Neutrophils	<4	Blast transformation; hemorrhage; infection

Not fully established; only 30 patients reported.

POLYCYTHEMIA VERA

Polycythemia vera, or PV, (*vera* is a Latin term meaning "true") is a clonal stem cell disorder characterized by panmyelosis (increase in all cellular bone marrow elements) and specifically by increased red cell mass (RCM). The condition also is known as "primary polycythemia." In PV, erythrocyte counts are increased to higher than 5.9×10^{12}/L in women and 6.6×10^{12}/L in men. A true increase in the RCM and the plasma volume is characteristic. A mild granulocytic leukocytosis and a considerable thrombocytosis also frequently occur.

If the cause for an erythrocytosis cannot be found, a stem cell-related disorder is usually suspected[1] and may be tentatively diagnosed as PV (see Differential Diagnosis section).

Clinical Presentation

Patients commonly complain of various combinations of headaches, vertigo, ringing in the ears, blurred vision, itching eyes, upper gastrointestinal pain (sometimes secondary to peptic ulcers), a feeling of fullness after eating small amounts (probably because of splenomegaly), and red, itchy skin (pruritus), especially after a hot bath. Thrombotic events, either venous or arterial, are common.[20]

Most patients are between 50 and 60 years of age; however, the condition has been seen in all age groups. The mucous membranes and skin have a ruddy cyanotic (reddish purple) appearance. Hypertension occurs frequently. Hepatomegaly and, more often splenomegaly, usually secondary to extramedullary hematopoiesis (cell formation outside the marrow), are common findings. Gout is also common because of the high uric acid levels caused by rapid cell turnover.[8]

Laboratory Findings

PERIPHERAL BLOOD

The most obvious finding in the peripheral blood is an extremely high erythrocyte count, which may reach 10×10^{12}/L. This leads to increased hemoglobin (Hb) levels (males greater than 17.5 g/dL; females greater than 15.5 g/dL) and Hcts (males greater than 0.55 L/L; females greater than 0.47 L/L). The mean cell volume (MCV) and mean cell hemoglobin concentration (MCHC) values are often low normal to slightly reduced because of the decreased or absent iron stores in the marrow as a result of chronic bleeding (possibly due to abnormal platelet function), and therapeutic phlebotomy, as well as increased RBC production and turnover. An occasional normoblast (NRBC) may be found. The reticulocyte count generally is not significantly increased. The leukocyte alkaline phosphatase (LAP) score usually is increased.

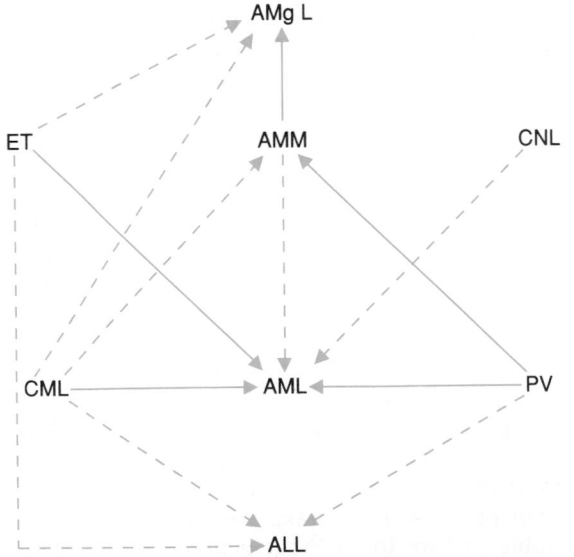

FIGURE 35-1. Transitions in chronic myeloproliferative disorders. CML, chronic myelogenous leukemia; AMM, agnogenic myeloid metaplasia; ET, essential thrombocythemia; PV, polycythemia vera; CNL, chronic neutrophilic leukemia; AML, acute myelogenous leukemia; ALL, acute lymphoblastic leukemia; AMgL, acute megakaryocytic leukemia; *solid arrow,* frequent; *dashed arrow,* infrequent.

Because panmyelosis is one of the distinguishing features of PV, the increase in RCM is only one element of this complex disorder. The patients also classically exhibit a granulocytic leukocytosis and thrombocytosis. Indeed, this is so often true that the absence of an increase in these components should alert the physician to the likelihood of a condition other than PV.[83] Leukocyte counts can go as high as 40 to 50 $\times$ 10^9/L. Occasionally, a slight left shift with a few metamyelocytes is seen. Basophil numbers frequently are elevated, and platelet counts can be as high as 2000 $\times$ 10^9/L. A moderate number of abnormal platelet forms may be present. Abnormal platelet aggregation and adhesiveness, as well as decreased levels of platelet factor 3 (PF3),[49] are frequently seen. It is often difficult to prepare a good peripheral blood film because of the increased blood viscosity. Even in the feather edge, the cells appear crowded. To make a better film, equal parts of the blood specimen and normal saline may be mixed in a small test tube to reduce blood viscosity. There is usually no sign of marrow fibrosis in the peripheral blood early in the disease and little if any at the time of diagnosis.

BONE MARROW

The marrow is hypercellular, with the fat spaces almost completely replaced by blood cells. Obvious features are increased megakaryocyte and normoblast numbers. Many megakaryocytes are large and abnormal in appearance. Basophils usually are increased, resulting in elevated levels of blood histamine, the probable cause of the itching that follows hot baths. Although little marrow fibrosis is seen early in PV, it tends to worsen as the disease progresses, possibly through the action of a number of factors, including megakaryocytic alpha granules releasing platelet-derived growth factor (PDGF).[16,91,94] Iron is decreased or absent.[76]

CHEMISTRY

Normal to elevated levels of serum vitamin B$_{12}$, increased B$_{12}$-binding capacity, and decreased serum iron and ferritin levels are present. Serum erythropoietin levels are decreased or normal in spite of the high RCM.

Differential Diagnosis

In 1967, the Polycythemia Vera Study Group was organized. One of its main goals was to develop a set of diagnostic criteria for PV. Table 35-2 summarizes the criteria recommended by this group.[11]

Increased RCM may be caused by conditions unrelated to a CMPD and may be categorized in one of two groups: secondary or relative. Both of these types of erythrocytosis are discussed in more detail in Chapter 10. A brief review is presented in the following.

In contrast to PV with its generally low erythropoietin levels, the *secondary polycythemias* show normal to increased erythropoietin production.[61] These *compensatory* erythrocytoses are associated with tissue hypoxia, which may result from living at high altitudes, cardiovascular or pulmonary disease, abnormal hemoglobins with an increased oxygen affinity (Chap. 14) or heavy smoking.[103] All of these disorders cause a decrease in the amount of oxygen delivered to the tissues, thereby stimulating erythropoietin production and increased erythrocyte production. Secondary polycythemia with *inappropriate* increases in erythropoietin is associated with some kidney diseases [72,92] and with erythropoietin-producing renal tumors, hepatocellular carcinoma,[80,95] ovarian tumors, uterine fibroids[81] and cerebellar hemangioblastoma.[51] In these conditions the RCM is abnormally increased.

Relative polycythemia is not associated with a true increase in RCM. Rather, RCM, as measured by the microhematocrit, is elevated because the plasma volume has decreased for some reason. Causes of relative polycythemia include plasma loss (*e.g.*, from severe burns) and dehydration from vomiting, severe diarrhea or lack of water.

The differential diagnosis between PV and secondary polycythemia is relatively simple from a clinical and laboratory viewpoint. Clinically, the spleen is rarely palpable in secondary polycythemia, but it is almost always palpable in PV. Thrombotic or hemorrhagic episodes are common in PV, but rare in secondary polycythemia. From a laboratory viewpoint, the combination of a granulocytic

TABLE 35-2
*Polycythemia Vera Study Group Criteria for Diagnosis of Polycythemia Vera**

Category A	Category B
1. Increased red cell mass 　Male >36 mL/kg 　Female >32 mL/kg	1. Thrombocytosis 　Platelets >400 $\times$ 10^9/L
2. Normal arterial O$_2$ saturation; 　>92%	2. Leukocytosis 　WBC >12 $\times$ 10^9/L with no fever or infection
3. Splenomegaly	3. Increased leukocyte alkaline phosphatase score 　(>100) with no fever or infection
	4. Increased serum B$_{12}$ (>900 ng/mL) or 　Increased unbound B$_{12}$ binding capacity 　(>2200 ng/mL)

* Diagnosis may be made if (1) all characteristics in category A are present or (2) category A characteristics 1 and 2 are present plus any two characteristics from category B. In addition, patients must have had the disease diagnosed no longer than 4 years and had no prior treatment except phlebotomy.
From Wasserman LR: The management of polycythemia vera. Br J Haematol 21:371, 1971, with permission.

leukocytosis, severe thrombocytosis, extreme erythrocytosis, and peripheral blood basophilia is so unusual that it almost always leads to the diagnosis of PV.

Testing for increased RCM may be performed in some suspected cases of PV. It also is helpful in distinguishing relative and absolute erythrocytosis. The test involves collection of a blood sample from which the red cells are separated and labeled with a small dose of radioactive chromium (^{51}Cr). After injection back into the patient, the labeled red cells are allowed to circulate for 15 minutes to allow them to disperse evenly in the circulation. At that point, a blood sample is removed and the amount of radioactivity in the erythrocyte portion determined. The lower the radioactivity measurement, the higher the blood volume. An RCM exceeding 36 mL/kg for males or 32 mL/kg for females is abnormally high and indicative of PV.[13] Plasma volume, which is normal or increased in PV, can be measured similarly using radioiodinated albumin. See Table 35-3 for other tests useful in the differential diagnosis of primary and secondary polycythemia.

Effects of Treatment on Laboratory Results

Because the cause of death is usually thrombotic events in patients treated only with phlebotomy, patients are usually treated with phlebotomy and radioactive phosphorus (^{32}P), myelosuppressive drugs, or a combination thereof. However, this mode of treatment has an unfavorable downside. Continued phlebotomy tends to worsen the iron deficiency and may aggravate the thrombocytosis. ^{32}P is given to reduce the proliferation of erythrocytes and platelets, but the long-term effect of ^{32}P is acute leukemia.[64] Although myelosuppressive drugs, such as busulfan and chlorambucil, have sometimes proved effective, they also have been associated with an increased incidence of acute leukemia and may cause the transformation of PV to acute leukemia.[98] A popular drug for the treatment of PV is hydroxyurea. Normalized blood counts were found in more than 80% of patients studied within 12 weeks of starting hydroxyurea treatment.[25] Hydroxyurea also appears to be less leukemogenic; therefore, it is the therapy of choice.[11,56]

Ideally, blood counts should approach normal within a short time. The ideal Hct is 0.45 to 0.50 L/L. The leukocyte count will usually approach normal, but the platelet count may remain in the high-normal range (350 to 500 × 10^9/L).[52] Granulocytes may be hypogranular. Some giant platelets may be present, and the patient may experience continued bleeding because of platelet hypofunction. If phlebotomy is continued, microcytic, hypochromic erythrocytes may be seen. An iron-deficient state is the desired effect, actually, because it limits the expansion of the RCM. The higher the RCM, the higher the chance of hemorrhage or thromboembolic episodes leading to stroke or myocardial infarction.[108]

Course of the Disease

The most obvious change in the peripheral blood in long-term PV (other than a decreasing MCV and MCHC) is the appearance of teardrop red cells on the blood film.[100] This change heralds the most common transition of PV, that of a secondary response causing increased and irreversible myelofibrosis and myeloid metaplasia. This is sometimes referred to as the "spent phase" (see Color Plate 35-1) of PV or postpolycythemic myeloid metaplasia (PPMM).[30] The latter is demonstrated in the bone marrow by increased reticulin content (marrow fibrosis).

Hepatosplenomegaly becomes more severe as the rate of extramedullary hematopoiesis accelerates. Splenectomy usually is recommended if splenic irradiation is ineffective and splenic enlargement causes increased red cell destruction and platelet sequestration. This operation does not, however, eradicate the myeloid metaplasia, which continues in the liver and other extramedullary sites.

As myelofibrosis and extramedullary hematopoiesis become more advanced, the blood film exhibits dramatic changes. Nucleated red blood cells increase out of proportion to the anemia and the low number of circulating reticulocytes. The differential shows a left shift in myeloid cells, including blast forms. Giant abnormal-appearing platelets increase in numbers, as do the numbers of micromegakaryocytes, micromegakaryoblasts, and megakaryocytic fragments on the peripheral blood film (see Color Plate 35-2). The leukocyte count is only moderately increased once corrected for NRBCs and megakaryocytes. Most patients in this phase have a poor prognosis. In some patients, platelet numbers increase to more than

TABLE 35-3
Findings in Primary and Secondary Polycythemia

	B$_{12}$ (ng/L)	LAP Score	Iron (μg/dL)	RBC Mass (mL/kg body wt)	Plasma Volume (mL/kg body wt)	Arterial O$_2$ Saturation
Reference range*	150–1500	11–95	40–140	Men: 25–35 Women: 20–30	Men and women: 40–50	≥92% of pO$_2$ (arterial)
Primary	>1500	Usually >100	<40	Men: >36 Women: >32	Men and women: N1 to ↑	≥92% of pO$_2$ (arterial)
Secondary	N1	N1	N1	N1 to ↑	↓	<92% of pO$_2$ (arterial)

Note that exact reference values for various tests may differ according to procedure used. However, the tendency toward abnormal values is apparent from this table. N1, normal; ↑, increased; ↓, decreased.

1000×10^9/L with only an occasional normal form seen, and megakaryocytic fragments and micromegakaryocytes reach high numbers.

Ultimately, normal forms of polymorphonuclear leukocytes, erythrocytes, and platelets may be eliminated with either concurrent increases in NRBCs coupled with increasing anemia (ineffective erythropoiesis) or a slow decrease in the number of NRBCs as abnormal megakaryocytes increase. In still other patients, the disorder transforms into a megakaryoblastic crisis, with platelet counts severely reduced. In any event, hemorrhage or infection is the usual cause of morbidity. Thrombosis and acute leukemia were reported as the most common causes of death in one study.[118] In a significant number of patients, PV transforms into AML and, in a few patients, to acute lymphoid leukemia. The increased numbers of acute leukemia transformations may be related, not to the CMPD, but to its treatment with leukemogenic drugs such as ^{32}P or the alkylating agents such as busulfan (Myleran) or chlorambucil.[12]

The Polycythemia Vera Study Group reported median survival times from diagnosis as 11.8 years for ^{32}P-treated patients, 8.9 years for those receiving chlorambucil, and 13.9 years for those treated by therapeutic phlebotomy.[11]

CHRONIC MYELOGENOUS LEUKEMIA

Chronic myelogenous leukemia (CML) is a malignant disorder characterized by leukocytosis, with an increase in mature and immature cells of the granulocytic series. Thrombocytosis is common. Splenomegaly, most likely attributable to extramedullary hematopoiesis, is frequent. An abnormal chromosome known as the Philadelphia chromosome (Ph[1]) may be found in cells of the malignant proliferating clone. Other chromosomal abnormalities have also been described. Ph[1] has been found in granulocytes, erythrocytes, megakaryocytes, and lymphocytes (B cells).

Chronic myelogenous leukemia is primarily a disease of adults, although it has been reported at all ages. The term "juvenile CML" is reserved for a Philadelphia-negative (Ph[1-]) CML-like disorder found in infants and very young children, usually younger than 2 years of age.

Clinical Presentation

The earliest and most common symptoms of CML are fatigue, shortness of breath after mild exertion, malaise, and fullness in the upper abdomen caused by hepatosplenomegaly. Patients often lose their appetite because of a sensation of fullness after they ingest even small quantities of food. This usually leads to anorexia and weight loss. Priapism (persistent penile engorgement) is another symptom associated with an extremely elevated leukocyte or platelet count. Signs of platelet abnormalities may be seen, such as retinal hemorrhage, hematuria, or epistaxis. Platelet abnormalities may occur because of functional or quantitative platelet disturbances.[48,107]

Sternal tenderness, warm, moist skin, pallor and a palpable spleen and liver are often detected. Occasionally, lymphadenopathy is present. In juvenile CML, patients usually present with severe splenomegaly and lymphadenopathy. Laboratory tests usually confirm an increased metabolic rate.[119] In adult CML, low-grade fever is common, although many patients have no fever until the terminal disease phase.[29]

Laboratory Findings

PERIPHERAL BLOOD

A marked leukocytosis is the obvious feature in the peripheral blood (see Color Plate 35-3). Generally, leukocyte counts range from 50 to 600×10^9/L before treatment. However, much higher counts have been reported: this author recalls a CML patient (who refused treatment) who had leukocyte counts exceeding 1500×10^9/L just before death.

If anemia is present, it is usually normocytic, normochromic. Platelet counts may be increased (approximately 600×10^9/L) or decreased, with occasional giant forms. Frequently, the leukocyte and platelet counts are inversely related: the higher the leukocyte count, the lower the platelet count. This effect is probably attributable to a "squeezing out" of marrow megakaryocytes by the overabundance of granulocytic cells. Leukocyte differential results approach the following: blasts 1% to 5%; promyelocytes 1% to 10%; myelocytes 10% to 20%; metamyelocytes 10% to 30%; bands 20% to 40%; neutrophils 30% to 50%; eosinophils 2% to 15% (including young forms); basophils 2% to 10% (including young forms); and normoblasts 2 to 4 per 100 leukocytes (see Color Plate 35-3). In my experience, dysplastic granulocytes and bizarre platelets are not characteristic of CML (see Chap. 33 on dysplasia) except under certain circumstances, such as impending myeloid blast transformation, Ph[1-] CML, or in patients first seen (by a physician) with CML in blast transformation (*i.e.*, CML in blast transformation de novo).

BONE MARROW

The marrow is markedly hypercellular with minimal fat, in large part because of myeloid hyperplasia. Most cells are in the granulocytic series. Marrow and peripheral blood differentials are similar except that the mean stage of maturity in the marrow is shifted to the left. Along with thrombocytosis, megakaryocytes frequently are increased, sometimes markedly. A reticulin stain on a biopsy specimen may demonstrate fibrosis.

CYTOGENETICS

The Philadelphia chromosome is one of the oldest known cytogenetic abnormalities in hematology. It is found in cells of the malignant proliferating clone in up to 95% of patients with CML.[31] The affected cells include granulocytes, erythrocytes, megakaryocytes and lymphocytes and are said to be Ph[1+]. The abnormality is the result of translocation of the long arm of chromosome 22 to the long arm of chromosome 9: t(9q$^+$; 22q$^-$) (Fig. 35-2).

The disease of adults and children (juvenile CML) whose cells are Ph[1-] has been suggested to be incorrectly

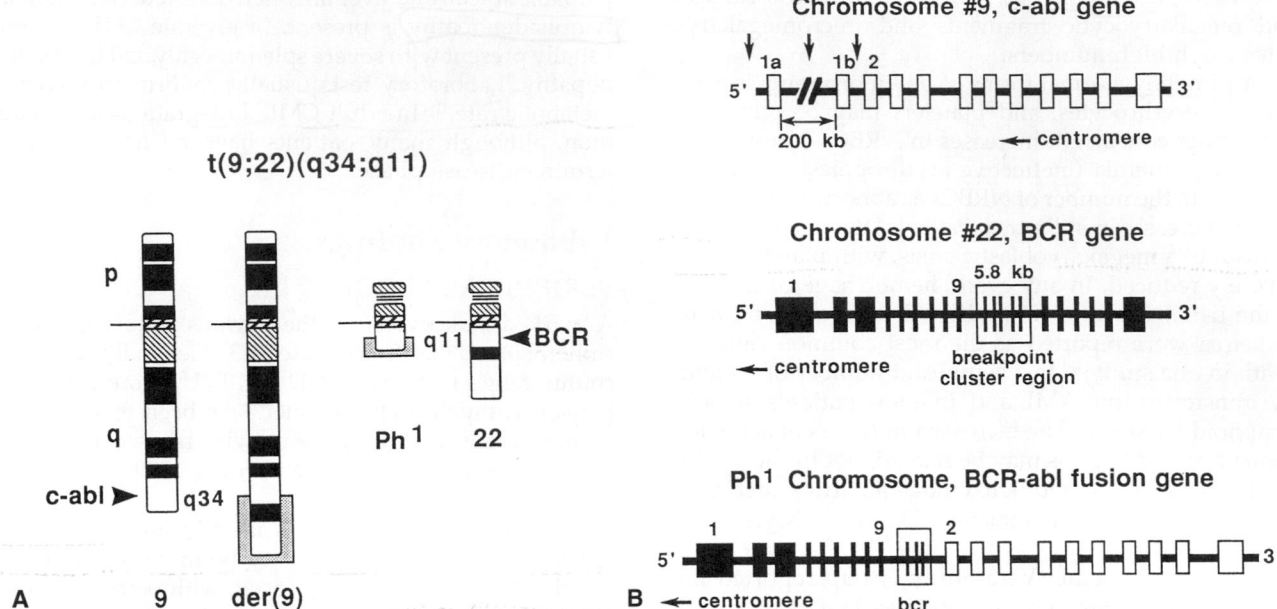

t(9;22)(q34;q11)

Chromosome #9, c-abl gene

Chromosome #22, BCR gene

Ph¹ Chromosome, BCR-abl fusion gene

FIGURE 35-2. (**A**) Ideogramic representation of Philadelphia translocation [t(9;22)] in CML indicating breakpoints at band q34 involving the c-*abl* proto-oncogene on chromosome 9, and q11 involving the *BCR* (breakpoint cluster region) gene on chromosome 22. Translocated segments on the derivative [der(9)] chromosome 9 and the Philadelphia (Ph¹) chromosome are *backshaded*. (**B**) Schematic representations at a molecular level of the c-*abl* gene on chromosome 9, the *BCR* gene on chromosome 22, and the *BCR–abl* fusion gene on the Ph¹ chromosome. *White boxes* are exons of the c-*abl* gene; *black boxes* are exons of the *BCR* gene. Breakage in the c-*abl* gene can occur at three sites indicated by *arrows* on the c-*abl* gene. In the *BCR* gene, the break occurs within the 5.8 kb breakpoint cluster region. The *BCR–abl* gene, as represented, includes the first 12 exons of the *BCR* gene and all exons distal to exon 1b on the c-*abl* gene. This fusion gene produces a fusion protein with enhanced tyrosine kinase activity.

classified as CML. One study[84] indicates that on the basis of the proposals by the French–American–British (FAB) group for the classification of dysmyelopoietic syndromes[9] (DMPS; Chap. 33), Ph¹⁻ CML probably belongs in the DMPS group, according to peripheral blood and bone marrow morphology. In this study, 17 previously diagnosed cases of Ph¹⁻ CML were reclassified as DMPS. It was demonstrated that myelodysplasia was rare in Ph¹⁺ CML if blast transformation occurred more than 12 months after initial diagnosis. Myelodysplasia was seen only when blast transformation occurred sooner than 12 months from initial diagnosis. Conversely, myelodysplasia occurred in all but one of the Ph¹⁻ group. Basophilia was not present in the Ph¹⁻ group, but it was consistently present in the Ph¹⁺ group. Finally, monocytosis seemed to be present in nearly all Ph¹⁻ cases but not in the Ph¹⁺ CML cases.

Another group of patients with Ph¹⁻ CML have a clinical picture indistinguishable from that of Ph¹⁺ CML, both in survival and in disease characteristics.[67] New findings in molecular genetics concerning Ph¹⁻ CML may explain this phenomenon. A study of 19 patients with Ph¹⁻ CML at the molecular level revealed that 7 patients had chromosome 9 and 22 rearrangement patterns thought to be pathognomonic for Ph¹⁺ CML, although the typical Ph¹⁺ rearrangement seen by standard cytogenetic techniques was not found. Specifically, these 7 patients had a rearrangement of the oncogene c-*abl* (from 9q34) translocating to the *bcr* region of 22q11.[7,40,74] This group of CML patients may be considered Ph¹⁺, albeit at the molecular level. Other studies using sophisiticated molecular techniques such as polymerase chain reaction agree that, except in rare cases, patients with CML will have some chromosomal alteration at the c-*abl* or *bcr* regions.[112]

Differential Diagnosis

The most common cause of leukocytosis with a left shift and mild thrombocytosis is infection or reaction to tissue necrosis or neoplasm. Because of confusion in the past between these reactions and CML, the term "leukemoid reaction" was developed to label any condition that mimicked leukemia but was, in fact, benign. However, differentiation between CML and a leukemoid reaction has been greatly simplified, and confusion is now less common. One of the tests used for differentiation is the leukocyte (or neutrophil) alkaline phosphatase (LAP/NAP) test. The LAP is normal or increased in a leukemoid reaction and decreased in CML unless there is a concurrent infection. Splenomegaly usually is absent with a leukemoid reaction, but is often present in CML (Table 35-4). The other disease most commonly confused with CML is myelofibrosis with myeloid metaplasia (see later discussion).

TABLE 35-4
Laboratory Features of CML and Leukemoid Reaction

Condition	Spenomegaly	WBC	Platelets ×10⁹/L	Left Shift	NRBCs per 100 WBC	Basophils and Eosinophils	LAP Score	Ph¹	Anemia
CML	Usually present	↑ ↑ ↑ ↑	>600 or <50	Back to blast (1–5%)	0–5	Normal or ↑ ↑ with young forms	↓*	+	Normocytic; normochromic
Leukemoid reaction	Usually absent	↑ ↑	200–450	Blasts seldom >0.5%	0–1	Normal	N1 to ↑	–	Not present

↑ ↑ ↑ ↑, *marked increase;* ↑ ↑, *moderate increase;* ↑, *slight increase;* ↓, *slight decrease; N1, normal.*
* Except in infection.

Effects of Treatment on Laboratory Results

Allopurinol is usually given before therapy, coupled with adequate hydration, to ameliorate the hyperuricemia caused by the rapid turnover and destruction of granulocytes by chemotherapy. Until recently, the traditional therapy for most CML patients was hydroxyurea or alkylating agents such as busulfan. These agents are myelosuppressive drugs used specifically to reduce the numbers of proliferating myeloid elements in an attempt to return the patient to a clinically normal state (*i.e.*, the elimination of anemia, splenomegaly, thrombocytosis and the marked leukocytosis with a left shift).

At least 75% of patients in the chronic phase of CML respond to single chemotherapeutic agents, such as busulfan, obtaining a peripheral blood remission.[60] Leukocyte counts can fall to and remain as low as 15 × 10⁹/L, often with only a slight left shift. However, it is not uncommon to find occasional myelocytes, promyelocytes, and even a rare blast even though the patient appears to be well. Platelet counts may remain in the high-normal range or be slightly increased. Basophilia (as much as 3%) is not uncommon in the treated CML patient. The Ph¹ chromosome seems to persist regardless of treatment. Drugs have little or no effect on cell morphology per se, although granulocytic hypogranulation is sometimes seen. The latest studies show that treatment with interferon-α as a more effective therapy than the alkylating agents or even hydroxyurea alone. The toxic effects appear reduced, although influenzalike symptoms, nausea, anorexia and a feeling of lethargy may cause cessation of the drug.[45]

Today, treatment for CML is not limited to chemotherapy. A highly popular therapy for CML in chronic phase or during first remission, resulting in potential cure, is allogeneic bone marrow transplantation.[21,41,44] Transplantation for CML patients in either the accelerated or the blast crisis phase has shown little therapeutic value.[33,105] Age is an important variable to transplant success. In patients older than 40 to 50 years of age, complications including relapse associated with depletion of T cells,[43] severe graft-versus-host disease (GVHD), an increase in the incidence of septic complications, and idiopathic interstitial pneumonitis are common and often fatal. As a result, 40 to 50 years is frequently the age limit for allogeneic marrow transplantation.[59] See Chapter 28 for a detailed discussion of bone marrow and stem cell transplantation. Unfortunately, autologous transplants do not promote long-term remission, because the patient's own marrow is rarely Ph¹⁻.[42,62] Use of autologous transplant may be more successful if the patient's bone marrow cells are permitted to stay in culture for longer periods. Observers have noted that after marrow cells from CML patients were cultured for 10 days, the Ph¹⁺ cells did not survive.[22] Based on this finding, clinical studies have followed a small group of CML patients transplanted with marrow autografts that were incubated in liquid culture for 10 days. Nearly all patients went into remission with Ph¹⁻ hematopoiesis. The longest complete remission in this study was 48 months posttransplant at the time of the report.[5] Of 40 CML patients treated with syngeneic marrow transplants, 65% remained disease-free at 6.6 years,[18,19] and 60% to 70% of more than 400 patients receiving allogeneic transplants during the chronic phase were surviving disease-free when examined after 3 years.[19,47]

Course of the Disease

Kamada and Uchino proposed a sequential process for CML on the basis of data from 20 patients.[55] It was noted that Ph¹⁺ patients showed no symptoms when the leukocytes were fewer than 50 × 10⁹/L. Increasing symptom severity coincided with disease progression and leukocyte count increases.[14,55] They concluded that there is a three-stage CML disease process: (1) proliferative and symptomless, lasting an average of 6.3 years; (2) preclinical, lasting approximately 19 months; and (3) terminal, advanced (accelerated), in which patients have symptoms and a 3-year mean survival. More clinical data are needed on a larger and less selected group before statistically valid conclusions can be reached.

For patients ineligible for bone marrow transplantation, the chronic phase generally responds to therapy and continues to do so for several years. However, within 2 to 4 years from the onset of symptoms, increasing marrow fibrosis is evidenced by the presence of approximately 5% teardrop-shaped red cells, abnormal platelets, and occasional megakaryocyte fragments. This blood picture is often confused with that of myelofibrosis with myeloid metaplasia.

The terminal accelerated phase is referred to as "blast transformation" or "acute exacerbation blast crisis." Several different patterns seem to emerge that herald blast transformation; these patterns may differ among patients. The patterns may include either evidence of dysplastic myelopoiesis (e.g., hypogranular and hyposegmented granulocytes, giant agranular platelets, and oval macrocytes) or development of an unexpected thrombocytopenia relative to the patient's standard counts during remission. Some patients show minimal dysplasia with the emergence of myeloid blast transformation. The only clue to blast transformation in these patients is a distinct decrease in the platelet count without a corresponding leukopenia and a slight (5% to 10%) increase in the blast count over previous numbers.

Not all CMLs transform directly into the myeloblastic phase. Some patients exhibit a marked basophilia (as much as 50%), show evidence of megakaryocytic blast crisis, and then develop a myeloid blast transformation. No matter how CML blast transformation emerges, the eventual outcome is the same. As transformation progresses, the leukocyte count and blast percentage rise, while thrombocytopenia becomes increasingly severe. The final blood picture may be indistinguishable from that of AML.

Transformation into lymphoblastic leukemia is more common than was once thought possible. In one study,[46] 30% of the subjects in CML blast transformation had a lymphoblastic transformation. Other transformations showed the phenotypes of erythroleukemia, mixed leukemia (having both myeloid and lymphoid blasts), and undifferentiated leukemia.

There are no clear prognostic indicators. For example, studies have agreed that certain findings indicate a poor prognosis. These include leukocytosis ($> 100 \times 10^9$/L); basophilia ($\geq 15\%$ to 20%); $> 1\%$ blasts in the peripheral blood or $> 5\%$ in the marrow; thrombocytosis ($> 700 \times 10^9$/L); thrombocytopenia ($< 150 \times 10^9$/L); splenomegaly; and karyotype abnormalities other than Ph^1 chromosome.[17,104,114] One study demonstrated that an increase in marrow myeloblasts and promyelocytes with a decreased number of mitotic cells also indicates a poor prognosis.[102] On the other hand, some investigators have reported that the prognosis is not affected by degree of leukocytosis,[54,73,115] a high percentage of blasts,[73] thrombocytosis,[73,115] or thrombocytopenia.[73,115] Likewise, disagreement exists between studies showing that severe anemia had no effect on prognosis,[73] and another study proposing that severe anemia indicated a poor prognosis.[54]

JUVENILE CHRONIC MYELOGENOUS LEUKEMIA

Juvenile CML, although not a CMPD, at one time was thought to be a CML variant with Ph^{1-} cells. The peak incidence occurs at 1 to 2 years of age.[3] The prognosis is extremely unfavorable. There is a dyserythropoiesis and a marked increase in serum and urine muramidase levels secondary to increased leukocyte destruction. Leukocyte counts are usually below 100×10^9/L and typically are lower than those in adult Ph^{1+} CML. Peripheral blood

and marrow monocytosis were reported in one study[2] but were not found in another.[87] Increased fetal hemoglobin (Hb F) is common; there are reports of 15% to 50%[2,65] and even 85%[96] Hb F. Other characteristics of fetal erythrocytes are also common, including a decreased Hb A_2 level and low levels of the enzymes G6PD, lactate dehydrogenase (LD), and pyruvate kinase (PK), among others.[28]

Although juvenile CML is still commonly referred to in older literature, the latest research indicates that, with rare exception, Ph^{1-} CML is better classified as a myelodysplastic syndrome (Chap. 33).

AGNOGENIC MYELOID METAPLASIA

Agnogenic myeloid metaplasia (AMM) or idiopathic myelofibrosis are terms used to describe a clonal chronic myeloproliferative disorder[53] characterized by increased collagen,[38] proliferation of fibroblasts, fibrosis, and granulocytic hyperplasia in the marrow and by proliferation of granulocytes in the spleen and liver.[34] Agnogenic myeloid metaplasia is found mostly in middle-aged to older persons. On rare occasions, it is found in children, either as a primary idiopathic disease or secondary to acute leukemia.[66] The fibrosis is believed to be a secondary reaction to the clonal proliferative disease, rather than the direct result of a clonal disorder. This conclusion is based on evidence that fibroblasts in heterozygous patients produce both G6PD isoenzymes A and B (enzyme mosaicism),[27,58] whereas the neoplastic hematopoietic cells of clonal disorders in similar patients produce only one isoenzyme. Megakaryocytes and platelets may contribute to fibrosis.

One of the most consistent findings in AMM is the increase in defective platelets as a consequence of dysplastic megakaryocytopoiesis. This results in premature death of these defective platelets and megakaryocytes and the release of their alpha granules, which contain platelet-derived growth factor (PDGF; Chap. 55). In vitro, the presence of increased alpha granules stimulates fibroblastic growth and secretion of collagen.[57,68] It is believed that in vivo, alpha granules stimulate marrow fibroblasts, which subsequently increase fibrous tissue, leading to myelofibrosis.[15] The chronic CMPDs are closely related; therefore, any of them may demonstrate various degrees of myelofibrosis as a secondary complication (see Fig. 35-1).

There are many synonyms for AMM, the two most common being myelofibrosis with myeloid metaplasia and idiopathic myelofibrosis. In AMM the marrow may become increasingly dominated by fibroblasts; thus the term myelofibrosis is also used in referring to this disorder. Myeloid metaplasia indicates that myeloid cells (granulocytes, erythrocytes and megakaryocytes) are produced in hematopoietic sites outside the marrow. Such production is also referred to as extramedullary hematopoiesis. These extramedullary sites are the same as those that formed blood cells in utero during the hepatic period of development (Chap. 5), including the liver, spleen, and reticuloendothelial system. Idiopathic (primary) myelofibrosis refers to fibrosis arising from an unknown cause.

Clinical Presentation

SYMPTOMS

The most common complaints are those relating to anemia, as well as abdominal pain, indigestion, and a fullness after eating small amounts secondary to splenomegaly. The latter results in anorexia and weight loss. Fever, night sweats, lethargy and weakness are common complaints.

PHYSICAL FINDINGS

Patients may appear ashen. Splenomegaly and sometimes hepatomegaly are evident. Petechiae may be present, and epistaxis may occur frequently.

Laboratory Findings

PERIPHERAL BLOOD

Leukocytes and platelets may be increased, normal, or decreased in number. A mild anemia may be present, and it is usually of the normocytic, normochromic type. Occasionally, a microcytic anemia is found, especially if patients have had repeated episodes of gastrointestinal bleeding. The blood film classically shows *dacryocytes* (*i.e.*, teardrop-shaped red cells; Fig. 35-3). The teardrops result from the cells' tortuous circulation through the enlarged spleen. Dacryocytes are a significant finding and should immediately alert the morphologist to search for conclusive evidence of myeloid metaplasia. The blood film usually reveals at least one other pathologic finding: (1) an occasional NRBC; (2) a giant, agranular platelet; (3) a rare megakaryocyte fragment; (4) an occasional immature myeloid cell; or (5) a rare myeloblast.

Although a mild reticulocytosis may be found, it is usually not as high as one would expect given the number of NRBCs found. The reticulocyte production index (Chap. 9) usually indicates ineffective erythropoiesis.

As the disease progresses, NRBCs, immature granulocytes (including myeloblasts), megakaryocytic fragments and micromegakaryocytes increase. Patients may become severely thrombocytopenic with increasing splenic sequestration, or the platelet count may become abnormally high with giant and bizarre forms.

BONE MARROW

Attempts to aspirate bone marrow are usually futile ("dry tap"), and only trephine biopsies are successful. On biopsy, moderate to marked amounts of reticular fibrosis or collagen deposition are found,[52] with hypocellularity, although normal or hypercellular areas can be found if, by chance, such an area of the bone marrow is sampled. Usually, increased numbers of megakaryocytes are found. The end stage of AMM usually shows increased osteosclerosis (hardening of the bone), and the marrow spaces are filled with enormous amounts of fibrotic tissue and small groups of megakaryocytes.[10]

OTHER LABORATORY VALUES

The LAP is normal to increased. Uric acid is increased, but serum albumin and cholesterol often are decreased. The LD is usually increased, probably because of ineffective myelopoiesis.[63,116]

Differential Diagnosis

Agnogenic myeloid metaplasia is most commonly confused with CML because of the similar immaturity of the peripheral blood leukocytes and the presence of all stages of myeloid maturation, including immature eosinophils and basophils. Several factors may assist in differentia-

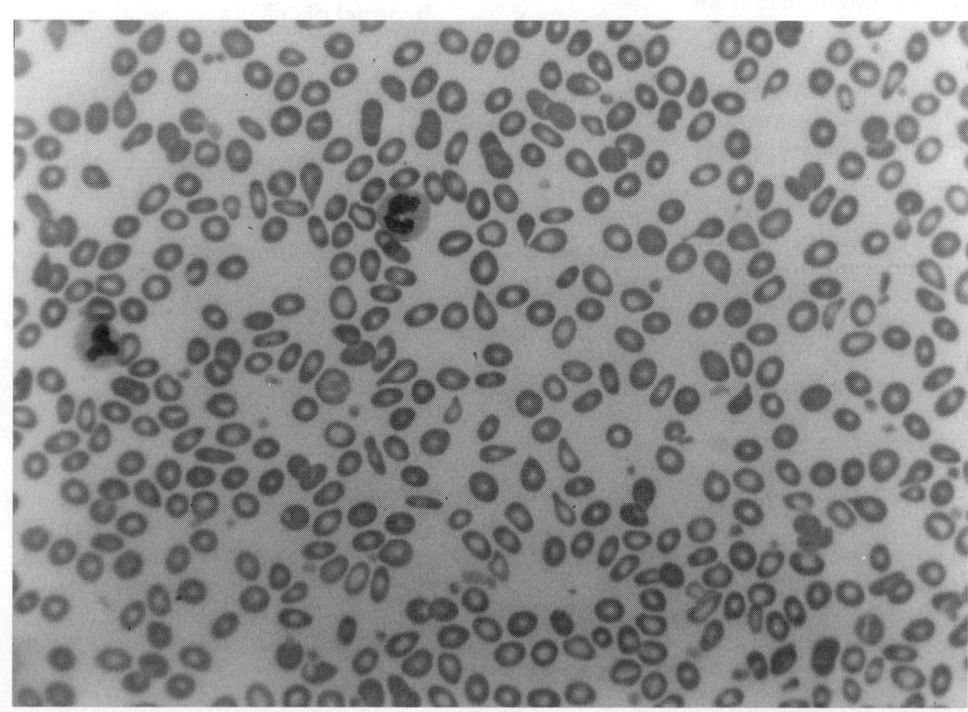

FIGURE 35-3. Note teardrop forms on peripheral blood film of patient with agnogenic myeloid metaplasia (original magnification ×500).

tion. The blood film in CML does not have the high numbers of NRBCs or dacryocytes seen in AMM, and although the CML film can have an occasional megakaryocytic fragment and a few abnormal-appearing platelets, the numbers do not approach those seen in AMM. The Ph[1] chromosome and an extremely low LAP are indicative of CML, whereas Ph[1] is not found in AMM and the LAP in AMM is usually normal or increased (see Table 35-7).

Cell immaturity, basophilia, eosinophilia, thrombocytosis, and the presence of splenomegaly may cause confusion between AMM and PV, particularly in those few AMM patients who are polycythemic, rather than anemic.[116] Significant numbers of dacryocytes and NRBCs with some megakaryocytic fragments indicate AMM. Splenomegaly generally is more pronounced in AMM than in PV, and the degree of fibrosis may be less in PV than in AMM at the time of diagnosis. However, in PV with advanced progression to AMM, the two are indistinguishable.

Confusion also arises when extramedullary hematopoiesis is demonstrated in other CMPDs and the bone marrow shows slight fibrosis. In such patients, several characteristics similar to those of AMM will be apparent, such as the appearance of a few dacryocytes, an occasional megakaryocytic fragment, and some bizarre platelets. However, none of the changes is as severe as in a moderately advanced AMM, except in PPMM, in which the changes are indistinguishable. Ferrokinetic studies using ^{52}Fe or ^{59}Fe may be performed to estimate the amount of extramedullary erythropoiesis in the spleen and liver. Extensive extramedullary erythropoiesis is indicative of AMM.

Agnogenic myeloid metaplasia may also be confused with myelophthisic anemia. The latter condition results from marrow replacement by malignant nonhematopoietic cells and may be accompanied by fibrosis, which leads to compensatory extramedullary hematopoiesis. From a pathogenic standpoint, AMM is a noncompensatory disorder that results from stem cell injury, rather than from marrow replacement.[89]

Differentiation of AMM from myelophthisic anemia can be difficult when looking at a blood film with no knowledge of the patient. Typically, this anemia demonstrates a leukoerythroblastic blood picture showing the same morphology as an early AMM; namely, normocytic, normochromic anemia with dacryocytes, a few NRBCs, a rare abnormal platelet, and immature granulocytes with an occasional myeloblast. Some conditions that may cause marrow infiltration and result in a leukoerythroblastic blood picture that may be confused with AMM are listed in Table 35-5. Dacryocytes seem to be most commonly associated with breast, bladder and prostate carcinomas.

A leukoerythroblastic reaction may also be seen without marrow infiltration. This occurs in normal newborns and in conditions for which a tremendous bone marrow response is present, such as severe hemolytic crisis (*e.g.*, thalassemia major),[8] hemorrhage (*e.g.*, gastrointestinal bleeding), postsplenectomy, and septicemia. Dacryocytes usually are not found in the leukoerythroblastic reaction associated with hemorrhage or infection, but they can be found in some congenital hemolytic conditions, such as thalassemia.

TABLE 35-5
Causes of Marrow Infiltration and Leukoerythroblastic Blood Picture That May Be Confused With Agnogenic Myeloid Metaplasia

Hodgkin's and non-Hodgkin's lymphoma

Infections (miliary tuberculosis, histoplasmosis)

Carcinoma, especially breast, prostate, lung, and bladder

Other neoplasms (neuroblastoma, carcinoma of the gastrointestinal tract, kidney, and thyroid)

Myelofibrosis:
   Primary: agnogenic or idiopathic
   Secondary: cancers or toxins (benzene, radiation)

Other chronic myeloproliferative diseases (PV, CML, ET)

Other hematologic disorders (hairy cell leukemia, ALL, multiple myeloma, acute myelofibrosis, AML)

Lipid storage diseases

Osteopetrosis

Adapted from Sun NCJ: Hematology—An Atlas and Diagnostic Guide, pp 158–163. Philadelphia, WB Saunders, 1983; and Peterson P, McIntyre OR: Myeloproliferative Disorders, pp 24–25. Publication for the ASCP National Meeting, 1987.

Effects of Treatment on Laboratory Results

Treatment generally is aimed at alleviating symptoms because there is no treatment that will affect the course or outcome of AMM. Splenectomy is not advised for patients who remain asymptomatic for long periods. Once the disease manifests itself, splenectomy is advised early because, during the advanced stage, this operation carries considerable hemorrhagic risk.[75] Splenectomy is particularly helpful if hemolytic anemia or thrombocytopenia persists despite use of chemotherapy or radiation to reduce splenic size.[101]

Normoblasts, abnormal platelets and megakaryocyte fragments increase after splenectomy, whereas dacryocytes virtually disappear. This finding upholds the traditional theory that the spleen is responsible for dacryocyte formation. Splenectomy causes the appearance of Howell-Jolly bodies, acanthocytes, spherocytes, and target cells on the blood film. In the absence of the spleen, platelet counts may exceed 1000×10^9/L, because the intact spleen normally pools many platelets; this increases the risk of thromboembolism. Standard myelosuppressive therapy with busulfan or hydroxyurea is used to decrease the platelet mass. At this point, the blood film is identical with the picture already described as PPMM.

Course of the Disease

Bone marrow transplantation is now the only hope for reversing myelofibrosis. Studies have demonstrated that marrow fibrosis is completely reversible, barring complications such as GVHD, after allogeneic transplantation that results in complete marrow engraftment.[24,38,69,78,88] In another report, no difference in engraftment time, rate of relapse, or survival was noticed in patients having extensive marrow fibrosis versus those with little or no fibrosis.[79] However, this finding is in complete contradiction with that of another study in which definite adverse effects were reported after bone marrow transplantation for patients with severe fibrosis.[86] Nonetheless, without transplantation, the prognosis is grave. Most patients die of complications from total marrow failure. Hemorrhage, infections, or cardiac complications are the immediate cause of death.[10] Approximately 5% to 8% terminate in AML or what appears to be a form of megakaryocytic leukemia. The blood film shows masses of abnormal platelet-producing micromegakaryocytes (see Color Plate 35-4) with few or no normal myeloid elements. Years ago, Hayhoe and Flemans referred to this pattern as "megakaryocytic myelosis."[50] There are reports, however, of patients who go into remission for periods as long as 22 months before transformation of the disease into AML.[85]

ESSENTIAL THROMBOCYTHEMIA

Primary or essential thrombocythemia (ET) is a CMPD characterized by a thrombocytosis in excess of 1000 × 10⁹/L, with spontaneous aggregation of functionally abnormal platelets. In this disorder there is no apparent cause for the thrombocytosis, whereas the cause usually is apparent in secondary thrombocytosis associated with splenectomy, chronic infections and other situations not related to CMPDs. Essential thrombocythemia is closely related to PV, the principal difference being that the diagnosis of PV requires an increase in total red cell mass, whereas that of ET requires an increase in platelet mass, without accompanying significant erythrocytosis. It is one of the least common of the CMPDs, second only to chronic neutrophilic leukemia, which is the least common.

Clinical Presentation

SYMPTOMS

There are frequent episodes of epistaxis, vomiting of blood, easy bleeding after minor dental surgery and gastrointestinal bleeding. Paradoxically, thrombotic events also are common. Fatigue is a frequent complaint.

PHYSICAL FINDINGS

Splenomegaly and, on occasion, hepatomegaly are detected. However, if the splenic blood supply is impeded by platelet aggregates in the microcirculation, the spleen may undergo a slow reduction in size as it atrophies secondary to lack of oxygen and nutrients. In these cases, the spleen is not palpable. There may be arterial or venous thrombosis involving the penile (resulting in priapism), hepatic, mesenteric, and portal vessels.[99] Pulmonary emboli and gangrenous toes are not uncommon.

Laboratory Findings

PERIPHERAL BLOOD

The most striking finding is the persistence of a marked thrombocytosis, with platelet counts exceeding 1100 × 10⁹/L. The highest count seen by this author was 8000 × 10⁹/L, but there are reports of counts as high as 14,000 × 10⁹/L.[32,48] Large masses of platelet aggregates are seen on the blood film, with many abnormal-appearing giant and bizarre forms. Marked platelet anisocytosis (large and small forms) and occasional megakaryocyte fragments are characteristic (Fig. 35-4).

The RBC count is occasionally slightly elevated. In the presence of chronic bleeding, microcytic, hypochromic erythrocytes indicate an iron deficiency anemia. Target

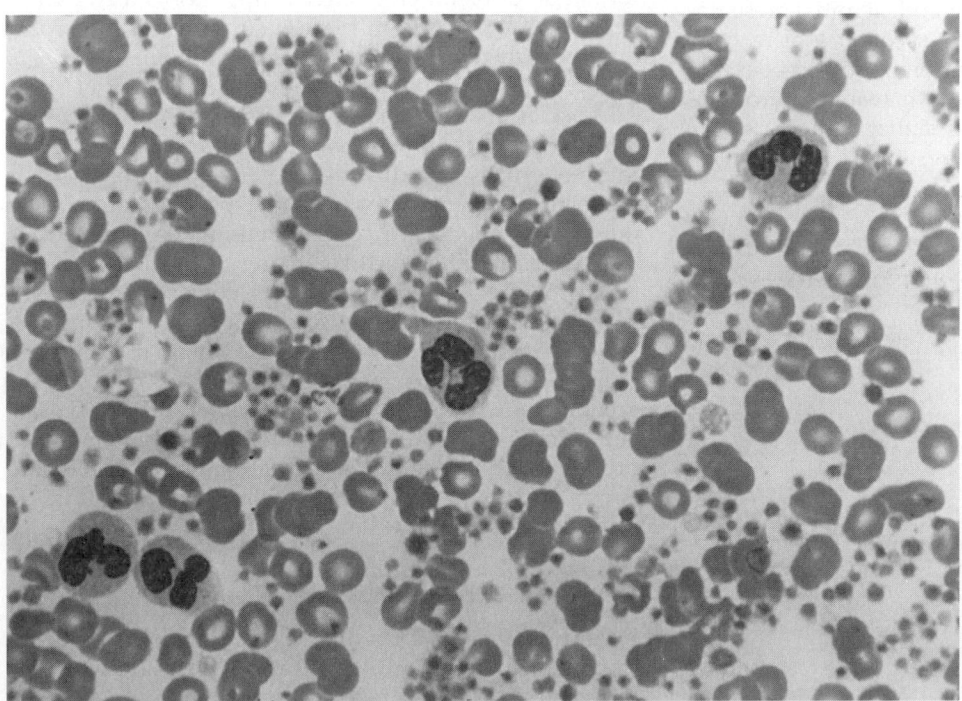

FIGURE 35-4. Essential thrombocythemia. Note granulocytosis, marked thrombocytosis and platelets that appear in clumps in this peripheral blood film (original magnification ×1000).

cells, acanthocytes and Howell-Jolly bodies will be found if splenic infarction occurs, causing poor splenic function.

The Polycythemia Vera Study Group[77] reported that the leukocyte count in 37 patients with ET ranged from 6 to 41×10^9/L with a median of 11.5×10^9/L and a neutrophilic left shift of mostly bands and metamyelocytes.

BONE MARROW

The marrow can be difficult to aspirate because of myelofibrosis; however, it may simultaneously be hypercellular, with a megakaryocytic hyperplasia and masses of aggregated platelets. The megakaryocytes may stick together as well, giving the whole marrow a "glued together" appearance. Some patients have a mild concurrent erythroid and granulocytic hyperplasia.

COAGULATION STUDIES

Platelet function studies are abnormal. Platelet aggregation (Chap. 56) is abnormal with ADP and epinephrine, but, oddly enough, when the platelet count is reduced to normal, platelet function returns to normal.[32] These patients probably have an acquired storage pool disease (Chap. 57), which is a common characteristic of the CMPDs.[82]

Differential Diagnosis

The most common condition confused with essential or primary thrombocythemia is a reactive or secondary thrombocytosis. Platelet aggregation studies are useful for differentiation because they are usually normal in secondary thrombocytosis but abnormal in ET.

A careful clinical evaluation of the patient is also helpful in differentiation. The Polycythemia Vera Study Group has published diagnostic criteria for ET (Table 35-6).[77] Patients with ET usually have some degree of splenomegaly or hepatomegaly or both at initial presentation, whereas this is unusual for a secondary or reactive thrombocytosis. Bleeding and thrombotic episodes are common with ET, but unlikely with reactive thrombocytosis unless the platelet count is higher than 900×10^9/

TABLE 35-6
Diagnostic Criteria for Essential Thrombocythemia

1. Platelet count $>600 \times 10^9$/L
2. Hemoglobin <13 g/dL or normal red cell mass
   Males <36 mL/kg
   Females <32 mL/kg
3. Stainable iron in marrow or failure of iron trial (<1 g/dL rise in Hb after 1 month of iron therapy)
4. No Ph[1] chromosome
5. Collagen fibrosis of marrow
   Absent *or*
   Less than one-third of biopsy area without both splenomegaly and leukoerythroblastic reaction
6. No known cause for reactive thrombocytosis

From Murphy S, Iland H, Rosenthal D, Laszlo J: Essential thrombocythemia: An interim report from the Polycythemia Vera Study Group. Semin Hematol 23:177, 1986, with permission.

L. Most helpful in differentiation is the platelet count itself, which usually is higher than 1500×10^9/L in ET, but rarely above 1000×10^9/L in reactive thrombocytosis.

The most common causes of reactive thrombocytosis are infection, chronic inflammation, neoplasms (including the lymphomas), and acute hemolytic crisis. It may also be found after surgery, including splenectomy, especially after an acute hemolytic crisis or when performed for treatment of idiopathic thrombocytopenic purpura (ITP).[89]

Essential thrombocythemia and PV may also be similar, as both exhibit microcytic, hypochromic red cells and thrombocytosis. By the time either of these disorders reaches this point, however, they usually have already been diagnosed. For the rare occasion when this is not so, the principal differentiating factor is the erythrocyte count. Generally, if the count is higher than 6.0×10^{12}/L and the cells in the blood film appear crowded despite the microcytic appearance of the red cells, odds are the disorder is a long-term treated PV. Also, ET rarely demonstrates the severe microcytic, hypochromic state that PV does. The MCVs in PV may fall to 59 fL or lower and the MCHCs to 30.5 g/dL routinely, whereas MCVs in ET usually do not fall below 70 fL. If time permits, iron replacement therapy with observation of patient response is helpful in this differential diagnosis, as indicated in criterion 3 of Table 35-6. No response to therapy (*i.e.*, no increase in Hb) is indicative of ET, whereas a response points to PV.

Effects of Treatment on Laboratory Results

Treatment of the symptomatic patient is still under investigation. Plateletpheresis can dramatically and swiftly reduce the platelet count.[111] Plateletpheresis alone is not sufficient because it may stimulate thrombopoiesis and formation of blood clots. Myelosuppressive therapy has been used for long-term platelet suppression. There is a question whether or not to treat asymptomatic patients (*i.e.*, patients who have no evidence or history of acute thrombosis or hemorrhage). This is based on the reasoning that there is no evidence supporting the degree of thrombocytosis as a direct cause of acute thrombosis or hemorrhage. Hence, lowering the platelet count, even those above 1500×10^9/L may be unwarranted.[90]

As in the other CMPDs, many cytotoxic agents are leukemogenic. Although busulfan has been the most common alkylating agent employed to reduce platelet mass, patients are increasingly being treated with hydroxyurea because its leukemogenic properties are less or with anagrelide, a new antiplatelet drug. To date, the clinical trials of anagrelide have demonstrated a lack of leukemogenic properties or mutagenic potential, although some side effects such as neurologic, gastrointestinal and cardiac problems have been of concern.[4,106]

Course of the Disease

As in the other CMPDs, the risk of transformation into acute leukemia is high. Whether this transformation is the result of cytotoxic therapy or the natural course of the disease is unclear. There also is a high risk of uncontrolled gastrointestinal hemorrhage, which has been the cause of high mortality rates. Patients whose hemorrhagic tendencies have been kept under control run the risk of acute leukemic transformation, most commonly to AML, although transformation into acute lymphocytic or megakaryocytic leukemia also are strong possibilities. The life expectancy is 1 to 5 years. Young patients (younger than 30 years of age) have a much better prognosis than older patients.[99] Patients who have had multiple splenic infarctions causing autosplenectomy may not fare as well as patients who present with and maintain splenomegaly.[99]

CHRONIC NEUTROPHILIC LEUKEMIA

Chronic neutrophilic leukemia is the rarest of the CMPDs, with relatively few cases reported.[6,26,35,70,97,109,120] The condition is of special interest because it may be confused, by the novice, with chronic granulocytic (myelogenous) leukemia, although there are many differentiating features. Cells from patients with chronic neutrophilic leukemia have reduced numbers of CFU-C (colony-forming units) when culture is attempted. In contrast, patients with CML or a reactive granulocytosis demonstrate increased CFU-C activity in both the bone marrow and peripheral blood.[70] Cytogenetic studies do not show any abnormal karyotypic pattern in chronic neutrophilic leukemia.

Clinical Presentation

The main complaints are the result of hepatosplenomegaly, including nausea, abdominal pain, and inability to eat normal quantities of food without a full feeling. Patients are afebrile and show no outward signs of infection. However, there may be mild to severe hemorrhagic episodes.

Laboratory Findings

PERIPHERAL BLOOD

Classically, there is a persistent neutrophilic leukocytosis *without* a left shift. Toxic granulation and a few Döhle bodies are present and, on rare occasions, an NRBC is found. Leukocyte counts may be as high as $100 \times 10^9/$L, with normal to slightly decreased platelet counts and mild anemia. Hemoglobin is usually close to 11 g/dL.

In one patient's case, the granulocytes, although able to phagocytize *Staphylococcus aureus* normally, had a 70% reduction in their ability to destroy the bacteria.[70] Electron microscopic observation of these neutrophils showed a reduction of both azurophilic and specific granulation that was not evident by light microscopy. This could explain why five patients with chronic neutrophilic leukemia reported have died of overwhelming bacterial infections.[26,35] Between 30 and 40 cases have been reported thus far, six of which have transformed into acute myeloblastic leukemia (AML).[121]

The LAP scores are extremely high, ranging from 350 to 400 (see Color Plate 35-5). The vitamin B_{12} levels and B_{12}-binding capacity are frequently markedly elevated.[120]

BONE MARROW

The marrow shows a marked cellularity. Although maturation in the granulocytic cell line is normal, there is a neutrophilic hyperplasia (*i.e.*, mature granulocytes generally make up 90% of the marrow's hyperplastic reaction). The marrow shows no signs of myelodysplasia. In contrast, although the marrow in CML also shows a myeloid hyperplasia, this usually consists of increases in both mature and immature myeloid cells. Patients with chronic neutrophilic leukemia are negative for the Ph^1 chromosome.

Differential Diagnosis

The main differential diagnosis to be made is between chronic neutrophilic leukemia and reactive granulocytosis; it is usually made through the process of elimination. There are many causes for neutrophilic granulocytosis (Chap. 25). Infection is one of the more common causes for a neutrophilia, but because patients with chronic neutrophilic leukemia are not febrile, infection is an unlikely cause for their disorder. Toxins, certain drugs, metabolic disturbances, and malignancy, all can cause a marked neutrophilia.[70] If all possible causative conditions can be ruled out and the neutrophilia persists, then a diagnosis of chronic neutrophilic leukemia should be considered.

Course of the Disease

Because relatively few cases have been reported, any judgment about prognosis is premature. Five patients died from infection[26,35] and two from hemorrhagic episodes.[120] Five patients had evidence of a myelodysplastic syndrome [121] and one patient was doing well 4 years after diagnosis.[70] Some patients originally believed to have chronic neutrophilic leukemia were found at autopsy to have a previously undiagnosed carcinoma metastatic to the bone marrow.[109]

DRUGS USED IN CHRONIC MYELOPROLIFERATIVE DISORDERS

Most patients with a CMPD will suffer from hyperuricemia (increased uric acid), a byproduct of cellular breakdown by cytotoxic agents. To prevent increased uric acid in the kidney, allopurinol, a xanthine oxidase inhibitor, is used.

Anagrelide is a quinazolin compound that is a strong inhibitor of platelet function, thereby decreasing aggregation. It also can cause thrombocytopenia, owing to its ability to inhibit the colony formation of megakaryocytes. Its apparent lack of leukemogenic properties will probably make this the drug of choice in the treatment of ET patients.

Busulfan was the traditional drug of choice for CML patients. It is a dual-function alkylating agent that is extremely useful in treating CML, except in cases of myeloid

TABLE 35-7

General Guide to Peripheral Blood Differences in the Chronic Myeloproliferative Disorders

	CML	PV	AMM	ET	CNL
WBC ($\times 10^9$/L)*	>50	15–50	Variable	6–41	30–100
Hb (g/dL)	N1 to ↓	↑↑↑	↓	Variable	↓
Plt ($\times 10^9$/L)*	Up to 800 or <50	>1000; usually not >2000	Variable	>1000	Low N1 to ↓
Marrow fibroblasts	N1 to ↑↑	N1 to ↑↑	↑↑ to ↑↑↑	N1 to ↑↑	No information
LAP	↓↓†	↑	N1 to ↑	N1 to ↑	↑↑↑
Ph¹	+(−)	−	−	−	−
Histamine	N1 to ↑	↑	N1	N1	N1
B₁₂	↑↑	N1 to ↑	N1 to ↑	N1 to ↑	↑↑↑
B₁₂-binding capacity	↑↑	N1 to ↑	N1 to ↑	N1 to ↑	↑↑↑

* *Reference ranges: WBC 5–10 $\times 10^9$/L; platelet 150–400 $\times 10^9$/L.*
† *Except when infection is present.*
↓, *slight decrease;* ↓↓, *moderate decrease;* ↑, *slight increase;* ↑↑, *moderate increase;* ↑↑↑, *marked increase;* N1, *normal.*

blast transformation. It serves to reduce the total granulocyte mass and thereby relieves symptoms. There seems to be a better response to busulfan than to ^{32}P, a radioisotope commonly used for myelosuppression. The leukemogenic properties of busulfan are of great concern. This concern has made busulfan less desirable especially in the face of the availability of less toxic drugs.

Hydroxyurea interferes with DNA synthesis (S-phase drug; Chap. 5) and seems to work well with patients having ET to reduce the total platelet mass. Because of its properties as an S-phase drug, patients taking hydroxyurea may show signs of megaloblastic erythropoiesis.

Interferon-α is an active glycoprotein that inhibits proliferation of cells *in vivo*. Myeloid cells have interferon (IFN) receptors. The IFN–receptor complex is internalized, which may cause the myelosuppression. The actual means by which IFN-α causes myelosuppresion, however, is not clear.

CHAPTER SUMMARY

The CMPDs are a unique group of disorders, each one being independent, although they are similar. To simplify, one could speculate that they are all the same basic disease, each with a slightly different manifestation. In other words the CMPDs all develop from a single abnormal hematopoietic stem cell and they all look similar, but each has its own individual idiosyncrasies. These disorders can take on similarities or transform into any other chronic CMPD or an acute leukemia or even overlap and take on the characteristics of two diseases. Table 35-7 provides a summary of the laboratory differences and similarities among the disorders.

Case Study 35-1

A 22-year-old man reported to the clinic in January complaining of abdominal discomfort, lethargy, fever, dizziness, anorexia and painful swelling in the genital region. Physical examination revealed priapism and moderate splenomegaly. He appeared pale. His skin was damp, and he exhibited sternal tenderness. Blood

test results were WBC, 587 $\times 10^9$/L; Hb, 9.8 g/dL; Hct, 0.305 L/L; platelets, 682 $\times 10^9$/L; vitamin B₁₂, 1800 ng/L (increased); histamine, 13 μg/dL (increased); uric acid, 9.8 mg/dL (increased). The differential revealed 34% neutrophils, 24% bands, 1% monocytes, 2% lymphocytes, 13% metamyelocytes, 9% myelocytes, 5% promyelocytes, 3% blasts, 4% eosinophils and 5% basophils. There were four normoblasts per 100 WBCs. Red cell morphology was unremarkable. Several abnormal-appearing platelets were noted

The patient underwent plasmapheresis to relieve his priapism. A bone marrow aspirate showed almost 90% cellularity, with myeloid hyperplasia. All forms of granulocytes, both mature and immature, were present in an orderly array. Megakaryocytes were increased with an occasional uninuclear form. The LAP score was 3. Cytogenetic studies revealed Ph¹⁺ cells.

A definitive diagnosis of CML was made, and the patient was started on a regimen of busulfan and allopurinol. He did well and was released. He maintained a leukocyte count of approximately 25 $\times 10^9$/L and a platelet count of 175 to 190 $\times 10^9$/L. In August his basophil count had risen to 31% and platelets were 350 $\times 10^9$/L with several "giant and bizarre" forms seen. In October, several cells similar to the ones shown in Color Plate 35-6 were seen on the blood film, coupled with a rising platelet count. Most platelets were abnormal in appearance. The following January, the patient was admitted for severe epistaxis, petechiae and gastrointestinal bleeding. His blood film showed a marked granulocytopenia. Most cells were of the type seen in Color Plate 35-6, all abnormal-appearing platelet precursors. The patient died in March of a cerebral hemorrage coupled with overwhelming infection.

1. What is the significance of the marked basophilia seen in August?
2. What are the cell types shown in Color Plate 35-6?
3. What is the final diagnosis of the disease in this patient? Can this condition usually be treated effectively?

Case Study 35-2

Over a period of several years four patients presented with severe dysplasia in the granulocytic line, blast counts between 10% and 20%, and markedly dysplastic thrombocytopenia. One patient had a marked increase in the number of eosinophilic myelocytes (more than 25%). The cells were Ph¹⁻. The patients did poorly with standard chemotherapy and their condition was diagnosed as Ph^{1-} CML.

1. Is the finding of Ph^{1-} cells generally consistent with the diagnosis of CML?
2. Do patients with CML generally do poorly with standard chemotherapy?
3. Is the prognosis less favorable for patients with Ph^{1-} or Ph^{1+} cells?

Case Study 35-3

A 77-year-old woman presented to an ophthalmologist complaining of itchy eyes. The ophthalmologist recommended treatment for allergies, which she received. However, her condition continued to worsen, so she obtained a second opinion. This ophthalmologist referred her to an internist, who, after reviewing the CBC results, referred her to an oncologist. On her first visit to the oncologist, it was noted that her complexion was purple.

Her presenting CBC was as follows: WBC, 18×10^9/L; RBC, 9.04×10^{12}/L; Hb, 20.8 g/dL; Hct, 0.64 L/L; MCV, 71 fL; MCHC, 32.5 g/dL; platelets, 406×10^9/L. Treatment first included therapeutic phlebotomy, with 4 units of blood being removed over approximately 10 days. After this her Hb was 18.5 g/dL, the Hct was 0.59 L/L and her platelet count had risen to 514×10^9/L. Blood volume measurements revealed the following: RCM, 43.6 mL/kg (reference range women: 20 to 30 mL/kg) and plasma volume, 30.9 mL/kg. Sixteen months after diagnosis, she was given radioactive phosphorus (^{32}P) to reduce her RCM. Four months later, her Hb and Hct had returned to the reference range 13.4 g/dL and 0.41 L/L, respectively.

1. What is the most likely diagnosis? Why?
2. Were any of the patient's symptoms or physical findings significant in the diagnosis?
3. What other tests might be useful in confirming the diagnosis?
4. Do all of the laboratory criteria fit the classic picture for the most likely diagnosis? If not, which do not and why?
5. Was the treatment unusual in this case?

Review Questions

35-1. The best description of polycythemia vera is that it is characterized by

A. thrombocytopenia.
B. increased red cell mass.
C. leukopenia.
D. increased myeloblasts.

35-2. An RBC poikilocyte that is considered to be the first sign of spent phase polycythemia is the

A. dacryocyte.
B. spherocyte.
C. target cell.
D. schistocyte.

35-3. In comparing CML and chronic neutrophilic leukemia, CML is more likely to exhibit

A. a left-shift in all granulocytes.
B. a hypercellular marrow.
C. complication by overwhelming bacterial infection.
D. all of the above.

35-4. _____ are the cells most responsible for the appearance of the marrow in agnogenic myeloid metaplasia.

A. Neutrophils
B. Erythrocytes
C. Lymphocytes
D. Fibroblasts

35-5. Hydroxyurea treatment may result in megaloblastic morphology because hydroxyurea is an

A. alkylating agent that damages DNA.
B. inhibitor of DNA replication.
C. inhibitor of platelet function.
D. inhibitor of maturation.

References

1. Adamson JW, Fialkow PJ, Murphy S et al: Polycythemia vera: Stem cell and probable clonal origin of the disease. N Engl J Med 298:913-916, 1976
2. Altman AJ, Baehner RL: In vitro colony-forming characteristics of chronic granulocytic leukemia in childhood. J Pediatr 86:221, 1975
3. Altman AJ, Palmer CG, Baehner RL: Juvenile "chronic granulocytic" leukemia: A panmyelopathy with prominent monocytic involvement and circulating monocyte colony-forming cells. Blood 43:341, 1974
4. Anagrelide Study Group: Anagrelide, a therapy for thrombocythemic states: Experience in 577 patients. Am J Med 92:69-76, 1992
5. Barnett MJ, Eaves CL, Phillips GI et al: Successful autografting in chronic myeloid leukaemia after maintenance of marrow in culture. Bone Marrow Transplant 4:345-351, 1989
6. Bareford D, Jacobs B: Chronic neutrophilic leukemia. Am J Clin Pathol 73:837, 1980
7. Bartram CR, Carbonell F: bcr rearrangement in Ph^1 negative CML. Cancer Genet Cytogenet 21:183, 1986
8. Beck WS: Hematology, 3rd ed. Cambridge, MIT Press, 1983
9. Bennett JM, Catovsky D, Daniel MT et al: Proposals for the classification of the myelodysplastic syndromes. Br J Haematol 51:189, 1982
10. Bently SA: Aplasia, hypoplasia, and myelofibrosis. In Koepke JA (ed): Laboratory Hematology, vol 1, p 129. New York, Churchill Livingstone, 1984
11. Berk PD, Goldberg JD, Donovan PB et al: Therapeutic recommendations in polycythemia vera based on Polycythemia Vera Study Group protocols. Semin Hematol 23:132, 1986
12. Berk PD, Goldberg JD, Silverstein MN et al: Increased incidence of acute leukemia in polycythemia vera associated with chlorambucil therapy. N Engl J Med 304:441, 1981
13. Berlin NI: Diagnosis and classification of the polycythemias. Semin Hematol 12:339, 1975
14. Brunning RD: Chronic myelogenous leukemia. In Koepke JA (ed): Laboratory Hematology, vol 1, p 289. New York, Churchill Livingstone, 1984
15. Castro-Malaspina H, Moore MAS: [Pathophysiological mechanisms operating in the development of myelofibrosis: Role of megakaryocytes.] Nouv Rev Fr Haematol 24:221, 1982
16. Castro-Malaspina H, Rabellino EM, Yen A et al: Human megakaryocyte stimulation of proliferation of bone marrow fibroblasts. Blood 57:781, 1981
17. Cervantes F, Roman C: A multivariate analysis of prognostic factors in chronic myeloid leukemia. Blood 60:1298, 1982
18. Champlin R, Mitsuyasu R, Elashoff R et al: The role of bone marrow transplantation in the treatment of chronic myelogenous leukemia. In Gale RP (ed): Recent Advances in Bone Marrow Transplantation, p 141. New York, Alan R Liss, 1983
19. Champlin RE, Gale RP: Role of bone marrow transplantation in the treatment of hematologic malignancies and solid tumors: Critical review of syngeneic, autologous, and allogeneic transplants. Cancer Treat Rep 68:145, 1984
20. Chievitz E, Thiede T: Complications and causes of death in polycythaemia vera. Acta Med Scand 172:513, 1962

21. Clift RA, Thomas ED, Buckner CD et al: Treatment of chronic granulocytic leukaemia in chronic phase by bone marrow transplantation. Lancet 2:623, 1982

22. Coulombel L, Kalousek DK, Eaves CL et al: Long term marrow culture reveals chromosomally normal hematopoietic progenitor cells in patients with Philadelphia-positive chronic myelogenous leukemia. N Engl J Med 308:1493,1983

23. Dameshek W: Some speculations on the myeloproliferative syndrome. Blood 6:372, 1951

24. Dokel I, Jones L, Deenmamode M et al: Allogeneic bone marrow transplantation for primary myelofibrosis. Br J Haematol 71:158, 1989

25. Donovan PH, Kaplan ME, Goldberg JD: Treatment of polycythemia vera with hydroxyurea. Am J Hematol 17:329, 1984

26. Dotten DA, Pruzanski W, Wong D: Functional characterization of cells in chronic neutrophilic leukemia. Am J Hematol 12:157, 1982

27. Douer D, Levin AM, Sparkes RS et al: Chronic myelocytic leukaemia: A pluripotent haemopoietic cell is involved in the malignant clone. Br J Haematol 49:615, 1981.

28. Dover GJ, Boyer SH, Zinkham WH et al: Changing erythrocyte populations in juvenile chronic myelocytic leukemia: Evidence for disordered regulation. Blood 49:355, 1977

29. Dutcher JP, Wiernik PH: Leukemia. In Spivak JL (ed): Fundamentals of Clinical Hematology, 2nd ed, p 229. Philadelphia, Harper & Row, 1984

30. Ellis JT, Peterson P, Geller SA et al: Studies of the bone marrow in polycythemia vera and the evolution of myelofibrosis and second hematologic malignancies. Semin Hematol 23:144, 1986

31. Eskola JU, Hamalainen M, Nanto V et al: Detection of Philadelphia chromosome using PCR and europium-labeled DNA probes. Clin Biochem 27:373, 1994

32. Fanger H, Cella LJ Jr, Litchman H: Thrombocythemia: Report of three cases and review of the literature. N Engl J Med 250:456, 1954

33. Fefer A, Cheever MA, Greenberg PD et al: Treatment of chronic granulocytic leukemia with chemoradiotherapy and transplantation of marrow from identical twins. N Engl J Med 306:63, 1982

34. Feldman F: Myelosclerosis in agnogenic myeloid metaplasia. Semin Roentgenol 9:195, 1974

35. Feremans W, Marceles L, Ardichvili D: CNL with enlarged lymph nodes and lysozyme deficiency. Am J Clin Pathol 36:324, 1983

36. Fialkow PJ: Clonal and stem cell origin of blood cell neoplasms. In Lobue J, Gordon AS, Silber R et al (eds): Contemporary Hematology/Oncology, vol 1, p 1. New York, Plenum, 1980

37. Franklin DZ, Greaves MF, Grossi CE et al: Atlas of Blood Cells, vol 2, p 605. Philadelphia, Lea & Febiger, 1981

38. Fruchtman SM, Berk PD: Polycythemia vera and agnogenic myeloid metaplasia. In Handin RI, Lux SE, Stossel TP (eds): Blood—Principles and Practice of Hematology, pp 439-453. Philadelphia, JB Lippincott, 1995

39. Fruchtman SM: Therapeutic implications of collagen metabolism in myelofibrosis. In Berk PD, Castro-Malaspina H, Wasserman LR (eds): Myelofibrosis and the Biology of Connective Tissue. Progress in Clinical and Biological Research, pp 154-467, 1995

40. Ganesan TS, Rassool F, Guo AP et al: Rearrangement of the *bcr* gene in Philadelphia-negative chronic myeloid leukemia. Blood 68:957,1986

41. Goldman JM, Apperley JF, Jones L et al: Bone marrow transplantation for patients with chronic myeloid leukemia. N Eng J Med 314:202-207, 1986

42. Goldman JM, Catovsky D, Goolden AW et al: Buffy coat autografts for patients with chronic granulocytic leukaemia in transformation. Blut 42:149, 1981

43. Goldman JM, Gale RP, Horowitz MM et al: Bone marrow transplantation for chronic myelogenous leukemia in chronic phase: Increased risk of relapse associated with T-cell depletion. Ann Intern Med 108:806-814, 1988

44. Goldman JM, Kearney L, Pittman S et al: Haemopoietic stem cell grafting for chronic granulocytic leukaemia: Clinical results and cytogenetic findings. Exp Hematol 10(suppl 10):76, 1982

45. Goldman JM, Marks DI: Chronic myelogenous leukemia. In Handin RI, Lux SE, Stossel TP (eds): Blood—Principles and Practice of Hematology, pp 457-470. Philadelphia, JB Lippincott, 1995

46. Griffin JD, Todd RF, Ritz J et al: Differentiation patterns in the blastic phase of chronic myelogenous leukemia. Blood 61:85-90, 1983

47. Grignani F: Chronic myelogenous leukemia. CRC Crit Rev Hematol Oncol 4:31, 1985

48. Gunz FW: Hemorrhagic thrombocythemia: A critical review. Blood 15:706, 1960

49. Hall R, Malia RG: Medical Laboratory Hematology, p 414. Boston, Butterworths, 1984

50. Hayhoe FGJ, Flemans RJ: An Atlas of Hematological Cytology, p 206. New York, John Wiley & Sons, 1970

51. Hennessy TG, Stern WE, Herrick SE: Cerebellar hemangioblastoma: Erythropoietic activity by radioiron assay. J Nucl Med 8:601, 1967

52. Hoffbrand AV, Pettit JE: Myeloproliferative disorders. In Essential Haematology, 2nd ed, p 182. Boston, Blackwell Scientific Ltd., 1984

53. Jacobson RJ, Salo A, Fialkow PJ: Agnogenic myeloid metaplasia: A clonal proliferation of hematopoietic stem cells with secondary myelofibrosis. Blood 51:189, 1978

54. Jacquillat C, Chastang C, Tanzer J et al: Facteurs prognostic de la leucémie myaeloid chronique. A propos de 798 observations. Nouv Rev Fr Hématol 15:229, 1975

55. Kamada N, Uchino H: Chronological sequence in appearance of clinical and laboratory findings characteristic of chronic myelogenous leukemia. Blood 51:843, 1978

56. Kaplan ME, Mack K, Goldberg JD et al: Long term management of polycythemia vera with hydroxyurea: A progress report. Semin Hematol 23:167, 1986

57. Kaplin DR, Chao FC, Stiles CD et al: Platelet alpha granules contain a growth factor for fibroblasts. Blood 53:1043, 1979

58. Kahn A, Bernard JF, Cottreau D et al: A deficient G-6PD variant with hemizygous expression in blood cells of a woman with primary myelofibrosis. Humangenetik 30:41, 1975

59. Klingemann HG, Storb R, Fefer A et al: Bone marrow transplantation in patients aged 45 years and older. Blood 67:770, 1986

60. Koeffler HP, Golde DW: Chronic myelogenous leukemia—new concepts. N Engl J Med 304:1269, 1981

61. Koeffler HP, Goldwasser E: Erythropoietin radioimmunoassay in evaluating patients with polycythemia. Ann Intern Med 94:44, 1981

62. Körbling M, Burke P, Braine H et al: Successful engraftment of blood derived normal hemopoietic stem cells in chronic myelogenous leukemia. Exp Hematol 9:684, 1981

63. Kough RH: Idiopathic myelofibrosis with myeloid metaplasia of the spleen: A disease entity being recognized with increasing frequency. Med Times 94:489, 1966

64. Landaw SA: Acute leukemia in polycythemia vera. Semin Hematol 13:38, 1976

65. Lanzkowsky P: Pediatric Hematology Oncology, p 338. New York, McGraw-Hill, 1980

66. Lascari AD: Hematologic Manifestations of Childhood Diseases, p 338. New York, Thieme-Stratton, 1984

67. Lawler SD: Significance of chromosome abnormalities in leukemia. Semin Hematol 10:257, 1982

68. Leeburg WT: Micromegakaryocytes: ASCP Check Sample. Hematology 25:1, 1983

69. McGlave PB, Brunning RD, Hurd DD et al: Reversal of severe bone marrow fibrosis and osteosclerosis following allogeneic bone marrow transplantation for chronic granulocytic leukaemia. Br J Haematol 52:189, 1982

70. Mehrotra DA, Winfield DA, Fergusson LH: Cellular abnormalities and reduced colony-forming cells in chronic neutrophilic leukaemia. Acta Haematol 73:47, 1985

71. Miale JB: Aplastic anemia, myeloproliferative disorders, leukemia, and lymphoma. In Laboratory Medicine, 6th ed, p 699. St Louis, CV Mosby, 1982

72. Mirand EA, Murphy GP, Steeves RA et al: Extra-renal production of erythropoietin in man. Acta Haematol 39:359, 1968

73. Monfardini S, Gee T, Fried J et al: Survival in chronic myelogenous leukemia: Influence of treatment and extent of disease at diagnosis. Cancer 31:492, 1973

74. Morris CM, Reeve AE, Fitzgerald PH et al: Genomic diversity correlates with clinical variation in Ph^l-negative chronic myeloid leukaemia. Nature 320:281, 1986

75. Mulder H, Steenberger J, Haanen C: Clinical course and survival after elective splenectomy in 19 patients with primary myelofibrosis. Br J Haematol 35:419, 1977

76. Murphy S: Hemopoietic stem cell disorders: Myeloproliferative disorders, polycythemia vera. In Williams WJ, Beutler E, Erslev AJ et al (eds): Hematology, 4th ed, p 193. New York, McGraw-Hill, 1990

77. Murphy S, Iland H, Rosenthal D et al: Essential thrombocythemia: An interim report from the Polycythemia Vera Study Group. Semin Hematol 23:177, 1986

78. Oblon DJ, Elfenbein GJ, Braylan RC et al: The reversal of myelofibrosis associated with chronic myelogenous leukemia after allogeneic bone marrow transplantation. Exp Hematol 11:681, 1983

79. O'Donnell MR, Nademanee AP, Snyder DS et al: Bone marrow transplantation for myelodysplastic and myeloproliferative syndromes. J Clin Oncol 5:1822, 1987

80. Okazaki N, Ozaki H, Arima M et al: Hepatocellular carcinoma associated with erythrocytosis: A nine year survival after successful chemotherapy and left lateral hepatectomy. Acta Hepato-Gastroenterol 26:248, 1979

81. Ossias AL, Zanjani ED, Zalusky R et al: Case report: Studies on the mechanism of erythrocytosis associated with a uterine fibromyoma. Br J Haematol 25:179, 1973

82. Pareti FI, Mannucci PM, Asti D et al: Acquired storage pool disease in myeloproliferative disorders. Thromb Haemost 42:44, 1979

83. Peterson P, McIntyre OR: Myeloproliferative disorders, p 6. Publication for the ASCP National Meeting, 1987

84. Pugh WC, Pearson M, Vardiman JW et al: Philadelphia chromosome-negative chronic myelogenous leukaemia: A morphological reassessment. Br J Haematol 60:457, 1985

85. Ragni MV, Shreiner DP: Spontaneous remission of agnogenic myeloid metaplasia and termination in acute myeloid leukemia. Arch Intern Med 141:1481, 1981

86. Rajantie J, Sale GE, Deeg HJ et al: Adverse effect of severe marrow fibrosis on hematologic recovery after chemradiotherapy and allogeneic bone marrow transplantation. Blood 67:1693, 1986

87. Rani S, Beohar PC, Mohanty TK et al: Chronic myelogenous leukaemia in infancy and childhood: A 10-year study at New Delhi, India. Acta Haematol 66:233, 1981

88. Rappeport J, Parkman R, Belli J et al: Reversibility of myelofibrosis (MF) after bone marrow transplantation (BM Tx). Blood 52(Suppl 1):271, 1978

89. Richards JD, Linch DC, Goldstone AH: A synopsis of haematology. In Myeloproliferative and Allied Disorders, p 116. Boston, Wright PSG, 1983

90. Rosenthal DS, Murphy S: Thrombocytosis. In Handin RI, Lux SE, Stossel TP (eds): Blood—Principles and Practice of Hematology, pp 439-453. Philadelphia, JB Lippincott, 1995

91. Ross R, Vogel A: The platelet-derived growth factor. Cell 14:203, 1978

92. Rosse WF, Waldmann TA, Cohen P: Renal cysts, erythropoietin, and polycythemia. Am J Med 34:76, 1963

93. Rowley JD: Nonrandom chromosome changes in hematologic diseases. In Franklin DZ, Greaves MF, Grossi CE et al (eds): Atlas of Blood Cells, vol 2, p 605. Philadelphia, Lea & Febiger, 1981

94. Scher CD, Shepard RC, Antoniades HN et al: Platelet-derived growth factor and the regulation of the mammalian fibroblast cell cycle. Biochim Biophys Acta 560:217, 1979

95. Scott D, Theologides A: Hepatoma, erythrocytosis and increased serum erythropoietin developing in long standing hemochromatosis. Am J Gastroenterol 61:206, 1974

96. Shapira Y, Polliack A, Cividalli G et al: Juvenile myeloid leukemia with fetal erythropoiesis. Cancer 30:353, 1972

97. Shindo T, Sakai C, Shibata A: Neutrophilic leukemia and blastic crisis. Ann Intern Med 87:66, 1977

98. Silverstein MN, Goldberg JD, Balcerzak SP et al: The incidence of acute leukemia in a randomized clinical trial for polycythemia vera. Blood(Suppl 1):209a, 1979 (abstr)

99. Silverstein M: Primary thrombocythemia. In Williams WJ, Beutler E, Erslev AJ, Lichtman MA (eds): Hematology, 3rd ed, p 218. New York, McGraw-Hill, 1983

100. Silverstein MN: Postpolycythemia myeloid metaplasia. Arch Intern Med 134:113, 1974

101. Silverstein MN, Remine WH: Splenectomy in myeloid metaplasia. Blood 53:515, 1979

102. Sjögren U, Brandt L, Mitelman F: Relation between life expectancy and composition of the bone marrow at diagnosis of chronic myeloid leukemia. Scand J Haematol, 12:369, 1974

103. Smith JR, Landaw SA: Smokers' polycythemia. N Engl J Med 298:6, 1978

104. Sokal JE, Cox EB, Baccarani M et al: Prognostic discriminators in "good risk" chronic granulocytic leukemia. Blood 63:789, 1984

105. Speck B, Gratwohl A, Osterwalder B et al: Bone marrow transplantation for chronic myeloid leukemia. Semin Hematol 21:48, 1984

106. Spencer CM, Brodgen RN: Anagrelide. A review of its pharmacodynamic and pharmacokinetic properties, and therapeutic potential in the treatment of thrombocythemia. Drugs 47:809-822, 1994

107. Spiers ASD: The clinical features of chronic granulocytic leukemia. Clin Hematol 6:17, 1977

108. Spivak JL: Erythrocytosis and polycythemia. In Fundamentals of Clinical Hematology, 2nd ed, p 115. Philadelphia, Harper & Row, 1984

109. Stein R: Granulocytosis and granulocytic leukemoid reactions. In Koepke JA (ed): Laboratory Hematology, vol 1, p 153. New York, Churchill Livingstone, 1984

110. Sun NCJ: Right lower lung infiltrate with leukoerythroblastosis. In Hematology—An Atlas and Diagnostic Guide, p 158. Philadelphia, WB Saunders, 1983

111. Taft EG, Nancock RB, Scharrfman WB et al: Plateletpheresis in the management of thrombocytosis. Blood 50:927, 1977

112. Toth FD, Kiss J, Kiss A et al: Co-expression of c-abl and c-myb oncogenes in Philadelphia chromosome-negative, bcr-negative chronic myeloid leukemia. Leuk Res 18:373, 1994

113. Tso SC, Hua ASP: Erythrocytosis in hepatocellular carcinoma: A compensatory phenomenon. Br J Haematol 28:497, 1974

114. Tura S, Baccarani M, Corbelli G et al: Staging of chronic myeloid leukaemia. Br J Haematol 47:105, 1981

115. Volkova MA: [Analysis of the factor influencing longevity in chronic myeloid leukemia.] Ter Arkh 48:61, 1976

116. Ward HP, Block MH: The natural history of agnogenic myeloid metaplasia. Medicine 50:357, 1971

117. Wasserman LR: The management of polycythaemia vera. Br J Haematol 21:371, 1971

118. Wasserman LR, Balcerzak SP, Berlin NI et al: Influence of therapy on causes of death in polycythemia vera. Trans Assoc Am Physicians 94:30, 1981

119. Wintrobe MM: Chronic myeloid leukemia. In Wintrobe MM, Lee GR, Boggs DR et al: Clinical Hematology, 8th ed, p 1565. Philadelphia, Lea & Febiger, 1981

120. You W, Weisbrot IM: Chronic neutrophilic leukemia. Report of 2 cases and review of the literature. Am J Clin Pathol 72:233, 1979

121. Zittoun R, Rea D, Ngoc LH et al: Chronic neutrophilic leukemia, a study of four cases. Ann Haematol 68:55, 1994

PART VIII

Malignant Lymphoproliferative Disorders

CHAPTER 36

Acute Lymphoblastic Leukemias

Anne S. Hobson

Clinical Manifestations

Causes of Death

Laboratory Findings
Peripheral Blood and Bone Marrow
Use of Laboratory Findings in ALL Classification
Use of Laboratory Findings in the Differential Diagnosis

Classification of Acute Lymphoblastic Leukemia

Morphologic Classification (FAB)
Cytochemical Classification
Immunologic Marker Classification
Cytogenetic Studies
New Approaches

Effects of Treatment on Laboratory Results
Chemotherapy
Bone Marrow Transplantation

Case Studies 36-1 and 36-2

3. List the surface markers used most frequently to classify the acute lymphoblastic leukemias into B-precursor, pre-B, B-cell and T-cell ALL.
4. Discuss the chromosomal abnormalities most often associated with subtypes of ALL.
5. Describe the two major therapeutic approaches to ALL.

Acute lymphoblastic leukemia (ALL) is a malignant disease of the lymphopoietic system that is manifested by the slow but uncontrolled growth of abnormal, poorly differentiated lymphoid cells whose DNA synthesis time is significantly longer than in normal tissues.[7] These abnormal lymphoid cells can be found in the bone marrow, spleen and lymph nodes. Normal bone marrow elements usually are replaced or displaced by the abnormal cells. Acute lymphoblastic leukemia is predominantly a disease of children, although improved immunologic and cytochemical methods of identification have increased the frequency of diagnosis in adults. Acute lymphoblastic leukemia is the most common malignant disease in children[10] and occurs most frequently between the ages of 2 and 10 years.

Objectives

1. List significant laboratory findings in the peripheral blood and bone marrow associated with acute lymphoblastic leukemia.
2. Describe the morphologic characteristics of the three FAB classifications of acute lymphoblastic leukemia.

This chapter will address the clinical manifestations, laboratory findings, and differential diagnosis of ALL, with a description of the various classification systems. Finally, therapy for ALL and its effects on laboratory results will be discussed.

CLINICAL MANIFESTATIONS

The clinical features of ALL do not differ substantially from those of other types of acute leukemia, but their onset is usually more sudden. Prodromal or preleukemic symptoms are more often associated with nonlymphocytic leukemias. Many of the signs and symptoms of ALL can be related to the replacement of normal hematopoietic elements in the bone marrow by abnormal lymphoid cells. This results in decreased red cells (anemia), phagocytes (granulocytopenia) and platelets (thrombocytopenia).

The most common presenting symptoms for ALL are malaise, fatigue and pallor that usually are related to the degree of anemia present. Granulocytopenia renders the patient vulnerable to infection that may be accompanied by chills and fever. Easy bruising, petechiae, epistaxis, and other hemorrhagic conditions related to the thrombocytopenia may also be presenting signs. The severity of the hemorrhagic complications correlates with the degree of thrombocytopenia. Generally there is weight loss, but it is not so severe that it causes the patient to see a physician. Bone pain, sternal tenderness and swelling, or tenderness of the large joints may occur. Cranial nerve paralysis, increased intracranial pressure, fundic (eye) hemorrhage, or other neurologic symptoms resulting from meningeal infiltration by leukemic cells may be present. Physical examination usually reveals enlargement of the superficial lymph nodes, as well as splenomegaly and hepatomegaly.

CAUSES OF DEATH

A serious complication in ALL is infection, a primary cause of death in ALL. The incidence of infection is directly related to the degree of granulocytopenia. Organisms causing sepsis during induction therapy (*i.e.*, therapy to induce a remission) include *Staphylococcus aureus*, *Pseudomonas aeruginosa*, *Candida albicans*, *Haemophilus influenzae*, *Proteus mirabilis*, and species of *Klebsiella*. With the use of more intense chemotherapy there has been an increased incidence of infection with *Pneumocystis carinii*, a parasite that causes a form of pneumonia, and in fungal infections with *Candida* and *Aspergillus*. Morbidity can be up to 20% with *Candida* and *Aspergillus* infections.[15] Patients receiving long-term immunosuppressive chemotherapy are at risk for infection by a wide variety of bacteria, viruses and fungi.

Bleeding is the second most significant complication, which usually results from thrombocytopenia. Spontaneous bleeding can occur when the platelet count falls below $50 \times 10^9/L$ but becomes more likely when the count is less than $20 \times 10^9/L$. The presence of a high blast count or infection tends to increase the risk of hemorrhage. Salicylates and other drugs that impair platelet function may be contributing factors. Leukemic infiltration of the liver may decrease hepatic function and interfere with the synthesis of the vitamin K–dependent clotting factors (Chap. 48).

LABORATORY FINDINGS

Peripheral Blood and Bone Marrow

The total leukocyte count is elevated (more than $10.0 \times 10^9/L$) in approximately 60% of patients. About 15% of patients have markedly increased leukocyte counts (more than $100.0 \times 10^9/L$), but approximately 25% are leukopenic (less than $4.0 \times 10^9/L$). The leukemic lymphoid blast is the predominant circulating cell except in leukopenic patients, in whom an aleukemic leukemia (*i.e.*, malignant cells are easily found in the bone marrow but not in the peripheral blood) may exist with few or no circulating lymphoblasts.

The bone marrow in ALL is almost always hypercellular and heavily infiltrated with, or even replaced by, lymphoid cells. Fibrosis is present in 10% to 15% of cases, particularly in patients with bone pain.[3] Thrombocytopenia and anemia are almost always present at the time of diagnosis, with normal marrow elements usually reduced in number or appearing to have been totally replaced.

Use of Laboratory Findings in ALL Classification

Laboratory findings are important in the French–American–British (FAB) morphologic and immunologic classifications of ALL. The FAB classification system depends on cell counts and microscopic observation of cytologic features. The immunologic classification system is based on cell surface marker patterns that may be identified using flow cytometry (Chap. 43). Immunoperoxidase staining using monoclonal antibodies (mAbs) may also be used to classify ALL.

Use of Laboratory Findings in the Differential Diagnosis

Acute lymphoblastic leukemia must be differentiated from other causes of lymphoid leukocytosis in the peripheral blood. Lymphoid leukocytosis or lymphocytosis occurs in pertussis, as well as in infectious lymphocytosis, infectious mononucleosis and other viral diseases (Chap. 25). These reactive disorders may also be accompanied by fever, enlarged superficial lymph nodes and splenomegaly. In general, however, the bone marrow is minimally affected in reactive conditions and does not contain a predominance of immature cells. Infectious mononucleosis (IM) may be associated with an autoimmune anemia and thrombocytopenia, with immature-appearing lymphocytes in the peripheral blood; however, the pleomorphic (variable) morphology of the reactive lymphocytes in IM (see Color Plate 25-5) and serologic tests for the heterophil antibody (positive in IM; negative in ALL) will help distinguish this condition.

Adult ALL differs from that seen most frequently in children in that adult ALL is more often associated with increased leukocyte counts, the Philadelphia (Ph[1]) chromosome, and the Type L2 morphologic classification (see later discussion). In addition, adult ALL cases are more frequently classified immunologically as null or unclassified because the cells demonstrate no definitive T or B cell markers. The differential diagnosis of ALL in the adult is difficult. The condition must be distinguished from such entities as leukemic lymphoma, blastic transformation in chronic lymphocytic leukemia, hairy cell leukemia and acute myeloid leukemia.

Occasionally, patients with solid tumors that metastasize to bone marrow, such as Ewing sarcoma, embryonal rhabdomyosarcoma and neuroblastoma (small-cell carcinoma; a disease primarily of infants and children), have bone marrow infiltration by tumor cells that are morphologically similar to those in ALL. The presence of leukoerythroblastic abnormalities in the peripheral blood and clumps or clusters of tumor cells in the marrow preparations may be helpful in identifying metastatic tumor.

In the past, the diagnosis of ALL required good bone marrow and peripheral blood preparations and was based solely on cell morphology in Romanowsky-stained preparations. Today, although these preparations are still important, the use of cytochemical and immunologic markers for the classification or subclassification of ALL has assumed equal importance. These techniques undoubtedly will have greater clinical application as knowledge of immature cells increases and the ability to target treatment for leukemic diseases is developed more fully.

CLASSIFICATION OF ACUTE LYMPHOBLASTIC LEUKEMIA

Morphologic Classification (FAB)

With the advent in the 1960s of chemotherapeutic drugs for the treatment of acute leukemia and the development of cytochemical stains to identify immature cells, a uniform system for the classification of acute leukemias became necessary. It was necessary to establish uniform criteria for the different types of acute leukemias so that responses could be correlated with treatment and prognosis in patients at various medical centers. The French–American–British (FAB) system was developed and has come into general use for the morphologic classification of acute leukemia.[1]

The FAB classification divides lymphoblastic leukemias into three types: L1, L2 and L3.[2] These types are defined according to two criteria: (1) the occurrence of individual cytologic features and (2) the degree of heterogeneity among the leukemic cells. The features considered are cell size, chromatin, nuclear shape, nucleoli, degree of basophilia in the cytoplasm and the presence of cytoplasmic vacuolation. As many as 10% of the cells are allowed to depart from the characteristics of the proposed cell type (Table 36-1).

It should be emphasized at this point that satisfactory blood films are imperative, because preparations that are too thick or not dried properly can mask the presence of lymphoblasts, the result being that they are misidentified as mature lymphocytes.

TYPE L1: SMALL CELL, HOMOGENEOUS

In L1 the blasts are predominantly small: up to twice the diameter of a small lymphocyte. They are generally uniform, and this lack of variation in size creates a homogeneous picture of similar cells. The chromatin is usually finely dispersed, but it may appear more clumped in smaller cells. Chromatin and cell size may show variation from case to case, but the homogeneous features within each particular patient are a primary feature. Nuclear shape is regular; however, there may be some degree of cleaving, folding or indentation. Nucleoli often are not visible or, if present, are small and indistinct. The cytoplasm is usually scanty (high nuclear:cytoplasmic ratio) and only slightly to moderately basophilic. Cytoplasmic vacuoles may or may not be present (see Color Plates 36-1 and 36-2). The L1 type is the acute leukemia that is common in childhood, with 74% of the cases occuring in children 15 years of age or younger.[2] Of the three classes

---

TABLE 36-1
Features of Acute Lymphoblastic Leukemias

Cytologic Feature	L1	L2	L3
Cell size*	Small cells predominate	Large, heterogeneous	Large and homogeneous
Chromatin	Homogeneous in any one case	Variable: heterogeneous in any one case	Finely stippled and homogeneous
Nuclear shape*	Regular; occasional clefting or indentation	Irregular; clefting and indentation common	Regular, oval to round
Nucleoli*	Not visible or small and inconspicuous	One or more present, often large	Prominent; one or more; vesicular
Amount of cytoplasm*	Scanty	Variable; often moderately abundant	Moderately abundant
Basophilia of cytoplasm	Slight or moderate; rarely, intense	Variable; deep in some	Very deep
Cytoplasmic vacuolation	Variable	Variable	Often prominent

Most useful features for differentiating L1 and L2 subtypes.
From Bennett JM, Catovsky D, Daniel MT et al: Proposal for the classification of adult leukaemia. Br J Haematol 33:451, 1976; by permission of Blackwell Scientific Publications Ltd.

of ALL, L1 generally has the best prognosis because it responds well to therapy.

TYPE L2: LARGE CELL, HETEROGENEOUS

In L2, most immature cells are more than twice the diameter of a small lymphocyte. Frequently, there is a marked heterogeneity of cell size. Chromatin ranges from fine and dispersed to coarse and condensed, thus presenting a mixed picture. Nuclear cleaving, indentation and folding are characteristic, and gross irregularities of nuclear shape are common. Nucleoli are nearly always visible and of various sizes and numbers. The degree of cytoplasmic basophilia is also variable (see Color Plate 36-3). Approximately 66% of the cases of ALL in patients older than 15 years are of Type L2.

A simple system for identification of Types L1 and L2 has been proposed based on four features: (1) nuclear:cytoplasmic ratio; (2) presence, prominence and frequency of nucleoli; (3) regularity of nuclear outline; and (4) cell size (see Table 36-1).[2] By using this system, correct classification of Types L1 and L2 was increased from 63% to 84% among trained hematologists.

TYPE L3: BURKITT TYPE

The Burkitt form is a relatively rare type of ALL (3% to 5% of cases). The blasts are large, primitive appearing and present a characteristically homogeneous picture. They have a rather finely stippled chromatin. The nucleus is oval to round, with a regular contour. One or more prominent vesicular nucleoli are visible in most cells. The cytoplasm is intensely basophilic and moderately abundant. Cytoplasmic as well as nuclear vacuolation is often prominent (see Color Plates 36-4 and 36-5). These vacuoles stain positively with oil red O, making this stain valuable in the diagnosis of Burkitt leukemia (L3) or lymphoma (Chap. 38). By immunologic markers, these are B-cell malignancies. A high mitotic index (approximately 5%) is characteristic. Patients with L3 leukemias generally have a poor prognosis because their disease responds poorly to chemotherapy.

Cytochemical Classification

In differentiating the ALLs from the acute nonlymphoblastic leukemias (ANLL), the Sudan black B or myeloperoxidase stains (Chap. 29) may be helpful. Abnormal lymphoid cells of ALL are Sudan black B– and myeloperoxidase-negative. Very immature myeloid blasts may also be negative; therefore, only positive myeloperoxidase staining is helpful in that it rules out lymphoblasts. However, some ALLs are weakly positive with Sudan black B.

The periodic acid–Schiff (PAS) stain has been important in the laboratory differentiation of ALL types. Staining is strongly positive in L1, being present as chunks or granules in a significant number of blasts. When scored from 1 to 4 on the basis of increasing granule size, L1 has a high score. In L2 the degree of positivity and the percentage of cells stained may be quite low—10% or less. L3 ALL is generally PAS negative.

Acid phosphatase is positive in ALL and has a localized pattern of positivity in the Golgi region in T-cell ALL. Otherwise, it shows a diffuse pattern that is also present in myeloid cells. Thus, the usefulness of this stain is limited.[5]

Nonspecific esterase (NSE) staining produces an area of focal positivity in T lymphocytes. The stain has diagnostic value in distinguishing M5 (acute monocytic leukemia) from L2, because in M5, the cytoplasm is diffusely stained.

Terminal deoxynucleotidyl transferase (TdT) is a unique intranuclear DNA polymerase enzyme because it does not require a DNA template to catalyze deoxynucleoside triphosphate to the 3′-hydroxy end of a primer DNA chain. TdT activity can be detected in human thymocytes, primitive lymphocytes and a small number of other cells in bone marrow.[4] Strong TdT activity is seen in approximately 90% of patients with ALL, as well as in lymphoblastic lymphomas. Because this enzyme is a helpful marker for primitive lymphoid cells, it is especially useful in the detection of "lymphoblastic transformation" of chronic myelogenous leukemia (CML).

Immunologic Marker Classification

Today, in addition to morphology, the classification of ALL is based on immunologic surface-marker patterns, gene rearrangement (DNA analysis) and cytogenetic studies.

Since the late 1970s, the development of mAbs toward cellular antigens has greatly increased our knowledge of cell differentiation and maturation. Initially, a large number of mAbs were developed by different investigators and given different names even though, in many instances, some were specific for the same antigen. This led to confusion until they were organized into groups of similar antigens and referred to as "clusters of differentiation" or CD. There are now at least 130 recognized human leukocyte antigens, each of which has been given a cluster differentiation (CD) number.[14]

A typical investigative panel of mAbs for a suspected case of ALL includes CD5, CD7, CD10, CD13, CD19, CD33, and HLA-DR. Thus, we have evolved from the use of only surface immunoglobulin (sIg) for the identification of B lymphocytes and sheep erythrocyte rosettes to detect T lymphocytes. Panels are now used to further differentiate subgroups of both B and T cells. SIg is now referred to as sCD22, and the sheep erythrocyte receptor is now known as CD2. A polyclonal antibody to what is known as common acute lymphoblastic leukemia antigen (CALLA), CD10, was produced by immunization of rabbits with sIg- and erythrocyte-rosette-negative ALL cells.[11] CD10 is present on the leukemic cells of 70% of patients with ALL.[19]

Using a combination of immunologic markers and flow cytometry, ALL has been found to be of either B-cell or T-cell lineage (Table 36-2). For prognosis and treatment, there are now four recognized classes (one T-cell and three B-cell) depending on the appearance of cell markers during maturation. The order of presentation of these classes will go from mature to immature, because our

TABLE 36-2
*Markers Useful for Subclassification of ALL**

Markers	Pro-B	Pre-B	B Cell	T Cell
CD2	−	−	−	+/−
sIg (sCD22)	−	−	+	−
cIg	−	+	−	−
TdT	+	+	−	+
HLA-DR	+	+	+	−
CD10	+	+	+/−	−
CD5	−	−	−	+
CD20	+/−	+	+	−
Focal Acid Phosphatase	−	−	−	+
Alpha Naphthyl-acetate esterase	−	−	−	+/−
Morphology	L1/L2	L1/L2	L3	L1/L2

*Note: The abnormal blasts of all subclassifications of ALL are myeloperoxidase-negative and usually Sudan black B-negative (some ALLs may have weakly positive SBB cells). Periodic acid–Schiff (PAS) is strongly positive in most cases of L1 ALL, but weakly positive in L2 ALL. A negative CD11 marker is expected in all subclassifications of ALL.

Modified to CD nomenclature from Sun T, Li CY, Yam LT: Atlas of Cytochemistry and Immunochemistry of Hematologic Neoplasms. Chicago, ASCP Press, 1985, with permission.

knowledge of poorly differentiated early cells is less well defined.

1. B-cell ALL: Cells of "Burkitt's" leukemia are positive for HLA-DR, CD19, sCD22 and CD24. Weak expression of CD10 (CALLA) is present in one-third to one-half of cases. Cytoplasmic immunoglobulin (cIg) and TdT are not present. This group accounts for less than 5% of ALL cases and corresponds to the FAB classification L3.

2. Pre-B cell ALL: These cells are characterized by the presence of HLA-DR, TdT, CD19, CD20, and CD24. CD10 (CALLA) may be present. They are capable of synthesizing μ-heavy chains and, therefore, cytoplasmic immunoglobulin (cIg) μ is present in the absence of sIg. This group accounts for 10% to 15% of ALL in children and adults, and a majority are classified morphologically as L1. A chromosomal abnormality, the t(1;19) translocation is associated with this group of lymphoid leukemias.

3. Pro-B (B-precursor) cell or common ALL (cALL): The leukemic cells in this group are characterized by the presence of HLA-DR, TdT, CD10, CD19, CD24, and sometimes CD20. These cells lack cIg, sIg, and μ heavy chains. This type accounts for approximately 85% of childhood and 75% of adult ALL. Common ALL has the highest remission rate and the longest initial remission with chemotherapy. About 5% of children and 20% of adults having common ALL have a translocation similar to the Philadelphia chromosome, t(9;22).[20]

The earliest recognizable stage of B-cell development is positive for HLA-DR, TdT, CD19 and CD34. CD34 is found on hematopoietic stem cells. This grouping has been referred to as pre (early)-B and occurs in about 5% of children and 11% of adults with ALL. In some instances this phenotype will show the presence of CD7, which is a T-cell marker and appears to be associated with a chromosomal translocation t(4;11).[17]

This latter immunophenotype frequently occurs in infancy and is associated with a very high WBC count and an extremely short survival time, and it is nonresponsive to chemotherapy.

4. T-cell ALL: Cells characteristic of this disorder should have more than one of the more sensitive T-cell antigens. These include CD7, CD5 and CD2. In general these three antigens are found in almost all cases of T-cell ALL. Other T-cell antigens such as cytoplasmic CD3 and CD6 may be found in some cases. A subclassification of T-cell ALL called pre-T cell has been proposed based on stages of cellular maturation. However, in the absence of clinical correlations or difference in survival time, this distinction does not appear to be significant. T-cell ALL accounts for about 15% of both childhood and adult ALL. The incidence is much higher in males, with a 5:1 ratio. About half the patients have a mediastinal (thymic) mass. Very high leukocyte counts are common in this group, and there is a higher incidence of central nervous system (CNS) involvement. T-cell ALL carries a much poorer prognosis.

Expression of T-lymphocyte antigens such as cytoplasmic CD3, surface CD2, CD7, or a combination thereof, may occur on leukemic cells that are predominantly myeloid and found in acute myeloid leukemia (AML). Approximately 5% to 10% of AMLs will express only a single T-cell antigen. Consequently, a battery of T-cell markers is needed for correct diagnosis. Because of the variability of immunophenotypes and cross-reactivity in mAbs for T cells, the morphology of cells in samples used in flow cytometry should be evaluated on a blood film made from the sample. For example, if a marrow specimen obtained from a child with pro-B cell ALL is contaminated with peripheral blood during collection, the predominant cells may be normal T lymphocytes. Should there be few blasts, the markers might be misinterpreted as a T-cell ALL if only flow cytometry is performed and a film of the sample is not examined to confirm morphology of the cells being analyzed.[16]

The terms *bilineage* (lineage infidelity) or *biphenotypic* (mixed lineage) may be used to denote cases where blasts express both myeloid and lymphoid antigens. *Bilineage* refers to the presence of two distinct blast populations (one lymphoid and one myeloid), whereas *biphenotypic* denotes the presence of both myeloid and lymphoid markers on the same blast cell. As leukemic blasts are being subjected to more extensive analysis, the incidence of bilineage and biphenotypic cases is rising to about 16% in children and 33% in adults.[22] It is important to identify acute lymphoblastic leukemias with myeloid markers (MY+ ALL), which in addition to markers specific for ALL, have one or more myeloid markers (*e.g.*, CD13, CD14, CD33 and CDw65). These MY+ ALLs may not respond well to standard treatment for myeloid leukemias, but will respond when the induction agents for ALL therapy are used.[15]

Cytogenetic Studies

The laboratory evaluation of karyotypes in ALL has been primarily used to predict therapeutic outcomes (prognosis). In about one-third of the cases of ALL, chromosomal translocations are associated with a poorer prognosis. Chromosomal translocations have been seen in about 50% of ALL cases, with half being random occurrences. As more cases have been analyzed, certain translocations are associated with specific immunologic subtypes of ALL. These include t(1;19), which has been associated with pre-B ALL; t(8;14), with B-ALL (Burkitt); t(4;11), with MY+ ALL; and t(9;22) or Ph[1](+) with pro-B ALL (cALL).

Evidence indicates that it is important to identify the breakpoint regions involved in the chromosomal translocations because the resulting protein formed may be related to the leukemic process and to response to therapy. As a case in point, the Philadelphia chromosome karyotype is found in both CML and Ph[1](+) ALL; however, there is a difference in where the chromosome breakpoint is located on chromosome 22 in the two disorders. This difference leads to the synthesis of different abnormal proteins and probably correlates with the fact that Ph[1](+) ALLs do not respond to standard ALL therapy.[14,15,21]

The presence of abnormal amounts of DNA in each cell (DNA aneuploidy) can also be detected using flow cytometry. The presence of an increased number of chromosomes per cell (hyperploidy) is seen more frequently in children and indicates a better prognosis.

New Approaches

Recent advances in DNA testing, especially in gene amplification analysis using the polymerase chain reaction (PCR; Chap. 31) have opened new areas for investigation. The use of DNA probes for B-cell immunoglobulin or T-cell receptor genes is important in recognizing clonal populations of malignant T and B cells and provides the means for early detection of lymphoid malignancies. Equally valuable is their use in the detection of residual disease after therapy. For example, if using older test procedures, the patient might appear to be in complete remission even though small numbers of leukemic cells are still present. It is at the molecular and genetic levels that most future discoveries will be made.

EFFECTS OF TREATMENT ON LABORATORY RESULTS

Therapy for ALL can be subdivided into chemotherapy and bone marrow transplantation. The goal is eradication of malignant cells. This is usually accompanied by severe pancytopenia.

Chemotherapy

Before the initiation of therapy, any physiologic imbalance is usually corrected. For example, correction of anemia and thrombocytopenia is accomplished by transfusion of packed red cells and platelets, antibiotic treatment is instituted for infection and intravenous supplements may be given to restore adequate hydration. Any of these measures may cause changes in cell counts and cellular morphology.

With the use of intensive multidrug regimens in treating ALL, nearly all children and more than 90% of adults will achieve remission with chemotherapy (Table 36-3). More than 80% of children who achieve a remission and finish 2 to 3 years of maintenance therapy are believed to be cured. Adults have only a 20% to 30% long-term survival rate. Patients who relapse will frequently achieve a complete remission with a repeat course of chemotherapy.[14]

In the past, approximately 50% of children with ALL who achieved a first remission and remained disease-free after 12 months, relapsed with CNS involvement. Such disease is an extension of the leukemic process with infiltration of the leptomeninges by leukemic cells. This occurs because most chemotherapeutic drugs do not pass the blood–brain barrier and malignant cells can thus ''escape'' the effects of chemotherapy by extending into the CNS. To prevent CNS involvement, children (but not adults) now receive prophylactic treatment with intrathecal drug injection and cranial irradiation. The use of a cytocentrifuge in the clinical laboratory to concentrate spinal fluid cells permits more sensitive detection of blasts to confirm CNS involvement (Chap. 30). With prophylaxis, the incidence of CNS relapse has been reduced to less than 5%. In addition to potential CNS involvement, males need to be carefully followed for evidence of any testicular involvement.[18]

Morphologic evidence of chemotherapy includes cytoplasmic fragmentation of lymphoid cells (Fig. 36-1), which may artificially elevate the results of electronic platelet counts. Another morphologic feature of chemotherapy is circulating necrotic lymphoid cells exhibiting nuclear lysis or dense pyknotic nuclei.

Purines are metabolized to uric acid. Therefore, hyperuricemia secondary to high purine turnover may result from increased leukocyte proliferation and from the de-

TABLE 36-3
Drugs Used in the Treatment of ALL

Drug	Class	Antitumor Action	Toxic Side Effects
Vincristine	Plant alkaloid	Inhibits RNA synthesis	CNS toxicity, peripheral nerve toxicity, reaction at injection site, baldness, diabetes, increased susceptibility to infection
Prednisone	Corticosteroid	Lysis of lymphoblasts	Personality changes, fluid retention, hypertension, osteoporosis, GI ulcerations
Methotrexate	Folic acid antagonist	Inhibits DNA synthesis	Myelosuppression, megaloblastic changes, oral and GI ulcerations, liver toxicity
6-Mercaptopurine (6MP)	Purine antagonist	Interferes with purine synthesis thus inhibiting RNA and DNA synthesis	Myelosuppression, liver toxicity
Cyclophosphamide	Synthetic alkylating agent	Inhibits DNA synthesis: arrests cells in mitosis	Severe myelosuppression, cystitis, baldness, increased susceptibility to infection
Daunorubicin	Antibiotic	Binds to DNA; inhibits DNA and RNA synthesis	Severe myelosuppression, cardiac toxicity, reaction to injection site, baldness, increased susceptibility to infection
L-Asparaginase	Enzyme (from a strain of *E. coli*)	Lysis of lymphoblasts, deprives the cells of L-asparagine	Allergic reaction, liver toxicity, acquired coagulation deficiencies, diabetes
Cytarabine (cytosine arabinoside; ara-C)	Pyrimidine antimetabolite	Inhibits DNA synthesis	Myelosuppression, immunosuppression, liver toxicity

struction of leukemic cells by chemotherapy and radiation. Renal failure may result because of uric acid nephropathy.

Bone Marrow Transplantation

The role of bone marrow transplantation in the treatment of ALL in refractory or in high-risk categories is still not established.[2a] Hillman and Ault[14] express the opinion that bone marrow transplantation should be considered in all patients who relapse and achieve a second remission, because response rates are high in ALL. A matched related donor for allogeneic transplant is preferred; if no match is available, autologous marrow that has been purged with anti-CD10 antibodies is preferable to marrow from an unmatched allogeneic donor.[14] More recently, stem cells harvested from peripheral blood have been used in place of marrow (Chap. 28). The laboratory must assist

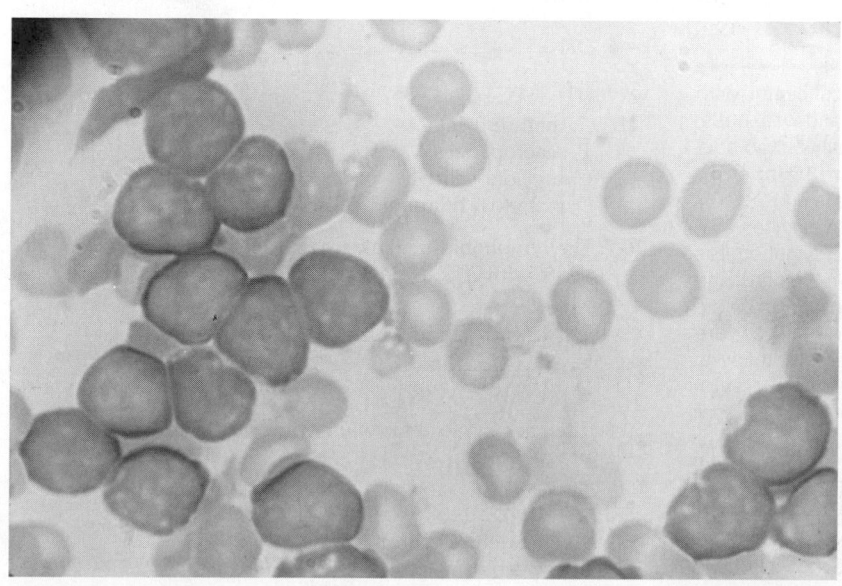

FIGURE 36-1. Cytoplasmic fragmentation in acute lymphoblastic leukemia. Note small, hyalinelike fragments of cytoplasm.

the physician in closely monitoring the patient's bone marrow and peripheral blood after transplantation.

CHAPTER SUMMARY

Acute lymphoblastic leukemia consists of three morphologic types (FAB classification) and four immunologic subclassifications have been identified: pro-B, pre-B, B-cell and T-cell ALL. Morphologic and immunologic classification, cytogenetic analysis and DNA studies are all valuable predictors for treatment and prognosis. Pro-B ALL has a good prognosis in children. T-cell ALL frequently occurs with a mediastinal (thymic) mass and carries a poor prognosis. Chromosomal translocations are now identified within certain immunologic groups. Biphenotypic and bilineage immunologic types may be seen. Therapy for ALL can cause significant changes in both cell counts and morphology. Death usually is caused by either infection or bleeding.

Case Study 36-1

A 3-year-old girl presented at an ambulatory care clinic with a 1-week history of vomiting, diarrhea and pallor. Easy bruising and petechiae on her face and trunk had been noted 2 days previously. On the day of her admission she felt warm and had been irritable, prompting her parents to take her to the clinic. Laboratory values were as follows: WBC, 105×10^9/L; Hb, 4.6 g/dL; Hct, 0.14 L/L; platelets, 23×10^9/L; differential: lymphocytes 10%, blasts 90%. The peroxidase stain was negative; acid phosphatase was positive in a diffuse pattern; PAS showed "chunky" positivity. The bone marrow aspirate was heavily infiltrated with lymphoid-appearing blasts. The morphology was described as consistent with L1. Immunologic marker studies showed: CD2, 9%; CD10, 90%; CD19, 92%; HLA-DR, 93%; cytoplasmic μ-positive, surface Ig negative. The patient responded well to vincristine and prednisone and is in remission.
1. The blasts in this case were said to be "consistent with L1." What does this mean?
2. What might have caused this patient's anemia and thrombocytopenia?
3. Is the child's age consistent with the diagnosis?
4. What is the immunologic classification of this ALL: pro-B, pre-B, B cell, or T cell ?

Case Study 36-2

A 20-year-old man was admitted to a local medical center with a 2- to 3-week history of left upper quadrant pain and weakness. The patient was noted to have hepatosplenomegaly but no adenopathy. Laboratory data included: WBC, 37×10^9/L; RBC, 2.14×10^{12}/L; Hb, 6.5 g/dL; Hct, 0.19 L/L; platelets, 112×10^9/L; differential: blasts 65%, myelocytes 1%, metamyelocytes 2%, band neutrophils 3%, segmented neutrophils 5%, lymphocytes 22%, and monocytes 2%; occasional NRBC were seen. The bone marrow was hypercellular with 74% blast forms. The blasts were consistent with L2 morphology; cytochemical stains were consistent with ALL. Immunologic markers were as follows: CD19, 58%; CD10, 54%; CD34, 56%; HLA-DR, 71%; cytoplasmic Ig was negative and surface Ig, CD13 and CD33 were less than 5%.

Despite treatment the blasts persisted in his peripheral blood. Ten months after diagnosis he was admitted to the bone marrow transplant unit and given an HLA-identical match from a sister. The patient continues to be well 18 months after transplant.

1. Contrast this case with Case 36-1 in terms of the peripheral blood findings, cytochemical stains, surface markers, morphology of the blasts, patient age and FAB classification.
2. What is the significance of finding CD34 surface markers?
3. What is the prognosis of ALL in children compared with adults? What treatments have improved survival in ALL?

Review Questions

36-1. The primary cause of death in patients with ALL is

    A. strokes.
    B. infection.
    C. bleeding.
    D. liver failure.

36-2. The major morphologic distinction between ALL and a reactive lymphocytosis such as infectious mononucleosis (IM) is the

    A. difference in size of the blasts.
    B. difference in nuclear:cytoplasmic ratio of the abnormal cell.
    C. pleomorphic morphology among reactive lymphocytes in IM.
    D. morphologic evidence that red cells are being destroyed in IM.

36-3. In the FAB classification of leukemias based on morphology, what percentage of cells may appear different from the proposed cell type of a specific classification?

    A. 1%
    B. 5%
    C. 10%
    D. 20%

36-4. The diagnosis of ALL in the adult must rule out

    A. leukemic lymphoma.
    B. blastic transformation of chronic lymphocytic leukemia.
    C. acute myeloid leukemia.
    D. all of the above.

36-5 The FAB classification type of acute lymphoblastic leukemia seen most commonly in children is

    A. L0
    B. L1
    C. L2
    D. L3

36-6 TdT activity is present in

    A. mature B cells.
    B. macrophages.
    C. myeloid cells.
    D. primitive lymphoid cells.

36-7. The lymphoblastic leukemia antigen found in 70% of patients with ALL is designated as CD

    A. 2.
    B. 10.
    C. 19.
    D. 22.

36-8. The karyotypic abnormality that carries a relatively good prognosis is

    A. t(8;14).
    B. t(9;22).
    C. Philadelphia chromosome.
    D. hyperploidy.

References

1. Bennett JM, Catovsky D, Daniel MT et al: Proposal for the classification of adult leukaemia. Br J Haematol 33:451, 1976
2. Bennett JM, Catovsky D, Daniel MT et al: The morphological classification of acute lymphoblastic leukaemia: Concordance among observers and clinical correlations. Br J Haematol 47:553, 1981
2a. Beutler E, Lichtman MA, Coller BS et al (eds): Williams Hematology, 5th ed. New York, McGraw-Hill, 1995
3. Boggs DR, Wintrobe MM, Cartwright CE: The acute leukemias: An analysis of 343 cases and a review of the literature. Medicine 41:163, 1962
4. Bollum FJ: Terminal deoxynucleotidyl transferase as a hematologic cell marker (review). Blood 54:1203, 1979
5. Catovsky A, Cherchi M, Greaves MF et al: Acid phosphatase reactions in acute lymphoblastic leukaemia. Lancet 1:749, 1978
6. Chessels JM: Acute lymphoblastic leukemia. Semin Hematol 19:155, 1982
7. Dosik GM, Barlogie B, Goehde W et al: Flow cytometry of DNA content in human bone marrow: A critical reappraisal. Blood 55:734, 1980
8. Foon KA, Todd RF III: Immunologic classification of leukemia and lymphoma. Blood 1:1, 1986
9. Fraumeni JF Jr, Miller RW: Leukemia mortality: Downward rates in the United States. Science 155:1126, 1967
10. Gale RP: Introduction: Leukemia. Semin Hematol 23:188, 1986
11. Greaves MF, Brown G, Rapson NT et al: Antisera to acute lymphoblastic leukemia cells. Clin Immunol Immunopathol 4:67, 1975
12. Greaves MF, Janossy G, Peto J et al: Immunologically defined subclasses of acute lymphoblastic leukaemia in children: Relationship to presentation features and prognosis. Br J Haematol 48:179, 1981
13. Guglielmi P, Preud'homme JL, Brouet JC: E-rosette receptor expression by chronic lymphocytic leukemia B lymphocytes. Eur J Immunol 13:641, 1983
14. Hillman RS, Ault KA: Hematology in Clinical Practice. New York, McGraw-Hill, 1995
15. Hoffman R, Benz EJ Jr, Shattil SJ et al (eds): Hematology, Basic Principles and Practices, 2nd ed. New York, Churchill Livingstone, 1995
16. Keren DF, Hanson CA, Hurtubise PE: Flow Cytometry and Clinical Diagnosis. Chicago, ASCP Press, 1994
17. Kocova M, Kowelezyk JR, Sandberg AA: Translocation 4;11 acute leukemia: Three case reports and review of the literature. Cancer Genet Cytogenet 16:21, 1985
18. Medical Research Council: Testicular disease in acute lymphoblastic leukaemia in childhood. Br Med J 1:334, 1978
19. Pui C-H, Behm FG, Christ WM: Clinical and biologic relevance of immunologic marker studies in childhood acute lymphoblastic leukemia. Blood 82:323, 1993
20. Rodenhuis S, Smets LA, Slater RM et al: Distinguishing the Philadelphia chromosome of acute lymphoblastic leukemia from its counterpart in chronic myelogenous leukemia. N Engl J Med 313:51, 1985
21. Sandberg A: The chromosomes in human leukemia. Semin Hematol 23:201, 1986
22. Secker-Walker LM, Swanbury GJ, Hardisty RM et al: Cytogenetics of acute lymphoblastic leukaemia in children as a factor in the prediction of long term survival. Br J Haematol 52:398, 1982
23. Sun T, Li CY, Yam LT: Atlas of Cytochemistry and Immunochemistry of Hematologic Neoplasms. Chicago, ASCP Press, 1985

CHAPTER 37

Chronic Lymphoproliferative Leukemic Disorders

Rita C. East

Objectives

1. Describe the morphology of the malignant lymphocytes in chronic lymphocytic, prolymphocytic and hairy cell leukemias.
2. Compare and contrast the bone marrow findings in chronic lymphocytic, prolymphocytic and hairy cell leukemias.
3. Describe the phenotypic information useful in diagnosing the chronic lymphoproliferative diseases.

The hematologic disorders known as chronic lymphoproliferative leukemic disorders (CLLD) are a heterogeneous group from which three distinct disease entities have emerged. Chronic lymphocytic leukemia (CLL), prolymphocytic leukemia (PLL) and hairy cell leukemia (HCL) are generally accepted as separate morphologic and clinicopathologic entities requiring different therapeutic approaches.[19]

Nearly all (99%)[17] of these leukemias are clonal B-lymphocyte diseases; that is, they involve proliferation and accumulation of clones of malignant B lymphocytes in the blood, bone marrow, lymph nodes or other organs.[34] A much smaller number of the CLLD are caused by T-lymphocyte proliferation. A reduced rate of cell death, rather than an increased rate of cell production, appears to account for the accumulation of these cells.[23] Research with polyclonal and monoclonal antibodies has shown that the B lymphocytes in CLL, PLL and HCL are malignant equivalents of different stages of normal lymphocyte development, with CLL being the least mature, HCL the most mature and PLL intermediate in maturity.[1,19,38,45]

It is important to distinguish B-cell malignancies from those caused by T cells because patients with T-cell disease tend to have a more aggressive disease and a poorer response to therapy.[32,46] It is interesting that cases of CLL[9] and HCL[74] have been reported in which the malignant cells possessed both B- and T-cell markers.

CHRONIC LYMPHOCYTIC LEUKEMIA

The first comprehensive study of CLL was published in 1924 by Minot and Isaacs.[57] This disease has since been recognized as the most common type of leukemia in the western hemisphere.

Among the important factors in the etiology of CLL are age, male gender and inherited or acquired immunologic defects that predispose some individuals to disease produced by certain leukemogenic agents. Not all leukemogenic agents cause CLL. For example, although ionizing radiation and alkylating agents are leukemogenic agents, they do not cause CLL. On the other hand, identification of the human T-cell leukemia virus (HTLV) indicates that the origin of certain lymphoid malignancies may be viral.[63] Genetic factors may play an important role in the etiology of some leukemias in humans, for multiple instances of leukemia have been reported in some families. Examples of such leukemias are CLL, acute leukemia and, less frequently, other lymphoproliferative diseases.[2,31,42,65,66]

In families in which more than one member has had CLL or another closely related lymphoproliferative disease, some of the apparently healthy relatives have immunoglobulin abnormalities or impaired lymphocyte transformation in response to phytohemagglutinin (PHA).[30,31] These immunoglobulin abnormalities may involve qualitative or quantitative changes in serum proteins, abnormal immune responsiveness and connective tissue vascular diseases.[3,77,87] Because not all individuals who are thus affected develop leukemia, the interaction of environmental and hereditary factors is probably necessary to produce leukemia.

Pathophysiology

Chronic lymphocytic leukemia is the proliferation and accumulation of lymphocytes (usually B cells) that are relatively unresponsive to antigenic stimuli. Consequently, they lie more or less dormant and accumulate in the peripheral blood, bone marrow, lymph nodes and spleen.[23] However, although earlier studies postulated that B-cell lymphocytes were arrested at an early stage of differentiation, there is now considerable evidence that these cells are able to differentiate.[4] Rarely, CLL is caused by T-cell proliferation. In such cases, epidermal sites (causing a rash) and the central nervous system (CNS) are more likely to become involved.

Clinical Presentation and Physical Findings

Chronic lymphocytic leukemia is primarily a disease of the elderly, with 90% of the patients being older than 50 years of age and nearly 65% older than 60.[18] Men are affected more than twice as frequently as women.

Symptoms of CLL usually develop so insidiously that the diagnosis is often made unexpectedly during routine or other examinations. Fatigue and reduced exercise tolerance are the most common presenting symptoms. Marked fatigue, bruising, pallor or jaundice associated with anemia, fever, recurrent or persistent infection, bone tenderness, weight loss and edema from lymph node obstruction may be seen in those patients with more advanced disease. Erythroderma with pruritus is common with T-cell CLL.

The clinical course of CLL may range from almost completely benign to severe. Approximately 10% to 15% of patients live 10 to 15 years in relatively good health with little or no treatment, whereas a slightly higher percentage have more aggressive disease and die within a year.[40,55] The median survival after diagnosis is 3 to 4 years.[40]

CLL is less likely to undergo acute exacerbation than are other leukemias, regardless of whether or not treatment has been instituted.[61] "Prolymphocytoid transformation" of otherwise typical B-CLL has been reported.[25] However, in cases of transforming CLL, the "prolymphocytes" may be morphologically and phenotypically different from the classic prolymphocytes seen in PLL.[15,25] In a small number of patients (3% to 10%) CLL may evolve to a more aggressive large cell lymphoma (Richter syndrome).[29] Whether Richter syndrome and other transformations are clonal evolutions of CLL or are independent disorders is presently unclear.

In the early presentation of CLL, the most common signs are enlarged lymph nodes and splenomegaly. As the disease progresses, the lymph nodes become larger, and new areas of nodal enlargement appear. Splenomegaly usually increases, and hepatomegaly develops. Lymphoid cells may infiltrate other organs such as the gonads, skin, prostate, kidney and walls of the gastrointestinal tract.

Laboratory Findings and Correlations with Disease

Chronic lymphocytic leukemia is commonly diagnosed by finding a persistent lymphocytosis in the peripheral blood. An absolute lymphocyte count between 10 and 150×10^9/L is usual with CLL, but counts as high as 1000×10^9/L may be encountered with untreated aggressive disease.[85]

Morphologically, these lymphocytes may appear virtually normal, especially in patients with mild disease. Usually, however, the lymphocytes are somewhat larger than normal, have nuclei with clumped or condensed chromatin, and may have prominent nucleoli. The cyto-

plasm may be abundant, nongranular and moderately basophilic, or it may be relatively scant. Patients with aggressive disease may have tiny lymphocytes with little cytoplasm and cleft nuclei suggesting a follicular cell origin.[56] The lymphocytes in CLL appear to be somewhat more fragile than normal, and blood films usually contain large numbers of "smudge" cells (lymphocytes broken when the film was made; see Color Plates 37-1 and 37-2). Although CLL lymphocytes can differ morphologically from patient to patient, they are usually monotonously similar in any given patient. This attests to the clonal origin of the disease.

The percentage of neutrophils is often decreased, but absolute numbers are usually normal or slightly increased, especially in the early stages of the disease.[8]

Patients with aggressive or advanced disease often have granulocytopenia, anemia or thrombocytopenia when lymphoid tissue fills 50% or more of the marrow space. These cytopenias are especially troublesome after blood loss, treatment with antineoplastic drugs or infection.

Besides decreased red cell production, anemia may be the result of splenic sequestration of red cells or of shortened red cell survival. Autoimmune hemolysis (Color Plate 37-2) is a third factor, which may account for anemia in 5% to 10% of those patients who have aggressive or advanced disease.[69,88] Such autoimmune responses may be triggered by viral infections, disease progression, therapeutic agents or membrane damage by abnormal proteins.[54,55,76,89] Laboratory findings in autoimmune hemolytic anemia include reticulocytosis, often spherocytosis, mild jaundice, shortened red cell survival, bone marrow erythroid hyperplasia and a positive direct antiglobulin test or DAT (formerly known as the Coombs' test).

In CLL, the lymphocytes contain more glycogen than usual, thus giving a positive-staining reaction with the periodic acid–Schiff (PAS) stain (Chap. 29).

Plasma immunoglobulins may be reduced, especially as the disease progresses. The gamma globulin levels may fall to 0.3 to 0.4 g/dL (reference range 0.8 to 1.6 g/dL), and patients become more susceptible to all types of infection.

Bone marrow aspiration and biopsy usually are not necessary for making the diagnosis of CLL except in those "aleukemic" or "subleukemic" cases with no nodal or splenic involvement and few or no abnormal cells in the peripheral blood. The marrow is sometimes the principal site of involvement in these patients.

Infiltration of the marrow usually occurs slowly with progression of disease, but 30% or more lymphocytes in the marrow, when accompanied by a sustained lymphocytosis in the peripheral blood, is considered diagnostic of CLL. Lymphocytes increase in number until normal marrow cells are crowded out. Eventually, the marrow becomes packed with lymphocytes.

Erythroid cells in the marrow may be megaloblastic, whereas an erythroid hyperplasia is suggestive of hemolytic complications. Mast cells may be increased in number.

Chromosomal abnormalities are detected in more than 50% of patients with CLL and indicate a worse prognosis.[43,51] The most frequently encountered (one-third of the cases) is trisomy 12 (+12).[50,51] The +12 abnormality is a marker for lymphocytic proliferation in general, not just CLL, and it appears to predict a progressive disease, with an early need for treatment.[68] Another cytogenetic abnormality found in a large cooperative study (41 of 433 patients) involves various translocations to the end of the long arm of chromosome 14 (14q⁺) at band 14q32.[51] Several chromosomes participate in the 14q translocation, but t(11;14) with the break in 11q13 seems the most common.[81] Other less frequently encountered alterations affect chromosomes 11, 6, 18, 3, 17, 7 and 8.[51] In most patients chromosomal abnormalities do not change throughout the disease. This is in contrast to what is observed in CML and myelodysplastic diseases.

Phenotypically, B-CLL cells differ from those of other B-cell malignancies and are characterized by the following:

1. B-CLL cells almost always express low amounts of surface immunoglobulin (sIg),[20,21,80] about one-tenth of that on normal B-lymphocytes.[80] Sometimes, however, they demonstrate increased amounts of intracytoplasmic Ig.[48]
2. B-CLL lymphocytes frequently (31% to 95%) form rosettes with mouse erythrocytes.[16,78]
3. In more than 90% of the cases, CLL lymphocytes express the CD5 antigen,[10,70,83] which was formerly thought to be a T-cell antigen. Cells from most cases of B-CLL also express CD19, CD24, CD37 and CD21 antigens. About 60% of CLL are positive for CD23[73] but infrequently demonstrate positivity for CD22.[59] (See Chap. 23 for a discussion of lymphoid surface markers.)

Effects of Treatment on Laboratory Results

The two goals of therapy in CLL are the relief of symptoms and the prevention of complications. Basically, there are three modes of therapy: chemotherapy, radiation and leukapheresis. Standard chemotherapy involves the use of alkylating agents such as cyclophosphamide or chlorambucil, either singly or in combination with vincristine (a plant alkaloid) and prednisone (a corticosteroid). Treatment with a new class of drugs known as adenosine deaminease (ADA) inhibitors has been promising, as has treatment with biologic response modifiers such as interleukin-2 (IL-2). Treatment with intravenous immunoglobulin (IV-Ig) has been used effectively as replacement therapy in CLL patients with hypoglobulinemia to treat and prevent infections, as therapy for autoimmune cytopenias and as therapy to suppress the leukemic process.[7]

Unfortunately, no treatment is without its risks to the patient, and one of the main risks with the use of chemotherapy is myelosuppression. Thus, these drugs, which are so effective in reducing both the tumor burden in the tissues and the number of abnormal lymphocytes in the peripheral blood, may also cause anemia, thrombocytopenia and granulocytopenia. Even the biologic treatments are not without side effects and IV-Ig becomes ineffective against leukemic activity as the disease progresses.

Radiation is used primarily to treat enlarged lymph nodes and splenomegaly that have proven resistant to chemotherapy. Radiation is an effective means of treating localized disease, but it does nothing to reduce the lymphocytosis in the peripheral blood and bone marrow.

Leukapheresis is especially useful in reducing the number of lymphocytes in the peripheral blood when the patient has symptoms of blood hyperviscosity because of the great number of lymphocytes. However, leukapheresis does not reduce the tumor burden elsewhere.

PROLYMPHOCYTIC LEUKEMIA

Prolymphocytic leukemia was first described by Galton and associates in 1974[35] in a study of 15 patients who had a "rare variant" of CLL. Those authors observed that PLL could be distinguished from other lymphoid diseases on the basis of the peculiar morphology of the lymphocytes as seen in blood and bone marrow films. It was also apparent that these patients, in addition to having similar lymphocyte morphology, all had certain other characteristics that differed from those seen in classic CLL.

Pathophysiology

The proliferation and accumulation of abnormal lymphoid cells in the spleen, bone marrow and, to a lesser extent, the liver account for the signs and symptoms of PLL. Immunologic deficiencies, such as low levels of gamma globulins and generally low levels of other immunoglobulins, are frequently found. Additionally, the number of T lymphocytes is below normal.[35]

Clinical Presentation and Physical Findings

Prolymphocytic leukemia shows a propensity for men in their 60s. Common symptoms are fatigue, weakness, weight loss, sweats and fever. In direct contrast to CLL, in which the onset may be insidious, the presenting symptoms in PLL are generally acute.[39]

The most common and most impressive physical sign is enormous enlargement of the spleen and, less often, the liver. Interestingly, lymphadenopathy is uncommon. The prognosis for PLL is considerably poorer than for either CLL or HCL. The mean survival is reported to be less than 1 year.[35]

Laboratory Findings and Correlations with Disease

The leukocyte count in the peripheral blood is typically high, from approximately 25 to 1000 × 10⁹/L.[35] The number of prolymphocytes in the blood differs from patient to patient, and these cells may constitute a small or large percentage of the differential leukocyte count. The prolymphocyte is a relatively large mononuclear lymphoid cell with an oval to round nucleus, coarse-appearing chromatin strands and one or two large vesicular nucleoli with perinuclear condensations of chromatin. The cytoplasm is usually agranular and is basophilic with Romanowsky stains (see Color Plates 37-3 and 37-4). Cells of similar morphology generally are not found in normal blood films. It has been suggested, on the basis of membrane phenotype, that the normal counterpart of the prolymphocyte in PLL can be found in B mantle zones (lymphocyte corona) of the peripheral lymph nodes.[36]

Absolute neutrophil counts can range from low (1 × 10^9/L) to high (20 × 10^9/L).[35] There may be an absolute monocytosis (higher than 0.8 × 10^9/L).[58] Nucleated red blood cells (NRBC) and immature granulocytes may be present on the blood film.

Bone marrow examination reveals almost total replacement of the marrow by prolymphocytic infiltration. Usually, only a few residual hematopoietic cells remain. Consequently, it is not uncommon for the patient to be both anemic and thrombocytopenic.

PLL occurs less frequently than CLL; accordingly, less is known concerning accompanying chromosomal anomalies. Of those 50 or so cases reported, the most frequent abnormality, present in about 50%, is a 14q⁺ marker with the breakpoint in band 14q32.[14,62] In most patients the translocated material has not been identified. Only two fully identified rearrangements have been detected more than once: t(11;14)(q13;q32) and t(14;17)(q32;q11). It is reasonable to hypothesize that all these 14q32 rearrangements are similar to those occurring in many other B-cell neoplasias.

Other chromosomal aberrations include trisomy 12; deletions of chromosomes 1 and 6, usually at bands q32 and q21, respectively; and terminal deletions of the short arm of chromosome 3, del(3)(p13) and chromosome 12, del(12)(p12-13).[14,49] Also reported is a 6;12 translocation, t(6;12)(q15;p13).[72]

Phenotypically, cells of PLL show increased expression of surface immunoglobulins, low formation of rosettes with mouse erythrocytes, low CD5 expression, and positivity for FMC7[22] (also known as B-Ly7 and recently renamed CD103), which is a marker of late differentiation rather than activation.[28]

Effects of Treatment on Laboratory Results

The goal of therapy is to reduce the lymphocyte mass in the blood, marrow and tissues; to reduce symptoms; and to improve hematopoiesis in those patients who are anemic or thrombocytopenic. Unfortunately, PLL generally responds poorly to the modes of therapy that are successful against CLL, such as alkylating agents and corticosteroids. Alkylating agents do not alleviate the disease symptoms and may, in fact, worsen myelosuppression. Prednisone may cause fluid and sodium retention, as well as increased excretion of calcium and potassium. It also may cause carbohydrate intolerance, glycosuria and hyperglycemia.[5] Occasionally patients may respond to combinations of chemotherapeutic agents such as cyclophosphamide, doxorubicin, vincristine, and prednisone.[29a]

HAIRY CELL LEUKEMIA

Hairy cell leukemia is a relatively rare neoplasm, accounting for only about 2% of all leukemias.[84] In 1923, Ewald[26] described a disease he called "leukemic reticuloendothe-

liosis." He considered two characteristics commonplace in this disease: a large spleen and circulating mononuclear cells with numerous cytoplasmic projections. Cases bearing similarity to Ewald's original description have appeared under many names, such as reticulosis,[27] aleukemic reticuloendotheliosis,[33] reticulum cell leukemia[53,79] and others. The term "hairy cell" leukemia, derived from the ultrastructural appearance of the cells, was first suggested by Schrek and Donnelly in 1966[75] and has since become accepted as the name of the disease.

Pathophysiology

Hairy cell leukemia has a rather indolent course in most patients. However, these patients are subject to many medical problems. The growth and accumulation of hairy cells in the spleen, blood and bone marrow account for the complications, which fall essentially into two groups: those related to cytopenias and splenomegaly, such as anemia, bleeding and infection; and paraneoplastic complications, including autoimmune syndrome and, less often, paraproteinemia (Chap. 39). The mean survival has been said to be 5 years, but one patient has been reported to be alive 27 years after diagnosis.[11]

Clinical Presentation and Physical Findings

Men are more often affected (4:1 to 5:1 male:female), with the median age at diagnosis being 55 years. Virtually no one younger than 20 is affected.[86] The symptoms are the same as those in many other hematologic neoplasms; namely bleeding, weakness and fatigue, infection and abdominal discomfort.

In HCL, the physical sign found most consistently is splenomegaly; approximately 90% of patients have splenomegaly, and the spleen is often enormous. Lymphadenopathy and hepatomegaly are seen less frequently.

Laboratory Findings and Correlations with Disease

Hairy cells are found in the peripheral blood in more than 90% of affected patients, but these cells usually account for fewer than 50% of the cells in the differential leukocyte count.[37] Hairy cells have scant to abundant, agranular, light grayish-blue cytoplasm. The plasma membrane appears irregular with hairlike or ruffled projections, which are seen more easily with phase microscopy on living cells, or by electron microscopy. These cells often have a round to oval nucleus; sometimes, the nucleus appears folded or bilobed. The chromatin is loose and lacy, and one or two nucleoli are commonly seen (see Color Plates 37-5 and 37-6).

Pancytopenia is the most consistent laboratory observation. Granulocytopenia and monocytopenia are the most common causes of the leukopenia seen in HCL. Cytopenias result from infiltration of the marrow with malignant cells and fibrous tissue, and the effect is augmented by sequestration of blood cells by an enlarged spleen.

Bone marrow aspiration often results in a "dry tap," because most HCL patients have marrow fibrosis. When an aspirate is obtained, an increase in moderately large (10 to 15 μm in diameter) lymphoid cells with relatively abundant cytoplasm is observed.

Histologically, the bone marrow biopsy shows a lymphoid infiltrate with a larger space between cell nuclei than in non-Hodgkin lymphomas because of the abundant cytoplasm of the hairy cell. Increased reticulin fibers are noted on the marrow biopsy in almost all patients.

The stain for tartrate-resistant acid phosphatase (TRAP; Chap. 29) will be positive in hairy cells, but negative in most other lymphoid cells.

Chromosomal abnormalities are thought to exist in most HCL patients. Numeric changes, clonal aberrations and structural changes have all been described. However, no consistent chromosomal anomalies have yet been identified.[6,13,24,41,44,60,71]

The most common phenotype is associated with expression of the following surface markers: CD19, CD20, CD22, CD25, CD103 and CD11c and negative for CD5.[47,67,82] However, B-HCL cells commonly express aberrant phenotypes with simultaneous expression of divergent markers of cell lineage and differentiation. In fact, phenotype data suggest that there may be a spectrum of HCL variants.[52]

Effects of Treatment on Laboratory Results

If the patient is asymptomatic, no therapy is needed. In the symptomatic patient, chemotherapy has not been very effective. Aggressive therapy with alkylating agents, which are so useful in treating many other lymphoid diseases, may reduce the tumor burden very little and, because of their toxicity may make cytopenias worse.[11,37] Corticosteroids have rarely been helpful in treating HCL because of the association of their use with serious infections.[12]

Splenectomy is one method of treatment, especially in those patients with severe cytopenias, which are attributable, at least partly, to splenic sequestration of cells. Removal of the spleen allows the volume of cells previously sequestered in the spleen to remain in the circulation and thus raises cell counts.

Hairy cell leukemia is especially problematic in those patients who do not improve after splenectomy. Successful treatment with interferons (IFN-α) has been reported.[64] The results compared favorably with the use of chemotherapy, without the toxicity of the latter. Other effective agents include pentostatin, 2-chlorodeoxyadenosine and a new agent called cladribine, which induces a partial or complete remission with very little toxicity.[29a]

CHAPTER SUMMARY

Chronic lymphocytic leukemia (CLL), prolymphocytic leukemia (PLL) and hairy cell leukemia (HCL) represent, for the most part, clonal B-lymphocyte chronic lymphoproliferative leukemic disorders (CLLD) with distinctive clinical, diagnostic, and prognostic features. Improved diagnostic techniques (*i.e.*, chromosomal banding and phenotypic analysis) facilitate faster, more accurate diagnosis. The CLLDs remain low-grade lymphocytic malignancies, which have little hope for cure; however recently, new drug therapies have given them a better prognosis with longer remissions.

Case Study 37-1

A 72-year-old retired man was seen because of fatigue, weight loss and fever. He had small nodes palpable bilaterally in the supraclavicular areas, a 3- by 2-cm node in the left axilla, and multiple palpable inguinal nodes. The liver was 3 cm below the right costal margin, and the spleen was enlarged to 8 cm below the left costal margin. Laboratory data included the following: WBC, 30.8 × 10⁹/L; Hb, 9.0 g/dL; Hct, 0.30 L/L; platelets, 215 × 10⁹/L; differential: segmented neutrophils 18%, lymphocytes 80%, and monocytes 2%. The reticulocyte count was 9%. The red cells were normocytic and normochromic. The serum bilirubin level was 2.1 mg/dL, and the direct antiglobulin test (DAT) was 4+ positive. The bone marrow showed 30% lymphocytes and erythroid hyperplasia. The patient was started on a therapeutic regimen of prednisone and was discharged 2 weeks later with a Hct of 0.33 L/L. After 4 weeks of prednisone, his Hct was 0.40 L/L. All medicines were discontinued.

One month later he was readmitted for fatigue and "blackout spells;" physical examination was unchanged. Laboratory data included the following: WBC, 139 × 10⁹/L; Hct, 0.20 L/L; platelets, 275 × 10⁹/L; and reticulocyte count 30%. The differential showed 88% lymphocytes. The serum bilirubin level was 9 mg/dL. The DAT remained 4+ positive. The patient was started on regimen of chlorambucil and prednisone daily. After 2 weeks in the hospital, his Hct had increased to 0.35 L/L, and his leukocyte count had decreased to 55 × 10⁹/L. Since then, he has been followed in the clinic on a regular basis, being maintained on 2 mg of chlorambucil and 20 mg of prednisone three times weekly. His DAT is still positive, although his Hct remains normal. Attempts to decrease steroids further have been unsuccessful. Signs of hypercorticism are minimal, and the patient does not have a cushingoid appearance.

1. What is the most likely diagnosis?
2. What complication is present?
3. How do we know that hemolysis is occurring in this patient?
4. In light of a 4+ positive DAT, how can the Hct remain normal?

Case Study 37-2

A 39-year-old policeman was admitted for evaluation of an inguinal hernia. Physical examination was otherwise unremarkable. Admission laboratory values included WBC, 10.6 × 10⁹/L; platelets, 109 × 10⁹/L; differential: segmented neutrophils 8%, band neutrophils 1%, lymphocytes 89%, monocytes 1%, and eosinophils 1%. Approximately one-third of the lymphocytes were noted to have fringed, wispy cytoplasm. A bone marrow examination showed mild hypercellularity and megakaryocytes that were present but decreased in number. The marrow was primarily filled with lymphoid cells, with round to oval nuclei having abundant clear to pale cytoplasm. TRAP stains on the bone marrow and peripheral blood were positive.

The patient received no treatment for his illness at that time, because he was asymptomatic. Two years later the patient was admitted for abnormal bruising. Significant was a platelet count of 68 × 10⁹/L. A computed tomography (CT) scan of the abdomen showed hepatosplenomegaly. A bone marrow aspirate could not be obtained owing to a dry tap. However, the bone marrow biopsy showed more than 90% abnormal lymphoid cells.

A treatment regimen of deoxycoformycin was initiated, after which the following laboratory values were noted: WBC, 4.3 × 10⁹/L; Hb, 16.7 g/dL; Hct, 0.49 L/L; platelets, 230 × 10⁹/L;

differential: segmented neutrophils 75%, band neutrophils 1%, lymphocytes 16%, monocytes 7% and basophils 1%. RBCs were normocytic and normochromic. No abnormal lymphoid cells were seen in either the peripheral blood or the bone marrow, which was again able to be aspirated. A CT scan of the abdomen revealed no hepatomegaly and only minimal splenomegaly. The patient remains in remission 4 years later.

1. What is the most likely diagnosis?
2. What is the significance of a dry tap in this patient?
3. Name two factors contributing to this patient's thrombocytopenia.
4. What does TRAP stand for and what is the significance of a positive TRAP stain?

Review Questions

37-1. The CLLDs share which of the following characteristics?

    A. The majority are clonal B-cell disorders.

    B. Insidious onset.

    C. Their malignant cells show strong positivity for surface immunoglobulin.

    D. All of the above.

37-2. Chronic lymphocytic leukemia

    A. often gives positive results with TRAP stains.

    B. commonly demonstrates CD5 positivity and trisomy 12.

    C. may only be diagnosed by bone marrow examination.

    D. All of the above.

37-3. Prolymphocytic leukemia

    A. is characterized by massive lymphadenopathy and hepatosplenomegaly.

    B. is characterized by almost total bone marrow replacement by prolymphocytes.

    C. has a comparable prognosis to CLL and HCL.

    D. All of the above.

37-4. Hairy cell leukemia is a disease in which the abnormal cells

    A. all have a scanty amount of cytoplasm.

    B. demonstrate positivity with tartrate-resistant acid phosphatase stain.

    C. express the CD5 surface marker.

    D. All of the above.

References

1. Aisenberg AC: Cell lineage in lymphoproliferative disease. Am J Med 74:679, 1983
2. Anderson RC: Familial leukemia: A report of leukemia in five siblings, with a brief review of the genetic aspects of this disease. Am J Dis Child 81:313, 1951
3. Axelsson U, Hallen J: Familial occurrence of pathological serum proteins of different gamma globulin groups. Lancet 2:369, 1965
4. Baldini L, Mozanna R, Cortelezzi A et al: Prognostic significance of immunoglobulin phenotype in B cell chronic lymphocytic leukemia. Blood 65:340, 1985
5. Becker TM: Cancer Chemotheraphy: A Manual for Nurses. Boston, Little, Brown & Co., 1981
6. Berger R, Bernheim A, Valensi F et al: 14q⁻ in two hairy cell leukemia patients [letter]. Cancer Genet Cytogenet 16:91, 1985
7. Besa E: Recent advances in the treatment of chronic lymphocytic leukemia: Defining the role of intravenous immunoglobulin. Semin Hematol 29(Suppl 2):14, 1992
8. Boggs DR, Sofferman SA, Wintrobe MM et al: Factors influencing the duration of survival of patients with chronic lymphocytic leukemia. Am J Med 40:243, 1966
9. Bona C, Fauci A: In vitro idiotype suppression of chronic lymphocytic leukemia lymphocytes secreting monoclonal immunoglobulin M anti-sheep erythrocyte antibody. J Clin Invest 65:761, 1980
10. Boumsell L, Bernard A, Lepage V et al: Some chronic lymphocytic leukemia cells bearing surface immunoglobulins share determinants with T cells. Eur J Immunol 8:900, 1978
11. Bouroncle BA: Leukemic reticuloendotheliosis (hairy cell leukemia). Blood 53:412, 1979
12. Bouza E, Burgaleta C, Golde DW: Infections in hairy-cell leukemia. Blood 51:851, 1978
13. Brito-Babapulle V, Pittman S, Melo JV et al: The 14q⁺ marker in hairy cell leukemia: A cytogenetic study of fifteen cases. Leuk Res 10:131, 1986
14. Brito-Babapulle V, Pittman S, Melo JV et al: Cytogenetic studies on prolymphocytic leukemia. I. B-cell prolymphocytic leukemia. Hematol Pathol 1:27, 1987
15. Caligaris-Cappio F, Janossy G: Surface markers in chronic lymphoid leukemias of B-cell type. Semin Hematol 22:1, 1985
16. Catovsky D, Cherchi M, Okas A: Mouse red-cell rosettes in B lymphoproliferative disorders. Br J Haematol 33:173, 1976
17. Catovsky D: Chronic lymphocytic, prolymphocytic and hairy cell leukemias. In Goldman JM, Preisler HD (eds): Leukemia, p 266. Sevenoaks, UK, Butterworths, 1984
18. Cutler SJ, Axtell L, Heise H: Ten thousand cases of leukemia: 1940–62. J Natl Cancer Inst 39:993, 1967
19. Den Ottolander GJ, Schmit HRE, Wayer JLM et al: Chronic B-cell leukemias: Relation between morphological and immunological features. Clin Immunol Immunopathol 35:92, 1985
20. Dighiero G, Follezou JY, Roisin JP et al: Comparison of normal and CLL lymphocyte surface Ig determinants using peroxidase labelled antibodies. II. Quantitation of light chain determinants in atypical lymphoid leukemia. Blood 48:559, 1976
21. Dighiero G, Bodega E, Mayzner R, Binet JL: Individual cell-by-cell quantitation of lymphocyte surface membrane Ig in normal and CLL lymphocytes and during ontogeny of mouse lymphocytes by immunoperoxidase assay. Blood 55:93, 1980
22. Dighiero G, Travade P, Chevret S et al: B-cell chronic lymphocytic leukemia: Present status and future directions. Blood 78:1901, 1991
23. Dormer P, Thelm H, Lau B: Chronic lymphocytic leukemia: A proliferative or accumulative disorder? Leuk Res 2:1, 1983
24. Emilia G, Torelli G, DiPrisco AU et al: Cytogenetic investigations in hairy cell leukemia: A survey of sixteen cases. Panminerva Med 27:175, 1985
25. Enno A, Catovsky D, O'Brien M et al: Prolymphocytoid transformation of chronic lymphocytic leukaemia. Br J Haematol 41:9, 1979
26. Ewald O: Die leukmische Reticuloendotheliose. Dtsch Arch Kinderheilkd Med 142:222, 1923
27. Farquhar JW, MacGregor AR, Richmond J: Familial haemophagic reticulosis. Br Med J 2:1561, 1958
28. Ferro LM, Zola H: Modulation of expression of the antigen identified by FMC7 upon human B-lymphocyte activation in vivo and in vitro. Immunology 69:373, 1990
29. Foon KA, Gale RP: Clinical transformation of chronic lymphocytic leukemia. Nouv Rev Fr Hematol 30:385, 1988
29a. Foon, KA, Gale RP: Chronic lymphoid leukemia. In Handin RI, Lux SE, Stossel TP (eds): Blood: Principles and Practice of Hematology, p 797. Philadelphia, JB Lippincott, 1995
30. Fraumeni JF Jr, Vogel CL, DeVita VT Jr: Familial chronic lymphocytic leukemia. Ann Intern Med 71:279, 1969
31. Fraumeni JF Jr, Wertelecki W, Blattner WA et al: Varied

manifestations of a familial lymphoproliferative disorder. Am J Med 59:145, 1975

32. Frei E, Sallan S: Acute lymphoblastic leukemia: Treatment. Cancer 42:828, 1978

33. Fukuda T: Malignant reticulosis. Tohoku J Exp Med 94:351, 1968

34. Galton DAG: The pathogenesis of chronic lymphocytic leukemia. Can Med Assoc J 94:1005, 1966

35. Galton DAG, Goldman JM, Wiltshaw E et al: Prolymphocytic leukaemia. Br J Haematol 27:7, 1974

36. Gobbi M, Caligaris-Cappio F, Janossy G: Normal equivalent cells of B-cell malignancies: Analysis with monoclonal antibodies. Br J Haematol 54:393, 1983

37. Golomb HM, Catovsky D, Golde DW: Clinical review: Hairy cell leukemia. Ann Intern Med 89:677, 1978

38. Gordon J, Aman P, Mellstedt H et al: In vitro differentiation of chronic lymphocytic leukemia cells with a small pre-B-like phenotype. Leuk Res 2:133, 1983

39. Gordon MY, Barrett AJ: Bone Marrow Disorders: The Biological Basis of Clinical Problems. Oxford, Oxford Scientific Publications, 1985

40. Green RA, Dixon H: Expectancy for life in chronic lymphatic leukemia. Blood 25:23, 1965

41. Gribbin TE, Glover T, Cody RL, Mitchell BS: Association of atypical hairy cell leukemia with a unique chromosomal abnormality and establishment of a cell line [abstr]. Proc Annu Meet Am Assoc Cancer Res 29:A116, 1988

42. Gunz FW, Fitzgerald PH, Crossen PE et al: Multiple cases of leukemia in a sibship. Blood 27:482, 1966

43. Han T, Henderson ES, Emrich LJ, Sandberg AA: Prognostic significance of karyotypic abnormalities in B cell chronic lymphocytic leukemia. Semin Hematol 24:257, 1987

44. Han T, Sadamori N, Block AM et al: Cytogenetic studies in chronic lymphocytic leukemia, prolymphocytic leukemia and hairy cell leukemia: A progress report. Nouv Rev Fr Hematol 30:393, 1988

45. Harden EA, Haynes BF: Phenotypic and functional characterization of human malignant T-cells. Semin Hematol 22:13, 1985

46. Heideman R, Falletta J, Mukhopadhyay N et al: Lymphocytic leukemia in children: Prognostic significance of clinical and laboratory findings at time of diagnosis. J Pediatr 92:540, 1978

47. Jansen J, LeBien TW, Kersey JH: The phenotype of the neoplastic cell of hairy cell leukemia studied with monoclonal antibodies. Blood 59:609, 1982

48. Johnstone AP: Chronic lymphocytic leukemia and its relationship to normal B lymphopoiesis. Immunol Today 3:343, 1982

49. Julisson G, Robert K-H, Ost A et al: Del(3)(p13) in B-prolymphocytic leukemia—a new nonrandom chromosomal aberration possibly related to the c-ras oncogene. Cancer Genet Cytogenet 14:191, 1985

50. Juliusson G, Robert K-H, Ost A et al: Prognostic information from cytogenetic analysis in chronic B-lymphocytic leukemia and leukemic immunocytoma. Blood 65:134, 1985

51. Julisson G, Oscier D, Fitchett M et al: Prognostic subgroups in B cell chronic lymphocytic leukemia defined by specific chromosomal abnormalities. N Engl J Med 323:720, 1990

52. Julisson G, Lenkei R, Liliemark J: Flow cytometry of blood and bone marrow cells from patients with hairy cell leukemia: Phenotype of hairy cells and lymphocyte subsets after treatment with 2-chlorodeoxyadenosine. Blood 83:3672, 1994

53. Lee SL, Rosner F, Rosenthal N et al: Reticulum cell leukemia. NY State J Med 69:422, 1969

54. Lewis FB, Schwartz RS, Dameshek W: X-radiation and alkylating agents as possible "trigger" mechanisms in the autoimmune complications of malignant lymphoproliferative disease. Clin Exp Immunol 1:1, 1966

55. Lockwood K, Stancke B, Clemmesen J: Survival rates for leukemia in various countries. Natl Cancer Inst Monogr 15:341, 1964

56. McKenna RW, Bloomfield CD, Brunning CD: Nodular lymphoma: Bone marrow and blood manifestations. Cancer 36:428, 1975

57. Minot GR, Isaacs R: Lymphatic leukemia: Age incidence, duration, and benefit derived from irradiation. Boston Med Surg J 191:1, 1924

58. Munan L, Kelly A: Age-dependent changes in blood monocyte populations in man. Clin Exp Immunol 35:161, 1979

59. Nadler LM: B cell/leukemia panel workshop: Summary and comments. In: Leukocyte Typing II. New York, Springer-Verlag, 1986

60. Ohyashiki K, Ohyashiki JH, Takeuchi J et al: Cytogenetic studies in hairy cell leukemia. Cancer Genet Cytogenet 24:109, 1987

61. Osgood EE: Contrasting incidence of acute monocytic and granulocytic leukemia in P^{32} treated patients with polycythemia vera and chronic lymphocytic leukemia. J Lab Clin Med 64:560, 1969

62. Pittman S, Catovsky D: Chromosome abnormalities in B-cell prolymphocytic leukemia: A study of nine cases. Cancer Genet Cytogenet 9:355, 1983

63. Poiesz BJ, Ruscetti FW, Gazdar AF et al: Detection and isolation of type-C retrovirus particles from fresh and cultured lymphocytes of a patient with cutaneous T-cell lymphoma. Proc Natl Acad Sci USA 77:7415, 1980

64. Quesada JR, Hersh EM, Gutterman JU: Hairy cell leukemia. Induction of remission with alpha interferon. Blood 62:207a, 1983

65. Reilly EB, Rappaport SI, Karr NW et al: Familial chronic lymphatic leukemia. Arch Intern Med 90:87, 1952

66. Rigby PG, Pratt PT, Rosenlof RC et al: Genetic relationships in familial leukemia and lymphoma. Arch Intern Med 121:67, 1968

67. Robbins BA, Ellison DJ, Spinosa JC et al: Diagnostic application of two-color flow cytometry in 161 cases of hairy cell leukemia. Blood 82:1277, 1993

68. Robert K-H, Gahrton G, Friberg K et al: Extra chromosome 12 and prognosis in chronic lymphocytic leukaemia. Scand J Haematol 28:163, 1982

69. Rosenthal MC, Pisciotta AV, Komninos ZD et al: The autoimmune hemolytic anemia of malignant lymphocytic disease. Blood 10:1978, 1955

70. Royston I, Majda JA, Baird SM et al: Human T-cell antigens defined by monoclonal antibodies: The 65000 dalton antigen of T cells (T65) is also found on chronic lymphocytic leukemia cells bearing surface immunoglobulin. J Immunol 125:275, 1980

71. Sadamori N, Han T, Block AW, Sandberg AA: Cytogenetic studies of stimulated lymphocytes in hairy cell leukemia. Cancer Genet Cytogenet 17:69, 1985

72. Sadamori N, Nishino K, Kusano M et al: Significance of chromosome 14 anomaly at band 14q11 in Japanese patients with adult T-cell leukemia. Cancer 58:2244, 1986

73. Sarfati M, Bron D, Lagneaux L et al: Elevation of IgE binding factors in serum of patients with B cell derived chronic lymphocytic leukemia. Blood 71:94, 1988

74. Saxon A, Stevens R, Golde D et al: T-lymphocyte variant of hairy cell leukemia. Ann Intern Med 88:323, 1978

75. Schrek R, Donnelly WJ: "Hairy" cells in blood in lymphoreticular neoplastic disease and "flagellated" cells of normal lymph. Blood 27:199, 1966

76. Schwartz RS, Costea N: Autoimmune hemolytic anemia: Clinical correlations and biological implications. Semin Haematol 3:2, 1966

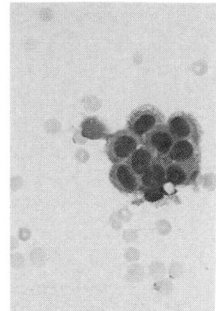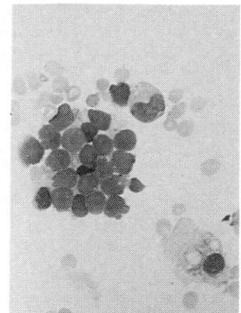

PLATE 30-1. (*Left*) Cluster of choroid plexus cells in CSF. (*Right*) Primitive cell cluster (PCC), of probable germinal matrix origin in CSF of premature infant. (*Courtesy of Diane Davey, M.D.*)

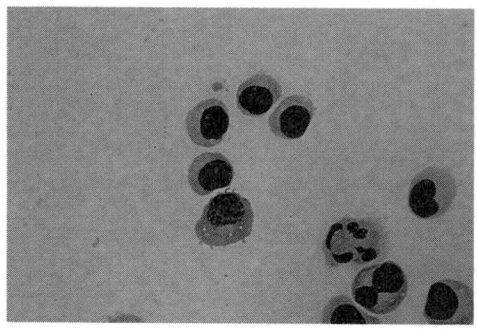

PLATE 30-2. A spectrum of reactive lymphocytes in meningitis. (*Courtesy of Diane Davey, M.D.*)

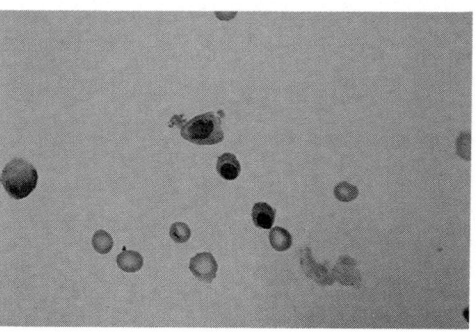

PLATE 30-3. Two pyknotic neutrophils resembling NRBCs in CSF. (*Courtesy of Diane Davey, M.D.*)

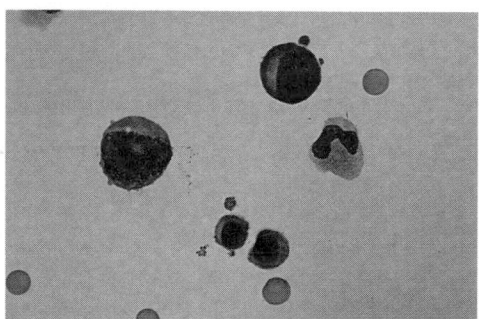

PLATE 30-4. Bone marrow contamination in CSF. (*Courtesy of Diane Davey, M.D.*)

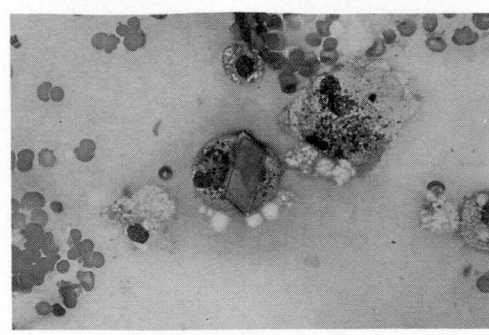

PLATE 30-5. Hematoidin crystal in a CSF macrophage. The other macrophage in the CSF contains hemosiderin (siderophage). (*Courtesy of Diane Davey, M.D.*)

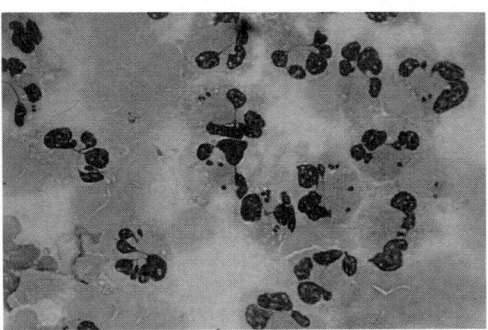

PLATE 30-6. Intracellular bacteria. Uniform size and pair formation differentiate bacteria from ingested cellular debris. (*Courtesy of Diane Davey, M.D.*)

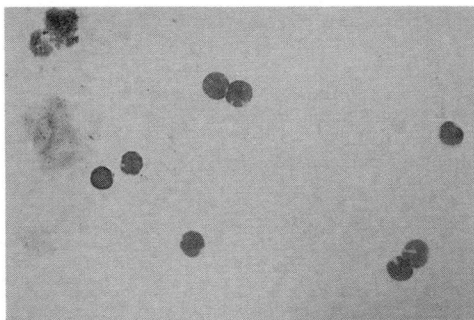

PLATE 30-7. Lymphoblasts in CSF in acute lymphoblastic leukemia (ALL). Note the characteristic scant cytoplasm, fine chromatin, and cleaved nuclei in a uniform population. (*Courtesy of Diane Davey, M.D.*)

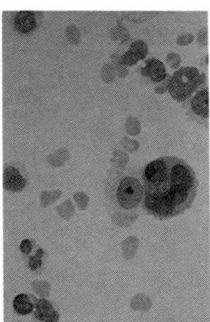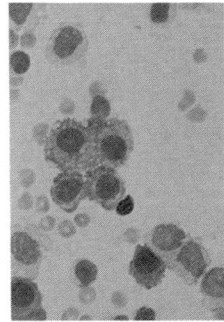

PLATE 30-8. (*Left*) Large, multinucleated mesothelial cell in serous fluid. (*Right*) Cluster of four mesothelial cells with "fried egg" appearance in serous fluid. (*Courtesy of Diane Davey, M.D.*)

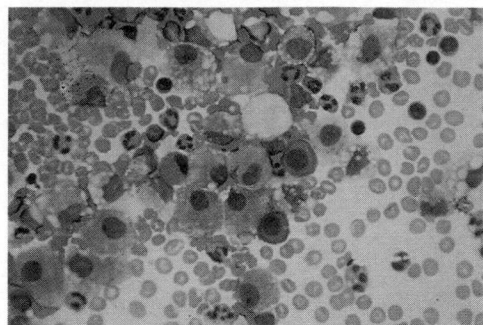

PLATE 30-9. Two mesothelial cells (large, dark blue) and numerous histiocytes (large, pale gray, some vacuolated) in serous fluid. (*Courtesy of Diane Davey, M.D.*)

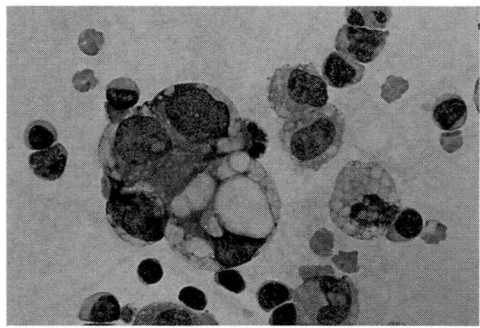

PLATE 30-10. Adenocarcinoma in peritoneal fluid. (*Courtesy of Diane Davey, M.D.*)

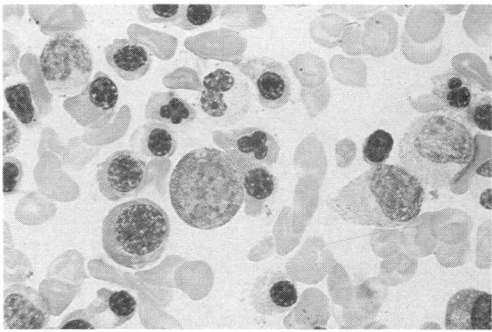

PLATE 33-1. Bone marrow from patient with refractory anemia. Note evidence of dyserythropoiesis, represented by multi lobed nucleated red cells (Wright stain; 1000×).

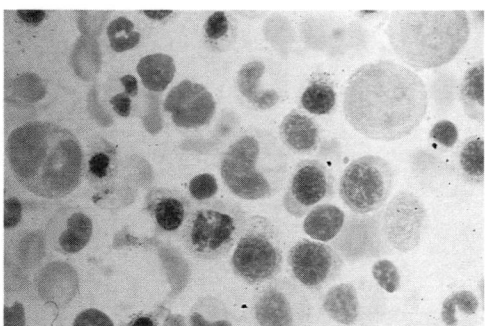

PLATE 33-2. Bone marrow from patient with refractory anemia with ringed sideroblasts (Prussian blue stain; 1000×). See also Color Plates 13-2 and 29-10.

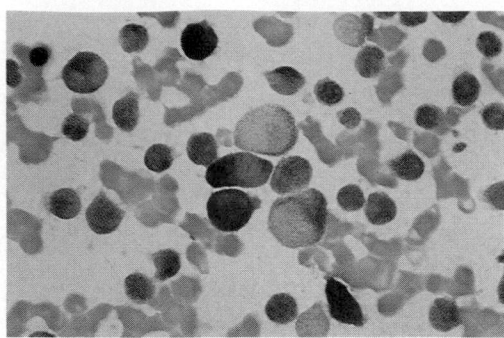

PLATE 33-3. Dual esterase stain. Blue reaction is chloroacetate esterase staining in neurophils or their precursors. Red staining represents butyrate esterase within monocytes and their precursors. (500×)

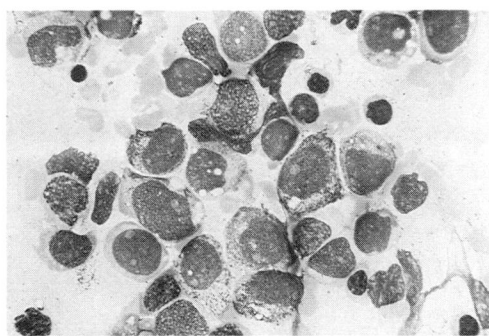

PLATE 33-4. Bone marrow from patient with refractory anemia with excess blasts in transformation. Note increased numbers of blast forms. (Wright stain; 1000×)

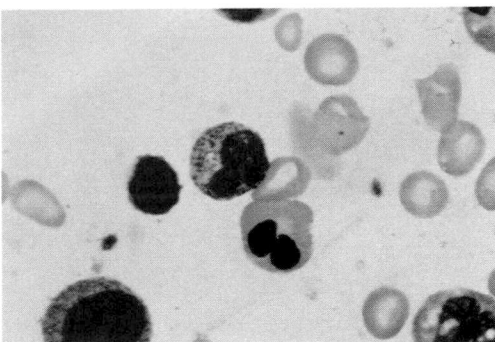

PLATE 33-5. Dyserythropoiesis caused by arsenic poisoning. Note the binucleated red cell. This patient was an elderly male who was initially thought to have refractory anemia. On further investigation, it was noted that he had abnormally high serum values for arsenic, and eventually it was determined that his wife had tried to poison him. (1000×)

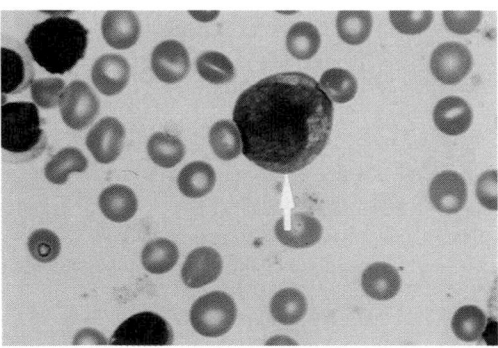

PLATE 33-6. Type I myeloblast (*arrow*). Note the smooth chromatin pattern and the presence of nucleoli. It is considered type I because of the lack of visible granules in the cytoplasm. See Color Plate 22-9 for another example of this cell. (1000×)

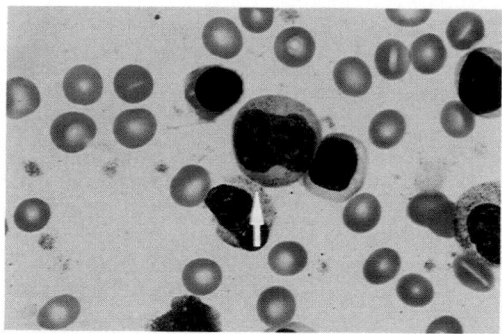

PLATE 33-7. Type II myeloblast (*arrow*). This cell is similar to the one in Color Plate 33-6, with the exception of the presence of a few primary granules visible in the cytoplasm. See Color Plate 22-10 for another example of this cell. (1000×)

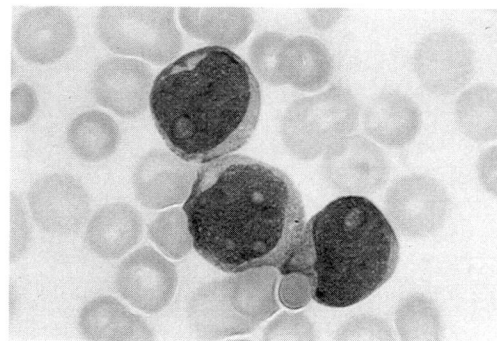

PLATE 34-1. M1 acute myelocytic leukemia without maturation. Blood film illustrates uniform population of type I blast cells. No cells with further granulocyte maturation are observed. (Wright stain; original magnification × 500)

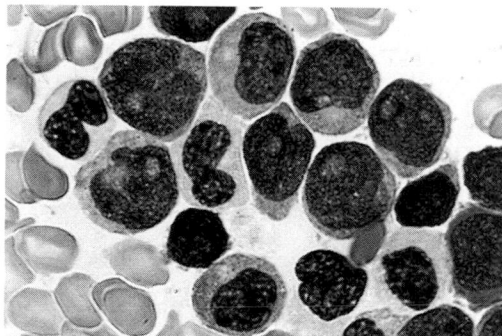

PLATE 34-2. M2 acute myelocytic leukemia with maturation. Bone marrow aspirate shows blasts and more differentiated granulocytic cells, including myelocytes, metamyelocyte, and neutrophil band cell. (Wright stain; original magnification × 500)

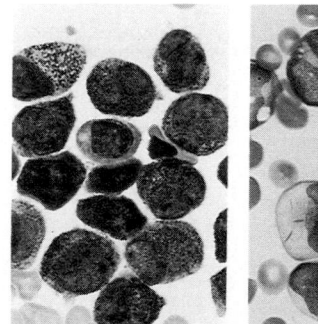
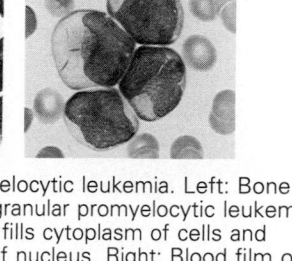

PLATE 34-3. M3 acute promyelocytic leukemia. Left: Bone marrow of patient with hypergranular promyelocytic leukemia. Note heavy granulation which fills cytoplasm of cells and sometimes obscures outline of nucleus. Right: Blood film of patient with microgranular variant of promyelocytic leukemia (M3m). Note that cells appear to be devoid of granules. Numerous Auer rods are present. (Wright stain; original magnification × 500)

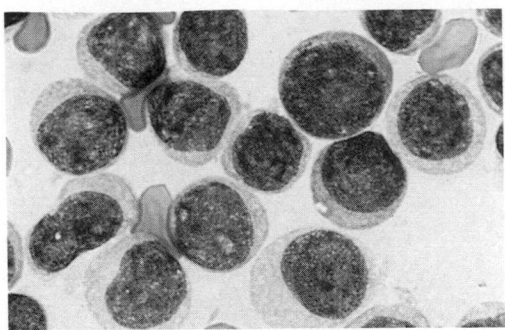

PLATE 34-4. M4 acute myelomonocytic leukemia. Bone marrow specimens stained with Wright stain such as this cannot differentiate adequately between abnormal granulocyte and monocyte precursors. Esterase stains are necessary. (Original magnification × 500)

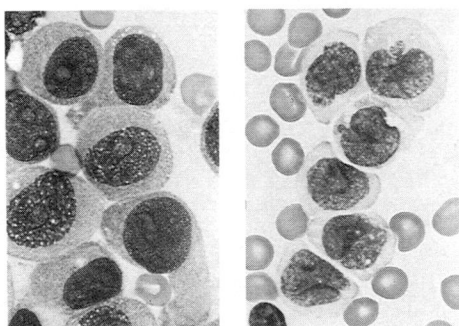

PLATE 34-5. M5 acute monocytic leukemia. (*Left*) Bone marrow from patient with poorly differentiated monoblastic leukemia (M5a). (*Right*) Peripheral blood from patient with differentiated monocytic leukemia (M5b). (Wright stain; original magnification × 500)

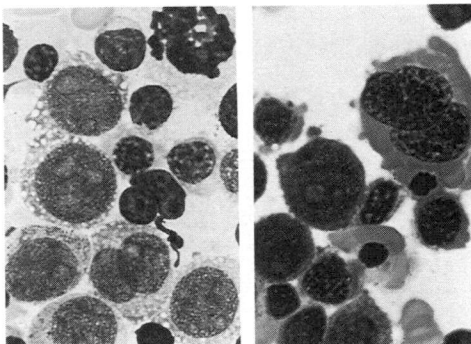

PLATE 34-6. M6 acute erythroleukemia. (*Left*) Bone marrow field illustrating highly vacuolated red cell precursors seen in some cases. (*Right*) This field is representative of bizarre, megaloblastoid red cell precursors characteristic of this leukemia. (Wright stain; original magnification × 500)

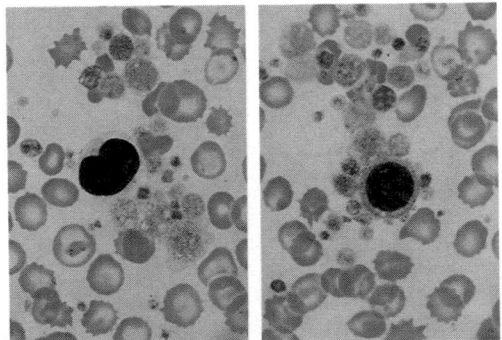

PLATE 34-7. M7 acute megakaryocytic leukemia. (*Left*) Abnormal micro (dwarf) megakaryocyte. Note the dense chromatin pattern. (*Right*) Cytoplasmic blebbing (source of abnormal giant platelets) that is commonly seen. (Wright stain; original magnification × 500)

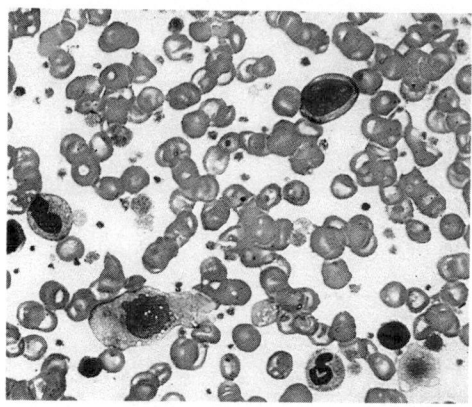

PLATE 35-1. Polycythemia vera in spent phase. Note micro-megakaryoblasts, myeloblasts, nucleated red blood cells and giant, bizarre platelets in the peripheral blood film. (Original magnification × 500)

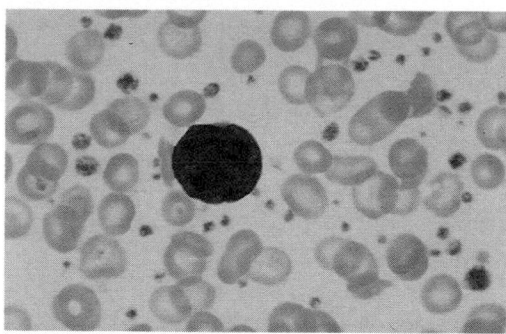

PLATE 35-2. Dwarf (micro) megakaryocyte. Note the density of the chromatin. This cell has only a small tag of visible cytoplasm; however, dwarf megakaryocytes may have more cytoplasm, and in some cases platelets may appear to be budding from the cytoplasm of the cell. (1000×)

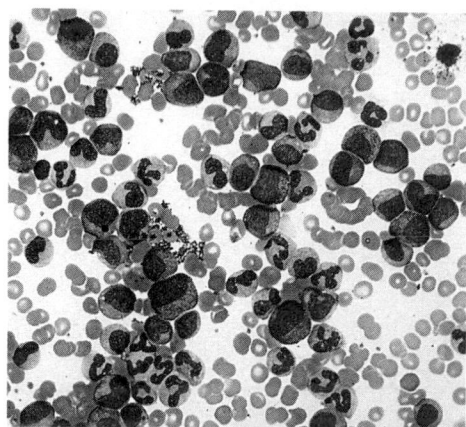

PLATE 35-3. Chronic myelogenous leukemia (CML). Note high leukocyte count and orderly left shift progression to blast in the peripheral blood film. (Original magnification × 500)

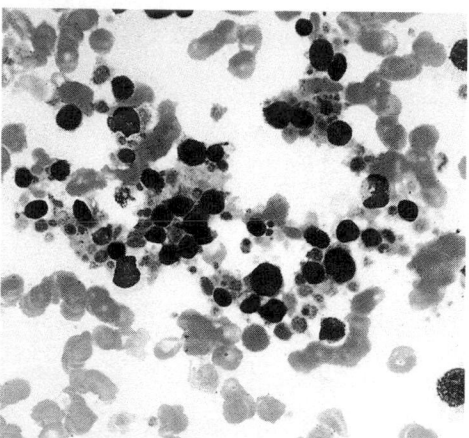

PLATE 35-4. Megakaryocytic leukemia. Megakaryocytic transformation of agnogenic myeloid metaplasia. Note multiple clumps of platelet-producing micromegakaryocytes in this peripheral blood film. (Original magnification × 500)

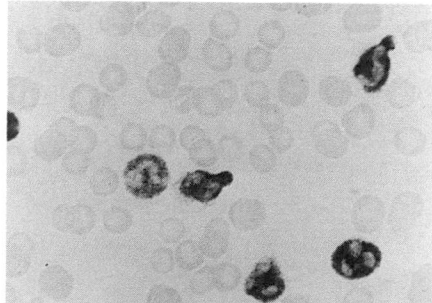

PLATE 35-5. Chronic neutrophilic leukemia (CNL). Peripheral blood film stained for leukocyte alkaline phosphatase (LAP). Note markedly increased LAP in neutrophils. (1000×)

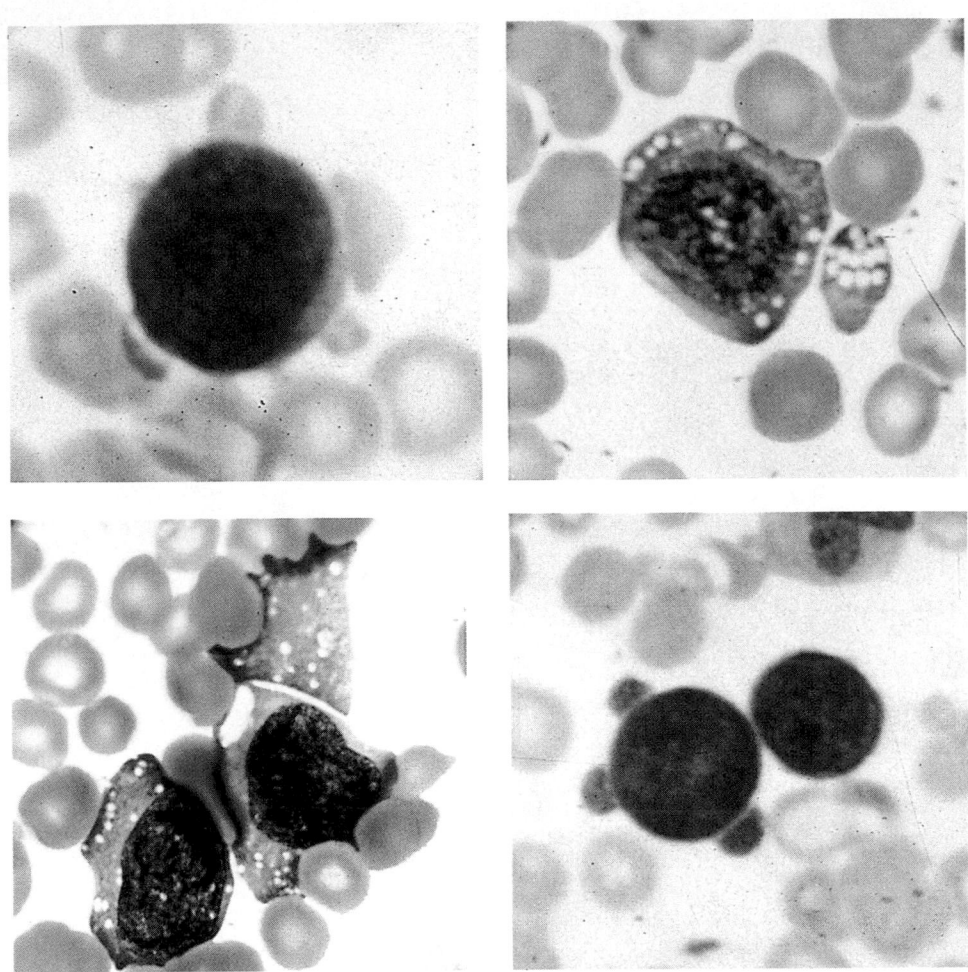

PLATE 35-6. Megakaryocytic blast transformation of CML. *(Top left)* Single micromegakaryocyte as evidenced by platelet blebs in cytoplasm. *(Top right)* Single megakaryoblast. Note the cytoplasmic fragment—a giant, abnormal platelet. *(Bottom left)* Two megakaryoblasts with a giant abnormal platelet. *(Bottom right)* Two micromegakaryoblasts. Note the platelet blebs. (1000×)

77. Seligmann M: A genetic predisposition to Waldenström's macroglobulinemia. Acta Med Scand Suppl 445:140, 1966

78. Stathopoulos G, Elliot EV: Formation of mouse or sheep red blood cell rosette by lymphocytes from normal and leukemic individuals. Lancet 1:229, 1974

79. Tedeschi LG, Lansinger DT: Sézary syndrome: A malignant leukemic reticuloendotheliosis. Arch Dermatol 92:257, 1965

80. Ternynck T, Dighiero D, Follezou JY, Binet JL: Comparison of normal and CLL lymphocytes surface Ig determinants using peroxidase labeled antibodies. I. Detection and quantitation of light chain determinants. Blood 43:789, 1974

81. Ueshima Y, Bird ML, Vardiman JW et al: A 14;19 translocation in B-cell chronic lymphocytic leukemia: A new recurring chromosome aberration. Int J Cancer 36:287, 1985

82. Visser L, Shaw A, Slupsky J et al: Monoclonal antibodies reactive with hairy cell leukemia. Blood 74:320, 1989

83. Wang CH, Good RA, Ammirak P et al: Identification of a p69,71 complex expressed on human T cells sharing determinants with B type chronic lymphatic leukemic cells. J Exp Med 151:1539, 1980

84. Westbrook CA, Golde DW: Clinical problems in hairy cell leukemia: Diagnosis and management. Semin Oncol 11:514, 1984

85. Williams WJ, Beutler E, Erslev AJ et al (eds): Hematology, 4th ed. New York, McGraw-Hill, 1990

86. Wintrobe MM, Lee GR, Boggs DR et al (eds): Clinical Hematology, 8th ed. Philadelphia, Lea & Febiger, 1981

87. Wolf JK: Primary acquired agammaglobulinemia with a family history of collagen disease and haematological disorders. N Engl J Med 266:473, 1962

88. Young LE, Miller G, Christian RM: Clinical and laboratory observations on auto-immune hemolytic disease. Ann Intern Med 35:507, 1951

89. Zuegler WW, Mastrangelo R, Stulberg CS et al: Autoimmune hemolytic anemia: Natural history and viral immunologic interactions in childhood. Am J Med 49:80, 1970

CHAPTER 38

The Lymphomas

Charles E. Manner

Objectives

1. Define the two principal classifications of lymphoma.
2. List the major clinical and laboratory findings in Hodgkin disease (HD) and non-Hodgkin lymphoma (NHL).
3. Describe the Reed-Sternberg cell, and state the type of specimen in which it is most frequently found.
4. Describe abnormal characteristics of lymphocytes in lymph node biopsies from NHL.
5. Summarize the effects of treatment on hematologic and chemical tests in HD and NHL.
6. Define mycosis fungoides and Sézary syndrome, and describe the peripheral blood cell that is pathognomonic for these disorders.

The lymphomas are a group of malignant diseases that originate from the uninhibited growth of cellular elements normally found in lymphatic tissue. The term "lymphoma" emphasizes the fact that the hallmark of these disorders is abnormal lymph node enlargement, with disruption or replacement of the normal histologic architecture. Although other malignant lymphoproliferative disorders such as acute lymphoblastic leukemia (Chap. 36) and plasma cell dyscrasias (Chap. 39) cause diffuse infiltration of the lymph nodes, the histologic structure of the nodes is still evident. Chronic lymphocytic leukemia can share with the lymphomas the feature of nodal involvement, but lymphomas ordinarily do not have peripheral blood involvement (*i.e.*, abnormal circulating cells) until late in the disease.

PRINCIPAL CLASSIFICATIONS OF LYMPHOMA

Lymphomas have traditionally been divided into two classes: Hodgkin disease (HD) and non-Hodgkin lymphomas (NHL). The cellular infiltrate in the lymph nodes of HD is much more variable or pleomorphic than it is in NHL. Many of the cells in nodes affected by HD are normal in appearance, and only a minor population of cells have neoplastic (*i.e.*, malignant) features.[10] In contrast, the infiltrates of NHL are more uniformly composed of similar-appearing neoplastic cells. To emphasize this distinction, the term "Hodgkin *disease*" is preferred to "Hodgkin *lymphoma*."

In NHL, the B lymphocyte is the neoplastic cell in roughly 95% of the cases; the T lymphocyte is the neoplastic cell in the remaining 5%.[38] In HD, the neoplastic cell generally is considered to be a multinucleated giant cell of distinctive appearance known as the *Reed-Sternberg cell*[29] (Fig. 38-1).

Diagnosis of the lymphomas is based on histologic examination of lymph node tissues. Hodgkin disease and NHL have been further subdivided into subtypes of distinctive histologic appearance, which will be addressed in this chapter. In the case of NHL, the histologic subclass has a much stronger bearing on the biologic behavior of the malignancy, and hence on patient prognosis, than is the case for HD.

Hodgkin disease probably is unifocal in origin. In other words, it starts in one lymph node group and spreads in a predictable fashion to adjacent lymph nodes; in very advanced cases, nonlymphatic tissue can be involved.[41] Non-Hodgkin lymphoma spreads in a much less predictable way. If NHL is ever unifocal, it remains so only briefly, as only 10% of patients present with truly localized disease.[6] Rather, the typical patient with NHL presents with involvement of multiple lymph node groups, which can be noncontiguous. Non-Hodgkin lymphoma also involves nonlymphatic tissue more commonly than does HD. Because of the more predictable biologic behavior of HD compared with NHL, the disease stage (a measure of disease extent) is more important prognostically for HD than for NHL.

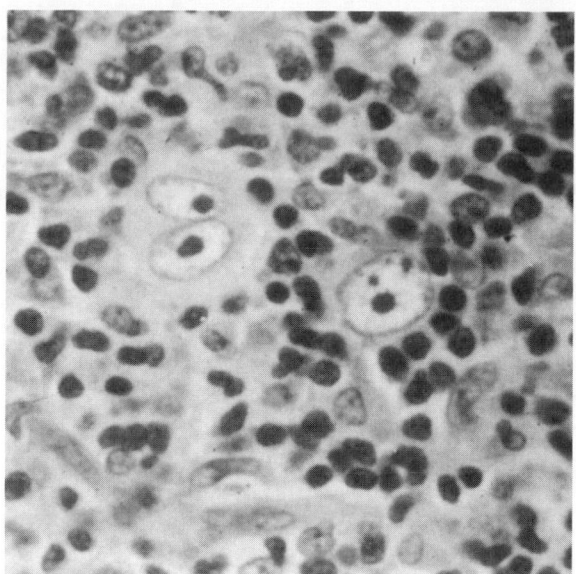

FIGURE 38-1. Characteristic Reed-Sternberg cell and mononuclear variant of Hodgkin disease (hematoxylin and eosin, magnification × 400). (From DeVita VT Jr, Hellman S, Rosenberg SA: Cancer Principles and Practice of Oncology, 3rd ed. Philadelphia, JB Lippincott, 1989, with permission.)

HODGKIN DISEASE

History

In 1832 Thomas Hodgkin first described the disease that bears his name.[23] The compound microscope and the histologic methods required to distinguish this disease from other causes of chronic lymph node enlargement were unavailable to Hodgkin. Full appreciation of the histologic features of HD and its characteristic giant cells did not come until the independent publications of Carl Sternberg in 1898[51] and Reed in 1902.[44] From the 1940s to the 1960s, various histologic classifications of HD were proposed. The four-part system in use today was agreed on at a symposium held in Rye, New York, in 1966.[36]

Epidemiology

The cause of HD, as is the case for many neoplasms, is unknown. A number of epidemiologic studies have proposed genetic influences,[18] exposures to environmental hazards,[19] or an infectious agent such as Epstein-Barr virus[39] as part of the pathogenesis. However, none of these hypotheses has been proven.

Taken together, HD and NHL are the seventh most common cause of death from cancer in the United States. Hodgkin disease accounts for roughly 25% of the cases, with NHL making up the remainder.[11] In economically developed countries, HD has a unique bimodal incidence curve.[37] The incidence begins to rise after the age of 10 years and peaks in the 20s, then declines to age 45, after which the incidence rises steadily with advancing age, as it does for NHL. Hodgkin disease is more common in men than in women, with a sex ratio of 3:2.[57]

Clinical Features

The most common presentation of HD is a painless enlarging lymph node, usually in the neck. In some cases, a routine chest radiograph discloses a mediastinal mass (one in the intervening space between the right and left lungs). Further examination may reveal enlarged cervical nodes. Occasionally, rapid enlargement of lymph nodes creates a painful mass.

The more ominous symptoms are fever, night sweats, or weight loss, or a combination thereof, which are referred to as the "B" symptoms. Such symptoms are important in disease staging. The stages of HD and NHL (discussed later in this chapter) can be denoted with the suffix "A" to indicate that the patient has no symptoms or "B" to indicate that the patient has one or more of the B symptoms. For example, Stage IVB is the most advanced stage of HD, the B denoting that the patient is suffering from one or more of the classic symptoms.

Over the course of weeks to months, the involved lymph nodes continue to enlarge. The disease spreads in an orderly fashion to adjacent lymph node chains. This orderliness of spread is reflected in the HD staging system (discussed below). In advanced cases, nonlymphatic tissue can be involved, presumably by metastases via the peripheral blood. Untreated patients die from recurrent infections or organ failure within a year or two of the onset of illness.

Laboratory Findings and Correlations with Disease

The only definitive test for HD is the lymph node biopsy. Other laboratory abnormalities are often nonspecific.

PERIPHERAL BLOOD

Early in the course of the disease, there may be an absolute increase in monocytes and eosinophils. Usually, there is no anemia, and platelets are normal in number. A transitory increase in lymphocytes may be noted. The blood film may show large, abnormal-appearing lymphocytes, which have very little cytoplasm and irregular nuclear chromatin.[54]

As the disease progresses, there often is a leukocytosis. Granulocytosis occurs in roughly 25% of patients, usually in the more advanced stages. In some cases, this change is extreme and mimics leukemia ("leukemoid reaction") (Chap. 25). Peripheral blood lymphocytopenia may develop with almost the same frequency as granulocytosis. Lymphocytopenia is a sign of a poor prognosis, as it is associated with advances stages of disease and with histologic subtypes that have poor prognoses.[53]

In advanced disease, granulocytes often display toxic granulation. The disease process may cause the production of large, bizarre platelets observable on the blood film.[4]

Plasma cells sometimes are observed on the peripheral blood film,[8] as, rarely, are Reed-Sternberg cells[48] (see Diagnostic Evaluation of Lymph Node Biopsy). Occasionally, another large (40 μm diameter) abnormal-appearing cell is seen.[20] It has moderately basophilic cytoplasm, and its nucleus is oval or lobulated with fine, reticular chromatin and one or more large nucleoli. Nonspecific abnormalities such as large monocytes with large vacuoles and large lymphocytes with deeply basophilic cytoplasm may also be seen on the blood film or on specially prepared leukocyte concentrate films.[21,22,48] It should be noted, however, that such abnormal cells may be associated with a number of other diseases such as viral infections.

Normochromic, normocytic anemia is a presenting feature in about 10% of patients.[7,54] Typically, the reticulocyte count is normal or low.

BONE MARROW

The bone marrow is seldom involved except in advanced (Stage IV) disease. Typically, films of the marrow aspirate are negative, and only the biopsy reveals disease, which usually is accompanied by marrow fibrosis. Even in positive marrows, the histologic class often cannot be determined, and it may not be possible to distinguish the condition from NHL. Again, the definitive diagnosis of HD depends on the lymph node biopsy.

OTHER LABORATORY FINDINGS

Commonly, the serum iron and total iron-binding capacity (TIBC) are reduced. These features, along with the anemia found in 10% of patients, are typical of the anemia associated with chronic disease (Chap. 13).[7,54] Rarely, the direct antiglobulin test (DAT) is positive, signifying a hemolytic component to the anemia.[34]

A variety of other laboratory abnormalities correlate with disease activity but are entirely nonspecific. These include elevations of the erythrocyte sedimentation rate, fibrinogen, haptoglobin, serum globulins, ceruloplasmin, and copper. Similarly, a number of serum enzymes have been reported to be elevated, including leukocyte alkaline phosphatase, lysozyme, lactic acid dehydrogenase (LD), and transaminases.[43]

Hyperuricemia may be found because of excess cell turnover. More importantly, with successful therapy, rapid tumor lysis may cause a marked increase in uric acid production with urate crystal deposition in the kidney tubules and urinary tract. Acute renal failure can result unless preventative measures are taken.

Diagnostic Evaluation of Lymph Node Biopsy: The Reed-Sternberg Cell

The diagnosis and classification of HD can be made only by lymph node biopsy (Fig. 38-2). The essential feature confirming the diagnosis is the presence of the Reed-Sternberg giant cell (see Fig. 38-1) in affected lymph nodes. This is a large cell, generally four to eight times the size of normal surrounding lymphocytes. It can be multinucleated or binucleated or may contain a single bilobed nucleus. Most often, the cell is binucleated with the two halves of the cell appearing as mirror images. The nuclear membrane is thick and well demarcated. The nucleoli are large and eosinophilic with a distinct halo, giving the cell what is typically referred to as an owl-eyed appearance (see Color Plate 55-14). Around the

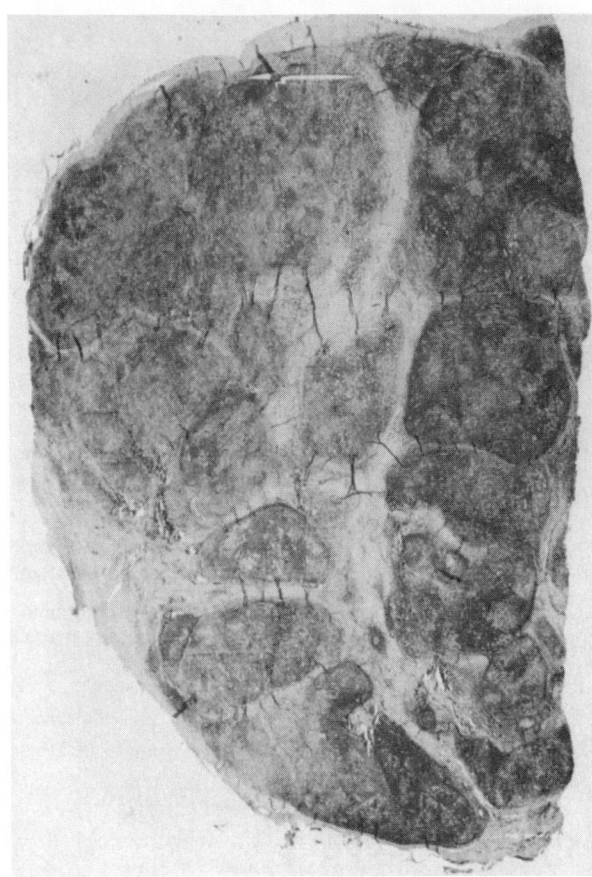

FIGURE 38-2. Lymph node, nodular sclerosing Hodgkin disease. Cellular nodules are surrounded by dense fibrous bands (hematoxylin and eosin, magnification × 8). (From DeVita VT Jr, Hellman S, Rosenberg SA: Cancer Principles and Practice of Oncology, 3rd ed. Philadelphia, JB Lippincott, 1989, with permission.)

nucleus is an abundant cytoplasm of amorphous consistency with a slight eosinophilia.

Immunohistologic techniques involving monoclonal antibodies have come into increasing use in the identification and classification of lymphomas.[40] The recent ability to isolate and even culture Reed-Sternberg cells from pathologic materials has made immunohistologic techniques even more useful in identifying HD.[49]

Table 38-1 profiles the antigenic and enzyme phenotype of the Reed-Sternberg cell. An understanding of the profile provides insight into the origin of this cell. It is apparent that the Reed-Sternberg cell has some features in common with monocytes and T and B lymphocytes. On the other hand, it distinctly lacks some antigens found on other T or B cells. It is no wonder, then, that the origin of the Reed-Sternberg cell has been a matter of controversy! It may be more practical to consider the Reed-Sternberg cell as a malignant cell with aberrant genetic expression that has no true counterpart among normal cells of the immune system.

Classification

RYE CLASSIFICATION

Hodgkin disease usually is classified into four histologic groups, as first proposed at the Rye Conference in 1965

TABLE 38-1
Immunohistologic Phenotype of Reed-Sternberg (RS) Cell

Antigenic Property Tested*	RS Cell Reaction	Other Cells Demonstrating the Property	Comments on Antigenic Property	References
CD15 (Leu M1)	+	Monocytes, granulocytes	Antigen	24
Fc receptors	+	B and T lymphocytes, monocytes	Receptors for Fc portion of immunoglobulins	29
C3 receptors	+	B and T lymphocytes, monocytes	Receptors for C3, the third component of complement	29
Ia†	+	B lymphocytes, monocytes, activated T lymphocytes	Immune response antigen	52
HLA-DR	+	B lymphocytes, monocytes, activated T lymphocytes	Major histocompatibility complex (MHC) Class II antigen	25, 52
CD25 (Tac)‡	±	T lymphocytes, monocytes, B lymphocytes	Receptor for the lymphokine interleukin-2 (IL-2)	25, 50
cIg	+	B lymphocytes	Cytoplasmic immunoglobulin	49
sIg	+	B lymphocytes	Surface immunoglobulin	49
CD20 (B1)	±	Immature B lymphocytes, B-cell malignancies	Antigen	50
CD19 (B4)	±	Immature B lymphocytes, B-cell malignancies	Antigen	50
CD22 (Leu 14)	−	B lymphocytes	Antigen found on 95% of B lymphocytes	50
CD3 (OKT3)	±	T lymphocytes	Antigen found on all T lymphocytes	50
Lysozyme	+	Monocytes, granulocytes	Enzyme	29
Esterase	+	Monocytes, granulocytes	Enzyme	28

* Note that antigen properties have been grouped according to common cell types with which they are associated. Where appropriate, the new cluster designation (CD) is given; these designations were established by an international panel and reflect reactivity with similar monoclonal antibodies.

† Ia is most abundant on B lymphocytes but can be found on monocytes and activated T lymphocytes.

‡ Tac is predominant on T lymphocytes but can be found on monocytes and B lymphocytes.

(Table 38-2).[32,35,36] The classification is based primarily on the extent of lymphocyte infiltration and the abundance of Reed-Sternberg cells. Even apart from disease stage, the histologic class correlates with prognosis: the lymphocyte-predominant class has the best outlook, whereas the lymphocyte-depleted class has the worst. Part of the relation of histologic class to prognosis has to do with the age of the patient and the stage of disease at the time of diagnosis. Younger patients and patients with earlier stages clearly do better, and these clinical features are seen in the two best prognostic patterns: lymphocyte predominant and nodular sclerosis.

ANN ARBOR STAGING SYSTEM

Hodgkin disease has a universally accepted staging system that was delineated at the Ann Arbor Conference in 1971.[5] The only modification that has been made to this

TABLE 38-2
Rye Classification of Hodgkin Disease

Pattern	Description	Reed-Sternberg (RS) Cells	Percent of Total Cases	Patient Age	5-Year Survival (%)
Lymphocyte predominant	Diffuse pattern of abundant lymphocytes; sparse granulocytes and plasma cells. No fibrosis	Scarce	5–10	Young	95
Nodular sclerosis	Nodularity with birefringent collagen bands; moderate lymphocytes, granulocytes, and plasma cells; RS cells sit in clear zones (lacunar RS cells)	Occasional	35–65	Young	85
Mixed cellularity	Moderate lymphocytes, granulocytes, and plasma cells in diffuse pattern	Many	20–40	Middle-aged to elderly	65
Lymphocyte depleted	Diffuse fibrosis with few lymphocytes	Abundant	1–5	Middle-aged to elderly	20

TABLE 38-3
Modified Ann Arbor Staging System for Hodgkin Disease and Non-Hodgkin Lymphoma*

Stage	Description
I	Involvement of a single lymph node region (Stage I) OR Involvement of a single extralymphatic organ or site (Stage I$_E$)
II	Involvement of two or more lymph node regions on the same side of the diaphragm alone (Stage II) OR With involvement of a contiguous extralymphatic organ or site (Stage II$_E$)
III	Involvement of lymph node regions on both sides of the diaphragm (Stage III). Stage III$_S$ indicates splenic involvement; Stage III$_E$ indicates involvement of an extralymphatic organ or site; Stage III$_{SE}$ indicates involvement of both spleen and an extralymphatic organ or site III$_1$ Abdominal disease limited to the upper abdomen, spleen, splenic hilar nodes, celiac nodes, or porta hepatis nodes III$_2$ Abdominal disease including para-aortic, mesenteric, iliac, or inguinal involvement with or without involvement of upper abdomen
IV	Diffuse involvement of one or more extralymphatic organs or sites not contiguous with lymphatic tissue

* Any stage can be given the additional suffix letters A or B or subscript letters E or S: A, no symptoms present; B, fever over 100.4°F, night sweats, or 10% weight loss in the preceding 6 months; E, extralymphatic involvement; S, splenic involvement.

scheme since 1971 has been a further breakdown of Stage III into Stage III$_1$ and Stage III$_2$. Stage III$_1$ represents disease confined to the upper abdomen above the renal artery. Stage III$_2$ signifies disease below this structure.[9] Table 38-3 outlines the modified Ann Arbor Staging System.

Stages may be given the additional suffix letters A or B. Suffix A denotes no symptoms. Suffix B indicates the presence of symptoms, specifically fever greater than 100.4°F, night sweats, or unexplained loss of 10% or more of body weight occurring within the preceding 6 months. Each stage also may be given a subscript of either E or S. Subscript E designates extralymphatic disease and S, splenic involvement (see Table 38-3).

One of the difficulties that can present when using this system is distinguishing either Stages II$_E$ or III$_E$ from Stage IV when a patient has only one extralymphatic site involved. Generally patients are classified as having E disease if the extent of the disease is limited enough that radiation therapy can most likely cure the patient. If this is not the case, the patient is considered to be in Stage IV.

Diagnosis and Treatment

Proper staging is essential for formulating the best treatment plan for a patient, as well as for evaluating the success of that treatment on followup examinations. The diagnostic methods employed are a mixture of clinical and pathologic methods (Tables 38-4 and 38-5). Implicit in the division of these tables is the fact that not every test needs to be done in each patient to stage the disease and plan treatment properly. The one fundamental principle that guides the use of diagnostic tests in a particular patient is that a procedure should be done if detection of disease by that method would change the stage assignment and therefore the treatment plan.

Effects of Treatment on Laboratory Results

Table 38-6 summarizes the treatments of choice for the various stages of HD according to the modified Ann Arbor staging system. It also lists their approximate cure rates.[13]

PHYSICAL EFFECTS

Effective therapy can dramatically reduce bulky adenopathy in a matter of days to weeks. Some patients will have no clinical evidence of disease within a month or so.

TABLE 38-4
Staging Procedures Essential in Hodgkin Disease and Non-Hodgkin Lymphomas Diagnosis

Thorough history and physical examination
Adequate surgical biospy reviewed by a hematopathologist
Routine laboratory tests
    CBC including platelet count
    Erythrocyte sedimentation rate
    Serum alkaline phosphatase
    Liver function tests
    Serum uric acid
    Blood urea nitrogen (BUN)
    Serum creatinine
Chest radiograph (posteroanterior and lateral views)
Bilateral core biopsy of marrow from posterior iliac crests
Bilateral lower extremity lymphangiogram
Computed tomographic (CT) scan of abdomen or equivalent study
Needle aspiration biopsy or surgical biopsy of any suspect extranodal lesions
Cytologic examination of any pleural effusion

Bone scan with plain skeletal radiographs of suspect areas
Laparoscopy and biopsies
Liver biopsy
Staging laparotomy and splenectomy
Intravenous pyelography
Radionuclide liver–spleen scan
Whole-body gallium-67 scan
CT scans of thorax

HEMATOLOGIC EFFECTS

Both radiation and chemotherapy are myelosuppressive. Thus, the main effect of treatment on laboratory values is reflected in the CBC. Generally, the effect of radiation in terms of myelosuppression depends on the size of the field treated. Treatment of the disease at an early stage, with radiation limited to the chest, neck, and upper thorax (the area known as a "mantle field") has a much milder effect on blood counts than does the total nodal radiation used in the treatment of intermediate stages of disease.

Combination chemotherapy has the most profound effect on blood counts, particularly the granulocyte and platelet counts. Generally, the lowest counts occur 10 to 15 days after the start of therapy. Granulocytopenia, often with absolute counts in the 0.5 to 1.0 $\times$ 10^9/L range (approximate reference range 1.8 to 7.7 $\times$ 10^9/L), is common. Platelet counts between 50 and 100 $\times$ 10^9/L are frequently seen; platelet counts below 20 $\times$ 10^9/L can be associated with spontaneous hemorrhage, which can be life-threatening, and usually are an indication for platelet transfusion. Depending on the regimen of chemotherapy used, recovery of granulocyte and platelet counts occurs by day 21 to 28 of the cycle, at which time more chemotherapy is given. Generally, the return of granulocyte counts to normal is heralded by a relative monocytosis 3 to 5 days earlier.

Because the erythrocyte is a much longer-lived cell than the granulocyte or platelet, the temperary cessation of production secondary to chemotherapy does not cause a significant decrease in erythrocytes during a single course of therapy. However, with repeated treatments, it is not unusual for patients to develop anemia severe enough to necessitate red cell transfusions. On achievement of remission of lymphoma and completion of chemotherapy or radiation therapy, the complete blood count returns to and remains normal.

CHEMICAL EFFECTS

Rapid tumor lysis by chemotherapy or radiation or both results in a release of intracellular substances such as uric acid, phosphate, and potassium, which can cause metabolic abnormalities (hyperuricemia, hyperphosphatemia, and hyperkalemia). High serum phosphate levels can lead to hypocalcemia because of precipitation of calcium phosphate salts. Renal failure, with elevated BUN and serum creatinine, can ensue because of uric acid and calcium phosphate deposition in the renal tubules. Management of this problem is preventive, with forced fluids, urine alkalization with bicarbonate, and blockage of uric acid production with allopurinol.

TABLE 38-6
Treatments of Choice for Hodgkin Disease by Stage and Approximate Cure Rates

Stage (Ann Arbor System)	Treatment of Choice	Approximate Cure Rate (%)	Comments
IA, IB, IIA	Radiotherapy	85–90	Early stages of disease respond well to radiotherapy alone (*i.e.*, chemotherapy is not needed)
IIIB, IVA, IVB	Combination chemotherapy	80	Using modern aggressive chemotherapy regimens, 55% to 70% of all patients with advanced disease can expect to be free of disease 5 years after diagnosis
IIB, IIIA$_1$, IIIA$_2$	Radiation alone or radiation plus chemotherapy	65–75	Radiation alone is associated with a higher relapse rate than that found in Stages IA, IB, and IIA. Chemotherapy is valuable in relapsing patients

From Fisher RI: Hodgkin's disease. In Wittes RE (ed): Manual of Oncologic Therapeutics 1989/1990, pp 370–373. Philadelphia, JB Lippincott, 1989.

NON-HODGKIN LYMPHOMAS

History

A few decades after the work of Thomas Hodgkin, Rudolph Virchow, the great pathologist, recognized the lymphomas.[55] Enlarging on his knowledge of leukemias, Virchow divided the lymphomas into two types: leukemic and aleukemic. The aleukemic lymphoma was called *lymphosarcoma*. This term was used by others in the latter part of the 19th century and came ultimately to designate a separate lymphoma subtype once specific histologic types were described.

The first comprehensive classification system for lymphomas was introduced by Gall and Mallory in 1942.[15] The true forerunner of modern schemes in use today was described by Rappaport and coworkers in 1956.[42] This system had two criteria, which are still in use in classifying lymphomas: the presence or absence of nodularity and the size of the cell involved in the infiltrates. This system was simple and prognostically relevant. Several other systems have been proposed to reflect our growing knowledge of lymphocytes and the origin of lymphomas. The most recent, the International Working Classification of Non-Hodgkin's Lymphomas, was proposed in 1982.[46]

Epidemiology

In the United States, NHL is three times as common as HD, with about 25,000 new cases diagnosed annually.[11] The incidence rises steadily with age starting around age 40. Non-Hodgkin lymphoma, like HD, is more common in men than in women, with a ratio of 3:2.

Congenital immunodeficiency diseases such as ataxia telangiectasia, the Wiskott-Aldrich syndrome, IgA deficiency, common variable immunodeficiency, and severe combined immunodeficiency have been associated with a 10,000-fold increase in the risk of developing cancer, of which the vast majority are NHL.[16] Acquired conditions of immune dysfunction also have been associated with an increased predisposition to NHL. Rhematoid arthritis, Sjögren's syndrome, and systemic lupus erythematosus are rheumatologic conditions associated with a 3- to 40-fold increase in the risk of lymphoma.[26,31,56] Organ transplant recipients taking immunosuppressive drugs to prevent graft rejection have a 40- to 100-fold increase in the risk of lymphoma.[33] This predisposed presentation is shared by the lymphoma associated with acquired immunodeficiency syndrome (AIDS).[17]

Viral agents may also be related to the development of NHL. The Epstein-Barr virus, the etiologic agent of infectious mononucleosis, which infects B lymphocytes, has been closely linked to the development of African Burkitt lymphoma (see below for definitions),[30] a form of small noncleaved-cell lymphoma. Human T-cell lymphocytotrophic virus (HTLV-1), a retrovirus that infects helper T cells, has been closely associated with the development of acute T-cell leukemia and lymphoma.[1]

One must recognize that for every virus-infected individual who has lymphoma, there are many more infected persons who do not develop lymphoma. Thus, any hypothesis of a viral etiology of lymphoma must invoke cocarcinogens. In summary, the exact etiology of NHL remains unknown.

Physical Findings

Painless lymph node enlargement is the most common presenting symptom. The cervical nodes are most often involved.

Symptoms

Systemic symptoms such as fever, weight loss, and night sweats are reported by approximately 30% of patients, particularly those with diffuse histologic patterns and advanced stages. It is more common for patients with NHL to present with more advanced stages (III or IV) than is the case in HD.

Laboratory Findings and Correlations with Disease

Blood counts are normal in most patients with NHL, even in those cases in which the bone marrow is involved.[47] Other laboratory findings often depend on the classification of the lymphoma (see next section for classifications). Some patients with small-cell or follicular lymphomas have a positive direct antiglobulin test and occasionally a consequent autoimmune hemolytic anemia. Sometimes, an autoimmune thrombocytopenia occurs as well.[27] Leukemic phases of disease can be seen with diffuse small-cell lymphocytic lymphoma and in lymphoblastic lymphoma.[14]

Serum chemistry abnormalities such as alkaline phosphatase, LD, and uric acid, as discussed for HD, may also occur in NHL.

Classification

The clinical pace of NHL depends heavily on the histologic pattern. In this regard, the histologic subtypes that make up the International Working Classification can be divided into three groups, ranked according to their aggressiveness as low, intermediate, and high (Table 38-7).

LOW GRADE

The low-grade lymphomas typically affect patients between the ages of 45 and 60 years. These are slow-growing lymphomas, and lymph node enlargement can be present for years before diagnosis. Often, patients can do well without treatment for 2 to 3 years. Most disease is in Stage III or IV at the time of diagnosis. Although the bone marrow frequently is involved, the peripheral blood often is normal. The median survival ranges from 5 to 7 years. In approximately 30% of these patients, the disease evolves into a diffuse large-cell lymphoma, which worsens the prognosis.[45]

INTERMEDIATE GRADE

The intermediate-grade lymphomas, like the low-grade varieties, affect individuals in later middle age. Patients present with a much more rapid lymph node enlarge-

TABLE 38-7
International Working Classification of Non-Hodgkin Lymphoma

Grade	Lymphoma Type	Mitoses in Microscopic Fields	Patient Median Age (Years)	Percent of Cases with Bone Marrow Involvement	Survival Median (Years)	Survival 5 Year (%)
Low	Small lymphocytic	Rare	60	71	5.8	59
	Follicular, small cleaved cell	Infrequent	54	51	7.2	70
	Follicular, mixed (small cleaved and large cells)	Infrequent	56	30	5.1	50
	Follicular, large cell	Usually numerous	55	34	3.0	45
	Diffuse, small cleaved cell	Variable	58	32	3.4	33
Intermediate	Diffuse, mixed (small cleaved and large cell)	Few to moderate	58	14	2.7	38
	Diffuse, large cell	Moderate	57	10	1.5	35
High	Immunoblastic (large cell)	Moderate	51	12	1.3	32
	Lymphoblastic	Numerous	17	50	2.0	26
	Small noncleaved cell (Burkitt and non-Burkitt types)	Numerous	30	14	0.7	23

From Rosenberg SA, Berard CW, Brown BW et al: National Cancer Institute sponsored study of classification of non-Hodgkin's lymphomas: Summary and description of a working formulation for clinical usage. Cancer 49:2112, 1982.

ment, and extranodal disease is more common. The only exception to this is the bone marrow, which is much less frequently involved than is the case in the low-grade lymphomas. Median survival ranges from 1.5 to about 3 years, although diffuse large-cell lymphoma is a potentially curable disease in as many as one third of the patients.[11]

HIGH GRADE

The high-grade lymphomas cause the most rapid enlargement of the lymph nodes and the fastest developing malignancies. Thus, if left untreated, these lymphomas are rapidly fatal.

Immunoblastic sarcoma usually occurs in adults over the age of 50. Advanced stage and systemic symptoms are common at presentation. Primary NHLs that arise in the central nervous system (CNS) are most often immunoblastic sarcoma. This disease responds poorly even to the most aggressive therapy, and short survivals (months to a year) are typical.

Lymphoblastic lymphoma is a T-cell malignancy typically seen in men in their teens or twenties. About half of these patients present with a large mediastinal mass, which disseminates rapidly to the bone marrow, peripheral blood, and CNS. This tumor may respond initially to chemotherapy, but relapse and a poor outcome are common.

Small noncleaved-cell lymphoma is an aggressive tumor of B lymphocytes. This disease affects a broad age range, from children to about age 30. It is further subdivided into the Burkitt type (which is common in African blacks) and the non-Burkitt type, depending on the cells found in the lymph node biopsy or bone marrow. There is a high rate of dissemination to bone marrow and the CNS. Patients often have bulky organ involvement with potential obstruction of the respiratory, gastrointestinal, or genitourinary tracts. This tumor is exquisitely sensitive to

chemotherapy, but early relapse after a complete remission foretells a poor prognosis.

Diagnostic Evaluation of Lymph Node Biopsy

The lymph node biopsy is the key diagnostic test in NHL. The histologic pattern has a much greater influence on the clinical course and treatment than is the case with HD. The International Working Classification organizes lymphomas by the pattern of lymph node infiltration—follicular (nodular) or diffuse—as well as by the types of cells involved in the infiltrate: small, large, or both. As can be appreciated from Table 38-7, the follicular lymphomas on the whole are less aggressive than the diffuse lesions, as shown by the median and 5-year survival rates.

Table 38-8 presents the characteristics of the various types of malignant cells that may be found in the lymph node biopsy. These are further described here.

Small lymphocytes are associated with low-grade small lymphocytic lymphoma. The nodal biopsy shows a diffuse pattern of small round lymphocytes with clumped chromatin, inconspicuous nucleoli, and scant cytoplasm; rare cells are in mitoses. This infiltrate is identical to that of chronic lymphocytic leukemia, and these cells are indistinguishable from normal peripheral blood lymphocytes. Roughly 95% of these infiltrates are B cell.[38]

The *small cleaved cell* is the same size to slightly larger than a normal peripheral blood lymphocyte (Fig. 38-3). Its cytoplasm is scant to almost nonvisible. The nucleus has coarsely condensed chromatin and prominent clefting or indentation.

The *large cell, cleaved* or *noncleaved,* is two to three times the size of a normal peripheral blood lymphocyte (Fig. 38-4). The nuclei are large and round to oval. The chromatin condensation is spotty such that the nucleus appears to have a lot of clear space. The nucleoli are

TABLE 38-8
Classification of Non-Hodgkin Lymphoma: Characteristics of Malignant Cells Found Predominantly in Lymph Node Biopsy

| Lymphocyte Type | Cell Size (μm) | Nucleus | | | Cytoplasm |
		Contour	*Chromatin*	*Nucleoli*	
Small	8–12	Round, regular	Dense to coarse	Inconspicuous	Scanty to almost nonvisible
Small cleaved	8–12	Angulated, folded	Coarse	Inconspicuous	Scanty to almost nonvisible
Large, noncleaved	>20	Round to oval	Spotty (vesicular to fine)	Prominent	Distinct but thin rim of cytoplasm
Large, cleaved	>20	Angulated, folded	Vesicular to fine	Inconspicuous	Distinct but thin rim of cytoplasm
Immunoblastic	>20	Round to oval	Fine	Prominent and central	Abundant, faint
Lymphoblastic	>20	Round to folded	Fine	Inconspicuous	Scanty
Small, noncleaved	15–30	Round to oval	Delicate to coarse	2–5 per cell; basophilic	Scanty, basophilic, vacuolated

large and prominent, numbering one to three per cell. The cytoplasm forms a distinct but thin rim around the nucleus.

The *immunoblastic large cell* is four to five times the size of a normal lymphocyte. The cytoplasm is abundant but stains much fainter than the large cell described above. The nucleus is large and round with prominent nucleoli.

The *lymphoblastic cell* has a large round or convoluted nucleus. The chromatin pattern is very fine, and nucleoli are indistinct. There are frequent mitotic forms in infiltrates involving these cells, and the majority are T cells. These cells are identical to those of T-cell acute lymphocytic leukemia.

The *small noncleaved cell* is misnamed. At 15 to 30 μm in diameter, it is a large cell but intermediate in size between the small cleaved lymphocytes (8–12 μm) and large lymphocytes (greater than 20 μm) described above. The cytoplasm is scant, deeply basophilic, and often vacu-

olated. The chromatin is coarse, and there are two to five prominent basophilic nucleoli. In the Burkitt type small noncleaved-cell lymphoma, the cells are uniform in size and shape, and mitotic figures usually are seen. In the non-Burkitt type small noncleaved-cell lymphoma, there is more heterogeneity in size and shape. The cells usually are larger than the Burkitt lymphocytes, and there usually are numerous mitotic figures.

These basic cell types are summarized in Table 38-8. In various patterns and mixtures, they account for all the subtypes described in the working formulation of Table 38-7.

Diagnosis and Treatment

The Ann Arbor staging system outlined in Table 38-3 is also used for NHL, and the diagnostic studies useful in staging are the same as those in Tables 38-4 and 38-5.

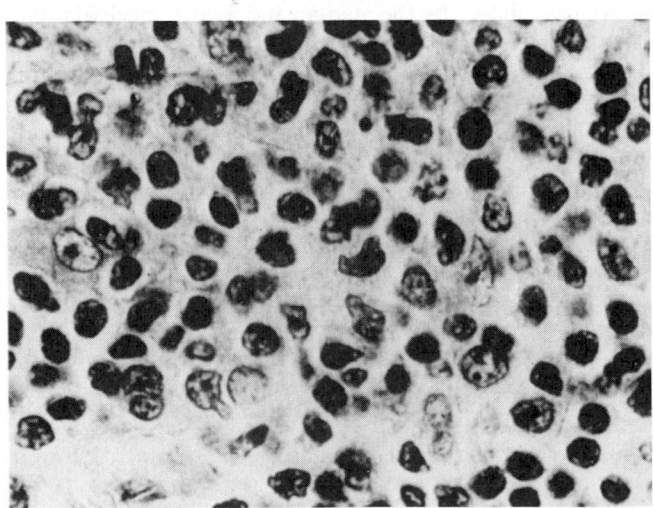

FIGURE 38-3. Follicular lymphoma, predominantly small cleaved cell. Atypical lymphocytes are indented and angular (hematoxylin and eosin, magnification × 1000). (From DeVita VT Jr, Hellman S, Rosenberg SA: Cancer Principles and Practice of Oncology, 3rd ed. Philadelphia, JB Lippincott, 1989, with permission.)

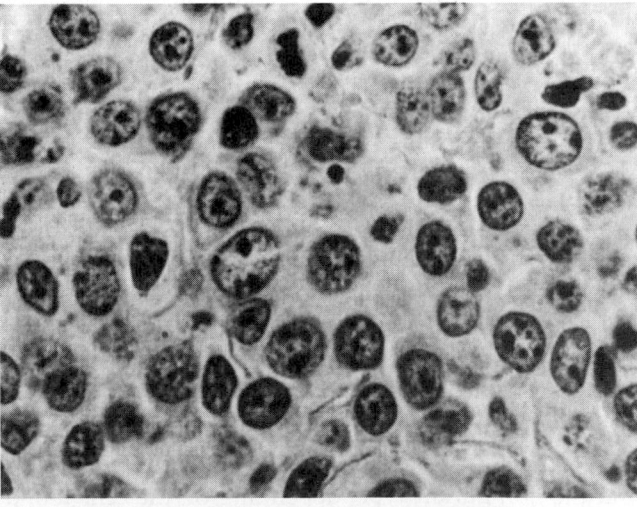

FIGURE 38-4. Malignant lymphoma, large cell type. Cells resemble large, noncleaved follicular center cells and have multiple prominent, often membrane-bound nucleoli (hematoxylin and eosin, magnification × 1000). (From DeVita VT Jr, Hellman S, Rosenberg SA: Cancer Principles and Practice of Oncology, 3rd ed. Philadelphia, JB Lippincott, 1989, with permission.)

Generally, the sequence of tests performed represents an attempt to demonstrate advanced disease, when present, early in the workup in order to spare the patient unnecessary tests. The bone marrow biopsy is especially useful in this regard because of the high frequency of positivity in the low-grade lymphomas and its effect on the staging of the intermediate- and high-grade lymphomas.

Effects of Treatment on Laboratory Results

As in HD, radiation and chemotherapy are used to treat NHL. The effects of these treatments on the laboratory results are the same as in HD, as discussed in the corresponding section earlier in this chapter.

Radiation therapy generally is given with curative intent for Stages I and II low-grade lymphomas and Stage I intermediate-grade lymphomas. Chemotherapy, usually with a combination of drugs, is used for all other types and stages. The prognosis with chemotherapy varies greatly, depending on the histologic subtype of the lymphoma.

Stages III and IV low-grade lymphomas readily go into remission with chemotherapy, but relapses are common. No currently available treatment is curative, but years of survival are nonetheless possible. The same applies to Stages III and IV follicular large-cell, diffuse small cleaved-cell, and diffuse mixed lymphomas within the intermediate grades. Stages III and IV diffuse large and diffuse small noncleaved-cell lymphomas, on the other hand, are potentially curable with aggressive chemotherapy regimens.

MYCOSIS FUNGOIDES AND SÉZARY SYNDROME

Mycosis fungoides and Sézary syndrome are rare lymphomas that represent different stages of a single neoplastic disorder. The neoplastic cell involved is the mature T-helper lymphocyte, which is produced in lymphatic tissue and migrates to the skin, which is the early primary site of involvement.

Epidemiology

It has been estimated that only 400 to 600 new cases of the conditions are diagnosed each year in the United States; thus, they account for only 2% of the annual incidence of lymphoma.[2] The typical patient is a man who is in late middle age or elderly.

Clinical Findings

The predominant early symptom is pruritus (severe itching), and the earliest lesions often are misdiagnosed as eczema, psoriasis, or other skin conditions. As the disease progresses, well demarcated reddened plaques form, or the skin can become diffusely thickened, especially about the face and in body folds. In some cases, most of the skin surface is involved, as it becomes red, thickened, and wrinkled; this process is referred to as "generalized

erythroderma." In these cases, the skin desquamates in large, dead flakes.

Diagnostic Evaluation of Skin and Lymph Node Biopsy

When the patient presents with the symptoms described above, and in some cases even prior to such a presentation, skin biopsy is diagnostic and will show the upper dermis to be involved with a dense, bandlike infiltrate of lymphocytes close to the epidermis. Characteristically, the epidermis is involved as well, with clusters of lymphocytes forming the so-called "Pautrier's microabscesses." Such a primary skin presentation is referred to as "mycosis fungoides" (although fungal infection is not present) and may exist for months to years before further progression occurs. As this condition evolves, lymph node infiltration and visceral involvement (liver, spleen, and lung) occurs, and a leukemic phase can be seen. This involvement beyond the skin with peripheral blood manifestations is referred to as Sézary syndrome. At this stage of the disease, the prognosis is worse, with survival between 12 to 15 months.[3]

Laboratory Findings and Correlations with Disease

Patients with mycosis fungoides or Sézary syndrome have laboratory abnormalities similar to those seen in other NHLs.

PERIPHERAL BLOOD

The laboratory scientist may be asked to search for cells thought to be pathognomonic of this condition. The lymphocyte involved is larger than normal with scanty cytoplasm, and the nucleus is large with clefting. Nuclear folding can be so extensive as to suggest an image of the brain, and these nuclei are thus described as cerebriform. The nuclear chromatin is fine with little condensation. There may or may not be visible nucleoli. These cells can be seen on the peripheral blood film in 15% to 20% of patients with plaque disease and in as many as 90% of those with generalized erythroderma.[2]

SPECIAL LABORATORY TESTS

Monoclonal antibody to surface markers will indicate the CD4+ subtype of helper lymphocyte. Because these disorders are fundamentally an excess of T-helper cells, it is common to see a polyclonal or monoclonal increase in immunoglobulins on serum protein electrophoresis.

Effects of Treatment on Laboratory Results

The skin infiltrative manifestation of this disorder can be treated with superficial electron-beam radiation, topically applied chemotherapy, or phototherapy with a combination of oral methoxsalen and long-wave ultraviolet light. These therapies are directed at alleviating skin symptoms and do not have the systemic effects previously described for radiation and chemotherapy of other lymphomas. Systemic combination chemotherapy is reserved for the treatment of lymph node, visceral, and leukemic manifestations. With current technology, these two conditions are treatable but not curable.

CHAPTER SUMMARY

Lymphomas are a group of malignant diseases with lymph node enlargement that disrupts the normal histology. Peripheral blood abnormalities are uncommon until advanced disease stages. The two principal classes of lymphomas are Hodgkin disease (HD) and non-Hodgkin lymphoma (NHL). Lymph node biopsy is the diagnostic tool. A biopsy in NHL shows uniformly malignant B lymphocytes with varying characteristics (see Table 38-8). In HD, there are mostly normal cells with a small number of Reed-Sternberg cells. The Reed-Sternberg cell is often binucleated with prominent, eosinophilic nucleoli and a perinucleolar halo, giving the cell its "owl-eyed" appearance (see Fig. 38-1).

In HD, there is usually no anemia and platelets are generally normal. Leukocytosis may appear in advancing disease, and abnormal-appearing lymphocytes with scant cytoplasm and irregular chromatin may be seen on the blood film. Lymphocytopenia heralds a poor prognosis. The bone marrow is seldom involved except in advanced cases. In NHL, blood counts are generally normal. Radiation and chemotherapy treatments for either NHL or HD suppress the marrow.

Mycosis fungoides and Sézary syndrome are rare T-cell lymphomas that cause skin lesions. Skin biopsy is the diagnostic tool. The laboratory abnormalities are similar to those of NHLs. The classic cell is a large lymphocyte with scant cytoplasm and a cerebriform nucleus.

Case Study 38-1

A 63-year-old woman was admitted with a 2-week history of a 102°F fever, drenching night sweats, and a 40-pound weight loss during the previous 4 months. She was obese and ill-appearing. Her neck was obviously asymmetric with a generalized fullness on the left that neither she nor her family had noticed. This fullness was caused by a matted mass of cervical lymph nodes approximately 6 cm in diameter. There were firm 3-cm lymph nodes under both axillae. The chest was clear, there was no hepatosplenomegaly, and there were no enlarged inguinal nodes.

A CBC revealed WBC 15.5×10^9/L with 6% eosinophils; platelets 475×10^9/L; Hb 12.6 g/dL; Hct 0.36 L/L. Both lactate dehydrogenase (LD) and alkaline phosphatase were elevated; all other chemistry tests performed were normal. A bone marrow film was normal, but a biopsy core revealed a lymphocytic infiltrate compatible with lymphoma. Biopsy of the left cervical nodes revealed mixed-cellularity HD. Because of her symptoms and bone marrow involvement, the disease was staged IVB, and no further tests were performed. Chemotherapy was initiated, and within the first week, the fever and night sweats abated. At 1 month, the patient was free of adenopathy. She received a total of six cycles of chemotherapy over 12 months with alternating combinations of eight drugs. Three years later, the patient remains disease free.

1. Are the patient's Hb and Hct unusual for such a diagnosis?
2. Is it common to find a normal bone marrow aspirate but an abnormal biopsy core in HD? Explain.
3. What effect might chemotherapy have had on her platelet, granulocyte, and erythrocyte counts?
4. If her platelet count had declined to 35×10^9/L, would a platelet transfusion have been appropriate?

5. Following chemotherapy, which leukocyte usually increases in relative numbers prior to granulocytosis, and how long before granulocyte recovery does this occur?

Case Study 38-2

A 38-year-old homosexual man with AIDS was admitted with a 2-week history of a 102°F fever, night sweats, and a 30-pound weight loss during the previous 2 months. The patient reported a gradual enlargement of the left side of his neck which had been painful for 1 week. On physical examination, there was bilateral adenopathy of the cervical node chains. A 5 × 7-cm mass was palpable on the left side of the neck and a 6 × 2-cm mass on the right. There was no hepatosplenomegaly. A chest radiograph was normal. Abdominal CT scan and a magnetic resonance imaging (MRI) scan of the brain were normal. The CBC, differential, and bone marrow biopsies were normal. The only chemical abnormality was a highly elevated LD. The CSF was accellular but positive for human immunodeficiency virus (HIV) antibody. Biopsy of the left neck mass showed diffuse large-cell lymphoma. The disease was staged IIB.

Chemotherapy was initiated with a combination that included methotrexate, a drug that crosses into the brain tissue and cerebrospinal fluid. The neck masses regressed dramatically, and within 1 month he was normal and returned to work. Four months later, he was readmitted for recurrent fever, lethargy, severe headaches, and slurred speech. By the second hospital day, he was confused and had experienced nerve paralysis. A CT brain scan demonstrated abnormal masses and an MRI brain scan showed multiple tumors. Toxoplasmosis serology studies were positive, and antibiotic therapy was given. By the sixth day, the patient was brain dead secondary to massive cerebral edema. He was taken off life support, and he died. Autopsy confirmed that he was free of lymphoma but died from the toxoplasmosis which had involved multiple organs, probably resulting from the effects of both chemotherapy and AIDS.

Review Questions

38-1. When Reed-Sternberg cells are found in a lymph node biopsy, they are indicative of

   A. Hodgkin disease.
   B. intermediate-grade non-Hodgkin lymphoma.
   C. Sézary syndrome.
   D. high-grade non-Hodgkin lymphoma.

38-2. The Reed-Sternberg cell is characterized as having

   A. a thin nuclear membrane.
   B. only one nucleus.
   C. large nucleoli with a distinct halo.
   D. a smaller size than normal lymphocytes.

38-3. The definitive diagnostic test for Hodgkin disease is a

   A. complete blood count.
   B. serum iron quantitation.
   C. bone marrow biopsy.
   D. lymph node biopsy.

38-4. Early in the course of Hodgkin disease, a complete blood count and/or differential may reveal

   A. anemia.
   B. thrombocytopenia.
   C. large lymphocytes with irregular nuclear chromatin.
   D. small lymphocytes with large amounts of cytoplasm.

38-5. Lymph node biopsies in non-Hodgkin lymphoma show mostly

    A. many normal cells mixed with a small number of neoplastic cells.

    B. many uniform, similar-appearing neoplastic cells.

    C. many Reed-Sternberg cells.

    D. malignant T lymphocytes.

38-6. During treatment for lymphoma, one common effect of a single course of combination chemotherapy includes a significant

    A. decrease in granulocytes.

    B. increase in platelets.

    C. decrease in erythrocytes.

    D. increase in leukocytes.

38-7. Mycosis fungoides and Sézary syndrome are rare lymphomas characterized by

    A. neoplastic B cell migration to the skin.

    B. small peripheral blood lymphocytes with small, clefted or folded nuclei.

    C. large peripheral blood lymphocytes with "cerebriform" nuclei.

    D. large peripheral blood lymphocytes with normal-appearing nuclei.

References

1. Blayney DW, Jaffe ES, Blattner WA et al: The human T-cell leukemia/lymphoma virus (HTLV) associated with American adult T-cell leukemia/lymphoma (ATL). Blood 62:401, 1983

2. Bunn PA Jr, Poiesz BJ: Cutaneous T-cell lymphomas (mycosis fungoides and Sézary syndrome). In William WJ, Beutler E, Erslev AJ, Lichtman MA (eds): Hematology, 3rd ed, p 1056. New York, McGraw-Hill, 1983

3. Bunn PA Jr, Huberman MS, Whang-Peng J et al: Prospective staging evaluation of patients with cutaneous T-cell lymphomas. Ann Intern Med 93:223, 1980

4. Bunting CH: The blood picture in Hodgkin's disease. Bull Johns Hopkins Hosp 22:369, 1911

5. Carbone PP, Kaplan HS, Musshoff K et al: Report of the Committee on Hodgkin's Disease Staging. Cancer Res 31:1860, 1971

6. Chabner BA, Johnson RE, Young RC et al: Sequential nonsurgical and surgical staging of non-Hodgkin's lymphoma. Ann Intern Med 85:149, 1976

7. Cline MJ, Berlin NI: Anemia in Hodgkin's disease. Cancer 16:526, 1963

8. Crowther D, Fairley GH, Sewell RL: Significance of the changes in the circulating lymphoid cells in Hodgkin's disease. Br Med J 2:473, 1969

9. Desser RK, Golomb HM, Ultmann JE et al: Prognostic classification of Hodgkin's disease in Stage III, based on anatomic considerations. Blood 49:883, 1977

10. DeVita VT Jr: Lymphocyte reactivity in Hodgkin's disease. A lymphocyte civil war. N Engl J Med 289:801, 1973

11. DeVita VT Jr, Jaffe ES, Hellman S: Hodgkin's disease and the non-Hodgkin's lymphomas. In DeVita VT Jr, Hellman S, Rosenberg SA (eds): Cancer: Principles and Practice of Oncology, 2nd ed, p 1623. Philadephia, JB Lippincott, 1985

12. DeVita VT Jr, Chabner B, Hubbard SP et al: Advanced diffuse histiocytic lymphoma, a potentially curable disease. Lancet 1:248, 1975

13. Fisher RI: Hodgkin's disease. In Wittes RE (ed): Manual of Oncologic Therapeutics 1989/1990, p 370. Philadelphia, JB Lippincott, 1989

14. Foucar K, McKenna RW, Frizzera G et al: Bone marrow and blood involvement by lymphoma in relationship to the Lukes-Collins classification. Cancer 49:888, 1982

15. Gall EA, Mallory TB: Malignant lymphoma: A clincial pathologic survey of 618 cases. Am J Pathol 18:381, 1942

16. Gatti RA, Good RA: Occurrence of malignancy in immunodeficiency disease. Cancer 28:89, 1971

17. Gill PS, Levine AM, Meyer PR et al: Primary central nervous system lymphoma in homosexual men: Clinical, immunologic, and pathologic features. Am J Med 78:742, 1985

18. Grufferman S, Cole P, Smith PG et al: Hodgkin's disease in siblings. N Engl J Med 296:248, 1977

19. Gutensohn N, Cole P: Childhood social environment and Hodgkin's disease. N Engl J Med 304:135, 1981

20. Halie MR, Huiges W, Nieweg HO: Abnormal cells in the peripheral blood of patients with Hodgkin's disease: I. Observations with light microscopy. Br J Haematol 28:317, 1974

21. Halie MR, Eibergen R, Nieweg HO: Observations on abnormal cells in the peripheral blood and spleen in Hodgkin's disease. Br Med J 2:609, 1972

22. Halie MR, Splett-Romascano M, Molenaar I et al: Abnormal cells in the peripheral blood of patients with Hodgkin's disease: II. Ultrastructural studies. Br J Haematol 28:323, 1974

23. Hodgkin T: On some morbid appearances of the absorbent glands and spleen. Med-Chir Trans 17:68, 1832

24. Hsu SM, Jaffe ES: Leu M1 and peanut agglutinin stain the neoplastic cells of Hodgkin's disease. Am J Clin Pathol 82:29, 1984

25. Hsu SM, Yang K, Jaffe ES: Phenotypic expression of Hodgkin's and Reed-Sternberg cells in Hodgkin's disease. Am J Pathol 118:209, 1985

26. Isomaki HA, Hakulinen T, Joutsenlahti U: Excess risk of lymphomas, leukemias, and myeloma in patients with rheumatoid arthritis. J Chronic Dis 31:691, 1978

27. Jones SE: Autoimmune disorders and malignant lymphoma. Cancer 31:1092, 1973

28. Kadin ME: Possible origin of the Reed-Sternberg cell from an interdigitating reticulum cell. Cancer Treat Rep 66:601, 1982

29. Kaplan HS, Gartner S: "Sternberg-Reed" giant cells of Hodgkin's disease: Cultivation *in vitro*, heterotransplantation, and characterization as neoplastic macrophages. Int J Cancer 19:511, 1977

30. Kaplan HS, Goodenow RS, Gartner S et al: Biology and virology of the human malignant lymphomas. Cancer 43:1, 1979

31. Kassan SS, Thomas TL, Moutsopoulos HM et al: Increased risk of lymphoma in sicca syndrome. Ann Intern Med 89:888, 1978

32. Keller AR, Kaplan HS, Lukes RJ et al: Correlation of histopathology with other prognostic indicators in Hodgkin's disease. Cancer 22:487, 1968

33. Kinlen LJ, Sheil AGR, Peto J et al: Collaborative United Kingdom-Australasian study of cancer in patients treated with immunosuppressive drugs. Br Med J 2:1461, 1979

34. Levine AM, Thorton P, Forman SJ et al: Positive Coombs' test in Hodgkin's disease: Significance and implications. Blood 55:607, 1980

35. Lukes RJ, Butler JJ, Hicks EB: Natural history of Hodgkin's disease as related to its pathologic picture. Cancer 19:317, 1966

36. Lukes RJ, Craver LF, Hall TC et al: Report of the Nomenclature Committee. Cancer Res 26:1311, 1966

37. MacMahon B: Epidemiologic evidence on the nature of Hodgkin's disease. Cancer 10:1045, 1957

38. Mann RB, Jaffe ES, Berard CW: Malignant lymphomas: A conceptual understanding of morphologic diversity. Am J Pathol 94:105, 1979

39. Munoz N, Davidson RJL, Witthoff B et al: Infectious mononucleosis and Hodgkin's disease. Int J Cancer 22:10, 1978

40. Nadler LM, Ritz J, Griffin JD et al: Diagnosis and treatment of human leukemias and lymphomas utilizing monoclonal antibodies. Prog Hematol 12:187, 1981

41. Peters MV, Alison RE, Buch RS: Natural history of Hodgkin's disease as related to staging. Cancer 19:308, 1966

42. Rappaport H, Winter WJ, Hicks EB: Follicular lymphoma: A reevaluation of its position in the scheme of malignant lymphomas, based on a survey of 253 cases. Cancer 9:792, 1956

43. Ray GR, Wolf PH, Kaplan HS: Value of laboratory indicators in Hodgkin's disease: Preliminary results. Natl Cancer Inst Monogr 36:315, 1972

44. Reed DM: On the pathological changes in Hodgkin's disease, with special reference to its relation to tuberculosis. Johns Hopkins Hosp Rep 10:133, 1902

45. Risdall R, Hoppe RT, Warnke R: Non-Hodgkin's lymphoma: A study of the evolution of the disease based upon 92 autopsied cases. Cancer 44:529, 1979

46. Rosenberg SA, Berard CW, Brown BW, and the Non-Hodgkin's Lymphoma Pathologic Classification Project Committee: National Cancer Institute sponsored study of classification of non-Hodgkin's lymphomas: Summary and description of a working formulation for clinical usage. Cancer 49:2112, 1982

47. Rosenberg SA, Diamond HD, Jaslowitz B et al: Lymphosarcoma: A review of 1269 cases. Medicine 40:31, 1961

48. Schiffer CA, Levi JA, Wiernik PH: The significance of abnormal circulating cells in patients with Hodgkin's disease. Br J Haematol 31:177, 1975

49. Silar G, Brusamolino E, Bernasconi C et al: Isolation of Reed-Sternberg cells from lymph nodes of Hodgkin's disease patients. Blood 73:222, 1989

50. Stein H, Mason DY, Gerdes J et al: The expression of the Hodgkin's disease associated antigen K_i-1 in reactive and neoplastic lymphoid tissue: Evidence that Reed-Sternberg cells and histiocytic malignancies are derived from activated lymphoid cells. Blood 66:848, 1985

51. Sternberg C: Über eine Eigenartige unter dem Bilde der Pseudoleukämie verlaufende Tuberculose des lymphatichen Apparates. Ztschr Heilk 19:21, 1898

52. Stuart AE, Jackson E, Morris CS: The reaction of xenogenic and monoclonal antisera with Reed-Sternberg cells. J Pathol 137:129, 1982

53. Tubiana M, Attie E, Flamant R et al: Prognostic factors in 454 cases of Hodgkin's disease. Cancer Res 31:1801, 1971

54. Ultmann JE, Moran EM: Clinical course and complications in Hodgkin's disease. Arch Intern Med 131:332, 1973

55. Virchow R: Gesammelte Abhandlungen zur wissenschaftlichen Medizin. Frankfurt, Meindinger, 1856

56. Wyburn-Mason R: SLE and lymphoma. Lancet 1:156, 1979

57. Young JL, Percy CL, Asire AJ (eds): Surveillance, Epidemiology, and End Results: Incidence and Mortality Data, 1973–77, Natl Cancer Inst Monogr 57. Washington DC, US Government Printing Office, 1981

Suggested Readings

Armitage JO (ed): Non-Hodgkins lymphoma. Hematol/Oncol Clin North Amer 5(5):845, 1991

Williams SF, Farah R, Goulumb HM (eds): Hodgkin's disease. Hematol/Oncol Clin North Amer 3(2):187, 1989

CHAPTER 39

Plasma Cell Disorders (Paraproteinemias)

Sandra R. Sommer

Objectives

1. Define monoclonal gammopathy and explain how it is identified and classified in the laboratory.
2. Compare and contrast the clinical and laboratory findings in multiple myeloma and Waldenström's macroglobulinemia.
3. Describe plasma cell leukemia, heavy chain disease, monoclonal gammopathy of uncertain significance (MGUS), and amyloidosis.

Earlier chapters have described leukemias characterized by the proliferation of immature lymphoid cells (acute lymphoblastic leukemias) and of more differentiated lymphocytes (chronic lymphoproliferative disorders). This chapter will address malignant diseases (dyscrasias) of the differentiated end cells of B lymphocytes: plasma cells and plasmacytoid lymphocytes. (See Chap. 23 for schema of normal B-lymphocyte maturation.)

Plasma cell disorders are sometimes referred to as *monoclonal gammopathies*. The term *monoclonal* is used because the malignant cells in these disorders represent a single clone, arising from a single abnormal parent cell. The term *gammopathy* refers to a disease in which plasma cells produce an increased amount of immunoglobulin (antibody) molecules. The proteins produced by malignant cells are called M (for monoclonal) proteins or paraproteins. Their concentration in serum becomes so great that it causes the appearance of a narrow peak or spike on serum protein electrophoresis. M proteins may be monomers, polymers, or fragments of immunoglobulins (see Review of Immunoglobulins, following).

REVIEW OF IMMUNOGLOBULINS

Plasma cells are capable of synthesizing heterogeneous proteins called immunoglobulins (Igs) or antibodies. Immunoglobulins have the capacity to bind the particular antigens that stimulated their production. Each cell produces a particular, specific Ig.

All Igs are composed of a basic structural unit of four polypeptide chains–two symmetrically arranged heavy (H) chains and two light (L) chains, which are linked with disulfide bonds (Fig. 39-1). There are two antigen-binding sites per unit. The variable regions on both the H and the L chains are specifically coded for antibody function and share this activity. The Fc portion of the H chains directs the biologic activity of the molecule, such as complement activation or adherence to surfaces of neutrophils, macrophages, and certain lymphocytes.

Although all Igs share a basic structural unit, there are five classes which differ in the amino acid sequence of their H chains and in their structural arrangement, making them functionally unique. The different H chains are designated gamma (γ), alpha (α), mu (μ), delta (δ), and epsilon (ε), and correspond to the five immunoglobulin classes IgG, IgA, IgM, IgD, and IgE. There are only two classes of L chains: kappa (κ) and lambda (λ). Any given molecule of an H-chain class will have either kappa or lambda L chains, never one of each.

Types

IgG exists as a monomer with a molecular mass of 150,000 daltons. It accounts for approximately 80% of the total Ig found in the blood and extravascular space. IgG is responsible for the secondary immune response, which occurs upon the second exposure to an antigen. IgG is produced in response to most bacterial and viral antigens and may be manifested as precipitating antibodies, virus-neutralizing antibodies, hemagglutinins, or hemolysins. Finally, IgG is also an activator of the classic complement pathway (see Fig. 19-1).

IgA often exists as a dimer, but monomers as well as polymers are found. Although IgA is the second most abundant immunoglobulin, it constitutes only 10% to 15%

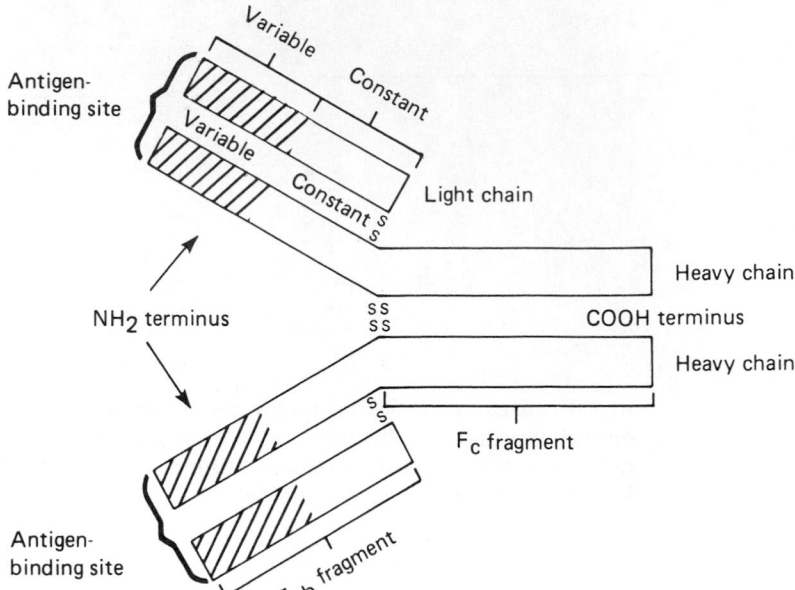

FIGURE 39-1. Immunoglobulin structure. (From Bishop ML, Duben-Von Laufen JL, Fody EP [eds]: Clinical Chemistry: Principles, Procedures, Correlations, p 154. Philadelphia, JB Lippincott, 1985, with permission.)

of the total amount. A slightly larger molecule than IgG (180,000 daltons), it is synthesized by plasma cells in the epithelium of the respiratory and gastrointestinal tracts and in most excretory glands. IgA provides the first line of defense on mucosal surfaces.

IgM, the largest Ig with a molecular mass of 900,000 daltons, has a circular pentameric arrangement. It makes up 5% to 10% of the total Igs and is localized in the blood. IgM is the first antibody to appear in response to antigenic challenge; that is, it is involved in the primary immunologic response.

IgD is a monomer with the lowest molecular mass (140,000 daltons) of the immunoglobulins. Only trace amounts are found in serum. IgD is a surface immunoglobulin on blood lymphocytes and may play a role in lymphocyte activation and suppression.

IgE is a monomer with a molecular mass of 200,000 daltons, only slightly greater than IgG and IgA. This is the "reaginic antibody" found mostly in the respiratory and gastrointestinal tracts. IgE attaches to mast cells and basophils. It mediates allergic reactions and plays a role in the response to parasitic infections.

Laboratory Measurement

Proteins have different net electrical charges owing to differences in amino acid composition. When placed in a supporting medium (*e.g.*, cellulose acetate) and exposed to an electrical field, they can be separated into various fractions. This process is called *electrophoresis*. These separated fractions are then stained and scanned densitometrically to obtain the relative percentage of each fraction. (This technique is also described in Chap. 14.) Serum proteins are commonly separated into albumin, alpha-1, alpha-2, beta, and gamma fractions. Most Igs migrate in the gamma fraction, although IgA also migrates in the beta fraction. Immunoglobulins make up approximately 12% to 20% of the total serum protein of normal individu-

als. A polyclonal increase is noted as a broad band uniformly larger than normal, representing an increase in heterogeneous immunoglobulins. A narrower, monoclonal peak occurs when molecules traveling at the same rate concentrate at the same point, suggesting activity of a single clone of plasma cells producing an M protein (a paraprotein). Figure 39-2 demonstrates examples of normal, polyclonal, and monoclonal patterns.

To detect an imbalance of Ig or the presence of free H or L chains, immunotechniques such as immunoelectrophoresis (IEP) or immunofixation electrophoresis (IFE) are used. Detailed discussions of these techniques may be found in immunology or clinical chemistry texts.

The following is a discussion of the more common plasma cell disorders. Table 39-1 summarizes the laboratory findings for each of these disorders.

MULTIPLE MYELOMA (PLASMA CELL MYELOMA)

Pathophysiology

Multiple myeloma is the most common malignant disease of plasma cells and generally affects older individuals (50–75 years). Twice as many African-Americans as whites are affected and it is somewhat more frequent in men than women. Although the etiology is unknown, genetics, radiation exposure, and chronic antigenic stimulation have been suggested as predisposing factors.[12] The transformation event probably occurs at the hematopoietic stem cell level, because malignant cells have been shown to express the pre–B cell antigen CALLA (CD10; Chap. 36), as well as megakaryocytic, myelomonocytic, and erythroid surface markers.[6]

Clonal proliferation of malignant plasma cells begins in the bone marrow. As the tumor grows, osteoclast activating factor is produced, leading to increased bone resorption (bone loss) and lytic bone disease. Pathologic

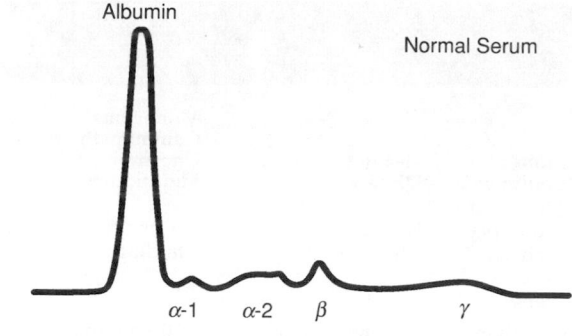

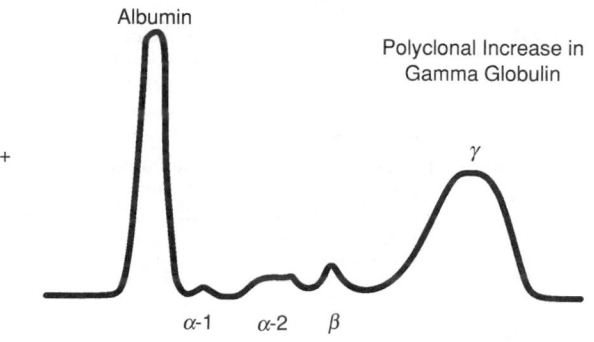

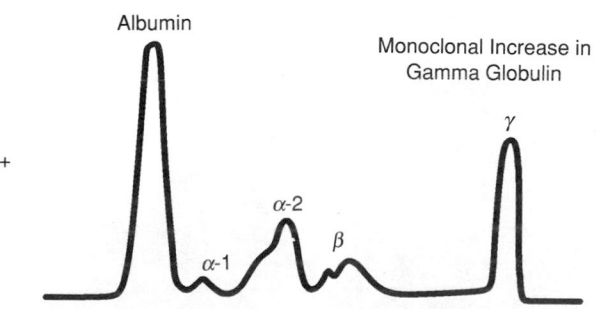

FIGURE 39-2. Electrophoretic patterns show separated serum fractions for normal serum and for polyclonal and monoclonal increases in gamma globulins.

bone fractures and vertebral collapse may occur as the bone is destroyed. Crowded by proliferating tumor cells, the marrow cannot continue normal production of other cellular elements, which leads to symptoms of anemia, infection, and/or bleeding. The cells may also infiltrate the lymph nodes, spleen, and other organs.

Increased risk of infection is also a result of the markedly decreased production of normal immunoglobulins, especially those associated with a primary immune response. Tumor cells suppress normal B and T lymphocyte functions, although cellular immunity is less affected than humoral.[16] Functional defects in phagocytic cells have also been reported.[7]

Properties of the M protein itself may lead to clinical manifestations. Low molecular weight L chains (Bence Jones proteins) are readily filtered out by the renal glomeruli, requiring massive reabsorption by the proximal tubules. In time, the entire nephron may be damaged, with resulting renal failure. Amyloid deposition is a further complication for about 15% of patients and is discussed later in this chapter. Some M proteins interfere with coagulation factors or platelet function.[8]

Clinical Presentation

The chief complaint of many myeloma patients is skeletal pain. Initial back pain and that associated with centrally located bones progresses to the severe pain of spontaneous (pathologic) bone fracture. Accompanying anemia and renal insufficiency cause patients to experience weakness and fatigue. There may be episodes of bleeding secondary to thrombocytopenia or coagulation abnormalities, as well as a greater susceptibility to infection.[16]

Laboratory Findings and Correlations with Disease

Peripheral Blood. The findings include normochromic, normocytic anemia with Hb levels between 7 and 12 g/dL. As expected, the erythrocyte sedimentation rate (ESR) is increased because of elevated serum globulins. Precipitates of the M protein may result in erroneous leukocyte or platelet counts or both, although this is more common in macroglobulinemia (described later).[10]

The blood film shows rouleaux and occasionally a pinkish background stain. Large amounts of M protein can cause the film to have a bluish tinge macroscopically. The differential may show a slight neutropenia with little or no evidence of abnormal plasma cells in the early stages. Later, a few abnormal plasma cells may be seen in the blood (Fig. 39-3). It should be noted that a benign reactive plasmacytosis may also result in a few circulating plasma cells and must be differentiated from multiple myeloma. Overpopulation of the marrow with abnormal plasma cells may produce pancytopenia and elicit a leukoerythroblastic response.

Bone Marrow. Bone marrow aspirate from an osteolytic site commonly reveals more than 10% to 15% abnormal plasma cells.[5] Within a specific specimen, most tumor cells will have a similar morphology, thus demonstrating their clonal nature. From specimen to specimen, however, there may be great diversity (see Color Plate 39-1). Abnormal cells may be large with immature-appearing chromatin or small with clumped chromatin. Prominent, large nucleoli can be seen. Cytoplasm may be pale or dark, depending on the amount of RNA. Occasionally, bizarre multinucleated plasma cells are encountered, whereas other cases present lobulated nuclei, all of which adds to the already confusing morphologic possibilities.[17] Cellular inclusions such as intranuclear (Dutcher) bodies, crystalline structures of abnormal immunoglobulin, or rounded accumulations of immunoglobulin in the cisternae of the rough endoplasmic reticulum of the cytoplasm (Russell bodies) are associated with multiple myeloma[11] (Fig. 39-4). A few IgA myelomas present flame cells characterized by abundant cytoplasm with a reddish tinge of ribosomal protein (see Color Plate 39-2).

TABLE 39-1
Laboratory Findings in Plasma Cell Disorders

	Multiple Myeloma	Plasma Cell Leukemia	Waldenström's Macroglobulinemia	Heavy Chain Diseases	Monoclonal Gammopathy of Uncertain Significance
Peripheral Blood	Rouleaux; rare abnormal plasma cells	Rouleaux; >2.0 × 10⁹/L abnormal plasma cells	Rouleaux; rare plasmacytoid lymphocytes or plasma cells	No significant findings	No significant findings
Bone Marrow	10%–15% abnormal plasma cells	Small-type abnormal plasma cells	Plasmacytoid lymphocytes, mast cells	Variant lymphocytes, plasma cells, vacuolated plasma cells	<10% plasma cells
Serum Proteins	Monoclonal peak	Monoclonal peak	Monoclonal IgM	Hypogammaglobulinemia; incomplete heavy chains of only one class	Monoclonal peak; concentration usually <30 g/L
Urine Protein	L chains occur in 80% of cases	—	L chains occur in 80% of cases	Heavy chains in the alpha and gamma subtypes; L chains in the mu subtype	Small amounts of L chains occur in 25%–40% of cases
Radiography	Significant osteoporosis; bone lesions	Slight osteolysis	—	—	—
Other	Amyloidosis develops in 15% of cases	—	Increased plasma viscosity; cryoglobulins	Mu subtype associated with CLL (Chap. 37)	—

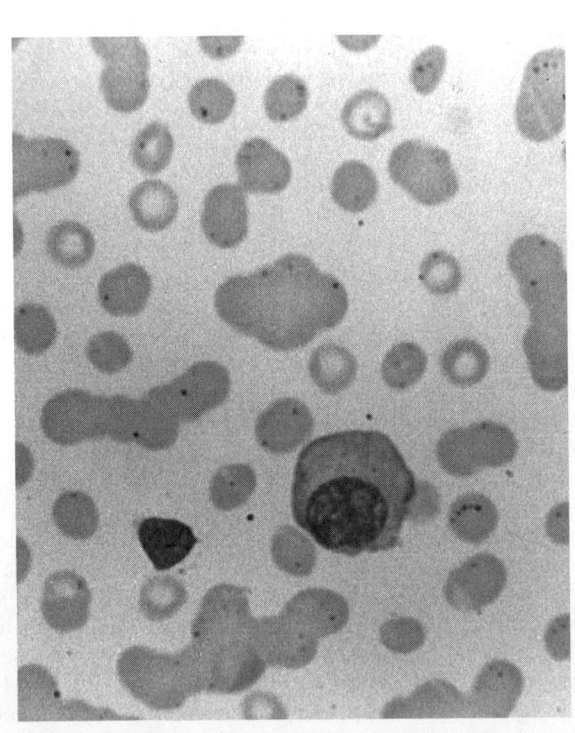

FIGURE 39-3. Peripheral blood sample of patient with multiple myeloma shows rouleaux and circulating plasma cell in center of field.

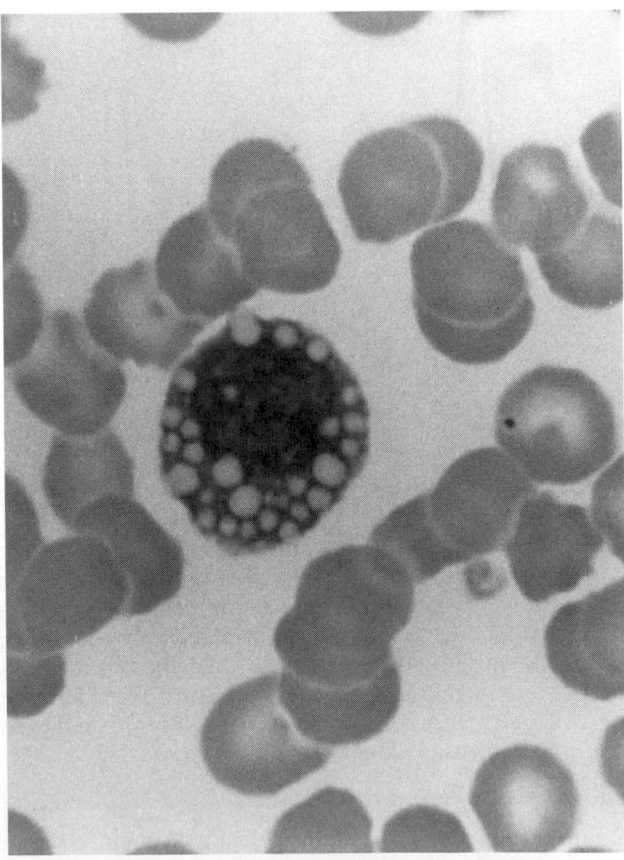

FIGURE 39-4. Abnormal plasma cell has immunoglobulin trapped in the cisternae of endoplasmic reticulum. This cell has been referred to as a Mott cell, grape cell, morula cell, or plasma cell with Russell bodies.

Urinalysis. Routine urinalysis may not determine the extent of proteinuria accurately because the reagent strip and sulfosalicylic acid tests are more sensitive to albumin than to globulin and L chains. Microscopic examination of urine sediment may reveal hyaline casts and evidence of renal tubular degeneration such as tubular epithelial cells embedded in the hyaline casts.

Chemistry. Protein electrophoresis reveals monoclonal immunoglobulin in both serum and concentrated urine. Immunotechniques using sensitive antisera are necessary to ascertain the immunoglobulin class and L-chain type. Either IEP or IFE of concentrated urine not only identifies the L chain (Bence Jones proteins) but, of more diagnostic importance, detects these proteins which are present in many patients with myeloma in the event of hypogammaglobulinemia or normal-appearing serum protein. Because they are readily filtered by the renal glomerulus, Bence Jones proteins are *not* found in significant amounts in serum.

More than 50% of the myelomas produce proteins of the IgG class. The second most frequent monoclonal protein is IgA, seen in about 20% of cases. IgD and IgE myelomas are rare, and IgM paraprotein is mostly associated with macroglobulinemia, although IgM myelomas have been described.[22] Clones producing only an L chain are a third significant group, comprising about 15%, and this class of myeloma is referred to as light chain disease or Bence Jones myeloma. Free L chains, more frequently kappa, can be detected in urine in about 80% of all myelomas.[14]

There may also be hyperuricemia, resulting from increased cellular turnover, and hypercalcemia from bone destruction. Serum alkaline phosphatase levels are normal because the enzyme is associated with osteoblast activity which is decreased in myeloma, causing the lack of compensation for osteoporosis. Radiologic evidence of osteoporosis and lytic bone lesions is of great diagnostic importance (see Color Plate 39-3).

Effects of Treatment on Laboratory Results

Chemotherapy is helpful in prolonging survival, but the overall prognosis is poor.[1] Patients responding to therapy (about 40%) live about 3 to 4 years after diagnosis. Median survival of nonresponders is less than 1 year.[12] Shorter survival has been reported when Bence Jones proteinuria is present, and Bence Jones myeloma has the worst prognosis.[15] Response to treatment is monitored by serum and concentrated urine protein studies, CBC, and radiographs. Further bone marrow studies usually have little value in therapeutic monitoring. Ideally, serum proteins return to normal levels with a concomitant decrease in the ESR. Likewise, bone lesions should decrease, reflecting decreased tumor cells, with associated resolution of cytopenias.

PLASMA CELL LEUKEMIA

A patient is said to have plasma cell leukemia when circulating plasma cells exceed 2×10^9/L.[5] A leukemic blood picture can occur as a late manifestation of multiple myeloma, also known as plasma cell myeloma, but plasma cell leukemia has also been reported as a discrete entity.[21]

Clinical Presentation

The patient with plasma cell leukemia is usually younger than one with multiple myeloma, complains less of bone pain, and shows less osteolysis. There is a greater incidence of lymphadenopathy and hepatosplenomegaly.

Laboratory Findings and Correlations with Disease

The peripheral blood demonstrates greater than 2×10^9 abnormal plasma cells/L, pancytopenia with leukoerythroblastic findings, and an elevated ESR. Morphologically, the abnormal plasma cells are small with little cytoplasm and pronounced nuclear/cytoplasmic asynchronism. Bone marrow infiltration is diffuse, and the proliferating cells exceed 45% of the population.[21] Serum and urine protein studies as well as morphology and cell markers will differentiate this disorder from the more common lymphocytic leukemias.

WALDENSTRÖM'S MACROGLOBULINEMIA

Pathophysiology

In 1944, Waldenström described a lymphoproliferative disorder characterized by a large concentration of monoclonal IgM. The abnormal B lymphocytes involved in this rare malignancy are transitional cells. They have the ability to differentiate into large plasmacytoid lymphocytes and plasma cells.[17] In classic Waldenström's macroglobulinemia, IgM exceeds 15% of the gamma globulin concentration (normal is 5%–10%). It is the increased concentration of these macromolecules that is responsible for the principal clinical manifestations. Unlike multiple myeloma, Waldenström's macroglobulinemia rarely causes osteolytic lesions. Renal consequences are less frequent than in multiple myeloma and are primarily glomerular lesions caused by deposition of IgM complexes of amyloid.[4]

Clinical Presentation

There is a gradual onset of symptoms as the IgM concentration mounts. Patients are more often men who are older than 50 years of age and complain of fatigue, weight loss, blurred vision, and bleeding episodes, especially epistaxis. Physical findings include hepatosplenomegaly and lymphadenopathy. Retinal abnormalities preceding retinal hemorrhage and neurologic changes are a result of hyperviscosity.

Laboratory Findings

Hemorrhage, hemodilution from hypervolemia, and decreased red cell survival contribute to the development of normochromic, normocytic anemia. The reticulocyte count usually is normal or decreased. The numbers of platelets and leukocytes are usually within reference ranges. An increased ESR secondary to rouleaux formation is expected. Bone marrow examination or biopsy reveals considerable variation in proportions of cell types (small lymphocytes, plasmacytoid lymphocytes, or plasma cells) among patients.[17] Mast cells may be increased, a helpful diagnostic feature if present. Malignant cells circulate in the peripheral blood only in the terminal stages.

Macromolecules at this concentration coat platelets and inhibit normal function, leading to increased bleeding time and abnormal platelet aggregation studies. Also, abnormal IgM can interact with coagulation factors and frequently produces prolonged activated partial thromboplastin and thrombin times. Artifactually low fibrinogen values may be encountered.

Differential diagnostic data for Waldenström's macroglobulinemia are obtained from serum protein electrophoresis, IEP, and IFE. An identifiable monoclonal peak frequently migrates in the beta–gamma region and constitutes greater than 15% of the total gamma globulin. Specific antisera verify the IgM class and L-chain type. About 80% of the patients produce small amounts of free L chains (Bence Jones proteins) in the urine.[14]

Other serum studies show greatly increased plasma viscosity. Significantly, monoclonal IgM may exhibit cryoglobulin activity demonstrated by precipitation or gel formation during refrigeration of serum at 4°C. Some of these IgM proteins possess antigenic specificity (anti-Ii) associated with Raynaud phenomenon and cold agglutinin disease resulting in an autoimmune hemolytic anemia. Occasionally these IgM proteins have an anti-IgG activity as well. Difficulties may occur with electronic cell counts on such specimens. Spuriously elevated platelet counts may indicate that plasma precipitates are being counted as platelets.[19] Depending on analytic conditions, leukocyte counts may also be affected.[10]

Effects of Treatment on Laboratory Results

If diagnosed in its early stages no treatment may be necessary. Immunoglobulin levels should be monitored as well as the monoclonal IgM level. Serum viscosity should also be measured periodically. Chemotherapy is required as the disease progresses. If needed, plasmapheresis is performed to reduce the M protein concentration and alleviate symptoms related to hyperviscosity. Survival in those who respond to therapy averages 4 years.

HEAVY CHAIN DISEASES

The heavy chain diseases (HCD) are rare immunoproliferative disorders characterized by abnormal synthesis of the Fc portion of a particular H chain. Incomplete H chains of three major classes of immunoglobulins are produced by the tumor cells: α, γ, or μ. The tumor cells involved resemble activated lymphocytes and plasma cells and cause a clinical picture similar to that of lymphoma.

Clinical Presentation

α-HCD, the most common of this group of gammopathies, is characterized by infiltration of plasmacytoid lympho-cytes into the duodenal or jejunal wall, producing malabsorption and abdominal distress. The respiratory tract, also a site for secretory IgA, is involved in a few cases. In contrast to the other plasma cell disorders, it has a predilection for young people. γ-HCD is found mostly in older men. μ-HCD, the rarest in this group, has been associated with chronic lymphocytic leukemia in more than half the known cases.[3]

Laboratory Findings

Because α-HCD does not usually involve the marrow, peripheral blood changes result from complications such as intestinal bleeding or malabsorption. A broad component migrating between the alpha-2 and beta regions may be found by serum electrophoresis (Fig. 39-2). However, serum protein electrophoresis is not helpful in more than half the cases.[18] Analysis of jejunal fluid or respiratory secretions by immunoelectrophoresis using H-chain-specific antisera produces more reliable evidence for alpha HCD.

In γ-HCD, variant (atypical) lymphocytes and plasma cells can be seen on peripheral blood films. Generally, there is a mixed population of lymphocytes, immunoblasts (plasma cell precursors), and plasma cells, morphologically similar to the picture in Waldenström's macroglobulinemia in the bone marrow.[18] A broad heterogeneous-appearing band or a sharp peak can be seen in the beta–gamma region of the electrophoretogram. Demonstration of gamma H chains by immunoelectrophoresis is diagnostic. There is no reaction with L-chain antisera.

Detection of mature, vacuolated plasma cells in the bone marrow provides a clue to μ-HCD in two-thirds of the cases. These large vacuoles do not contain immunoglobulin.[18] Serum protein electrophoresis shows a hypogammaglobulinemia. If an abnormal fraction appears, it is small and migrates in the alpha-2 region. Immunoelectrophoresis demonstrates free μ chains in the serum but not in the urine. This is the only HCD in which L chains (Bence Jones protein), usually kappa, are secreted in the urine. The abnormality on the H chain prevents H- and L-chain assembly.

Treatment is relatively unsatisfactory except for α-HCD, which may respond to antibiotics in some cases.[2] Life expectancy ranges up to 5 years from the onset of symptoms.

AMYLOIDOSIS

Amyloidosis is a condition in which proteinaceous deposits (amyloid) occur throughout the body, producing symptoms and clinical disease. *Primary* amyloidosis is closely associated with plasma cell disorders such as multiple myeloma, although a few patients with polyclonal plasma cells have been described.[20] Amyloid is composed of L-chain fragments from the variable region of immunoglobulin. Lambda chains are more often involved than kappa chains.[9] *Secondary* amyloidosis is associated with chronic illness, and the amyloid protein is unrelated to immunoglobulin.

Diagnosis is made after biopsy of involved tissue. Treatment addresses the associated plasma cell dyscrasia or underlying disease to control further amyloid deposition and subsequent loss of organ function.

MONOCLONAL GAMMOPATHY OF UNCERTAIN SIGNIFICANCE

A surprisingly frequent finding, especially with increasing age, is the presence of a monoclonal protein on electrophoresis with no other clinical or laboratory evidence of the plasma cell disorders described above. This M protein concentration remains stable over many years. The presently preferred term for this condition is monoclonal gammopathy of uncertain (undetermined, unknown) significance (MGUS); an older name is "benign" monoclonal gammopathy. As many as 1% of those older than 25 years and up to 3% of those over 70 have been found to have MGUS.[13]

Diagnosis is based on exclusion. Typically the M protein is less than 30 g/L, and remains below this level. Fewer than 10% plasma cells are seen in the bone marrow. These patients must be followed indefinitely because up to 25% will develop one of the malignant disorders, most commonly multiple myeloma.[13]

CHAPTER SUMMARY

Alterations of normal B-lymphocyte maturation by malignant transformation are responsible for the plasma cell disorders. In addition to morphologic identification, essential diagnostic information is obtained by detecting and identifying the monoclonal immunoglobulin by serum and urine protein studies using electrophoresis and immunotechniques.

Case Study 39-1

A 51-year-old woman was admitted through the emergency room with complaints of fever and chills, neck pain and stiffness, and photophobia. Her medical history was unremarkable. The following laboratory data were obtained: CBC: WBC 4.7 × 10⁹/L; RBC 2.77 × 10¹²/L; Hb 8.5 g/dL; Hct 0.23 L/L; PLT 67 × 10⁹/L; differential: segmented neutrophils 38%; band neutrophil 18%; lymphocytes 37%; monocytes 4%; metamyelocytes 1%; plasma cells 2%; NRBC/100 WBC 2; RBC morphology: marked rouleaux formation. The CSF showed RBC 5.2 × 10⁹/L; WBC 0.6 × 10⁹/L; mononuclear cells 18%; polynuclear cells 82%. The ESR was 72 mm/hour. The serum chemistry findings were albumin 2.8 g/dL (reference range 3.5–5.0 g/dL) and total protein 13.2 g/dL (reference range 6.0–7.8 g/dL). Serum protein electrophoresis demonstrated a monoclonal spike in the gamma region. On the urine electrophoretogram two sharp peaks were observed in the gamma region. The patient, who was deteriorating rapidly, was plasmapheresed and treated with antibiotics and packed cell transfusions. Two days later, 13% plasma cells were reported in the patient's leukocyte differential.
1. From the admission data, what prompted further serum and urine protein studies?
2. What is a likely diagnosis?
3. Is the difference between 2% and 13% plasma cells significant?

Case Study 39-2

A 63-year-old man was seen for severe epistaxis. There was no family history of bleeding disorders. Physical examination revealed lymphadenopathy and splenomegaly. No evidence of osteolytic lesions was found in the bone radiographs. The following laboratory results were reported: CBC: WBC 5.6 × 10⁹/L; RBC 2.44 × 10¹²/L; Hb 7.3 g/dL; Hct 0.23 L/L; MCV 94.2 fL; MCH 29.9 pg; MCHC 31.7 g/dL; PLT 180 × 10⁹/L; PTT 52 sec (reference range 21–31 sec); PT 18 sec (reference range 9.2–12.7 sec); ESR 74 mm/hr. Platelet aggregation studies revealed decreased aggregation with collagen and ADP. Serum protein electrophoresis demonstrated a large monoclonal peak in the gamma region.
1. The monoclonal protein in this patient is most likely to be of what immunoglobulin class? Why?
2. Which laboratory results in addition to the serum protein electrophoresis are abnormal? Why?
3. Although not seen in this case, what other laboratory tests may be affected in this disorder? Why?

Review Questions

39-1. At the time of diagnosis, the peripheral blood film of a patient with multiple myeloma typically shows

A. greater than 10% plasma cells.
B. marked lymphocytosis.
C. neutrophilia.
D. rouleaux.

39-2. A patient is suspected to have multiple myeloma. Serum protein electrophoresis appears to be normal. The laboratorian should

A. examine the urine for Ig light chains.
B. repeat the serum protein electrophoresis.
C. measure plasma viscosity.
D. perform an erythrocyte sedimentation rate.

39-3. A patient's bone marrow is found to have increased numbers of plasma cells, plasmacytoid lymphocytes, and mast cells. The patient's serum most likely has an M protein composed of

A. IgA.
B. IgG.
C. IgM.
D. heavy chains only.

39-4. The following hematology results were obtained from a patient known to have Waldenström's macroglobulinemia: WBC, 6.1 × 10⁹/L; RBC, 3.44 × 10¹²/L; Hb, 8.8 g/dL; Hct, 0.28 L/L; MCV, 82 fL; MCH, 25.6 pg; MCHC, 31.3 g/dL; PLT, 687 × 10⁹/L.

Which laboratory result is most likely in error?

A. Hb
B. MCV
C. PLT
D. WBC

References

1. Alexanian R, Dimopoulos M: The treatment of multiple myeloma. N Eng J Med 330:484, 1994
2. Barlogie B, Alexanian R, Jagannath S: Plasma cell dyscrasias. JAMA 268:2946, 1992
3. Brouet J, Seligmann M, Danon F et al: μ-Chain disease: Two new cases. Arch Intern Med 139:672, 1979
4. Deuel TF, Davis P, Avioli LV: Waldenström's macroglobulinemia. Arch Intern Med 143:986, 1983
5. Dick FR: Plasma cell myeloma and related disorders with monoclonal gammopathy. In Koepke JA (ed): Laboratory Hematology, vol 1, pp 449, 464. New York, Churchill Livingstone, 1984

6. Epstein J, Xiao H, He X: Markers of multiple hematopoietic-cell lineages in multiple myeloma. N Eng J Med 322:664, 1990

7. Foerster J: Multiple myeloma. In Lee GR, Bithell TC, Foerster J, Athens JW, Lukens JN (eds): Wintrobe's Clinical Hematology, 9th ed, pp 2222, 2223. Philadelphia, Lea & Febiger, 1993

8. Glaspy JA: Hemostatic abnormalities in multiple myeloma and related disorders. Hematol Oncol Clin North Am 6:1301, 1992

9. Glenner GG: Amyloid deposits and amyloidosis: The β-fibrilloses. N Engl J Med 302:1283, 1980

10. Gulati GL, Piao YF, Song AS, Kim WB, Hyun BH: Interference by cryoproteins in the blood with automated CBCs. Lab Med 26:138, 1995

11. Hsu SM, Hsu PL, McMillan PN et al: A light and electron microscopic immunoperoxidase study. Am J Clin Pathol 77:26, 1982

12. Hussein M: Multiple myeloma: An overview of diagnosis and management. Cleve Clin J Med 61:285, 1994

13. Kyle RA: Diagnostic criteria of multiple myeloma. Hematol Oncol Clin North Am 6:347, 1992

14. Kyle RA, Garton JP: The spectrum of IgM monoclonal gammopathy in 430 cases. Mayo Clin Proc 62:719, 1987

15. Merlini G, Waldenström JG, Jayakar SD: A new improved clinical staging system for multiple myeloma based on analysis of 123 treated patients. Blood 55:1011, 1980

16. Paglieroni T, MacKenzie MR: Studies of the pathogenesis of an immune defect in multiple myeloma. J Clin Invest 59:1120, 1977

17. Reed M, McKenna RW, Bridges R et al: Morphologic manifestations of monoclonal gammopathy. Am J Clin Pathol 76:8, 1981

18. Seligmann M, Mihaesco E, Preud'homme J et al: Heavy chain diseases: Current findings and concepts. Immunol Rev 48:145, 1979

19. Waldenström JG, Raiend U: Plasmapheresis and cold sensitivity of immunoglobulin molecules. I: A study of hyperviscosity, cryoglobulinemia, euglobulinemia, and macroglobulinemia vera. Acta Med Scand 216:449, 1984

20. Wolf BC, Kumar A, Vera JC et al: Bone marrow morphology and immunology in systemic amyloidosis. Am J Clin Pathol 86:84, 1986

21. Woodruff RK, Malpas JS, Paxton AM et al: Plasma cell leukemia (PCL): A report of 15 patients. Blood 52:839, 1978

22. Zarrabi MH, Stark RS, Kane P et al: IgM myeloma, a distinct entity in the spectrum of B-cell neoplasia. Am J Clin Pathol 75:1, 1981

CHAPTER 40

Systematic Laboratory Evaluation of Leukocyte Abnormalities

John A. Koepke

Objectives

1. Define reactions and disorders and list the four types of clinical leukocyte responses.
2. List several conditions that may be indicated by monocytosis and eosinophilia.
3. Identify the laboratory tests most frequently used by physicians to diagnose leukocyte abnormalities.
4. Use the leukocyte abnormality decision tree to give examples of myeloproliferative and lymphoproliferative disorders and reactions.
5. State the indications for a bone marrow examination or lymph node biopsy.

They come to me, and I manage to put them on the right scent. They lay all the evidence before me, and I am generally able, by the help of my knowledge of the history of crime, to set them straight. There is a strong family resemblance about misdeeds, and if you have all the details of a thousand at your finger ends, it is odd if you can't unravel the thousand and first (from Sherlock Homes, *A Study in Scarlet*).

The chapters in the preceding two sections of this book provide detailed discussions of malignant myeloproliferative and lymphoproliferative disorders. They also discuss benign conditions that may mimic these diseases because the two must be differentiated in the diagnosis for proper treatment.

The goal of this section's concluding chapter is to put these diseases and conditions into perspective by focusing on laboratory methods used to evaluate the various leukocyte abnormalities when such a disorder is first discovered but not yet definitively diagnosed. Ideally, the physician and the laboratory scientist should have a similar systematic approach to the evaluation of these disorders and work together to diagnose and monitor them most efficiently.

The deliberations of Sherlock Holmes are exemplified in the foregoing quotation from *A Study in Scarlet*.[1] In fact, he and Dr. Watson did perform some laboratory studies on blood that helped them solve the strange murder of Mr. Strangerson. Laboratory scientists and physicians might think of their deliberations in hematologic diagnosis in a similar manner.

The value of laboratory studies, including bone marrow and lymph node biopsy, in the diagnosis of these diseases is probably best exemplified by the clinical staging of their extent and gravity.

REACTIONS AND DISORDERS

The term *reaction* is used here to designate the expected physiologic proliferation of either myeloid or lymphoid elements in response to a stimulus such as infection or inflammation. The term *disorder* is reserved for malignant proliferation of these cells. Thus, four types of leukocyte responses are seen clinically: benign reactions and malignant disorders of myeloproliferation and benign reactions and malignant disorders of lymphoproliferation.[7] The late hematologist Dr. William Dameshek must be credited with the initial popularization of these unifying concepts in modern hematology.[4] These are symbolized in Figure 40-1 by the four main branches of the "tree of leukocyte abnormalities."

MYELOPROLIFERATION

At times, the myeloid cell compartment produces either increased numbers of normal myeloid cells as a response or reaction to some stimulus[9] or increased numbers of abnormal myeloid cells as part of a malignant process or disorder.[4] This process can involve any or all of the myeloid elements—granulocytic, megakaryocytic, or erythrocytic. The process frequently evolves over time. The myelodysplastic syndrome with its several variants is an especially interesting example of this evolution. Most often, the bone marrow is the first organ involved, but extramedullary tissues (*i.e.*, the liver, spleen, or lymph nodes) may subsequently participate in this proliferation. Hepatosplenomegaly more often signals the progression of a malignant process, although it may indicate a benign infectious process.[4]

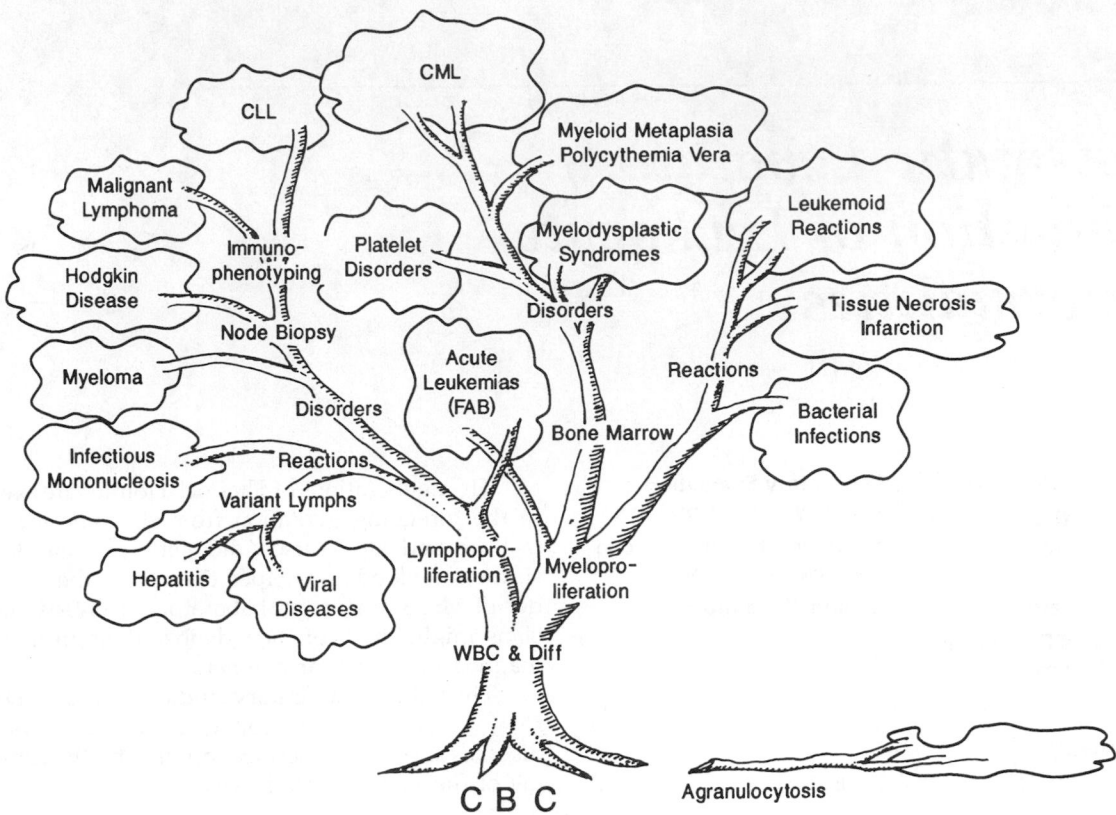

FIGURE 40-1. Decision tree for leukocyte reactions and disorders, both myeloproliferative and lymphoproliferative. The complete blood count (CBC) and evaluation of the peripheral blood film are the primary tests, but additional studies, such as bone marrow or lymph node biopsy, are frequently necessary for diagnosis.

Monocytosis and Eosinophilia

Increased numbers of monocytes are a feature of a number of infections as well as a harbinger of several premalignant conditions. In addition, acute and chronic monocytic leukemias have evident increases in monocytes. Morphologic differentiation of benign from malignant monocytes may be difficult unless the cells are frankly malignant.[10]

Eosinophilia is associated with infestations of parasitic helminths and protozoa, especially during the visceral (tissue) phases of such infestation. The intensity of the eosinophilic response is variable, but tends to decrease as the disease becomes more chronic. A wide variety of additional diseases have been associated with eosinophilia, such as acute and chronic allergic reactions. Increased eosinophils may be found in malignant conditions such as chronic myelogenous leukemia or eosinophilic leukemia.

LYMPHOPROLIFERATION

Increased production of lymphoid cells, either abnormal numbers or abnormal types of lymphocytes, can occur as a response to certain agents (*e.g.*, viruses) or conditions. This proliferation is evident in lymph nodes as well as in lymphoid tissue in the liver, spleen, or bone marrow. The process can be either benign or malignant. Lymphoproliferation may be confined to the tissues (*i.e.*, lymphoma), with little if any peripheral blood involvement, or it may be manifested primarily by peripheral blood changes (*i.e.*, leukemia).[6]

Malignant lymphoproliferation can be a continuum from frank lymphocytic leukemia to tissue lymphoma and any blend of these two extremes. Late in the disease process, lymphomas sometimes evolve into a frankly leukemic picture. These interrelations are understandable if one appreciates the broad scope of the term *lymphoproliferative disorder*. It therefore follows that the apparent evolution of the disease from primary tissue involvement to evident leukemia is not unusual; in fact, it occurs frequently.

THE PHYSICIAN'S ROLE IN THE DIAGNOSTIC PROCESS

Determination of the etiology of leukocyte abnormalities is made by integrating clinical information with laboratory data.[4] In addition to ordering appropriate tests initially, the physician plays a key role in evaluating the information obtained from a medical history and a physical examination of the patient and in interpreting laboratory data. These studies include the leukocyte count and differential, sometimes leukocyte cytochemical or monoclonal antibody studies, and a bone marrow examination or lymph node biopsy when necessary.

The etiology of the patient's problem is not always obvious. Table 40-1 presents examples of clues from the

TABLE 40-1
Examples of Common Signs and Symptoms Associated with Leukocyte Reactions and Disorders

Signs and Symptoms	Associated With
Lymph node enlargement	Lymphoma, metastatic tumor, chronic leukemia
Hepatosplenomegaly	Chronic leukemia, lymphoma
Fever	Infection; less often, malignancy
Petechiae	Acute leukemia
Rashes	Viral infection
Swollen gums	Monocytic leukemia
Bone pain	Acute leukemia, myeloma
Ruddy complexion	Polycythemia vera

patient's history or physical examination that may help one make the diagnosis or at least suggest helpful laboratory tests. For instance, the patient may recount a history of an infection, which becomes a stimulus for granulocyte production. On the other hand, leukemia manifests itself as anemia or bleeding tendencies, both reactions being secondary to the primary leukemic process. A patient with agranulocytosis often may be unaware of exposure to toxic drugs or chemicals. Thus, the patient's history may or may not be helpful.

The most important abnormal physical findings in patients with leukocyte disorders are related to liver and spleen size and lymph node size and consistency. Lymphadenopathy (palpable lymph nodes) may be generalized or localized. Hepatic or splenic enlargement or both also provide clues to the cause of leukocyte changes.

Laboratory evidence of anemia and thrombocytopenia usually indicates significant bone marrow replacement by neoplastic cells. Thrombocytopenia without significant evidence of anemia is characteristic of an acute and rapid growth of neoplastic cells in the marrow.

LABORATORY EVALUATION OF LEUKOCYTE ABNORMALITIES

In Chapter 21, the "anemia tree" was introduced as a logical approach to the laboratory evaluation of anemia. The decision tree for leukocyte abnormalities in Figure 40-1 can be applied in a similar fashion. This tree is based on the division of leukocyte proliferation into benign reactions and malignant disorders. It illustrates the subgroups with some of the more common clinical entities involving leukocytes, which have been discussed in earlier chapters.

PERIPHERAL BLOOD AND BONE MARROW EVALUATION

The so-called complete blood count (CBC) is the basic and primary laboratory test in hematology. The results of the automated analysis and, in particular, the total

leukocyte count and the leukocyte differential form the trunk as we begin to "climb the tree." This information provides the leads for the careful examination of the blood film, much as Sherlock Holmes and Dr. Watson pieced together disparate information to solve a case. The blood film is examined thoroughly in an effort to discover additional clues, with emphasis on leukocytes, both number and morphology. A recent publication provides many helpful suggestions for examining the blood film and the interested reader is encouraged to study the referenced chapter.[8]

Other tests on blood and bone marrow films may be very helpful in the diagnostic process. Special studies of the leukocytes may be required to differentiate the various leukemias. The French–American–British (FAB) classification scheme for myeloid as well as lymphoid leukemias has made a great contribution to the exact diagnosis of leukemia.[2] Cytochemical stains also contribute greatly to the diagnoses of leukemias[3]; and more recently, immunophenotyping and sophisticated molecular techniques have added very powerful tools. But because these molecular techniques are highly specific for the various types of leukemia, careful attention to physician's practice guidelines can help practitioners to avoid the unnecessary use of these costly tests.

Patients with leukocyte reactions or disorders may be candidates for a marrow study. The cause of an unexplained leukocytosis may become evident during careful study of the bone marrow. The diagnosis of leukemia and the assessment of the response to therapy rely heavily on the status of the marrow compartment. In the patient case depicted in Figure 40-2, for example, six marrow biopsies or aspirates were obtained during the course of diagnosis and treatment of acute myelocytic leukemia. These specimens are used to assess the need for additional therapy as well as to determine prognosis.

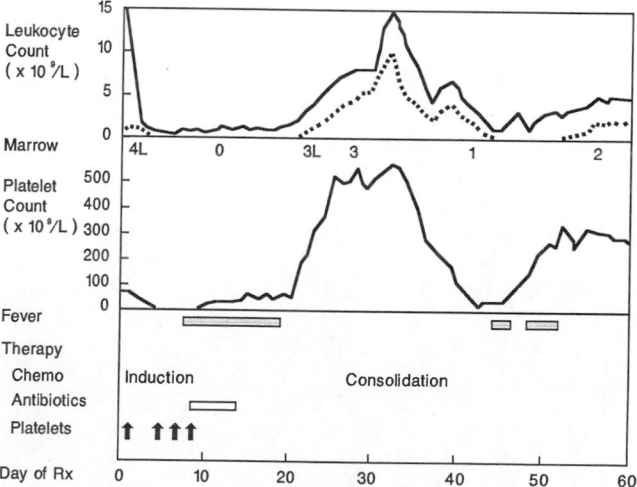

FIGURE 40-2. Characteristic clinical course of a patient with acute myelogenous leukemia receiving induction and consolidation chemotherapy. Note leukopenia and thrombocytopenia after therapy. *Solid line*, total leukocyte count; *dotted line*, granulocyte count. Platelet transfusions were given when count was fewer than 10 × 10⁹/L. Marrow examinations show estimated cellularity, 4 being packed marrow and 0 being acellular; *L* indicates presence of leukemic infiltrate.

LYMPH NODE BIOPSY

In lymphoproliferative disorders as well as reactive conditions that may mimic malignant lymphoma or non-Hodgkin lymphoma, the lymph node biopsy is a key study in the differential diagnosis. In addition to the usual hematoxylin and eosin-stained histologic sections, various special preparations (*e.g.*, the immunoperoxidase stain or monoclonal antibodies) are helpful in differentiating these diseases. The exact roles of some newer procedures (*e.g.*, DNA probes) are still being determined, but the results are quite promising.

Review Questions

40-1. The myeloproliferative response to infection may be called a

    A. disorder.
    B. malignant process.
    C. reaction.
    D. myelodysplastic syndrome.

40-2. Lymphoproliferation may be evident in the

    A. peripheral blood and bone marrow only.
    B. peripheral blood only.
    C. bone marrow only.
    D. peripheral blood, bone marrow, and lymphoid tissues.

40-3. Infectious mononucleosis is a

    A. lymphoproliferative disorder.
    B. lymphoproliferative reaction.
    C. myeloproliferative disorder.
    D. myeloproliferative reaction.

40-4. Of the following four tests, the one that is least likely to be required for the *diagnosis* of leukemia is

    A. molecular studies.
    B. a complete blood count.
    C. a bone marrow biopsy.
    D. bone marrow cytochemical stains.

References

1. Baring-Gould WS (ed): The Annotated Sherlock Holmes, A Study in Scarlet, vol 1, p 160. New York, Clarkson N Potter, 1967
2. Bennett JM, Catovsky D, Daniel MT et al: Proposals for the classification of acute leukaemias. Br J Haematol 33:451, 1976
3. Bennett JM, Catovsky D, Daniel MT et al: Proposed revised criteria for the classification of acute myeloid leukemia. Ann Intern Med 103:626, 1985
4. Dameshek W: Some speculations on the myeloproliferative syndromes. Blood 6:372, 1951
5. Dacie JW, Lewis SM: Use of haematological techniques in clinical work. In Practical Haematology, 6th ed, p 132. Edinburgh, Churchill Livingstone, 1984
6. Dick FR: Chronic lymphocytic leukemia, prolymphocytic leukemia and leukemic non-Hodgkin's lymphoma. In Koepke JA (ed): Laboratory Hematology, p 325. New York, Churchill Livingstone, 1984
7. Koepke JA, Koepke JF: Leukemia and leukemoid reactions. In Guide to Clinical Laboratory Diagnosis, 3rd ed, p 189. Norwalk, CT, Appleton & Lange, 1987
8. Shively JA: Interpretive aspects of hematology tests with a focus on the blood film. In Lewis SM, Koepke JA (eds): Hematology Laboratory Management and Practice, p 12. Oxford, Butterworth-Heinemann, 1995
9. Stein RB: Granulocytosis and granulocyte leukemoid reactions. In Koepke JA (ed): Laboratory Hematology, p 153. New York, Churchill Livingstone, 1984
10. Stein RB, Linder J: Mononuclear leukocytosis and infectious mononucleosis. In Koepke JA (ed): Laboratory Hematology, p 189. New York, Churchill Livingstone, 1984

PART IX

Instrumentation for Hematologic Evaluation

CHAPTER 41

Introduction to Hematologic Automation

E. Anne Stiene-Martin

Objectives

1. Describe the first two principles of cell counting that were sufficiently accurate and practical to be used in the clinical laboratory.
2. Discuss the differences and similarities between single and multiple parameter cell counters.
3. Describe the various principles of cell counting and differentiation.

The concept of counting blood cells automatically began in the mid-1930s with a report describing a photoelectric method for counting cells passing through a capillary tube using darkfield optics.[10] Later, darkfield optics or light scatter were proposed to scan hemocytometer chambers in an attempt to bypass human error.[6] Endeavors to correlate the RBC count with the turbidity of cell suspensions were also proposed.[13] Instruments manufactured on these principles did not gain wide acceptance at that time because of their inaccuracy, lack of sensitivity, or lack of practicality.

In the late 1940s and early 1950s, two instruments were introduced that proved to be accurate as well as practical. The first was a modification of the original capillary method using darkfield optics. A suspension of cells was pumped through a narrow capillary tube in the path of darkfield lighting.[3] Light pulses reflected by the cells were collected with a series of mirrors and lenses into a photomultiplier tube. This information was then converted to cells per microliter.[8] The original instrument (Fisher Autocytometer) is no longer in production, but the principle of darkfield optical scan or light scatter is still used today in other instruments.

The second instrument was based on a completely new non-optical principle of cell counting: electrical gating or electrical impedance.[9] This instrument was introduced by Coulter Electronics, Inc., and the counting principle was patented, so no other manufacturer in the United States could produce such an instrument for 17 years. The patent restrictions were not applicable outside this country, however, and several European companies developed similar instruments (Celloscope, Microscal), and at least one instrument (TOA) was manufactured in Japan.[5]

Electrical impedance measurement is based on the fact that cells are relatively poor conductors of electricity. If two electrodes conducting an electrical current through an electrolyte solution such as saline are separated so that the only connection is through a tiny aperture, any interference (such as a blood cell passing through the aperture) will change the conductance. As cells are pulled by vacuum through the aperture, the changes in voltage that occur as the cells increase resistance to the current

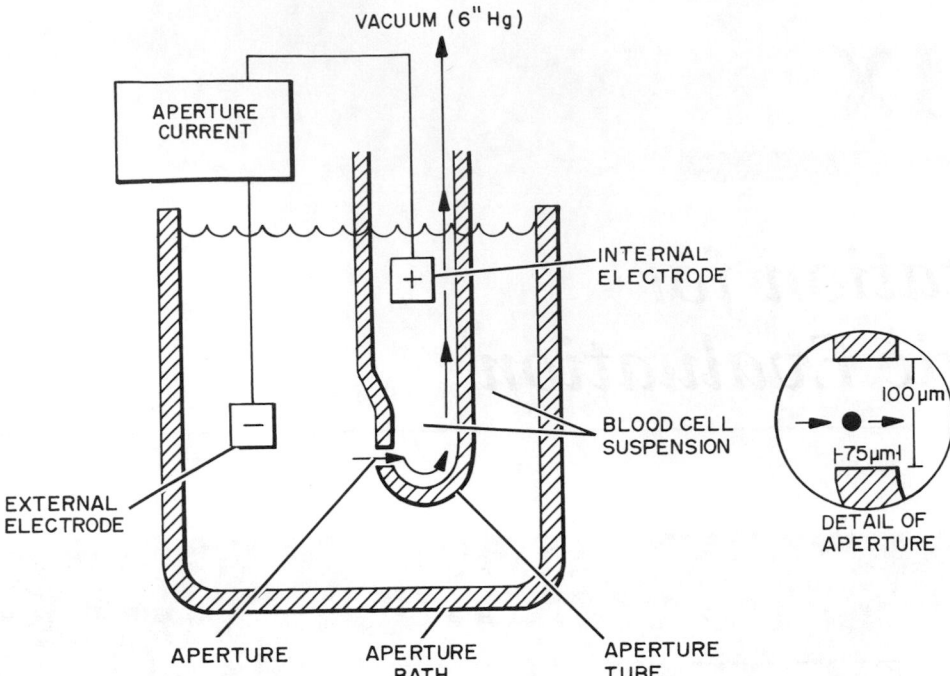

FIGURE 41-1. Aperture tube (Courtesy of Coulter Electronics, Inc.)

are sensed by the instrument (Fig. 41-1). This is a good illustration of Ohm's Law: voltage = current × resistance. The magnitude of the voltage pulses produced by cells is directly related to cell size, a fact that has been used in subsequent clinical instruments for direct measurement of cell volume.

In order for these instruments to count and size particles accurately, a means of discriminating between particle sizes had to be developed. Thus, the concept of "thresholds" was born. A *threshold* is a voltage limit with which a pulse is compared. Only pulses that exceed the threshold are sized or counted. Both a lower and an upper threshold can be set. Figure 41-2 is a diagrammatic representation of one of these instruments. Increasing the lower threshold eliminates unwanted small pulses such as those caused by debris. An upper threshold eliminates large pulses. By manipulating the upper and lower thresholds, it is possible to produce a "window," a specific particle size range. Because these instruments have adjustable thresholds, they are capable of being calibrated and of producing accurate cell counts. Thus, they can be considered to be reference methods and are unique.

Since the instruments described above are not capable of counting erythrocytes, leukocytes, and platelets simultaneously, they are sometimes referred to as "single-parameter" instruments. At the present time, the Coulter single-parameter instruments (Z series) are the only ones being used to any extent. Their use is mostly in research laboratories where their versatility is very important. By simply changing the size of the aperture, the amount of aperture current, the threshold, and the amount of sample that is pulled through the aperture, these instruments can count any type of particle, from fungal spores to spermatozoa or from carbon particles to latex particles. Occasionally, one may find a single-parameter instrument

in a clinical laboratory where it might serve as a reference or back-up instrument. The clinical use of single-parameter instruments, however, has become very limited in the past decade, and for that reason, they will not be addressed any further in this text.

In the mid-1960s, Coulter Electronics introduced a new instrument capable of simultaneous RBC and WBC counts, as well as determinations of hemoglobin (Hb) concentration and mean corpuscular volume (MCV). Using these data, the instrument calculated the hematocrit (Hct), mean corpuscular Hb (MCH), and mean corpuscular Hb concentration (MCHC; Chap. 9). This instrument was the Model S and was one of the pioneering "multiparameter" instruments.[11] The Model S has since undergone several modifications (S Sr, S Jr, S Plus series I through VI, STKS, and most recently, GEN S) leading to increased capacity, new determinations, and subsequent decreased cost per determination. These instruments are discussed in Chapter 42.[4]

At about the same time (mid-1960s) Technicon Instruments Corporation introduced a multiparameter instrument based on darkfield optical scanning using the same continuous-flow mechanisms that had become popular in the clinical chemistry laboratory. This instrument was referred to as a *sequential multiple analyzer* (SMA). A problem soon surfaced relative to the method Technicon had chosen to determine Hct (electrical resistance of a suspension of blood cells) when it was discovered that inaccurate results were obtained in certain patients with plasma conductivity abnormalities. The SMA instruments remained in production only a few years and were replaced by a new instrument called the Hemalog that was capable of performing a CBC and platelet count.[2] Blood coagulation tests, including prothrombin times and partial thromboplastin times, were also included in early models. A centri-

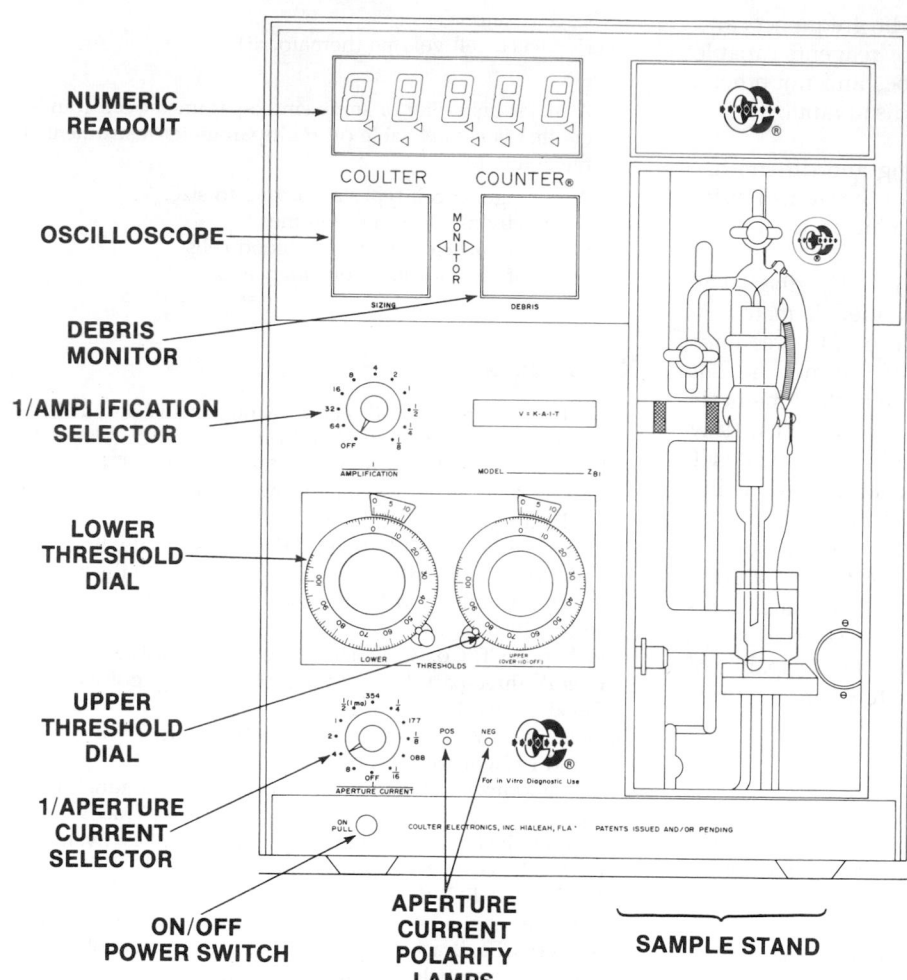

NUMERIC READOUT

OSCILLOSCOPE

DEBRIS MONITOR

1/AMPLIFICATION SELECTOR

LOWER THRESHOLD DIAL

UPPER THRESHOLD DIAL

1/APERTURE CURRENT SELECTOR

ON/OFF POWER SWITCH

APERTURE CURRENT POLARITY LAMPS

SAMPLE STAND

FIGURE 41-2. Front panel of Coulter ZBI showing threshold and aperture current controls. (Courtesy of Coulter Electronics, Inc.)

fuged Hct as well as one based on electrical conductivity was available with this instrument. Technicon also produced another instrument named the Hemalog D that determined leukocyte differential counts based on cellular cytochemistry.[1] Subsequent models, the most recent called the H·3, have combined blood cell counts with the leukocyte differential count. The more recent models offer additional determinations, including the reticulocyte count. These instruments are discussed in Chapter 42.

The mid-1970s saw a new entry into the multiparameter instrument market. Ortho Diagnostic Systems introduced a cell-counting instrument based on laser light scatter. In addition to the use of a laser beam as a means of cell detection, this instrument introduced the concept of hydrodynamic focusing to routine cell counting. Hydrodynamic focusing generates an extremely narrow channel through which cells may proceed in single file, thus avoiding a problem that had plagued cell counters until that time: the inability to size individual cells accurately because of the random coincidental passage of more than one cell through the orifice simultaneously resulting in a negative error (coincidence counting or coincidence loss).[7] The Ortho instrument is no longer in production, but the concepts of hydrodynamic focusing and laser scatter have been incorporated into numerous instruments

including those made by Coulter and Technicon, and the Cell-Dyn instrument produced by Abbott Laboratories.

After the Coulter Electronics patent on electrical impedance counting expired, a large number of cell counters were introduced to the marketplace by several companies, some of which have since been purchased by other companies. The result has been a bewildering array of multiparameter cell counters based on electrical impedance or a combination of electrical impedance and other cell counting principles. The situation is so fluid that it would be impractical to list the companies involved; such a list would be outdated within months. The resulting competition in the market has been beneficial, yielding a wide range of instruments with various capacities that are able to fit the needs of laboratories ranging from large, high-volume laboratories to physician offices.

Most larger automated hematology systems are now capable of generating a leukocyte differential. Methods for differentiating the five types of normal circulating leukocytes have varied according to manufacturer and tend to be based on a combination of principles. These principles include (1) determination of cell volume (electrical impedance or forward scatter of laser light), (2) cytochemistry (peroxidase staining), (3) evaluation of internal cellular organelles and nuclear characteristics (90°

laser scatter, polarizing laser light, radio frequency, and electromagnetic pulses), and (4) use of reagents capable of differentially lysing certain cell types and not others. Each method has advantages and disadvantages and these are covered in Chapter 42.

A unique principle of cell counting and differentiation based on expansion and analysis of the stained buffy coat in a centrifuged specimen has been introduced.[12] This also is described in Chapter 42.

In Chapter 43, the flow cytometer is described. The flow cytometer is essentially an expanded hematology instrument that has incorporated the use of fluorescence for cell identification. In fact, some of the more recent hematology systems are now offering cytoflow methods for reticulocyte counting using fluorescent dyes. The flow cytometer is capable of analyzing single cells, such as T and B lymphocytes, for a particular characteristic using fluorescent-tagged monoclonal antibodies.

In summary, the majority of instruments produced today are multiparameter. There is an extensive variety of instruments with differing capabilities from small, portable instruments used in point-of-care testing to large, sophisticated (and very expensive) systems capable of generating over two dozen parameters on a single blood sample.

Review Questions

41-1. The first two principles of cell counting that were sufficiently accurate and practical for the clinical laboratory were

  A. electrical impedance and laser scatter.
  B. darkfield optical scan and electrical impedance.
  C. darkfield optical scan and laser scatter.
  D. cytochemistry and electromagnetic pulse.

41-2. Hydrodynamic focusing results in decreased

  A. electrical interference.
  B. false counts caused by debris.
  C. sensitivity.
  D. coincidence counting.

41-3. Ninety-degree laser scatter will provide information on

  A. cellular organelles.
  B. cell number.
  C. cell volume.
  D. packed cell volume (hematocrit).

41-4. A major capability of some single-parameter cell counters that is *not* available on multiparameter instruments is the ability to

  A. distinguish cell types according to size.
  B. directly measure cell volume.
  C. count particles other than blood cells.
  D. count cells without coincidence loss.

References

1. Ansley H, Ornstein L: Enzyme histochemistry and differential white cell counts on Technicon Hemalog D. Automated Analysis, vol 1. Tarrytown, NY, Mediad, Inc, 1971
2. Brittin GM, Dew SA, Felwell EK: Automated optical counting of blood platelets. Blood 38:422, 1971
3. Gagon TE, Atherns JW, Boggs DT et al: An evaluation of the variance of leukocyte counts as performed with the hemacytometer, Coulter and Fisher instruments. Am J Clin Pathol 46:684, 1966
4. Haberman T, Cox C, Pierre R: Evaluation of the Coulter S-Plus IV three-part differential as a screening tool (abstract). Blood 62:80a, 1983
5. Helleman PW, Benjamin CJ: The TOA micro cell counter. Scand J Haematol 6:69, 1969
6. Langerkranz C: Photoelectric counting of individual microscopic plant and animal cells. Nature 161:25, 1948
7. Lewis SM: Hemacytometry by laser beam optics: Evaluation of the Hemac 630L. J Clin Pathol 30:54, 1977
8. MacFarlane RG, Payne AM, Poole JCF et al: An automatic apparatus for counting red blood cells. Br J Haematol 5:1, 1959
9. Mattern CFT, Bracket FS, Olson BJ: Determination of number and size of particles by electrical gating: Blood cells. J Appl Physiol 10:56, 1957
10. Moldavan A: Photoelectric technique for the counting of microscopical cells. Science 80:188, 1934
11. Pinkerton PH, Spence I, Oglivie JC et al: An assessment of the Coulter counter model "S." J Clin Pathol 23:68, 1970
12. Wardlaw SC, Levine RA: Quantitative buffy coat analysis: A new laboratory tool functioning as a screening complete blood count. JAMA 249:617, 1983
13. Whitlock JH: The use of photoelectric turbidimetry in the determination of red blood count, hematocrit and hemoglobin. Blood 2:463, 1947

CHAPTER 42

Multiparameter Hematology Instruments

*Mary Ann Dotson**

Objectives

1. Explain electronic impedance technology used for blood cell counting.
2. Explain principles of light scatter cell counting technology to include two properties of laser light; hydrodynamic focusing; and principle of laminar flow.
3. Name cell characteristics identified by forward light scatter; 90° light scatter; and radio frequency.
4. List those instruments that use stain to help identify cell characteristics and describe which cells take up the specific stain.
5. Define "screening differential" and list two advantages and two disadvantages.
6. List two sample conditions that may cause interference with platelet counting.
7. List two sample conditions that may cause interference with WBC counting.
8. List at least two WBC types that are not identified and counted in an automated "screening" differential.
9. Compare unknown histogram/scattergram patterns to "normal" patterns and recognize abnormalities.

* The author gratefully acknowledges the following individuals and institutions who generously supplied some of the scattergrams used in this chapter: Connie Bishop and Sandra Ratliff, University of North Carolina Hospital, Chapel Hill, NC; Rick Grooms, Wake Medical Center, Raleigh, NC; Colleen Miller, Rex Hospital, Raleigh, NC; and Jerri Walters, Sinai Samaritan Medical Center, Milwaukee, WI.

Instruments capable of measuring more than one hematologic parameter at a time were introduced in the mid-1960s by two manufacturers using different principles of cell counting. Technicon Instruments offered the SMA 4, capable of providing simultaneous white blood cell (WBC) and red blood cell (RBC) counts as well as hemoglobin (Hb) and hematocrit (Hct) determinations. Coulter Electronics introduced a seven-parameter instrument, the Model S, which was capable of performing the four studies listed above plus three red cell indices plus mean cell volume (MCV), mean cell hemoglobin (MCH), and mean cell hemoglobin concentration (MCHC). In 1966 Technicon added the three indices to their system to produce the SMA 7. The Technicon instruments were based on darkfield optical scanning, whereas the Coulter instruments utilized electronic impedance for cell counting. Other manufacturers soon followed with their own seven-parameter instruments. Ortho Diagnostic Systems introduced a laser-based optical instrument in 1975.

Over the years, the microscopic examination of leukocytes, erythrocytes, and platelets on a blood film—better known as the manual leukocyte differential count—has been recognized as the foundation for diagnosis of hematologic abnormalities. Manual differentials, however, are labor intensive, expensive, and tedious and they require a highly skilled laboratorian. Even with a highly skilled individual, the test procedure has a relatively high inherent error rate primarily due to sampling, because only 100 cells are routinely identified.[12,32,33] Preparation technique, fatigue and subjectivity also play a role in the poor reproducibility of the 100-cell manual differential.[32,40,44]

Not until companion technologies of integrated circuits, computers, artificial intelligence, cytochemical techniques, flow-through systems and computer-assisted image analysis were developed could automated differential systems be realized.[2,40] A fortunate byproduct of the automation of the differential count has been the standardization of blood film processing, as well as nationally recognized definitions of standard cell types.[36]

Automated systems using cytochemical flow-through technology and computer-assisted image analysis (pattern recognition) were developed in the early 1970s. Automated systems based on computer-assisted image analysis helped reduce the subjectivity and fatigue factors but did not significantly improve precision. Pattern recognition systems were slow and counted only 100 cells (or increments of 100). Five different manufacturers produced instruments based on pattern recognition during the 1970s and 1980s.[33] These systems are no longer being manufactured. Flow-through technology using cytochemical staining and light scatter detection methods developed by Technicon (now Bayer) will be discussed later in this chapter.

Separation of leukocyte subpopulations using electronic impedance (volume) analysis began with the identification of lymphocyte percent and number. Development of special lysing reagents that remove or shrink the cytoplasm soon provided the so-called "three-part-differential" by detecting cells with small, medium, and large nuclei. These automated three-part leukocyte differentials were used as "screening" differentials. They were initially designed to identify samples with normal ratios of lymphocytes, monocytes/mononuclear cells, and granulocytes so as to reduce the number of manual, routine microscopic differentials. Further development has produced five-part screening differentials capable of determining absolute numbers and percentages for five leukocyte types (neutrophil, lymphocyte, monocyte, eosinophil, and basophil).

Most instruments that generate leukocyte differentials have "flagging" analysis programs to identify variations from expected cell patterns. Such flags alert the laboratory to samples which may contain qualitative or quantitative abnormalities and which should be subjected to microscopic evaluation of a stained blood film by a morphologist. Some of the flags suggest interference that could render the flagged count incorrect. Further study of these specimens is required before release of a report. According to the National Committee for Clinical Laboratory Standards (NCCLS), the "automated differential" must be at least as good as the manual method in flagging and identifying abnormalities, whether they are distributional or morphologic.[36]

Today's marketplace has a variety of multiparameter instruments from several manufacturers. These instruments may be subdivided into two basic principles of operation: electronic impedance (or resistance) and light scatter (both laser and nonlaser light) with or without the use of specific stains or dyes. A new instrument using centrifugal force was introduced in the early 1980s, but it does not count individual cells. Most manufacturers offer several instruments of increasing complexity and sophistication that differ in the number of tests available and the degree of automation, ranging from discrete analyzers to walkaway instruments.

In this chapter the development of various technologies will be presented, and the evolution of the complete blood count (CBC) will be described. The general principles of cell counting and characterization will be detailed. The particular characteristics of each of the principal systems will be described with consideration given to interferences and review criteria. Several illustrations of histograms and scattergrams from the principal systems will be discussed. Finally, guidelines and considerations helpful in selecting instruments will be reviewed for various types of laboratories.

DEVELOPMENT OF AUTOMATED ANALYZERS

Development of the automated hematology analyzer has been continuous, with each step increasing the number of tests performed simultaneously, increasing the speed, and decreasing the required sample size.

All multiparameter instruments use colorimetric methodology to measure hemoglobin. The cyanmethemoglobin method has been modified by each instrument manufacturer to speed the reaction time for rapid sample analysis. One company has developed a hemoglobin method that does not use a cyanide-based reagent. This noncyanide method is reported to be comparable to the reference method.[34,39] Calibration of the hemoglobin channel is performed using calibration material that is traceable back to the reference method (cyanmethemoglobin) as required for College of American Pathologists (CAP) accreditation.

Current multiparameter hematology instruments report hematocrit values that are not obtained by centrifugation. They use the individual RBC volume analysis, RBC histogram, and the RBC count to calculate the "packed red cell volume" (PCV). The area of the pulse generated as a cell passes through a sensing zone represents the cell's volume.[46] The areas are "summed." These measurements and a calibration factor (constant) are used to determine the hematocrit in percentage or L/L. The calibration constant takes into account the dilution factor and the volume of sample analyzed. All instruments automatically correct for coincidence (defined as more than one cell in the sensing zone), which is mathematically predictable based on particle concentration. The volume measurement of a cell is affected by its path through the sensing zone. Centered cells produce "clean" pulses that represent the cell's volume. Cells that do not traverse the central path produce unusual pulses that do not truly represent the cell's volume. Editing of unusual pulse shapes is programmed into systems that do not employ hydrodynamic focusing (to be described later). All cells are counted for the RBC count while editing identifies only clean pulses for use in the determination of the MCV and Hct. The volume measurement of a red cell is affected by the relative osmotic pressure of the cell and its surrounding medium (plasma or diluting fluid). The red cell's response (volume change) to the diluting fluid of an automated instrument depends on the osmotic differences between the cell and the diluting fluid. Several plasma conditions (i.e., hyper-, hyponatremia; hyper-, hypo-osmolality) affect cell volume responses owing to increased osmotic differences. Increased amounts of urea or glucose make cells hyperosmolar. Excess ethylenediaminetetraacetic acid (EDTA) causes red cell (osmotic) shrinkage.[20] In conclusion, automated hematocrits are calculated from RBC counts and RBC volume measurements and, except in relatively rare conditions just described, they correlate quite well with spun hematocrit values.

CBC parameters starting with the basic four are listed in Table 42-1. After the addition of red cell indices and platelet counts, the list includes parameters that were developed as computer programs became more sophisticated. Some parameters that are instrument specific are noted in the table.

Automation of some measurements, such as the addition of platelet enumeration in the presence of RBCs, came in response to diagnostic needs. Of the laboratories reporting in the 1986 CAP Comprehensive Hematology Survey, 92% were using an automated method for plate-

TABLE 42-1
Evolution of Parameters That Are Included in a CBC

1. Hgb, Hct, RBC, WBC	1950s
2. MCV, MCH, MCHC	
3. PLT, RDW, (PDW, MPV, PCT, P-LCR, RDW-SD)	
4. LUC, CHCM, HDW, LI, MPXI Technicon™ only	1960s
5. LYM, MONO, GRAN (% & #)	1970s
6. NEUT, EOS, BASO (% & #)	1980s
7. Flagging messages for all parameters (definitive & suspect)	
8. Reticulocyte counts	1990s

when counting ends. However, if the size of the channel in which each pulse occurs is identified, the pulses can be counted and stored in memory in their appropriate channel. Plotting the number of pulses on the Y axis and the cell size (channel number) on the X axis produces a histogram (Fig. 42-1) that depicts the volume distribution of the cell population. Two-dimensional cytograms (scattergrams) represent two cell properties or characteristics, and cell types appear as clusters, the number of dots in each cluster denoting the concentration of that cell type. Figure 42-2 compares a cytogram/scattergram and a histogram of unstained normal WBCs. The X axis of the scattergram is internal cell complexity, and the Y axis is relative size.

lets,[11] up from 12% in 1977.[10] Today only 3% of laboratories routinely report manual phase platelet counts, although the phase count may be used as a back-up method or when automated platelet counts are suspect.[31] Other new tests were developed as a result of engineering developments and advances in computerization. One example is the measurement of the coefficient of variation (CV) of volume distribution within a population of RBCs; this CV is reported as the red cell distribution width (RDW). This value is proposed as an indicator of anisocytosis. Together with the MCV, the RDW has been used as a means of classifying anemias.[8] Similar volume measurements and calculations have been extended to platelets as a mean platelet volume (MPV) and platelet distribution width (PDW). Studies have linked platelet measurements to clinical states,[7] but to date such measures have not been widely used.

Oscilloscope displays have been part of clinical instruments since the time of the first Coulter counters. They show the pulses that are created by the cells as they interrupt the current, but as real-time displays, they cease

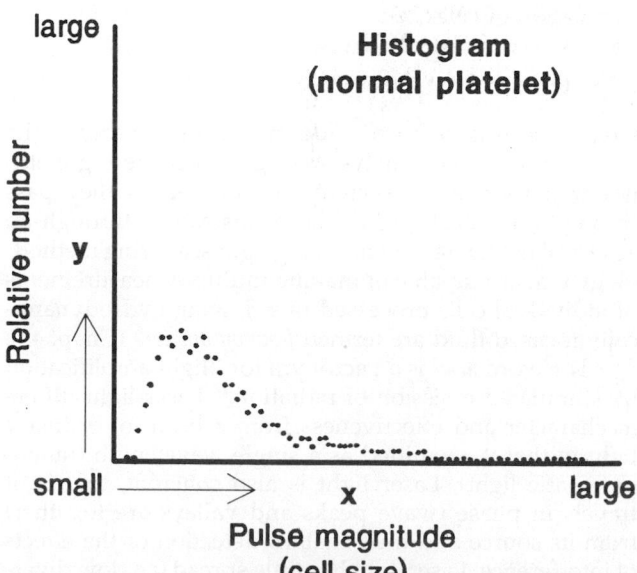

FIGURE 42-1. Visual display of one cell characteristic and cell frequency as a histogram with X axis being pulse magnitude (cell size/volume) and Y axis being relative number (cell concentration).

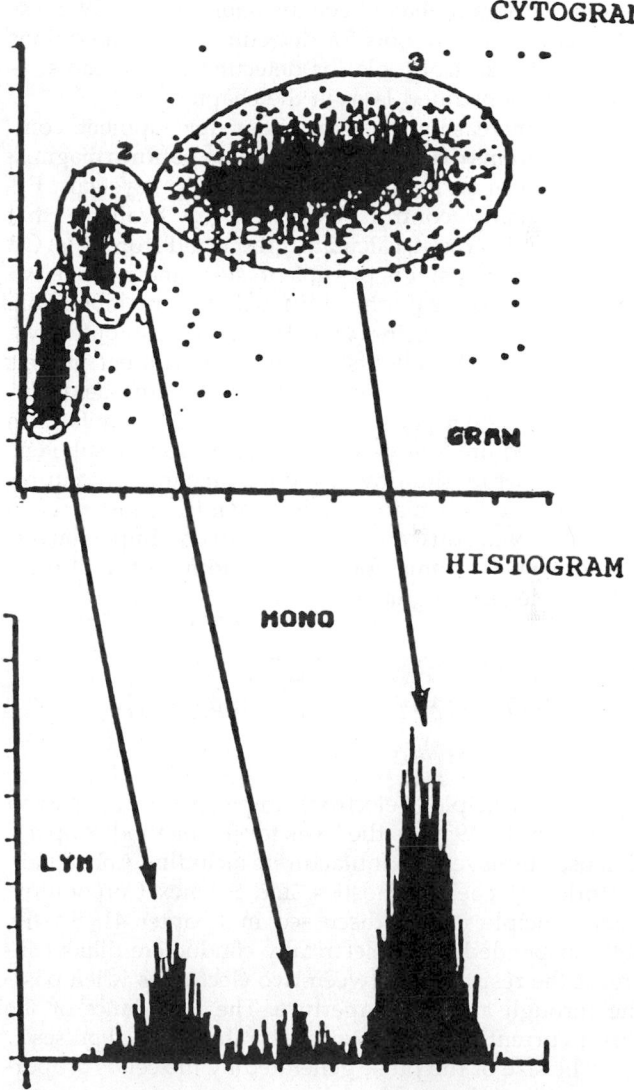

FIGURE 42-2. Visual display of two cell characteristics as cytogram (or scattergram) and histogram. This example is a normal unstained whole blood sample. Normal human leukocyte light scatter signals produce three distinct clusters on the forward *versus* right-angle scattergram display. By mathematically transforming this information into a one-dimensional histogram, three peaks (*arrows*) are derived, corresponding uniquely to each of the three clusters. Peaks, from left to right, are lymphocytes, monocytes, and granulocytes. (ELT, courtesy of Ortho Diagnostic Systems Inc.)

The ability to produce histograms brought with it the ability to count the number of cells within selected size ranges. This capability, in concert with new lysing agents, has allowed subsequent instruments to generate data on relative and absolute numbers of small, medium, and large leukocytes, or the "three-part differential." The result of all of these advances has been a redefinition of the CBC, which may now include more than 24 measurements and calculations that characterize the RBC, WBC, and platelet populations in approximately 60 seconds using 100 μL of whole blood. The latest technologic developments analyze cells simultaneously using two or more methods. These advancements in technology have produced a "five-part differential."

Automation brought significant improvement in counting precision; and, as each method was automated, it became a more valuable diagnostic tool. Volume distribution histograms have been available since 1979; these offer useful clinical tools for detecting certain conditions and quality control tools for detecting interferences, as will be demonstrated later in the chapter.

With increasing microprocessor development, computer programs direct the instrument to perform diagnostic self-checks on the electronic and optical systems. Extensive quality control (QC) files are available that automatically accept, calculate, graph, and store data. On many instruments, it is possible to store and retrieve patient results, some with additional data manipulation. Bidirectional interfacing with laboratory computer systems allows delta checks by some instrument models (Chap. 46). Analysis of bar-coded samples provides walkaway systems with positive patient sample identification that only require follow-up on abnormals and result verification. Startup, shutdown, and maintenance procedures are automated on many models, requiring just a touch on the keypad. Software enables relatively simple conversion of some systems, for example, to report in SI units or in a selected language.

GENERAL PRINCIPLES OF INSTRUMENT OPERATION

Electronic Impedance

The basic principle of electronic impedance developed by Coulter in the 1950s is the basis for the method of operation used by several manufacturers including Abbott Laboratories, Roche Diagnostics, and Sysmex Corporation. This principle is also discussed in Chapter 41. Briefly, cells suspended in an electrically conductive diluent increase the resistance between two electrodes when passing through a sensing aperture. The impedance of the direct current (DC) creates measurable voltage pulses.

The size of the pulse generated by the cell is proportional to its volume. The cell count is determined by the number of pulses generated. Separate channels are used for WBC and RBC counting. The WBCs are counted in a dilution in which the RBCs have been lysed. In the RBC channel, the dilution is great enough to make the number of WBCs negligible and thus not a source of interference except when they are present in extremely high numbers. In the more advanced models, platelets and RBCs generally are counted together and the counts separated by computer analysis of pulse heights.

In first-generation electrical impedance instruments, several things were found to affect volume measurements. The "coincidence" of more than one cell arriving at the orifice at the same time or the position of the cell with respect to the center of the orifice may create an artificially large pulse. Also, cells recirculating back into the sensing zone can create erroneous pulses. These problems have been addressed in newer generations of instruments. To manage orientation and coincidence, Coulter Electronics employed sophisticated circuitry to electronically "edit" out anomalously shaped pulses as described above. A backwash of diluting fluid is used to prevent recirculation of cells into the counting zone. This reduces red cell interference with platelet counting. To increase platelet counting sensitivity, the RBC/PLT aperture size was decreased.

Taking another approach, Sysmex instruments use hydrodynamic focusing to force red cells and platelets into single-file-passage through the center of the sensing zone. The fluid aperture produced through hydrodynamic focusing minimizes the protein buildup and plugs that are inherent to small rigid apertures. (See next section for detail.)

In recent generations of instruments employing electronic impedance, these methods have been extended to leukocyte differential analysis. With the aid of lysing agents that strip away or shrink the cells' plasma membrane and cytoplasm, leaving "bare" nuclei, the cells are counted and sized as they pass through the aperture. The various size determinations have been related to WBC types: small—lymphocytes; medium—mononuclear cells and eosinophils; large—granulocytes. Enumeration of these three subpopulations of cells can be used as a screening differential. Further classification of the granulocytes into neutrophils, eosinophils, and basophils occurs in the newest instruments. These instruments use a more controlled alteration of the cell nucleus and cytoplasm and employ multiple analytic methods to characterize each population of cells.

Light Scattering

Great strides have been made in just a few years in the development of cell analysis using light scattering methodology. Cells are detected and counted as they pass through a focused beam of light instead of through an electrical field. Instruments using light scattering methodology that are capable of making multiple measurements of individual cells processed in a flowing hydrodynamically focused fluid are termed *flow cytometers* (Chap. 43).

The word *laser* is an acronym for "**l**ight **a**mplification by **s**timulated **e**mission of **r**adiation." Laser light differs in character and effectiveness from a beam of ordinary light in that it is emitted as a single wavelength (monochromatic light). Laser light is also coherent; that is, it travels in phase (wave peaks and valleys are together) from its source and thus enables detection of the effects of interference. Laser light has little spread (*i.e.*, low divergence). The fourth characteristic of laser light is its brightness. Noncoherent light sources are present in some instruments that use filters to obtain appropriate wavelengths instead of the more expensive lasers.

Light scatter by cells is the summation of three independent processes: *diffraction* (bending around corners),[63] *refraction* (bending because of a change in speed),[62] and *reflection* (light rays turned back by the surface or boundary of an obstruction).[60,61] Cells scatter light in all directions, with diffraction generally dominating at small angles relative to the incident light, reflection dominating at larger angles, and refraction generally dominating at intermediate angles.[45,57]

Flow cells are made of quartz rather than glass because quartz is transparent and does not bend the light that passes through it. It also allows ultraviolet (UV) light to pass, whereas glass blocks the passage of UV light. The flow cell is where the cells are sensed and counted, and where cell characteristics are measured. The light source is focused on a small area of the flow cell, and the sample stream is directed through this area (sensing zone) for analysis.

Sheath fluid is the fluid that fills a flow cell and surrounds the sample stream as it passes through the flow cell. It prevents the flow cell from being coated by reagents, cell stroma, or any other substance that would artifactually bend the rays of light as they enter the flow cell. Sheath fluid also facilitates laminar flow and hydrodynamic focusing.

Laminar flow describes the flow properties of a fluid moving relatively constantly through a long channel or pipe. When laminar flow conditions exist, all particles flow in parallel lines as they travel through the channel (flow cell). Under these conditions, a second fluid containing the sample does not mix with the surrounding sheath fluid. Laminar flow is dependent on flow velocity, channel diameter, fluid density, and the fluid viscosity coefficient. These factors are used in a formula to calculate the *Reynolds number*, which must be below the critical value of 2300 for laminar conditions to exist.[27,57] Flow becomes turbulent when the critical value is exceeded.

Hydrodynamic focusing of the sample stream is produced by symmetrically decreasing the cross-sectional area of the fluidic channel in the flow cell and reducing the area in which the fluid is flowing. This results in faster-flowing central fluid with narrowing of the central sample stream. The design is such that the sample stream is sufficiently narrowed to separate and align the cells into a single file for passage through the sensing zone.[27,57]

Light scattered by a particle in the sensing zone of the flow cell is detected by appropriately placed *photodetectors (scatter detectors)*. Photodiodes and photomultiplier tubes (PMT) are commonly used for this purpose. Photodiodes are light detectors that are not very sensitive but are sufficient to detect forward scatter, which has a relatively strong light level. On the other hand, PMTs are sensitive to weak light levels and, as the name implies, multiply weak signals into stronger, useful signals. PMTs are used to detect 90° (right-angle) scatter and staining or fluorescence, which is also measured at 90°.

Blocker bar (Fig. 42-3), *obscuration bar*, or *darkfield stop* are names given to the barriers that prevent direct (unscattered) light from reaching (and "blinding") the light scatter detectors.

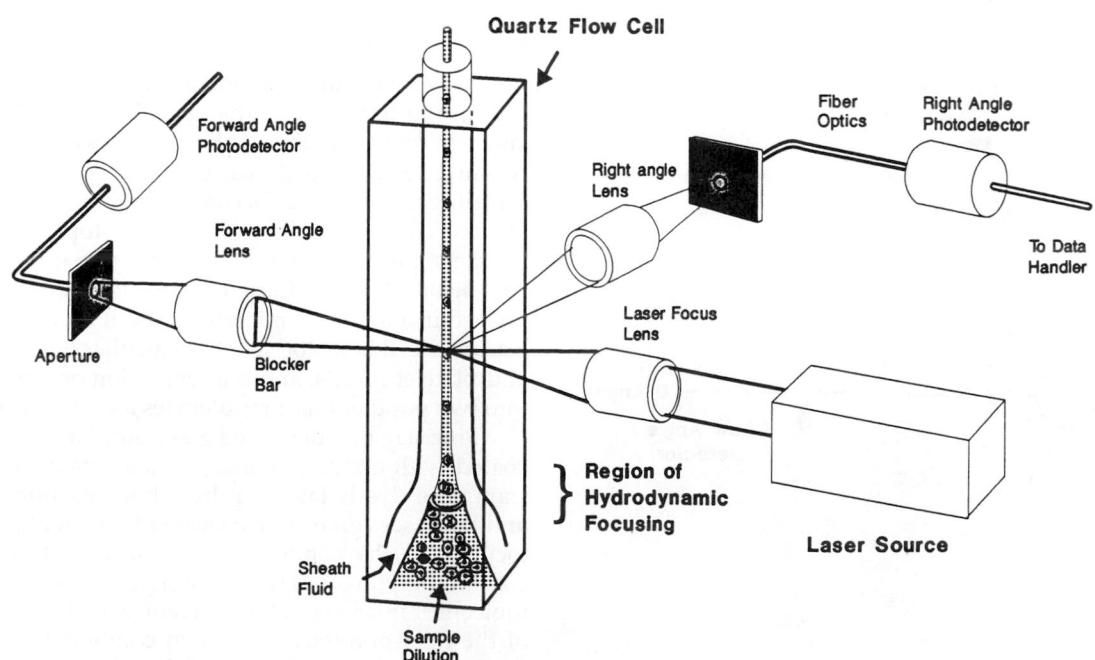

FIGURE 42-3. Basic concepts of "cytometers" employing light scattering principles for cell analysis are shown. Labels identify the light source (laser), quartz flow cell, blocker bar (obscuration bar), photodetectors (at various angles), sheath, sample stream, region of hydrodynamic focusing in flow cell, and concept of laminar flow. (ELT Optics Bench, courtesy of Ortho Diagnostic Systems Inc.)

TABLE 42-2
Data Obtained from Light Scatter Cell Analysis of Technicon

H-Series	Angle 1	Angle 2
Cell counts	Low forward scatter (size)	
Differential	Low forward scatter AND	90° (right-angle) scatter absorbance (stain)
RBC analysis	Low forward scatter 2°–3° (RBC volume)	High-angle forward scatter (H_gb conc.) 5°–15°
Lobularity index	Low forward scatter 2°–3° (size)	High-angle forward scatter (internal complexity) 5°–15°

Forward low-angle light scatter correlates with cell volume primarily because of diffraction of light (bending by the outside surface of a cell).[45] Figure 42-3 depicts photodetectors in an optical system. *Forward high-angle light scatter* measurements depict the degree of structure inside the cell.[26] *Differential scatter* is the combination of low- and high-angle forward scatter. This scatter analysis is used to analyze RBC (volume versus Hb concentration) and WBC (volume *versus* nuclear lobularity) properties[35] (Fig. 42-4). The intensity of light scatter at larger angles is attributable primarily to refraction and reflection of light from larger structures inside the cell. Structures such as nuclei and cytoplasmic granules determine the intensity of light scattering at right angles.

A *beam splitter* separates different wavelengths of light for collection by different photosensing devices and for analysis. *Mia analysis* is a light scattering technique in which RBC volume and Hb concentration are determined by analyzing scattered monochromatic light from individual sphered RBCs at two carefully chosen angular intervals.[56]

Absorbance Combined with Light Scatter

The darkfield optical method of light scatter combined with light absorbance measurements used by Bayer Diagnostics (Technicon) counts and classifies the WBC. With this method, when no cells are present in the scatter channel, the darkfield disc prevents the light from hitting the photodetector. As each cell passes through the sensing zone, light is scattered through the opening around the darkfield disc, hitting the photodetector and generating signals or pulses, which are summed for the cell counts. In the absorbance channel, when either unstained cells or no cells are passing, there is no light absorbed by stain; therefore, the photodiode receives maximum light. As a stained cell passes, it absorbs a portion of the light, decreasing the amount hitting the photodetector (photodiode). The amount of light absorbed is proportional to the amount of staining. Cell types may be differentiated on this basis.[49] Table 42-2 summarizes the use of light scatter for cell analysis by Bayer (Technicon) hematology instruments.

Centrifugal Analysis

An innovative centrifugal method does not actually count cells but rather analyzes the red cell layer and buffy coat layers in centrifuged whole blood samples. The technique was first described in the early 1980s.[58] Whole blood, when centrifuged, will layer according to the specific gravity of each component (from bottom to top: RBCs, WBCs, platelets, plasma). Quantitative buffy coat (QBC; Becton Dickinson Primary Care Diagnostics) analysis is performed in a modified microhematocrit tube and provides a centrifuged hematocrit value, calculated total leukocyte and platelet counts, and the separation of the white cells into two populations: granulocytes and nongranulocytes.

Precisely manufactured glass capillary tubes are precoated with acridine orange, which acts as a supravital stain. The dye is taken up by white cell nucleoproteins and fluoresces green when excited by violet light. Granulocytic cells have numerous granules that contain glycosaminoglycans. Acridine orange absorbed by these molecules fluoresces at a different wavelength than that of the nucleoproteins and when combined with nuclear fluorescence, makes this part of the white cell layer appear bright orange. The granulocytic cell layer is the heaviest component of the buffy coat and layers immediately on top of the RBCs. Cells lacking granules with glycosaminoglycans (lymphocytes and monocytes) remain above

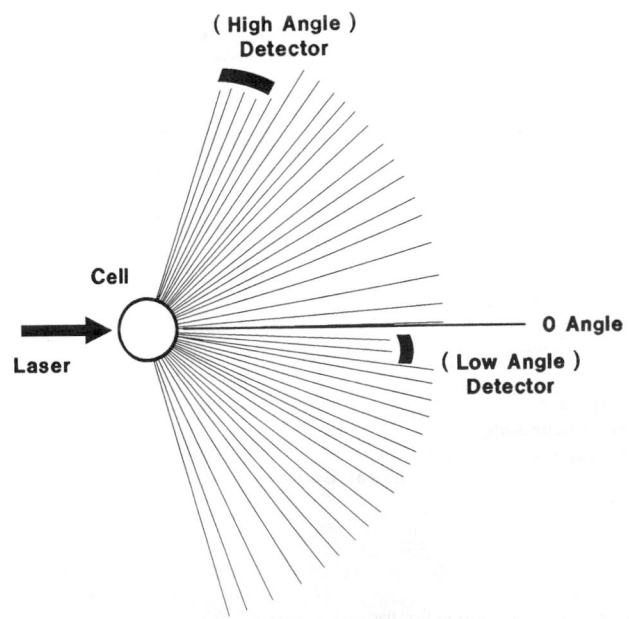

FIGURE 42-4. Differential scatter detection. Low forward-angle scatter and high forward-angle scatter detection used by Bayer Diagnostics H·Series for red cell and white cell analysis.

the granulocytes in a single layer and fluoresce a brilliant emerald green. Platelets, fluorescing yellow, form the top cell layer. Cell-free plasma fluoresces green.

Analysis of each layer is possible because of a solid cylindrical plastic float that expands the buffy coat layer (Fig. 42-5). The plastic cylinder has a specific gravity between that of plasma and RBCs. It becomes positioned at the top of the RBC layer during centrifugation and is surrounded by the expanded buffy coat layers. These layers are expanded by a factor of 10.71 and are only two to three cells thick, which is optimum. An optical device with a UV light source, appropriate filters, and a micrometer is used to measure the length of each layer. Precise measurements of the tube's longitudinal movement are made from interface to interface, and the band (layer) lengths are converted into count equivalents. QBC

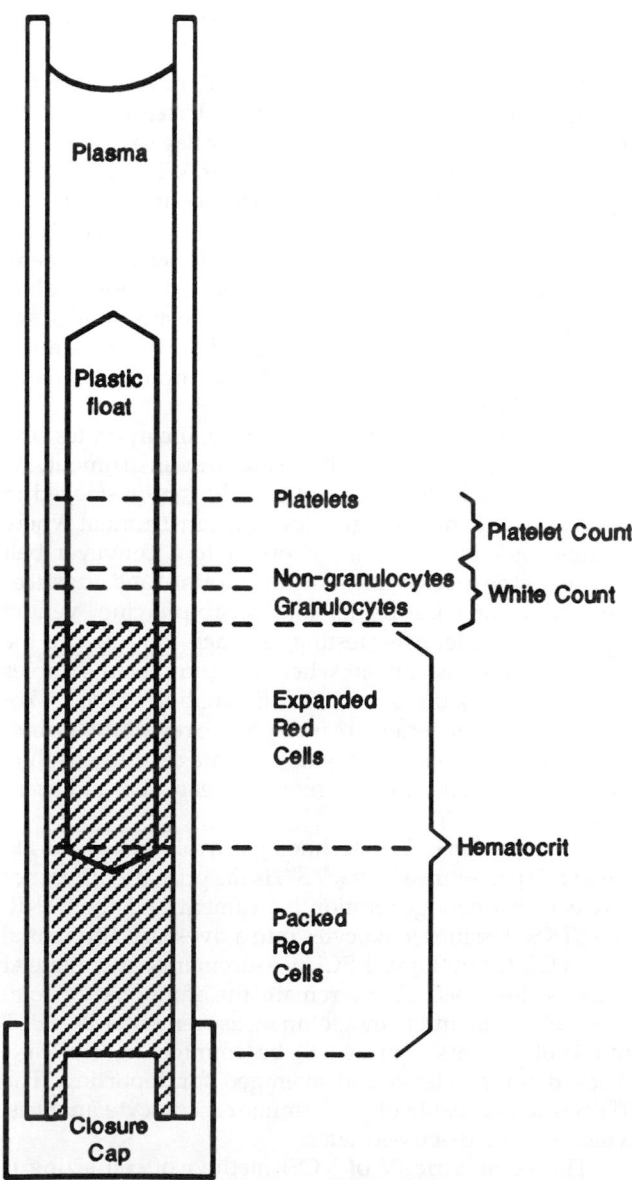

FIGURE 42-5. Whole blood layers in centrifugal analyzer tube. Cell counts are derived from expanded and nonexpanded layers as indicated.

AUTOREAD produces a report printout following automatic instrument identification of the layer interfaces. This analysis takes 90 seconds and printing takes another 30 seconds. The report includes Hct, WBC count, platelet count, granulocyte count and percentage, lymphocyte/monocyte count and percentage, a derived Hb value, and an MCHC.

QBC instruments were designed primarily for use in physician offices. Successful operation does not require extensive training or a background in laboratory techniques. The instrument provides accurate and rapid screening CBC results, with less than 5% unreadable samples from populations seen in an outpatient setting. A study comparing buffy coat analysis results and standard hematology testing methods showed good correlation.[58] The authors of this study recommend that platelet values less than 80×10^9/L be confirmed by an independent method such as blood film examination. If a hematologic dyscrasia is suspected, referral for a blood film examination is essential, and cell counts may need to be determined by another method. Buffy coat analysis provides rapid results but is not designed to detect red cell abnormalities (*e.g.*, hypochromia), increases in cell types (*e.g.*, eosinophils), or abnormal (leukemic) white cells. Samples from inpatient populations tend to have more frequent streaming problems (poor separation of layers) in the instrument than samples from an outpatient setting. A recent study showed good correlation between QBC Autoread System results and the hospital laboratory CBC analysis. Proportional and intercept biases found in this study are reported not to be clinically significant.[38] The ideal setting for this instrument is in the routine outpatient clinic or doctor's office.

PRINCIPAL INSTRUMENT SYSTEMS

Electronic Impedance Instruments

COULTER ELECTRONICS

The basic components of a hematology instrument such as the Coulter S-Plus series are a power unit, an analyzer, a diluter, and a data terminal. A ticket printer prints the determined values, and a printer-plotter provides a hard copy of the data displayed on the terminal.

The power unit consists of a pneumatic portion (vacuum and pressure pumps), which move fluids through the diluter and an electronic portion that provides regulated voltages for the system's circuitry. The diluter unit has an aspiration tip, sample valve, mixing chambers, WBC and RBC sensing apertures, and the hemoglobinometer. The analyzer module contains electronic and computing circuitry that controls the sequence of operations in the diluter and processes the data generated. The information from the analyzer is received by the data terminal, where results and histograms are displayed.

The aspirated whole blood sample is divided into two aliquots, and each is mixed with isotonic diluent. One dilution is delivered to the RBC aperture bath for information about RBCs and platelets. The other is delivered to the WBC bath, where a lytic reagent is added to break down the RBC membrane and release Hb. There are three sensing apertures in each of the counting baths.

Count and size information is generated in triplicate in the form of pulses. After the leukocyte information is obtained, the diluted specimen is delivered to the hemoglobinometer that measures light transmittance at a wavelength of 525 nm. The information is sent to the analyzer.

Three values are considered to be measured directly: RBC, WBC and hemoglobin concentration. Other values are calculated.

The platelet count is determined from pulses in the RBC analysis within the range of 2 to 20 fL. The pulses obtained in this range are classified as platelets for the raw count. To obtain an accurate platelet count in the presence of red cells, a mathematical model is applied to the raw data. Histograms of the raw count (data) are fitted to a lognormal curve ranging from 0 to 70 fL. The extended curve eliminates particles interfering at both ends, such as debris (low end) or microcytic RBCs (high end). The final platelet count is derived from this fitted curve. If certain criteria for curve fitting and platelet data are not met, the count is flagged and not reported.[14]

Size distribution histograms of WBC, RBC, and platelet populations are established by pulse height analysis. When a histogram does not reach one-half scale (Y axis), it is automatically scaled to one-half height on the Y axis for evaluation of the cell distribution pattern. Thus, cell counts cannot be estimated from these histograms. (Fig. 42-6A illustrates patterns from a normal sample.) The MCV and RDW are derived from the RBC histogram, whereas the MPV and PDW are derived from the platelet histogram. Triplicate counting of RBC/PLT and WBC with statistical analysis for agreement of the independent counts ensures precision. In addition, the microprocessing capabilities have been expanded, permitting three-part (and five-part interpretive) leukocyte subpopulation analysis. Patient record, histogram and scattergram storage, sorting files by parameters (e.g., all samples with abnormal platelet values), QC files for commercial and patient controls with Levey-Jennings charts, the use of the Bull algorithm for moving averages (Chap. 45), and an automated calibration procedure are some features offered on various analyzer models. Walkaway automated cap-piercing is available on many models.

The Coulter Counter S-Plus series (models IV through VI and STKR) provide (in addition to routine 10-parameter profiles) percentages and absolute values of lymphocytes, mononuclear cells, and granulocytes, as well as leukocyte, erythrocyte, and platelet histograms (Fig. 42-6A). Leukocytes are sized electronically after they have had their cytoplasm and nucleus differentially shrunken by a special lysing agent and reagent system.[15] The cells are then classified as lymphocytes (small cells), mononuclear cells (medium cells), and granulocytes (large cells). A relative-size histogram is constructed and smoothed, and mathematical equations are applied to it looking at peaks and valleys. Internal flags (e.g., region "R" flags; Fig. 42-6B), backlighting of values, or instrument data rejection (dots or dashes instead of a numerical result) may occur if the values or shapes of the curves are not acceptable according to preset tolerances.[15,41] In Figure 42-6B, the R₁ flag denotes interference in the valley to the left of the lymphocyte subpopulation at approximately 35 fL. This interference could be caused by clumped or giant platelets, nucleated RBC (NRBC), non-lysed red cells (e.g., sickled red cells), malarial parasites, fibrin strands, cryoglobulin, or fat globules attributable to total parenteral nutrition.[41] The R₂ flag indicates excessive number of cells at the lymphocyte-mononuclear boundary (approximately 90 fL). Cell types that could be present are variant lymphocytes, abnormal lymphocytes (e.g., plasma or hairy cells) and blasts. Eosinophilia, monocytosis, and basophilia will also generate an R₂ flag.[41] The R₃ flag indicates an overlap of cells at the mononuclear-granulocyte boundary (approximately 160 fL). Many of these are false-positive flags, but they may indicate neutrophilia, neutrophilic left shift, eosinophilia, or a sample processed less than 30 minutes after collection. An R₄ flag indicates truncation of the distribution at the upper leukocyte threshold (450 fL) and is most often triggered when granulocyte numbers are increased. Each flag will appear simultaneously next to the percentage and the absolute values of the cell type(s) in question. "RM" indicates interference at multiple regions. Incomplete computation (. . .) may or may not appear in place of the numerical value simultaneously with R flags.

Backlighting of the leukocyte count indicates that the histogram curve does not start on the baseline below 35 fL (the lower leukocyte threshold). This flag can be caused by the same interferences as the R₁ flag. When backlighting occurs behind the total leukocyte count, it will also appear behind all the absolute numbers for each cell type, because the total leukocyte count is used to calculate them. Such backlighting indicates a possible erroneous value. Backlighting sometimes occurs only on relative and absolute numbers of mononuclear cells. This event is automatic when the absolute mononuclear number exceeds $1.5 \times 10^9/L$.[15,16]

The STKR (pronounced "stacker"), incorporates several new features to make it a walkaway instrument. As many as 12 racks (of 12 samples each) can be stacked in the loading bay on the right side of the instrument where a single rack automatically drops onto a conveyer belt that mixes the tubes (with a rocking motion) and advances them to a bar code reader and a cap-piercing, vented aspiration needle. After testing, the rack continues to the left side of the instrument where the completed samples once again stack up for removal. Evaluation of the leukocyte histogram generates an interpretive report for eosinophils and basophils along with percentages and absolute counts for the lymphocytes, mononuclear cells, and granulocytes.

The addition of VCS technology (triple transducer) to the STKS (pronounced "stack S") is the primary difference between this new generation instrument and the STKR. The STKS classifies leukocytes into a five-part differential with VCS technology. RBC measurements and platelet analysis described above remain the same, as do total WBC cell count and hemoglobin measurement. RBC/PLT and WBC counts continue to be counted in triplicate, checked for precision and averaged for reporting. The STKS is also capable of performing reticulocyte analysis, which will be discussed later.

The volumetric (V of VCS) method of cell sizing is combined with laser light scatter (S of VCS) and conductivity (C of VCS) measurements. The differential portion

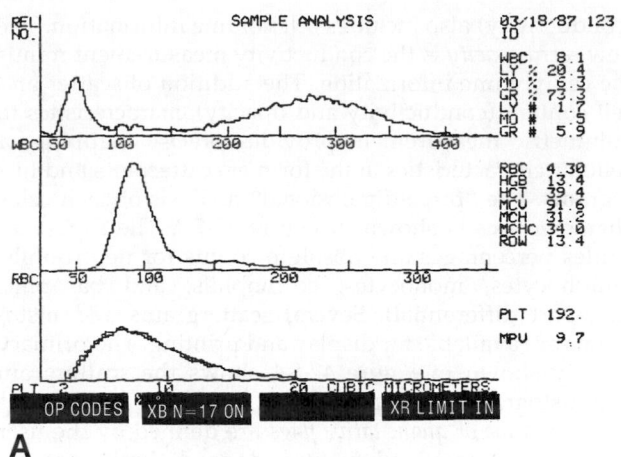

A

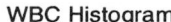

WBC Histogram

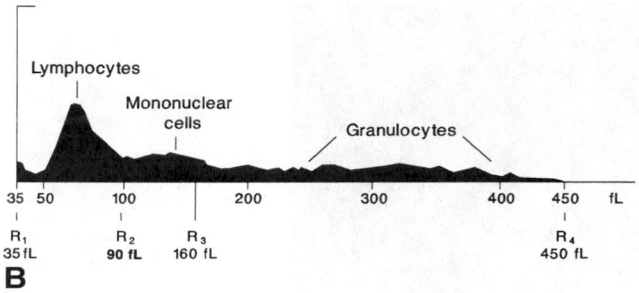

B

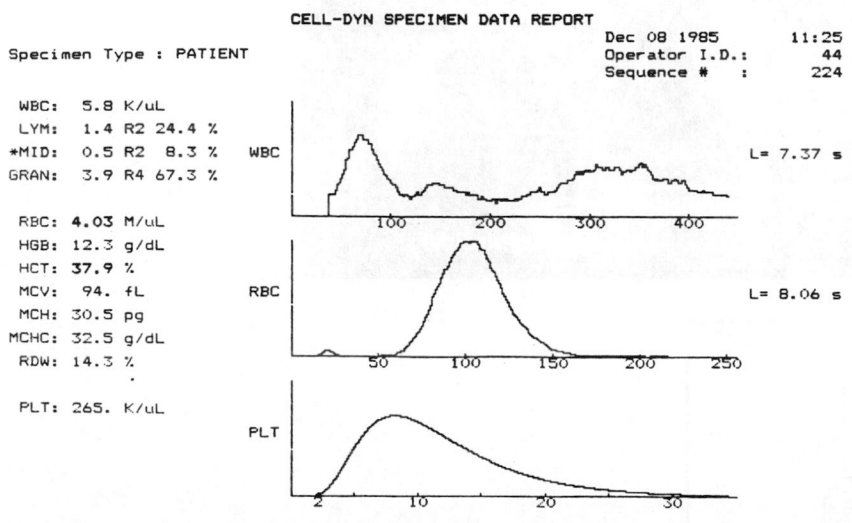

* MID cells include less frequently occurring and rare cells correlating to monocytes, eosinophils, basophils, blasts and other precursor white cells.

C

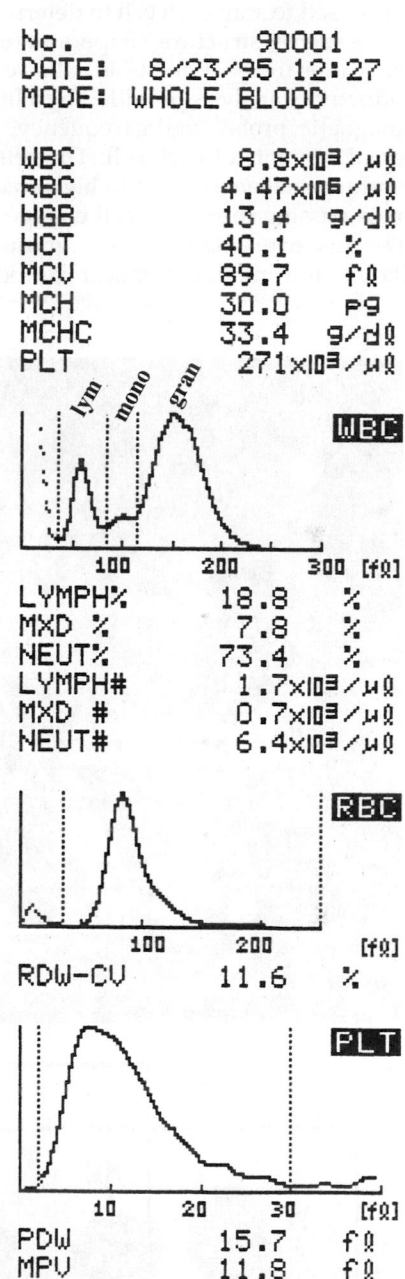

D

FIGURE 42-6. Normal composite histogram printouts from instruments with three-part differentials. (*A*) Normal example from Coulter S-Plus. (*B*) Normal WBC histogram display of Coulter S-Plus series showing leukocyte subpopulation locations and indicating locations of region ("R") flags. (*C*) Normal example from Unipath Cell-Dyn 2000. Note different terminology and reporting units for differential, RBC, and PLTs. (*D*) Normal example from Sysmex K-1000.

of each sample is directed through the flow cell with the use of hydrodynamic focusing and laminar flow fluidic technology (described earlier in this chapter). Therefore each white cell in its near-native state is analyzed individually as it passes through the "sensing zone" where VCS signals are simultaneously generated. Figure 42-7A depicts the three measurements taken for each cell. Laser light is used to scan each cell to determine surface characteristics such as structure, shape, and reflectivity. Forward light scatter from 10° to 70° is collected for this analysis. Conductivity analysis provided by a high-frequency electromagnetic probe (radio frequency, RF) measures the internal contents of each cell. The cell wall itself acts as a conductor when exposed to high-frequency current. RF signals passing through a cell change in response to the cell's nuclear composition, granular (cytoplasmic) makeup, and interior chemical composition. This signal

(conductivity) also includes cell volume information. The new term *opacity* is the conductivity measurement minus the cell volume information. The addition of scatter and cell content (conductivity and opacity) characteristics to volumetric measurement provides precise mapping of cellular characteristics in the form of scatterplots and histograms. The "three-dimensional" analysis of each cell's characteristics is shown in Figure 42-7B. The report includes percentages and absolute counts for neutrophils, lymphocytes, monocytes, eosinophils, and basophils (five-part differential). Several scattergrams and histograms are available for display and printing. The primary display shown in Figure 42-8A shows the scattergram and histograms from a "normal" sample.

Definitive or quantitative flags are defined by the user and are generated when (user-defined) limits are exceeded by numeric data (*e.g.*, thrombocytopenia, leukocy-

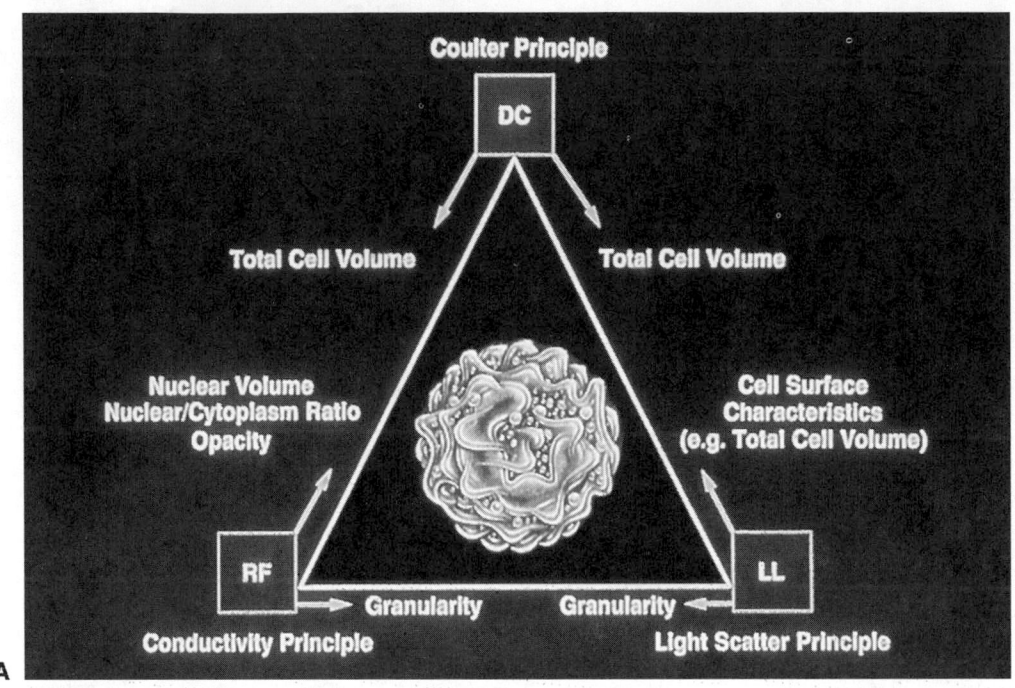

A

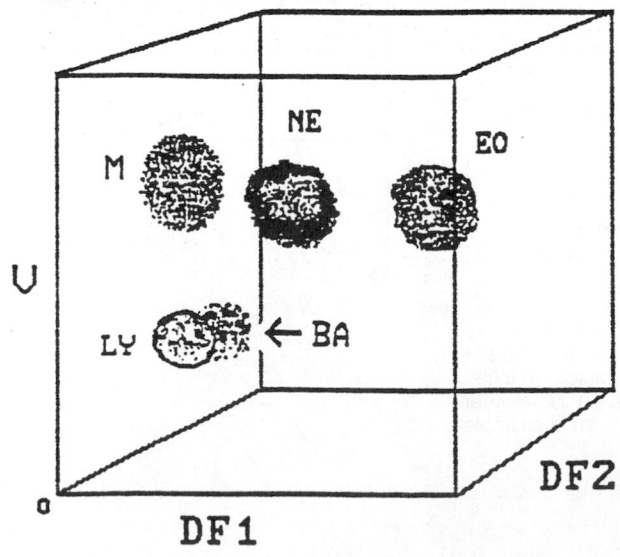

B

FIGURE 42-7. (*A*) Three technologies used by Coulter are altered as each cell passes through the VCS flow cell. Cell classification is based on cell volume, content, morphology, granularity, and surface characteristics. The triangle represents the cell characteristic measurements taken as each cell traverses the "sensing zone." DC = Direct current (total cell volume); RF = high frequency radio waves which measure each cell's internal content; LS = laser light scatter analysis measuring surface characteristics, morphology, and granularity. (*B*) The three-dimensional cube display shows cell placement in relation to volume (V), light scatter (DF1), and conductivity (DF2) or internal content. M = Monocyte; NE = neutrophil; EO = eosinophill; LY = lymphocyte; BA = basophil (partially hidden behind the lymphocytes). (Courtesy of Coulter Corporation.)

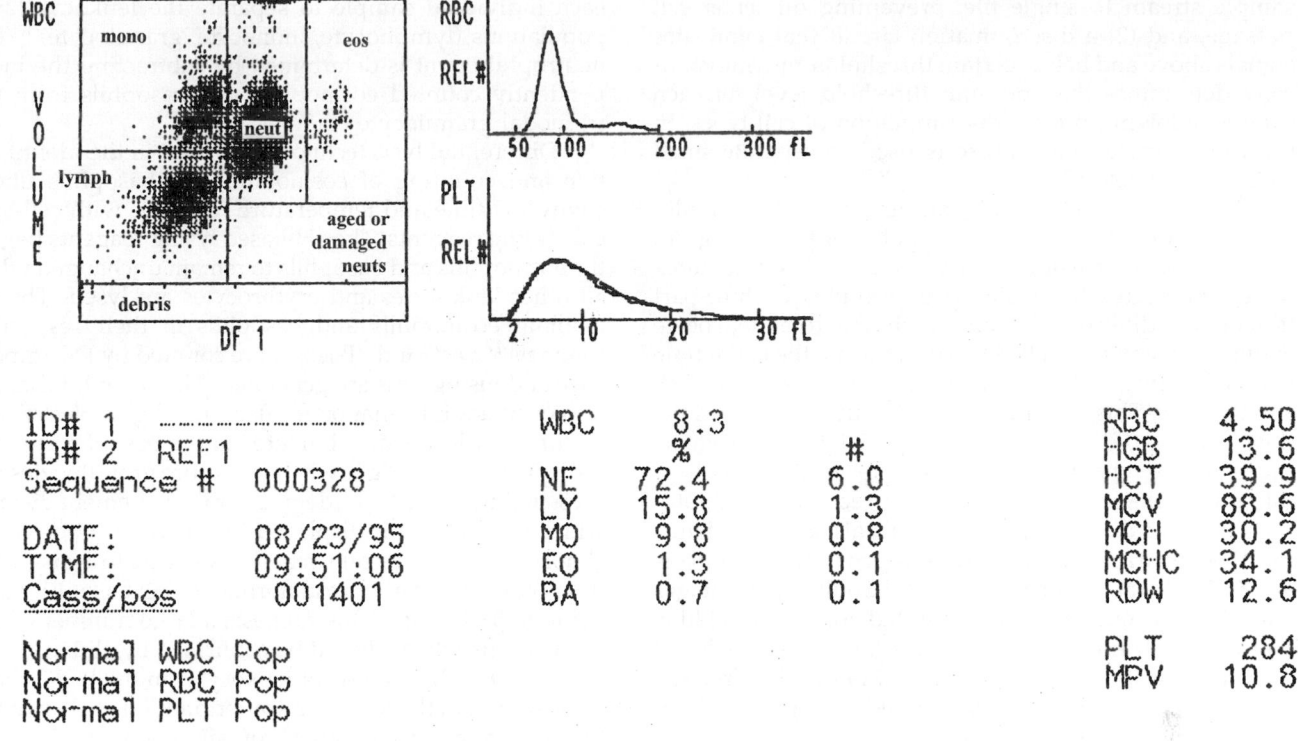

ID# 1   ——————————   WBC   8.3
ID# 2   REF1

Sequence #   000328   NE   72.4   6.0

DATE: 08/23/95   LY   15.8   1.3
TIME: 09:51:06   MO   9.8   0.8
Cass/pos   001401   EO   1.3   0.1
   BA   0.7   0.1

Normal WBC Pop
Normal RBC Pop
A Normal PLT Pop

RBC   4.50
HGB   13.6
HCT   39.9
MCV   88.6
MCH   30.2
MCHC   34.1
RDW   12.6

PLT   284
MPV   10.8

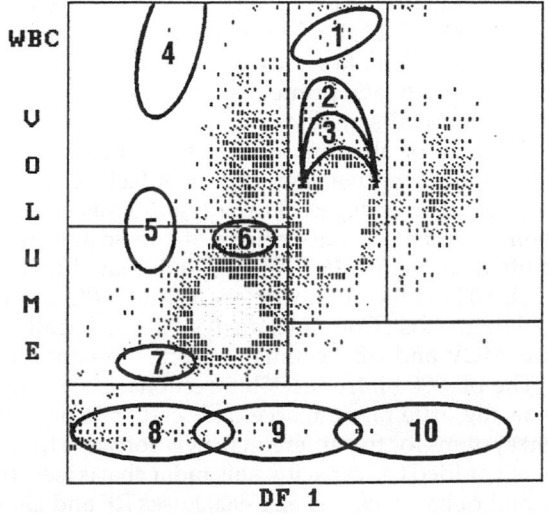

1. Suspect Blasts
2. Suspect Immature Granulocytes
3. Suspect Bands
4. Suspect Blasts
5. Suspect Blasts
6. Variant Lymphocytes
7. Variant Lymphocytes
8. Nucleated Red Blood Cells
9. Giant Platelets
10. Platelet Clumps

B

FIGURE 42-8. (*A*) Example of Coulter STKS display of scattergram, histograms and data. Name of each cell population has been added. This is a normal sample with no flags. The default display is DF1; others may be selected for review. DF2 rotates the cube and looks at conductivity *versus* volume and DF3 electronically subtracts out neutrophils and eosinophils from the DF2 data to "uncover" basophils. (*B*) Abnormal cell regions are outlined and defined in this DF1 display from the STKS. These regions are analyzed for each patient and flags are set/displayed/printed when significant activity is present in these gated regions. (*B*, courtesy of Coulter Corporation.)

tosis, eosinophilia). *Suspect or qualitative flags* are instrument-generated messages from defined "abnormal" areas of the scattergrams and histograms. Suspect messages may represent potential analysis interference (*e.g.*, platelet clumps, micro RBCs/RBC fragments) or suggest morphologic abnormalities (*e.g.*, blast, variant lymphs), which require review of a stained blood film. Figure 42-8*B* indicates flagging regions of the WBC differential scattergram analysis. Guidelines and follow-up actions for suspect flag messages will be discussed later.

SYSMEX (TOA MEDICAL ELECTRONICS CO., LTD.)

There is a full line of Sysmex instruments with 18 to 23 parameters based on the electronic resistance (impedance) detection method for counting and sizing the WBCs, RBCs, and platelets. These instruments have three primary hydraulic subsystems: WBC, RBC/PLT, and Hb. There are two unique features: (1) the use of hydrodynamic focusing in the RBC/PLT subsystem to narrow the sample stream to single file, preventing off-center cell passage, and (2) a discrimination circuit that eliminates signals above and below certain thresholds and automatically determines the optimum threshold level for each sample, allowing precise discrimination of cell types. In the RBC sample, this feature is used to separate small RBC from platelets.[54]

The E-5000 model is fully automated with a sampler and bar-code ID reader and is capable of processing 116 samples per hour using 200 μL samples. A single transducer (aperture) for leukocytes provides a three-part (screening) differential along with the total leukocyte count. Precision is checked by subdividing the count time and comparing the number of particles counted in each subdivision. This monitors for interruptions of sample flow during the count period. Special lysing reagents cause enough change in the leukocytes to separate them into three subpopulations, which are recognized by automatic floating discriminators. Abnormals are flagged during this separation and analysis procedure. These flags are similar to the region flags used by Coulter. Percentages and absolute numbers are generated for small, middle, and large cell ratios. Lymphocytes fall in the small cell region, neutrophils (or granulocytes) fall in the large cell region, and monocytes fall in the middle region. Eosinophils and basophils may fall in either the middle or large cell regions but more often fall in the middle cell group.[42] Other special features include warming of the RBC diluent to 37°C and the option to relocate the threshold (discriminator) levels to isolate a special population of cells, such as separating two RBC populations to measure number and volume of native and transfused red cells. In addition, computer memory can store complete data including histograms from 300 samples. Data manipulation, such as retrieval of selected abnormals, also is possible. Quality control options include a moving average formula for patient samples, multiple files for Levey-Jennings or duplicate sample analysis, and automatic calibration.

The K-1000 and the fully automated version (K4500) are the Sysmex models that provide 8- to 18-parameter results with or without a three-part automated differential count. The technology is the same as that used in the E-5000 described above. A K-1000 printout from a normal sample is shown in Figure 42-6D.

New technology has been added to the E-Series instrument to produce the NE-8000, which generates a five-part differential count. Hemoglobin analysis is based on a noncyanide method, sodium lauryl sulfate (SLS), which has been equated to the traditional cyanmethemoglobin methodology.[34,39] New lysing reagents slightly alter the leukocytes for counting and classification of subpopulations. Radio frequency (RF) analysis has been combined with direct current (DC) volumetric sizing for simultaneous measurement of each white cell. DC is low-frequency direct current, whereas RF is high-frequency alternating current. The DC method sizes the entire cell, including the nucleus and the cytoplasm, whereas the RF method detects and sizes the cell on the basis of the overall density.[17] Changes in the RF signal correlate with the overall cell density, including nuclear and granular density.

Eight floating discriminators automatically adjust to each individual sample to separate the leukocyte subpopulations (lymphocyte, monocyte, granulocyte).[17] The neutrophil count is determined by subtracting the independently counted eosinophils and basophils from the tri-modal granulocyte count.

Differential lysis technology is used in the identification and counting of eosinophils and basophils under controlled time and temperature reactions with cell-specific lysing reagents. The pH-based lysing reagents permit the eosinophils and basophils to remain unchanged while all other leukocytes and erythrocytes are lysed. The remaining eosinophils and basophils in their respective channels ("Eos" and "Basos") are counted by DC impedance and histograms are generated. The basophil channel also provides information for flagging of granulocyte immaturity. A lower discriminator in the basophil channel is displaced to the right when immature granulocytes are present (Fig. 42-9C). The degree of this movement dictates which suspect flag is displayed/printed.[17] In some cases, abnormal immature cells may be resistant to lysis in the Baso channel and give an abnormally high basophil number (e.g., 58% Baso). This suggests a large number of abnormal cells which should be confirmed by slide review.

The DC/RF analysis of leukocytes in the WBC channel is shown in the form of a scattergram for each sample. In addition the patient report contains a volume distribution histogram of the tri-modal analysis along with histograms for RBC, PLT, Eo, and Baso. These pattern displays and the numeric data for each sample are displayed on the color monitor and printed automatically. Figure 42-9A is from a normal sample.

Flagging of abnormal samples includes laboratory-set limits, or definitive flags, and manufacturer-set limits, or suspect flags. Suspect flags are not adjustable by the customer. (Suspect flag regions of the scattergram are identified in Fig. 42-9B.) Another automated feature on the NE-8000 is the automatic analysis of RBC when two populations exist. Computer analysis automatically documents MCV and RBC counts for each subpopulation.

The SE-9000 introduces bidirectional host computer interfacing, true random access, discrete testing, new reagent systems for the differential, new software for cluster analysis, added QC capacity, new radar charts (see following) and delta checks. The SE-9000 uses RF and DC technology for the differential (diff) channel and the IMI (immature information) channel.[55] Figure 42-10 is a normal sample display. The WBC count reagent eliminates the lyse resistance problems encountered in the NE model. Granulocytes, lymphocytes, and monocytes are identified in the diff channel using newly developed reagents and software for "cluster analysis" as opposed to linear discrimination used in the NE-8000.[23]

The newly developed IMI channel identifies immature granulocytes based on their special cytochemical makeup and response to the lysing reagent used in this channel. Significant differences in patterns of lipid composition exist between red cells, mature leukocytes, and immature leukocytes. Immature cells are resistant to lysis, whereas the lysing reagent in the IMI channel lyses the red cells and the mature leukocytes based on the difference in their lipid makeup.[21,22] The response of immature cells to the IMI reagent is shown by their location on the RF-DC

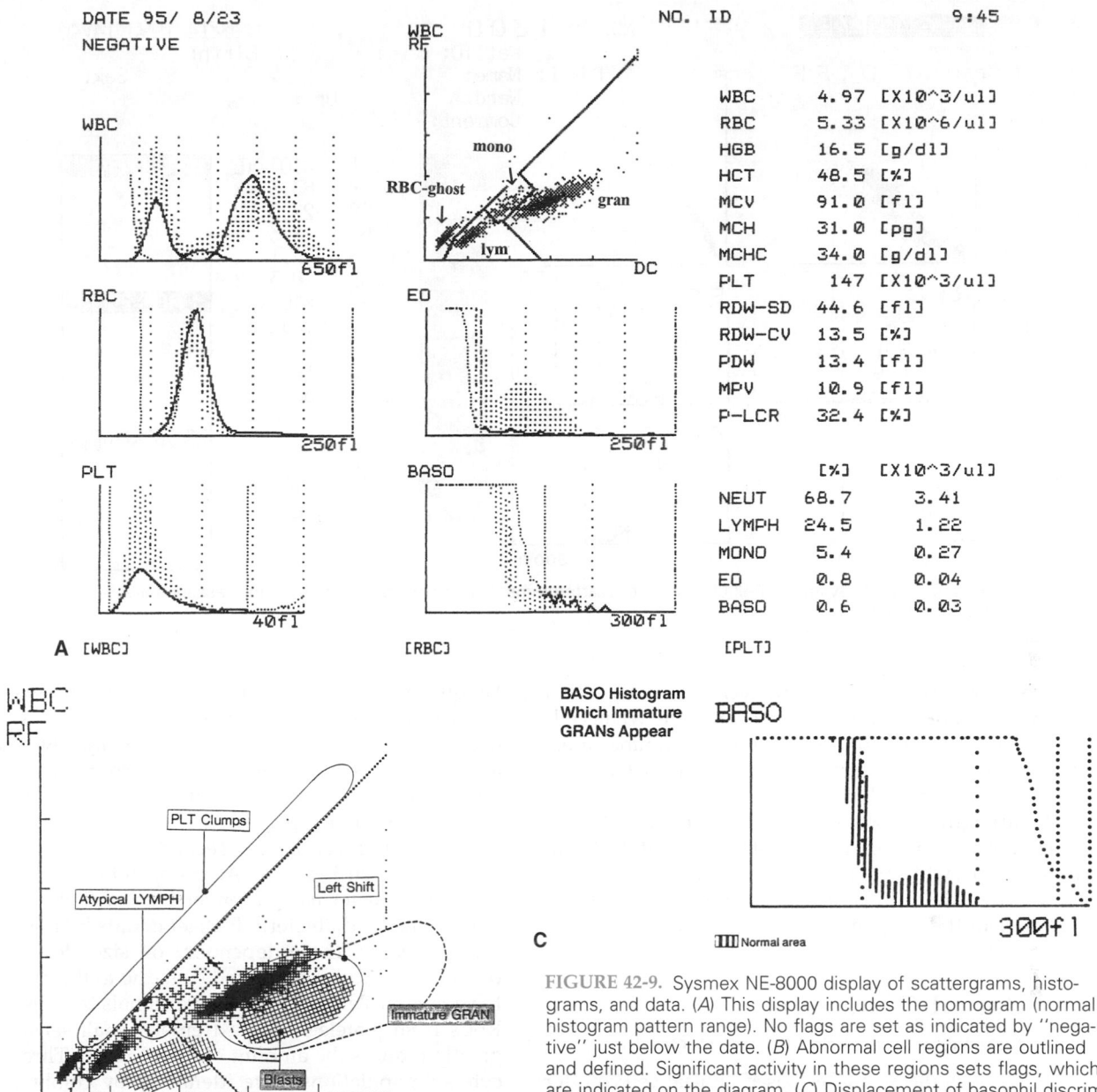

FIGURE 42-9. Sysmex NE-8000 display of scattergrams, histograms, and data. (*A*) This display includes the nomogram (normal histogram pattern range). No flags are set as indicated by "negative" just below the date. (*B*) Abnormal cell regions are outlined and defined. Significant activity in these regions sets flags, which are indicated on the diagram. (*C*) Displacement of basophil discriminator in the presence of immature granulocytes. (Courtesy of Sysmex Corporation.)

plot, which triggers appropriate suspect flags when preset limits are exceeded. In Figure 42-11, *A* and *B* show the now suspect flag regions of the diff and IMI scattergrams.[55] All of the other flags and user-defined flag capabilities of the NE remain on the SE model.

Radar plots graphically display individual patient results in relation to normal values and to each other. Scattergram patterns along with histograms and radar plot changes may be followed through a patient's course of treatment.[55] Figures 42-12, *A*, *B*, and *C* show a radar plot from a normal sample and two abnormal ones.

Discrete testing coupled with bidirectional host inquiry permit reagent savings when only selected parameters are requested by a physician. Auto-differential testing does not occur unless an instrument differential is or-

dered, thus eliminating differential reagent consumption. Unordered test results (that could be abnormal) do not appear on display or on the printed report, which means the laboratory is not required to establish policies for unrequested data that fall out of the normal range. The new Diff and IMI channels are reported to improve the sensitivity and specificity of abnormal flagging.[23]

COBAS-HELIOS (ROCHE DIAGNOSTICS)

The Cobas-Helios is based on electrical impedance technology and includes a three-part differential. The Cobas-Argos 5 Diff combines impedance technology with cytochemical staining and optical absorbance to provide 26 parameters including a five-part differential in this closed-

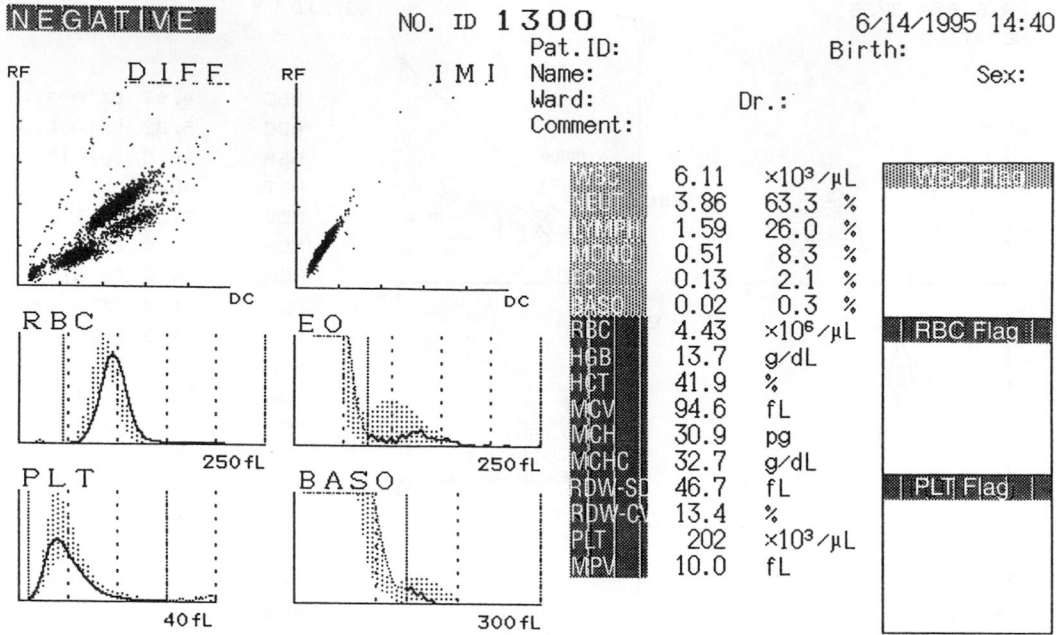

FIGURE 42-10. Sysmex SE-9000 display of scattergrams, histograms, and data. No flag messages are set on this normal sample.

tube analyzer.[3,4] The white cell analysis differs from that of other automated differential analyzers. The white cells are analyzed by variation of impedance (volume) measurements, light scatter staining (absorbance) measurements and differential lysis.[3]

The strengths and weaknesses of each manufacturer's instruments and of a particular instrument within an instrument series will have to be determined by each potential user. A guide for this process is described and referenced later in the chapter.

Laser Optical Counters

ORTHO DIAGNOSTIC SYSTEMS INC.

The Hemac was the first laser-based clinical cell counter and part of the ELT series of instruments (ELT is an acronym for **e**rythrocyte, **l**eukocyte, **t**hrombocyte).[37]

Unique features of these instruments at the time of development included: sample size of 100–120 μL, use of hydrodynamic focusing, and laminar flow for RBC and PLT analysis. Red cells and platelets were counted simultaneously, using three variables (volume, refractive index, and time of flight) to distinguish these two cell types. *Time of flight* is the number of microseconds it takes a cell to pass through the sensing zone. At a constant speed, cells with a larger diameter have a longer time of flight than cells with a smaller diameter.[45] Platelet counts by this method are superior to those dependent on size alone because the refractive index of the red cell, due to the presence of Hb, plays a role in the distinctive signals that distinguish RBCs from platelets. The extremely small sensing zone greatly reduces the amount of interference. Three leukocyte subpopulations were identified by combining forward light scatter volume information with right-angle scatter "internal complexity" information. This was the

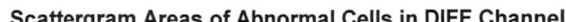

FIGURE 42-11. Sysmex SE-9000 abnormal cell regions identified for the Diff channel (*A*) and the IMI channel (*B*). Flagging occurs when significant cell activity is identified in these regions. (Courtesy of Sysmex Corporation.)

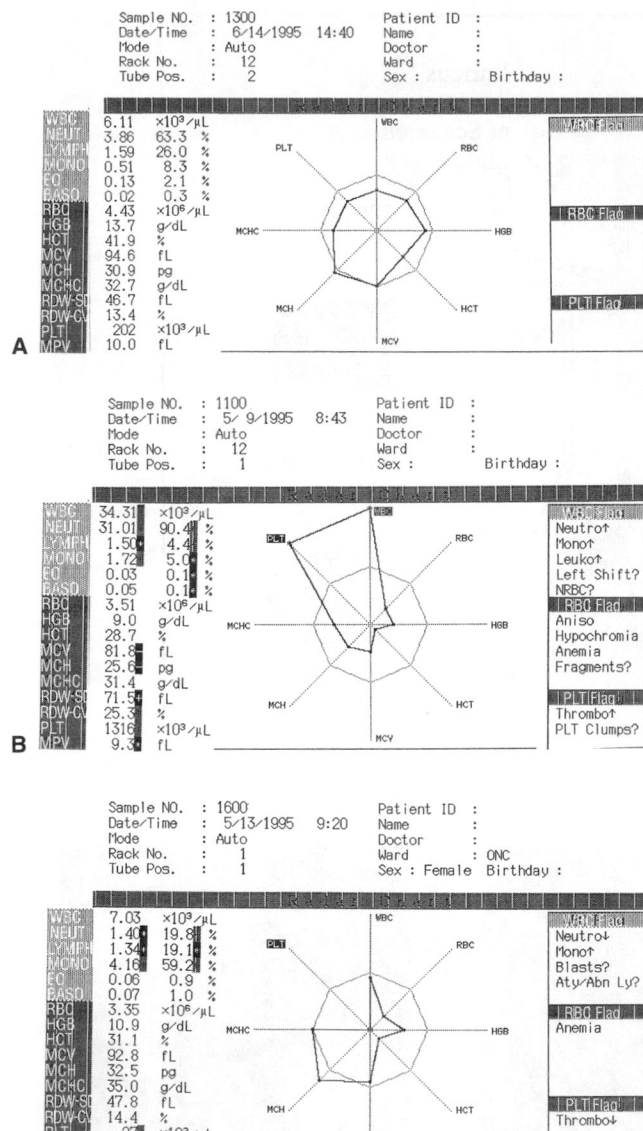

FIGURE 42-12. Sysmex SE-9000 Radar plots have been altered to include the numeric data (*left panel*) and flagging information (*right panel*). (*A*) Normal plot. (*B*) Red cell parameters (approaching center of circle) are decreased while elevated WBC and PLT have extended well beyond the limits of normal. (*C*) Evidence of anemia and extremely low platelets.

first automated differential that was developed without staining the cells. In addition, this system did not have any carryover from one sample to another. Production of these instruments ceased when the instrument division was sold by its parent company.

ABBOTT LABORATORIES

Abbott Laboratories combined impedance and optical laser technology in their Cell-Dyn 3000 series instruments. The Cell-Dyn 3500 features include closed sample aspiration (<355 μL), bar-code reader for positive patient sample identification, 22 parameters, impedance and optical WBC counts (with cross-check for interference), as well as solid-state LED readout of hemoglobin measurement

(540 nm) using a modified cyanmethemoglobin method. RBC and PLT are sized and counted using the impedance method in a patented transducer chamber. Use of the patented von Behrens transducer plate minimizes the effect of interference from recirculating cells. Counts from the 60 × 70 micrometer aperture are automatically corrected for coincidence passage and edited. The editing function includes all cells in the RBC count but also excludes red cells from the MCV determination when they traverse the aperture in a nonaxial manner. Nonaxial transit through the aperture falsely increases the cell volume signal due to broadening of the pulse. This would falsely elevate the MCV value if those signals were included in the averaging calculations.[1]

Impedance WBC counts (WIC) are performed on the same sample used for Hb determination. The RBCs are lysed for Hb reaction and the WBCs are stripped of their cytoplasm, leaving only the nuclei. The WIC aperture is 100 × 77 μm and the von Behrens transducer plate is used in the transducer chamber to minimize the effect of interference from recirculating cells. A WIC histogram is generated. Coincidence passage is automatically corrected and the WIC and WOC counts (impedance and optical) are compared. If preset tolerance limits are exceeded, the delta flag is added to the display and the report. Extended lyse mode, if selected by the operator, increases the sample/lyse reagent reaction time prior to counting a sample with lyse-resistant RBCs.[1]

Optical WBC counts (WOC) and the five-part differential are performed using multi-angle polarized scatter separation technology (MAPSS). Sheath fluid surrounds the sample stream for laminar flow and hydrodynamic focusing of the cells into single file for passage through the optically clear quartz flow cell where the vertically polarized helium neon laser beam is interrupted by passage of each individual cell (Fig. 42-13*A*). The light scattered by cell passage through the laser beam is collected by sensors at different angles. Forward scatter measurements are taken at 1° to 3° and is referred to as 0° (scatter). Scattered light is collected at 7° to 11° and this narrow-angle light scatter is referred to as 10°. Ninety-degree (70°–110°) (right-angle or orthogonal) scatter measurements primarily represent internal complexity (internal structure) with cell surface information. Ninety-degree depolarized scatter is referred to as 90°D. The analysis of these signals provides information about each cell's size, granularity, internal structure, and surface characteristics.[53] The four measurements from each cell are stored for step by step analysis and cell identification for the five-part differential and total leukocyte count.[1] Table 42-3 lists the scatter angle comparisons that sequentially separate cells into one of five classifications for reporting. Figure 42-13*B* shows the first step in cell analysis; parts *C* and *D* show the remaining steps of scatter analysis used to identify the leukocyte cell types. Figure 42-14 is a normal sample with scattergrams, histograms, and numeric data from the Cell-Dyn 3500. The measured angle of light scatter is indicated on each axis of each scattergram.

White blood cells remain close to their native state following dilution for WBC analysis. The basophils, however, do change slightly owing to the water soluble nature

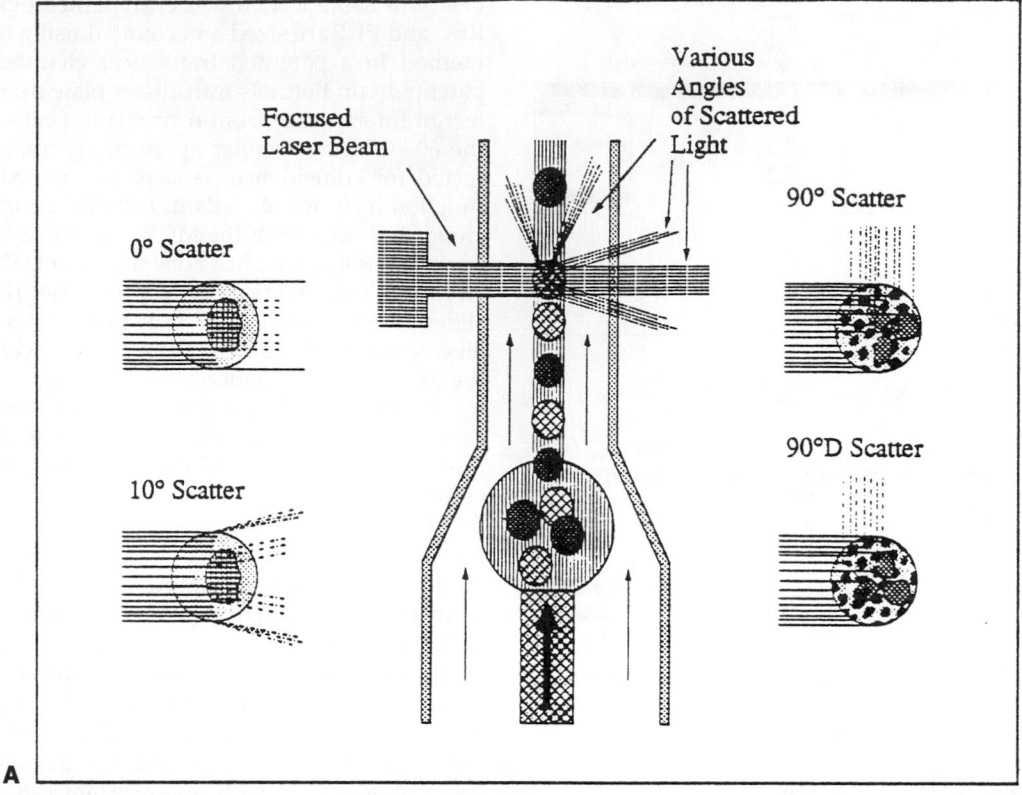

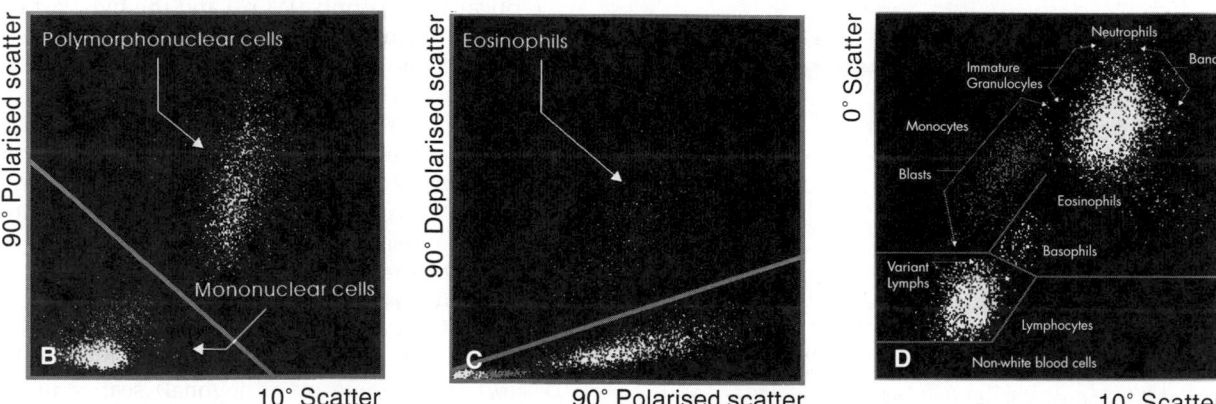

FIGURE 42-13. Optical analysis and MAPSS technology. (*A*) Diagram of WBC light scatter includes the flow cell and use of hydrodynamic focusing of the sample stream for single cell passage through the focused laser beam. Four light scattering characteristics of each cell are measured. (*B*) MAPSS technology analysis of list mode cell characteristics. Mononuclear cells are separated from polynuclear cells based on 10° scatter (X axis) and 90° polarized scatter (Y axis) signals. (*C*) The polynuclear cells identified in *B* are then characterized by analysis of 90° polarized (X axis) and 90° depolarized scatter (Y axis) to separate eosinophils from neutrophils. (*D*) The mononuclear cells identified in *B* are further characterized by 10° scatter (X axis) and 0° scatter (Y axis) to identify the lymphocytes, monocytes, and degranulated basophils. This display also includes the previously identified neutrophils and eosinophils. (Approval to reproduce figures from Cell-Dyn 3500 Operator's Manual Abstracts and MAPSS Case Study Atlas has been granted by Abbott Laboratories, all rights reserved by Abbott Laboratories.)

of their granules. The red cells are altered by the WOC reagent such that the hemoglobin diffuses out of the cell and the remaining intact red cell membrane takes on water from the reagent. The red cell then has the same refractive index as the reagent and is rendered invisible to the detection system. The laser beam is vertically polarized and focused into an ellipse so that the sample stream may vary slightly and still pass through the focused laser beam.[1]

The 90° scatter detection system uses a beam splitter to direct scattered light into two separate PMTs. Part of the scattered light goes directly to the 90° scatter PMT for analysis while another part of the scattered light is sent through a horizontal polarizer. Thus, only depolarized light reaches the 90° depolarized scatter PMT (90°D). The granules in the eosinophil have the unique characteristic of changing the polarization of the laser light. The depolarization of the laser light by the eosinophils separates

TABLE 42-3
Data Obtained from Light Scatter Cell Analysis of Abbott Cell-Dyn 3500

Angle	Characteristic	Cell Identified	Figure
90° *vs* 10°	Lobularity *vs* complexity	Mononuclear *vs* polynuclear	42-13*B*
90°D *vs* 90° (polynuclear from 90° *vs* 10° analysis)	Granularity *vs* lobularity	Neutrophil *vs* eosinophil	42-13*C*
0° *vs* 10° (mononuclear from 90° *vs* 10° analysis)	Size *vs* complexity	Lymphocyte, monocyte and (degranulated) basophil	42-13*D*

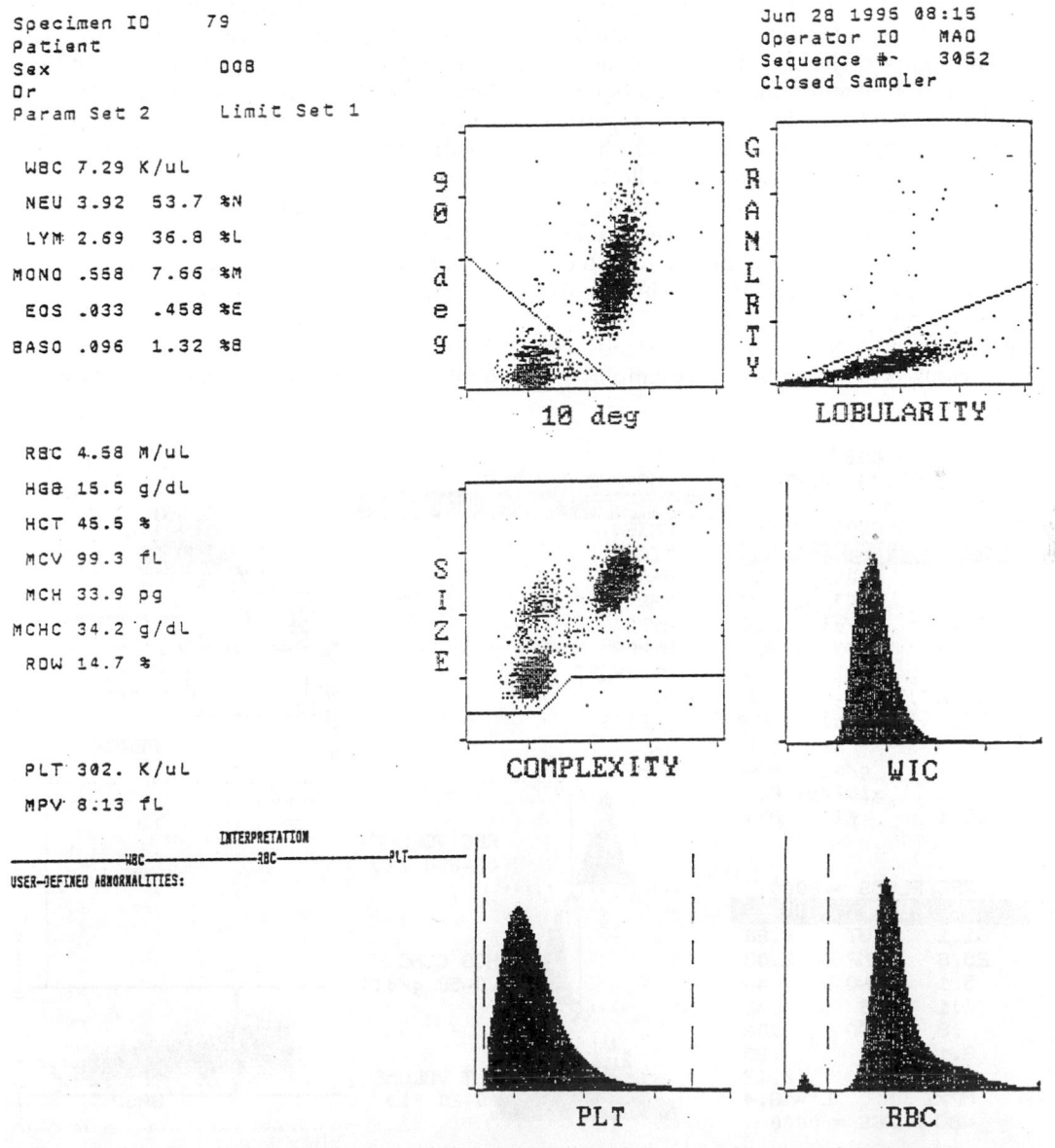

FIGURE 42-14. Abbott Cell-Dyn 3500 data from a normal sample. Several combinations of displays may be selected by the operator to show sets of four patterns. This display pattern has been altered to include six of the scattergram and histogram patterns.

them from the other polynuclear cells (neutrophils) in the 90° *vs* 90°D analysis, as shown in Figure 42-13C.[53]

Operational messages and data flagging alert the operator to conditions that require follow-up action. Messages include suspect parameter and suspect population flags (see Fig. 42-13D) as well as user-defined interpretive messages. Suspect message responses are discussed later in the section on interferences and limitations.

Optical Plus Cytochemical Counters

The darkfield optical method of cell analysis employed by Bayer (Technicon Systems) has been modified through several generations of instruments. The H6000 combines the leukocyte differential analysis of the earlier D-90 and the CBC of the Hemalog 8 into one operation in a continuous-flow analyzer. The H·series (H·1, H·2, H·3) of instruments features reduced instrument size, reduced reagent volumes, improved flagging of abnormals, measurement cross-checks, reagent modifications, software package enhancements, autosampling, positive patient identification, and faster throughput. The H·2 differs from the H·1 primarily in the addition of autosampling. Additionally, the peroxidase channel can be used for an immunoperoxidase method of lymphocyte subset analysis, which is of interest in certain laboratories. This feature allows the laboratory to extend its testing capability to lymphocyte T- and B-cell analysis without investing in a second flow cytometer. The H·3 includes walkaway cap-piercing technology and reticulocyte counting capability, which is discussed later in this chapter.

In general, the H·series of instruments extends the technology of previous systems while greatly simplifying the operation of the hydraulics. They are discrete analyzers in three modules: the electronics and analytic modules and the data terminal. A 100-μL whole-blood sample is aspirated and split four ways: one portion is analyzed spectrophotometrically for hemoglobin concentration using modified cyanmethemoglobin methodology; a second portion is used for RBC and platelet counting; a third is cytochemically stained for myeloperoxidase for leukocyte differential analysis,[43] and the final portion is analyzed in a basophil and lobularity channel. Figure 42-15 illustrates a composite of a normal sample.

The primary technology of this instrument series is based on differential light scattering (defined earlier). Two sources of light are used: a helium laser, which is used for counting RBCs and platelets and for detecting nuclear lobularity, and a tungsten lamp, which is used in the counting of leukocytes and for differentiating the granulocyte populations in the alkaline peroxidase channel. Sheath fluid and laminar flow conditions hydrodynamically focus the sample stream into the center of the flow cell for single-file passage of cells through the sensing zone of the focused light (tungsten or laser light). Scattered light detected by the sensors at various angles is converted into digital form and sent to a microprocessor for display and output on a printer or into a laboratory information system.

The laser channel has two scatter detectors, which are sensitive to light scattered at two separate angles (see earlier and Fig. 42-4A). RBC reagents in this channel "sphere" and fix the red cells,[28] which are then counted and sized according to their light scattering properties. A PMT permits quantitation of platelets, which scatter light at low levels. The hematocrit is the sum of the signals

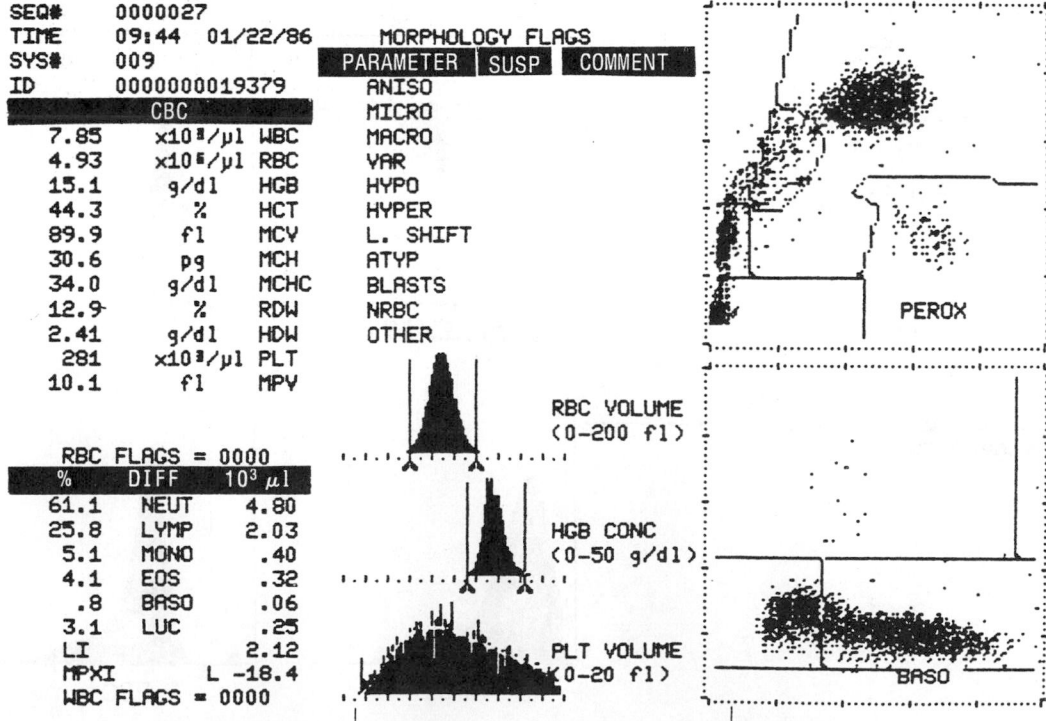

FIGURE 42-15. Normal example from Technicon H·1 (now Bayer H·Series) showing scattergrams, histograms, and data.

from the detected RBC population. RBC light scatter analysis produces a two-dimensional cytogram, plotting volume *versus* hemoglobin concentration (Fig. 42-16*A*). Computer analysis of this cytogram enables RBC enumeration plus independent measurements of RBC volume and direct measurement of individual red cell hemoglobin concentration. An MCHC value is calculated in the traditional manner (from Hb and Hct). The direct measurement of Hb concentration, termed the *CHCM* (**c**ellular **h**emoglobin **c**oncentration **m**ean), is unaffected by lipemia and icterus. The instrument performs an internal cross-check between the MCHC and the CHCM and flags any discrepancy. Histograms of both RBC volume and the Hb concentration distribution are generated. The dispersion of each distribution curve is reported as RDW and HDW, respectively. Further computer analysis of this information provides morphology flags for microcytosis, macrocytosis, anisocytosis, hypochromia, hyperchromia, and anisochromia. Figure 42-16*B* is an example of an abnormal patient sample and shows the independent variation of the RBC volume and Hb concentration and the morphology reports.

The peroxidase cytochemistry is similar to that in the H6000, with a shortened reaction time and more sophisticated analysis.[50] The computer establishes floating thresholds that fit around the population clusters and identify the cell types (Fig. 42-17*A*). The thresholds differ for each individual sample.[52] Total leukocyte, neutrophil, lymphocyte, monocyte, and eosinophil counts are determined in this channel. The tungsten lamp is used in counting the leukocytes and for differentiating the granulocyte populations using an alkaline peroxidase stain to detect cell volume and light absorption. On the basis of these properties and the count from the basophil channel, the WBCs are differentiated into the five traditional categories. In addition, large unstained cells (LUCs) and cells with high peroxidase activitiy (HPX) are identified. The LUCs correspond to variant lymphocytes, blasts, or any large cell devoid of peroxidase activity. The HPX relates to immature neutrophils, although not necessarily to morphology.[6] Flagging limits for film review of samples with an increased HPX index and LUCs must be developed by each laboratory. These instrument parameters may be helpful in identifying low concentrations of abnormal cells, since several thousand cells are analyzed in the peroxidase as well as in the basophil-lobularity channels.

In the basophil-lobularity channel, the WBCs are selectively stripped of their cytoplasm using an acid with a buffer that enhances the natural resistance of the basophils. Only the basophils are resistant to the lysing agent. Using the RBC laser optics with two-angle light scatter to analyze the effluent, leukocyte subpopulations can be identified on the basis of the scatter information from the nuclei.[51] In the basophil/lobularity cytogram (see Fig. 42-17*B*) the basophils are much larger than the nuclei of other leukocytes and can be detected as those cells above a set (volume) scatter threshold. The two-angle laser scatter detection method separates the nuclei of the remainder of the leukocytes according to their degree of lobation. Segmented neutrophils, which have a large amount of high-angle scatter, fall to the right on the X axis, and mononuclear cells fall to the left. When neutrophils are less mature (band and metamyelocyte forms), their scatter

signature is different, and the cells move to the left on the X axis. Blasts give a somewhat lower amount of high-angle forward scatter based on their chromatin texture and are separated from the mononuclear cells at the extreme left of the X axis. The instrument keeps track of

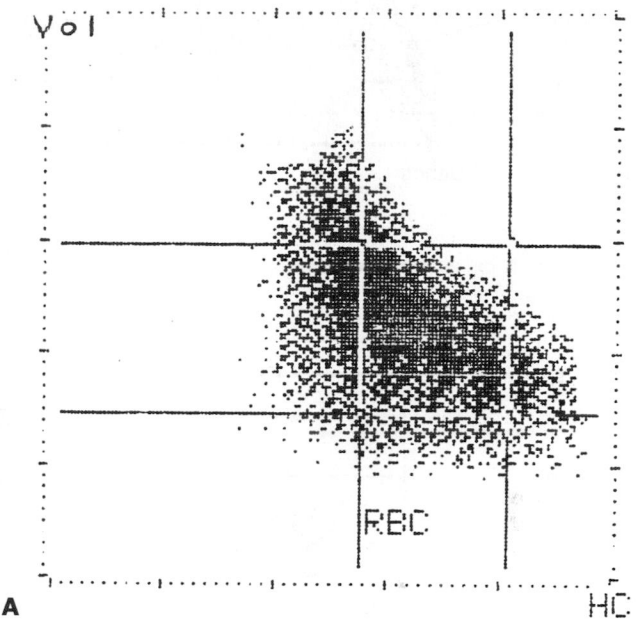

A

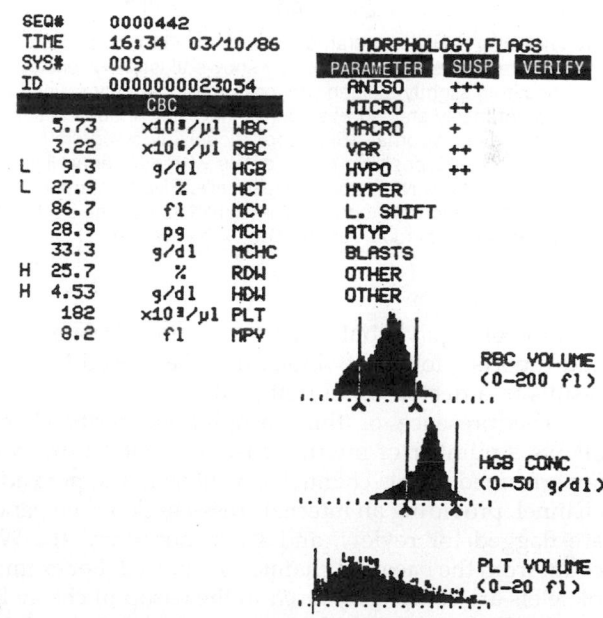

B

FIGURE 42-16. Cytogram/scattergrams from Technicon H·1 (now Bayer H·Series). (*A*) Linear analysis display. Cytogram from the RBC channel plotting RBC volume *versus* hemoglobin concentration. Majority of cells are normocytic and normochromic. (*B*) Data display of abnormal sample demonstrates independent measurements of RBC volume and hemoglobin concentrations shown in histogram form. Morphology flags are generated by computer analysis of numeric and histogram data. (Copyright 1986 by the Technicon Instruments Corporation; reproduced with permission.)

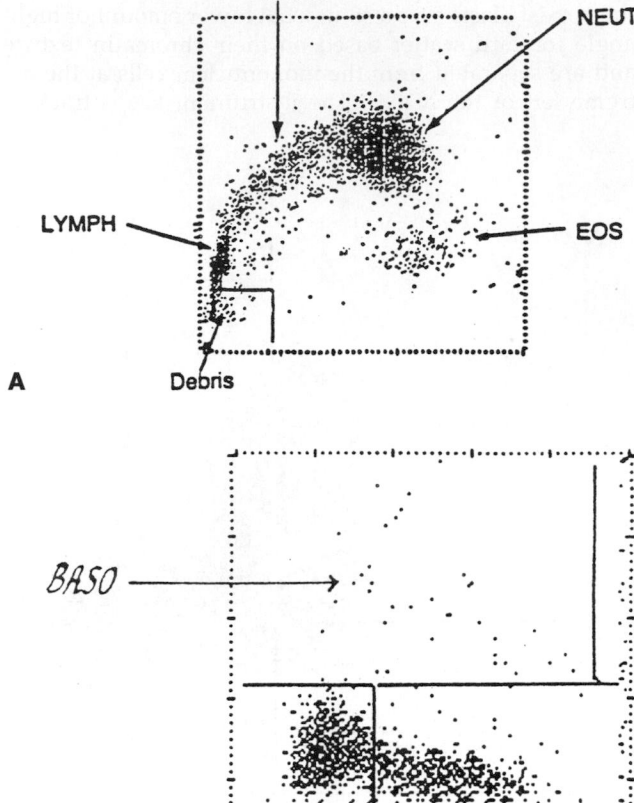

A

B

FIGURE 42-17. H·1 cytograms (normal stained whole blood sample). (*A*) Peroxidase channel display shows clusters of unstained lymphocytes, slightly stained monocytes, moderately stained neutrophils, intensely stained eosinophils, and unstained debris (platelets and red cell stroma). (*B*) Basophil/lobularity cytogram shows detection of cell types using laser optics with differential light scatter. BL = blasts; MN = mononuclear cells; PMN = combination of neutrophils and eosinophils. (Copyright 1986 by the Technicon Instruments Corporation; reproduced with permission.)

the ratio of highly lobulated nuclei to nonlobulated nuclei and reports a lobularity index (LI). Decreased lobularity results in a decreased LI (left shift).[33]

The presence of this basophil/lobularity channel allows a number of internal checks. A total WBC count is performed in this channel as well as in the peroxidase channel, providing an internal cross-check. Discrepancies are flagged for review, and when necessary, the WBC count from the basophil channel is reported. For example, platelets are completely lysed in the basophil channel, so the WBC count from this channel is unaffected by platelet clumps or giant platelets, which would alter the WBC count from the peroxidase channel. Other discrepancies can occur in the presence of nucleated or lysis-resistant RBCs.[59] NRBC areas from the lobularity and peroxidase channels are compared and a flag set when preset tolerance limits are exceeded. The blast flag is set when a comparison of the number of "blasts" detected by nuclear

shape and the LUC number in the peroxidase channel suggests that blasts are likely. Additional flags are set when analysis tolerance limits are exceeded for "left shift" and atypical lymphocytes.

Automated Reticulocyte Counting

In the early 1990s automated reticulocyte counting became available to the clinical laboratory.[18,24] Flow cytom-

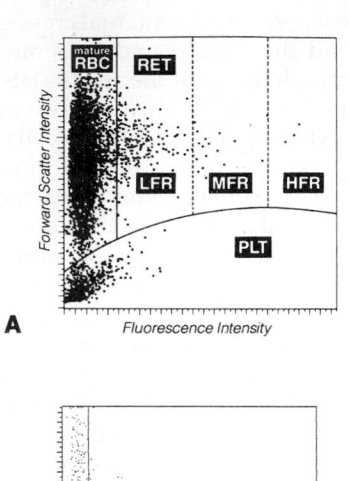

A

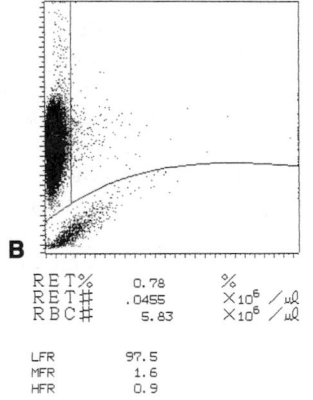

B

R E T %	0.78	%
R E T #	.0455	×10⁶ /µℓ
R B C #	5.83	×10⁶ /µℓ

LFR	97.5
MFR	1.6
HFR	0.9

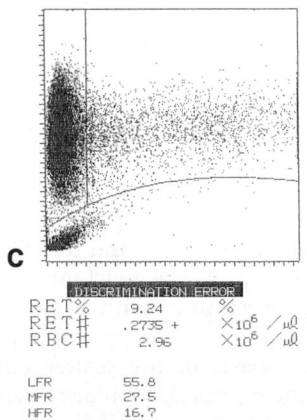

C

DISCRIMINATION ERROR		
R E T %	9.24	%
R E T #	.2735 +	×10⁶ /µℓ
R B C #	2.96	×10⁶ /µℓ

LFR	55.8
MFR	27.5
HFR	16.7

FIGURE 42-18. Sysmex R-1000 scattergrams. (*A*) Mature RBC, reticulocytes (RET), and platelets (PLT) are identified. Fluorescence intensity is on the X axis and cell volume is on the Y axis. Fluorescence intensity is expressed as **l**ow, **m**edium, or **h**igh fluorescence **r**atio (LFR, MFR, HFR). (*B*) Display with low numbers of mostly low fluorescence staining reticulocytes is from a patient with β-thalassemia trait. (*C*) Display of increased reticulocytes shows increased staining intensities (MFR and HFR). This sample is from a patient showing marrow response to a sickle cell crisis. (*A*, courtesy of Sysmex Corporation, with permission.)

eter reticulocyte analysis was available prior to the 1990s, but flow cytometers were not usually found in the routine clinical laboratory. The improvement in precision by automated methods is a giant leap forward for the clinical laboratory. In addition to the percent and absolute numbers of reticulocytes, added information about reticulocyte maturity is available. By using staining or fluorescence intensity information, a reticulocyte maturation index (RMI) measurement is possible. There are three manufacturers with automated reticulocyte counting capabilities. Sysmex has a dedicated counter, R-Series, while Coulter and Bayer (Technicon) have added the capacity for reticulocyte counting to their newer automated hematology analyzers. The increased precision brought about by automation and enumeration of tens of thousands of red cells offers improvements in anemia classification, detection of bone marrow transplant engraftment, and response to erythropoietin therapy.[19]

The Sysmex R Series instruments analyze 100 μL of whole blood, counting about 30,000 RBCs and measuring the relative fluorescence intensity of each reticulocyte. The sample is hydrodynamically focused to pass through an argon laser beam for single-cell analysis. Forward light scatter analysis counts and measures cell volume, while 90° scatter analysis detects and quantifies staining (with auramine O) intensity. Auramine O stains nucleic acid (RNA) in cells. Floating discriminators adjust and separate platelets from red cells, and mature red cells from reticulocytes. Figure 42-18*A* shows a Sysmex scattergram display of the RBC and reticulocyte areas. Beyond the reticulocyte upper threshold are the NRBCs and WBCs that are "gated out" (ignored) as a consequence of the upper threshold. The reticulocyte area is subdivided into three areas of fluorescence intensity: low (LFR), medium (MFR), and high (HFR). The concentration of reticulocytes in each area is indicated in the report. Numerous investigators have studied reticulocyte maturation. These studies have been thoroughly reviewed by Houwen.[24] Figure 42-18*B* is a reticulocyte scattergram from a patient with β-thalassemia trait and Figure 42-18*C* represents a sickle cell crisis. Note the differences in RBC number, reticulocyte percentage, and absolute number and the fluorescence intensity differences between these two samples.

Briefly, the reticulocyte analysis performed on the Coulter STKS or MAXM is done on a manually prepared, incubated sample. An aliquot of whole blood is incubated with Coulter ReticPrep Reagent A (modified new methylene blue stain) for at least 5 minutes. A portion of this first mixture is diluted with ReticPrep Reagent B and incubated for 30 seconds before aspiration into the instrument for analysis. VCS measurements are used to identify and count mature RBCs and reticulocytes. Red cell count as well as reticulocyte percentage and absolute numbers are reported.[18]

The H·3 (Bayer) uses an aliquot of whole blood plus a reticulocyte reagent (nucleic acid dye, oxazine 750). These are incubated for 15 minutes prior to analysis by the H·3. The erythrocytes are isovolumetrically sphered and fixed and RNA remaining in the RBCs is stained. Analysis of each sample includes automatic calculation/ placement of thresholds; high- and low-angle scatter measurements; absorption measurements; and scattergram

display. Reticulocyte percentage is the only clinical parameter reported, since other parameters generated (staining intensities and ratios) are for research purposes and laboratory use only.[18] Reticulocyte analysis displays from the STKS and H·3 are shown in Figure 42-19, *A* to *C*.

GENERAL CONSIDERATIONS
Interferences, Limitations, and Flagging

Each system or methodology has its own unique set of special features as well as limitations. Although a laboratory with instruments based on differing methodologies has problems of reconciling calibration, there are interesting possibilities for crosschecks on abnormal samples and values. Some of the top-of-the-line instruments have their own built-in crosschecks (and delta flags). These checks help identify samples that produce problems with some of the special reagent systems required by the multiparameter analyzers.

Today many instruments have two sets of flagging criteria. One set is user defined (adjustable) and the other set (usually called "suspect") is defined by the manufacturer. Each laboratory must define the flagging limits to which their staff must respond with appropriate follow-up action to verify or validate data or questionable results before reports are released from the laboratory. Quantitative flags are usually set by the laboratory. They may be based on age, gender, or special clinic area (*e.g.*, emergency room, pediatric). The College of American Pathologists accreditation checklist recommends that the laboratory has upper and lower range limits of performance defined for each instrument. Sample values beyond the upper limit would require dilution and repeat for confirmation. Low values (*e.g.*, WBC or PLT) may need repeating through the instrument following zero background documentation and then a blood film review to confirm the low value. Another method of checking unusual results is to check previous individual patient results when they are available (delta check; Chap. 46). Each laboratory must define its own set of limits by parameter for delta checking. This is best performed by a computer program if available.

Recognition of abnormal histogram and scattergram patterns along with instrument flags can be used together to reduce the possibility of sending out erroneous data. Unusual/abnormal samples may cause erroneous results. The operator must be familiar with the instrument operation and recognize those factors leading to and suggesting sample or instrument error. Instruments that generate three-part automated differentials have flags for each region that separates the cell populations. Coulter region flags (R_1, R_2, R_3, R_4, RM with suggested interferences listed earlier) can be translated to the terminology used by other manufacturers of instruments with three-part differentials. Each manufacturer defines each population and the type of cells that brings about overlap between those populations. For example, the Coulter R_1 flag represents interference with the total leukocyte count determination and with the lymphocyte analysis. The same sample problem will cause interference in those areas on all instruments performing three part-differentials. Similar prob-

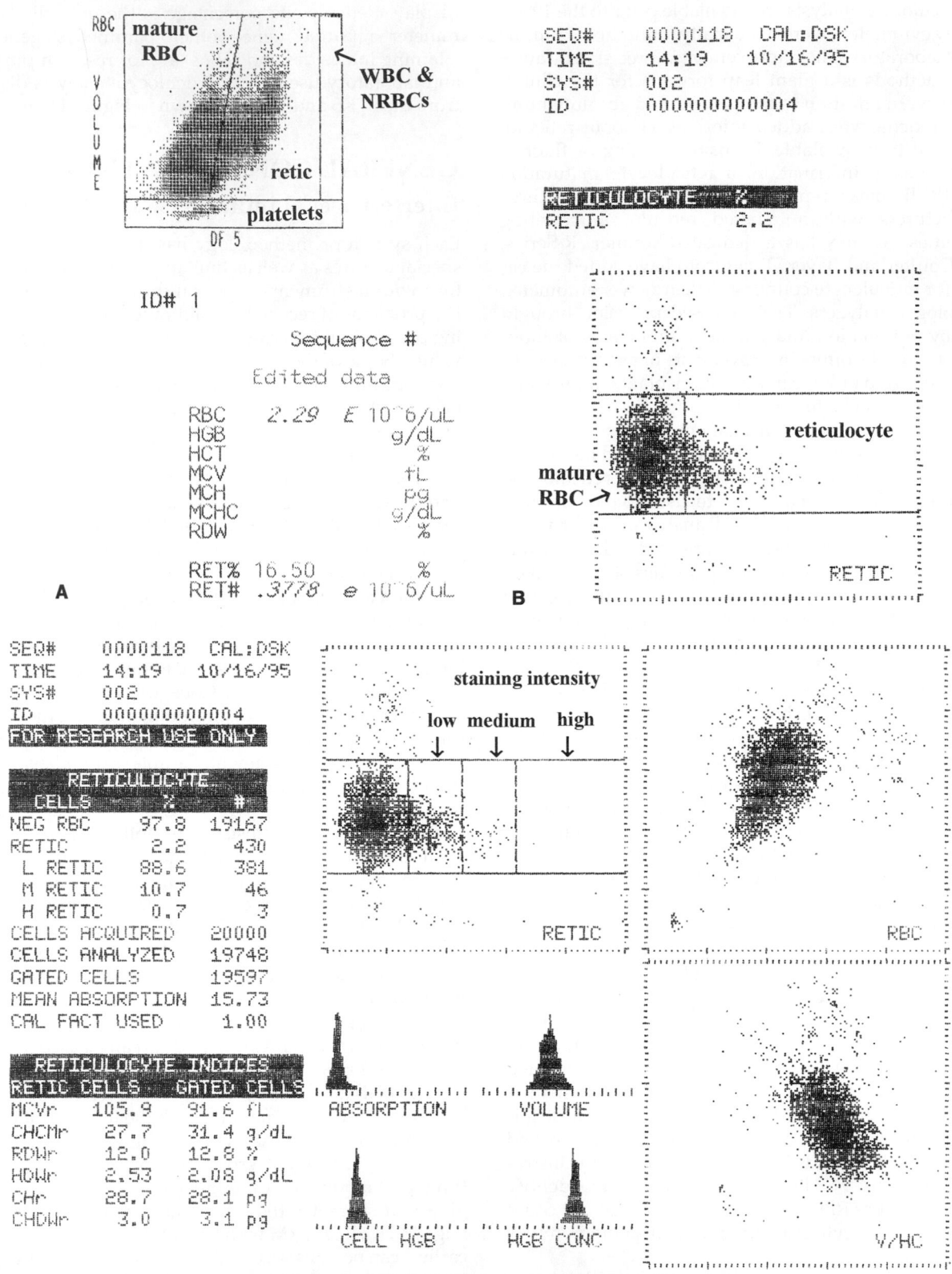

FIGURE 42-19. Reticulocyte scattergrams. (A) STKS scattergram pattern with increased reticulocytes (16.5%) (B) Technicon (Bayer) H·3 result screen. X-axis is staining intensity and Y-axis is cell volume. (C) H·3 reticulocyte research screen for laboratory research use only. Here absorbance is separated into low-, medium-, and high-staining intensity. (A, B and C, courtesy of Bayer Corporation Diagnostics Division, Tarrytown, NY.)

lems are also encountered in the five-part differential analysis.

Limitations and interference affect several parameters. Table 42-4 lists the flags considered to be suspect. The names used in the table are names selected by this author to describe a general interference/problem rather than specific flag names used by each manufacturer.

Lyse-resistant RBCs were discovered when special lysing reagent systems for leukocyte analysis ("diff reagents") were changed to permit classification of WBC subpopulations. The new reagent systems were less lytic to "save the leukocyte cytoplasm" for whole cell analysis to enhance the differences between lymphocyte, monocyte, and granulocyte. It was found that some red cells are resistant to these diff reagents. Sickle cells are frequently resistant to lysis in the "diff channel." This causes interference not only in the differential analysis but also in the total WBC count. See WBC count interference section below.

Instrument suspect flags for distribution abnormalities require a blood film review for significant morphology that should be reported. The RBC count, Hb and Hct relationships (rule of three), and RBC indices (Chap. 9) are useful tools to help evaluate and correlate instrument data and blood film morphology. Hemoglobin interference, RBC agglutination, and/or RBC destruction are suspected when the Hb and Hct do not match or the MCHC is more than 37%. MCHCs below 31% should correspond to hypochromic RBC on film review.

RBC PARAMETER INTERFERENCE

A *dimorphic red cell population* flag prompts blood film review and reporting of significant morphology. Because the MCV is an average number, it does not reflect the presence of two different populations of RBCs; however, the RDW (if given) will be elevated. *Microcytosis* and *red cell fragments/schistocytes* will falsely lower the RBC count if they are small enough to be excluded by the lower RBC counting threshold. Anytime the RBC count is falsely lowered, the MCH and MCHC are affected also. Spinning a microhematocrit determines whether the loss of RBCs in the count is significant. Interference with the platelet count can be caused by these small particles.

The red cell count is falsely lowered by *RBC agglutination*. MCH and MCHC will be unusually high numbers and the MCV may also be elevated (see Fig. 42-21). Warm-

ing the sample to 37°C for 10 minutes before repeat analysis may correct this problem. A blood film using a warmed glass slide should also be prepared from the warmed sample for microscopic examination. Falsely lowered RBC and Hct may be caused by *hemolysis*, since the Hb and Hct will not correlate. Spinning a microhematocrit will identify hemolysis (discolored plasma) and a new sample should be requested to obtain valid results.

Elevated WBC counts (>100 × 10⁹/L) may impact RBC counts, MCV, and possibly the hemoglobin reading (interference or lack of it is instrument specific). Dilution prior to recounting is necessary to bring the leukocyte count into linearity range. Corrected RBC count (subtract WBC) and spun hematocrit are used to calculate the MCV.

Lipemia (depending upon instrument reagent system and lipemia severity) may falsely increase the Hb value causing Hb and Hct values not to correlate. A falsely high Hb will result in the MCH and MCHC being falsely elevated. This picture is similar to the one seen with RBC agglutination, except that the RBC count should be accurate in the presence of lipemia. Spinning a microhematocrit will identify lipemic (cloudy or milky) plasma and the microhematocrit usually matches the instrument hematocrit. In the case of RBC agglutination, the microhematocrit is usually higher than the instrument value but correlates with the instrument Hb value. In order to obtain an accurate Hb, an aliquot of a lipemic sample can be treated in one of two different ways: (1) removing a precisely measured volume of plasma and replacing it with saline for retesting; and (2) spinning an aliquot of the well mixed sample and performing an Hb test on only the plasma. This gives the "plasma interference" level. This plasma value is adjusted based on the patient Hct level and the adjusted value is subtracted from the original Hb reading. Plasma interference level equals plasma value multiplied by the decimal plasma fraction. For example, if the Hct = .37 L/L, the plasma fraction is 1.0 − .37, or .63. The plasma Hb value multiplied by the plasma fraction (.63) is subtracted from the original whole blood Hb value. Regardless of the method used to adjust the hemoglobin value, the adjusted value should correlate with the Hct value.

PLATELET COUNT INTERFERENCE

Morphology or distribution flags and the other flags suggesting platelet count interference prompt the same fol-

TABLE 42-4
Suspect Flags by Parameter

RBC	PLT	WBC/DIFF
RBC morph/distribution	PLT morph/distribution	WBC morph/distribution
NRBC	PLT clumps	Left shift
Dimorphic population	Giant/large platelets	Immature granulocytes
Micro RBC/fragments		Blast
RBC agglutination		Atyp/variant lymphocytes
Turbidity/Hgb interference		Review slide/delta check
RBC lyse resistant		

low-up actions: Blood film preparation and examination including platelet count estimation. Blood film estimates and instrument counts should agree within ± 20%.

Micro RBC/fragments or *schistocytes* suggest a falsely increased platelet count. Likewise, fragments of leukocyte cytoplasm as may be found in some leukemias may interfere with the platelet count. Blood film evaluation and estimate are appropriate follow-up actions and usually confirm platelet count interference. Accurate quantitative platelet counts may require a manual phase platelet count. The accuracy of a phase chamber count is directly related to the experience of the laboratorian. If experience in chamber counts is lacking, a film estimate is probably as good as an attempt at phase counting.

Giant platelets may *not* be included in the platelet count, thus falsely lowering the value.

Platelet clumps falsely lower the count and may be induced by EDTA. *Platelet satellitism* (platelets clinging to the edges of leukocytes) also results in a falsely low platelet count and also may be induced by EDTA. The only clue for platelet satellitism may be an unexpectedly low platelet count. Low power scanning of a blood film is the only means of positively identifying platelet satellitism. Collection of a new sample in sodium citrate may eliminate the problem. The count is repeated on the citrated sample, and a blood film review, including a platelet estimate, should be performed.

WBC COUNT INTERFERENCE

NRBC interference with WBC counting is instrument system dependent. Some instruments automatically eliminate NRBCs from the leukocyte count, some count all of the NRBCs as leukocytes and require WBC correction, and other instrument systems require case by case review. In general, a NRBC flag should prompt a blood film review, WBC count estimation, and counting and reporting of the number of NRBCs per 100 WBCs. See Chapter 24 for a description of how to correct a leukocyte count for NRBCs.

Lyse resistant RBCs interfere with WBC counting on some systems that perform screening differentials. Incubating equal parts of 1% ammonium oxalate and a blood sample for 5 minutes prior to analysis usually clears up this problem. A film review and WBC count estimation should also be performed.

Fibrin strands and *platelet clumps* may also trigger WBC count interference flags. Both can be identified by low power scanning of a good blood film. (See earlier platelet interference section for suggested action.) *Megakaryocyte fragments* and *micromegakaryocytes* may interfere with WBC counting when present in sufficient quantities. Correction of the WBC count for megakaryocyte interference can be accomplished using the same formula as for NRBC correction.

WBC/diff suspect flags should be followed up by evaluating a blood film for significant morphology. Performance of a 100-cell manual differential count may be indicated by the film review. All film evaluations should include an estimation of the WBC count, platelet count, and RBC morphology review.

The instruments that perform automated differentials are approved by the Federal Drug Administration (FDA) to identify and count neutrophils, lymphocytes, monocytes/mononuclear/mixed, eosinophils, and basophils. Manual 100-cell count differential performance was defined by a study done in the early 1980s.[32] Automated instrument differentials must perform as well as or better than the routine manual 100-cell differential and they must identify or flag abnormals (or suspected abnormals). Many single-instrument evaluations have been done over the years. A few studies have been done using the same set of samples on multiple instruments.[5,9,13,48] When reviewing these studies one must be cautious in evaluating the study and instrument performance because of several factors. The case mix of normals and abnormals is critical to the outcome of a study. The outcome may differ each time a study is performed if a different patient sample mix is used or if the instrument configuration is changed (*e.g.,* upgraded). False-positive and false-negative rates should only be determined using the local patient population. This is a difficult, time-consuming undertaking that most laboratories cannot afford to do. Single-instrument study outcomes cannot be compared. Multiple-instrument studies are frequently used by instrument manufacturers to identify areas that can be improved with hardware or software modifications.

Instrument Selection

The last 10 years have seen a proliferation of instruments on the market, which may be overwhelming to the prospective buyer. How does one sort through this plethora? First, the buyer's priorities should be outlined.[29] The particular patient mix served by the laboratory and the need for screening *versus* diagnosis should be considered. For example, a large oncology service may require an instrument that can identify abnormal cells within low WBC counts, not merely flag these for the less precise and tedious microscopic counts. Second, throughput requirements will differ depending on the percentage of emergencies (STATs) and on whether analysis is performed in batches. For example, a throughput of 120 samples an hour will not be important if only 200 samples are analyzed a day. Third, the values to be measured should be evaluated. Some of the more esoteric, such as MPV, may have little relevance to a particular laboratory. Optional functions should be weighed. Are cap-piercing, walkaway, and computer-interface capabilities needed? Other questions to ask include, what are the maintenance requirements and are they automated? What technical skills are needed to operate the instrument and what are those needed to interpret results and instrument flags? Is discrete testing capability needed? What do operators in laboratories that have already purchased a system think of it? A list of all system users can be obtained from the manufacturer. A few should be selected and direct communication should be initiated. A careful review of the professional literature can provide valuable information about instrumentation currently on the market, as well as studies or reviews of new products. Finally, be wary of salespeople who downgrade a competitor rather than sell their system on its own merits. Careful selection will save money and reduce headaches in the long run.

Calibration and Installation

There are a few instances with all systems when performance of calibration procedures is imperative. Initial installation of the instrument will require verification of the calibration. Most instruments are calibrated by the service people during installation using commercial calibration material. The 1994 CAP Hematology Checklist used for laboratory accreditation inspections includes requirements for new methods introduced after September 1992. These include laboratory evaluation and documentation of accuracy, precision, sensitivity, specificity, reportable range, and reference range. Calibration must be checked and confirmed at least every 6 months or whenever major parts are changed, optical alignment is adjusted, critical length tubing is changed, or other parts that directly affect calibration are replaced. Most hematology analyzers are very stable and usually have routine preventive maintenance visits (at least) every 6 months by service representatives. Service calls and the calibration material results provide the necessary documentation to comply with regulatory requirements for calibration checks every 6 months. Calibration monitoring is discussed in more detail in Chapter 45.

Film Review Criteria

The goal in setting blood film review criteria for an instrument is to ensure the accuracy of patient results while fully utilizing the potential of automation. This requires a hard look at the strengths and limitations of the instrument and the imprecision of the microscopic method. For instance, most of the more sophisticated instruments count several thousand cells for a WBC count and differential. Thus, no purpose would be served in trying to recheck the precise numbers generated solely on the basis of a count outside normal limits. Normal samples can be screened out, and the laboratorian's time can by spent more productively in examining blood films that require an experienced morphologist's interpretations of abnormalities. Scrutinize all data: values, histogram patterns, scattergram patterns, instrument function flags, and interpretive flag messages. Flagging limits on specific parameter data in combination with instrument limits and histogram and scattergram pattern flags allow detection of samples that may have significant morphologic findings. Once identified, an abnormality can be reviewed periodically. If a significant morphologic change is identified during a film review, a manual differential count may be performed and added to the final laboratory report. Each laboratory must establish its own rules and limits to be used in the flagging system that prompts blood film review and, at times, the addition of a manual differential count.

With each generation of instruments the laboratory scientist is required to be more expert in interpretation of computer-analyzed electronic data including scattergram and histogram patterns. Once it is accepted that this information is a valuable adjunct to the blood film, the information made available to the clinician is greatly expanded.[25,30,47]

Film reviews are standard operating procedure for

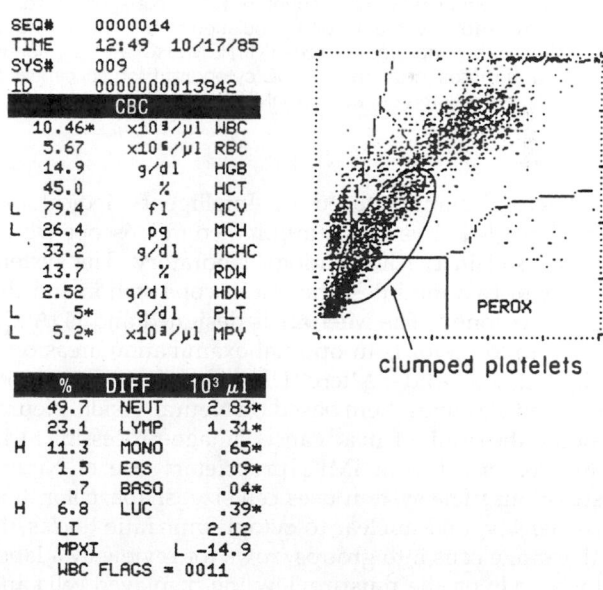

FIGURE 42-20. Platelet interference apparent in histogram and cytogram patterns. (*A*) Coulter S-Plus WBC histogram showing increased debris at 50 fL on X axis (arrow); clumped platelets falsely elevate total WBC count and cause vote-out of platelet and differential counts. Platelet histogram (no-fit) shows tailing (arrow) up at 20 fL on X axis. (*B*) Technicon H·1 peroxidase cytogram shows clumped platelets (arrow) causing characteristic pattern and falsely elevating WBC count. White count measurements in basophil channel are unaffected by platelet clumping (platelets are lysed) and can be used to replace peroxidase WBC count.

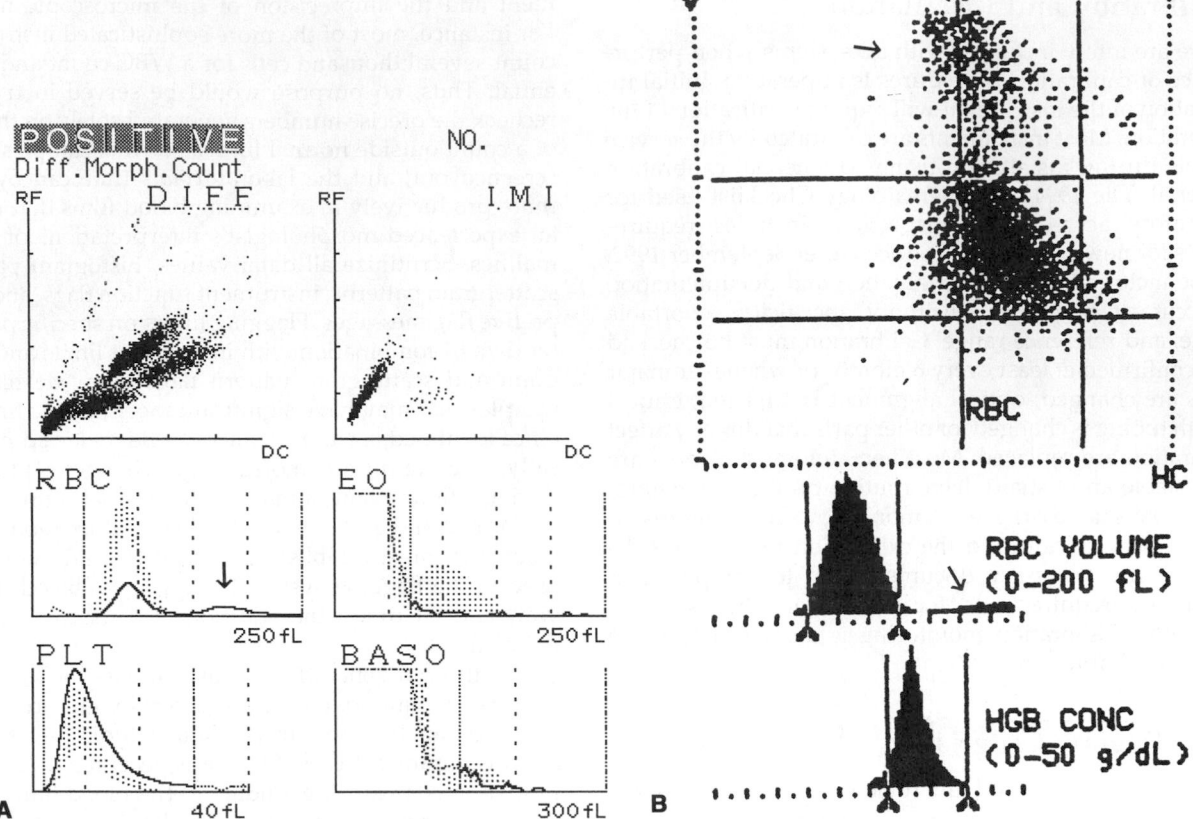

FIGURE 42-21. Cold agglutination. (*A*) Results from a room temperature sample tested on Sysmex SE-9000 indicate unusually low RBC count, low Hct that does not agree with Hgb value, very high MCV, and abnormal indices. Histogram pattern shows low RBC peak with second population to the right (arrow between 150–200 fL). This second (larger cell) peak represents the groups of RBCs that are not being individually counted due to the agglutination. (*B*) Technicon H·1 gives a similar RBC histogram pattern with a second population to the right of the main RBC histogram peak. The MCV is reasonable but the other indices (MCH, MCHC) are very abnormal. The agglutinated cells are (characteristically) represented on the RBC cytogram (Hgb concentration *vs* cell volume) by the cluster of cells falling above the dense normal RBC population (arrow center of display).

the Micro21 manufactured by Intelligent Medical Imaging, Inc (IMI). It is a fully automated microscope which can be used in the hematology laboratory. The system consists of two modules: the microscope station and the review station(s). The Micro21 is designed and FDA approved to locate cells in optimal examination areas on a Wright stained slide. Micro21 searches for cells, counts them, and classifies them based on Neural Vision. Neural Vision is the result of an advanced image-processing technique combined with IMI's proprietary use of Neural Networking. The system uses cell size, shape, color, texture, density, and nuclear to cytoplasmic ratio to classify and arrange cells into groups/rows for review by a laboratorian. He or she must review the displayed cells and confirm the classification of each cell processed by Micro21. A morphologist must identify "bands" and "variant lymphocytes." Cell classification is verified by the reviewing morphologist or pathologist and may be changed if needed. Troublesome cells may be selectively grouped with other cells for comparison and an on-board atlas (text and pictures) may be consulted to aid in the identification of abnormal cells. Programming with this instrument continues to evolve. Multiple fields are available for review of RBC morphology and PLT morphology. The instrument is designed to reduce time at the microscope searching for cells (especially when WBC count is very low). The ability to select specific cells for side by side comparison is very helpful when reactive or abnormal cells are present. Multiple review stations may be connected to the microscope station; one may be in the pathologist's area for consultation and the Micro21 can be directly interfaced with a laboratory information system. Reports may include a color printout of selected cells from the display screen.

UTILIZATION OF COMPUTER DATA

Histograms and Scattergrams

Histogram and scattergram analyses provide valuable information. Normal histogram and scattergram pattern examples are shown in the following figures: Abbott, Figure 42-14; Coulter, Figures 42-6*A* and 42-8*A*; Sysmex, Figures 42-6*D*, 42-9*A*, and 42-10; and Technicon, Figure 42-15. Refer to these normal patterns to help in recognizing

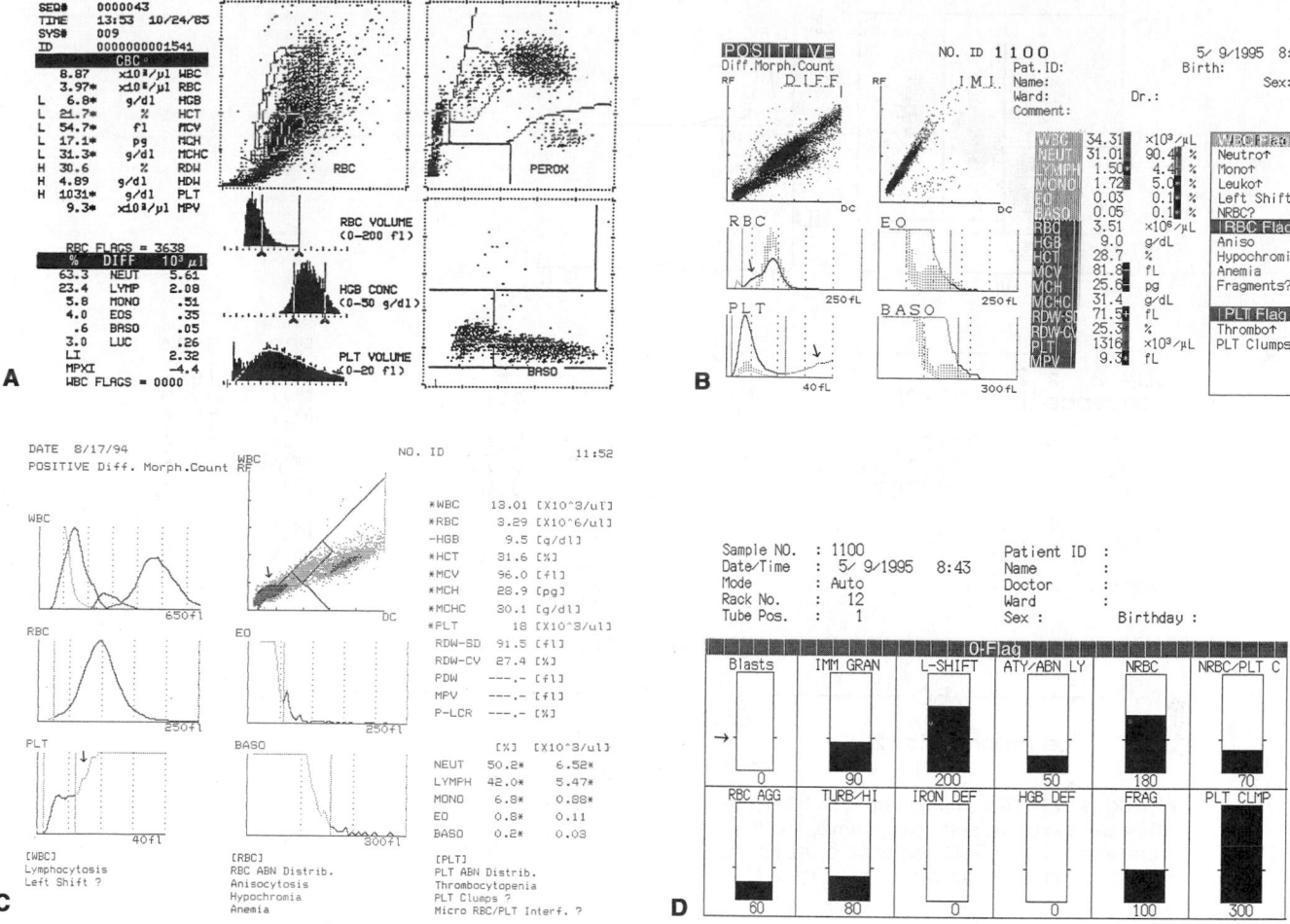

FIGURE 42-22. Platelet interference caused by red cell fragments (schistocytes). (*A*) Technicon H·1 sample has low MCV with schistocytes on blood film examination. Schistocytes falsely increase platelet count and may reduce red cell count. RBC indices calculated from red cell count are also affected. RBC pattern shifted to the left edge of the histogram display agrees with the MCV of 54.7 fL. (*B*) A sample tested on the Sysmex SE-9000 has a normal RBC population with an extended shoulder to the left, indicating smaller or fragmented cells (schistocytes) which generated the "fragments?" and "aniso" flags. The schistocytes can be seen along the right side of the platelet histogram. Film examination is required to estimate platelet count to determine impact of schistocytes on the platelet analysis. (*C*) Sysmex NE-8000 example shows schistocyte interference with platelet enumeration ("micro RBC/ PLT Interf.?" flag). Blood film platelet estimate was 31 × 10⁹/L. Platelet and schistocyte overlap on this sample made it impossible to count electronically. The WBC scattergram pattern also shows debris crossing the WBC threshold into the lymphocyte region. This generated the "PLT Clumps?" flag, which indicates WBC count interference and suppresses the NRBC flag. This sample had many NRBCs, 208 per 100 WBCs and an alternate method WBC count of 12.9 × 10⁹/L. Scattergram and histogram patterns and instrument flags alert the instrument operator to possible interference with sample analysis. (*D*) Sample shows the level of abnormality for the suspect flags on the SE-9000 (in *B*). The flagging rate or sensitivity of these flags is adjustable. The bar graphs range from 0% to 300%. The small marks on the bars indicate the level dividing negative and flagged values.

the abnormal pattern examples that are discussed in this section. Figure 42-6*B* shows the region flag locations for the Coulter three-part differential. Scattergram locations monitored for suspect flags are shown in the following figures: Abbott, Figure 42-13*D*; Coulter, Figure 42-8*B*; and Sysmex (5-part diff) instruments, Figures 42-9*B* and 42-11*A* and *B*.

Abnormal patterns may suggest anomalous cell distributions, problems with the sample or with the instrument. Abnormal patterns may be explained by careful blood film examination. For example, platelet clumping in EDTA usually produces a very low platelet count, a distinctive WBC histogram (or scattergram) pattern with increased debris, and a falsely elevated WBC count (Fig. 42-20*A* and *B*). Sufficient numbers of giant platelets may affect histogram and scattergram patterns and if above the platelet threshold, they are not included in the platelet count. Similarly, red blood cells that resist lysis, such as sickle cells, can also produce falsely elevated WBC counts and falsely increased numbers of lymphocytes in the automated differential. Another sample problem reflected in scattergram and histogram patterns is RBC cold aggluti-

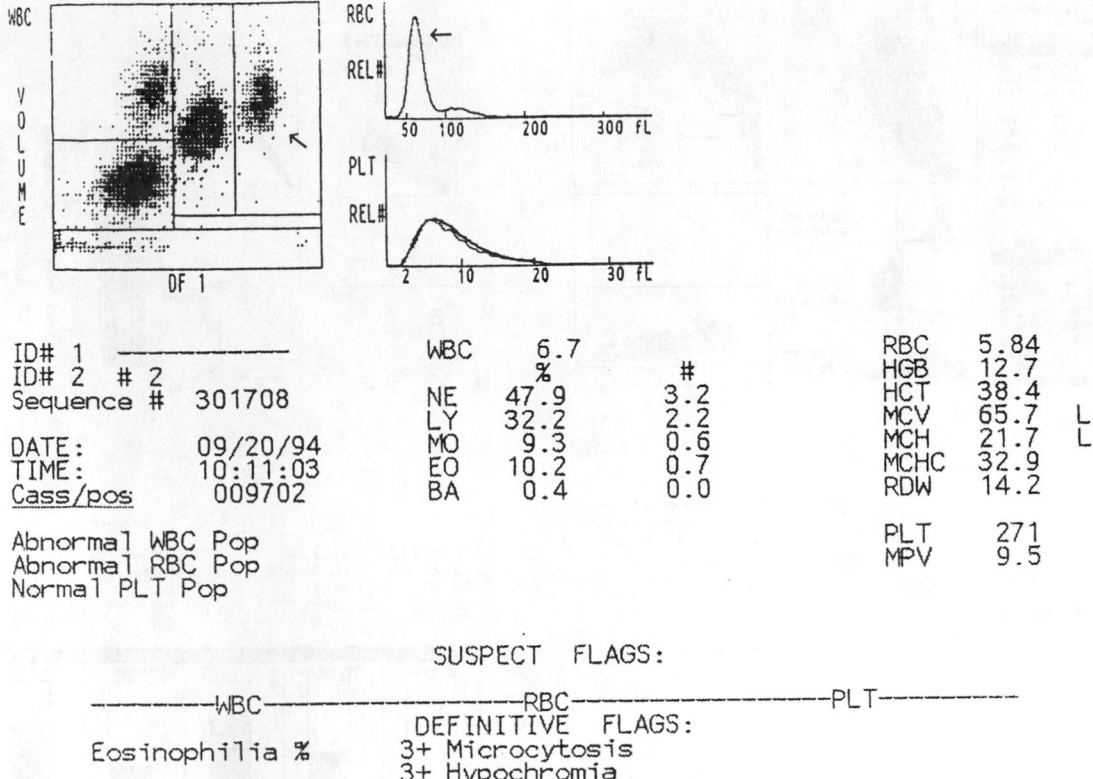

```
ID# 1  ───────────        WBC    6.7                      RBC   5.84
ID# 2  # 2                        %            #          HGB   12.7
Sequence # 301708         NE    47.9          3.2         HCT   38.4
                          LY    32.2          2.2         MCV   65.7   L
DATE:       09/20/94      MO     9.3          0.6         MCH   21.7   L
TIME:       10:11:03      EO    10.2          0.7         MCHC  32.9
Cass/pos    009702        BA     0.4          0.0         RDW   14.2

Abnormal WBC Pop                                          PLT   271
Abnormal RBC Pop                                          MPV    9.5
Normal PLT Pop
```

```
                       SUSPECT  FLAGS:

──────────WBC──────────────────RBC──────────────────PLT──────────
                       DEFINITIVE  FLAGS:
        Eosinophilia %      3+ Microcytosis
                            3+ Hypochromia
```

FIGURE 42-23. This example from the Coulter STKS is from a patient with β thalassemia trait. The RBCs are microcytic and hypochromic, and the eosinophils (arrow) are increased. The microcytosis is represented on the RBC histogram by its position near the left edge of the X axis. Reticulocyte analysis of this same sample is shown in Figure 42-18B.

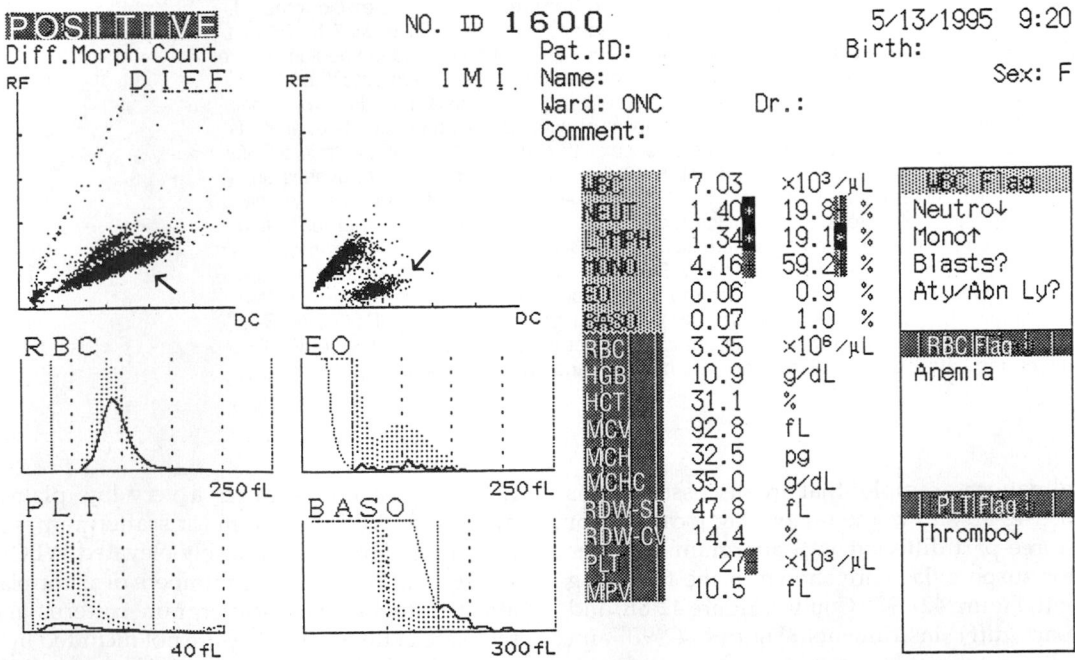

FIGURE 42-24. Example of leukemia sample from the Sysmex SE-9000. Compare the scattergram patterns to the normal example shown in Figure 42-10. Diff display shows small cluster of cells near the granulocyte area with a larger extended cluster of "abnormal" cells in the lymphocyte and monocyte areas. A large population of immature cells is seen in the IMI channel, and the "Blasts?" flag is set. This is an FAB M-2 (acute leukemia).

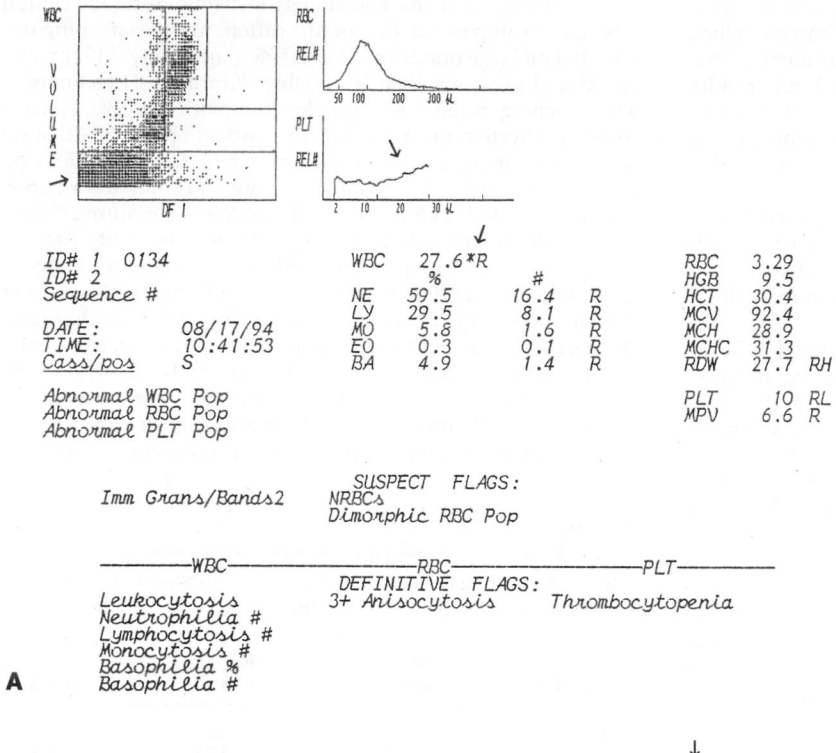

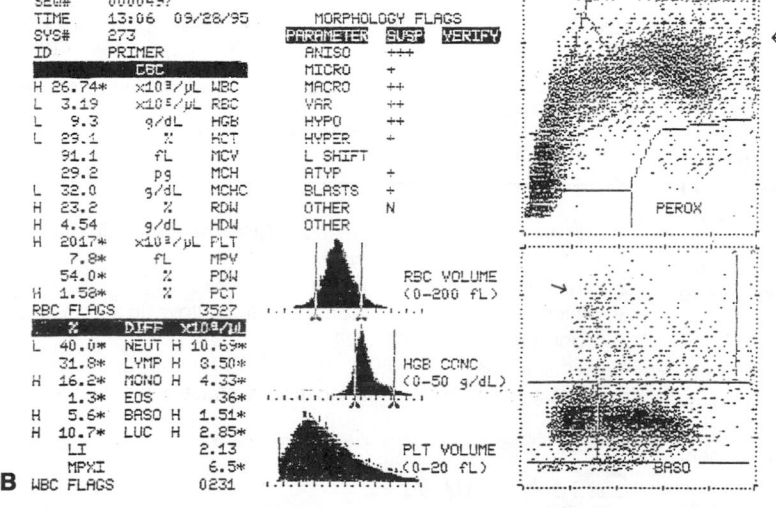

FIGURE 42-25. (*A*) Coulter STKS sample with a diagnosis of myelofibrosis. WBC (impedance count) interference (*R) is from the 208 NRBCs (per 100 WBCs). Corrected WBC count is 9×10^9/L. No-fit platelet count with interference (R) flag. Platelet count film estimate is 29×10^9/L. Immature granulocytes were reported on the manual differential. (*B*) Technicon H·2 sample with diagnosis of chronic granulocytic leukemia (CGL). The peroxidase cytogram is characteristic of CGL with large variation of cell volumes and staining intensities. This represents the variety of immature stages of granulocytes present in this sample. Increased number of basophils is also characteristic and is shown in the basophil channel scattergram. Most parameters are beyond reference ranges as indicated by L (low) and H (high). Compare these patterns to normal patterns found in Figure 42-15.

nation (Fig. 42-21*A* and *B*). Increased abnormal plasma proteins may precipitate with lysing reagents and produce abnormal WBC patterns (increased debris) and give invalid white cell counts. Nucleated RBCs and red cell fragments (schistocytes; Fig. 42-22*A–C*), may produce invalid counts and recognizable histogram/scattergram patterns affecting the WBC (NRBC interference) and platelet counts (schistocyte interference). Specific unusual histogram/scattergram patterns that occur repeatedly on sequential patient samples strongly suggest an instrument problem that needs to be identified and fixed. Thus, information provided by histogram patterns, scattergram patterns, and instrumentation flagging program messages can be used as a quality control tool in the identification of sample or instrument problems. Figures 42-23 through 42-25 are examples of abnormal scattergram patterns from

patients with hematologic abnormalities (*i.e.*, anemia, leukemias). These are examples of the data, histogram, and scattergram interpretation required of laboratory scientists operating complex multiparameter hematology instruments.

CHAPTER SUMMARY

Continued advancements in technology and computerization have increased precision and analysis speed, decreased sample (size) requirements, and have added new parameters to hematology instruments. Available instruments range from those offering a few parameters to the very sophisticated analyzers that are approaching 30 parameters. Built-in quality control programs are comprehensive and include the Bull moving average program (Chap. 45). They monitor instrument functions (such as counting time) and flag sample analysis when specific functions fall out of range. They permit the use of patient samples along with commercial control materials to monitor instrument calibration and precision. These programs flag out-of-limits results, chart data, and permit editing of data for statistical purposes without erasing the data from a file. Some programs include ability to mark data when a new vial of control material is opened. These features are very helpful in meeting documentation requirements for laboratory certification. Several instruments include the ability to check individual patient results against previous results (delta checking). Some maintenance procedures are now programmed to be performed automatically at the touch of the keypad.

Impedance and optical methods have continued to be refined. With the development of laser technology and advances in fluidic processes such as hydrodynamic focusing and laminar flow management came the ability to count platelets accurately and precisely at extremely low concentrations (1.0×10^9/L). Continuing advances have provided more information about cell maturity and RBC morphology. Screening blood samples rapidly for clinically significant morphology and numeric abnormalities is possible with these multiparameter instruments. The most popular instruments provide visual as well as numeric information about each sample. Histogram and cytogram (or scattergram) patterns can be valuable when an experienced eye analyzes them for suggestions of cellular abnormality as well as sample or instrument problems. Instrumentation has gone beyond the point where an operator simply processes samples with the touch of a button. A sound background in instrument theory and clinical hematology is necessary to analyze and interpret the complex numeric and graphic data generated by these sophisticated instruments.

Following the introduction of the automated (screening) differential, flagging programs for identification of abnormalities have continued to improve by reducing the number of false-positive flags and maintaining the number of false-negatives at a very low level. Each laboratory must develop its own set of parameter limits that require confirmation of results before release of the data. Instrument interference flags must also be appropriately addressed before reporting patient results. Instrument manufacturers and laboratories are working together to safely reduce the number of interferences and flags that require follow-up procedures.

Advances in technology have improved reticulocyte counting precision to the point of detecting slight changes in marrow activity that were lost in the imprecision of the manual counting method. These changes are important in detecting engraftment of bone marrow transplants. The staining intensity of the reticulocyte (although not yet standardized from manufacturer to manufacturer) is being related to the age of the reticulocyte producing a new term, *reticulocyte maturation index* (RMI). Some manufacturers are adding reticulocyte analysis to the routine hematology analyzer's menu of parameters.

The QBC (Becton Dickinson) screening instrument, which is based on centrifugation of whole blood, does not actually count cells and yet is small, inexpensive, rapid, and quite useful in settings such as point-of-care testing, physician offices, or outpatient clinics.

Before choosing a new instrument for a hematology laboratory, a major question should be answered: What information is needed in this setting? An instrument with additional features or information that will not be used should not be purchased. Unused features are expensive. The medical community and government regulations leave little room for extravagance. Discrete testing and bidirectional interfacing of instruments are newer advances in hematology instrumentation. Robotic sample preparation and delivery to the testing station is being developed.

Currently, available hematology instruments for the clinical laboratory can perform the routine differential or screening differential on large numbers of leukocytes accurately with greater speed and precision than is possible with manual techniques. The screening differential, in conjunction with the CBC, appears to be an effective means to identify patient specimens that do not require more extensive testing and to flag specimens on which more testing is valuable. As more and more information about a sample is being generated, the laboratorian must keep up with the advances in technology and be able to interpret the data as well as histogram and scattergram patterns. Many of these advances are helping to reduce the number of film reviews that are necessary. Thus, the laboratory can more readily meet the needs of cost containment and efficiency. Lastly, as technology develops, so does the sophistication of laboratory equipment. New advances seem to be in the direction of extended leukocyte classification, more sophisticated sample handling systems, and patient data integration and processing systems.

Case Study 42-1

The following instrument results were obtained on an EDTA anticoagulated whole blood sample:

Parameter	Original Results	Repeat Results	Units
WBC	30.82	34.39	$\times 10^9$/L
RBC	1.76	2.88	$\times 10^{12}$/L
Hb	9.6	9.6	g/dL
Hct	0.185	0.273	L/L
PLT	376	338	$\times 10^9$/L

Follow-up action: No instrument maintenance or adjustments were necessary. Following sample preparation (original sample tube), the sample was repeated and the values obtained are found in the column of data labeled "Repeat results" above.

1. Calculate the MCV, MCH, and MCHC for the original test results.
2. Which indices are unreasonable?
3. Which measured parameter(s) need(s) follow-up action before reporting any patient results?
4. Calculate the MCV, MCH, and MCHC for the repeat testing.
5. What sample preparation most likely caused the change in results?

Case Study 42-2

The following instrument results were obtained on a patient sample:

Parameter	Original Results	Repeat Results of Dilution and Film Examination	Units
WBC	21.27*	11.18 ammonium oxalate	$\times 10^9$/L
RBC	3.00		$\times 10^{12}$/L
Hb	12.2		g/dL
Hct	0.28	Spun Hct 0.28	L/L
MCV	93.7		fL
MCH	40.7		pg
MCHC	43.4		g/dL
PLT	161	Manual diff.%	$\times 10^9$/L
NEUT %	43.4*	75	
LYMPH %	44.6*	20	
MONO %	11.5*	5	
EOS %	0.3*		
BASO %	0.2*	WBC film estimate 12.0	$\times 10^9$/L

Two problems are present in this case. The original test results had interference flags for WBC (indicated by *) and autodiff results. An ammonium oxalate dilution gave a lower WBC count as indicated in the column of repeat test results. The latter value has been corrected for the dilution factor. This WBC agreed with the blood film estimate of the WBC count.

1. What other parameters need further follow-up?
2. What clue can be obtained from the microhematocrit determination?
3. Why are the manual differential results so different from the original results?
4. An aliquot of the plasma from this whole blood sample was tested on the hematology analyzer and a hemoglobin value of 4.0 g/dL was obtained. What does this suggest?
5. How can the information given in question 4 be used to complete the follow-up action required before reporting the results for this patient sample?

Review Questions

42-1. Coulter impedance technology uses _____ to count and measures _____ cell volume.

  A. laser light scatter; overall
  B. low frequency direct current; nuclear
  C. low frequency radio waves; nuclear
  D. low frequency direct current; overall

42-2. Impedance technology is based on the fact that leukocytes are

  A. good conductors of electrical current.
  B. volumetrically sphered.
  C. poor conductors of direct current.
  E. uniformly sized and nucleated.

42-3. Counters based on the laser light scatter detection method protect the forward scatter sensors from direct laser light by

  A. using a focusing lens.
  B. using a blocker bar.
  C. using a series of filters.
  D. using opposite polarizing lenses.

42-4. Hydrodynamic focusing and laminar flow are used by Coulter for

  A. red cell analysis.
  B. platelet analysis.
  C. MCV and RDW analysis.
  D. differential analysis.

42-5. Hydrodynamic focusing does not

  A. dilute the sample.
  B. cause cells to line up in single file.
  C. narrow the sample stream.
  D. center cells in the flow cell.

42-6. Automated screening (WBC) differentials are capable of identifying and counting

  A. immature granulocytes.
  B. blasts.
  C. variant lymphocytes.
  D. lymphocytes.

42-7. Match the analysis method and cell characteristics identified.

___1. overall cell volume	A. radio frequency signals
___2. internal complexity	B. forward light scatter
___3. opacity	C. 90° light scatter
___4. eosinophil granules	D. 90° depolarized scatter
___5. fluorescent staining	

42-8. Match the technology with the instrument manufacturer/instrument.

___ 1. Sweep flow	A. Abbott Cell-Dyn® 3500
___ 2. von Behrens transducer plate	B. Bayer H·3
___ 3. IMI analysis	C. Becton Dickinson QBC®
___ 4. Isovolumetric sphering	D. Coulter STKS, MAXM
___ 5. VCS	E. Sysmex E-Series (NE or SE)
___ 6. Basophil lobularity	F. Sysmex R-Series
___ 7. RF-DC tri-modal analysis	
___ 8. Mia analysis	
___ 9. Noncyanide Hb analysis	
___10. 90° polarized/depolarized laser scatter analysis	
___11. Auramine O fluorescence	
___12. Acridine orange fluorescence	

Use the following to answer questions 42-9, 42-10 and 42-11

  A. 1 and 3 are correct
  B. 2 and 4 are correct
  C. 1, 2, and 3 are correct
  D. Only 4 is correct
  E. All are correct

42-9. Automation of reticulocyte counting has resulted in the ability to

  1. detect response to erythropoietin therapy.
  2. identify immature reticulocytes by staining intensity.
  3. detect bone marrow engraftment.
  4. improve precision.

42-10. Leukocytes that stain positively for peroxidase in the Bayer H·Series instruments are

  1. lymphocytes and blasts.
  2. monocytes and neutrophils.
  3. atypical lymphocytes and basophils.
  4. eosinophils.

42-11. Instruments that use a modified cyanmethemoglobin method for hemoglobin measurement are

  1. Coulter S-Plus Series instruments.
  2. Abbott Cell-Dyn Series instruments.
  3. Technicon H-Series instruments.
  4. Sysmex E-Series instruments.

References

1. Abbott Cell-Dyn 3500 Operator's Manual. Abbott Park, TX, Abbott Laboratories 97-9634/R1-4-Sept 1994
2. Bacus JW: The development of automated differential systems. In Koepke JA (ed): Differential Leukocyte Counting, p 95. Skokie, IL, College of American Pathologists, 1978
3. Bas BM, Catsberg MJ, de Kamp SLK: A short evaluation of a new haematological analyzer: The Cobas Argos 5-Diff. Eur J Clin Chem Biochem 31:603, 1993
4. Bentley SA, Johnson TS, Schier CH et al: Flow-cytochemical differential leukocyte analysis with quantitation of neutrophil left shift. An evaluation of the Cobas-Helios analyzer. Am J Clin Pathol 102(2):223, 1994
5. Bentley SA, Johnson A, Bishop CA: A parallel evaluation of four automated hematology analyzers. Am J Clin Pathol 100:626, 1993
6. Bentley SA, Pegram MD, Ross DW: Diagnosis of infective and inflammatory disorders by flow cytometric analysis of blood neutrophils. Am J Clin Pathol 88:177, 1987
7. Bessman JD: New parameters on automated hematology instruments. Lab Med 14:488, 1983

8. Bessman JD, Gilmer PR, Gardner FH: Improved classification of anemias by MCV and RDW. Am J Clin Pathol 80:322, 1983

9. Buttarello M, Gadotti M, Lorenz C et al: Evaluation of four automated hematology analyzers. Am J Clin Pathol 97:345, 1992

10. College of American Pathologists: Comprehensive Hematology Survey: Limited Coagulation Module. Participant Summary, Set H-1A. Skokie, IL, CAP, 1977

11. College of American Pathologists: Comprehensive Hematology Survey: Limited Coagulation Module. Participant Summary, Set H-1C. Skokie, IL, CAP, 1986

12. Connelly DP, McClain MP, Crowson TW et al: Use of the differential leukocyte count for inpatient case finding. Hum Pathol 13:294, 1982

13. Cornbleet PJ: Hematology update: The five-part differential. ASCP Workshop, Boston, April 1992

14. Coulter Electronics, Inc: Coulter Counter Model S-Plus IV Operator's Manual, PN 4235360. Hialeah, FL, Coulter Electronics, Sept 1983

15. Coulter Electronics, Inc: Coulter Counter Model S-Plus IV with Three-Population Differential and Auto Transfer: Product Reference Manual 4235328B. Hialeah, FL, Coulter Electronics, Nov 1983

16. Cox CJ, Habermann TM, Payne BA et al: Evaluation of the Coulter Counter Model S-Plus IV. Am J Clin Pathol 84:297, 1985

17. Culp NB, Fritsma G: NE-Series User's Guide. A Practical Approach to Interpreting NE-Series Scattergrams and Histograms. Los Alamitos, CA, Clinical Applications Division, TOA Medical Electronics (USA), 1991

18. Davis BH, Bigelow NC: Automated reticulocyte analysis. Clinical practice and associated new parameters. Hem Onc Clin N Am 8(4):617, 1994

19. Davis BH, Bigelow NC, Koepke JA, et al: Flow cytometric reticulocyte analysis. Multi-institutional interlaboratory correlation study. Am J Clin Pathol 102:468, 1994

20. England JM: Blood cell sizing. In Koepke JA (ed): Practical Laboratory Hematology, p 111. New York, Churchill Livingstone, 1991

21. Gottfried EL: Lipids of human leukocytes: Relation to cell type. J Lipid Res 8:321, 1967

22. Gottfried EL: Lipid patterns in health and disease. Semin Hematol 9:241, 1972

23. Houwen B et al: Performance evaluation of the Sysmex SE-9000 hematology workstation. Sysmex Journal International, vol 4, p 5. Kobe, Japan, TOA Medical Electronics Co, 1995

24. Houwen B: Reticulocyte maturation. Blood Cells 18:167, 1992

25. Hoyer JD: Leukocyte differential. Mayo Clin Proc 68:1027, 1993

26. Jovin TM, Morris ST, Striker G et al: Automated sizing and separation of light scattering intensities. J Histochem Cytochem 24:269, 1976

27. Kachel V, Menke E: Hydrodynamic properties of flow cytometric instruments. In Melamed MR, Mullaney PF, Mendelsohn HL (eds): Flow Cytometry and Sorting, p 41. New York, Wiley Medical, 1979

28. Kim YR, Ornstein L: Isovolumetric sphering of erythrocytes for more accurate and precise cell volume measurement by flow cytochemistry. Cytometry 3:419, 1983

29. Koepke JA: Fitting the cell counter to the bed count. Clin Lab Med 13:4, 1993

30. Koepke JA: Let's improve the flagging of abnormal hematology specimens. Medical Laboratory Observer Nov:22, 1994

31. Koepke JA: Quantitative blood cell counting. In Koepke JA (ed): Practical Laboratory Hematology, p 48. New York, Churchill Livingstone, 1991

32. Koepke JA, Dotson MA, Shifman MA: A critical evaluation of the manual/visual differential leukocyte counting method. Blood Cells 11:173, 1985

33. Krause JR: The automated white blood cell differential. A current perspective. Hem Onc Clin N Am 8(4):605, 1994

34. MacLaren IA, Conn DM, Wadsworth LD: Comparison of two automated hemoglobin methods using Sysmex SULFO-LYSER and STROMATOLYSER C. Sysmex Journal International 1:59, 1991

35. Mohandas N, Kim YR, Tyeko DH et al: Accurate and independent measurement of volume and hemoglobin concentration of individual red cells by laser light. Blood 68:506, 1986

36. National Committee for Clinical Laboratory Standards: H20-A: Approved standard for reference leukocyte differential counting and evaluation of methods. Villanova, PA, NCCLS, 1990

37. Ortho Diagnostic Systems Inc: Ortho ELT 15 Advanced Hematology Analyzer with Screening Differential: Operator Reference Manual. Westwood, MA, Clinical and Research Laboratory Instrument Systems (410 University Ave, Westwood, MA 02090), Dec 1985

38. Paul RI, Badgett JT, Buchino JJ: Evaluation of QBC® Autoread performance in an emergency department setting. Pediatr Emerg Care 10:359, 1994

39. Pearson RW, Houwen B, Mast B: SULFOLYSER Automated Hemoglobin Reagent—Introduction of a New Cyanide-Free Method. Monograph. Los Alamitos, CA, TOA Medical Electronics (USA), Inc, 1991

40. Pierre RV: Leukocyte differential counting. In Koepke JA (ed): Practical Laboratory Hematology, p 131. New York, Churchill Livingstone, 1991

41. Pierre RV: Seminar and Case Studies: The Automated Differential (Medical Education Program). Hialeah, FL, Coulter Electronics, 1985

42. Pierre RB, Payne BA, Lee WK et al: Comparison of four leukocyte differential methods with the National Committee for Clinical Laboratory Standards (NCCLS) reference method. Am J Clin Pathol 87:201, 1987

43. Ross DW, Bardwell A: Automated cytochemistry and the white cell differential in leukemia. Blood Cells 6:455, 1980

44. Rumke CL: The statistically expected variability in differential leukocyte counting. In Koepke JA (ed): Differential Leukocyte Counting. Skokie, IL, College of American Pathologists, 1978

45. Salzman GC, Mullaney PF, Price BJ: Light scattering approaches to cell characterization. In Melamed MR, Mullaney PF, Mendelsohn ML (eds): Flow Cytometry and Sorting, p 106. New York, Wiley Medical, 1979

46. Savage RA: The red cell indices. Yesterday, today and tomorrow. In Ward PCJ (ed): Routine hematology testing. Clin Lab Med 13(4):773, 1993

47. Shively JA: Interpretive aspects of hematology tests with a focus on the blood film. In Lewis SM, Koepke JA (eds): Hematology Laboratory Management and Practice, p 12. Oxford, Butterworth-Heinemann Ltd, 1995

48. Simson E, Groner W: The state of the art for the automated WBC differential. Part I: Analytic performance. In: Laboratory Hematology. International Society for Laboratory Hematology, vol 1, no 1. Kluge, Carden, Jennings Publishing Co Ltd, 1995

49. Technicon Instruments Corp: Technicon H6000 System Product Labeling. Technicon Publications No. UA81-443-00. Tarrytown, NY, Technicon, May 1981

50. Technicon Instruments Corp: Technicon H·1 System Operator's Guide. Technicon Publications No. TA8-5588-10. Tarrytown, NY, Technicon, Oct 1985

51. Technicon Instruments Corp: Proceedings of the Technicon H·1 Hematology Symposium. Tarrytown, NY, Technicon, Oct 1985

52. Technicon Instruments Corp: Technicon H·System Operator's Guide, Technical Publication No. TAB-5588. Tarrytown, NY, Technicon, Oct 1985

53. Terstappen LWMM: Flow cytometric characterization of white blood cells of healthy donors and patients with lymphocytic diseases. Mountain View, CA, Sequoia-Turner Corporation, p 11, 1988

54. TOA Medical Electronics Co., Ltd: Sysmex Operator's Manual Model E-5000. Code No 461-2104-2. Kobe, Japan, TOA, April 1985

55. TOA Medical Electronics Co., Ltd: Sysmex Operator's Manual Automated Hematology Analyzer SE-9000. Code No 461-2456-2. Kobe, Japan, TOA, Dec 1994

56. Tycko DH, Metz MH, Epstein EA et al: Flowcytometric light scattering measurements of red blood cell volume and hemoglobin concentration. Appl Optics 24:135, 1985

57. Van Dilla MA, Mendelsohn ML: Introduction and resume of flow cytometry and sorting. In Melamed MR, Mullaney PF, Mendelsohn ML (eds): Flow Cytometry and Sorting, p 14. New York, Wiley Medical, 1979

58. Wardlaw SC, Levine RA: Quantitative buffy coat analysis. JAMA 249:617, 1983

59. Watson JS, Davis RA: Evaluation of the Technicon H·1 Hematology System. Lab Med 18:316, 1987

60. Williams JE, Tinklein FE, Metcalfe HC (eds): The nature of light: Waves and particles. In: Modern Physics, p 279. New York, Holt, Rinehart and Winston, 1979

61. Williams JE, Tinklein FE, Metcalfe HC (eds): Reflection. In: Modern Physics, p 313. New York, Holt, Rinehart and Winston, 1979

62. Williams JE, Tinklein FE, Metcalfe HC (eds): Refraction. In: Modern Physics, p 329. New York, Holt, Rinehart and Winston, 1979

63. Williams JE, Tinklein FE, Metcalfe HC (eds): Diffraction and polarization: Interference and diffraction. In: Modern Physics, p 357. New York, Holt, Rinehart and Winston, 1979

CHAPTER 43

Flow Cytometry

Jeffrey Louie
John W. Parker

Objectives

1. Describe the major features of a flow cytometer.
2. Discuss the technical and safety precautions related to the use of the flow cytometer.
3. Describe how flow cytometry may be applied in the clinical laboratory—both now and in the near future.

Flow cytometry (FCM) is a technology that analyzes thousands of cells individually and rapidly for various physical and other properties. By using flow cytometry, one is able to perform quantitative multiparameter characterization of cells in heterogeneous populations and thus identify specific subpopulations. This technology has produced significant diagnostic and prognostic information and has had a major impact on immunology and hematology. It also has increased our understanding of the normal development of human blood cells.

HISTORY

The basic principle of flow cytometry was incorporated into the first Coulter counter. In that instrument, individual cells were counted and sized as they flowed in a conduction liquid through a small orifice between two electrodes. The change in voltage that occurred as each cell passed through the sensing zone was detected and counted.[4]

In 1953, Crossland-Taylor described a technique capable of directing cells to the center of a flow stream in single file.[5] This technology is variously known as *laminar sheath flow* or *hydrodynamic focusing* (Chap. 42) and is a fundamental feature of most cytometers today. In 1965, a flow cytometer capable of discriminating cells based on their light scattering properties and of measuring more than one property of each cell was introduced.[17] The technology was further advanced by the introduction of the first instrument able to separate and sort cells.[11]

The complexity and expense of early fluorescence-activated cell sorters made it impractical for these instruments to be used routinely in the clinical laboratory and serious clinical application did not appear until the 1980s. Parallel developments in instrumentation, fluorochrome chemistry, monoclonal antibody production, and computer hardware and software made it feasible to develop clinical flow cytometers. Antibodies conjugated to fluorescein-isothiocyanate (FITC) for use in the immunophenotyping of lymphomas and leukemias and dyes with varying degrees of affinity for DNA were introduced. However, it was the finding that enumeration of CD4- and CD8-positive T lymphocytes in blood was of value in the diagnosis and monitoring of patients with HIV/AIDS that caused the use of clinical flow cytometry to "take off."

It became apparent that more than one fluorochrome could be analyzed with single laser cytometers because different dyes (*e.g.,* FITC, phycoerythrin) could be stimulated at one wavelength (488 nm) but emit at different wavelengths. This has had a major impact on the extent to which one can characterize a cell population and has emphasized the value of multiparameter analysis. With the commercial development of automated samplers and increasing automation of cytometers, the value of the clinical flow cytometer has continued to increase, particularly in those laboratories which analyze large numbers of specimens. However, automation has not relieved laboratories of the necessity of providing well-trained technologists in this still rapidly developing and complex field.

PRINCIPAL FEATURES OF FLOW CYTOMETRY

The most important feature of flow cytometers is their capacity for multiparameter analysis of cells or particles as they pass through a beam of laser light. A fundamental

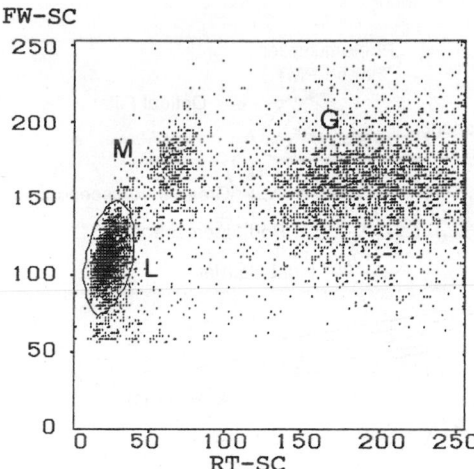

FIGURE 43-1. Forward (FW-Sc) *versus* side (RT-Sc) scatter histogram of peripheral blood. Lymphocytes (L), monocytes (M), and granulocytes (G) are clearly delineated and each can be selected ("gated") for analysis. Lymphocytes have been electronically gated.

Optics

Detecting fluorescence of small particles requires intensely bright illumination. Therefore the light sources of choice in flow cytometry are mercury arc lamps or lasers. The mercury arc lamp radiates multiple wavelengths of light in all directions which provide a wide spectral range for excitation of fluorochromes. Mercury lamps have not been used as much as lasers because of difficulties in achieving sufficient light intensity at selected wavelengths. Other disadvantages are the requirement for relatively elaborate power supplies, short lamp life, a somewhat complicated lens system for selecting specific excitation and emission wavelengths, and the need for frequent alignment of the lamp for optimal light focusing. However, these lamps are much less expensive than lasers and there is a resurgence of interest in them by manufacturers.

Laser light sources are more popular. The emitted laser light is extremely bright, coherent (waves of light are parallel and unidirectional), and monochromatic (the frequency of light represents a single wavelength or color). The laser light beam, with its stability and spectral purity, can be directed at cells without a need for additional complex lens focusing systems or constant adjustments of the light beam.

The air-cooled argon laser, emitting a 488-nm wavelength with 15 mW of power, is the most common clinical flow cytometer light source. These newer, air-cooled lasers are smaller, require less current (standard 115-V outlet), have a longer life, are less expensive, and require less maintenance than the older, larger, water-cooled, gas ion lasers found on research instruments. The argon laser

component of this analysis is the use of the light scatter of particles to help characterize them. Although cells scatter the incident laser light in all directions, the measurement of light scatter is routinely made at two positions relative to the cell as it passes through the laser beam. Forward-angle light scatter (FALS) is measured along the incident laser light path (2° to 10°) and increases with cell size. Orthogonal or side scatter (SSC) is measured between 70° to 90° from the incident light path and increases with cytoplasmic and nuclear complexity. Light scatter signals are amplified by photomultiplier tubes (PMTs) and converted from analog to digital signals. FALS and SSC results can be plotted to form a scattergram which, in the case of leukocytes, will separate granulocytes, monocytes, and lymphocytes from whole blood into separate cell clusters (Fig. 43-1). The cells of interest can then be electronically selected or "gated" for specific analysis.

In addition to their light scatter characteristics, cells and other particles can be analyzed for the presence or absence of fluorescence (Fig. 43-2). Cells are labeled with specific probes (antibodies, ligands, molecular probes) conjugated to fluorochromes that fluoresce when excited by the incident light. The flow cytometer measures the fluorescence intensity of each cell at an extremely high rate of speed (thousands of events per second). Depending on the wavelength(s) of the light source, emitting wavelength(s) of the fluorochrome(s), and the number of probes used, viable, intact cells can be analyzed for the presence or absence of a variety of surface antigens, receptors, enzymes, and other molecules. Cell membrane permeability can be increased by chemical fixation and/or the use of detergents, which allows staining of internal (cytoplasmic/nuclear) components.

Analytical flow cytometers have four major components: optics, fluidics, pneumatics, and data processing (Fig. 43-3), each of which is discussed here. More complete information may be found in various reference textbooks (see Suggested Reading).

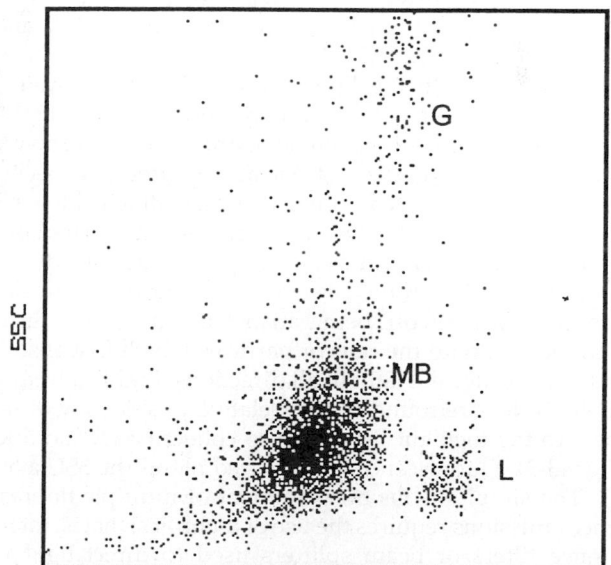

FIGURE 43-2. CD45-FITC (FL1) *versus* side scatter (SSC) histogram of peripheral blood in a case of acute myeloid leukemia. Lymphocytes (L) stain intensely for CD45 and show low side scatter. Granulocytes (G) have high side scatter and less CD45 intensity. Because of low intensity CD45 and low side scatter, myeloblasts (MB) stand out from the other more mature cells.

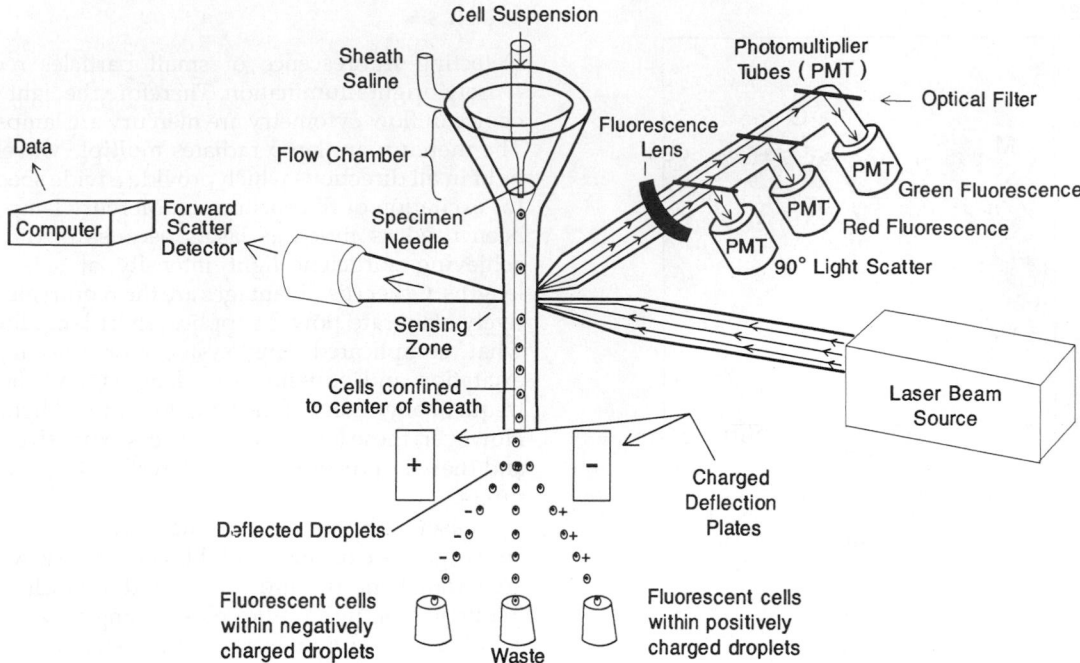

FIGURE 43-3. Diagram of operation of flow cytometer and cell sorter.

is quite useful for excitation of many common fluoro-chromes, including FITC (green) and phycoerythrin (PE) (orange), which are commonly conjugated to monoclonal antibodies for immunophenotyping. Lasers other than argon are also available, including krypton-ion, helium-neon, and helium-cadmium, which, when used in tandem with argon, allow for three or more color analyses. However, three-color analysis is also possible using a single argon laser because of the availability of "third" color dyes such as peridinin chlorophyll protein (PerCP) and energy coupled dye (ECD).

In addition to the light source, the optical system comprises a system of lenses and filters designed to focus, direct, and selectively screen out extraneous wavelengths of light. This allows the intrinsic light scatter and specific fluorescence associated with each probe attached to cells or particles to be directed to a light detector. The laser light first passes through beam-shaping optics that define the configuration of the laser beam to suit the particular size of particle or cell being analyzed. The laser light is then focused onto the cells or particles which first absorb and then scatter the light in all directions. Light collecting photodiodes are found in two relative positions with respect to the incident light path to collect FALS and SSC (Fig. 43-3). Fluorescence is measured along the SSC axis.

The simultaneous measurement of multiple fluores-cence emissions requires the use of dichroics; that is, inter-ference filters or beam splitters used to direct light in different spectral regions to different detectors. These are usually of the long bandpass type, causing short wave-length light to be reflected while longer wavelengths out-side the bandpass are transmitted. Use of a combination of dichroic filters directs emitted light from specific dyes to photodetectors for amplification. In addition bandpass filters are placed before each photomultiplier tube to

allow only a specified wavelength to be collected for pro-cessing (Fig. 43-3).

Single laser systems (argon) commonly used in the clinical laboratory can excite multiple dyes such as FITC and PE. However, the emission spectra of these and other dyes often overlap and require electronic fluorescence compensation to reduce the unwanted signals of one flu-orochrome from interfering with that of another. Light signals that represent debris, dead cells, or nonspecific fluorescence can also be eliminated from signal processing by electronic circuitry that sets a threshold voltage for signal acceptance. If the signal does not exceed the preset threshold, then it is eliminated from the display and analysis.

Fluidics/Pneumatics

The fluidics system of flow cytometers is composed of a series of fluid valves, pumps, and/or syringes which transport cells to a flow chamber. *Hydrodynamic focusing* refers to the mechanism by which one smoothly flowing stream of fluid containing the sample (the sample or core stream) is injected into the center of another larger smoothly flowing stream of fluid (the sheath stream). By gradually narrowing the physical area through which the two streams must pass, the cells or other particles in the sample stream will line up in single file in the very center of the flow chamber without mixing with the outer cell-free sheath stream. This condition is called *laminar flow* and must remain stable throughout sample analysis in order to maintain maximum exposure of the cells to the laser beam. Any disruption in the flow stream from clogs, air bubbles, or fluctuations in pressure will cause subse-quent measurements to be imprecise and inaccurate.

The sample and sheath streams may be driven by

either gas under pressure (air or nitrogen), a vacuum, or syringe-like pumps. The latter allows delivery of a known volume of sample per unit of time which, when the sample flow rate is known, can be used to calculate absolute numbers of cells per unit volume. Currently most clinical flow cytometers report only % positive cells (*e.g.*, CD4 T-cell enumeration in HIV immunophenotyping) and must rely on hematology cell counters to provide the absolute number of lymphocytes in order to calculate the number of CD4 T-lymphocytes per cubic millimeter. This creates major difficulties in quality control and the proficiency testing of laboratories because the intrinsic errors of two different instruments are compounded.

Flow Chambers and Cell Sorting

Flow chambers (flow cells) are of two types. The more common type used in bench-top clinical flow cytometers is a flat-sided rectangular quartz flow cell. The other is a stream-in-air type that allows the sample to exit the flow cell in a thin stream. The advantage of the enclosed quartz cell is that it prevents exposure of the operator to the potentially biohazardous sample stream (*e.g.*, HIV-positive samples for CD4 surface marker testing; blood from hepatitis B patients), because the sample stream exits the flow cell through enclosed tubing to a closed waste container. In addition, the quartz flow cells allow the sample to remain in the laser beam longer, resulting in greater sensitivity in the detection of dimly fluorescing cell markers. On the other hand, the stream-in-air flow cell allows the direct analysis of the sample stream without the interference of the light refracting properties of the quartz crystal, which may become dirty or scratched. Cell sorting is only possible with the stream-in-air flow chamber, and since it is not a closed system, it requires careful biohazard monitoring.

Flow cytometers with cell-sorting capacity were once only found in research laboratories. Because of the user friendliness of present day sorters, clinical laboratories can now take advantage of this unique capability. Cells that meet preselected "sort gating" criteria can be physically segregated from unwanted cells by breaking the cell-containing sample stream into fine droplets. The droplets containing the cells of interest are then electrically charged and deflected away from the remaining sample stream in an electromagnetic field and collected into a tube, onto a slide, or into microtiter wells for further studies.

Data Analysis

Analytical flow cytometers can analyze as many as 5000 cells or events per second. Newer cell sorters can sort up to 15,000 cells per second. Each individual cell can have two light scatter properties (FALS and SSC) and three or more fluorescent parameters measured simultaneously. This rapid multiparameter analysis of events requires computer-assisted signal processing. Light scatter signals are first amplified through photodiodes and photomultiplier tubes; run through spectral compensation and signal threshold circuitry; converted from analog to digital signals; and displayed as single- or dual-parameter histograms. These histograms can be log or linear displays.

Typically, inherent light scatter properties are presented linearly while fluorescence is presented in log form. Log presentation of fluorescence allows amplification of dim signals while keeping brightly staining events from appearing off-scale.

One of the more powerful aspects of data analysis is the concept of *gating*. Computer software allows flow operators to electronically separate or "gate" cell populations that have any assortment of measurable parameters, such as FALS (cell size), SSC (cell complexity), and FL1, FL2, and FL3 (three fluorescent colors). In this way a gated cell population can be analyzed separately from the rest of the cells in the sample.

Fluorochromes

The development of a variety of fluorescent dyes (fluorochromes) has expanded the number of cell parameters that can be measured simultaneously with one laser, because they emit over a range of wavelengths. For example, the argon laser which excites at 488 nm can stimulate different fluorochromes to emit at 530 nm (FITC), 580 (PE), and 620 (PerCP). Thus two or more antibodies or other probes can be conjugated to these different fluorochromes resulting in two- to four-color phenotyping of a cell population. The addition of other lasers (*e.g.*, HeNe [633 nm]) further expands this capability by making it possible to use other fluorochromes as well. Multicolor analysis requires that the cytometer be equipped with appropriate filters. Also, because there is always some emission spectrum overlap, this must be compensated for electronically.

QUALITY ASSURANCE
Technical Precautions

As with other instruments that count and characterize cells, flow cytometers require systematic and regular (laser) alignment, calibration, and cleaning. Unlike automated hematology analyzers, most clinical flow cytometers require significant operator involvement and judgment in selecting analysis gates and in recognizing problems with cell dispersion, cell viability, instrument settings, fluidics, and so forth. However, manufacturers are producing increasingly automated, walkaway instruments that stain samples, introduce them to the instrument (auto-biosamplers), select gates, and make appropriate adjustments. These still involve operator monitoring and manual manipulations for problem samples, but the degree of automation may soon approach that of hematology analyzers. Interpretation of results will continue to require experienced professional personnel.

Safety

Because specimens from HIV-infected patients are the most frequently analyzed specimens in many clinical flow laboratories, the potential for operator infection exists, not only by HIV but also by other organisms with which these patients are infected. All human material prepared for flow analysis should be prepared in a biohazard hood and the flow cytometer must be a closed system. The operator must not be exposed to aerosols, and liquid waste must be collected in a sealed container and be disposed of as biohazardous material. The fluidics system must be rinsed with a disinfectant (10% bleach) at least once daily. Centrifuges used for preparing specimens must be equipped to prevent aerosol leakage.

Instrument Selection

The selection of a flow cytometer for clinical laboratory use depends on several factors, including cost of the instrument and of maintenance contracts; types and numbers of assays to be analyzed; ease of learning and use by operators; and the desired degree of flexibility, software packages, and reporting formats. There are currently three major vendors of flow cytometers. These instruments have many common features, but each has advantages and disadvantages. The major similarity is that they use single laser (argon) light sources.

Large medical center laboratories may need two-laser instruments for combined clinical diagnostic use and clinical research. Smaller laboratories can perform two- and three-color phenotyping, DNA cell cycle analysis, and most other applications with a single argon laser instrument. Recent technologic developments may renew interest in the manufacture of relatively inexpensive mercury arc cytometers for clinical use.

CLINICAL APPLICATIONS

The range of fluorochromes and the number of monoclonal antibodies commercially available has led to an explosion in the amount of data made available to clinicians, so much so that validation of the clinical value of this data has proved to be a barrier in implementing new applications. Flow cytometry technology has progressed at a rapid rate, along with the development of new reagents and proposed clinical applications. However, the long-term clinical trials needed to validate their diagnostic and prognostic value prevent their immediate use.

This is just the beginning of increasingly complex data analysis and interpretation. The ability of a single laser to stimulate three or more different fluorochromes and the potential for innumerable probes (antibodies, lectins, and molecular probes) have made it feasible to perform multicolor immunophenotypic analyses with the commonly used clinical cytometers. The use of multiple lasers compounds the amount of data available which, in turn, must be interpreted in a clinical context.

The number of current and potential clinical applications, beyond DNA analysis, leukemia/lymphoma phenotyping, and CD4 lymphocyte surface marker quantitation in HIV disease is impressive. Some of these applications are discussed here and others are listed in Table 43-1.

HIV Immunophenotyping

Currently the most widely used clinical application of flow cytometry is in the quantitation of CD4+ T cells in patients with HIV infection. The quantitation of CD4+

TABLE 43-1
Clinical Applications of Flow Cytometry

IN CURRENT WIDESPREAD USAGE

Surface Immunophenotyping
    Quantitation of CD3, CD4, CD8 lymphocytes in HIV infection
    Leukemia
    Lymphomas
Measurements of DNA Content of Tumors
    Ploidy, S phase, proliferation associated markers

EXPANDING USAGE

Cross-matching in organ transplantation

Reticulocyte counts and reticulocyte maturation

Detection of anti-platelet antibodies

Intracytoplasmic immunophenotyping in leukemia

Bone marrow transplantation–stem cell quantitation, purification, and post-transplant monitoring

TdT measurements in leukemias and lymphomas

Detection of small numbers of leukemic cells in blood and bone marrow

EMERGING USAGE

Blood transfusion typing and cross-matches

Detection of small numbers of cells or organisms
    Fetal cells in maternal circulation
    Microorganisms

Platelet phenotyping and function

Detection of cell membrane phenomena
    Drug uptake
    Tumor cell drug resistance: P-glycoprotein, MDR*
    Membrane turnover
    Membrane potential

Detection of antibodies, antigens, microorganisms by immunobead–flow cytometry technology

Evaluation of leukocyte function
    Neutrophil oxidative metabolism in evaluation of phagocytosis gene defects (CGD†)

Molecular biology: *in situ* hybridization for detection of gene products, viruses, *etc.*

Apoptosis

Rapid measurement of lymphocyte activation and proliferation
    Expression of CD69 and other activation antigens
    Ki-67

Evaluation of intracellular metabolism
    pH
    Enzyme function
    Calcium transport

Cytogenetics
    Karyotyping

Semen analysis

MDR = Multidrug resistance
†CGD = Chronic granulomatous disease

lymphocytes in HIV antibody-positive patients is used in conjunction with other laboratory measurements (*e.g.*, viral load) and with clinical signs and symptoms to monitor the disease. As the disease progresses, relative and absolute values for CD4+ lymphocytes decrease until, in advanced AIDS, they may no longer be detectable. The number of CD8+ lymphocytes generally increases as CD4+ cells decrease, and a pronounced increase in the former may indicate a better prognosis. Patients with advanced AIDS and opportunistic infections may show a decrease in CD8+ lymphocytes.

CD4 quantitation in HIV disease has been made more specific by two-color flow cytometric analysis. Only cells that express both CD3 and CD4 are CD4 T lymphocytes (Fig. 43-4). Those cells expressing CD4 without CD3 are usually monocytes. By phenotyping lymphocytes from HIV patients with antibodies that recognize subsets of the CD4 and CD8 populations, additional prognostic information may be obtained. A recent example is the report by Liu and coworkers describing the prognostic value of CD38 intensity on CD8+ T lymphocytes.[20]

A significant problem in evaluating absolute CD4/CD8 counts lies in the inability of clinical flow cytometers, until recently, to provide absolute cell counts directly. This is because these instruments have not been equipped with precise and reliable volumetric sample delivery systems. They can provide accurate percentages of cell subsets, but absolute values are calculated from the absolute lymphocyte counts obtained from hematology analyzers. Thus, any instrument errors are compounded and comparisons of results between laboratories using different cytometers and different hematology analyzers reveal major discrepancies. Newer flow cytometers on the market have attempted to address this problem with varying degrees of success. Parallel studies of absolute CD4 counts obtained using flow cytometers plus hematology analyzers *versus* cytometers with absolute CD4 count capacity are in progress.

Leukemia/Lymphoma Immunophenotyping

Immunophenotyping leukemias and lymphomas with monoclonal antibodies was one of the first clinical applications of flow cytometry. Such phenotyping has become an important component of the diagnosis of these neoplasms. However, unlike many other diagnostic laboratory tests, phenotyping results require significant interpretation. This is because of variability in the expression and relative surface density of the markers by which cells of interest can be selected for analysis. In addition, except for CD3 on T lymphocytes, surface antigens identified by monoclonal antibodies on leukemia/lymphoma cells are not specific for a particular cell lineage. These cells typically do not express a single phenotypic marker which is diagnostic for the disease. Therefore an interpretation of the pattern and relative intensity of staining with large panels of antibodies is necessary to accurately identify the cell lineage of poorly differentiated leukemia/lymphoma cells.

An even more fundamental question is whether the population studied is neoplastic or reactive. With B lymphocyte proliferations this may appear obvious, in that only one light chain (kappa or lambda) expressed on B lymphocytes (CD19, CD10), represents a clonal and thus neoplastic expansion of one class of cells.[10]

Clonality in T lymphocyte and monocyte/myeloid proliferations is less clearly apparent. Therefore, panels of antibodies are used to detect aberrant antigen expression and to identify the cell type[27] and lineage. Results must be correlated with morphology and clinical features for diagnosis. Use of DNA/ploidy analysis may help if the cells in question are aneuploid (*i.e.*, not containing the normal number of chromosomes).

Because morphologically abnormal cells cannot be selected visually for analysis by flow cytometry, electronic gating (light scatter) alone or in conjunction with antibodies is used to isolate abnormal cells for phenotyping.[19] Laboratories vary greatly in the way they gate cells, in the antibodies they use, and in the way they interpret results.[12] However, regardless of the range of opinions as to how to phenotype leukemia and lymphoma cells, it is frequently essential for accurate diagnosis[2,9] and for detection of small numbers of leukemia cells in blood and bone marrow, pre- and post therapy.

The advantages of FCM immunophenotyping over immunohistochemical staining (Chap. 29) include (1) small sample requirement; (2) the ability to identify multiple cell markers on the same cell, such as surface immunoglobulin (sIg) kappa or lambda on CD19+ B cells for detecting clonality in B-cell neoplasms[10] (Fig. 43-5); (3) the ability to analyze any specimen from which single-cell suspensions can be prepared (blood, bone marrow, body fluids, solid tumors, etc.); (4) the ability to assess differentiation/maturation in addition to cell lineage, such as pre-B ALL *versus* B-CLL; and (5) rapid turnaround time (hours rather than days). Disadvantages of FCM include the need for live (non-fixed) cells for surface immunophenotyping and the need to select cells for study electronically rather than morphologically. Nevertheless, an FCM immunophenotype involving a two- or three-color panel of antibodies can aid in specific cell type identification of leukemias or lymphomas, which are difficult to classify by morphology and special stains alone.

Because of the lack of consensus among laboratories as to how leukemias and lymphomas should be analyzed by flow cytometry, several groups are attempting to develop consensus guidelines regarding selection of antibody panels, gating strategies, interpretation and reporting of data, and quality control.

DNA Cell Cycle Analysis

DNA cell cycle analysis by flow cytometry has become a routine method for assessing the ploidy (DNA content) of tumors. With the use of DNA fluorochromes, which bind quantitatively to the DNA of cells, the measurement of ploidy and proliferation (S-phase fraction—the DNA synthesis phase) can be determined. Tumors can be demonstrated to be either diploid (normal number of chromosomes) or aneuploid (abnormal number of chromosomes), the latter usually indicating a worse prognosis or greater possibility of relapse. In general, tumors with a high fraction of cells in S phase have a worse prognosis than those with a low fraction in S phase. On the other hand, rapidly dividing leukemia/lymphoma cells are frequently more susceptible to radiation and chemotherapy. The ploidy status and S-phase fraction must be used in conjunction with other prognostic factors such as tumor size, tumor stage, histologic grade, and hormone receptor status, in order to maximize their prognostic value. DNA cell cycle analysis is currently most commonly applied to tumors

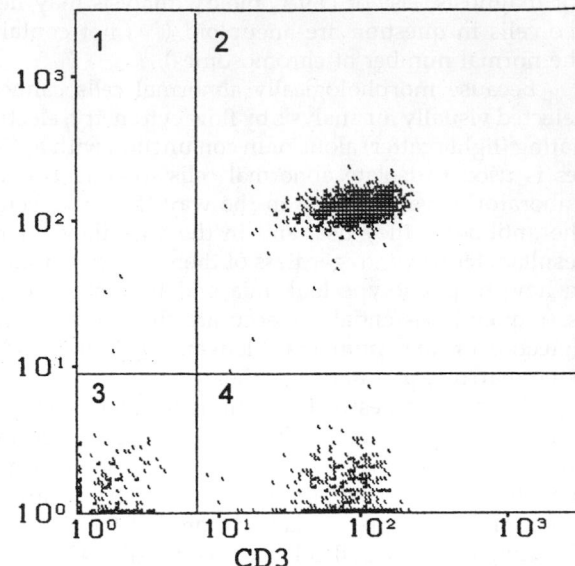

CD4

REG -+ 3 0.2 %	REG ++ 1,045 63.0 %
REG -- 154 9.3 %	REG +- 456 27.5 %

CD3 : 90.5 % 1,501 cells
CD4 : 63.2 % 1,048 cells

FIGURE 43-4. CD3/CD4 two-color histogram from three-color staining of peripheral blood for CD3(PerCP)/CD4(FITC)/CD8(PE). The double stained CD3+/CD4+ cells (quadrant 2) are true CD4 lymphocytes. The CD3+/CD4− cells (quadrant 4) are primarily CD3+/CD8+ lymphocytes. Quadrant 1 contains CD3−/CD4+ cells, which are monocytes found in the lymphocyte light scatter gate. Quadrant 3 contains CD3−/CD4− cells, which are most likely B lymphocytes and NK cells.

of the breast, but increasing analysis of tumors of the colon, ovary, prostate, and bladder indicates prognostic value.[15]

Hematology Applications

RETICULOCYTE COUNTS

Reticulocytes are young erythrocytes that contain residual ribosomes, mitochondria, and centrioles with accompa-

nying RNA and DNA, but no nuclei (Chap. 6). Because these organelles are absent in mature erythrocytes, their presence in RBCs in the peripheral blood may be an indication of premature release and, in turn, increased erythropoiesis—a feature of some forms of anemia.[18]

Reticulocytes traditionally have been detected and quantitated by staining with new methylene blue or brilliant cresyl blue and counting with a microscope (Chap. 9). Recently, fluorescent dyes (acridine orange, ethidium

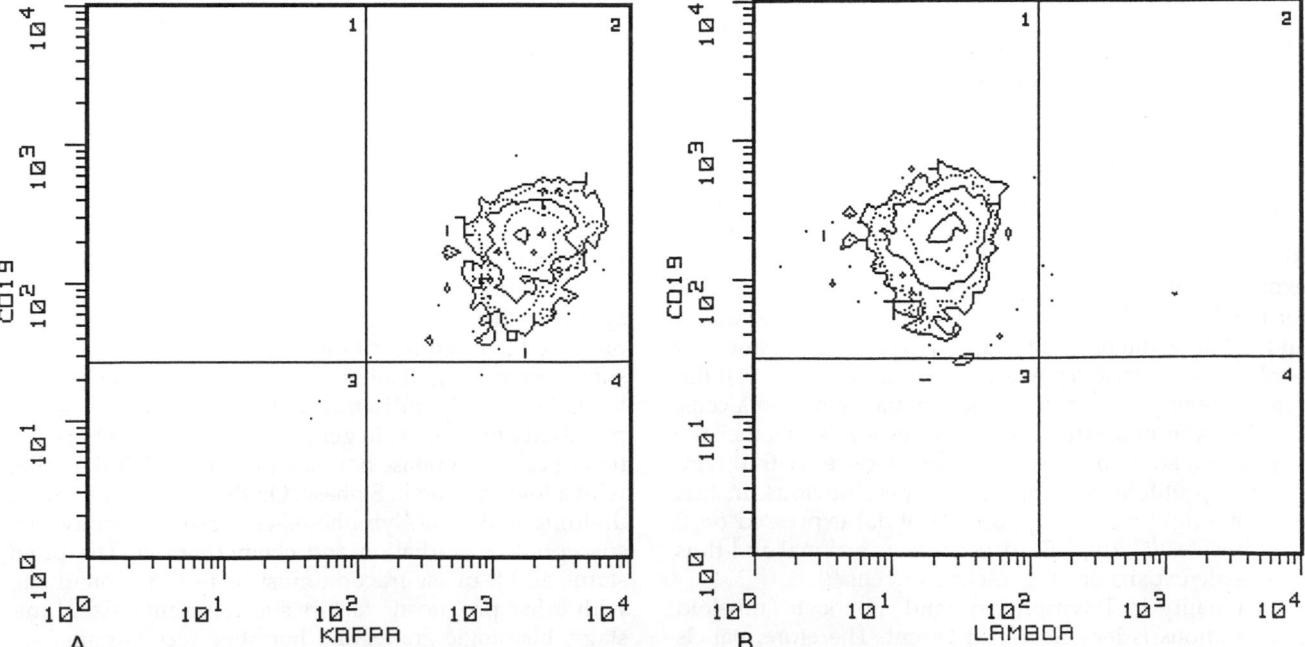

FIGURE 43-5. Dual-color histograms of CD19 *versus* sIg kappa (*A*) and lambda (*B*). The CD19 B lymphocytes are positive for sIg kappa but negative for sIg lambda. This light chain restriction or monoclonality strongly supports a diagnosis of a B-cell neoplasm.

bromide, pyronin Y, thioflavin T, and thiazole orange) have been used with flow cytometry to count reticulocytes because they stain RNA. Thiazole orange appears to be the dye of choice because it (1) binds to RNA, but does not precipitate it; (2) gives a high quantum yield with high resolution between reticulocytes and background RBCs; (3) is stable; (4) excites at 488 nm (argon); and (5) correlates well with microscope counts and is simple to use. However, thiazole orange also (1) binds to DNA; (2) stains some WBCs and giant platelets; (3) does not distinguish Howell-Jolly bodies; and (4) may bind to cytometer tubing with subsequent leaching into other samples. Flow cytometry reticulocyte counts have the additional advantages of speed, sample size (thousands *vs* hundreds of cells counted), and uniformity of cell distribution.

Another important advantage is that flow cytometry can distinguish between early and late reticulocytes. *Early* reticulocytes, generally released during a hemolytic episode, contain more RNA and thus show greater staining intensity than "common" or late reticulocytes (Fig. 43-6). This fluorescence intensity difference allows for calculation of the **reticulocyte maturation index** (RMI) or the immature reticulocyte fraction (IRF). The IRF has proved clinically useful not only in hemolytic anemia but also following bone marrow transplantation and chemotherapy as an early indicator of recovering hematopoiesis.[6,7]

PLATELETS

The detection of anti-platelet antibodies by flow cytometry is proving to be reliable in the different types of thrombocytopenia, such as idiopathic thrombocytopenic purpura (ITP), thrombotic thrombocytopenic purpura (TTP), transfusion allosensitization, and drug-induced thrombocytopenia (Chap. 57). Circulating and platelet-bound antibodies can quickly be detected and the type of antibody simultaneously determined.

For detection of circulating anti-platelet antibodies (indirect), patient's serum is reacted with platelets from a healthy donor. Anti-platelet antibody is bound to the normal platelets and detected with FITC-labeled anti-human immunoglobin (IgG, A or M). Platelet-bound antibodies (direct) are detected by FITC conjugated anti-human Ig. In both instances the presence of the antibodies is measured with a flow cytometer and compared to a negative platelet control.

Although not widely used clinically, other features of platelets can be measured by flow cytometry, such as platelet activation and platelet phenotyping. Platelet membrane glycoproteins (GP) I, II, and III are present on normal platelets. Decreases in GPIb and GPIIIa have been reported in diseases such as acute leukemia, Glanzmann's thrombasthenia, and the Bernard-Soulier syndrome (Chap. 57).[1]

TERMINAL DEOXYNUCLEOTIDYL TRANSFERASE (TdT)

The nuclear enzyme TdT is used as an ancillary diagnostic indicator in certain types of leukemia, such as acute lymphocytic leukemia (ALL), both T and pre-B, T lymphoblastic lymphoma, and small numbers of cases of acute and chronic myeloid leukemia (AML and CML) in blast crisis. Although not very useful in distinguishing the types of poorly differentiated leukemias, it is used by some in monitoring therapy and detecting small numbers of leukemic cells in early relapse.

Measuring TdT enzyme activity is impractical for a variety of reasons. However, the use of anti-TdT antibodies and flow cytometry has made the assay quite practical for use in the clinical laboratory. Because TdT is intranuclear, cells must be fixed and made permeable to allow entry of the anti-TdT antibody into the cell and its nucleus. A variety of techniques have been used, but those which use two-color staining and allow the simultaneous detection of TdT and a surface antigen that identifies the leukemic cell type appear to be most useful (Fig. 43-7).[8,13]

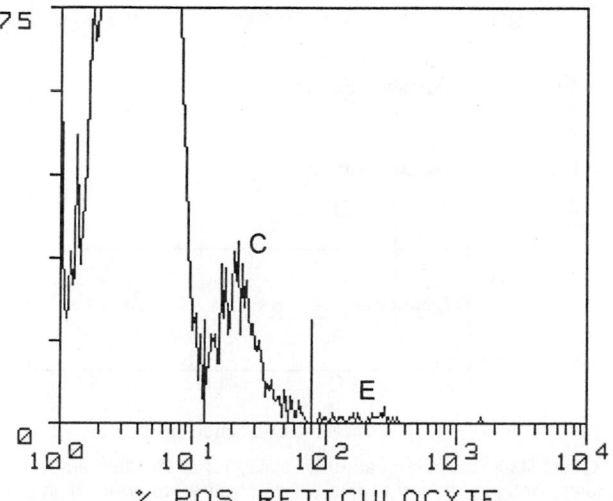

FIGURE 43-6. Single-color display of reticulocyte histogram. Peak C represents the late or common reticulocytes; peak E, the early reticulocytes which contain more RNA. The difference is used to calculate the reticulocyte maturation index (RMI).

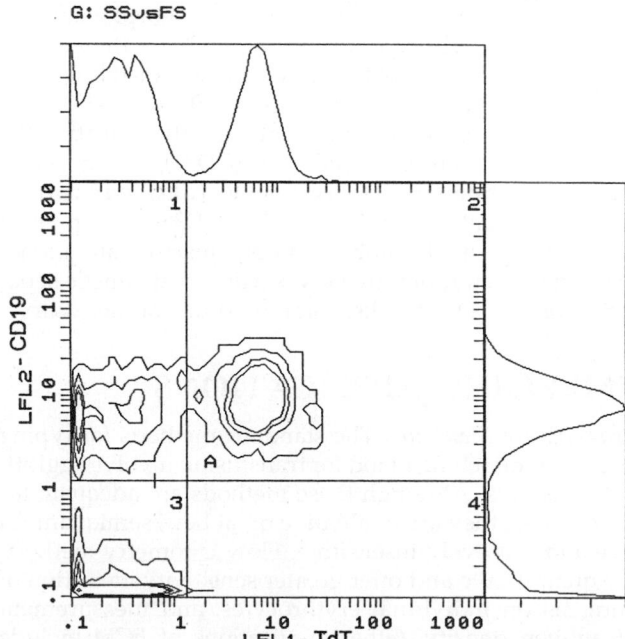

FIGURE 43-7. Two-color histogram of CD19 (FITC) *versus* TdT (PE). Quadrant 2 contains the double-labeled pre-B ALL cells which are TdT positive.

Transplantation

Flow cytometry has been used in a variety of ways in organ transplantation in pre- and post-transplant evaluation.[23] Traditionally, human leukocyte antigen (HLA) tissue typing and cross-matching has been performed by the microlymphocytotoxicity assay. This is complex, time-consuming, and somewhat subjective. Although HLA typing can be performed by FCM, the FCM cross-match is the most commonly used clinically.

In contrast to the standard microcytotoxicity assay, FCM is rapid, objective, and highly sensitive. An additional advantage is that it can determine, in the same assay, the class of the potential organ recipient's preexisting antibodies and whether they are directed against donor T or B lymphocytes, platelets, other leukocytes, endothelial cells, or other cell types. Recipient serum is incubated with donor cells, followed by the addition of FITC-labeled anti-human IgG and flow cytometry. If the donor cells are lymphocytes, fluorochrome-labeled anti-T and anti-B monoclonal antibodies can be added to determine whether the recipient's antibody(ies) is/are directed at T or B lymphocytes or both.

The FCM cross-match will detect low-titer, non-complement fixing, noncytotoxic antibodies, which are not detected by the standard cytoxicity assays, as well as anti–B cell and non-HLA antibodies. However, the clinical importance of these noncytotoxic antibodies has not been fully determined. Other current and potential uses of FCM in the transplantation field include the cell-mediated immune assay (mixed lymphocyte culture); post-transplant monitoring for anti-donor antibodies and antibodies to the OKT3 immunosuppressive agent; phenotyping of lymphocytes infiltrating grafts; and lymphocyte subset analysis.

Flow cytometry offers a rapid method for quantitating stem cells prior to bone marrow transplantation.[25] Cells which are CD34+ but CD38− possess many of the features of stem cells in that they are morphologically primitive, capable of self-renewal, and committed to a number of hemopoietic lineages, as determined by *in vitro* colony formation.[26] Cells which are CD34+/CD38+ are committed, expressing other antigens that identify the lineage, for example, erythroid (CD71), B lymphoid (CD10), T lymphoid (CD7), or myeloid (CD33). The primitive pluripotent stem cells (CD34+/CD38−) are present in extremely small numbers in bone marrow and blood, making concentration by FCM sorting or magnetic separation of all CD34+ cells, committed or not, necessary.

EMERGING APPLICATIONS

Transfusion Medicine. The standard methods for typing and cross-matching blood for transfusion involve agglutination assays. Although these methods are adequate for routine use, they are qualitative or, at best, semiquantitative and relatively insensitive. Flow cytometry methods are quantitative and offer greater sensitivity, detection of antigens on individual erythrocytes, and measurement of antigen density. Other applications of FCM include confirmation of parentage; family and population genetic studies; zygosity[21]; and quantitation, sorting, and pheno-

typing of small numbers of fetal erythrocytes in maternal blood. The latter provides a safer method for prenatal diagnosis (*e.g.*, sex determination, karyotyping, and detection of abnormal hemoglobin and cellular enzyme deficiencies) by avoiding the risks of amniocentesis.[3]

Enzyme Analysis. Standard measures of cellular enzyme activity involve multicellular assays using colorimetric techniques. Utilization of enzyme substrates, which are acted upon by a specific cellular enzyme with the resulting appearance or disappearance of fluorescence or a change in the emission wavelength, provides a means by which enzyme activity can be measured in individual cells by FMC.[22] These cells can also be simultaneously immunophenotyped.

Antigen–Antibody Detection. Recently, a method called *immunobead technology* using FCM and beads coated with antigens or antibodies to detect a specific antibody or antigen in serum has been used in clinical FCM laboratories.[16] Serum antibody that has bound to antigen-coated beads is detected by fluorochrome-labeled anti-human immunoglobulin. Because flow cytometers can detect and display particle size differences as well as fluorescence, several different antibodies or antigens can be detected in serum simultaneously (Fig. 43-8).[14] This same technology can be used for *in situ* hybridization.

Molecular Biology. Because the flow cytometer is a particle counter and measures fluorescence, any probe which fluoresces can be detected. This capacity has resulted in flow karyotypic analysis (Chap. 5) and chromosome sorting, as well as fluorescence *in situ* hybridization (FISH) and polymerase chain reaction (PCR) (Chap. 31).

Although this methodology is currently used primar-

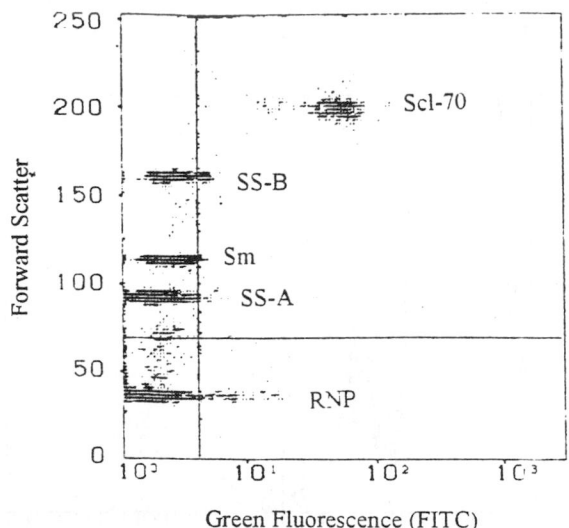

FIGURE 43-8. Immunobead–flow assay for antinuclear autoantibodies. Antigens bound to five beads of different sizes, all in one tube, have been exposed to serum from a patient with autoantibodies to Scl-70. The beads that bind these antibodies fluoresce when anti-human Ig-FITC is added. In this example the test is strongly positive for Scl-70, negative for the others.

ily in research, there is great interest in its clinical potential (*e.g.*, oncogene and virus detection) because of its great sensitivity, particularly when used in conjunction with PCR.[24]

CURRENT USE

In the past few years the number of reported clinical applications of flow cytometry has greatly increased, but their exploitation in the clinical laboratory has been slow. In part this reflects the fact that new flow cytometers, cytometer software, and computers, fluorochromes, monoclonal antibodies, molecular probes, and ideas for applications have far exceeded the capacity of clinical laboratories to utilize them in a time of budget constraints. Much of this has to do with the expense of research and development, the slowness with which these applications are accepted by the clinical community, the rate of approval by regulatory agencies and third-party insurance carriers, and the need for curtailing health care costs. The clinical utility of new applications may be obvious and published pilot studies indicate practicality and even cost savings, but the collection of enough clinical validating data for each new application to convince the above communities is slow.

CHAPTER SUMMARY

Clinical flow cytometry is a rapidly developing field. Advances in instruments, fluorochromes, antibodies and other probes, computer hardware and software, and the appearance of new applications make it difficult for clinical flow cytometry laboratories to keep abreast with the "state of the art." This is compounded by the increasing activities of regulatory and accreditation agencies involved in the field. It is a time of maximum growth but diminishing financial resources for most laboratories. Nevertheless, flow cytometry has proved to be an important clinical laboratory technology with a broad range of applications of diagnostic, prognostic, and monitoring value.

Case Study 43-1

A reticulocyte count was ordered on a patient with sickle cell anemia and poor splenic function. A review of the patient's blood film revealed the presence of numerous Howell-Jolly bodies. A manual reticulocyte count was reported as 3.2%, whereas the percentage of reticulocytes by flow cytometry using thiazole orange was 5.0%.
1. What is a possible cause for the discrepancy between the manual and FCM reticulocyte counts?
2. In the majority of cases, a reticulocyte count performed by flow cytometry is statistically superior to manual methods. Explain why this is the case.
3. On what is an IRF (immature reticulocyte fraction) based?

Case Study 43-2

A patient sample was submitted to the laboratory for quantitation of CD4+ T lymphocytes.
1. What disorder is usually monitored by this test?
2. What is a significant problem in evaluating CD4+ counts generated by many flow cytometers?
3. What safety precautions should be taken?

Review Questions

43-1. In order to direct scattered light to various photodetectors, the flow cytometer uses interference filters that are usually of the _____ type.

   A. long bandpass
   B. short bandpass
   C. monochromatic
   D. polychromatic

43-2. Cell sorting requires a _____ type of flow cell.

   A. closed system
   B. quartz
   C. stream-in-air
   D. sheath stream

43-3. One advantage of flow cytometric immunophenotyping is the ability to

   A. identify several cell markers on the same cell.
   B. evaluate fixed cells.
   C. select cell types based on morphology.
   D. generate a result in 3 to 5 days.

43-4. The purpose of analyzing the DNA cell cycle is to

   A. detect cells in proliferation.
   B. assess the ploidy of tumor cells.
   C. indicate prognosis.
   D. all of the above.

43-5. Flow cytometry is useful in bone marrow transplantation because of its ability to quantitate small numbers of

   A. granulocyte precursors.
   B. pluripotential stem cells.
   C. erythroid precursors.
   D. CD10-positive cells.

43-6. The major similarity between the available clinical flow cytometers on the market is the fact that most utilize

   A. single laser (argon) light sources.
   B. cell sorters.
   C. mercury arc lamps.
   D. cell counting devices.

References

1. Adelman B, Michelson AD, Handin RI et al: Evaluation of platelet glycoprotein Ib by fluorescence flow cytometry. Blood 66:423, 1985
2. Braylan RC, Benson NA, Iturraspe I: Analysis of lymphomas by flow cytometry: Current and emerging strategies. Ann NY Acad Sci 677:364, 1993
3. Chueh J, Golbus MS: Prenatal diagnosis using fetal cells in the maternal circulation. Semin Perinatal 14:471, 1990
4. Coulter WH: High speed automated blood cell counter and cell size analyzer. Proc Natl Electron Conf 12:1034, 1956
5. Crossland-Taylor PG: A device for counting small particles suspended in a fluid through a tube. Nature 171:37, 1953
6. Davis BH, Bigelow NC: Clinical flow cytometric reticulocyte analysis. Pathobiology 58:99, 1990
7. Davis BH, Bigelow HC: Clinical flow cytometric reticulocyte analysis. In Coon JS, Weinstein RS (eds): Diagnostic Flow Cytometry, pp 103–114. Baltimore, Williams and Wilkins, 1991
8. Drach J, Ettringer C, Hubs H: Combined flow cytometric assessment of cell surface antigens and nuclear TdT for the detection of minimal residual disease in acute leukemia. Br J Haematol 77:37, 1991

9. Duque RE: Flow cytometric analysis of lymphomas and acute leukemias. Ann NY Acad Sci 677:309, 1993

10. Duque RE: Interactive data analysis for evaluation of B-cell neoplasia by flow cytometry. Methods Cell Biol 42:231, 1994

11. Fulwyler MJ: Electronic separation of biological cells by volume. Science 150:910, 1965

12. Hassett J, Parker JW: Laboratory practices in the reporting of flow cytometry results for leukemia and lymphoma specimens: Results of a survey. Cytometry 22(4):264, 1995

13. Hechinger MK, Hernandez AM, Barr NJ et al: A clinical laboratory approach to the evaluation of terminal deoxynucleotidyl transferase (TdT) by flow cytometry (FCM). J Clin Lab Anal 8:211, 1994

14. Hechinger MK, Parker JW, Clark K: Immunobead/flow cytometry detection of antinuclear antibodies. Cytometry (abstr) 26(1):302, 1996

15. Hedley DW, Shankey TV, Wheeless LL: DNA cytometry consensus conference. Special report. Cytometry 14:471, 1993

16. Horan PK, Sehenle EA, Abraham GN et al: Fluid phase particle fluorescence analysis: Rheumatoid factor specifically evaluated by laser flow cytophotometry. In Nakamura RM, Dito WR, Tucker EA (eds): Immunoassay in the Clinical Laboratory, pp 185–198. New York, Alan R Liss, 1979

17. Kamentsky LA, Melamed MR, Derman H: Spectrophotometer: New instrument for ultra rapid cell analysis. Science 150:630, 1965

18. Koepke JF, Koepke JA: Reticulocytes. Clin Lab Haematol 8:169, 1986

19. Kramer E, Grossmüller F: Light scatter based lymphocyte gate—Helpful tool or source of error? Cytometry 15(1):87, 1994

20. Liu Z, Hultin LE, Cumberland WG et al: Elevated levels of CD38+, CD8+ T cells in HIV infection add to the prognostic value of low CD4+ T cell levels: results of 6 years of follow-up. The Los Angeles Center, Multicenter AIDS Cohort Study. J Acquir Immune Defic Syndr 6(8):904, 1993

21. Oien L, Nance S, Arndt P et al: Determination of zygosity using flow cytometric analysis of red cell antigen strength. Transfusion 28:541, 1988

22. Rice GC, Bump EA, Shrieve DC et al: Quantitative analysis of cellular glutathione by flow cytometry utilizing monochlorobimane: Some applications to radiation and drug resistance *in vitro* and *in vivo*. Cancer Res 46:6105, 1986

23. Riley RS, Thomas JM, Ross W: Applications of flow cytometry in organ transplantation. In Riley RS, Makin EJ, Ross W (eds): Clinical Applications of Flow Cytometry, pp 635–703. New York-Tokyo, Igaku-Shoin, 1993

24. Riley RS, Ross W: Applications of flow cytometry in genetics and molecular biology. In Riley RS, Makin EJ, Ross W (eds): Clinical Applications of Flow Cytometry, pp 705–752. New York-Tokyo, Igaku-Shoin, 1993

25. Siena S, Bregni M, Brando B et al: Flow cytometry for clinical estimation of circulating hematopoietic progenitors for autologous transplantation in cancer patients. Blood 77:400, 1991

26. Terstappen L, Huang S, Safford M et al: Sequential generations of hematopoietic colonies derived from single nonlineage-committed CD34+ CD38− progenitor cells. Blood 77:1218, 1991

27. Terstappen LW, Safford M, Unterhalt M et al: Flow cytometric characterization of acute myeloid leukemias: IV. Comparison to the differentiation pathway of normal hematopoietic progenitor cells. Leukemia 6(10):993, 1992

Suggested Reading

Keren DF, Hanson CA, Hurtubise PE (eds): Flow Cytometry and Clinical Diagnosis. Chicago, ASCP Press, 1994

Riley RS, Makin EJ, Ross W (eds): Clinical Applications of Flow Cytometry. New York-Tokyo, Igaku-Shoin, 1993

Shapiro HM: Practical Flow Cytometry. New York, Wiley-Liss, 1995

PART X

Quality Control and Quality Assurance

CHAPTER 44

Introduction to Quality Control and Quality Assurance in Hematology

John A. Koepke

Objectives

1. Define quality control (QC), quality assurance (QA), total quality management (TQM), and continuous quality improvement (CQI).
2. List and briefly describe several factors upon which the feasibility and analytic reliability of a method or instrument are based.
3. Define precision and accuracy and briefly explain how they are monitored in the hematology laboratory.
4. Define random and systematic error, primary and secondary standard, calibration, and control.
5. Define and calculate median, mode, mean, range, variance, standard deviation, and coefficient of variation for a data set.
6. Describe the procedure for determining a population reference range and the most common frequency distribution of such a range.

The clinical hematology laboratory is an integral part of contemporary medical practice because its comprehensive analyses of body fluids are used in diagnosis and treatment. As the usefulness of laboratory tests and the reliability of the results have improved, clinicians have become increasingly dependent on these hematologic results in making critical decisions on therapeutic interventions for their patients.[37] This reliance has greatly increased the responsibility of the clinical laboratory to ensure the quality of its analyses.

The methods used to assure reliable test results are collectively referred to as a *quality assurance program*. The term *quality assurance* (QA) encompasses comprehensive concepts, including components of *quality control* (QC), which are primarily quantitative and statistical, and those aspects of laboratory management that impart perceptions of credibility and medically useful results to the clinician. The goal of QC is the reduction of both systematic and random errors to zero. In Japan, this concept is called *zero defect*.[35] Although QC is invaluable in the laboratory setting, it serves only as a foundation for a comprehensive program of assuring high-quality patient care. The Joint Commission on Accreditation of Healthcare Organizations (JCAHO) defines QA as a "well-defined, organized program designed to enhance patient care through the ongoing objective assessment of important aspects of patient care and the correction of identified problems."

Many services within the health care field, including clinical laboratories, are now modifying their operations to incorporate quality concepts and methods developed by industry. Such concepts and methods include total quality management (TQM) and continuous quality improvement (CQI) programs. Such TQM and CQI programs include the need for coordination and cooperation among hospital departments as well as with clinicians, as for example, in the development and monitoring of blood transfusion practices. The hematology laboratory performs blood counts, the coagulation laboratory performs coagulation tests, and then the transfusion service releases appropriate blood products, all following previously agreed upon practice guidelines.

Additionally, TQM programs are being used to set priorities for the laboratory service (*e.g.*, improving outpatient turnaround times). Finally, the CQI programs, after documenting present practices, are being established to develop achievable goals that are then continuously monitored in an effort to document improving laboratory services.

HISTORY OF LABORATORY QUALITY CONTROL

The concept of the quality of workmanship of any kind has always been present, but it was not until the emergence of industries and mass production that the term quality control was used.[14] In the late 1920s and early 1930s, Dodge and Shewhart of the Bell Telephone Company originated a systematic approach to QC that used statistics.[14,36] It was a few decades later, however, that clinical laboratories adopted similar programs for their routine analyses. Before 1950, there were few QC programs established in the clinical laboratory. The first reported survey, by Belk and Sunderman in 1947, revealed enormous disagreement in the results of different clinical chemistry laboratories.[5] This finding triggered a great deal of interest in devising methods for producing high-quality analytical results. In 1950 the idea of analyzing a control serum daily and plotting the results graphically was introduced by Levey and Jennings.[30] In 1953 control sera for use in clinical chemistry laboratories were made available commercially.

Several years passed before any type of commercial control material or QC program was used in the clinical hematology laboratory. A standard cyanmethemoglobin solution certified by the College of American Pathologists (CAP) was available in 1959 for standardization of spectrophotometers used in the measurement of hemoglobin (Hb) concentration.[26] However, control of this test procedure was achieved only by using a normal donor blood or hemolysate specimen for comparison with the patient specimens. Commercial control materials for all hematologic measures were not readily available until the first automated hematology analyzers were introduced in the late 1960s. Furthermore, it was not until 1967 that the hemiglobincyanide (HiCN) standard solution and methodology, described in 1961,[42] was adopted as a reference procedure by the International Committee for Standardization in Haematology (ICSH).[23]

Unfortunately, in contrast to the clinical chemistry laboratory, where the approach to QC is relatively well established and straightforward, many areas of QC in hematology still lack clear-cut standardized approaches, to a great extent because the measurements in hematology involve living cellular components.[12] This fact results in specific problems, such as a lack of stable materials for use as standards or controls.[38] This chapter will deal with several strategies and statistical tools available for use in hematology QA and QC programs. If these tools are diligently applied, reliable test results can be obtained.

METHOD AND INSTRUMENT EVALUATION AND SELECTION

The appropriate choice of instruments and analytic methods is a critical first step in the assurance of accurate and precise laboratory testing.[28] An *analytic method* is defined as "a set of instructions which describe the procedure, materials, and equipment which are necessary for the analyst to obtain a result."[9] A comprehensive QA program should include procedures to be used in the evaluation and selection of analytic instruments and methods. In this manner, a consistent and objective evaluation can be performed, resulting in selection of methods of suitable quality and reliability. The evaluation results show laboratory personnel both the strengths and weaknesses of each method or instrument, and provide standards for comparing alternatives. Information about the performance of an analytic method or instrument should be obtained before purchase or use in the processing of patient specimens. This performance is judged on both the *feasibility* and *analytic reliability* of the method.

Feasibility

Feasibility is evaluated on the basis of speed, cost, technical skill required, dependability, and safety. Table 44-1 outlines several aspects of such studies. *Speed* encompasses both turnaround time (the time needed for analysis of one specimen) and throughput (the number of specimens that can be analyzed per unit of time under routine conditions). The *cost* per assay includes both the cost of all materials, reagents and quality control materials as well as an estimated value for laboratorian time for required maintenance, reagent preparation, calibration, quality control and troubleshooting.

Analytic Reliability

The reliability of a proposed method is judged on the basis of many factors (Table 44-1). The magnitude of analytic variation is one of the factors that reflects reliability, and it requires further explanation. Analytic variation can be divided into two types: random (Chap. 46) and systematic (Chap. 45). Random analytic variation is often referred to as *precision*, whereas systematic analytic variation is often referred to as *accuracy*.

RANDOM ANALYTIC VARIATION—PRECISION

The precision of a method is assessed by performing replicate analyses of a biologic specimen containing stable amounts of a constituent and is expressed as the magnitude of error inherent in the method. The National Com-

mittee for Clinical Laboratory Standards (NCCLS)[31,32] has published protocols for establishing the precision of automated analytic systems in which a distinction is made between the total random analytic variation and the within-run or within-day variation (short-term imprecision). The total variation includes all components that affect method performance, including within-run, run-to-run and day-to-day variation, as well as the stability of materials and calibration factors.

Hackney and Cembrowski[21] have made recommendations for measurement of within-day and day-to-day imprecision. Both measurement types may be performed during the same period. For measurement of within-day imprecision, those authors recommend ten replicate analyses of five to ten samples that represent the various levels of medical interest. The samples should be a mixture of patient and control specimens. Tests of within-day imprecision should be run over a 3- to 5-day period (using different samples) to avoid bias on any given day. For measurement of day-to-day imprecision, those same authors recommend that two or three levels of control material be analyzed three or four times per day, these levels being normal, low abnormal and high abnormal.[21] Because such a study should extend over at least 7 days and, if possible, 20 days using the same material, stabilized control material is used; patient specimens are stable for only 24 hours at best. Hackney and Cembrowski[21] recommend analysis of each control level four times per day for the 7- to 20-day period. CLIA '88, the Clinical Laboratory Improvement Amendment passed by Congress in 1988, requires each control to be run once per shift.

To evaluate the data for imprecision, the mean value of the data for the within-day and day-to-day categories is calculated, and the associated dispersion is calculated as the standard deviation (SD) and coefficient of variation (CV). These values may then be compared with the known SD and CV for the reference or current method. The calcu-

---

TABLE 44-1
Factors To Be Considered in Method and Instrument Evaluation and Selection

FEASIBILITY	Speed	Turnaround time; throughput
	Cost	Materials; technologist time
	Technical skill required	Higher skill levels cost more money
	Dependability	Average frequency and duration of breakdowns
	Safety	Avoidance of biohazards
ANALYTIC RELIABILITY	Sensitivity	Minimum concentration of constituent method is capable of measuring; reliability of test being positive when condition to be detected IS present
	Specificity	Extent to which test measures only single constituent; reliability of test being negative when condition to be detected is NOT present
	Dynamic range	Range of test linearity without specimen dilution
	Freedom from interference	Effects of interfering substances and factors (*e.g.*, hemolysis, lipemia, cold agglutinins, platelet clumps)
	Magnitude of analytic variation	Random variation (precision); systematic variation (accuracy)

lation of mean, SD and CV is reviewed in the following section of this chapter.

SYSTEMATIC ANALYTIC VARIATION—ACCURACY

Systematic analytic variation or analytic bias is the accuracy of a proposed method and is defined as the extent to which measurements approach the "true value" of the constituent being analyzed. The magnitude of analytic bias for any given laboratory procedure may be measured in several ways. These include (1) the use of control specimens assayed by different methods, (2) comparison of the new method with a proven method using both "normal" donor specimens and patient specimens, and (3) the use of recovery experiments.[3,43,44] Recovery experiments are rarely, if ever, used in hematology and so will not be discussed.

In the first approach, commercial calibration materials with a stated value for the constituent in question are obtained.[18] The calibration specimens should cover a broad range of values and must be compatible with the manual or automated methods in use. With linear regression analysis (see discussion later in this chapter), the relation between the observed values and the stated values may be assessed for all methods and the magnitude of any bias determined.[34] Both constant (*y* intercept) and proportional (slope of the regression line) biases can be detected by this method (see Fig. 44-9).

When using the technique of comparison with a proven method, a number of specimens are assayed using the new method and a comparison method. About 40 patient specimens spanning the entire analytic range are assayed by the two methods. If the study is to be published in a medical journal, at least 100 specimens should be analyzed to ensure adequate data.[21] The selection of the comparison method is important.

Selection of Instrumentation and Reagents

An integral part of method evaluation is the use of high-quality materials. These include everything from expendables used for specimen collection, processing, storage, and preservation, to reagents and standards, to miscellaneous equipment, such as centrifuges and thermometers, to the instruments themselves.

The selection of reagents and instrumentation should be made based on the unique requirements of the individual laboratory, as well as the general performance characteristics of the product. In the case of reagents and controls, these general characteristics are included in the manufacturer's data sheet. If an in-house evaluation is not possible, it is best to base the decision on results obtained at a reliable institution.

The results from a widely used comprehensive proficiency survey (*e.g.*, the CAP surveys)[11] may also be helpful. But remember, surveys use stabilized specimens, which may introduce other problems. Selection of analytic instrumentation is particularly important and usually is based on several factors, including those listed in Table 44-1, and manufacturer support and reputation. Certain

intangible factors relating to how the proposed system fits with existing space, personnel, preferences and equipment (*e.g.*, laboratory information systems) cannot be ignored.

CONCEPTS AND STATISTICAL METHODS USED IN QUALITY CONTROL

Variations and Errors in Laboratory Measurements

Every measurement performed in the hematology laboratory contains an inherent variability. These variations result in two types of errors—*random* and *systematic* (Fig. 44-1). Random (indeterminate) errors affect precision, because repeated measurements increase the scatter of values about the true value. Random errors are the result of chance and sampling errors; they generally do not affect an entire batch of specimens and, therefore, cannot be detected by testing control specimens.

In contrast, systematic or determinate errors (sometimes referred to as bias) affect accuracy and all determi-

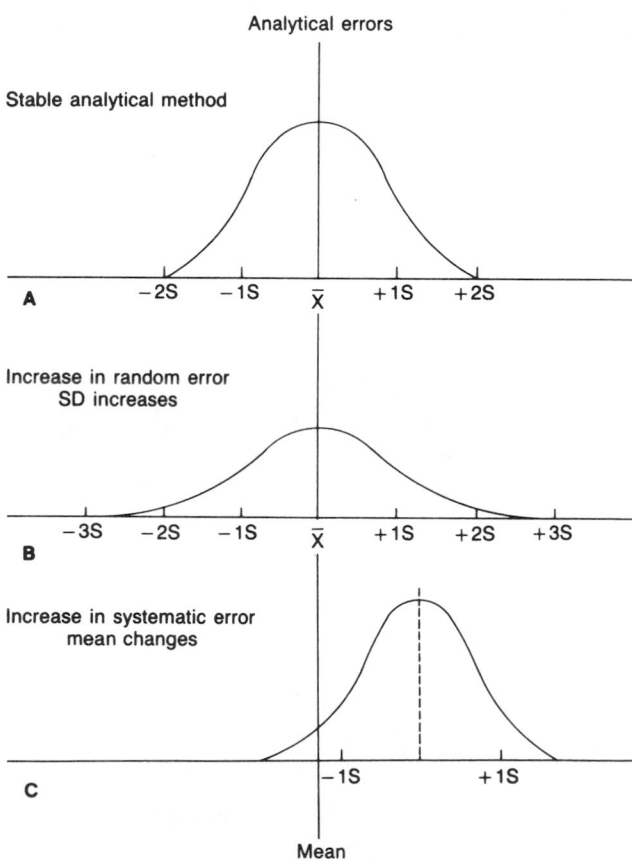

FIGURE 44-1. Schematic representation of distributions of control data: **(A)** Situation with no analytic error; **(B)** increased random error, which causes increased standard deviation (s or SD); **(C)** systematic error causing shift in mean ($\bar{x}$). (From Cembrowski GS, Sullivan AM: Quality control and statistics. In Bishop ML, Duben-Engelkirk JL, Fody EP, eds: Clinical Chemistry—Principles, Procedures, Correlations, 3rd ed, p 82. Philadelphia, JB Lippincott, 1996, with permission.)

nations in a batch equally. They can usually be detected by testing control specimens. Systematic errors are attributable to causes other than chance, such as deteriorating reagents or an instrument that has lost calibration. Random errors (Chap. 46) introduce increased *variability* into an analysis, whereas systematic errors (Chap. 45) introduce a *bias*. Both types of analytical errors and the methods used to control them are discussed in detail in Chapters 45 and 46.

Assessments of the Quality of Laboratory Measurements— Precision and Accuracy

Two terms used in conjunction with laboratory measurements to define the quality of the analyses are *precision* and *accuracy*. The precision of a test is its reproducibility or the variation among duplicate or replicate measurements of the same analyte; for example, the consistency of a cell count between the first and second measurement or on two different days. The statistical means by which the precision of a quantitative analysis is expressed is described later in this chapter under Frequency Distributions and Associated Statistical Terms. Accuracy, on the other hand, refers to the closeness with which measured values agree with the true values. Accuracy has been defined by the ICSH as "agreement between the best estimate of a quantity and its true value."[40]

Precision is possible without accuracy. The difference between the two is graphically represented in Figure 44-2, in which ten gunshots are shown on each of three targets. Just like the performance of the hypothetical marksman shooting at the targets in Figure 44-2, the quality of an analysis can be described in one of three ways: (1) neither accurate nor precise; (2) precise but lacking accuracy; or (3) both accurate and precise.

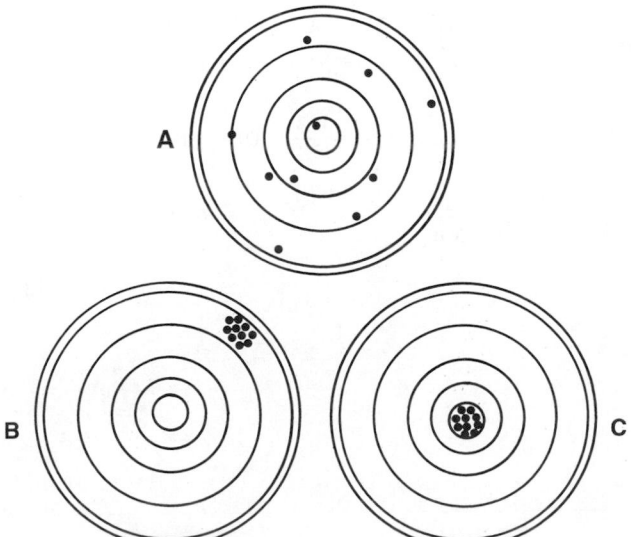

FIGURE 44-2. Accuracy versus precision: Bullseye represents accurate shot. **(A)** Shots are neither accurate nor precise; **(B)** shots are precise (all clustered in one area), but not accurate; **(C)** shots are both precise and accurate.

Initial Establishment of Accuracy in Hematology by Calibration

Establishment of the accuracy or true value of an analysis begins with calibration of the method using a standard or calibrator.[34] Ideally, a stable material of precise concentration and purity of the analyte to be measured is used to prepare a *primary standard* for use in the calibration procedure. For example, in the chemistry laboratory, a sample of chemically pure glucose may be carefully weighed and dissolved in chemically pure water to make a primary glucose standard.

The International Haemoglobin Standards are the *only* primary standards used in hematology, having been designated by the World Health Organization (WHO) as primary hemoglobin reference materials.[41] However, these preparations are only available to approved national groups for the assignment of hemoglobin values to preparations which are used, in turn, for the assignment of hemoglobin values to whole blood calibrators using the hemiglobincyanide reference method. These whole-blood preparations thus become *secondary standards*. A reference method is defined as one that is specific for the analyte and that quantitates the true concentration of the analyte. It may require instrumentation not available in many laboratories. The International Federation of Clinical Chemistry defines a *reference method* as one which, after exhaustive investigation, has been found to have negligible inaccuracy in comparison with its degree of random analytical variation.[39]

The only reference method in hematology that has been formally accepted nationally and internationally is the photometric measurement of hemiglobincyanide for determination of Hb concentration in human blood.[24] This method is calibrated using a hemiglobincyanide secondary standard, as discussed in the foregoing. Reference methods for other hematologic measures[6,17,18,25,27] are discussed in Chapter 45.

Use of Controls for Monitoring Precision and Accuracy

Once accuracy has been established for a particular method, precision and accuracy are monitored with stabilized control materials. The ICSH definition states that a *control material* is "a substance used in routine practice for checking the concurrent performance of an analytical process or instrument. [Controls] must be similar in properties to, and be analyzed along with, patient specimens."[40] Commercial control products, patient specimens, or both can be used in many ways for this purpose,[6] as discussed later in this chapter under Establishment of Control Procedures and also in more detail in Chapters 45 and 46.

Measures of Frequency Distributions and Associated Statistical Terms[2]

When a number of analytical values or observations are plotted against the frequency of their occurrence, a distribution curve is obtained. A common distribution curve

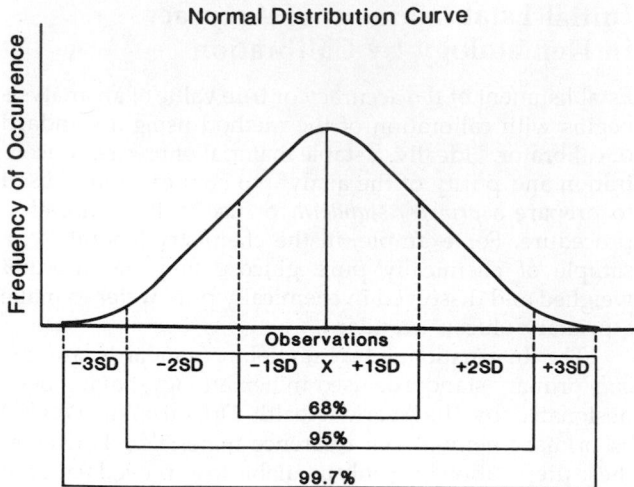

FIGURE 44-3. Normal curve, known as a Gaussian distribution; it is characteristically symmetric about the center and bell-shaped.

is a normal, or Gaussian, distribution, which is symmetric about the center and bell-shaped (Fig. 44-3). The distribution can be described in terms of where its center (mean) value is, how dispersed it is, how symmetric or skewed it is and how broad it is. Precision is measured by data dispersion, whereas bias (accuracy) is measured by the agreement of the mean value with the true value.

Median, mode and mean are the three measures generally used to indicate the midpoint of a distribution (Table 44-2).

Median. The median is simply the middle value of a set of numbers arranged according to size; therefore, 50% of the observations lie below the median and 50% above it. When the number of observations is even, the median is the average of the two values closest to the middle.

Mode. The mode is the value occurring most frequently. When a distribution has two values with the same fre-

TABLE 44-2
Calculation of Various Values From a Hypothetical Reference Range Study of Hemoglobin Values

Value	$(x - \bar{x})$*	$(x - \bar{x})^2$		
14.5	−0.9	0.81		
14.5	−0.9	0.81		
14.6	−0.8	0.64		
14.6	−0.8	0.64		
14.7	−0.7	0.49		
14.8	−0.6	0.36		
14.8	−0.6	0.36		
14.8	−0.6	0.36		
14.9	−0.5	0.25		
15.0	−0.4	0.16		
15.2	−0.2	0.04		
15.3	−0.1	0.01	VARIANCE (s^2)	$\dfrac{\Sigma(x - \bar{x})^2}{n - 1} = \dfrac{11.58}{(30 - 1)} = 0.4$
15.3	−0.1	0.01		
15.4	0.0	0.00	STANDARD DEVIATION (s)	$\sqrt{\dfrac{\Sigma(x - \bar{x})^2}{n - 1}} = \sqrt{0.4} = 0.63$
15.5	0.1	0.01		
15.5	0.1	0.01		
15.5	0.1	0.01	COEFFICIENT OF VARIATION (CV)	$\dfrac{s}{\bar{x}} \times 100\% = \dfrac{0.63}{15.4} \times 100 = 4.1\%$
15.6	0.2	0.04		
15.6	0.2	0.04	STANDARD ERROR OF THE MEAN (SEM)	$\dfrac{s}{\sqrt{n}} = \dfrac{0.63}{\sqrt{30}} = 0.12$
15.6	0.2	0.04		
15.6	0.2	0.04		
15.9	0.5	0.25		
16.1	0.7	0.49		
16.2	0.8	0.64		
16.2	0.8	0.64		
16.3	0.9	0.81		
16.3	0.9	0.81		
16.3	0.9	0.81		
16.4	1.0	1.00		
16.4	1.0	1.00		
Σ (sum) = 463.4		Σ = 11.58		

* Mean $(\bar{x}) = \dfrac{\Sigma x}{n} = \dfrac{463.4}{30} = 15.4$; median (middle value) = 15.5; mode (most common value) = 15.6; range 14.5–16.4

quency, indicating two populations, the distribution is termed bimodal.

Mean. The arithmetic mean ($\bar{x}$) is the average value of a group of observations. It equals the sum (Σ) of all the values (Σx), divided by the number of observations (n), as shown in Table 44-2. The mean is the most reliable measure of the center of a distribution and uses all of the information in the data set, but it is markedly affected by extreme values. In contrast, the median is not affected by extreme values. In a normally distributed set of data, the mean (average value), the median (central value), and the mode (most frequent value) are identical.

SKEWNESS

When the values are not distributed evenly about the mean, the lack of symmetry is known as skewness (Fig. 44-4). Frequency distributions that are not symmetric extend farther in one direction than in the other. A distribution with extreme values on the high side is skewed to the right and is said to have positive skewness. It has a mean larger than the median and a median greater than the mode. A distribution with extreme values on the low side is skewed to the left and said to have negative skewness. It has a mean smaller than the median and a median smaller than the mode.

Measures of Data Variation

Just as there are three measures of the middle of a distribution, there are three measures of variation or dispersion of a distribution: range, variance (s^2) and standard deviation (SD). Measures of variation are used to indicate the spread of the curve.

Range. The range is the difference between the largest and the smallest values in a data group (Table 44-2). This is a simple but weak measure, because it fails to give any consideration to the array of values between the two extremes and is greatly influenced by extremely large or small values.

Variance. The variance (s^2), another measure of variability, is computed as the sum of the squared deviation of each observation (x) from the mean ($\bar{x}$) divided by the number of observations (n) minus 1 (n − 1). Table 44-2 provides an example of the calculation of variance. The deviations of each observation from the mean are squared

before summation to resolve the possible problem of cancellation by an equal number of positive and negative deviations which could result in a meaningless value.[16]

Standard Deviation. Although the variance is an accurate measure of dispersion, it is still the square of the deviations. The square root of the variance is called the standard deviation (SD, s or σ). The formula, shown in Table 44-2, is used to calculate the SD when replicate determinations are performed on the same sample and, in some cases, for determining the population reference range. As with the formula for variance, the denominator can be represented by either n or n − 1, depending on the number of observations. If fewer than 30 replicates are tested, the n − 1 denominator is used.

Standard Deviation in Duplicate Sample Testing. When one or more samples in a batch are tested in duplicate, a second equation is used to calculate s. The summation of the square of the differences between the duplicate analyses (Σd^2) is divided by the number of analyses, and the square root of this number is determined. The following formula is used, where n − 1 is the number of samples minus 1, 2n − 1 represents the actual number of analyses minus 1, and Σd^2 is the summation of the difference between duplicate measurements of each sample[12]:

$$s = \sqrt{\frac{\Sigma d^2}{2n - 1}}$$

For example, five samples were run in duplicate in testing the prothrombin time, with the following results:

Test 1	Test 2	d	d^2	2n − 1
11.5	11.4	0.1	0.01	2(5) − 1 = 9
11.6	11.7	−0.1	0.01	
11.4	11.6	−0.2	0.04	
11.2	11.3	−0.1	0.01	
11.5	11.2	0.3	0.09	
			$\overline{0.16}$ = Σd^2	

For this example:

$$s = \sqrt{\frac{0.16}{9}} = 0.13$$

In the clinical hematology laboratory, the standard deviation is an extremely helpful measure, and it is used more extensively than the variance. When the standard deviation is used together with the mean, the shape of the normal distribution curve is completely defined. When the normal curve is drawn on the standard deviation scale in positive and negative directions from the mean (Fig. 44-3), 68.27% of the values fall within the area under the curve that is enclosed by lines 1 SD from the mean, 95.45% of the values fall within the area that is 2 SD from the mean, and 99.73% of the values fall within the area 3 SD from the mean. This principle is embodied in a large portion of all QC programs in the clinical laboratory. Analytical values outside 3 SD are ordinarily statistically unacceptable; they should be within 3 SD when the analysis is properly performed and in control.

Skewness Curves

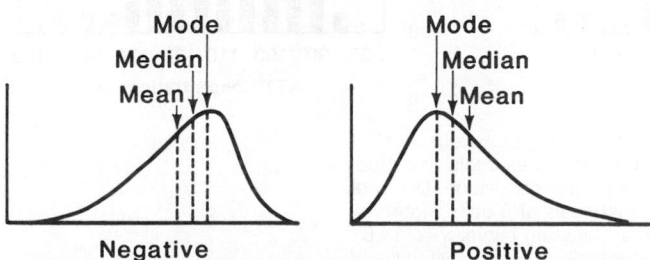

FIGURE 44-4. Distribution curves with extreme values on the low side have negative skew (*left*). Curves with extreme values on the high side have positive skew (*right*).

COEFFICIENT OF VARIATION

The coefficient of variation (CV) is calculated as the SD (s) divided by the mean ($\bar{x}$) and is expressed as a percentage (see Table 44-2 for the formula). The CV gives a more understandable picture of the deviation than SD regardless of the nature of the measurement or method or the units used for reporting a measurement.

In contrast to CV, SD is expressed in the same units of measurement as the value being analyzed. It can be expected to increase as the concentration of the analyte increases. It is, therefore, impossible to compare the variation between methods that use different units for reporting results. It is likewise impossible to compare the variation between methods if specimens of different concentration are used to evaluate the methods. For example, an SD of $5.0 \times 10^9/L$ does not give any idea of the quality of the measurement unless one knows the mean cell count for the measurements from which the SD was derived. If the mean were $7.0 \times 10^9/L$, an SD of $5.0 \times 10^9/L$ would indicate poor precision for the method evaluated, whereas if the mean were $300 \times 10^9/L$, the SD of $5.0 \times 10^9/L$ would be excellent. This dilemma is solved by expressing the SD as a fraction of the mean; that is, by converting the SD into CV which is expressed in percentage form.

STANDARD ERROR OF THE MEAN

Commonly, the standard deviation of a sampling distribution of a statistic is referred to as the standard error of that statistic. When a sample of a population is taken to make an inference about that population, the standard error of the sample mean is referred to as the standard error of the mean (SEM) and is calculated as shown in Table 44-2. Note that as the standard deviation (s) decreases and the number of observations in the sample (n) increases, the SEM decreases. The lower the SEM, the less a sample mean varies owing to chance. Thus, it is advisable to have as large a sample as possible in any statistical study of this nature.

With a sample size of at least 30, the SEM may be used to calculate the 95% confidence limits (approximately ±2 SD of the mean) commonly used for determining reference ranges. This range is calculated as:

$$\bar{x} \pm \frac{2s}{\sqrt{n}}$$

For the study in Table 44-2, the 95% confidence limits based on the SEM would be 15.2 to 15.6 g/dL according to the following calculations:

$$15.4 - \frac{2(0.63)}{\sqrt{30}} = 15.2 \text{ and } 15.4 + \frac{2(0.63)}{\sqrt{30}} = 15.6$$

The 95% confidence limits predict a range of values within which the true population mean will fall 95% of the time.

Determining Population Reference Ranges[33]

The purpose of most statistical studies is to make accurate and unbiased generalizations about measurements on the basis of samples taken from certain populations. A population is the whole group about which specific information is required, whereas the sample is any portion of the fully defined population. Most of the time, a sample is the only means by which inferences about the population as a whole can be made.[19]

In hematology and hemostasis testing, the most important application in selecting a population sample is in the determination of reference ranges, which is required in all laboratories to establish what is "normal" for

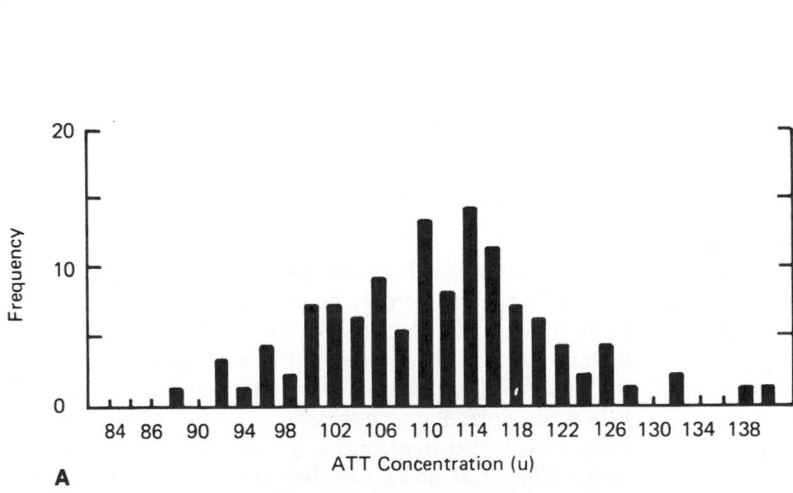

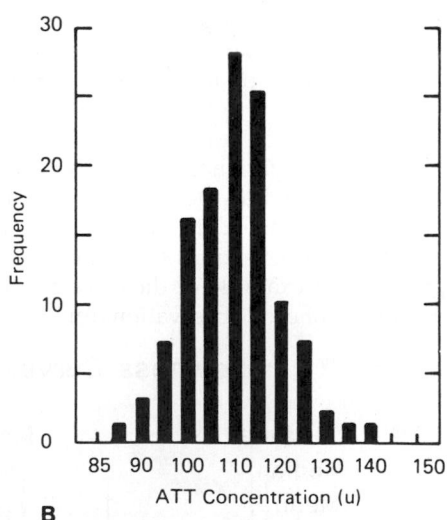

FIGURE 44-5. Frequency distribution histograms show the number of results falling at various intervals across the range of values obtained in any given reference range study. In this example, the study of antithrombin III was performed to obtain the reference range for a local patient population. **(A)** Data have been grouped in intervals of 2 units. **(B)** Data have been grouped in intervals of 5 units; note how same data can look different graphically, although both form a normal Gaussian curve. $\bar{x} = 111.6$; s = 9.5 units. (From Cembrowski GS, Sullivan AM: Quality control and statistics. In Bishop ML, Duben-Engelkirk JL, Fody EP, eds: Clinical Chemistry—Principles, Procedures, Correlations, 3rd ed, p 63. Philadelphia, JB Lippincott, 1996, with permission.)

healthy persons in the population from which the patients come. The concept of a reference range is now used in laboratories to indicate that a reported patient value falling within this range corresponds with those values in a reference group that is presumed to be free of any condition that might distort the measurement. The use of reference ranges is important to both clinicians and laboratorians, especially in hematology, where multiple values are measured simultaneously and the coordinated interpretation of more than one test frequently is used in diagnosis and treatment. Reference ranges include the expected intraindividual and interindividual nonpathologic sources of variation and help to discern whether a patient's value is pathologic or simply indicative of the usual physiologic variations of the analyte in that patient population.

It is recommended that each laboratory establish its own reference ranges for all tests performed, both when tests are introduced and when they are modified. In designing a statistical study to obtain reference ranges based on samples, it is important to establish the method of sampling to be used before data collection. Once data are collected, the frequency distribution curve of that data indicates the type of statistical analysis required. Unfortunately, the process of obtaining and characterizing reference values is fraught with problems both in selecting the population samples and in the methods of statistical analysis. These problems can be overcome for the most part, however, and valid reference ranges can be determined.

SELECTING AND TESTING SAMPLES FROM THE POPULATION TO DETERMINE THE REFERENCE RANGE

Ideally, one should use at least 40 subjects, and preferably more, who provide the necessary variety of demographic factors (*e.g.*, sex, age and race) and who do not have any conditions that might influence the measurement under study. Of course, data from populations that are expected to be different, such as adults and children, should not be mixed, because the reference ranges are expected to be different. It is often difficult for a laboratory to obtain a suitable subject population.

All personnel normally responsible for specimen analysis should be involved in determination of the reference range, and the samples collected for this determination should be treated just the same as the patient specimens.[8] Only five to ten samples should be drawn and tested per day; if all samples are drawn and analyzed at the same time, an erroneous reference range may be determined because of transient instrument or reagent differences, which cannot be accounted for when analyzing samples over a short time period. The reader is referred to Chapter 58 for a discussion of factors that must be considered in selecting subjects for a reference range study for hemostasis tests and for further details on the general rules for testing specimens in a reference range study.

SELECTING STATISTICAL METHODS TO DETERMINE THE REFERENCE RANGE

Once sufficient data have been obtained, the frequency distribution histogram may be plotted (Fig. 44-5) to determine whether the data have a Gaussian (normal; Fig.

44-3) or skewed (lognormal; Fig. 44-4) distribution. If any outliers are found among the data, these should be investigated further to see if there is any explanation for them, such as a previously undiagnosed abnormal hematologic condition. If an explanation is found, these data should not be used in the determination of the reference range.

From the distribution curve, the method of statistical analysis may be chosen. In the unusual event that the curve is Gaussian, as in Figure 44-5, the mean ±2 SD may be calculated, as explained earlier in this chapter, to obtain the reference range. If a frequency histogram is only slightly skewed, the reference range may be determined simply by excluding 2.5% of the values at the lower end and 2.5% of the values at the upper end of the range of values obtained.[19] Thus, in this procedure, the 95% range of values is taken as representing the reference range. Table 44-3 presents an eosinophil reference range study for which this procedure was used to determine the popu-

TABLE 44-3 *Eosinophil Reference Range Data for Frequency Histogram* and Cumulative Frequency Histogram***			
Eosinophil Interval (%)	No. of Subjects	Cumulative Number	Cumulative Percent
0.0	5	5	2.9–2.5%
0.5	10	15	8.8
1.0	28	43	25.3
1.5	21	64	37.6
2.0	25	89	52.4
2.5	16	105	61.8
3.0	14	119	70.0
3.5	19	138	81.2
4.0	9	147	86.5
4.5	7	154	90.6
5.0	6	160	94.1
5.5	4	164	96.5
6.0	0	164	96.5–97.5%
6.5	3	167	98.2
7.0	0	167	98.2
7.5	0	167	98.2
8.0	0	167	98.2
8.5	0	167	98.2
9.0	1	168	98.8
9.5	1	169	99.4
10.0	0	169	99.4
10.5	1	170	100.0

Reference range is determined by the eosinophil interval percentage closest to 2.5% and 97.5% cumulative percent. In this study, the population reference range is 0.0% to 6.0% eosinophils. Cumulative number represents a running total of the number of subjects. Cumulative percent represents the cumulative number divided by the number of subjects in the study (n = 170). For example, 10 subjects had an average of 0.5 eosinophils per 100 leukocytes differentiated. The cumulative number at that point is 15 (10 + 5 subjects who had 0% eosinophils on the differential) and the cumulative percent is 8.8 [(15/170) × 100%]. Courtesy of Duke University Department of Laboratory Medicine, Durham, NC.
* See Figure 44-7.
** See Figure 44-8.

lation reference range, even though the data are skewed (see Fig. 44-7).

If the curve is skewed, calculation of the reference range is a little more complicated. Most biologic measurements do not fit Gaussian frequency distributions[3]; rather, they often form a skewed curve.[15] Several common hematology studies result in characteristically skewed distributions. These include eosinophil, basophil and monocyte counts in the differential leukocyte count and the prothrombin time and partial thromboplastin time in coagulation testing.

If the mean and SD are calculated from data that are not Gaussian, the mean ±2 SD may give a reference range with a lower limit that is a negative number—no hematologic measure has a negative value. In a study of the mean ±2 SD for the erythrocyte sedimentation rate (ESR) reference range, the calculation might well yield a range of −6 to 18 mm in 1 hour, whereas the lowest possible true result is 0 mm in 1 hour. Therefore, to apply parametric statistical analysis (*e.g.*, mean, median, mode, SD and CV), the raw data must be transformed to fit a distribution that is Gaussian.

Such a transformation of data may be performed in several ways. One method, applicable for slightly skewed distribution curves, requires plotting a cumulative fre-

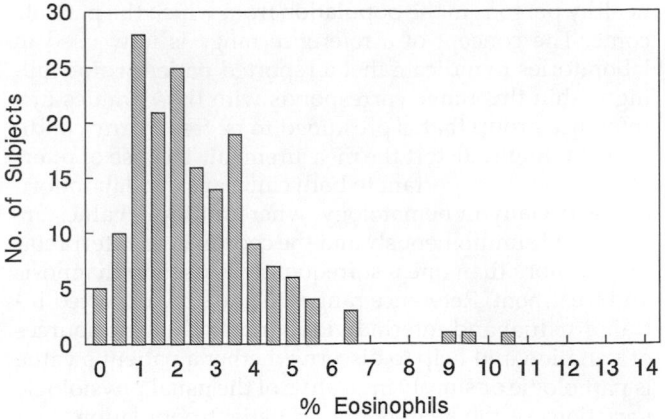

FIGURE 44-7. Skewed frequency histogram from an eosinophil reference range study. The corresponding probability plot is shown in Figure 44-8. (Courtesy of Duke University Department of Laboratory Medicine, Durham NC.)

quency histogram on probability paper, as shown in Figure 44-6. Note that this method makes the Gaussian distribution linear and allows drawing the best-fit line. From this curve, the values that correspond to 2.5% and 97.5% cumulative frequency determine the 95% confidence limits and thus the reference range for that measure. For the antithrombin III study in Figure 44-6, the 95% limits for the reference range are 92.5 U and 129 U.

For significantly skewed distributions, such as that in Figure 44-7 (for which the raw data are shown in Table 44-3), which result in a curved cumulative frequency histogram when plotted on probability paper (Fig. 44-8), it is difficult to draw a best-fit line. However, determination of the 95% confidence limits using this probability plot is still valid because the percentiles are unaffected by the curved form of the graph. From Figure 44-8 and Table 44-3, the 2.5 and 97.5 percentile limits that establish the overall 95% confidence limits are 0 to 6 eosinophils.

As an alternative, skewed data distributions can occasionally be transformed to normal distributions using a lognormal data transformation. This may be accom-

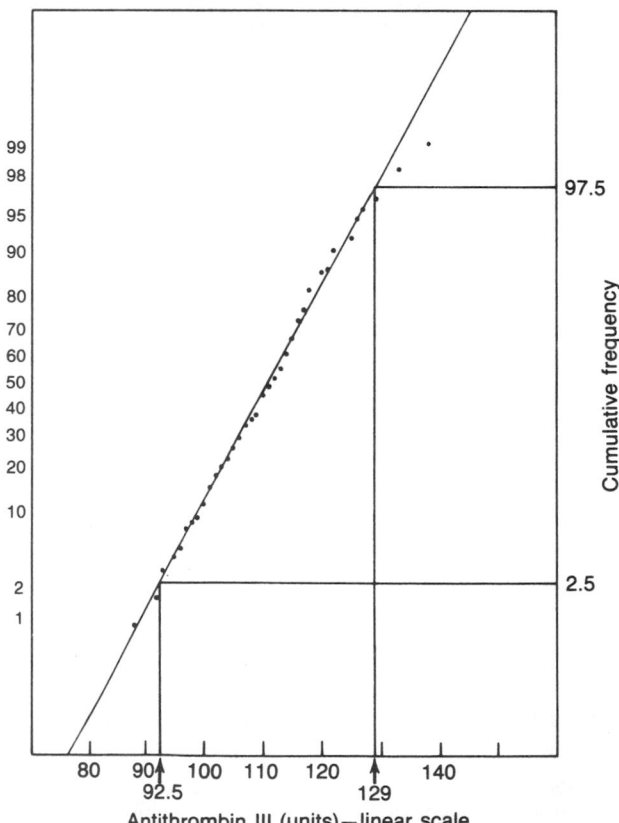

FIGURE 44-6. Cumulative frequency histogram or probability plot for antithrombin III using a linear scale. The line represents the best-fit; 92.5 and 129 units represent the 2.5 and 97.5 percentiles, respectively, and indicate the 95% reference range values. (From Cembrowski GS, Sullivan AM: Quality control and statistics. In Bishop ML, Duben-Engelkirk JL, Fody EP, eds: Clinical Chemistry—Principles, Procedures, Correlations, 3rd ed, p 70. Philadelphia, JB Lippincott, 1996, with permission.)

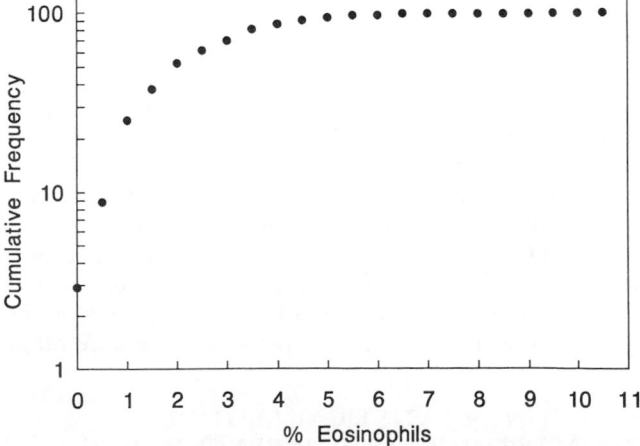

FIGURE 44-8. The linear scale probability plot from an eosinophil reference range study (see also Fig. 44-7). (Courtesy of Duke University Department of Laboratory Medicine, Durham NC.)

plished by using graph paper with a logarithmic scale on one axis and a normal-probability scale on the other. Because a skewed distribution curve is not always indicative of a lognormal distribution, the assumption of a lognormal distribution must be tested. On testing the data from Figure 44-8, there was no significant improvement in the linearity of the data. The 95% reference range using the lognormal transformation method was 0.5 to 7, not a clinically significant difference from the range determined by the probability plot in Figure 44-8.

Lognormal data transformation may also be performed by converting all data to logarithmic form, then plotting the cumulative frequency against these values on a linear scale. If the resulting best-fit line is linear, the log values of the 2.5 and 97.5 percentiles indicating the 95% reference range may be determined. The antilog of these values is then taken to obtain the final reference range.

Frequently, transformation by any of the foregoing methods still cannot change the data enough to fit a Gaussian distribution. Alternatively, nonparametric statistics may be used, which are not as dependent on the distribution of the data being normal or Gaussian as are the parametric statistics such as mean and standard deviation. Refer to standard statistical texts for further information on nonparametric analysis.[3]

The choice of statistical analysis method can greatly affect the reference range. Thus, it can be seen that reference ranges do not provide final definitive diagnostic guidelines; rather, they provide 95% interval estimates for biological measures.

Statistical Measures of Correlation Between Two Methods

Part of laboratory QA and QC involves the evaluation and selection of satisfactory instrumentation and methodologies for measurement of one or more values. For example, a new instrument may be advertised to be faster, less expensive, more precise, and more accurate than other instruments for performing complete blood counts. Many aspects must be considered in such an evaluation, and these were discussed earlier in this chapter (see Table 44-1).

Whenever comparing two methods or instruments, it is important to include patient specimens covering the range of expected results to include normal results and mildly, moderately and markedly abnormal results. For tests that become abnormal in only one direction (*e.g.,* prothrombin times) the study population should be divided into quartiles of equal size so that the statistical analyses are not unduly influenced by an excessivley large normal group. For tests such as hemoglobin, for which results can be greater or less than the normal range, both anemic and polycythemic specimens should be included in sufficient numbers, again, to avoid undue influence by the normal values.

At this point, the statistical tools for evaluation of a new method or instrument will be discussed. Statistical analysis is required for the comparison-of-methods study, which is one of the last steps in the method or instrument

TABLE 44-4
Statistical Analysis of Paired Samples Recommended in Method Comparison*

Analytical Method	Comments
Scatter plot	Graph results of each specimen using reference (or currently used) method and new test method (Fig. 44-9)
Linear regression analysis	Use 100 samples, if possible, 5 per day over 20 days
Slope	Proportional systematic error
y intercept	Constant systematic error
$s_{y/x}$ (SD of regression line)	Intermethod random error

* These tests are a part of the total procedure required for comparison of a new test method with a reference method or the method currently in use in a laboratory, as outlined in Table 44-1.

evaluation process. If all other aspects of an instrument or method are satisfactory, such as precision and accuracy, then the laboratory must compare the new method with the current method or, if possible, a reference method, to determine whether the two methods agree.[4]

The recommended statistical tools for comparison of methods to be discussed in the following are (1) regression analysis and (2) the standard deviation of the regression line, also called the standard error of estimate, abbreviated as $s_{y/x}$ (Table 44-4). Another statistical tool with limited use in comparison of methods is the correlation coefficient.

REGRESSION ANALYSIS

When two methods are compared, the strength of the association between their results is indicated in terms of correlation. The same variables from each method are represented by paired data points. Traditionally, data from the current or reference method are plotted on the x axis and data from the new method on the y axis to produce a scatter plot (Fig. 44-9). Although the best-fit line may be drawn visually to estimate the agreement between the two methods, a more accurate calculation of the agreement may be obtained through *regression analysis.* A straight line through the points, called the *linear regression line* or *least-squares line,* is obtained. This line of best-fit is calculated so that the sum of the squares of the deviations from the points to the line is the least. This line may be represented by the formula:

$$y = y_0 + bx$$

where y_0 is the y intercept (the value of y at $x = 0$) and b is the slope of the line.

The y intercept is an indication of one form of systematic error called *constant error.* The slope determines the other type of systematic error, called *proportional error.* Both of these errors are discussed later and shown in Figure 44-9.

Calculation of the regression line slope b usually is performed by a computer using the following formula:

$$b = \frac{n\Sigma x_i y_i - \Sigma x_i \Sigma y_i}{n\Sigma x_i^2 - (\Sigma x_i)^2}$$

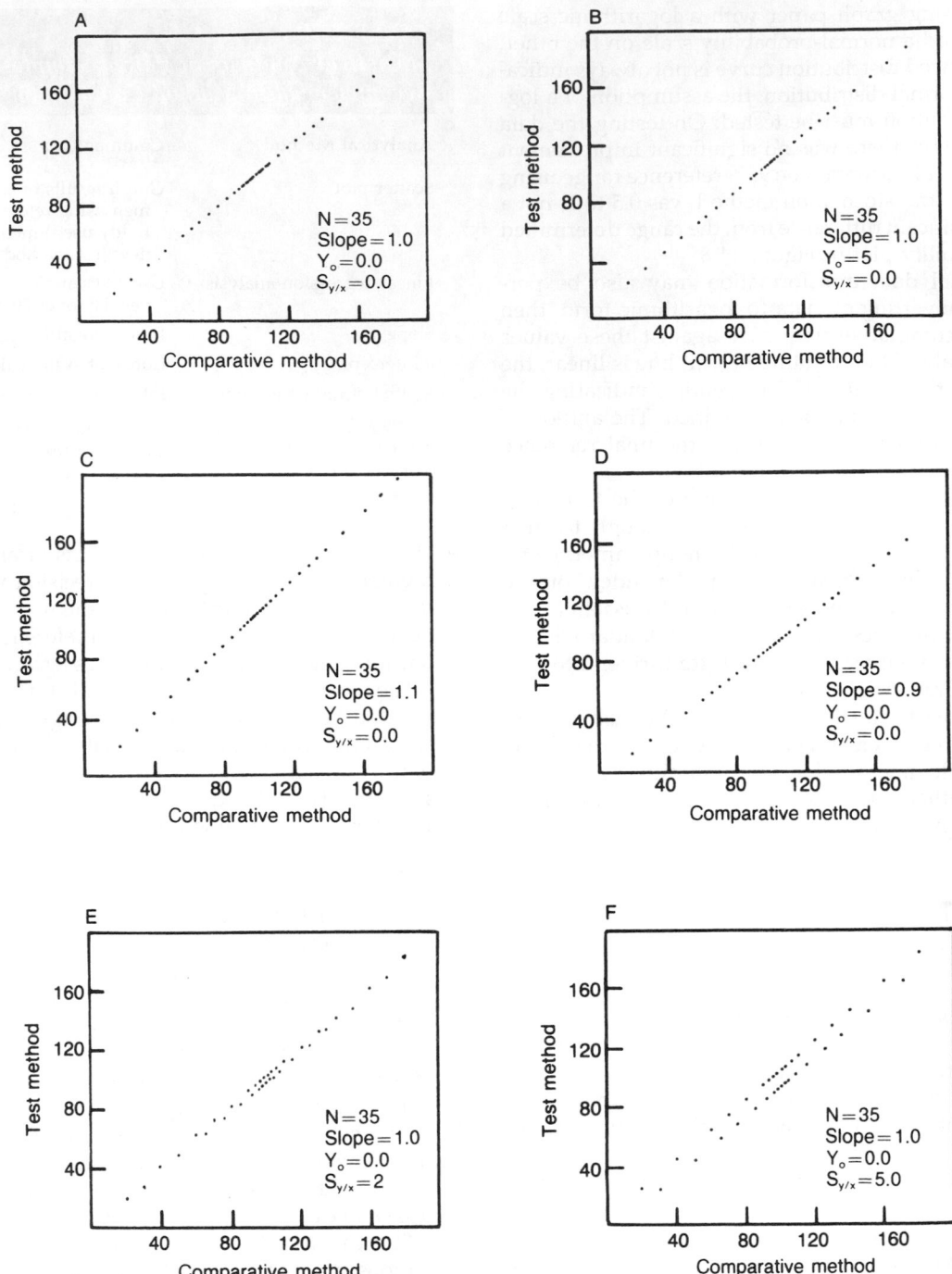

FIGURE 44-9. Comparison-of-methods experiments using simulated data: **(A)** No error; **(B)** constant error ($Y_o = 5$); **(C,D)** proportional error (slope 1.1 and 0.9, respectively; **(E,F)** random error ($S_{y/x} = 2$ and 5, respectively). (From Cembrowski GS, Sullivan AM: Quality control and statistics. In Bishop ML, Duben-Engelkirk JL, Fody EP, eds: Clinical Chemistry—Principles, Procedures, Correlations, 3rd ed, p 66. Philadelphia, JB Lippincott, 1996, with permission.)

The y intercept is calculated based on the slope b and the means of all observations in each method:

$$y_o = \frac{\Sigma y_i}{n} - \frac{b\Sigma x_i}{n}$$

OR

$$y_o = \bar{y} - b\bar{x}$$

Figure 44-9 demonstrates the hypothetical results of six comparison-of-methods regression analysis studies

that illustrate various kinds of error. Figure 44-9B through 44-9F should be compared with Figure 44-9A which shows perfect agreement between two methods because the y intercept is 0 and the slope is 1.0. Figure 44-9B illustrates a test method with a constant systematic error: it has consistently higher measurements than the reference method, as indicated by the y intercept of 5.0. Figure 44-9C shows a y intercept of 0 but a slope of 1.1, indicating that unless the analyte being measured has a value of 0, the test method measures are higher than those of the reference (comparative) method. Figure 44-9D illustrates a test method for which the measures are lower than those of the comparative method for all nonzero values, as the y intercept is again 0, but the slope is 0.9 (*i.e.*, less than 1). Both Figures 44-9C and 44-9D reflect proportional systematic error because the difference between the test and the reference method is proportional to the analyte value.

STANDARD DEVIATION OF THE REGRESSION LINE (STANDARD ERROR OF ESTIMATE)

One statistical measure of the degree of scatter about the regression line is the standard error of estimate, which is denoted $s_{y/x}$. This is defined as the average SD of the y values for a given x in a comparison-of-methods experiment (*i.e.*, the standard deviation around the regression line in the y direction) and is expressed in the units of measurement contained in the data groups. It is calculated as follows:

$$s_{y/x} = \sqrt{\frac{1}{n-2}\left[\left[\Sigma y_i^2 - \frac{(\Sigma y_i)^2}{n}\right] - \frac{\left[\Sigma x_i y_i - \frac{(\Sigma x_i)(\Sigma y_i)}{n}\right]^2}{\Sigma x_i^2 - \frac{(\Sigma x_i)^2}{n}}\right]}$$

The $s_{y/x}$ is a measure of random error (*i.e.*, error attributable to chance). It measures intermethod imprecision.

Figure 44-9E and 9F graphically demonstrate the effects of a nonzero $s_{y/x}$. When this value is 0 as it is in Figure 44-9A through 44-9D, there is no scatter about the regression line. In Figure 44-9E and 44-9F, the values of 2 and 5, respectively, were alternately added and subtracted from each value in Figure 44-9A, where there was a perfect correlation between methods, causing the scatter shown on each graph and increased $s_{y/x}$ values.

CORRELATION COEFFICIENT

The Pearson correlation coefficient (r) may be used in method comparisons for measuring how closely the points cluster about the regression line.

The calculation is:

$$r = \frac{n\Sigma x_i y_i - \Sigma x_i \Sigma y_i}{\sqrt{[n\Sigma x_i^2 - (\Sigma x_i)^2] \times [n\Sigma y_i^2 - (\Sigma y_i)^2]}}$$

The r value has been popular because it is a straightforward measure of correlation between two methods with values ranging from -1 (perfect negative correlation) through 0 (no correlation) to $+1$ (perfect positive correlation). Although the r often has been used in method comparisons, it is not advisable to rely on this value alone for conclusive information. Other statistical measures such as $s_{y/x}$ and visual inspection of the regression line should also be used to make valid conclusions in method comparisons.

The disadvantages of the correlation coefficient include its sensitivity to random error, outliers and the range of concentration of the analyte.[44] Sensitivity to these factors can be considered a drawback in method comparison.[21] Furthermore, the correlation coefficient is not sensitive to constant or proportional error,[21] which are important factors in a method comparison. The correlation coefficient may, however, be helpful in determining when an alternative method of regression analysis is necessary, such as weighted regression or transformation of the data (*e.g.*, logarithmic transformation or square root transformation).[13]

T-TESTS AND F RATIOS

The t-test and F ratio are two inferential values that are discussed in most standard statistical texts. These values have been and continue to be used by some investigators in comparing methods; however, their real value in such comparisons is questionable.[21]

The t-test is used to determine whether there is a statistically significant difference between the actual means of two groups of data.[10] The *paired* t-test is used to compare the mean of the differences between positively correlated pairs of results such as the results in a comparison-of-methods study, the results being obtained on the same blood specimen using the two methods or instruments. An important reason that the t-test is not recommended for use in comparative studies is that it may show a statistically significant bias between two methods that may *not* be clinically significant.

The F ratio is used in method comparison to determine whether there is a statistically significant difference between the standard deviations of two methods. Similar to the t-test, it may indicate statistical significance that does not indicate clinical significance. Indeed, Westgard and Hunt state that the F ratio should not be used to determine whether a test or method is acceptable.[44]

COMMENTS ON STATISTICAL ANALYSIS IN COMPARISON OF METHODS

Regression analysis frequently is used in method comparisons, because it quantitates the correlation between two data groups and can indicate the positive or negative bias of one group compared with the other. It is important to note, however, that *all* summary statistics (*i.e.*, y intercept, slope and $s_{y/x}$) obtained from the linear regression analysis should be used to describe the association between two methods to prevent an erroneous interpretation of the data. Helpful guidelines for method comparisons have been proposed by the NCCLS.[31,32]

COMPONENTS OF A QUALITY ASSURANCE PROGRAM

Basic Requirements

Meaningful QA in hematology, as in all other areas of the laboratory, requires an appreciation that many of the activities occur away from the laboratory. Therefore, monitoring the processing of test measurements is only a part of the program. The laboratory must design a program that encompasses all activities, rather than limiting its scope to data acquisition. These activities can be divided into two basic types, nonanalytic control and analytic QC, both of which are important in QA.

NONANALYTIC CONTROL FUNCTIONS

Nonanalytic activities encompass all those not directly related to the performance of the clinical assay itself. These include control procedures for preanalytic functions such as test ordering; patient preparation and identification; and specimen collection, identification, transport, accession, and handling before analysis.[20] Also included are control procedures for such postanalytic functions as reporting results and test charging mechanisms. A procedure manual concerning all nonanalytic activities should be available to appropriate laboratory personnel.

ANALYTIC QUALITY CONTROL FUNCTIONS

Analytic activities and their control are discussed in detail in the remainder of this chapter and in Chapters 45 and 46.

Establishment of Control Procedures

When a new analytic test is introduced to the clinical laboratory, it is imperative that its performance reliability be maintained under day-to-day operating conditions. Various control protocols should be established to involve all laboratory personnel responsible for performing the procedure. The purpose of these control procedures is threefold: (1) to assess the laboratory's usual analytic performance realistically and establish acceptable limits of error; (2) to identify significant problems or errors; and (3) to document all QC results and any corrective action taken. With these objectives in mind, the statistical control procedures should be designed so that the expected frequency of analytic errors is taken into consideration for each individual method or instrument. Ideally, a control procedure should be designed to have a very low probability for false rejections (rejection of a run with no errors) and a very high probability for error detection.

BIOLOGIC CONTROLS

The widely accepted practice of running whole-blood controls along with patient samples provides the most common means by which clinical laboratories maintain performance reliability and identify significant problems. These biologic control materials can be used in a number of ways (Chaps. 45 and 46) and can be of two types (*i.e.*, commercial stabilized control products or retained patient specimens for repeat testing). The concurrent statistical evaluation of specimen data using the Bull testing algorithm (Chap. 45) is also a very good method, but requires a significantly large testing workload so that contemporary quality control information (*i.e.*, sufficient data gathered in the same time period) is available for evaluation.

CONTROL RESULT LIMITS REQUIRING STAFF ACTION

Control procedures establish the methods by which abnormal, erroneous, or out-of-control results can be detected. When control limits are exceeded (*i.e.*, the control value falls outside of the 3 SD range), action is mandatory. Tolerance limits must be established for each of the following aspects of a QC program: biologic control materials (commercial controls and retained patient specimens), instrument function checks, interlaboratory comparisons, and proficiency testing. If the tolerance limits are too narrow, an inordinate amount of time and effort will be spent pursuing insignificant problems. If the limits are too broad, significant problems may go uncorrected. Specific

methods used for these different aspects of a QC program are discussed in Chapters 45 and 46.

Once out-of-control situations or abnormal patient results have been identified, action must be taken according to an established procedure. This protocol should delineate the steps to be followed by personnel to differentiate the specimens involved in an out-of-control situation from those that are clinically abnormal. If the test system is out of control, procedures must be in place either to rectify the problem or to employ an alternative (backup) method to obtain accurate results on the samples incorrectly analyzed. Likewise, for an abnormal specimen or one containing interfering substances, specific procedures should be written that include the abnormal indicators to identify such a specimen as well as the action to be taken to obtain accurate results.

Monitoring and Documenting Control Results

A monitoring program should be established to evaluate, display, organize, summarize, and statistically document the results obtained from control procedures. This type of program usually involves one or more charting techniques, sophisticated statistical analyses and data management systems, multirule QC algorithms, and the Bull algorithm.[8] These are discussed in Chapter 45.

The expansion of quality control and quality assurance programs to include total quality management (TQM) systems (discussed earlier in this chapter) has led to the development by the Joint Commission on Accreditation of Healthcare Organizations (JCAHO) of a program to monitor laboratory medicine practices using so-called indicators. A variety of specific laboratory quality indicators have been proposed including estimates of laboratory data reliability, evaluation of quality laboratory management, and measures of appropriate laboratory utilization. These indicators can be used to estimate the quality of the laboratory service.

Laboratory data reliability, in addition to being monitored on a real-time basis with comprehensive quality control programs, has also been checked for many years with proficiency-testing programs.[11] Participant summary reports together with the participating laboratory's results document data accuracy.

Workload recording and productivity or the assessment of test turnaround times are examples of indicators of quality management. Many of these have been the subjects of the College of American Pathologists Q-Probes program which was begun in 1988.[1] More than 600 laboratories have enrolled in this program and submit detailed data on the particular subject of the Q-Probe. The data are collated and evaluated statistically and a percentile ranking is indicated for each participant laboratory. Each laboratory can then assess its own level of compliance with national laboratory practices.

Laboratory utilization indicators are to a degree beyond the control of the laboratory service. However, the laboratory is in a strategic position to monitor testing patterns, especially with the increasing sophistication of laboratory and hospital information systems. For example, a review of the ratio of automated blood counts (without a manual differential count) to so-called complete blood counts (which include a complete manual/visual differential count and blood film review) may indicate inappropriate ordering of complete blood counts when only one or a few of the parameters in the automated count would be sufficient. By gathering such data and analyzing it together with the hospital clinical staff, more appropriate laboratory utilization can be obtained.[29]

CHAPTER SUMMARY

In the last 20 years, the clinical hematology laboratory has seen tremendous changes in all aspects with the advent of fully automated, multiparameter, high-speed hematology analyzers. Nationwide, standardization techniques have been increasingly accepted, and significant improvements have been made in reagent and control stability.

Although many powerful techniques and procedures have been developed recently for assessing and monitoring the quality of all these changes, a complex job still exists for the laboratorian within the hematology area. The supervisor is well challenged when establishing a QC program for formative instrumentation and new analytic measurements to ensure the highest quality results. To increase the challenge, the laboratory may be forced to develop such a program within narrow financial constraints. To meet this challenge the laboratory scientist must be constantly aware of new developments in laboratory hematology and be prepared to implement innovative techniques in a constantly evolving, dynamically changing QA program.

Review Questions

44-1. The closeness with which a measured value agrees with the true value is referred to as

A. standard deviation.
B. standard error of the mean.
C. accuracy.
D. precision.

44-2. The average value of a group of observations is known as the

A. standard deviation.
B. mean.
C. median.
D. mode.

44-3. When reviewing quality control results, analytical values outside the _____ range are ordinarily *un*acceptable.

A. $\bar{x} \pm 0.5$ SD
B. $\bar{x} \pm 1$ SD
C. $\bar{x} \pm 2$ SD
D. $\bar{x} \pm 3$ SD

44-4. The range of values commonly used as a population reference range in a Gaussian or slightly skewed data distribution is

A. $x \pm 20$.
B. $x \pm 1$ SD.
C. $x \pm 2$ SD.
D. $x \pm 3$ SD.

44-5. The frequency distribution of most biologic measurements is

A. Gaussian.
B. skewed.

C. impossible to determine.
D. symmetric about the center and bell-shaped.

44-6. The reliability of a test being positive when a condition to be detected is present is called the test's

A. dynamic range.
B. sensitivity.
C. specificity.
D. analytic variation.

44-7. Perfect correlation between two methods or instruments in a comparison-of-methods study using regression analysis is indicated by a linear slope of _____ and a y intercept of _____.

A. 1, 0
B. 0, 1
C. 1, 1
D. -1, 0

For the following questions, choose from these answers:
A. 1 and 3
B. 2 and 4
C. 1, 2 and 3
D. 4 only
E. all of the above

44-8. It is possible for automated analytic measurements, to be

1. precise but not accurate.
2. both accurate and precise.
3. neither accurate nor precise.
4. found outside of an established reference range.

44-9. Establishment of instrument or method accuracy for hemoglobin can be accomplished by calibration using

1. secondary standards.
2. commercial calibrators.
3. primary standards.
4. commercial control products.

44-10. When determining a population reference range for adult hemoglobin,

1. at least 40 subjects should be used.
2. specimens from all subjects should be analyzed on the same day.
3. all personnel involved in specimen analysis should assist in the determination.
4. an approximately equal number of males and females should be included and the results merged.

44-11. The statistical measure $s_{y/x}$ indicates the

1. degree of scatter about a regression line.
2. error caused by chance in a test method.
3. intermethod imprecision.
4. systematic error in a test method.

References

1. Bachner P, Howanitz PJ: Q-Probes. A tool for enhancing your lab's QA. Med Lab Obs November, 111, 1991
2. Bahn AK: Basic Medical Statistics. New York, Grune & Stratton, 1972
3. Barnett RN: Clinical Laboratory Statistics, 2nd ed. Boston, Little, Brown & Co, 1979
4. Barnett RN, Youden WJ: A revised scheme for the comparison of quantitative methods. Am J Clin Pathol 54:454, 1970
5. Belk WP, Sunderman FW: A survey of the accuracy of chemical analyses in clinical laboratories. Am J Clin Pathol 17:853, 1947

6. Bollinger P, Drewinko B: A quality control program for a computerized, high-volume, automated hematology laboratory. Am J Med Technol 49:9, 1983

7. Brittin GM, Brecher G, Johnson CA et al: Stability of blood in commonly used anticoagulants. Am J Clin Pathol 52:690, 1969

8. Bull BS, Elashoff RM, Heilbron DC et al: A study of various estimators for the deviation of quality control procedures from patient erythrocyte indices. Am J Clin Pathol 61:473, 1974

9. Buttner J, Borth R, Boutwell JH et al: Provisional recommendations on quality control in clinical chemistry. 2: Assessment of analytical methods for routine use. Clin Chim Acta 69:F1, 1976

10. Castle WM: Statistics in Small Doses. New York, Churchill Livingstone, 1977

11. College of American Pathologists: Summing Up: A publication of the Surveys Committee of the College of American Pathologists 14(3):6, 1984

12. Dharan M: Total Quality Control in the Clinical Laboratory. St Louis, CV Mosby, 1977

13. Dixon WJ, Massey FJ: Introduction to Statistical Analysis, p 323. New York, McGraw-Hill, 1969

14. Dodge HF: Using inspection data to control quality. Manuf Ind 16:517, 1928

15. Flynn FV, Piper KA, Garcia-Webb P et al: The frequency distribution of commonly determined blood constituents in healthy blood donors. Clin Chim Acta 52:163, 1974

16. Freund JE: Statistics—A First Course. Englewood Cliffs, NJ, Prentice-Hall, 1970

17. Gilmer PR Jr, Williams LJ: The status of methods of calibration in hematology. Am J Clin Pathol 74:600, 1980

18. Gilmer PR Jr, Williams LJ, Koepke JA et al: Calibration methods for automated hematology instruments. Am J Clin Pathol 68:185, 1977

19. Golob JK: Normal ranges in clinical work: Their uses and methods of determination. Am J Med Technol 26:167, 1960

20. Gulati GL, Hyun BH: Quality control in hematology. Clin Lab Med 6:675, 1986

21. Hackney JR, Cembrowski GS: Need for improved instrument and kit evaluations. Am J Clin Pathol 86:391, 1986

22. Hackney JR, Cembrowski GS, Carey RN: Quality control in hematology. In Cembrowski GS, Carey RN (eds): Laboratory Control Management. Chicago, ASCP Press, 1989

23. International Committee for Standardization in Haematology: Recommendation for haemoglobinometry in human blood. Br J Haematol 13(suppl):71, 1967

24. International Committee for Standardization in Haematology: Recommendations for reference method for haemoglobinometry in human blood. J Clin Pathol 31:139, 1978

25. International Committee for Standardization in Haematology: Recommended Methods for the Determination of Packed Cell Volume. Geneva, World Health Organization, 1980

26. King JW, Willis CE: Cyanmethemoglobin certification program of the College of American Pathologists. Am J Clin Pathol 54:496, 1970

27. Koepke JA: The calibration of automated instruments for accuracy in hemoglobinometry. Am J Clin Pathol 68:180, 1977

28. Koepke JA: Fitting the cell counter to the bed count. Clin Lab Med 13:817, 1993

29. Koepke JA, Bull BS: The intralaboratory control of quality. In Lewis SM, Koepke JA (eds): Hematology Laboratory Management and Practice. Oxford, Butterworth-Heineman, 1995

30. Levey S, Jennings ER: The use of control charts in the clinical laboratory. Am J Clin Pathol 20:1059, 1950

31. National Committee for Clinical Laboratory Standards: User comparison of quantitative clinical laboratory methods using patient samples, EP9-P, Vol 6, p 1. Villanova, PA, NCCLS, 1986

32. National Committtee for Clinical Laboratory Standards: Preliminary evaluation of quantitative clinical chemistry methods, 2nd ed; tentative guideline EP10-T2. Villanova, PA, NCCLS, 1993

33. National Committee for Clinical Laboratory Standards: How to define, determine and utilize reference intervals in the clinical laboratory; approved guideline C28-A. Villanova, PA, NCCLS, 1995

34. Savage RA: Calibration bias and imprecision for automated hematology analyzers: An evaluation of significance of short-term bias resulting from calibration of an analyzer with S-Cal. Am J Clin Pathol 84:186, 1985

35. Schonberger RJ: Japanese Manufacturing Techniques: Nine Hidden Lessons in Simplicity. New York, Free Press, 1982

36. Shewhart WA: Economic Control of Quality of Manufactured Products. New York, Van Nostrand Reinhold, 1931

37. Skendzel LP, Barnett RN, Platt R: Medically useful criteria for analytic performance of laboratory tests. Am J Clin Pathol 83:200, 1985

38. Statland BE, Westgard JO: Quality control: Theory and practice. In Henry JB (ed): Clinical Diagnosis and Management by Laboratory Methods, 17th ed, p 74. Philadelphia, WB Saunders, 1984

39. Statland BE, Winkel P: Sources of variation in laboratory measurements. In Henry JB (ed): Clinical Diagnosis and Management by Laboratory Methods, 16th ed. Philadelphia, WB Saunders, 1979

40. van Assendelft OW, England JM: Terms, quantities and units. In: Advances in Hematological Methods: The Blood Count. Boca Raton, FL, CRC Press, 1982

41. van Assendelft OW, Horton BR, Parvin RM: Calibration and control in haemoglobinometry. Clin Lab Haematol 12(suppl):31, 1990

42. van Kampen EJ, Zijlstra WG: Standardization in hemoglobinometry. II: The hemiglobincyanide method. Clin Chim Acta 6:538, 1961

43. Wakkers PJM, Hellendoorn HB, Op-de-Weegh GJ et al: Applications of statistics in clinical chemistry: A critical evaluation of regression lines. Clin Chim Acta 64:173, 1975

44. Westgard JO, Hunt MR: Use and interpretation of common statistical tests in method comparison studies. Clin Chem 19:49, 1973

CHAPTER 45

Methods to Monitor and Control Systematic Error

Mary Ann Dotson

Objectives

1. Name two methods used for instrument calibration and list two disadvantages for each method.
2. List three disadvantages of commercial control materials for monitoring instrument calibration.
3. List four hematology procedures for which commercial control materials are not available.
4. Describe three methods of charting control results and draw a diagram showing the characteristics of each method.
5. Describe a statistical method using patient indices as a QC tool and name and explain two functions of the algorithm used in this method.
6. Name the agencies that set standards, accredit laboratories through inspections, and regulate the laboratory and medical device industries.

A systematic error affects all samples equally in a proportionate or constant manner. Improper instrument calibration or loss of calibration secondary to malfunction are causes of systematic errors. Such errors are detected and corrected by a quality control (QC) program, a series of activities performed to ensure accuracy and precision of results. A QC program includes calibration, internal and external monitoring of accuracy and precision, documentation, preventive maintenance, and troubleshooting–all of which are essential.

CALIBRATION

Calibration involves any adjustments made to an instrument to correct the results recovered so that they match "truth," which is defined by standards or reference procedures.

Standards: Primary *versus* Secondary

A *primary standard* is a pure chemical substance that can be weighed and placed in solution. The International Haemoglobin Standards are the only primary hematology standards, having been designated by the World Health Organization (WHO) as primary hemoglobin reference material. These preparations, however, are only available to approved national groups for the assignment of hemoglobin values to preparations which are used, in turn, for the assignment of hemoglobin values to whole blood callibrators using the hemoglobin cyanide (methemoglobin) reference method. These whole blood preparations, thus, become secondary standards. A *secondary standard* is a biologic specimen in which the analyte in question is measured by an accurate reference method such as the International Council for Standardization in Haematology (ICSH) cyanmethemoglobin reference method. Secondary standards may be used to make instrument calibration adjustments. Fresh whole blood samples drawn from healthy donors become secondary standards when tested by reference methods.

Reference Methods

Reference methods that are acceptable for instrument calibration have been selected by the ICSH and by the National Committee for Clinical Laboratory Standards (NCCLS). A reference method is one whose accuracy has been well established over the years by independent means. When a reference method is used on a sample of blood, that sample becomes a secondary standard with a known value that is a reasonable estimate of "truth." However, the reference method is accurate only if it is performed correctly. The NCCLS has published detailed documents outlining the correct procedures for hematologic methods, including proper calibration. These documents are also referred to as standards (written standards). Selected committees of the NCCLS may spend as long as 3 years in the development of a document or standard. Each written standard goes through two to three consensus levels of development: proposed, tentative, and approved. Some noncontroversial documents may go directly from proposed to approved, thus speeding up the time required to develop a new standard. Approved documents undergo periodic review and updating. An up-to-date list of these documents can be obtained on request from the NCCLS.*

Calibration by Reference Methods Using Fresh Whole Blood

The ideal method for first-time calibration of hematology cell counters uses fresh whole blood and reference methods. Hemoglobin reference values are obtained through photometric measurement of cyanmethemoglobin using a spectrophotometer that has been calibrated with a cyanmethemoglobin secondary standard.[7] Reference erythrocyte and leukocyte counts are determined using a single-channel semi-automated electronic counter that has been calibrated by threshold curve methods.[5,8] Packed cell volume (PCV) or hematocrit (Hct) is determined using the microhematocrit method without correction for trapped plasma.[10] The reference platelet count method is phase microscopy counting, which is very demanding (Chaps. 24 and 56).[1] Monitoring the RBC/PLT ratio along with the RBC count is suggested as a method to evaluate platelet calibration when RBC and PLT counting is performed in the same chamber on the same dilution.[1]

The numbers of fresh normal whole blood samples and number of required replicate tests are given in each reference method procedure. Calibration of multiparameter cell counters using reference methods and fresh whole blood specimens usually is reserved for the initial calibration of a new instrument when no other calibrated multiparameter instrument is available. Other simpler and less time-consuming methods which will be described are utilized to recalibrate instruments and to calibrate second- or third-generation instruments.

National Committee for Clinical Laboratory Standards (NCCLS), 940 West Valley Rd, Suite 1400, Wayne, PA 19087-1898.

Preserved Cells as Calibrators for Cell Counters

In the past, a common calibration procedure for cell counters was to adjust the instrument to target values on the insert sheet of a commercial control product. This practice is no longer acceptable. Although calibration procedures and control procedures share much in the way of materials and methods, they are fundamentally different. If the reference method results on fresh whole blood are not available or another calibrated instrument does not exist in the setting, commercial calibration material is available for purchase. *Commercial calibration material* has assigned values for each parameter with very narrow tolerance limits. These values are obtained by the manufacturer under strictly controlled conditions using instruments calibrated by whole blood reference methods and are specific for individual instrument–reagent systems. The manufacturers monitor their calibration products throughout the dated period (time prior to expiration) of each lot number. *Control material,* in contrast, is not as carefully monitored and does not have assigned values. Rather, controls have *ranges* for each measurement.

If commercial calibrating material is used to calibrate an instrument, the following precautions are recommended:

1. The manufacturer of the calibrating material should be different from the manufacturer of the control material to be used.
2. The directions from the manufacturer must be followed carefully.
3. The purchase of calibrating material should be handled differently from that of control material to avoid inadvertently keeping calibration material past its expiration date.

Statistical System for Calibration of Cell Counters

A statistical formula referred to as the *Bull algorithm*[3] (discussed later in this chapter) has been proposed as capable of acting as a calibrator. The algorithm is programmed into computers to perform a statistical analysis on patient red cell indices. The proposal to use this algorithm for instrument calibration is predicated on the predictability and stability of the sum total of patient red cell indices.

Calibration and Control of Other Equipment

Other equipment used in the hematology laboratory, such as centrifuges, balances, and dilutors, must also be properly calibrated and controlled. It is beyond the scope of this chapter to describe these procedures. Calibration of microscopes is covered in Chapters 4 and 24, Hct centrifuge and spectrophotometer calibration are discussed in Chapter 9, and detailed calibration and control methods for dilutors and balances may be found in standard reference texts for clinical chemistry.

The College of American Pathologists (CAP) publishes the *Laboratory Instrument Verification and Mainte-*

nance Manual, which includes information on requirements, regulations, and standards of the CAP, the Joint Commission on Accreditation of Healthcare Organizations (JCAHO), and NCCLS.[12] Sample forms for documentation, frequency, and type of maintenance required for all laboratory equipment are outlined in this publication.

Instrument Linearity

A part of overall instrument calibration should include an evaluation of linearity. That is, is there a quantitative value below or above which results are not reliable? An example might be that cell counts below $0.4 \times 10^9/L$ or above $100 \times 10^9/L$ are not accurate or reliable. Cell counts of very high levels are impacted by coincidence, whereas very low count recovery is impacted by background counts and increased imprecision. Increased statistical variation is a result of smaller and smaller numbers of cells being counted at the very low end of the count range. In-house linearity studies can be very time consuming. Most laboratories rely on linearity ranges published by the instrument manufacturer. Regardless of whether linearity ranges are established in-house or by the manufacturer, every laboratory should have written policies and procedures indicating the protocol to be followed for values exceeding the set ranges. For example, very high counts should be diluted to within the linear range and repeated and very low counts may be repeated using an instrument with a very low background count followed by a blood film review for verification.

USE OF CONTROLS

Any material used as a control for a test procedure should be as nearly identical as possible to the material being tested. Fresh whole blood is stable for only a short period before cell deterioration and death alters the results. Many routine hematology procedures can be performed on blood samples for up to 24 hours if the samples are refrigerated. Sample requirements, storage instructions, stability, and limitations should be written into the laboratory procedure manual.

Commercial Control Material

Automated cell counters prompted the development of commercially prepared control materials, which subsequently became the backbone of most hematology QC systems. Controls are also available commercially for sickle cell testing and Hb electrophoresis. Commercial controls and QC methods for coagulation are discussed in Chapter 58.

Commercial control material consists of blood cells (human, avian, porcine, and others) that have been altered to delay deterioration. The terms *fixed, buffered, stabilized,* or *preserved* have been used to describe this process. Nucleated avian red cells are used as "white cells" in some control material. Each manufacturer provides an expiration date for each lot number of control material, which refers to stability of the *unopened* bottle or vial. The information sheet that comes with each package indicates how long a vial should remain stable once it has been opened,

but this period will be greatly decreased if the material is not handled or stored properly. Evaporation and contamination must be avoided.

The primary function of commercial controls is to monitor the performance of automated cell counters on a continuing, long-term basis. Modifications of the manufacturing process have been made to include leukocyte subpopulations to monitor automated (2 to 6 part) differentials. The principal drawback of these materials is their relatively short shelf life. Month-to-month continuity in monitoring is difficult. Most hematology controls have a shelf life of at least 4 weeks. Further modification of the manufacturing process has extended the shelf life of some control materials to 2 months.

Control Levels

Most commercial hematology controls are available at three levels: normal, low, and high, based primarily on red cell parameters. Having three levels of control is a conceptual carryover from the chemistry laboratory, where it is necessary to check for appropriate substrate availability in enzyme testing, and the levels are relevant in the hemostasis laboratory. Substrate concentration is not a concern in cell counting or colorimetric tests such as Hb measurement and therefore, a single level of control material, preferably within the normal range, should be sufficient for these tests. Nevertheless, the CAP checklist for accreditation requires that at least two levels of controls be tested every 8 hours of operation.

The use of three levels of control material for cell counts may increase the chance of error secondary to improper handling or storage of the control. Questions that are raised include, what is done when one control level is "out of control" and the others are "in control"? How many times does an abnormal-level control detect a problem with the instrument that is not detected by the normal-level control? Moreover, a high- or low-level control value that is beyond acceptable limits frequently is attributable to production problems of the control, especially when the normal-level control is within range.[9]

Target Values in Commercial Control Material

Producers of commercial controls supply an insert or assay sheet with statistical data for each lot number. The mean and range for each measurement are usually listed by instrument type regardless of the reagent system in use. Some companies determine the assay or target values in-house using their own reference methods, whereas other companies send their material to reference laboratories to gather a consensus for each instrument type represented on the assay sheet. The values that are recovered for each measurement differ from instrument to instrument of the same model, from one model to another (same company), and among instruments from different companies. In addition, the values may be reagent system dependent. Each individual instrument "sees" the altered blood product in its own manner, resulting in the generation of different target values and ranges. The method for target value assignment should be noted. Control limits are usually 2 standard deviations (SD) from the mean, but this should be confirmed.

Commercial material does deteriorate, even though it is common to think that it is perfectly acceptable until the expiration date. Shipping conditions and delivery can affect the status of the cells, and original target values may no longer be recovered. Once opened, contamination from the sampling tip (diluent) or flakes of dried control material (from lid) may alter value recovery. Improper storage also affects stability.

Procedures for Ensuring Validity with Commercial Controls

It is appropriate to overlap the use of old and new control lots when changing lots, because most control products change lots every 4 to 8 weeks. New lots should be validated before the old lot expires. Product changes attributable to shipping and delivery, as well as inaccurate target value assignment, may be detected during this overlap period. Assuming the new lot evaluation is performed using an instrument that is "in control," the mean of the control sample values represents the laboratory's target value for the new control lot. The new control lot is acceptable as long as this value is within the range printed on the manufacturer's assay sheet (preferably near the middle of the range).

The laboratory's target values do *not* have to match the manufacturer's target or mean values, but if target values outside the manufacturer's suggested ranges are recovered, either the new lot has deteriorated, it is incorrectly labeled, or the instrument is malfunctioning. The manufacturer should always be notified when control material is suspect, and that lot should not be used. If the laboratory's target values are within the specific range but are not the same as the mean specified by the manufacturer, the laboratory should adopt its own target values obtained during the control overlap testing period plus or minus the manufacturer's standard deviation range for that control. Instrument recalibration is not required. If control values continue to differ from the assayed values, then the laboratory's standard deviation index (SDI) should be checked. This appears on a monthly report generated by some commercial control manufacturers that compares results among peer laboratories. An SDI should remain less than 2.0 on primary measurements. If it is greater, a possible calibration bias should be investigated.

Additionally, a microhematocrit test should be performed on a random bottle from a new shipment of commercial control to evaluate the amount of color in the plasma. A pale pink color is not uncommon, but without a baseline color evaluation it is difficult to tell later if hemolysis caused by red cell destruction has occurred. Another clue to the acceptability of the control product is the histogram pattern produced on many multiparameter instruments. Abnormal patterns may indicate deterioration. If a platelet value is generated on a control product that does not contain platelets, the "platelets" are actually representative of debris, which is an indication of control

deterioration. All the above information, taken together, is useful in evaluating each bottle as well as the entire lot of control material.

Use of Unassayed Control Products

Some companies offer unassayed control products, although these products are not yet widely used. A concept being evaluated by the NCCLS and the manufacturing community proposes that the manufacturer stop assaying and including target means and ranges with control materials. This change has been suggested because every laboratory should establish its own values on each new lot number of control material when it is received.

Fresh Whole Blood Controls

There are several hematology procedures that must be controlled with fresh (less than 1-hour old) whole blood which cannot be purchased commercially. Examples of such procedures include the osmotic fragility and autohemolysis tests, the Kleihauer-Betke stain for fetal Hb, and the heat precipitation test for demonstration of unstable hemoglobin. Special staining procedures require slide preparations of fresh normal blood as controls. In recent years, some innovative methods of monitoring instrument stability have been developed using data from patient samples of fresh whole blood.

Fresh whole blood is the ideal control, because it is identical to the material being tested. Hemoglobin is stable for a number of days, but platelet and leukocyte counts are affected quickly by aging unless the sample is refrigerated, in which case fresh whole blood can safely be used as a control for 24 hours. It should be noted, however, that leukocyte subpopulations in fresh whole blood (five-part differentials) are stable for only 4 to 8 hours, depending on the instrument used. The reproducibility of the five-part differential will deteriorate as the sample ages. Sample age is critical because leukocyte subpopulations are identified according to how they are altered by the reagent system. Finally, platelet clump development over a 24-hour period may lower a platelet count.

WITHIN-DAY MONITORING

A small number of patient blood specimens should be tested repeatedly throughout a 24-hour day to monitor the reproducibility of all values, particularly those for leukocytes and platelets. Standard deviation (SD) and coefficient of variation (CV) information must be interpreted according to the number of observations (n) over the 24-hour period (*i.e.*, from all shifts) and the level or concentration of the values being measured. Repeat testing at least every 4 hours provides a minimum n of 6. If time permits, duplicate testing is encouraged to provide paired data, as well as to increase n to 12.

The concentration of cells greatly influences the SDs and CVs recovered for leukocyte and platelet counts. For example, if the CV limit is 3.0% for the leukocyte count precision check, this limit may be exceeded with a very low leukocyte count while the SD is well within the acceptable limits. A solution for this problem is to use only the SD for evaluation of low mean values. A second choice is to establish another set of limits for SD and CV for low values.

DAY-TO-DAY MONITORING

Fresh patient specimens that are tested, refrigerated for 24 hours, returned to room temperature, mixed, and tested again can also serve as a check on instrument reproducibility. These samples may be split and a portion used for within-day testing while the other portion is used for 24-hour testing. Five samples should be tested, and a mean for each determination should be established before refrigeration. The 24-hour mean is calculated and compared with the original mean. Differences between the two means are dependent on concentration. The original mean, plus or minus a variable percentage of the mean (which is determined by the laboratory), establishes the limits of acceptability. Plus or minus 0.5 g/dL should be the maximum limit of acceptability for Hb, which changes minimally over 24 hours. Deterioration of leukocyte or platelet counts is not uncommon and should be taken into account to avoid the incorrect conclusion that the instrument is out of control or has lost calibration. Leukocyte subpopulations (five-part differential) are *not* stable for 24 hours and cannot be controlled in this manner.

Frequency of Control Testing

Controls are used to monitor the calibration of instruments from day to day. Repeat testing of patient samples can be used to check instrument function from batch to batch, especially if an hour or more elapses between batches. In laboratories that have large workloads, repeat testing of the same patient sample (so-called secondary controls) should be done every 2 to 3 hours. More frequent checks are provided when a laboratory uses a moving average program (see later). Commercial material is too expensive to use as a batch-to-batch check. Testing of control material (commercial and/or patient) may be as frequent as each batch, every 2 to 3 hours, every shift, or from one 24-hour period to the next, or even less frequently in certain cases. When more than 100 patient samples are tested every 24 hours, the moving average program can provide sufficient information to allow commercial control testing to be done once per shift.

Procedures Without Controls

Despite all the technical advances of the last two decades, there remain hematology procedures that are difficult to control because appropriate control materials are not available. These include the erythrocyte sedimentation rate (a commercial control for ESR has recently been marketed but is not totally evaluated as yet) and manual leukocyte differential counts, eosinophil counts, and spinal fluid cell counts. In such cases, accuracy and reproducibility are maintained through strict attention to procedure and adequate testing and education of personnel. Manual reticulocyte counts were on this list until recently. Commercial controls are now available for manual and automated reticulocyte counting methods.

QUALITY CONTROL CHARTS AND THEIR INTERPRETATION

Many of the multiparameter hematology instrument systems include computer programs ("QC package") that automatically store and chart data for control materials. This is done for each control level, lot number, and test value. Instruments without QC packages may have QC data transferred to a personal computer for generation of monthly statistics and charts. Manual charting of the data may be required when a personal computer is not available and the instrument does not have an internal QC program. The mean ±2 SD range of a specific control lot is drawn on manually prepared charts. Every time values are determined on the control material, the results are plotted. The results and the charts should be reviewed regularly. Each lot of control must have its own set of charts.

Levey-Jennings Charts

Levey-Jennings charts are the most commonly used QC charts and consist of parallel lines representing the mean ± 1, 2, and 3 SD limits for a single control parameter (Fig. 45-1). Time is plotted along the horizontal axis and analyte concentration along the vertical axis. New charts must be prepared each time a new lot is placed in service.

When a particular determination is "in control," the data points fall within the ±2 SD limits and are scattered equally above and below the mean. Five percent of the data points are expected to fall between the 2 SD and 3 SD limits. When this occurs, repeating the control once should bring it back within the ±2 SD limits as long as an in-control situation exists. When two or more consecutive values fall between the 2 SD and 3 SD limits, the instrument is considered to be out of control. Any single value beyond ±3 SD is out of control. The problem and all corrective action taken must be recorded in a problem logbook, and controls should be tested after completion of maintenance or repair work to confirm that the problem has been resolved. Patient testing must stop immediately when control data indicates that the instrument is out of control. The problem log notations should include the time and date the instrument was taken out of service and (after successful repair and confirmation of being

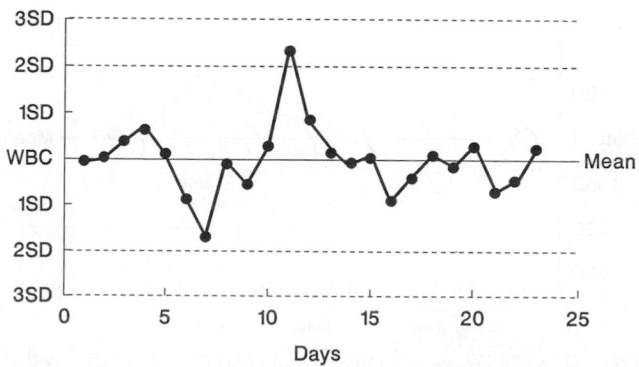

FIGURE 45-1. Levey-Jennings chart of WBC control results for 23 days with mean and 1, 2, and 3 SD limits indicated. Distribution is normal and in control.

back in control) the time and date the instrument was fixed and put back in service for patient testing. Patient samples tested just prior to detection of the problem must be retested (after repair). Sample retesting must identify samples with results that were affected by the problem and reports must be corrected.

Out-of-control situations may also be identified when reviewing control charts for trends or shifts, either of which suggests a change in instrument function or calibration. An example of a Levey-Jennings chart with acceptable results is shown in Figure 45-1. A downward shift is shown in Figure 45-2. An upward trend is also shown in the same figure with the successive data points being increasingly farther from the mean. Some situations that may cause a determination to be out of control are mechanical failure, power surges, improper equipment calibration, technical error, and reagent deterioration or contamination.

Youden Plots

Youden plots may be appropriate when two levels of control are used; however, these plots are not easily done without a computer program. A modified Youden plot displays single-parameter results from two different levels of control. The chart design is shown in Figure 45-3: a square with the center being the mean of both levels of control. The scaling is difficult to do manually. When both control results are acceptable, the data points will fall along a diagonal line from the lower left (2 SD) corner, as shown by the shaded area in Figure 45-3.

Plots that fall in the upper right or the lower left corner suggest random error, which usually is corrected by a single repeat of the control material. Plots falling in the upper left or lower right corners of the chart need immediate attention, because one control is reading too high and the other is reading too low. Patient results should not be reported until corrective action has fixed the problem and the patient samples have been retested under an in-control situation. Control results that fall in any of the four corners indicated as shaded areas on Figure 45-4 also mandate immediate corrective action on the instrument, because results in these areas indicate that

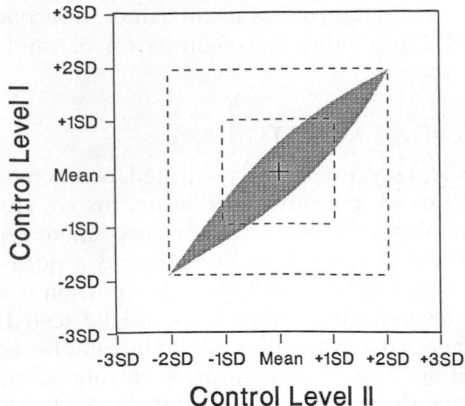

FIGURE 45-3. Modified Youden plot for two levels of control material, one plotted on X-axis (abscissa) and the second plotted on the Y-axis (ordinate). Mean 1, 2, and 3 SD are indicated. Shaded area indicates where results should fall to be in control.

both control results are beyond 2 SD. Only 1 in 20 test results is allowed to fall between the 2 SD and 3 SD limits.

Upward shifts and trends are identified on the Youden plot by the accumulation of dots above horizontal line A and to the right of vertical line B (see Fig. 45-4). Downward shifts and trends would be indicated by most dots falling below line A and to the left of line B.

Cumulative Sum Charts

A cumulative sum chart is another monitoring technique consisting of the summation of the differences of each control material test value from the expected value. This charting technique, commonly called *Cusum*, is not widely used. Once a target value or mean is established for a measurement, this value is subtracted from each subsequent value obtained. The difference is then added to the total of the previous days' differences to calculate the cumulative sum of the differences from the mean. Table 45-1 demonstrates the Cusum technique using a WBC control with a mean value of $4.7 \times 10^9/L$. This value may be plotted daily on a chart with a zero line and the Cusum

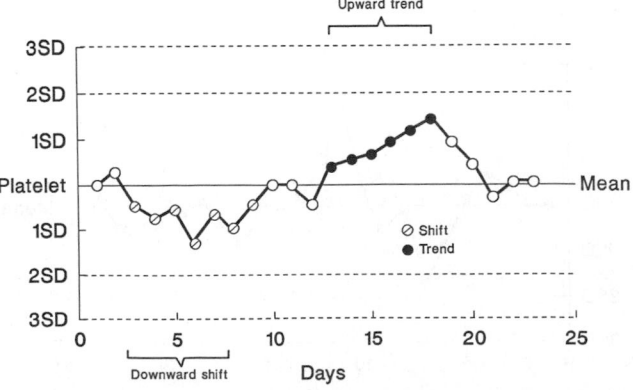

FIGURE 45-2. Levey-Jennings control chart of platelet data with downward shift and upward trend indicated. Trend is indicated by six successive data points with increasing (or decreasing) values relative to mean.

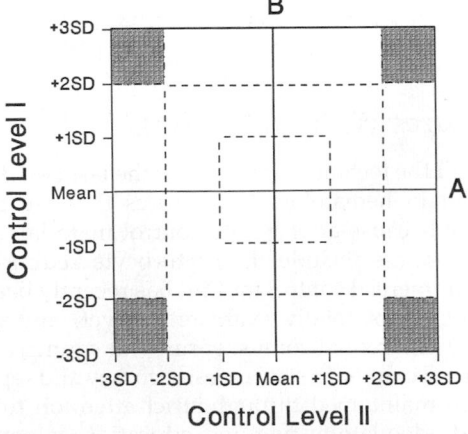

FIGURE 45-4. Youden plot with shaded areas indicating where both control values are beyond 2 SD. Such a result means stop immediately and troubleshoot to correct instrument problem before resuming patient testing.

TABLE 45-1
Calculation of Cumulative Sum (Cusum) During First 18 days of January for Normal WBC Count Control*

Date	WBC Control Results ($\times 10^9$/L)	Difference from Mean ($\bar{x} = 4.7 \times 10^9$/L)	Cumulative Sum (Cusum) of Differences from Mean
1	4.8	0.1	0.1
2	4.7	0.0	0.1
3	4.7	0.0	0.1
4	4.5	−0.2	−0.1
5	4.6	−0.1	−0.2
6	4.7	0.0	−0.2
7	4.6	−0.1	−0.3
8	4.9	0.2	−0.1
9	4.8	0.1	0.0
10	4.8	0.1	0.1
11	4.7	0.0	0.1
12	4.5	−0.2	−0.1
13	4.5	−0.2	−0.3
14	4.6	−0.1	−0.4
15	4.9	0.2	−0.2
16	4.6	−0.1	−0.3
17	4.5	−0.2	−0.5
18	4.7	0.0	−0.5

* *Results are plotted in Figure 45-5.*

plotted as shown in Figure 45-5. Ideally, the Cusum of the differences remains around zero, as the Cusum will alternate in sign (positive and negative). An out-of-control situation may be indicated when the Cusum constantly falls on one side of the zero line, indicating a shift or trend. A statistically significant difference is not necessarily medically significant. The Cusum chart is very sensitive to systematic errors but not to random errors (Chap. 46). Therefore, another monitoring device such as the

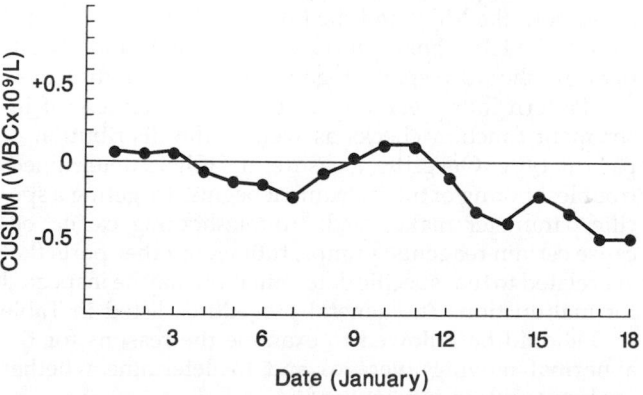

FIGURE 45-5. Cumulative sum (Cusum) difference graph for WBC count control for first 18 days of month. (Calculations are shown in Table 45-1). Days 12 through 18 show downward shift, indicating that WBC is out of control. Problem must be determined and corrected before running any more patient samples.

Levey-Jennings chart should be used in conjunction with the Cusum.

Monthly Control Performance Reports

Monthly control performance reports should be generated for each lot number of commercial control to summarize its performance. The report should include charts for each measurement and level of control material tested and the final mean, SD, and CV for each parameter. Many vendors provide a computer service for their customers that generates monthly reports that include all of this information plus comparisons with other laboratories using the same lot number and instrumentation. Monthly statistics are required by CAP for laboratory accreditation. Evidence of data/report review is also required by CAP along with documentation of corrective action taken for each point on each chart (*e.g.*, Levey-Jennings) that is out of control.

STATISTICAL SYSTEM FOR QUALITY CONTROL

A statistical formula known as the Bull algorithm was developed by Bull and colleagues in 1974[3] as an alternative method for monitoring instrument accuracy. Other names for this algorithm include moving average indices, moving averages, and $\bar{x}_B$ (pronounced x-bar-b).

The rationale for the Bull algorithm is based on the following findings:

1. Analysis of erythrocyte indices from various hospitals in different regions of the United States and the world revealed that the mean MCV, MCH, and MCHC are similar for the various population groups.
2. The average indices from acute care facilities were shown to be stable from day to day, week to week, and month to month, and the mean values of the indices were found to be the same in a study of acute care centers in the United States, Japan, and Wales. The "international" means are MCV = 89.5 ± 1.5 fL, MCH = 30.5 ± 0.5 pg, and MCHC = 34 ± 0.5 g/dL.[2]
3. The mean values may differ if the patient population mix is not similar to that found in an acute care center. For example, oncology or pediatric patient populations may have different mean values from those predicted for an acute care center; therefore, every laboratory must establish its own mean indices values.

The target values of the indices should be established using an instrument whose calibration is carefully controlled. One thousand patient samples is ideal, but as few as 250 will suffice to establish the mean index values *if* the resulting values correspond to the international mean index values. Once the mean value for each red cell index has been established for a given laboratory's patient population, the Bull algorithm is applied to evaluate the indices of consecutive groups of patient specimens as they are processed. The algorithm analyzes the data and provides the operator with an error message or flag when abnormalities in the moving averages are detected.

The Bull algorithm provides a sensitivity of 1% to changes in instrument calibration or patient population when the batch size is set at 20 samples.[11] The principal functions of the algorithm are to "smooth" and "trim" the data in each new batch. Smoothing is accomplished by incorporating previous batch data in the formula, giving it a weight of 40%, and giving new batch data a weight of 60% on the new mean. Trimming is accomplished by using the square root function. This proportionately decreases the effect of outliers within a batch, thus reducing the possibility of abnormal samples causing the moving averages to be out of control.

The beauty of the moving average program is that the control material *is* the tested material (*i.e.*, patient samples become control samples) making this control material *identical* rather than similar to the tested material. Laboratories that test more than 100 patient samples daily should consider the purchase of a hematology cell counter that incorporates the Bull algorithm program. The purchase of a computer into which patient data can be transferred is an alternative means for a laboratory with sufficient workload but having an instrument that is not already programmed for moving average indices.

Calculation of each RBC index is based on two measurements, either RBC count, Hb, or Hct, as shown in Table 45-2. This pairing, combined with the narrow range of indices values compatible with life, leads to the unique monitoring system described by Bull. The limits of acceptable operation are set at 3% of the mean. Sample testing must stop and corrective action must be taken when two consecutive batch calculations are beyond the limits on two determinations simultaneously.

Figure 45-6 is an example of moving average indices charts representing data analyzed by an instrument computer program over 10 days of sample testing. The pattern displayed for MCH is the expected normal pattern, with all dots within the 3% limit and with bounding above and below the mean. The patterns for MCV and MCHC both show a drift toward the 3% limit. The MCV has remained within the limit; however, the most recent plots were above the mean rather than both above and below it, reflecting an upward shift. One dot on the MCHC chart has dropped below the lower limit, and the MCHC plots reflect a downward shift. The upward shift of the MCV, combined with the downward shift of the MCHC, points to a problem with the measurement that is common to both of these indices—the Hct. Looking again at Table 45-2, it would appear from the formulas for MCV and

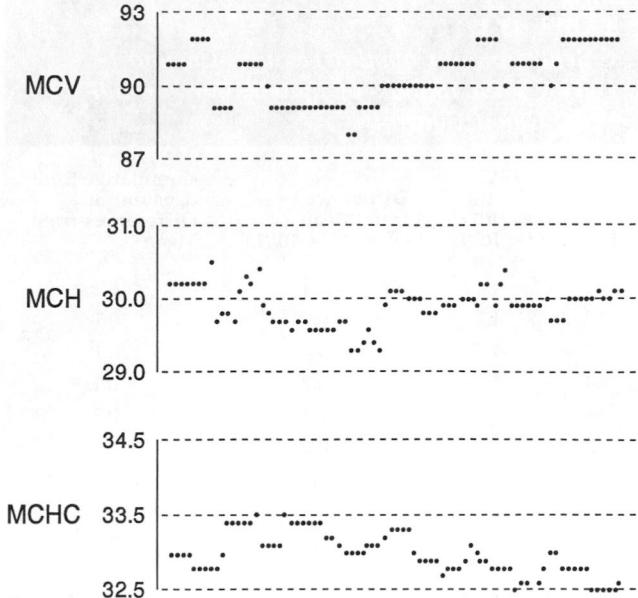

FIGURE 45-6. Charts of moving average indices (Bull moving averages). New moving average calculation of each batch of 20 patients is represented by successive dots. Only one dot (MCHC chart) is out of limits, but a pattern that warrants investigation is developing with MCV and MCHC. Situation is still in control, as only one dot of one indice has gone beyond 3% of mean limit. Measure of concern is Hct, because it is common to MCV and MCHC formulas (see Table 45-2). Retesting a few samples from earlier in-control batch may help confirm or rule out instrument problem involving Hct.

MCHC that the Hct value has shifted upward, causing the MCV to shift upward. In other words, because the Hct is in the numerator of the MCV formula and in the denominator of the MCHC formula, a change in Hct calibration will cause these indices to respond in opposite directions.

The RBC count is common to the MCV and MCH formulas, and because it is the denominator in both formulas, a change in RBC measurement will result in changes in the same direction for MCV and MCH. For example, an upward shift in the calibration of RBC would cause both the MCV and the MCH to show a downward shift. If the Hb calibration changes, the MCH and MCHC patterns should respond together in the same direction.

Pattern interpretation must include a review of instrument function checks as well as the distribution of patient type. Once the measure at fault is determined, troubleshooting of the instrument begins. Targeting a specific parameter makes such troubleshooting easier, because certain reagents, pumps, tubing, or other parts that are related to that specific determination may be inspected for malfunction. The general procedures listed in Table 45-3 should be followed to examine the reasons for the abnormal moving averages and to determine whether corrective action is required.

Finally, as mentioned in the section on calibration, it should be noted that although the Bull algorithm was developed as a monitoring (control) device, the mean target values of the indices program are so predictable

---

TABLE 45-2
Erythrocyte Indices Formulas

$$MCV = \frac{Hct \times 10}{RBC}$$

$$MCH = \frac{Hb \times 10}{RBC}$$

$$MCHC = \frac{Hb \times 100}{Hct}$$

Note that each index is calculated from two measured parameters: either Hct, RBC count, or Hb. These formulas are used both in the diagnosis of hematologic abnormalities and as a monitoring system for instrument malfunction.

TABLE 45-3
Procedures for Determining Cause of Abnormal Moving Averages

1. Check type of samples run in batch in question.
2. Check instrument calibration and precision with a control.
3. Visually inspect reagents and instrument.
4. Troubleshoot instrument.
5. Rerun samples from batch with moving averages error flag.

TABLE 45-4
Steps for Troubleshooting a Malfunctioning Instrument

1. Rerun last sample tested.
2. Rerun previously run normal control specimen.
3. Review maintenance logbook.
4. Inspect visually for leaks, disconnected tubes, wires, reagent depletion.
5. Observe for persistent abnormality.
6. Review QC data (*e.g.*, look for shifts or trends).
7. Identify specific nature of problem.
   a. Search problem logbook for similar problems in past.
   b. Check troubleshooting section of instrument manual.
8. Notify supervisor and manufacturer's service department as needed.
9. Complete all necessary adjustments to correct problem(s).
10. Document all symptoms and corrective action taken; note duration of down time.
11. Repeat controls to ensure return to proper functioning state.

and stable that it has since been proposed that they can also be used for instrument calibration. In conjunction with reference Hb or Hct determinations, they are proposed for use in calibration of red cell parameters.

INSTRUMENT MAINTENANCE

Routine maintenance procedures are outlined in each manufacturer's instrument manual. Proper routine maintenance of all instruments such as cell counters, stainers, centrifuges, refrigerators, and automatic pipettes is essential to keep a laboratory functioning smoothly and to ensure reporting of accurate results. The key to the longevity and proper functioning of any instrument is good routine preventive maintenance. This point cannot be overemphasized. The best way to ensure proper care of an instrument is to follow the recommendations of the manufacturer for cleaning, lubrication, and replacement of expendable parts. This maintenance will minimize instrument down time and decrease the frustration of personnel. The CAP publishes guidelines for routine maintenance of laboratory instruments.[12] CAP accreditation checklists also require that the various maintenance procedures be documented and reviewed (at least monthly) by a supervisor to meet Health Care Financial Administration (HCFA) and the Clinical Laboratory Improvement Amendments (CLIA) requirements. See Federal Regulation of Clinical Laboratories at the end of the chapter.

TROUBLESHOOTING PROCEDURES

Difficulties encountered in troubleshooting an instrument problem are greatly reduced when a comprehensive preventive maintenance program and a reliable and sensitive QC program are in place. Problems must be approached calmly and in an orderly manner. Prompt identification of the true nature of the problem is essential. All symptoms must be recognized, and the order in which the events occurred must be established and documented. A sixth sense, intuition, should not be ignored; some individuals develop an uncanny sense for how an instrument is working. Familiarity with the instrument and experience are the best training available for instrument troubleshooting.

Diagnosis of a problem will be easier if the step-by-step approach outlined in Table 45-4 is taken.[4] All of these observations and, especially, observation of the exact sequence of events are crucial to a successful and rapid solution to an instrument problem. All of this information documented in a problem logbook can be used by company engineers to solve problems and as a reference when a problem recurs.

QUALITY CONTROL DOCUMENTATION

Laboratories must maintain records in accordance with accreditation requirements; documentation is the backbone of quality control programs. Procedure, safety, and laboratory policy manuals must be complete, reviewed yearly, and updated periodically. Patient result records and QC results, charts, and summaries with timely reviews documented are necessary for accreditation. Instrument maintenance records should include documentation of routine maintenance, periodic manufacturer preventive maintenance, and instrument problems, as well as the corrective actions taken. An instrument problem logbook is a vital part of a complete QC program. Step-by-step documentation of a problem is critical to the quick solution of an instrument problem. The following information should be included[4]:

1. Record the exact nature and frequency of the problem. Note whether it is consistent or sporadic.
2. Record the sequence of events. The sequence is important, especially when a second problem develops.
3. Identify measurements involved in the problem: are the cell counts involved, the Hb, the Hct, or the indices? If all measurements are affected, this may indicate a dilution malfunction, whereas a problem with a single measurement can eliminate certain malfunctions from consideration.
4. Identify the segment of the instrument cycle involved.

Is the problem in the diluting, counting, or calculating phase of the cycle?

5. Record all corrective actions. If several things appear to need fixing, fix one at a time and observe the effect on specimen results before fixing another. If several items are changed simultaneously, it is difficult to tell what solved the problem. Jumping in and fixing everything without documentation can lead to further problems.

A written record of all QC measures taken must be available for evaluation by accreditation inspectors. If a review or action taken is not documented, it did not take place, and the inspector will cite the laboratory for a deficiency.

INTERNAL LABORATORY MONITORING

Exchanges of patient samples and blood films between instruments within the same institution or between institutions in the local area constitute internal laboratory monitoring of hematology instruments and provide valuable QC information. Any laboratory that has at least two similar instruments in operation can set up an exchange of samples, which provides cross-comparison of results. The frequency of exchanging samples will differ depending on the distance separating the instruments, the type of transport system available, and the overall QC program that is in place. The use of some method to monitor consistency between instruments is a CAP requirement.

Blood film exchange on a weekly or bimonthly basis will identify areas of disagreement in cell type and morphology identification. This should prompt establishment of continuing education sessions that standardize the criteria for cell identification such as segmented *versus* band neutrophils, normal *versus* variant lymphocytes, or variant lymphocytes *versus* monocytes. The preparation of extra films and their subsequent exchange provides interesting, unusual, and stimulating cases from which individuals from several laboratories or shifts can learn. A method or program to monitor consistency between individuals performing manual WBC differentials (and body fluid differentials) is a CAP requirement.

When evaluating the results of sample exchange, it must be realized that results will differ somewhat from instrument to instrument. How much variation can be expected must be determined when all instruments are in control. There will be more variation among instruments from different manufacturers than among instruments of the same type and model. The main purpose of monitoring patient cell counts is to identify clinically significant changes. Within-instrument and instrument-to-instrument variation must remain below the clinically significant variation that prompts physician intervention.[6] Normal cell counts differ depending on the time of sample collection in relation to meals, physical activity, hydration, and other variables. Surgical trauma and medications also affect cell counts. A good QC program attempts to minimize the variations between instruments so that they do not mask these physiologic and pathologic variations.

EXTERNAL LABORATORY MONITORING

Regional Programs

Most large manufacturers of commercial controls offer free QC programs that monitor data from program participants. These data are analyzed, and a monthly report is distributed to the participating laboratories. The report usually includes mean, SD, and CV based on the laboratory's data. It also compares results from laboratories using the same instrumentation or methods. This peer group comparison provides one more piece of the puzzle for the overall picture of the QC program being used.

State Programs

Regulations concerning laboratory testing and personnel differ widely from state to state. Requirements range from none to proficiency testing or licensing requirements for laboratory personnel. The terms *proficiency testing* or *proficiency survey* refer to the practice of sending aliquots of the same sample (plasma, serum, preserved cells, blood films, or photomicrographs of cells) to all participating laboratories and collecting data for analysis and evaluation. Regulations differ according to the type of laboratory being evaluated (*i.e.*, state, independent or commercial, physician's office, or hospital). The state department of health usually is the branch of state government that provides proficiency testing, continuing education programs, and enforcement of existing regulations.

Federal Programs

The United States Centers for Disease Control and Prevention (CDC) offers limited continuing education programs and workshops for laboratory personnel but no longer provides interlaboratory survey programs. There are, however, federal regulations for clinical laboratories wishing to receive Medicare and Medicaid payments, which will be discussed.

Professional Programs

Hospital and laboratory accreditation is voluntary, but accreditation by the JCAHO is required for a hospital to receive Medicare and Medicaid payments. A JCAHO hospital inspection includes a review of the laboratory unless it is accredited by the CAP (JCAHO accepts CAP accreditation as comparable). CLIA'88 and HCFA rules have been incorporated into CAP checklist questions in order for CAP to obtain "deemed status" (*i.e.*, be a federally approved accrediting agency). Accredited laboratories participate in a proficiency survey program. Results from each laboratory are compared with those of other laboratories using the same methods. These surveys provide laboratories with an accuracy check. The mean of all participants is considered to be "truth." Acceptable performance guidelines (CLIA'88) are published in the *Federal Register* and in the *CAP Survey Manual* (published every year).

Evaluation of External Laboratory Monitoring Results

State-of-the-art information is provided by regional, state, federal, and professional programs. Analyses of these data provide valuable information about the performance of the various clinical laboratory services throughout the United States. As a general rule, good and acceptable performance by a laboratory on unknown samples includes all reported values that are within 2 or 3 SDs of the method mean. Data that fall beyond are judged as unacceptable performance. It is very important that one keep in mind the fact that statistically, 1 in 20 values should fall outside a 2 SD range. For the most part, the statistical limits are much tighter than the limits of variation that constitute a clinically significant change in the condition of a patient. When referees or referee laboratories do not agree or provide wide variation in results, that sample or parameter is not graded.

CLIA'88 (see following) rules now use proficiency testing as a regulatory tool. Tracking of the samples through the laboratory (receipt, storage, preparation, testing, *etc.*) is required. Survey samples are to be tested with the regular workload by regular testing personnel with a signed statement to that affect being part of the final report. In the past many laboratories handled survey samples with special care that did not reflect routine testing conditions under which patient samples were tested. This practice is no longer acceptable.

Federal Regulation of Clinical Laboratories

Throughout this chapter reference has been made to CLIA'88 (Clinical Laboratory Improvement Amendments of 1988), and the various agencies and programs that monitor the quality of service provided by laboratories. CLIA'88 is the result of continued evaluation and development of regulations and standards for the clinical laboratory and associated industries. These regulations began with CLIA'67. The government agencies responsible for regulating clinical laboratory services are the Healthcare Financial Administration (HCFA) and the Food and Drug Administration (FDA) with advice from the CDC. HCFA has the responsibility and authority to monitor the use of medical devices as they are used by laboratories providing services to the medical community. This is done through various regulations and standards that define the quality control requirements and personnel requirements in certain instances that must be met by the laboratories. FDA regulates manufacturing by the medical device industry. Regulations cover market entry, production and distribution of instruments, reagents, and systems used in the clinical laboratories. CDC provides technical and scientific expertise for HCFA and the FDA. Laboratory accreditation is accomplished by meeting the standards and regulations set forth by HCFA and CLIA'88. Laboratory inspection is carried out by a recognized accrediting agency with deemed authority from HCFA or by HCFA. Several state agencies, JCAHO, CAP, American Association of Blood Banks (AABB), and other agencies unrelated to laboratory hematology have authority to evaluate and accredit laboratories. CAP checklists (beginning in 1994) have "new standards" that meet those set forth by CLIA'88. Regulations and standards of practice will most probably continue to evolve over time.

CHAPTER SUMMARY

Two fundamental areas of quality control (QC) for systematic error are calibration of instruments so that they generate accurate data and monitoring (controlling) the instruments over time to be sure they remain accurate. Three monitoring methods are frequently used: (1) commercial control materials; (2) blood samples from patient sources; and (3) the Bull algorithm. The latter incorporates patient data into a statistical formula and updates the data after every batch of 20 patient samples. Combinations of these three procedures provide most laboratories with an effective and cost-manageable means of detecting a systematic error.

If a computerized system for maintaining records of control material results is not available, the laboratory may choose to plot control results using Levey-Jennings charting methods (see Figs. 45-1 and 45-2) which may be supplemented by charts using the cumulative sum (Cusum) method (see Fig. 45-5 and Table 45-1). A more difficult manual charting system is the Youden plot, which is used to plot a normal and abnormal level control on the same chart (see Figs. 45-3 and 45-4). Study of the patterns of these charts indicates whether the instrument is in control. When it is out of control, instrument troubleshooting is required before patient samples may be run.

Documented instrument maintenance and troubleshooting are critical components of any QC program. Internal and external monitoring systems provide the final component of a total QC program. Frequent exchanges among laboratories within the same or closely located institutions constitute internal systems; subscription external programs at the state, regional, and federal levels provide information regarding accuracy among laboratories across the United States.

JCAHO, CAP, and several other agencies are federally approved to inspect and accredit clinical laboratories. Performance of QC activities, documentation and documented review of procedures, logs, and charts are critical to successful laboratory inspection and accreditation as well as to the reporting of accurate patient results.

Case Study 45-1

A fresh whole blood sample was selected as an in-house control to monitor instrument precision for 24 hours. It was refrigerated and tested every 3 hours during the 24-hour period. The following results were obtained:

Time Tested	WBC ($\times 10^9$/L)	RBC ($\times 10^{12}$/L)	Hb (g/dL)	Hct (L/L)	MCV (fL)	PLT ($\times 10^9$/L)
08:00	8.53	3.32	10.3	0.297	89.5	188
11:00	8.51	3.31	10.2	0.296	89.4	180
14:00	8.62	3.36	10.3	0.298	88.7	164
14:03	8.67	3.33	10.3	0.297	89.2	162
17:00	8.70	3.34	10.2	0.296	88.6	153

The target values for the counts were established at 07:00 a.m. as follows: WBC 8.58; RBC 3.33; Hb 10.2; Hct 0.298; MCV 88.6; and PLT 190. The expected performance limits are: WBC ±0.5; RBC ±0.07; Hb ±0.2; Hct ±0.006; MCV ±1; and PLT ±10.

1. Are there sufficient data to evaluate for trends or shifts?

2. Evaluate each set of results. Is any parameter out of control? If so, which parameter(s) and why?
3. List at least one disadvantage and one advantage of using fresh whole blood as control material.

Review Questions

45-1. Calibration of a new hematology analyzer is easily and quickly accomplished using

    A. fresh whole blood and reference count methods.
    B. commercial calibration material.
    C. unassayed control material.
    D. assayed control material.

45-2. Purchased quality control materials for hematology analyzers are primarily used to monitor

    A. control parameter tolerance limits.
    B. fresh whole blood response over time.
    C. expected target value changes of parameters over time.
    D. reproducibility of parameter values over time.

45-3. Charting of hematology QC data is most frequently done using

    A. Cusum charts.
    B. scatter plots.
    C. Youden plots.
    D. Levey-Jennings charts.

45-4. The square root function of the moving average algorithm of Bull

    A. diminishes the effect of outliers.
    B. weights previous batch data.
    C. eliminates outliers from the mean.
    D. identifies outliers for further evaluation.

45-5. HCFA is the federal government regulatory agency that oversees clinical laboratory compliance with regulations and standards set forth by the

    A. College of American Pathologists (CAP).
    B. Clinical Laboratory Improvement Amendments of 1988 (CLIA'88).
    C. Centers for Disease Control and Prevention (CDC).
    D. American Society for Clinical Laboratory Science (ASCLS).

References

1. Bull BS: Quality assurance strategies. In Koepke JA (ed): Practical Laboratory Hematology, pp 12–14. New York, Churchill Livingstone, 1991
2. Bull BS, Hay KL: Are red cell indices international? Arch Pathol Lab Med 109:604, 1985
3. Bull BS, Elashoff RM, Heilbron DC et al: A study of various estimators for the derivation of quality control procedures from patient erythrocyte indices. Am J Clin Pathol 61:473, 1974
4. Dotson MA: Troubleshooting multichannel hematology instruments. Lab Perspect 1:9, 1982
5. Groner W: Standardization of multiparameter instruments for blood cell counting and sizing. In Cavill I (ed): Quality Control, 2nd ed, pp 39–42. New York, Churchill Livingstone, 1990
6. Groner W: Standardization of multiparameter instruments for blood cell counting and sizing. In Cavill I (ed): Quality Control, 2nd ed, pp 46–48. New York, Churchill Livingstone, 1990
7. International Committee for Standardization in Haematology: Recommendations for reference method for haemoglobinometry in human blood, ICSH Standard EP 6/2, 1977; and Specifications for international hemiglobincyanide reference preparation, ICSH Standard EP 6/3, 1977. J Pathol 31:139, 1978
8. Koepke JA: Quantitative blood cell counting. In Koepke JA (ed): Practical Laboratory Hematology, pp 51–52. New York, Churchill Livingstone, 1991
9. Levy WC, Bull BS, Koepke JA: The incorporation of red blood cell index mean data into quality control programs. Am J Clin Pathol 86:193, 1986
10. National Committee for Clinical Laboratory Standards (NCCLS): Procedure for Determining Packed Cell Volume by the Microhematocrit Method—Second edition, Approved Standard H7-A, vol 5, no 5. Villanova, PA, NCCLS, 1993
11. Skonie V: Hematology quality control–A continuing education course in print. Lab World 29:14, 1978
12. Sodeman TM, Floering DA, Mozdzem JJ Jr et al: Laboratory Instrument Verification and Maintenance Manual, 4th ed. Skokie, IL, College of American Pathologists, 1989

Recommended Reading

College of American Pathologists: CAP Survey Manual. Northfield, IL, CAP, 1995

Gilmer PR, Williams JL: The status of methods of calibration in hematology. Am J Clin Pathol 74:600, 1980

Gilmer PR, Williams JL, Koepke JA et al: Calibration methods for automated instruments. Am J Clin Pathol 68:185, 1977

Lewis SM, Koepke JA (eds): Hematology Laboratory Management and Practice. Oxford, Butterworth-Heinemann Ltd, 1995

National Committee for Clinical Laboratory Standards (NCCLS): Performance Goals for the Internal Quality Control of Multichannel Hematology Analyzers, Approved Standard H26-A. Wayne, PA, NCCLS, 1996

CHAPTER 46

Methods to Monitor and Control Random Error

John A. Koepke

Definition

Quality Control and Random Error
Controlling Minor and Major Random Error
Strategies for the Prevention of Random Error
Strategies for the Detection of Random Error

Use of Instrument and Laboratory Information Systems for the Detection of Random Errors
Detection of Unusual Results
Detection of Data Entry Errors
Delta Checks
Computer-Generated Reports

A System for the Detection and Control of Laboratory Errors

Objectives

1. Define random errors and give at least five examples.
2. List six strategies for prevention and detection of random errors and give examples of each.
3. Define multivariate check and give four examples.
4. Discuss the advantages of a laboratory information system in detecting random errors.
5. Define delta check, state two methods for its calculation and two methods for its determination, and list several laboratory values for which it is useful.
6. Describe the four categories of laboratory errors.

DEFINITION

Laboratory errors can be defined simply as mistakes; random errors are mistakes that occur without a definable pattern or frequency. In a perfect world, no errors are made, and the results of a laboratory analysis are always accurate and precise. Unfortunately, we do not live in a perfect world and our quality control programs may not always discover laboratory errors.[4] Systematic errors (Chap. 45) differ from random errors in that the former are regularly occurring deviations in a test "system," in contrast to the haphazard nature of random errors. Random errors may affect quantitative or qualitative tests. Errors affecting quantitative tests have a varying impact on patient care, primarily depending on the degree of error. However, errors affecting qualitative

tests, which may simply indicate either a yes–no answer (a normal or an abnormal result), can be more problematic. This chapter will focus on the detection of random errors (both quantitative and qualitative) and their prevention.

Each laboratory procedure has intrinsic imprecision or, in other words, *minor random errors* caused by factors beyond the laboratory scientist's control, which therefore cannot be avoided. These imprecisions are continuously operative and are caused by small fluctuations in the analyzing system. Examples include the inherent unpredictable motion of particles in a suspension (*e.g.*, blood cells in a diluting fluid) moving rapidly in a flowing stream through a flow cell or over the surface of a glass slide.

A test method's inherent imprecision or random error is demonstrated numerically when a specimen is repeatedly analyzed and a standard deviation (SD) is calculated. The SD expresses a method's variability in absolute terms while a coefficient of variation (CV) expresses the variation in proportional terms (Chap. 44). Both SD and CV describe the dispersion of individual values around the mean value and are indicative of the method's reproducibility. Larger SDs or CVs indicate poor precision. It is the goal of the laboratory to be sure that the amount of error is limited as much as possible to the inherent imprecision and is not increased by other errors.

Major random errors are mistakes or blunders that occur haphazardly and can have a significant impact on patient care. These errors cause a greater loss of precision and accuracy than normal and occur in an unpredictable fashion that differs from one sample to the next. Some examples are listed in Table 46-1.

QUALITY CONTROL AND RANDOM ERROR

Controlling Minor and Major Random Error

Although most quality control (QC) procedures in hematology adequately measure the amount of small inherent random error and systematic error in a test procedure, they do not detect or control the major random errors. Systematic errors are detected and measured using com-

TABLE 46-1
Some of the Random Errors Observed in Clinical Laboratories

1. Specimen is labeled with wrong name, and results are reported on wrong patient.
2. Results are recorded on wrong requisition and reported on wrong patient.
3. Air bubble is trapped in bottom of sample cup of an analyzer that samples from bottom, resulting in a short sample.
4. EDTA-anticoagulated specimen is not mixed well at the time of collection, resulting in formation of a fibrin clot and platelet clumping. Specimen is not checked for fibrin and is used for a platelet count.
5. While a specimen is held for sampling on an automated cell counter, the sample probe is not placed deep enough during aspiration, resulting in a short sample.
6. An EDTA-anticoagulated specimen is not mixed well prior to sampling, resulting in a concentration of cells in the lower portion of the collection tube. The aliquot for counting is collected from the upper portion of the tube.
7. While recording a prothrombin time from the printout of an automated coagulation instrument, the technologist reads 12.8 seconds but writes 18.2 seconds.
8. While performing a manual WBC count on a serous fluid, the technologist misreads the meniscus in the pipette and underdilutes the specimen by 10 μL.

mercially prepared control materials and patient samples that are analyzed periodically and compared with established control ranges. Random errors, by their unpredictable nature, will not be detected with control samples unless the error happens to occur while analyzing the control. Therefore, other strategies must be employed to prevent and detect potentially harmful random error.

Strategies for the Prevention of Random Error

LABORATORY STAFF SENSITIVITY

The best defense against a significant random error is an alert laboratory staff. If the analyst knows where the pitfalls and problems may be in a procedure and is vigilant in guarding against their occurrence, the chance of an accident or error greatly decreases. There can be no substitute for this, nor can its importance be overemphasized. All of the quality control and quality assurance programs that have been and will be instituted to prevent errors and mistakes are no better than the laboratory workers who perform the analyses and produce the results. Continuing education programs are useful in keeping levels of awareness of potential problems high and should be regularly scheduled.

CURRENT PROCEDURE MANUALS

Clearly written and comprehensive specimen collection and technical procedure manuals provide the blueprints for a well-structured error prevention program. Procedure manuals outlining the materials required in a technical procedure and the step-by-step instructions for per-

forming it will help to reduce errors caused by ignorance. Careful adherence to instructions by the staff is required for consistent performance.

PROPER INSTRUMENT MAINTENANCE

Properly maintained instruments are less likely to be the source of random and systematic errors than are marginally maintained instruments. The manufacturer's instructions and recommendations for routine preventive maintenance should be incorporated into a documented daily, weekly, and monthly schedule and logged when such maintenance is performed. All auxiliary equipment such as pipettes, dilutors, and waterbaths should also be maintained to deliver reliable service. Well-maintained instrumentation will increase the confidence of the operator in its abilities to produce error-free results.

Strategies for the Detection of Random Error

EVALUATE REASONABLENESS OF TEST RESULTS

For each sample, the operator should review the result to consider whether it is a reasonable value, one that is compatible with life or at least with the patient's state of health.[1] For example, an erythrocyte count of $0.70 \times 10^{12}/$ L is unreasonably low and should be investigated to see whether there was short sampling, the specimen was diluted with intravenous fluid, or the specimen is not peripheral blood but some other type of fluid such as a bloody abdominal or cerebrospinal fluid incorrectly labeled and processed as whole blood. Simple evaluation of the reasonableness of a value is the first step in detecting an error. The flow chart in Figure 46-1 outlines a simple strategy which the instrument operator can use for determining whether or not an individual test result is reasonable. With laboratory computerization, such strategies can be more fully implemented to cover the complete analytic process.

SPECIMEN INTEGRITY

The following list details actions, in addition to those in Figure 46-1, that can be taken at the time of analysis to reduce random errors.

1. Double check the name on the specimen requisition against the name label on the specimen at the time of analysis to avoid sample mix-ups, one of the more common random errors.
2. Use a wooden applicator stick or toothpick to stir all specimens prior to analysis on an automated cell counter. The wood may pick up small pieces of fibrin that could be present and make the sample unacceptable for analysis. Cell counts inadvertently performed on samples containing clots will be falsely decreased because of entrapment of cells in the clot. Also, small fibrin clots aspirated into the analyzer may clog sample tubing, causing the analyzer to perform inaccurately.
3. Inspect all pipetted specimens visually to see if it appears that the appropriate volume of sample has been delivered and that inappropriate air bubbles have not

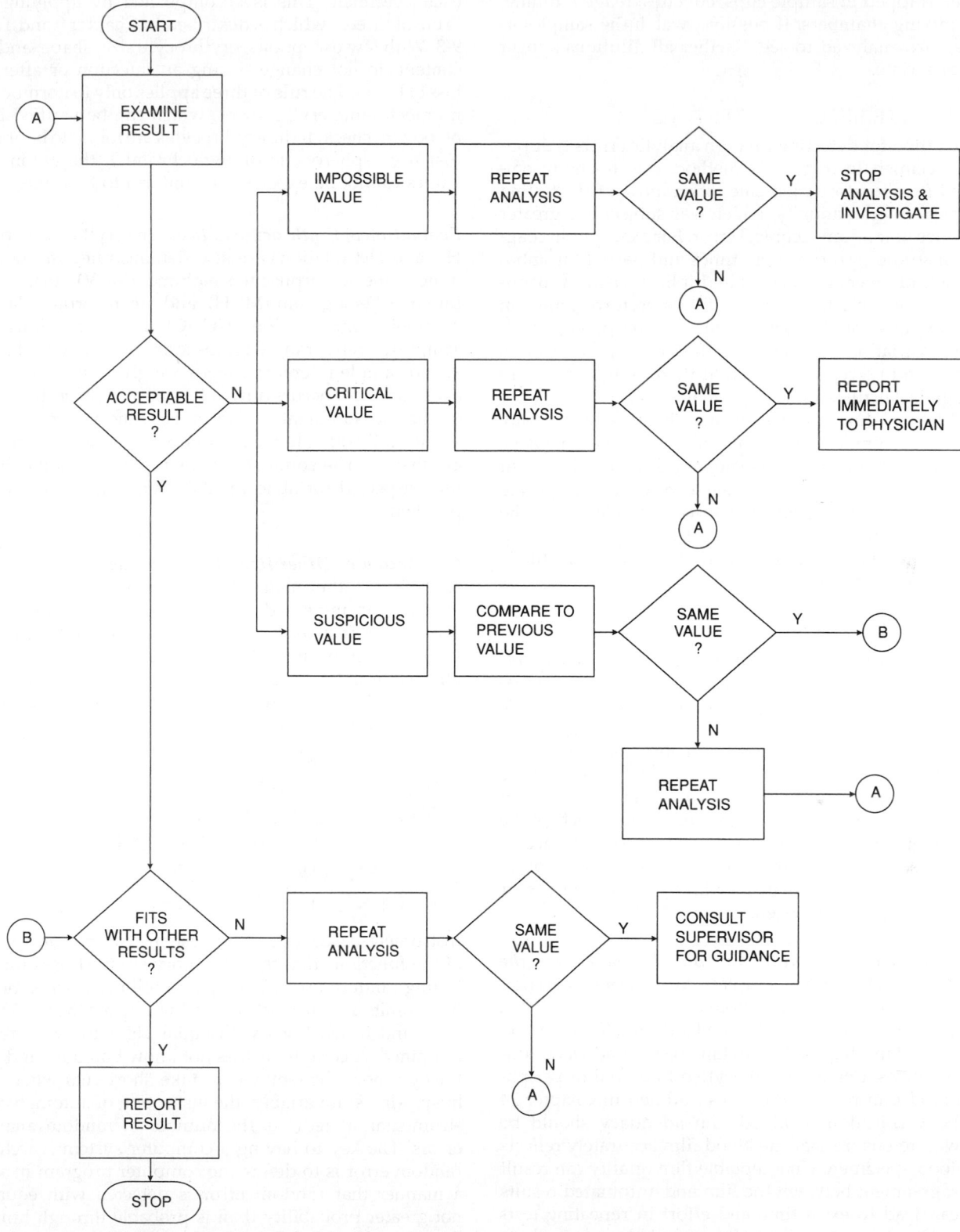

FIGURE 46-1. Flow chart for evaluation of test result for random error: A simple strategy for determining whether individual test result is reasonable and correlates with other results. Y, yes; N, no. Symbols *A* and *B* show interconnection between results of evaluation of repeat testing and where decision-making strategy should resume (far left). For example, if an impossible value is obtained, and repeat analysis does not show same value, uppermost horizontal line of chart says that testing procedure should return to symbol *A*, where the steps are begun again with EXAMINE RESULT. Adapted from Cembrowski GS: Use of patient data for quality control. Clin Lab Med 6:715, 1986, with permission.

been trapped in sample cups, cuvettes, reagent tubing, or mixing chambers. If possible, watch the samples as they are analyzed to see whether all dilutions appear appropriate.

DUPLICATE SPECIMEN TESTING

One method for detecting random analytic errors is duplicate specimen testing. This method was formerly employed in laboratory medicine when more of the testing was performed manually, which was subject to a greater incidence of random technical error. For example, in coagulation studies, prothrombin times and partial thromboplastin times were performed in duplicate using a coagulometer. Some electronic cell counters perform counts in duplicate or triplicate. The counts are compared, and if there is variation outside a specified range, the result is rejected and no report is given. If there is agreement, an average is calculated and reported.

Whereas duplicate testing may be an effective way to discover significant random errors, it can be expensive and time-consuming and may not be justified with current highly precise analyzers. When considering duplicate testing, the time and effort involved in relation to the number of random errors detected by duplicate testing should be weighed and compared to alternative methods for eliminating random errors.

MULTIVARIATE CHECKS

Multivariate checks are a form of QC in which the interrelations (correlations) between different tests and the measurements within a test are compared with acceptable limits to detect random errors. Certain hematologic tests lend themselves to comparison with other measurements, and when these comparisons are performed on a routine basis, many spurious results can be detected. Some of these comparisons can be performed at the bench as the specimen is analyzed, whereas others require either access to the medical record, the patient's physician, or other laboratory results as available through a laboratory or hospital information system.

Comparison of the Automated Blood Count with the Blood Film. One of the simplest correlations is accomplished by comparing the automated leukocyte, platelet, and differential counts with the blood film. This method is discussed in Chapter 24 in detail. Every time a laboratorian performs a manual leukocyte differential or peripheral blood film review, the steps outlined in Chapter 24 for the verification of blood film adequacy should be followed to ensure that the blood film accurately reflects the blood specimen. Unacceptable film quality can result in disagreement between the film and automated results and can lead to extra time and effort in repeating tests for results that were originally correct. In cases where there is disagreement between the automated blood count and the film estimate, a new blood film should be prepared and reviewed and the automated count should be repeated.

Rule of Three. Another correlation that can be checked is that of the erythrocyte count, Hb, and Hct agreement for each specimen. This is accomplished by applying the "rule of three," which is described in Chapter 9 and Table 9-3. With few exceptions, erythrocyte size, shape, and Hb content do not change during an infection or after the loss of blood. The rule of three applies only to normocytic, normochromic erythrocytes, which can be verified by a blood film check. If the erythrocytes are found to be abnormal (*e.g.,* spherocytic or hypochromic), the automated values cannot be expected to conform to this rule.

Evaluation of Erythrocyte Indices. The erythrocyte count, Hb, and Hct relations are also demonstrated in the RBC indices mean corpuscular volume (MCV), mean corpuscular hemoglobin (MCH), and mean corpuscular hemoglobin concentration (MCHC). The calculations and sample reference ranges for these are reviewed in Chapter 9, and sample reference ranges are given in Table 9-1. If a random error occurs during the counting of erythrocytes or the measurement of Hb or Hct, the indices will be significantly outside the reference ranges, and the results are suspect. The count should be repeated and the blood film inspected for abnormalities that might point to the problem.

Correlation of Other Hematology Values. Correlation of results with other hematology values can be helpful. For example, an increased reticulocyte count should correspond with increased polychromasia on the blood film. If there is a computer information system that can supply other clinical data, or if there is good communication with the physician, correlations can also be established with other clinical information.

USE OF INSTRUMENT AND LABORATORY INFORMATION SYSTEMS FOR THE DETECTION OF RANDOM ERRORS

Instrument-based operating systems can perform many of the functions that the laboratory scientist uses for detecting random error. The system follows a series of defined limits and instructions and will apply these calculations and instructions with equal vigor to every result examined. A computer does not know boredom and distraction, nor is it tempted to take short cuts when it is busy. Almost invariably, the institution of automated instrumentation reduces the number of random analytic errors. The key to having a computer system search for random error is to define the computer program in such a manner that random error is detected with equal if not greater probability than is probable through human detection. Much of the same logic used to contemplate the validity of a test result can be used in defining the program instructions. However, a word of caution: computer detection of random error is no better than the thought and logic put into the program. Computers will be just as consistent in not detecting errors as they are in detecting errors if the programming is not comprehensive.

Detection of Unusual Results

The computer can check each result to establish whether it is reasonable, *i.e.*, to see if the value falls within the physiologic range compatible with life. If not, the value is flagged to alert the operator, and automatically the value is rejected. For example, a Hb of 1.0 g/dL for a whole blood specimen would be rejected because it is not compatible with life (see Fig. 46-1). This practice should be extended, not only to computer-interfaced analyzers, but also to results entered manually on the computer. The individual responsible for entering a rejected result after it has been verified as correct must take some distinct action to force acceptance of the value by the computer system if it falls outside the specified limits.

Detection of Data Entry Errors

To detect random data entry errors, the laboratory information system can be programmed to check the validity of entered data by performing a variety of calculations and other checks. For example, a search for correct decimal placement in the entries can be performed on each blood count. A manual differential count can be checked by the computer to see if it equals 100%. Many other calculations can be used to detect data entry errors.

A laboratory information system can perform sophisticated multivariate checks. Samples with a low MCV can be flagged, and the erythrocyte morphology report from an accompanying blood film review can be checked to see whether the cells are indeed microcytic. A specimen with low serum iron levels can be checked to see whether the Hb and RBC indices are also low. Because of access to a larger database and the computer's ability to process information rapidly, the computer-generated multivariate check is more sophisticated than a human one. Multivariate checks are more useful when reviewing the patient's cumulative laboratory report than when reviewing any individual laboratory result.

Delta Checks

Perhaps the most dramatic impact of a laboratory information system on detection of random error is in the capability of performing delta checks. The *delta check* is a technique for the detection of random errors by comparison of a current result with the most recently reported result for any given patient. This method has been greatly advanced with the improvement of laboratory computer information systems. By accessing the laboratory patient database, the computer can rapidly perform a delta check on the measurements of each sample for each patient. Test-specific rules can be defined that spell out the maximum allowable differences in consecutive results on a single patient based on various defined time limitations between analytical tests. These rules determine whether the computer will flag a result and when.

One of the first manual delta check systems was described in 1974.[6] Today, delta checks for a specific patient involve either a manual or a computerized calculation of the difference between a current measurement and a previous measurement of an analyte or blood component and then a comparison of this difference with a predefined maximum allowable difference limit for that component.[2] When calculating the difference between consecutive measurements, the time that has elapsed between the measurements must be taken into consideration. For example, the operator or computer must consider whether the time lapse has been only hours, days, or months. The computer may be programmed to consider the time factor and compare the difference with a certain maximum allowable difference set by the laboratory on the basis of a given time lapse between consecutive measurements. In this way, results that are correct usually will not be flagged as possible errors. If various time frames and maximum allowable difference limits for the delta check are properly assigned, then the most frequent causes of delta check rejection of an individual specimen will be specimen mix-up or random sampling and processing errors.

When the delta check limits are exceeded, the operator should first review the specimen identification information to ensure that it is definitely the specimen of the patient in question. Next, the patient's cumulative result record should be reviewed. If possible, the patient's current medical condition should be checked for clues to the significant change in values, *e.g.*, recent surgery, bleeding, or dehydration. If necessary, the specimen should be retested, using a different method if possible.[1] If both the specimen identification and the retesting yield no clues to the delta check failure, improper collection of the specimen should be suspected, and another sample should be requested. If no errors are found, the results should be reported with a comment on the report indicating that the unusual result has been checked and verified to ensure the physician of the result's validity. It is possible that the *previous* determination was in error.

The delta check difference between consecutive measurements can be determined as either (1) delta check as a difference in the absolute value, *i.e.*, result 2 − result 1 = delta in test units; or (2) delta check as a percentage difference, *i.e.*, ([result 2 − result 1]/result 1) × 100% = delta percent. Once determined, this difference must be compared with a predefined maximum allowable difference. There are two methods to determine the maximum allowable difference for the delta check. The more analytic approach is to collect a minimum of 20 paired consecutive test runs on the analyte in question and determine the deltas (differences between each consecutive test) for each pair. The deltas are then plotted as a frequency histogram, and either a 95% or a 99% confidence limit is determined. The other approach is to estimate the delta limit on the basis of clinical experience and expected intraindividual variation. This approach is empirical but is also much easier to determine. Regardless of the method used, the delta limit should be adjusted so that the majority of the real changes in patient test values are not flagged as failure of the delta limits.

Hematology tests that lend themselves to delta checks have little intraindividual variation over a short period of time. Red cell parameters, platelet counts, prothrombin time, and other coagulation studies are more adaptable to delta checking than are leukocyte counts and WBC differentials, which can have significant physiologic variation over short time periods.

Computer-Generated Reports

Computers can generate a variety of reports from their accumulated databases. For example, an "abnormal patient report" can list all patient results that exceed defined limits, such as alert or so-called "panic" values. This report can be generated on a next-day basis for review by the clinical laboratory supervisor or medical director. This procedure will detect random errors whose magnitude would not cause rejection by a reasonable value rule but for which there are no previous results with which to perform a delta check. The report permits comparison of exception results with the patient's chart and clinical symptoms.

A SYSTEM FOR THE DETECTION AND CONTROL OF LABORATORY ERRORS

Laboratory accreditation regulations include a requirement for a system for the detection of analytic and clerical errors. Many different "systems" are undoubtedly used in laboratories. A study was done in the United Kingdom to analyze random errors in two clinical chemistry departments. This study indicated an error rate of less than 0.1% among all results obtained. Almost half of the errors were detected before the final reports were issued, while the remainder were detected in a number of different ways. The errors were divided basically into three groups: preanalytic, analytic, and postanalytic.[5]

In a recent College of American Pathologists (CAP) Q-Probe, investigators studied reporting errors in more than 600 laboratories in the United States and made a series of useful recommendations.[3] The analysis of the CAP data included a division of the errors into four categories. The rare category A errors were serious errors likely to cause deleterious actions in patient care. Category B (by far the most common) were serious errors which were unlikely to cause untoward effects on patient management. Category C (the next most common) errors were defined as minor clerical errors. Finally, Category NL were nonlaboratory errors such as improper specimen collection by nonlaboratory personnel or incorrect patient demographic data.[3]

At least one study showed that the usual quality control procedures may not detect these errors, indicating that other methods are necessary.[4] As noted earlier in this chapter, the sensitivity of the laboratory staff to error detection is probably the single most important factor. The staff should be encouraged to report and log all errors that are detected. More importantly, these errors should be analyzed on a real-time or at least on a monthly basis to find ways to prevent their future occurrence.

The error detection and analysis process should become an integral part of the overall laboratory quality assurance program. Analysis may uncover certain problem areas where changes in specimen collection techniques could eliminate many errors. Certain individuals (phlebotomists, nurses, or physicians) may be "error prone," and education and counseling may be indicated.

Perhaps the single greatest factor in reducing random errors is the implementation of automation and a laboratory information system. As compared to referral laboratories, physicians' office laboratories have higher error rates, probably owing to the relative paucity of automation and laboratory information systems.[6] In our laboratory, the low rate of errors (which we continually log) was halved after the information system was activated. Such systems reduce the preanalytic and postanalytic error rates in particular.

CHAPTER SUMMARY

Random error is unpredictable and is generally not detected by conventional quality control methods using commercial controls or patient specimens. An alert and vigilant laboratory scientist is the best insurance against random error. A variety of strategies can be used to detect its occurrence, including checking test results to ensure that they are reasonable and performing duplicate analyses, multivariate checks, and delta checks. The use of laboratory computers and information systems can increase the efficiency of random error detection, because computers can perform truly consistent analysis of results, thus preventing most mistakes.

Review Questions

46-1. All of the following are examples of random error *except*

    A. a decreasing Hb value on six consecutive hourly analyses of a control value.

    B. a manual Hb value measured as 15.2 g/dL but reported as 12.5 g/dL.

    C. short sampling of a specimen due to an air bubble in a sample cup.

    D. improper specimen labeling causing results to be reported on the wrong patient.

46-2. Random error may be prevented or detected by

    A. checking to see whether a laboratory value is reasonable.

    B. checking specimens for fibrin clots prior to analysis.

    C. performing multivariate checks.

    D. all of the above.

46-3. Multivariate checks for random error include all of the following *except*

    A. the rule of three.

    B. calculation of the difference in consecutive individual patient Hb values.

    C. evaluation of erythrocyte indices.

    D. correlation of the automated blood count with the blood film.

46-4. Delta checks provide a method to

    A. correlate the Hb and Hct in a patient specimen.

    B. correlate erythrocyte indices with peripheral blood film erythrocyte morphology.

    C. monitor differences in analytic values between two different patients.

    D. monitor differences in analytic values for consecutive specimens from a given patient.

46-5. Delta checks can be used to check all of the following parameters for random error *except*

 A. Hb and Hct.
 B. RBC and platelets.
 C. WBC and differentials.
 D. prothrombin and partial thromboplastin times.

46-6. The first key to the success of a laboratory information system in detecting random error is

 A. laboratory staff awareness.
 B. generation of valuable reports for management review.
 C. a comprehensive computer program.
 D. proper instrument maintenance.

References

1. Cembrowski GS: Use of patient data for quality control. Clin Lab Med 6:715, 1986
2. Houwen B: Random errors in haematology tests: A process control approach. Clin Lab Haematol 12(Suppl):157, 1990
3. Howanitz PJ, Walker K: Reporting Error—Data Analysis and Critique. Q-Probe 15A. Northfield IL, College of American Pathologists, 1990
4. Kazmierczak SC, Catrou PG: Laboratory error undetectable by customary quality control/quality assurance monitors. Arch Path Lab Med 117:714, 1993
5. Lapworth R, Teal TK: Laboratory blunders revisited. Ann Clin Biochem 31:78, 1994
6. Nosanchuk JS, Gottmann AW: CUMS and delta checks. Am J Clin Pathol 62:707, 1974
7. Nutting PA, Main DS, Fischer PM et al: Problems in laboratory testing in primary care. JAMA 275:635, 1996

Recommended Reading

Iizuka Y, Kume H, Kitamura M: Multivariate delta check method for detecting specimen mix-up. Clin Chem 28:2244, 1982

Ladenson JH: Patients as their own controls: Use of the computer to identify "laboratory error." Clin Chem 21:1648, 1975

Sheiner, LB, Wheeler LA, Moore JK: The performance of delta check methods. Clin Chem 25:2034, 1979

Stewart CE, Koepke JA: Basic Quality Assurance Practices for Clinical Laboratories. Philadelphia, JB Lippincott, 1987

Van Kampen EJ: Throwing a curve at laboratory error. Diagn Med 3:54, 1980

PART XI

Hemostasis

CHAPTER 47

Introduction to Hemostasis

Cheryl A. Lotspeich-Steininger

Objectives

1. Define and briefly explain the three hemostatic components; primary hemostasis; secondary hemostasis; contact phase; hypocoagulation; hypercoagulation; and the intrinsic, extrinsic, common, and alternate coagulation pathways.

2. Discuss the various hemostatic roles of endothelial cells.

3. List at least six substances found in platelet α-granules and two substances found in platelet dense bodies, and briefly state their roles in hemostasis.

4. List five important roles of platelets in hemostasis.

5. State the function of fibrinolysis in hemostasis, and briefly define the roles of plasmin, tissue plasminogen activators, and the protein C–S complex.

6. List three types of vascular abnormalities, and give examples of associated conditions and any significant laboratory findings.

The word *hemostasis* is derived from a Greek word meaning "the stoppage of blood flow." This chapter provides a brief introduction to the concepts of hemostasis. The coagulation and fibrinolytic mechanisms, as well as platelets, are introduced. In addition, the contribution of blood vessels to hemostasis and the vessel abnormalities that interfere with hemostasis are addressed. (These two topics are not covered at length in any other chapter.)

The next 11 chapters in this section of the text address the theories of coagulation and fibrinolysis (Chap. 48), as well as disorders related to abnormalities of the coagulation and fibrinolytic mechanisms (Chaps. 52 and 53). Laboratory procedures for the evaluation of hemostatic abnormalities and their treatment are discussed in detail (Chaps. 49–51 and 54). The structure and function of platelets, qualitative and quantitative abnormalities of platelets, and laboratory evaluation of platelets are also discussed (Chaps. 55–57). The final chapter in this section

(Chap. 58) presents concepts of instrumentation and quality control (QC) as they relate uniquely to the hemostasis laboratory.

THE THREE HEMOSTATIC COMPONENTS

There are three basic components of hemostasis: the extravascular, vascular, and intravascular components.

Extravascular Component

The extravascular hemostatic component involves the tissues surrounding blood vessels. These tissues become involved in hemostasis when a local vessel is injured. Extravascular mechanisms play a part in hemostasis by providing back pressure on the injured vessel through swelling and the trapping of escaped blood. The increased tissue pressure tends to collapse venules and capillaries. The ability of the surrounding tissues to aid in hemostasis depends on the following factors:

1. The bulk or amount of surrounding tissue. A wound in the fleshy part of the thigh will not bleed as profusely as an identical wound in the scalp.
2. The type of tissue surrounding the injured vessel. For example, skeletal muscle is more absorbent and effective in arresting hemorrhage than is loose connective tissue.
3. The tone of the surrounding tissue. The amount of tissue elasticity correlates with the amount of bleeding. Thus, identical wounds in a 17-year-old individual with great tissue elasticity tend to bleed less than those in a 71-year-old with less tissue elasticity.

Vascular and Intravascular Components

The vascular hemostatic component involves the vessels through which blood flows. The role played by vessels in hemostasis depends on their size, the amount of smooth muscle within their walls, and the integrity of the endothelial cell lining (see Role of Blood Vessels in Hemostasis).

The key components in intravascular hemostasis are platelets and many biochemicals (procoagulants) in the plasma. These components are involved in either coagulation (clot or thrombus formation) or fibrinolysis (clot or thrombus dissolution), the two essential processes of hemostasis.

CONCEPTS OF NORMAL HEMOSTASIS, HYPOCOAGULATION, AND HYPERCOAGULATION

Normal Hemostatic Balance

Prior to the many advances in biomedical research and laboratory techniques of recent decades, hemostasis was understood simply as the normal process by which bleeding from injured blood vessels was stopped through blood coagulation. Today, hemostasis is more thoroughly understood as a complex interaction between blood vessels, platelets, and biochemical reactants or coagulation factors in the plasma (Fig. 47-1). These interactions not only create clots that stop bleeding through the coagulation process but also dissolve clots through the fibrinolytic process as injured vessels are healed.

Under normal conditions, the formation and dissolution of thrombi is maintained in a delicate balance (see Fig. 47-1). Without this balance, an individual may experience either excessive bleeding (as a result of poor clot formation or excessive fibrinolysis) or thrombosis (uncontrolled formation of thrombi in the vascular system that blocks vessels and deprives organs of blood). Conditions associated with excessive bleeding are referred to as *hypocoagulable* states. Conditions in which there is uncontrolled thrombosis are called *hypercoagulable* states. Both abnormal states can be fatal if not controlled promptly.

Hypocoagulation

Many clinical conditions, both inherited and acquired, are associated with hypocoagulation or abnormal bleeding. Several of these conditions are readily diagnosed by laboratory tests, particularly coagulation factor assays that measure factor activity. Hemophilia is a well-known example of an inherited hypocoagulable disorder (Chap. 52). Patients with hemophilia have a defective coagulation mechanism that is unable to form adequate clots, resulting in excessive bleeding from trauma. Acquired conditions associated with hypocoagulation generally involve many clinical problems in addition to bleeding (Chap. 52). Examples include liver and kidney disease as well as disseminated intravascular coagulation (DIC). In DIC, excessive formation of thrombi results in consumption of coagulation factors and platelets and ultimately leads to hypocoagulability.

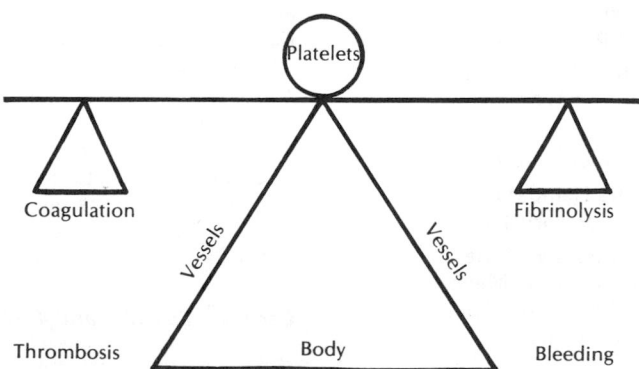

FIGURE 47-1. Balance of hemostasis. Vessels, coagulation and fibrinolytic proteins, and platelets all work together toward thrombus formation in a well-orchestrated, carefully balanced process. Platelets are the center of clot formation. A swing of the balance to the right, *i.e.*, excessive fibrinolysis or inadequate coagulation, can result in bleeding. A swing to the left, *i.e.*, excessive coagulation or inadequate fibrinolysis, can result in pathologic clotting (thrombosis). (From Corriveau DM, Fritsma GA [eds]: Hemostasis and Thrombosis in the Clinical Laboratory, p 9. Philadelphia, JB Lippincott, 1988, with permission.)

Hypercoagulation

Hypercoagulation or thrombosis is associated with the inappropriate formation of thrombi in the vasculature, which occlude normal blood flow. Thrombi generally consist of leukocytes, platelets, and erythrocytes held together by fibrin. Thrombi can be painful and cause a number of symptoms and abnormal physical findings, as well as abnormal laboratory results. Thrombi can even be life-threatening if the blood supply to a vital organ is cut off. Hypercoagulation is caused by a defect in one or more regulatory systems of coagulation or a lack of activation of the fibrinolytic system.

Most hypercoagulable states are associated with acquired diseases or altered physiologic states (see Table 53-2). Malignancy[22] and surgical procedures[18,26] are the most frequent stimuli for hypercoagulation. Unfortunately, it is difficult to predict the risk or anticipate the development of thrombosis by the more common laboratory tests. Hypercoagulable states are discussed in Chapter 53 and specialized laboratory tests for detection of thrombosis are presented in Chapter 51.

HISTORICAL BACKGROUND OF HEMOSTASIS

The study of hemostasis dates to the time of Aristotle and Plato.[36] The bleeding disorder hemophilia was the first coagulation disorder to be recognized, being described during the second century AD, although its pathophysiology was not understood. In the fifth century Talmud,[41] two male children were described who had died from excessive bleeding after circumcision. It was recommended that any male child not be circumcised if he was born to a mother who had previously given birth to two infants who had died from such a bleeding disorder; otherwise, he was also likely to die.

Clinical descriptions of families with the hemophilia disorder were first published by Otto in 1803.[32] The disorder was given the name hemophilia, which means "love of hemorrhage," by Schönlein.[44] The disorder was first described as hemophilia in a thesis by Hopff published in 1828.[16]

HISTORICAL DEVELOPMENT OF CLINICAL HEMOSTASIS

It was not until 1913 that a laboratory test to evaluate the clotting mechanism was described in the literature. This test was the Lee-White whole blood coagulation (clotting) time (WBCT; Chap. 49).[19] The WBCT is an *in vitro*, visual, qualitative assessment of blood clotting capability. It is seldom performed today.

As recently as the 1940s, there were only a few routine tests for evaluating the hemostatic mechanism: the platelet count, bleeding time, WBCT, and the prothrombin time (PT). The PT was developed by Quick in the 1930s.[38] Even though it is somewhat misnamed, being dependent on more than prothrombin, slightly modified versions are still in use today.[39]

THE HEMOSTASIS LABORATORY TODAY

Over the past few decades, many tests of the coagulation and fibrinolytic system have been developed and automated, and test reagents have been made commercially available. Consequently, many clinical hemostasis laboratories now operate independent of the hematology laboratory. Visual examination of clot formation has been replaced in large part by mechanical or photo-optical clot detection. In addition, quantitation of substances involved in enhancement or inhibition of coagulation as well as fibrinolysis may now be performed by both immunoassay and by spectrophotometric measurement using synthetic substrates (Chap. 58). Automation has considerably improved the precision and accuracy of coagulation testing.

OVERVIEW OF THE HEMOSTATIC MECHANISM

Primary and Secondary Hemostasis

Hemostasis involves the interaction of blood vessels, platelets, the coagulation mechanism, fibrinolysis, and tissue repair. Hemostasis occurs in two phases, primary and secondary (Table 47-1). Primary hemostasis involves the vascular and platelet response to vessel injury. Secondary hemostasis includes the response of the coagulation process to such injury. These processes ultimately lead to the formation of a stable fibrin–platelet plug at the site of injury, which permits vessel healing. At the same time, fibrinolysis is initiated, allowing for gradual clot dissolution.

Role of Blood Vessels in Hemostasis

INTACT VESSELS

Blood flows through the vascular system to and from all parts of the body. The vascular system consists of capillaries, arteries, and veins (Fig. 47-2).

Capillaries. Every cell in the body is within 0.13 mm of one or more capillaries which are the smallest and most numerous blood vessels in the body. Metabolic exchange between the blood and tissues takes place in thin-walled capillaries, which are lined with a single continuous endothelial cell layer that is attached to a supportive basement membrane (see Fig. 47-2). The capillary lumen is just large enough for a single erythrocyte or leukocyte to pass. There are openings called *junctions* along the capillary wall that allow the passage of leukocytes, oxygen, and nutrients into and out of the blood as necessary. Also, waste may pass from the tissues into the blood through these junctions. Erythrocytes and platelets usually do not leave the intravascular system. Pericytes are cells that lie beneath the endothelium of capillaries, arteries, and veins; they may differentiate into vessel-related cells when needed.

Arteries and Veins. The physical capabilities of arteries and veins include constriction and dilation, which are controlled by the smooth muscle in these vessels. Vaso-

TABLE 47-1
Basic Sequence of Events in Primary and Secondary Hemostasis After Vessel Injury

	Event	Comments
Step 1	Vasoconstriction (P)	Controlled by vessel smooth muscle; enhanced by chemicals secreted by platelets
Step 2	Platelet adhesion (P)	Adhesion to exposed subendothelial connective tissue
Step 3	Platelet aggregation (P)	Interaction and adhesion of platelets to one another to form initial plug at injury site
Step 4	Fibrin–platelet plug formation (S)	Coagulation factors interact on platelet surface to produce fibrin; fibrin–platelet plug then forms at site of vessel injury
Step 5	Fibrin stabilization (S)	Fibrin clot must be stabilized by coagulation factor XIII

Key: (P) = primary hemostasis; (S) = secondary hemostasis.

constriction and vasodilation provide the means for control of blood flow rate and blood pressure. Arteries and veins are larger than capillaries. Their structure includes three layers: (1) the *tunica adventitia* or outer part of the vessel wall, which consists of connective-tissue fibroblasts and collagen fibers; (2) the *tunica media*, composed of smooth muscle cells and connective tissue, including collagen fibers and occasional fibroblasts; and (3) the *tunica intima* or inner endothelial lining, which comes into contact with blood cells and separates them from a subendothelium composed of a basement membrane, elastic connective tissue, and collagen fibers (see Fig. 47-2).

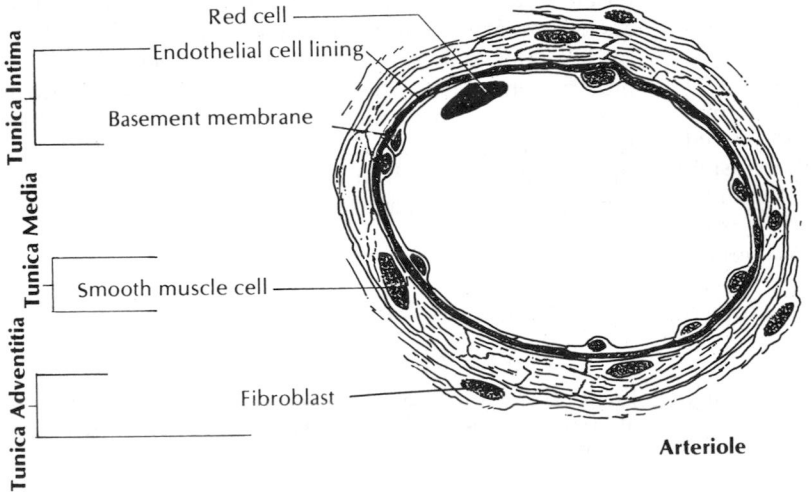

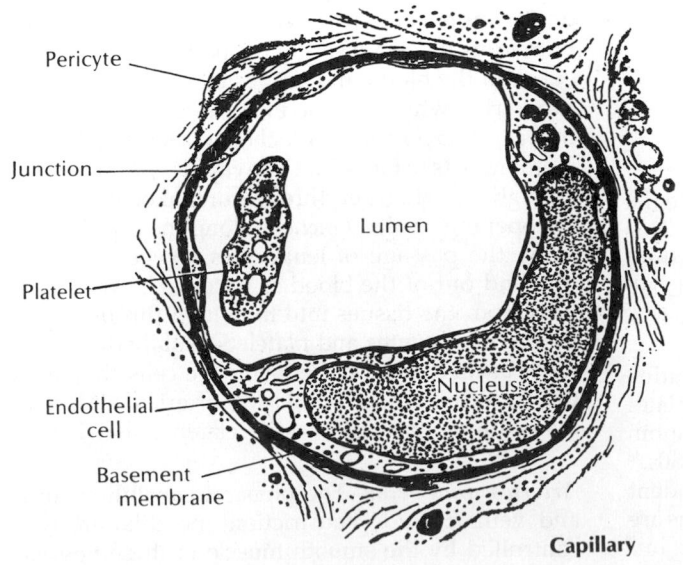

FIGURE 47-2. Comparison of capillary and arteriole structure viewed through vessel lumen. Capillary is shown at higher magnification than arteriole to display details. (From Corriveau DM, Fritsma GA [eds]: Hemostasis and Thrombosis in the Clinical Laboratory, p 15. Philadelphia, JB Lippincott, 1988, with permission.)

TABLE 47-2
Antithrombotic, Fibrinolytic, and Coagulant Substances Released from or Found on the Surface of Intact Endothelial Cells

Substance	Action	Hemostatic Role
Prostacyclin (prostaglandin I$_2$ [PGI$_2$])	Inhibits platelet adhesion and aggregation; stimulates vasodilation	Anticoagulant Reduces blood flow rate
Adenosine (metabolic product of ATP and ADP)	Stimulates vasodilation	Reduces blood flow rate
ADPase	Destroys ADP, limits platelet activation	Anticoagulant
Thrombomodulin	Endothelial surface receptor for thrombin Binds and inactivates thrombin and enhances anticoagulant and fibrinolytic action of protein C found in the plasma (see Fig. 53-1)	Anticoagulant Fibrinolytic
Heparan sulfate	Coats the endothelial cell surface and weakly enhances activity of antithrombin-III, a plasma anticoagulant	Anticoagulant
Tissue plasminogen activator (TPA)	Converts plasminogen to plasmin, which plays important role in fibrinolysis Released only on appropriate stimulus, such as vessel injury, to prevent excessive clot formation at the site of injury and begin slow clot dissolution as the injured vessel heals	Fibrinolytic
Plasminogen activator inhibitor-1	Regulatory protein for fibrinolytic system	Antifibrinolytic
von Willebrand factor (vWF)	Protein produced in endothelium and stored in subendothelium (in the form of Weibel-Palade bodies) before secretion into the plasma and attachment to factor VIII:C	Coagulation and platelet adhesion

The endothelium plays multiple roles to promote normal blood flow and prevent thrombotic episodes and to prevent excessive clot formation at the site of vessel injury. On the other side of the hemostatic spectrum, endothelial cells produce vWF, which promotes platelet adhesion to exposed collagen on vessel injury.

The intact endothelial lining of blood vessels is antithrombotic: it does not activate platelets or promote coagulation. This lining provides a smooth surface that facilitates blood flow and reduces turbulence since turbulence promotes thrombosis. Substances released from the endothelial cells and subendothelial smooth muscle also contribute to normal blood flow and prevent abnormal formation of clots in blood vessels. These substances influence coagulation, fibrinolysis, and platelets (Table 47-2 and Chap. 48). For example, endothelial cells produce von Willebrand factor (vWF, a protein that is required for normal platelet adhesion to injured tissue) and store it in the subendothelial matrix where vWF binds to collagen.

DAMAGED VESSELS

Blood is maintained in a fluid state as it flows through intact vessels. On vessel injury, vasoconstriction occurs as a neurogenic response. Injury breaks the smooth endothelial lining, exposing collagen, a surface that promotes thrombus formation by causing the adhesion of platelets to the area of injury.

Endothelial damage also exposes tissue factor (TF, factor III). TF is a receptor protein found in the plasma membrane of many cell types (but not normally in endothelial cells). On exposure to TF, plasma factor VII binds with high affinity to TF forming the TF:VII complex. This complex initiates the *extrinsic coagulation pathway* (see Role of Coagulation in Hemostasis).

In contrast to its role in coagulation promotion, vessel injury also initiates fibrinolysis (see Fibrinolysis in Hemostasis) through endothelial cell release of tissue plasminogen activators (TPAs). This response provides one of the necessary checks and balances on the coagulation system to ensure that excessive coagulation does not occur. The physiologic responses to vessel injury are summarized in Figure 47-3.

Role of Coagulation in Hemostasis

Coagulation is the process whereby, on vessel injury, plasma coagulation proteins, tissue factor, and calcium (Ca^{2+}) interact on cell surfaces to form a fibrin clot. Platelets provide a surface for the coagulation reaction and interact with fibrin to form a stable platelet-fibrin clot. Table 48-1 (Chap. 48) lists the coagulation factors with their preferred names and synonyms. Most are referred to both by Roman numerals and by names assigned by the International Committee on Nomenclature of Blood Coagulation Factors.[50] These factors (except Ca^{2+} and tissue factor) normally circulate in the plasma as inactive proteins. On activation, some factors form enzymatic proteins known as *serine proteases* that activate other specific factors in the coagulation sequence.

Basically, there are three interrelated pathways of coagulation, each representing a unique series of biochemical reactions (Fig. 47-4). These include the intrinsic, extrinsic, and common pathways. The extrinsic pathway is now thought to be the primary mechanism by which coagulation is initiated *in vivo*. However, part of the intrinsic pathway is still recognized to be important for *in vivo* coagulation (factors XI, IX, and VIII). It is also important to understand the complete intrinsic pathway because it is evaluated in the commonly performed and diagnostically valuable partial thromboplastin time (PTT) test. The ex-

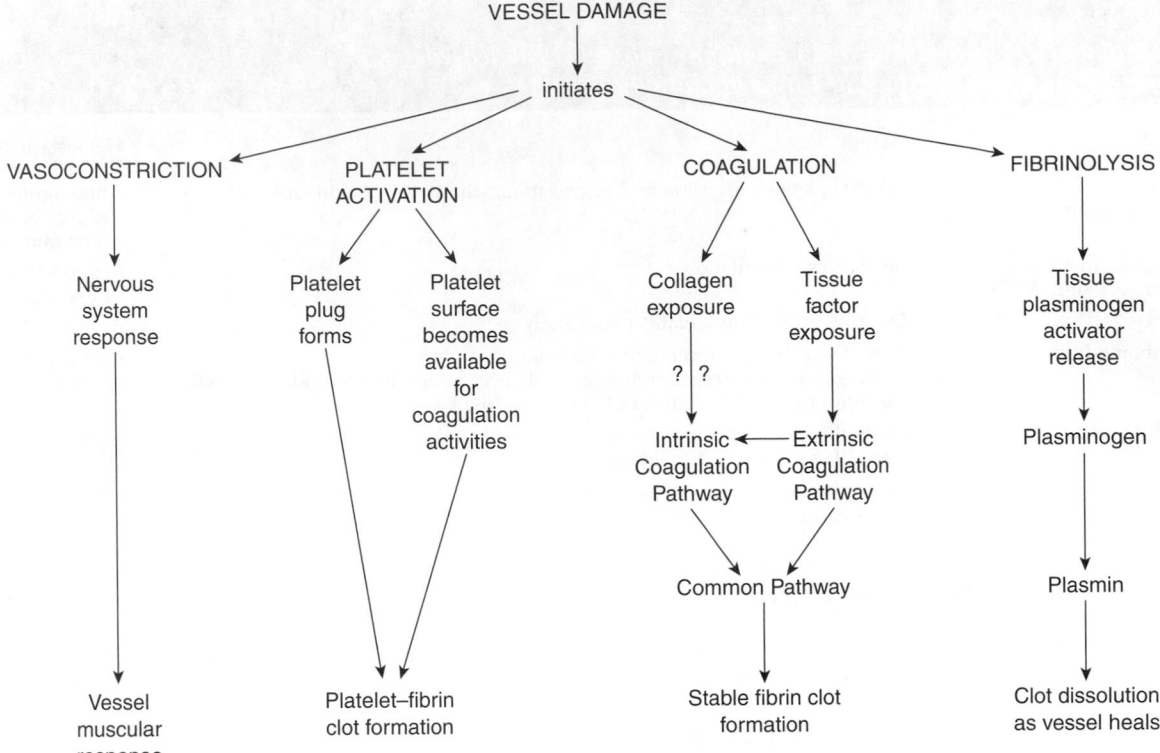

FIGURE 47-3. Physiologic response to vessel injury.

trinsic and intrinsic pathways ultimately come together to initiate the common pathway, which leads to stable fibrin clot formation.

THE EXTRINSIC PATHWAY

The extrinsic coagulation pathway is activated following vascular endothelial cell injury. Such injury causes the exposure of TF, a receptor protein on cells that underlie the endothelium. TF and plasma factor VII bind to form the TF:VII complex which itself is enzymatic, but is made more enzymatically active by the activation of factor VII, resulting in the TF:VIIa complex. A number of substances are reported to activate factor VII to the serine protease VIIa, including factors IXa and Xa, among others (Chap. 48). The ''a'' that accompanies the Roman numeral indicates the activated state of the factor. The TF:VIIa complex, along with Ca^{2+}, activates factor X to the serine pro-

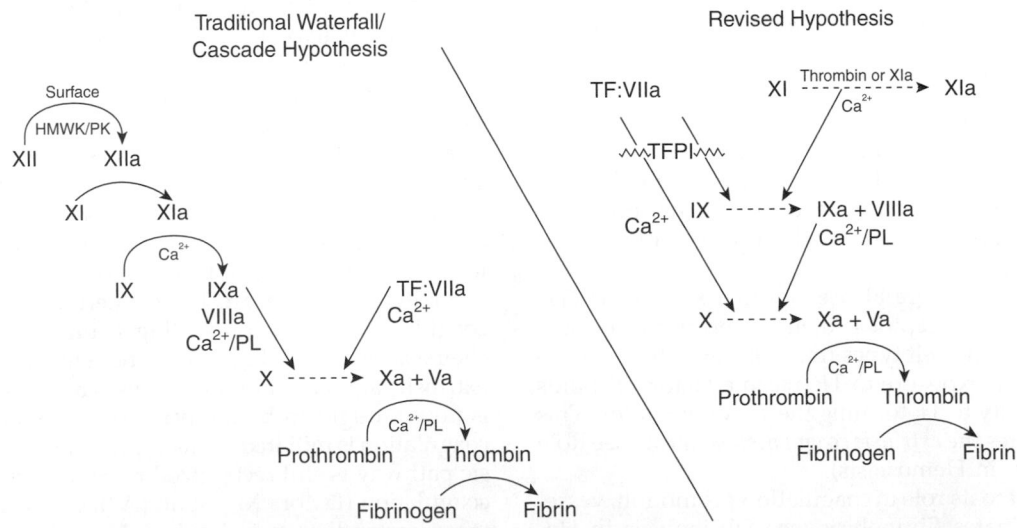

FIGURE 47-4. Comparison of the traditional waterfall/cascade hypothesis to the recently revised hypothesis for *in vivo* coagulation. Note revised hypothesis does *not* include the contact factors XII, HMWK, or PK. Key: HMWK, high-molecular-weight kininogen; PK, prekallikrein; TF, tissue factor; PL, phospholipid; TFPI, tissue factor pathway inhibitor (TFPI inhibits the TF:VIIa complex [Chap. 48]).

tease Xa in the common pathway (see Fig. 47-4). The extrinsic and common pathways are evaluated in the prothrombin time (PT) test.

THE INTRINSIC PATHWAY

Activation of the intrinsic pathway *in vitro* occurs when factor XII is exposed to a negatively charged surface such as glass or kaolin. This initiates the *contact phase* of coagulation and involves the so-called contact factors XII, XI, high-molecular-weight kininogen (HMWK), and prekallikrein (see Fig. 47-4). The contact factors XII and XI are converted to the serine proteases XIIa and XIa. Factor XIa, with Ca^{2+}, in turn converts factor IX to the serine protease IXa. Factor IXa, with platelet phospholipid, Ca^{2+}, and a cofactor, factor VIIIa, converts factor X to Xa in the common pathway. The intrinsic and common pathways are evaluated in the PTT. Patients with factor XII, HMWK, or prekallikrein deficiencies do not have bleeding abnormalities. On the other hand, the role of the contact phase factors does appear to be important in the *in vivo* initiation of the inflammatory response, complement activation, and fibrinolysis (Chap. 48).[6]

THE COMMON PATHWAY

The common pathway begins with activation of factor X to Xa by either the intrinsic or the extrinsic pathway (see Fig. 47-4). Factor Xa with a cofactor, Va, lipid, and Ca^{2+} converts prothrombin (II) to thrombin (IIa). Factor IIa converts fibrinogen (I), to fibrin. Factor XIII then stabilizes the fibrin clot.

ALTERNATE PATHWAYS

It is now recognized that *alternate pathways* of coagulation exist that link the extrinsic, intrinsic, and common coagulation pathways, *i.e.*, the three are no longer thought of as separate entities into which the coagulation factors neatly fit. In the early 1990s, a revised scheme for the *in vivo* pathways of coagulation was proposed[4,30a,49] which is depicted in Figure 47-4. This model stands in contrast to the traditional "waterfall"[7] or "cascade"[24] theories proposed over 30 years ago. The linkages among the three pathways are discussed in detail in Chapter 48.

Role of Platelets in Hemostasis

HISTORY OF CLINICAL RECOGNITION AND INVESTIGATION

Platelets were described by several investigators in 1842,[1,8,11] although no one at that time knew the origin of platelets. In 1878, it was recognized that platelets, like erythrocytes and leukocytes, are unique elements of the blood.[14] Much later, it was discovered that platelets originate from large cells in the bone marrow called megakaryocytes. In the 1940s, researchers were first able to begin studying platelet structure using the electron microscope. It has become clear that platelets play a vital role in hemostasis, and that qualitative or quantitative platelet abnormalities can cause hypocoagulation or hypercoagulation disorders. Normal hemostatic function requires peripheral blood platelets that are normal in number (approximate reference range 150–400 x 10^9/L) and function.

Quantitation of platelet numbers has been performed since the early part of the 20th century using a hemocytometer, microscope, and platelet-specific stain. In 1950, a method for counting platelets was described that involves phase-contrast microscopy[3] (Chap. 56). Today, platelets are routinely enumerated using automated methods.

Qualitative (functional) platelet evaluation was first available with the introduction of the *bleeding time test* by Duke in the early 1900s.[9] A prolonged bleeding time can indicate either a thrombocytopenia (decreased platelet count; Chap. 57) or thrombocytopathy (abnormal platelet function; Chap. 57). Although the bleeding time is still the only *in vivo* screening test for platelet function, more specific tests such as *platelet aggregation studies* (Chap. 56) are now available. It has been suggested that the bleeding time is *not* an appropriate screening test for platelet function in patients with no personal or family history of bleeding.[21]

PLATELET MORPHOLOGY AND FUNCTION IN HEMOSTASIS

As shown in Table 47-1 and Figure 47-3, platelets play a central and immediate role in the response to vessel injury. Platelets are the smallest microscopically visible cellular element on the peripheral blood film. They are 2 to 4 μm in diameter and approximately 7 fL in volume and have a discoid shape. With Wright stain, platelets have a light violet-purple granular appearance (see Color Plate 47-1). They have a life span of 9 to 10 days.[13] The stages of platelet maturation and platelet function are presented in Chapter 55. Platelets play the following important roles in hemostasis: (1) adhesion to injured vessels; (2) aggregation at the injury site; (3) promotion of coagulation on their phospholipid surface; (4) release of biochemicals important to hemostasis from their α granules and dense bodies (Table 47-3); and (5) induction of clot retraction.

Clot retraction is the last act of platelets within a platelet-fibrin clot. This requires Ca^{2+}, thrombin, and a tremendous amount of energy (ATP). It can be observed *in vitro* when blood clots in a test tube after a few hours, leaving clear serum adjacent to the test tube walls. The exact purpose of clot retraction is unclear; hypotheses include participation in pulling the sides of an injured vessel together or debulking of the clot to help reestablish blood flow.

Fibrinolysis in Hemostasis

Fibrinolysis is the system whereby the temporary fibrin clot is systematically and gradually dissolved as the vessel heals in order to restore normal blood flow. Recognition of this system goes back to the late 1700s when John Hunter reported the unexplained finding that blood from people who had died as the result of accidents or some trauma did not clot.[17] In 1937, MacFarlane reported that damaged tissues release a substance (plasminogen activator) that activates the inert and circulatory precursor called plasminogen to its active form, plasmin. Plasmin is capable of degrading fibrin as well as factors I, V, and VIII.[25] The process of fibrinolysis has since been elucidated extensively (Fig. 48-3) and its laboratory evaluation greatly advanced (Chap. 50).

TABLE 47-3
Summary of Important Substances Secreted by Platelets and Their Role in Hemostasis

Role in Hemostasis	Substance*	Source	Comments on Principal Function**
Promote coagulation	HMWK	α-granules	Contact activation of intrinsic coagulation pathway
	Fibrinogen	α-granules	Converted to fibrin for clot formation
	Factor V	α-granules	Cofactor in fibrin clot formation
	vWF	α-granules	Assists platelet adhesion to subendothelium to provide coagulation surface
Promote aggregation	ADP	Dense bodies	Promotes platelet aggregation
	Calcium	Dense bodies	Same
	Platelet factor 4	α-granules	Same; also inhibits heparin
	Thrombospondin	α-granules	Same
Promote vasoconstriction	Serotonin	Dense bodies	Promotes vasoconstriction at injury site
	Thromboxane A_2 precursors	Membrane phospholipids	Same; promotes platelet release reaction
Promote vascular repair	Platelet-derived growth factor	α-granules	Promotes smooth muscle growth for vessel repair
	β-thromboglobulin	α-granules	Chemotactic for fibroblasts to help in vessel repair[45]; inhibits heparin
Other systems affected	Plasminogen	α-granules	Precursor to plasmin, which induces clot lysis
	α_2-antiplasmin	α-granules	Plasmin inhibitor; inhibits clot lysis
	Protease nexin II	α-granules	Inhibits factor XIa and thus factor IX activation[49]
	Platelet inhibitor of factor XI (PIXI)	α-granules	Inhibits factor XIa and thus factor IX activation[49]
	C1 esterase inhibitor	α-granules	Complement system inhibitor

* Other substances are secreted from platelets in addition to those listed here.
** Functions other than those listed also exist for some substances.

BASIC TERMINOLOGY FOR CLINICAL FINDINGS IN BLEEDING DISORDERS

The reader should be familiar with the meanings of terms describing the clinical findings associated with bleeding disorders caused by abnormal vessels or platelets or an abnormal coagulation or fibrinolytic mechanism. The following is a short list of basic clinical terms that are used in this and later chapters to describe such clinical findings; their meanings may be found in the glossary at the back of this textbook: petechiae, purpura, ecchymosis, epistaxis, hemarthrosis, hematemesis, hematoma, hematuria, hemoglobinuria, hemoptysis, melena, and menorrhagia.

BLEEDING DISORDERS CAUSED BY VASCULAR DEFECTS

Many types of vascular defects result in hemostatic abnormalities. Often, these defects are initially diagnosed because a patient has a bleeding tendency or a specific type of skin lesion, in spite of platelet number and function as well as coagulation factor activity being normal. There are no characteristic laboratory findings; however, the finding of normal results can help to rule out other diagnoses. Fortunately, there is usually some clinical sign or symptom that assists in the diagnosis. Vascular defects may be categorized by a variety of methods. Table 47-4 divides vascular abnormalities into hereditary and ac-

quired defects causing bleeding secondary to vascular defects of several types.

Hereditary Connective Tissue Defects

Connective tissue is found in all three layers of the vessel wall; thus, hereditary connective tissue defects affect vessels in all three layers of their structure. Connective tissue provides support for vessels as well as other structures of the body. A more detailed review of these disorders may be found elsewhere.[37]

EHLERS-DANLOS SYNDROME

The Ehlers-Danlos syndrome is a heterogeneous group of nine rare disorders with different modes of genetic transmission. The connective tissue of the skin, vasculature, and bones is adversely affected, causing a lack of structural tissue support and great tissue fragility. The defect can lie in (1) a peptidase enzyme that converts procollagen to collagen[35]; (2) the procollagen structure itself[5]; or (3) the crosslinking of mature collagen.[34] The affected individual has hypermobile joints and hyperextensible skin which can be stretched much more than normal skin but returns to normal on release. There may be large skin ecchymoses and hematomas, bleeding from the gums, excessive postpartum bleeding, and gastrointestinal bleeding. Patients often report easy bruisability. Coagulation and structural and functional platelet abnormalities may contribute to bleeding.[10] In spite of the com-

TABLE 47-4
*Principal Hereditary and Acquired Bleeding Disorders Associated
With Vascular Abnormalities*

Abnormality	Hereditary	Acquired
Connective tissue defects	Ehlers-Danlos syndrome Pseudoxanthoma elasticum	Vitamin C deficiency (scurvy) Senile purpura Corticosteroid purpura Cushing disease Others
Altered vessel wall structure	Hemorrhagic telangiectasia Cavernous—hemangioma congenital (Kasabach-Merritt syndrome)	Diabetes mellitus Amyloidosis Others

Vascular damage		Infectious purpura
		    Bacterial: tuberculosis, scarlet fever, typhoid fever, diphtheria, endocarditis, others
		    Viral: smallpox, influenza, measles, others
		    Rickettsial: Rocky Mountain spotted fever, others
		    Protozoal: malaria, others
		Autoimmune vascular purpura
		    Allergic purpuras: Henoch-Schönlein purpura
		    Drug-induced purpuras: quinine, procaine penicillin, aspirin, sulfonamides, sedatives, coumarins, others

Miscellaneous abnormalities causing purpura secondary to vessel damage		Waldenström's macroglobulinemia Kaposi's sarcoma Certain skin diseases Hemochromatosis Snake venom Others

Modified from Bithell TC: Bleeding disorders caused by vascular abnormalities. In Lee GR, Bithell TC, Foerster J et al (eds): Wintrobe's Clinical Hematology, 9th ed, (p. 1375.) Philadelphia, Lea & Febiger, 1993, with permission.

plications, these patients generally have a normal life span. There is no known therapy.

PSEUDOXANTHOMA ELASTICUM

This is a rare connective tissue disorder that is transmitted as an autosomal recessive trait. The elastic fibers of the skin are abnormal, which causes the skin to be lax. The connective tissue elastic fibers in small arteries are calcified and structurally and functionally abnormal. Easy bruisability and hemorrhagic episodes are common. Subarachnoid and gastrointestinal bleeding are the most common causes of death. Laboratory tests are not usually helpful in the diagnosis except to rule out other causes of the clinical abnormalities. There is no known therapy for the disorder.

Acquired Connective Tissue Defects

VITAMIN C DEFICIENCY (SCURVY)

Scurvy is an acquired disorder caused by dietary deficiency of vitamin C (ascorbic acid), which is required for the formation of intact, stable collagen, particularly in blood vessels. Without vitamin C, there is a deficiency of the intercellular cement substance that holds endothelial cells together. Also, hydroxylation of the amino acids proline and lysine cannot take place and collagen cannot be formed properly. This deficiency causes capillary fra-

gility and serious bleeding problems. Vitamin C is also important in the body's iron absorption process. In the United States, two populations are reported to be increasingly at risk—the institutionalized elderly and alcoholics.[31] The RDA for ascorbic acid is 60 mg.[30] Dietary deficiency was historically identified on a large scale in British sailors who developed bleeding gums and other hemorrhagic manifestations secondary to lack of dietary vitamin C while at sea for lengthy periods. On the basis of the observations of James Lind, sailors began eating limes to relieve the symptoms; thus, the sailors' nickname "limeys."

Gingival (gum) bleeding, coiled hairs, ecchymoses, purpura, and hemorrhage into subcutaneous tissues and muscles are characteristic. Petechiae often develop on the thighs and buttocks, particularly around the hair follicles (perifollicular petechiae). Large hemorrhagic areas may develop just below the eyes, particularly in affected infants.

Although patients with vitamin C deficiency do have abnormal laboratory findings, the best and most cost-effective way to confirm this diagnosis is by observation of the clinical response to vitamin C replacement therapy (see Treatment). There may be anemia, a mild thrombocytopenia, and a low plasma ascorbic acid level. Measurement of ascorbic acid in the platelet-leukocyte layer obtained by centrifugation of a heparinized peripheral blood sample,[20,33] although time-consuming, is a more reliable indicator of vitamin C deficiency and body stores than the plasma or whole blood levels, which more closely reflect recent dietary intake. The reference range for leukocyte vitamin C is 20 to 53 $\mu g/10^8$ leukocytes (deficiency, less than 10) and for plasma, 0.5 to 1.5 mg/dL (deficiency, less than 0.2).[48]

The bleeding time and coagulation tests are usually normal in patients with scurvy, although tests of platelet function may sometimes be abnormal.[2] The other exception is the *tourniquet test* for capillary fragility, which is usually positive (*i.e.*, petechiae are found on the skin after the test).[12,27] However, the tourniquet test is rarely performed to diagnose vitamin C deficiency as it is not specific for this disorder and can be positive in many qualitative and quantitative platelet disorders.

Administration of ascorbic acid usually brings the plasma level of vitamin C and the vascular integrity back to normal and rapidly eliminates the hemorrhagic manifestations in this disorder.

SENILE PURPURA

Senile purpura is a benign, acquired, and chronic disorder of the elderly. The aging process brings about a progressive degeneration and loss of collagen, elastin, and subcutaneous fat.[2] There may also be a defective cross-linking of collagen.[46] Characteristically, patients demonstrate red to purple ecchymotic spots on the forearm and on the backs of the hands and neck secondary to loss of skin and vascular elasticity.[47] Often the area retains a permanent brownish color, possibly because the hemoglobin is not properly removed by the aging macrophage system.

The bleeding time is normal or only slightly prolonged, and other coagulation tests are normal. No treatment of any real value has been found.[2] Corticosteroid therapy, Cushing disease, and other debilitating disorders can induce formation of purpura similar to that seen in senile purpura.[2]

Hereditary Alterations of Vessel Wall Structure

HEREDITARY HEMORRHAGIC TELANGIECTASIA

An autosomal dominant trait, hereditary hemorrhagic telangiectasia is characterized by bleeding that occurs from telangiectasias—vascular malformations of thin, dilated small vessels in the skin and mucosae. The small blood vessels are focally disorganized and dilated throughout the body, their wall support is poor, and their ability to contract is diminished; therefore any trauma to the vessels causes them to bleed readily and for a prolonged period.

This disorder is most often found in Anglo-German, Latin, Scandinavian, and Jewish populations.[2] Although relatively uncommon, it is the most commonly inherited vascular bleeding disorder.[23]

The lesions range from pinpoint size to 3 mm, are red to violet, and may be raised or flat, and round or spider-like. They may bleed either spontaneously or from minor trauma. They appear most commonly on the face, lips (Fig. 47-5), tongue, mucous membranes of the mouth and nose, ears, conjunctivae, and palms of the hands and

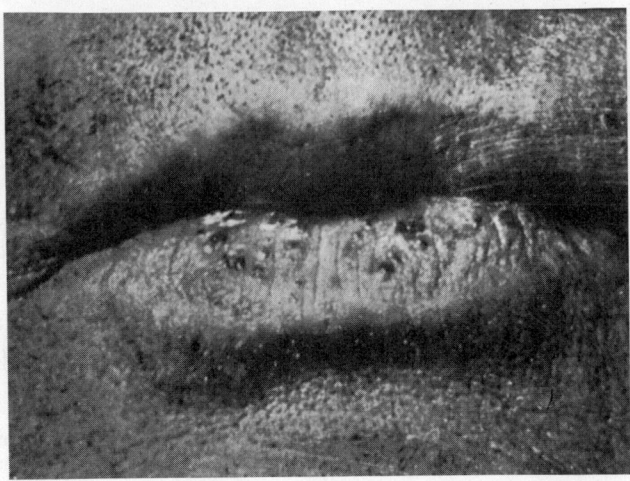

FIGURE 47-5. Hereditary hemorrhagic telangiectasia; characteristic lesions on the lips. (From Bithell TC: Bleeding disorders caused by vascular abnormalities. In Lee GR, Bithell TC, Foerster J et al [eds]: Wintrobe's Clinical Hematology, 9th ed, p 1381. Philadelphia, Lea & Febiger, 1993, with permission.)

soles of the feet. Although they may be detected in childhood, the number of lesions increases with advancing age, and bleeding usually begins during the second or third decade. Epistaxis and alimentary bleeding are the most common symptoms, but patients may also present with symptoms of anemia. Telangiectasias are permanent; they do not disappear with time. Ecchymoses and purpura are not seen in this disorder.

Anemia is seen in many cases, depending on the degree of bleeding. An iron deficiency anemia may develop from either gastrointestinal bleeding or other chronic blood loss. There are no characteristic laboratory findings. Usually, the bleeding time, platelet function tests, tourniquet test, and coagulation tests are normal. The diagnosis is based largely on the finding of telangiectasias. The oral administration of iron may be used to alleviate iron deficiency anemia. Generally, treatment is given only based on symptoms. A number of therapeutic drugs and surgical techniques may be required to stop or prevent bleeding episodes.[2] The offspring of two affected parents die at an early age.[29]

CAVERNOUS HEMANGIOMA (KASABACH-MERRITT SYNDROME)

The cavernous or "strawberry" (for its red-blue color) hemangioma is a tumor that encloses large vascular spaces and is partly or completely filled with blood. It is usually present at birth or soon thereafter. Such tumors are composed of soft vascular malformations that commonly swell and bleed at the surface and range in size from small to enormous lesions that protrude from the skin surface. They generally require surgical removal.

Formation of fibrin clots, platelet consumption, and red cell destruction secondary to vascular obstruction occur at the site of the tumor. This leads to laboratory test results indicative of diffuse intravascular coagulation (DIC) (Chap. 52), which is found in association with a variety of disorders.

Acquired Alterations of Vessel Wall Structure

A number of other disorders may damage the vessel wall structure, *e.g.*, *diabetes mellitus* and *amyloidosis*. In diabetes mellitus, the large vessels may become atherosclerotic and the capillary basement membrane may thicken, thus blocking normal blood flow. Amyloidosis involves the abnormal deposition of the fibrillar protein amyloid, which obstructs the function of many organs including the vascular system. It weakens vessels and causes hemorrhaging. There are no characteristic hematologic or hemostatic abnormalities associated with either of these disorders.

Other Causes of Vascular Damage

Many autoimmune or infectious agents (*e.g.*, rickettsia) are responsible for vascular damage. This damage can lead to either hypocoagulation or hypercoagulation. Hypertension may also damage the endothelium, resulting in a microangiopathic hemolytic anemia.

AUTOIMMUNE VASCULAR PURPURA

Autoimmune vascular purpura may be drug induced or caused by an allergic reaction.

Drug-Induced Purpura. Table 47-4 lists some of the more common drugs that induce purpura in susceptible patients. Such purpura disappears on discontinuance of the drug.

Allergic Purpura. This purpura includes a broad group of disorders resulting from what is presumed to be an autoimmune process that is not clearly understood. Patients with allergic purpura develop vascular inflammation due to an immune disturbance which leads to characteristic purpuric eruptions on the skin surface. The tissues below the surface are also affected to some degree. The lesions may be accompanied by swelling, and in some cases ulcers develop at the lesion sites. Most commonly, lesions develop on the arms and legs (Fig. 47-6). The lesions begin as small, round, raised, pink areas that within hours turn to a darker red and begin to coalesce into larger patches. In the recovery phase, the area turns purple and then brown.

Children are the most frequently affected by allergic purpura. Adolescents are affected less often and adults rarely.[2] Patients may complain of headaches, abdominal or joint pain, anorexia, nausea and vomiting, or fever. They may also report an itching, tingling, or a numb sensation at the lesion sites.

Henoch-Schönlein Purpura. Two specific types of allergic purpura have been recognized since the 1800s. Purpura associated with abdominal pain secondary to gastrointestinal hemorrhaging is called Henoch's purpura.[15] When associated with joint pain, especially in the knees, ankles, and wrists,[40] the disorder is called Schönlein's purpura.[43] Abdominal and joint pain related to allergic purpura may occur together, thus the designation Henoch-Schönlein

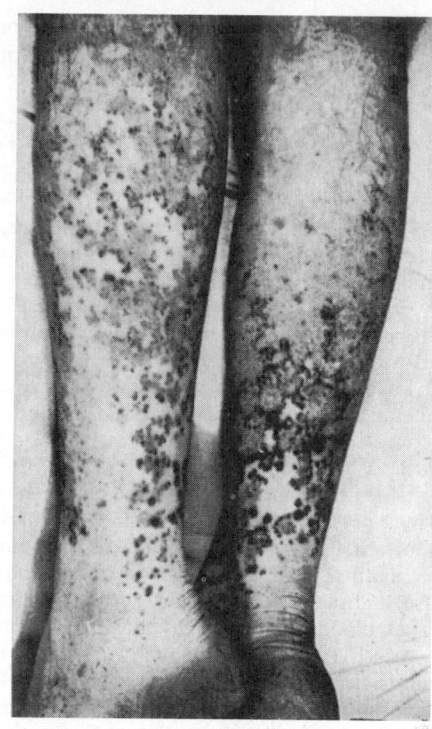

FIGURE 47-6. Henoch-Schönlein purpura; note ecchymoses and erythematous lesions on both legs. (From Bithell TC: Bleeding disorders caused by vascular abnormalities. In Lee GR, Bithell TC, Foerster J et al [eds]: Wintrobe's Clinical Hematology, 9th ed, p 1377. Philadelphia, Lea & Febiger, 1993, with permission.)

purpura (see Fig. 47-6). In this disorder, IgA, IgG, and C3 are deposited in the cutaneous and renal vasculature.[42]

Usually, there is no anemia, but there may be a modest neutrophilia or eosinophilia.[2] The tourniquet test may be positive, but other tests of coagulation, platelet number, and platelet function usually are normal. IgA immune complexes can be detected in the serum. The stools may be positive for blood. In some cases, there is renal involvement which leads to proteinuria, hematuria, and casturia.[23]

The diagnosis can be difficult because purpura is not always obvious, and other disorders may produce similar symptoms, particularly joint and abdominal pain, which are associated with a number of conditions. Treatment is usually limited to symptomatic therapy, as the purpuric episodes begin and subside spontaneously; most patients recover within a month, although lesions may recur over a period of weeks to months.[23] Any recognized allergen should be avoided. Deposits of IgA in vasculitic lesions have been associated with a longer clinical course and a high incidence of systemic involvement.[28]

INFECTIOUS PURPURA

As listed in Table 47-4, vascular damage can be caused by a number of infectious agents, which may produce purpura as well as petechiae. The purpura may form as a result of an inflammatory response to the infectious process, an autoimmune response, bacterial products, toxins, or direct injury by the infectious agent. In some disorders, there is concurrent thrombocytopenia and DIC that contribute to the formation of purpura. When an infectious agent is suspected, laboratory tests are performed to identify the infectious agent and select appropriate antibiotic treatment, when possible.

CHAPTER SUMMARY

Hemostasis involves the interaction of blood vessels (see Fig. 47-2 and Table 47-2), platelets, plasma procoagulants, fibrinolysis, and tissue repair. Abnormalities in any of these components may result in mild to life-threatening bleeding or clotting. Upon vessel injury, four sequential events occur (see Fig. 47-3) including vasoconstriction, platelet activation, activation of coagulation factors, and fibrinolysis.

The extrinsic coagulation pathway is now considered dominant *in vivo* (see Fig. 47-4). It involves the tissue factor:factor VIIa–Ca^{2+} complex activation of factor X in the common pathway (factors X, V, II, I, and XIII), and it is here that the final reactions in stable fibrin clot formation take place. The *in vivo* role of some intrinsic pathway factors (XI, IX, and VIII) in coagulation remains important. Contact activation seems to be unimportant to *in vivo* coagulation; nevertheless, it does initiate the inflammatory response, complement activation, and fibrinolysis.

Peripheral blood platelets may be increased (thrombocytosis), decreased (thrombocytopenia), or normal in number but abnormal in function (thrombocytopathy). Platelets secrete many substances that are important to hemostasis (see Table 47-3). Fibrinolysis begins to dissolve a clot as soon as it is formed; the enzyme responsible for this is plasmin. A lack of fibrinolysis results in thrombotic disorders; excessive fibrinolysis, in bleeding disorders. Hereditary and acquired vascular abnormalities cause many types of bleeding disorders (see Table 47-4), the most common hereditary condition being hemorrhagic telangiectasia (see Fig. 47-5).

Case Study 47-1

A small group of physicians, laboratory scientists, and nurses set up a clinic in a developing country plagued by famine. In one particular village, the group noticed that many of the children and adults had bleeding gums and petechiae on the buttocks. A few of the children had hemorrhagic areas below their eyes.

1. What is the most likely cause of these abnormal physical findings?
2. What is the name of this disorder, and how does it affect the vascular system?
3. What is the easiest and most cost-effective diagnostic approach when this disorder is suspected?
4. With successful treatment, what are the effects on abnormal laboratory findings and patient physical findings relating to this disorder?

Case Study 47-2

A 9-year-old black girl with a markedly prolonged PTT (58.0 sec, control 28.0) was referred to a hematologist for evaluation of her coagulation abnormality in preparation for a dental extraction. The patient's PT (11.4 sec, control 11.3) and bleeding time (6.5 min; normal 2–7) were normal. She had undergone an appendectomy at 2 years of age without any bleeding complications. There was no family history of a bleeding disorder on the paternal side; however, no information was available on the maternal side.[1]

[1]Case study obtained from DeLa Cadena RA: Fletcher factor deficiency in a 9-year-old girl: Mechanisms of the contact pathway of blood coagulation. Am J Hematol 48:273, 1995. Reprinted by permission of Wiley-hiss, Inc., a subsidiary of John Wiley & Sons, Inc.

1. Which of the classic coagulation systems appears to be affected in this case? Why?
2. What coagulation factors could be deficient?
3. Given her abnormal PTT, is it surprising that she had no bleeding problems associated with her appendectomy? Explain.
4. What coagulation factors are more likely to be deficient given that this child does not appear to have bleeding problems?
5. What coagulation tests might be recommended to evaluate this child's abnormal PTT?
6. Would she be expected to have bleeding complications from a dental extraction?

Review Questions

47-1. Factor I is commonly known as

    A. tissue factor.
    B. prothrombin.
    C. antihemophilic factor.
    D. fibrinogen.

47-2. The traditional intrinsic coagulation pathway includes factors

    A. X, V, IV, III, II, and I.
    B. XII, XI, IX, VIII, prekallikrein, and HMWK.
    C. IX, X, XII, XIII, prekallikrein, and HMWK.
    D. VII and tissue factor.

47-3. A substance released from platelets that promotes their aggregation is

    A. HMWK.
    B. ADP.
    C. factor V.
    D. α_2-antiplasmin.

47-4. Epistaxis means

    A. nosebleed.
    B. vomiting of blood.
    C. excessive menstrual bleeding.
    D. blood in the urine.
    For the following questions choose from these answers:
    A. 1 and 3
    B. 2 and 4
    C. 1, 2, and 3
    D. 4 only
    E. all are correct

47-5. A normal hemostatic mechanism depends upon the normal structure and function of

    1. tissues surrounding the blood vessels.
    2. platelets.
    3. blood vessels.
    4. plasma coagulation proteins.

47-6. In the disorder called scurvy,

    1. bleeding abnormalities are unusual.
    2. plasma ascorbic acid levels are usually decreased.
    3. several laboratory tests are required for the diagnosis.
    4. a dietary vitamin C deficiency is the cause.

References

1. Addison W: On the colorless corpuscles and on the molecules and cytoblasts in the blood. London Med Gaz (New Series) 30:144, 1842
2. Bithell TC: Bleeding disorders caused by vascular abnormalities. In Lee GR, Bithell TC, Foerster J (eds): Wintrobe's Clinical

Hematology, 9th ed, pp 1375, 1378-9, 1382-4. Philadelphia, Lea & Febiger, 1993

3. Brecher G, Cronkite EP: Morphology and enumeration of human blood platelets. J Appl Physiol 3:365, 1950

4. Broze GJ Jr: The role of tissue factor pathway inhibitor in a revised coagulation cascade. Semin Hematol 29(3):157, 1992

5. Byers PH, Holbrook KA: Ehlers-Danlos syndrome. Prin Pract Med Genet 1:1065, 1990

6. Colman RW: Surface mediated defense reactions: The plasma contact activation system. J Clin Invest 73:1249, 1984

7. Davie EW, Ratnoff OD: Waterfall sequence for intrinsic blood clotting. Science 145:1310, 1964

8. Donné AD: L'origine des globules der sang de leur mode de formation et de leur fin. Comp Rend Acad Sci 14:366, 1842

9. Duke WW: The pathogenesis of purpura haemorrhagica with especial reference to the part played by the blood platelets. Arch Intern Med 10:445, 1912

10. Estes JW: Platelet abnormalities in heritable disorders of connective tissue. Ann NY Acad Sci 201:445, 1972

11. Gerber F: Elements of General and Minute Anatomy of Man and Mammals. London, G Gulliver, 1842

12. Hare FW Jr, Miller AJ: Capillary resistance tests. Arch Dermatol Syph 64:449, 1951

13. Harker LA: Platelet survival time: Its measurement and use. In Spaet TH (ed): Progress in Hemostasis and Thrombosis, p 321. New York, Grune & Stratton, 1978

14. Hayem G: Recherches sur l'évolution des hématies dans le sang del'homme et des vertébrés. Arch Physiol Norm Pathol 5:692, 1878

15. Henoch E: Über eine eigenthümliche Form von Purpura. Berlin Klin Wochenschr 11:641, 1874

16. Hopff F: Über die Hämophilie oder die erbliche Anlage zu todtlichen Blutungen [thesis]. Würzburg, Germany, 1828

17. Hunter J: A Treatise on the Blood, Inflammation, and Gun-Shot Wounds, 3rd ed. London, Sherwood, Gilbert, and Piper, 1828

18. Kakkar VV: The diagnosis of deep vein thrombosis using the ^{125}I-fibrinogen test. Arch Surg 104:152, 1972

19. Lee RI, White PD: A clinical study of the coagulation time of blood. Am J Med Sci 145:495, 1913

20. Lee W, Hamernyik P, Hutchinson M et al: Ascorbic acid in lymphocytes: Cell preparation and liquid-chromatographic assay. Clin Chem 28:2165, 1982

21. Lind SE: The bleeding time does not predict surgical bleeding. Blood 77:2547, 1991

22. Lipinska I, Lipinski B, Gurewich V et al: Fibrinogen heterogeneity in cancer, in occlusive vascular disease, and after surgical procedures. Am J Clin Pathol 66:958, 1976

23. Lowe GDO: Vascular disease and vasculitis. In Ratnoff OD, Forbes CD (eds): Disorders of Hemostasis, p 5. Philadelphia, WB Saunders, 1991

24. MacFarlane RG: The basis of the cascade hypothesis of blood clotting. Thromb Diath Haemorrh 15:591, 1966

25. MacFarlane RG: Fibrinolysis after operation. Lancet 1:10, 1937

26. Madden JL, Hume M: Venous Thromboembolism: Prevention and Treatment. New York, Appleton-Century-Crofts, 1976

27. Miale JB: Laboratory Medicine Hematology, 6th ed, p 916. St Louis, CV Mosby, 1982

28. Mills JA, Michel BA, Bloch DA et al: The American College of Rheumatology 1990 criteria for the classification of Henoch Schönlein purpura. Arthritis Rheum 33:1114, 1990

29. Muller JY, Michailov T, Izrael V et al: Maladie de RenduOsler dans une grande famille saharienne. Presse Med 7:1723, 1978

30. National Research Council (U.S.): Recommended Dietary Allowances, 10th ed. Washington, DC, National Academy Press, 1989

30a. Nemerson Y: The tissue factor pathway of blood coagulation. Semin Hematol 29(3):170, 1992

31. Oeffinger KC: Scurvy: More than historical relevance. Am Fam Physician 48(4):609, 1993

32. Otto JC: An account of an hemorrhagic disposition existing in certain families. Med Resposit 6:1, 1803

33. Pachla LA, Reynolds DL, Kissinger PT: Analytical methods for determining ascorbic acid in biological samples, food products, and pharmaceuticals. J Assoc Off Anal Chem 68:2, 1985

34. Pasquali M, Dembure PP, Still MJ et al: Urinary pyridinium cross-links: A noninvasive diagnostic test for Ehlers-Danlos syndrome type VI. N Engl J Med 331(2):132, 1994

35. Petty EM, Seashore MR, Braverman IM et al: Dermatosparaxis in children. Arch Dermatol 129:1310, 1993

36. Plato: Timaeus. In Jewett B (ed): The Dialogues of Plato, 3rd ed, vol 3, p 339. New York, Macmillan, 1982

37. Prokop DJ, Kiririkko KI: Heritable diseases of collagen. N Engl J Med 311:376, 1984

38. Quick AJ: The prothrombin in hemophilia and obstructive jaundice. J Biol Chem 109:73, 1935

39. Quick AJ: The development and use of the prothrombin tests. Circulation 19:92, 1959

40. Rogers PW, Bunn SM Jr, Kurtzman NA et al: Schönlein-Henoch syndrome associated with exposure to cold. Arch Intern Med 128:782, 1971

41. Rosner F: Hemophilia in the Talmud and Rabbinic writings. Ann Intern Med 70(4):833, 1969

42. Schneiderman P: The vascular purpuras. In Beutler E, Lichtman MA, Coller BS et al (eds): Williams Hematology, 5th ed, p 1408. New York, McGraw-Hill, 1995

43. Schönlein JL: Allgemeine und specielle. Patholgie und Therapie 2:45, 1837

44. Schönlein JL: Hämorrhaphilie (erbliche Anlage zu Blutungen) in Allgemeine und specielle Pathologie und Therapie. In Nach JL: Schönleins Vorlesungen niedergeschrieben und herausgegeben von einem seiner Zuhörer, 2nd ed, vol 2, p 88. Würzburg, Germany, Etlinger, 1832

45. Senior RM, Griffin GL, Huang JS et al: Chemotactic activity of platelet alpha granule proteins for fibroblasts. J Cell Biol 96:382, 1983

46. Shiozawa S, Tanaka T, Miyahara T et al: Age-related change in the reducible cross-link of human skin and aorta collagens. Gerontology 25:247, 1979

47. Tattersall RN, Seville R: Senile purpura. Q J Med 19:151, 1959

48. Tietz NW: Clinical Guide to Laboratory Tests, 2nd ed, p 584. Philadelphia, WB Saunders, 1990

49. Walsh PN: Factor XI: A renaissance. Semin Hematol 29(3):189, 1992

50. Wright IS: The nomenclature of blood clotting factors. Thromb Diath Haemorrh 7:381, 1962

CHAPTER 48

Mechanisms of Coagulation and Fibrinolysis

Muriel I. Jobe

Objectives

1. Identify the name, Roman numeral designation, active form, site of production, and location of pathway participation for each of the clotting factors.
2. List the coagulation factors that are vitamin K dependent.
3. Name the inheritance pattern, inherited coagulopathy, and at least one acquired coagulopathy for each clotting factor.
4. List the properties of the contact, the prothrombin, and the fibrinogen groups of coagulation factors.
5. Identify the mode of inheritance, parts, and function of the factor VIII complex.
6. Explain the intrinsic, extrinsic, common, and alternate pathways of coagulation.
7. Explain the mechanisms of fibrinolysis.
8. Name and describe the action of the coagulation and fibrinolytic inhibitors.

Blood extravasation (the escape of blood from vessels into surrounding tissues) normally is controlled or prevented by the delicate balance among at least five systems and their biochemical reactions: (1) the lining of endothelial cells in the blood vessels (Chap. 47); (2) platelets (Chap. 55); (3) plasma coagulation proteins; (4) physiologic and naturally occurring protease inhibitors; and (5) the fibrinolytic system. These systems work together when the blood vessel endothelial lining is disrupted by mechanical trauma (*e.g.*, surgery), physical agents (*e.g.*, heat), or chemical injury (*e.g.*, bacterial endotoxins or drugs). The emphasis in this chapter is on the coagulation proteins, inhibitors, and fibrinolysis. In addition, the kinin and complement systems will be discussed as they relate to coagulation.

HEMOSTASIS OVERVIEW

Hemostasis can be divided into two stages: primary and secondary. *Primary hemostasis* includes the platelet and vascular response to vessel injury. *Secondary hemostasis* includes the coagulation factor response to such injury. Together, platelets, vessels, and coagulation factors combine to stop bleeding and allow for vessel repair through formation of a stable fibrin–platelet plug at the site of injury.

Primary Hemostasis

Primary hemostasis is initiated by the exposure of platelets to the subendothelial connective tissue components (see Fig. 47-2) of blood vessels (collagen, microfilaments, basement membranes, von Willebrand factor, and others). If acute injury occurs, the small vessels constrict, and platelets immediately adhere to the exposed surfaces. Next, reversible primary platelet aggregation takes place, during which platelets adhere to one another. Platelets also change shape, and their organelles become centralized. At this point, platelets may disaggregate in the absence of further stimulation. However, with continued stimulation, secondary, irreversible platelet aggregation characteristically occurs (see Table 47-1). Important substances released during platelet aggregation include ADP,

ATP, thromboxane A$_2$ and serotonin (see Table 47-3). ADP promotes secondary platelet aggregation and recruits additional platelets to the site of injury. ATP may play a role in limiting the size of the platelet plug by inhibiting excessive platelet aggregation.[33] Thromboxane A$_2$, in addition to being a potent vasoconstrictor, induces and maintains the platelet shape change as well as the platelet release reaction. Serotonin also promotes platelet aggregation and further vasoconstriction, although a lack of platelet serotonin does not impair vasoconstriction[116] or prolong the bleeding time.[97] During aggregation, phospholipid becomes available on the platelet membrane surface (Chap. 55), providing a site for thrombogenesis (the formation of fibrin blood clots).

Secondary Hemostasis

Secondary hemostasis includes the response of the coagulation process to vessel injury (see Table 47-1). In Chapter 47 the intrinsic and extrinsic pathways of coagulation, which involve various proteins and other substances, were introduced. To review, the intrinsic system is activated *in vivo* by the contact of certain coagulation proteins with subendothelial connective tissue, which sets the secondary hemostatic mechanism into motion (Fig. 48-1). The extrinsic coagulation pathway, in contrast, is initiated with the release of *tissue factor* (TF) from injured vessel endothelial cells and subendothelium into the vessel lumen. TF, a high-molecular-weight lipoprotein, is found in most organs as well as in large blood vessels such as the vena cava and aorta. Especially high concentrations are found in the lungs, brain, and placenta. Both intrinsic and extrinsic coagulation pathways lead to the activation of the common pathway and the formation of a stable fibrin clot. The clot includes both fibrin formed in secondary hemostasis and the platelet plug formed in primary hemostasis. This chapter will provide a detailed explanation of the factors and reactions of the intrinsic, extrinsic, and common coagulation pathways.

THE COAGULATION PROTEINS

The coagulation pathways are a series of reactions that involve coagulation factors known as enzyme precursors (*zymogens*), nonenzymatic cofactors, calcium (Ca^{2+}), the substrate protein fibrinogen (factor I), and phospholipid. All coagulation factors except TF are normally present in the plasma, and phospholipid is provided by platelets. The zymogens are factors II, VII, IX, X, XI, XII, XIII, and prekallikrein; the cofactors are factors V and VIII, TF, Ca^{2+}, and high-molecular-weight kininogen (HMWK). Zymogens are substrates that have no biologic activity until converted by enzymes to active enzymes. With the exception of factor XIII, the zymogen factors are converted to enzymes called *serine proteases*, which have exposed, serine-rich, active enzyme sites. Serine proteases selectively hydrolyze arginine- or lysine-containing peptide bonds of other zymogens, thus converting them to serine proteases.[18] When converted to its active enzyme form, factor XIII has an active enzyme site containing cysteine rather than serine.

Zymogen activation may involve either: (1) a confor-mational change (*e.g.*, twist, turn, or bend) in the zymogen molecule or (2) hydrolytic cleavage of a specific zymogen peptide bond by a serine protease. Initially, coagulation reactions occur on the injured, exposed endothelial surfaces of blood vessels and consist of zymogen activation by conformational changes. Later, coagulation reactions occur on the phospholipid surfaces of aggregated platelets and involve hydrolytic cleavage of the next sequential zymogen to an active enzyme.

Activation of factor X requires both factor IXa and the nonenzymatic cofactor VIII. Activation of factor II requires both factor Xa and the nonenzymatic cofactor V. To perform their functions, these cofactors must be activated (VIIIa and Va) by trace amounts of thrombin (factor IIa). On the other hand, high concentrations of thrombin *inhibit* VIII and V activity. Cofactors assist in activation of zymogens by either altering zymogen conformation to permit more efficient cleavage by the serine protease, or binding the zymogen and appropriate serine protease on a platelet phospholipid surface to enhance and accelerate the zymogen activation process, or both. The transformation of zymogens to active serine proteases causes biochemical amplification of the coagulation process; that is, the production of serine proteases increases the rate of further transformation of zymogens and the activity levels of cofactors. For example, traces of thrombin increase the activity of factor VIII 80-fold.[84]

The hemostatic process simultaneously provides amplification of the control mechanisms that prevent excessive clotting and clot lysis. Inhibitors and thrombolytic factors maintain a balance in the system between adequate and excessive clotting. While tissue is being repaired, the clot is slowly dissolved by the fibrinolytic system, which depends upon the glycoprotein enzyme plasmin (also called fibrinolysin). Although plasmin is capable of digesting many proteins (fibrin, fibrinogen, factors V and VIII), it is regulated by several inhibitors discussed later in this chapter.

COAGULATION AND THE KININ SYSTEM

Kinins are peptides of low molecular weight. They are involved in chemotaxis and the sensation of pain. They mediate inflammatory responses, increase vascular permeability, cause vasodilation and hypotension, and induce contraction of smooth muscle. The *kinin system* contains factors that are also activated by the coagulation and fibrinolytic systems (see Fig. 48-1). These factors are important in coagulation as well as in complement system activation.

The kinin system factors involved in coagulation do not have assigned Roman numerals. They include (1) prekallikrein (Fletcher factor); (2) kallikrein (the serine protease or activated form of prekallikrein); and (3) high-molecular-weight kininogen (HMWK [Fitzgerald factor]). Other substances in the kinin system include the kinins which are produced through conversion of kininogens by the enzyme kallikrein. One example is bradykinin, which has no apparent effect on coagulation.[43,44]

Prekallikrein circulates in plasma as a complex with the cofactor HMWK. Prekallikrein is converted to the

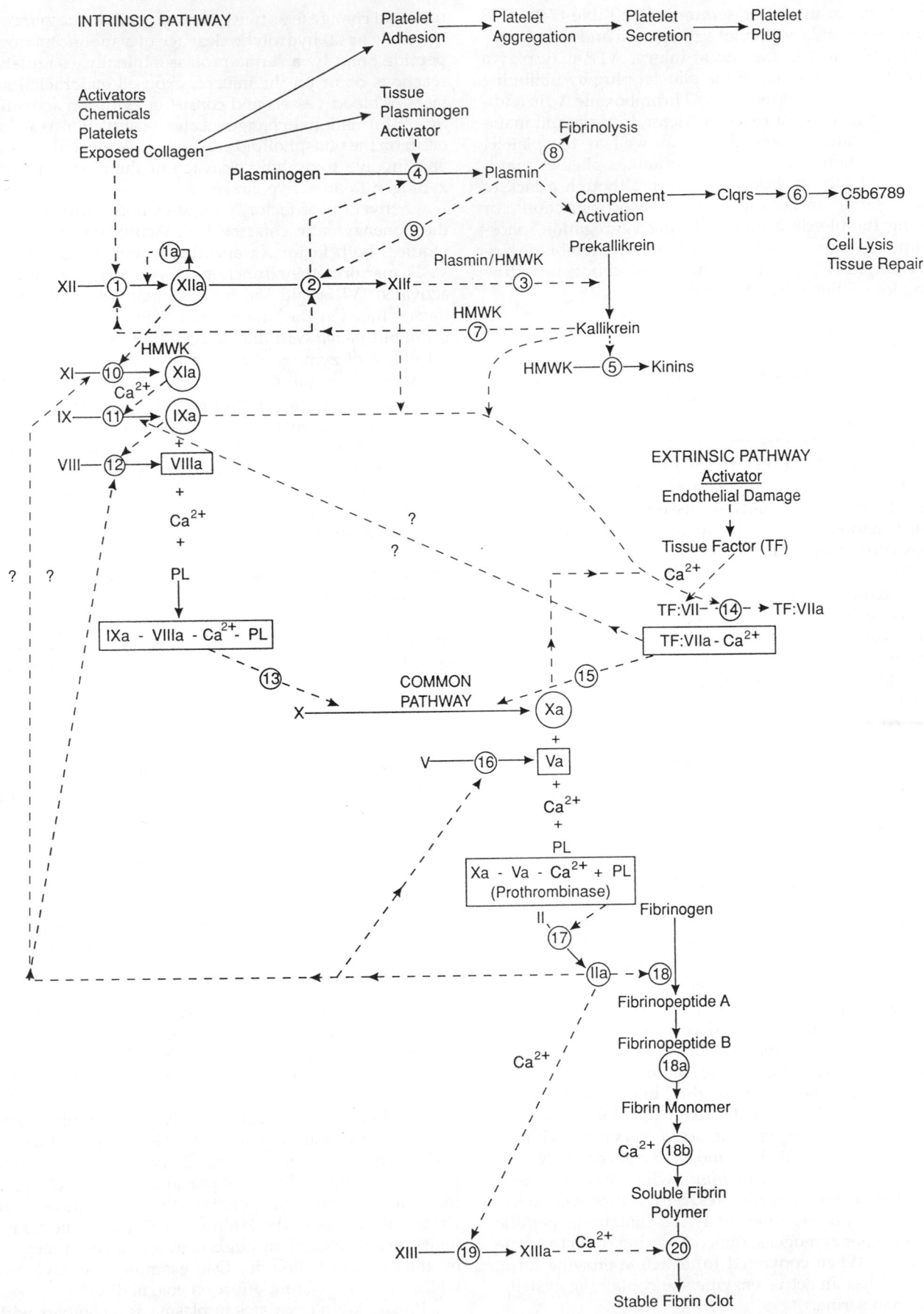

FIGURE 48-1.

serine protease kallikrein in the presence of factors XIIa and XIIf, plasmin, and HMWK. Kallikrein converts HMWK to kinins and accelerates factor XII activation. Kallikrein is also involved in the fibrinolytic system. Kallikrein and activated factor XII (XIIa) form a complex known as a "plasminogen activator," which converts plasminogen to its active form *plasmin* (see Fig. 48-3). Plasmin dissolves fibrin clots.

COAGULATION AND THE COMPLEMENT SYSTEM

The complement system, which is important in the mediation of immune and allergic reactions, is activated by plasmin during coagulation and fibrinolysis (see Fig. 48-1, Rxn 6). Plasmin, in the presence of antibody–antigen complexes to which complement has bound, can directly activate the first component in the complement cascade, C1 (also known as C1 esterase). C1 is composed of the proteins C1q, C1r, and C1s and causes cleavage of C3 to C3a and C3b (see Fig. 19-1). C3a is an anaphylatoxin that causes increased vascular permeability, which can lead to hypotension and shock. These clinical findings are common in diffuse intravascular coagulation (DIC) and other thrombohemorrhagic disorders.[89] C3b causes immune adherence of erythrocytes to neutrophils and macrophages, thus enhancing their phagocytosis.

Plasmin can also directly activate C3 in the absence of antibody in what is known as the alternate (properdin) complement pathway.[31] In any case, complement system activation is held in check by an inhibitor known as C'1 inactivator (see Table 48-7), which binds to C1r and C1s and prevents their activation of C3. C'1 inactivator also inhibits complement activation by inhibiting factors XIIa, plasmin, and kallikrein, which can activate the complement system (see Fig. 48-1). Refer to Chapter 19 for details on the complement system.

THE COAGULATION FACTORS

Factor Nomenclature

The nomenclature of coagulation factors includes (1) those referred to by Roman numerals assigned by the International Committee on Nomenclature of Blood Coagulation Factors[117]; and (2) the two factors in the kinin system, prekallikrein and HMWK, which are referred to by name only. Each Roman numeral was assigned in the order of factor discovery, not its place in the reaction sequence. These factors are listed in Table 48-1 with their preferred names and other synonyms.

An important aspect of coagulation factor nomenclature is the "a" that sometimes accompanies a Roman numeral (*e.g.*, factor XIIa). It denotes the activated serine protease form of that factor rather than the zymogen (except in the case of cofactors V and VIII, discussed earlier). An "f" refers to fragmented factor XII (XIIf).

Tissue factor (TF) is sometimes referred to as factor III and the calcium ion (Ca^{2+}) as factor IV (see Table 48-1). However, *tissue factor* and *calcium* are the generally accepted terms today, and these terms will be used in the various figures in this chapter demonstrating the coagulation process. What was once called factor VI was discovered to be activated factor V; therefore, "factor VI" is nonexistent.

Characteristics of the Coagulation Factors

Table 48-2 provides information concerning the characteristics of the active form of each coagulation factor. The presence of certain coagulation factors and the absence of others in barium sulfate ($BaSO_4$)-adsorbed plasma is a characteristic that allows laboratories to screen for factor deficiencies using substitution (mixing) studies (Chap. 49, Table 49-1). However, substitution studies are being replaced in many institutions by factor assays that can specifically identify a factor deficiency. Table 48-2 also presents a list of chromosomes determined to be responsible for production of the coagulation factors. Table 48-3 presents an overview of the mode of inheritance for each factor deficiency. It also gives the names of the coagulopathies associated with both inherited and acquired deficiencies of each factor (see Chap. 52 for details).

THE COAGULATION FACTOR GROUPS

The properties of the coagulation and kinin factors have similarities that allow for convenient division of these factors into three groups: (1) the contact group; (2) the prothrombin or vitamin K-dependent group; and (3) the fibrinogen group. The features common to each group are listed in Table 48-4. The reader should become familiar with the properties that distinguish the three coagulation groups.

Contact Group

Prekallikrein and HMWK of the kinin group, along with factors XII and XI, make up the contact group. The contact group is activated by contact with a negatively charged

---

FIGURE 48-1. Pathways of coagulation (intrinsic, extrinsic, and common) and fibrinolytic systems and their interaction with the kinin and complement systems. Circles containing Roman numeral factor numbers are serine proteases; kallikrein and plasmin are also serine proteases. Factors within a square are cofactors (Va and VIIIa). Rectangles are coagulation complexes. Numbers for various reactions in small circles are referred to in text as reaction (Rxn) numbers. Solid arrows indicate factor transformation. Dashed arrows indicate action. PL, platelet phospholipid. See Fig. 19-1 for details on the complement pathway; all reactants are not shown. ?? = The activation of XI to XIa by thrombin and of IX to IXa by TF:VIIa — Ca^{2+} has been shown *in vitro* but remains uncertain *in vivo*.

TABLE 48-1
Coagulation Factor Nomenclature With Preferred Names and Synonyms

Numeral	Preferred Name	Synonyms
I	Fibrinogen	
II	Prothrombin	Prethrombin
III	Tissue factor	Tissue thromboplastin
IV	Calcium	Ca^{2+}
V	Proaccelerin	Labile factor Accelerator globulin (AcG)
VII	Proconvertin	Stable factor Serum prothrombin conversion accelerator (SPCA) Autoprothrombin I
VIII:C	Antihemophilic factor (AHF)	Antihemophilic globulin (AHG) Antihemophilic factor A Platelet cofactor 1
IX	Plasma thromboplastin component (PTC)	Christmas factor Antihemophilic factor B Platelet cofactor 2
X	Stuart-Prower factor	Stuart factor Prower factor Autoprothrombin III Thrombokinase
XI	Plasma thromboplastin antecedent (PTA)	Antihemophilic factor C
XII	Hageman factor	Glass factor Contact factor
XIII	Fibrin stabilizing factor	Laki-Lorand Factor (LLF) Fibrinase Plasma transglutaminase Fibrinoligase
—	Prekallikrein	Fletcher factor
—	High-molecular-weight kininogen (HMWK)	Fitzgerald factor Contact activation cofactor Williams factor Flaujeac factor

surface such as glass *in vitro* or collagen or the subendothelium *in vivo*. The role of contact activation in physiologic hemostasis is uncertain (see Intrinsic Coagulation Pathway). The contact factors are also involved in kinin formation and activation of fibrinolysis and the complement system (see Fig. 48-1).

Prothrombin (Vitamin K-Dependent) Group

The prothrombin group contains the vitamin K-dependent coagulation factors II, VII, IX, and X. Vitamin K is fat soluble and normally ingested in the diet. It is also manufactured by the gut flora. There is no substantial storage of vitamin K in the body.

Vitamin K is necessary to γ-carboxylate the glutamic acid residues at the N-terminal or amino- (NH_2) end of the enzyme precursors.[103] This allows the factors to bind Ca^{2+} and form *calcium bridges* with the acidic phospholipid surface of activated platelets. Both Ca^{2+} and platelet surface phospholipid are essential for enzyme and substrate functions in the coagulation pathways.[53]

Vitamin K-dependent reactions may be decreased or inhibited by several mechanisms: (1) dietary vitamin K deficiency; (2) diseases causing malabsorption of vitamin K (*e.g.*, sprue, celiac disease, and ulcerative colitis); (3) administration of antibiotics that sterilize the intestinal tract, where normal flora usually synthesize vitamin K; or (4) oral anticoagulant therapy, such as with the coumarin drug warfarin, which interferes with γ-carboxylation.[5,72] Any of these mechanisms can cause the formation of nonfunctional vitamin K-dependent coagulation factors. When such factors are released to the circulation, they cannot bind to the platelet phospholipid surface and ultimately prevent prothrombin activation, causing a coagulation deficiency.[37]

Fibrinogen Group

The fibrinogen group includes factors I, V, VIII, and XIII. These factors have the highest molecular weights of all the factors, are the most labile, are consumed in coagulation, and are the only group that act as substrates for the fibrinolytic enzyme plasmin (*i.e.*, they are destroyed by plasmin). Factors I and V are found in platelet α-granules and factor XIII is found in the general platelet cytoplasm.

TABLE 48-2
Characteristics of Clotting Factors

Factor	Active Form	Molecular Weight (×10³)	Pathway Participation	Site of Production	Vitamin K Dependent?	In Vivo Half-Life (Hours)	Plasma Concentration (µg/mL)	Minimum Hemostatic Level (%)*	Chromosome Coding for Production[63,93]
I	Fibrin clot	340	Common	Liver	No	72–120	160–415▲	100 mg/dL	4q23-q32
II	Serine protease	72	Common	Liver	Yes	67–106	100	20–40	11
V	Cofactor	330	Common	Liver	No	12–36	7	10–25	1q21-25
VII	Serine protease	63	Extrinsic	Liver	Yes	4–6	0.5	5–10	13
VIII:C	Cofactor	267 (VIII/vWF >1000)	Intrinsic	Uncertain for (VIII:C)**	No	10–12 / 22–40†	1–8 (VIII/vWF)	25–30	Xq28
IX	Serine protease	55	Intrinsic	Liver	Yes	18–40	5	15–25	X
X	Serine protease	55	Common	Liver	Yes	24–60?‡	10	10–20	13q32-qter
XI	Serine protease	160	Intrinsic	Liver	No	48–84?‡	4–6	10–20	4q35
XII	Serine protease	80	Intrinsic	?‡	No	52–60	30–45	0–5	5q33-qter
XIII	Transglutaminase	320	Common	Liver	No	3–7 days?‡	25	2–3	XIIIa: 6p-24-25 XIIIb: 1q31-q32.1
Prekallikrein	Serine protease	85	Intrinsic	?Liver‡	No	35?‡	35–50	?‡	4[35a]
HMW Kininogen	Serine protease	120	Intrinsic	?Liver‡	No	6.5 days?‡	70–90	?	3q[35a]

*Approximate minimum plasma concentration required for normal coagulation. Note that minimum hemostatic level for factor XII is 0–5% (i.e., factor XII may not be required for normal coagulation).

**vWF portion synthesized by endothelial cells and megakaryocytes.

†22–40 hours for high-molecular-weight subunit of factor VIII.

?‡ Insufficient data or significant disagreement exists among published values; for minimum hemostatic level, none reported.

▲ Fibrinogen reported as 160–415 mg/dL.

TABLE 48-3
Disorders of Coagulation Causing Clotting Factor Deficiencies

| Factor | Inherited Coagulopathies | | Acquired Coagulopathies |
	Inheritance Pattern	*Coagulopathy*	
I	Autosomal recessive	Afibrinogenemia	Severe liver disease Diffuse intravascular coagulation Fibrinolysis†
	Autosomal dominant	Dysfibrinogenemia	
II	Autosomal recessive	Prothrombin deficiency	Liver disease Vitamin K deficiency Anticoagulant therapy
V	Autosomal recessive	Factor V deficiency	Severe liver disease Diffuse intravascular coagulation Fibrinolysis†
VII	Autosomal recessive	Factor VII deficiency	Liver disease Vitamin K deficiency Anticoagulant therapy
VIII	X-linked recessive	Hemophilia A	Diffuse intravascular coagulation Fibrinolysis†
	Autosomal dominant	von Willebrand's disease	
IX	X-linked recessive	Hemophilia B	Liver disease Vitamin K deficiency Anticoagulant therapy
X	Autosomal recessive	Factor X deficiency	Liver disease Vitamin K deficiency Anticoagulant therapy
XI	Autosomal recessive	Hemophilia C	Severe liver disease
XII	Autosomal recessive	Factor XII deficiency	?*
XIII	Autosomal recessive	Factor XIII deficiency	Liver disease Diffuse intravascular coagulation Fibrinolysis†
Prekallikrein	Autosomal recessive	Fletcher trait	?
HMWK	Autosomal recessive	Fitzgerald trait	?

* *It is unclear whether any acquired disorders cause factor XII deficiency or prekallikrein or HMWK deficiency.*
† *Clotting factor may or may not be deficient in abnormal fibrinolysis.*

However, factor VIII:C, the coagulant portion of factor VIII, is *not* found in platelets (see Table 48-4).

Factor VIII (VIII/vWF) is a large, multimeric molecule that has two principal parts: the coagulant portion (VIII:C), which acts as a cofactor in the intrinsic coagulation pathway, and also the von Willebrand portion (vWF), which is important to normal platelet function. *In vitro* the molecule can be separated into low-molecular-weight and high-molecular-weight parts (Fig. 48-2). Factor VIII:C, which probably is produced in the liver, has also been called *antihemophilic factor*, because it is defective in patients with hemophilia A, the best known of all bleeding disorders (Chap. 52). The high-molecular-weight portion of factor VIII is a large polymer that is synthesized by endothelial cells and megakaryocytes and is referred to as vWF or as vWF:Ag if measured immunologically. The International Committee on Thrombosis and Haemostasis has proposed a nomenclature for factor VIII and its various parts (see Table 52-1). This nomenclature reflects the different laboratory methods used to detect functional and physical abilities of the factor VIII complex.

PHOSPHOLIPIDS CONTRIBUTING TO COAGULATION

Tissue Factor

The existence of a substance called tissue thromboplastin was first recognized in 1905, when Paul Morawitz presented his classic theory of coagulation.[65] Morawitz theorized that blood remained fluid because a thromboplastic factor was not found in plasma. This factor was believed to remain inside cells until tissue injury occurred.

Today, Morawitz's proposed thromboplastic factor is known to be a phospholipid-containing, membrane-bound glycoprotein called *tissue factor* (TF, tissue thromboplastin, or factor III). TF is found in the plasma membrane of many cell types except endothelial cells, which have little or no TF. TF is important for activation of the extrinsic coagulation pathway. It binds both factors VII and VIIa on cell surfaces and has two cofactor roles in coagulation: (1) it potentiates the enzymatic activity of factor VIIa on factors IX and X; and (2) it accelerates

TABLE 48-4
Properties of the Coagulation Groups

	Contact	Prothrombin	Fibrinogen
FACTORS	XII, XI, prekallikrein, HMWK	II, VII, IX, X, protein C, protein S	I, V, VIII, XIII
FUNCTION	Serine proteases: XII, XI, prekallikrein Cofactor: HMWK	Serine proteases: II, VII, IX, X, protein C Cofactor: protein S	Precursor of fibrin: I Cofactors: V, VIII Transamidinase: XIII
MOLECULAR WEIGHT (DALTONS ×10³)	Medium (80–160)	Low (55–70)	High (>250)
STABILITY	Fairly stable	Heat labile: VII, IX, X Well preserved in stored plasma	Heat labile: I, V, VIII Storage labile: V, VIII
VITAMIN K DEPENDENT FOR SYNTHESIS?	No	Yes	No
ADSORBED BY $BaSO_4$, $Al(OH)_3$ AND OTHER SALTS?	Partially	Yes	No
CONSUMED IN COAGULATION?	Partially	No (except II)	Yes
SITE	Plasma or serum	Plasma or serum (except II is not present in serum)	Plasma
DESTROYED BY PLASMIN OR HIGH CONCENTRATIONS OF THROMBIN?	No	No	Yes
FOUND IN PLATELETS?	No	No	α-granules: I, V, vWF General cytoplasm: XIII Not present: VIII:C
ACUTE-PHASE REACTANTS?	No	No	Yes
PRODUCTION REDUCED BY ORAL ANTICOAGULANTS?	No	Yes	No

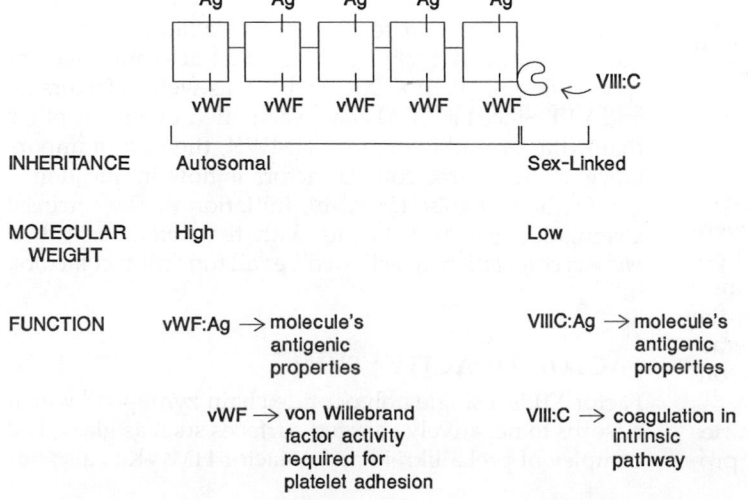

INHERITANCE	Autosomal	Sex-Linked
MOLECULAR WEIGHT	High	Low
FUNCTION	vWF:Ag → molecule's antigenic properties	VIIIC:Ag → molecule's antigenic properties
	vWF → von Willebrand factor activity required for platelet adhesion	VIII:C → coagulation in intrinsic pathway

FIGURE 48-2. The factor VIII molecule (VIII/vwF) is a polymer with multiple subunits composed of vWF(vWF:Ag) connected to a small coagulant unit known as VIII:C. See Table 52-1 for a detailed explanation of the nomenclature of the factor VIII molecule.

the feedback activation of factor VII by factor Xa (see Fig. 48-1).

The term *extrinsic* was applied to the extrinsic coagulation pathway because TF does not normally circulate in the peripheral blood. The prothrombin time (PT) test evaluates the extrinsic and common pathways by adding TF and calcium to plasma followed by measurement of the time necessary for clot formation.

Partial Thromboplastin and Platelet Phospholipid

Partial thromboplastin is a reagent used as a platelet substitute in evaluating the intrinsic and common coagulation pathways (Chap. 49) with a test appropriately called the partial thromboplastin time ("partial" because the reagent contains only the phospholipid portion of TF). In addition to the contact factors, the intrinsic system requires a complex of phospholipid, Ca^{2+}, activated factor IX (IXa), and cofactor VIII (VIIIa) in order to activate factor X in the common pathway. *In vitro* tests of the intrinsic system require the use of platelet-poor plasma to avoid test variation attributable to the patient's platelets; the partial thromboplastin reagent provides the necessary platelet phospholipid substitute.

PHYSIOLOGIC VARIATIONS OF THE COAGULATION FACTORS

The concentration of various coagulation factors depends on the patient's age and physical condition. At birth, infants normally are deficient in vitamin K owing to a sterile gut and an immature liver. Therefore, a moderate deficiency exists in the vitamin K–dependent factors.[1] Newborn infants are frequently given vitamin K supplements to correct this deficiency.

Among adults, physiologic variations of coagulation factors are most commonly associated with increases in concentrations (Table 48-5). These variations generally do not cause coagulation abnormalities. A few conditions are associated with decreases in coagulation factor concentrations that are not clinically significant, as they do not cause abnormal hemostasis. When factor abnormalities are the primary cause of clinical disorders, they are classified as acquired (*e.g.*, liver disease) or inherited (*e.g.*, hemophilia) coagulation disorders, which are discussed in Chapters 52 and 53 and summarized in Table 48-3.

THE PROCESS OF FIBRIN CLOT FORMATION

In 1964, two theories for the coagulation mechanism were presented, the "cascade"[52] and the "waterfall."[17] These theories (introduced in Chap. 47) presented the intrinsic and extrinsic coagulation pathways, both activating the common coagulation pathway without any other interaction among the pathways. The intrinsic pathway was considered the primary initiator of coagulation.

Today, highly modified versions of these theories have become the accepted models. Currently, it is pro-

TABLE 48-5
Conditions Most Often Associated With Physiologic Variations in Coagulation and Fibrinolytic Factors

Condition	Related Factor Increases	Related Factor Decreases
Stress[8]	I	
Tissue necrosis[8]	I	
Inflammation[8]	I	
Pregnancy[15,30,42,79]	I, VIII, IX, X	XIII, XI, AT-III
Oral contraceptives[10,16]	I, VIII, VII, IX, X	
Hypermetabolism (*e.g.*, hyperthyroidism)[6,38]	I, VIII, plasminogen	
Vigorous exercise[40,86]	VIII, XI, XII	
Chronic thrombocytopenia[48]	VIII	
Hypothyroidism[6,50,99]		IX, XI, plasminogen
Childbirth[48,51]*	I, VIII	
Surgical procedures[48,51]*	I, VIII	
Trauma[48,51]*	I, VIII	
Myocardial infarction[48,51]*	I, VIII	
Acute illness[48,51]*	I, VIII	

Temporary elevations associated with acute conditions. Once the acute reaction has subsided, factor concentration usually declines to normal.

posed that TF in the extrinsic pathway is the primary initiator of coagulation upon its exposure to factor VII in plasma. Modern theories also emphasize the importance of factors VIII and IX from the intrinsic pathway in the clot-formation process.

Intrinsic Coagulation Pathway

The term *intrinsic* is used to describe this pathway because all the components are found in the circulating blood. The intrinsic pathway includes the contact activation factors (prekallikrein, HMWK, XII, and XI), as well as factors IX and VIII. Since factor XI can be activated by means other than XIIa, prekallikrein, and HMWK, the *in vivo* importance of these three contact factors is now in question.

In the test tube (*in vitro*), initiation of the intrinsic coagulation pathway begins with the *contact activation phase of coagulation*, which involves all four contact factors.

FACTOR XII ACTIVATION

Factor XII is a single polypeptide chain zymogen[25] which adsorbs to negatively charged surfaces such as glass. The complex of prekallikrein and cofactor HMWK is also adsorbed to the negatively charged surface with factor XII. Factor XI also complexes with HMWK on the surface.

Once the contact group is assembled, *in vitro* studies show that factor XII undergoes a conformational change (Rxn 1; see Fig. 48-1) in the presence of kallikrein, with enhancement by HMWK (Rxn 7). Factor XII can be autoactivated, *i.e.*, activated by trace amounts of its own activated form (XIIa) without stimulation from HMWK; however, this is an extremely slow reaction (Rxn 1a).

Factor XIIa is cleaved into fragments called XIIf (Rxn 2). This is achieved by a number of proteolytic enzymes, including plasmin (Rxn 9) and, probably most importantly, kallikrein. The HMWK enhances the proteolytic effect of kallikrein on factor XIIa (Rxn 2). Both factors XIIa and XIIf activate prekallikrein to kallikrein (Rxn 3).

Factors XIIa and XIIf play several roles in hemostasis, although again, their physiologic significance remains unclear.[98]

1. *Factor XIIa is an initiator of the intrinsic coagulation pathway.* In the presence of HMWK, XIIa converts the zymogen factor XI to the serine protease XIa (Rxn 10). Note that factor XIIf is a very poor activator of factor XI and XIIf does not activate factor XII.
2. *Factors XIIa and XIIf can initiate the extrinsic coagulation pathway.* In an alternate coagulation pathway, factors XIIa and XIIf can activate the tissue factor:factor VII (TF:VII) complex to TF:VIIa in the extrinsic coagulation pathway (see Fig. 48-1).[81,119]
3. *Factors XIIa and XIIf initiate fibrinolysis.* Factor XIIa and kallikrein together (Rxn 2) form the complex required for conversion of the zymogen plasminogen to the serine protease plasmin (Rxn 4), which is fibrinolytic (Rxn 8). Factor XIIf can also cause conversion of plasminogen to plasmin.
4. *Factor XIIf initiates the kinin and complement systems.* The conversion of prekallikrein to kallikrein by XIIf and HMWK (Rxn 3) causes the conversion of HMWK to kinins (Rxn 5) such as bradykinin. The plasmin formed as a result of kallikrein can also initiate the complement system (Rxn 6). Factor XIIf (not XIIa) can directly activate the first component of the complement system.

Kallikrein plays three roles during contact activation (see Fig. 48-1).

1. It perpetuates factor XII activation and its own production (Rxns 2, 3, and 7).
2. It initiates the kinin system (Rxn 5).
3. It initiates the fibrinolytic (Rxns 2 and 4) and complement systems (Rxn 6) together with factor XIIa.

Plasmin, which is formed as a result of contact activation, plays three major roles in contact activation (see Fig. 48-1).

1. It promotes clot dissolution (fibrinolysis) (Rxn 8). Plasmin in a clot begins the fibrinolytic process of gradual blood clot dissolution.
2. If plasmin is not destroyed as it should be by plasma antiplasmins, it cleaves factor XIIa to XIIf (Rxn 9), thus inhibiting further contact activation since XIIf is a very poor activator of factor XI.
3. It can activate the kinin and complement systems.

See The Fibrinolytic System for the roles of plasmin in other parts of the hemostatic mechanism.

FACTOR XI ACTIVATION

Factor XIIa, with HMWK, activates factor XI to the serine protease XIa (Rxn 10). It appears that factor XI, like factor XII,[111] can be activated directly by contact activation and that factor XIa also activates plasminogen; thus, both XIa and XIIa are involved in initiation of the fibrinolytic and complement systems.

Since people with factor XII deficiency do not have bleeding abnormalities, but people with factor XI deficiency may have mild bleeding abnormalities, there must be an alternate pathway for factor XI activation.[110a] Two alternate pathways that do not involve factor XIIa contact activation have been proposed. One pathway involves a positive feedback in which thrombin activates factor XI in the presence of a charged surface like that required for contact activation. Thus, thrombin could accelerate its own formation.[27] This mechanism has been demonstrated in purified systems, but it has not been demonstrated in plasma, perhaps because plasma contains fibrinogen which reportedly blocks thrombin activation of factor XI.[92]

The second alternate pathway of factor XI activation involves activation by its immediate product—factor XIa (autoactivation). This also requires a charged surface and is blocked by fibrinogen.[92] Both of these pathways remain hypothetical until further research confirms their existence *in vivo*.

FACTOR IX ACTIVATION

The activation of factor IX to the serine protease IXa by factor XIa requires Ca^{2+} (Rxn 11). Kallikrein is also capable of directly activating factor IX.[76] Factor IXa combines with the factor VIII cofactor (VIIIa) and Ca^{2+} on the platelet phospholipid surface. Factor VIII, although not a zymogen, must be modified to its functional form (VIIIa) by thrombin (Rxn 12). The platelet provides a surface for the formation of the multimolecular IXa-Ca^{2+}-VIIIa complex, which binds with platelet phospholipid and together converts factor X to Xa (Rxn 13). This complex causes the conversion rate to be accelerated several thousand times beyond the reaction rate associated with factor IXa acting alone.[39] The coagulation cascade continues on the platelet surface (see Fig. 55-12).

Extrinsic Coagulation Pathway

The extrinsic pathway is much less complex than the intrinsic, although it is considered the dominant pathway *in vivo*. It was named "extrinsic" because factors other than those normally found in the plasma are required for initiation. This pathway consists only of tissue factor (TF or factor III), factor VII, and Ca^{2+}.

TF is a receptor protein (containing both lipid and carbohydrate) that is present in the plasma membrane of many cell types and has a high affinity for plasma factor VII. When vascular endothelium is injured, the exposure of TF to plasma factor VII allows the formation of a Ca^{2+}-

dependent tissue factor:factor VII (TF:VII) complex on the cell surface. Ca^{2+} acts as a bridge between factor VII and TF.

Factor VII is vitamin K dependent and circulates as a single-chain glycoprotein. The zymogen form is believed to have some enzymatic activity,[120] which makes it unique among the zymogens, however this remains to be confirmed. The exact mechanisms causing factor VII activation *in vivo* are still uncertain. *In vitro*, the TF:VII complex is activated to TF:VIIa (Rxn 14) by cleaving VII into one light and one heavy chain that are linked by a disulfide bond. Substances reported to activate factor VII include kallikrein,[95] thrombin, and factors XIIa, XIIf,[81,119] IXa, and Xa.[60,80,83] Plasmin may also be involved.[95] The TF:VIIa-Ca^{2+} complex on a cell surface converts factor X to Xa in the common pathway (Rxn 15). It is also reported[56,59,69] to be able to convert factor IX to IXa in the intrinsic coagulation pathway *in vitro*, and this is thought to occur *in vivo* (see Fig. 48-1). TF:VIIa has considerably more enzymatic activity than the factor VII zymogen or TF:VII complex.[2]

A control mechanism for the extrinsic pathway exists in that large concentrations of factor Xa cleave factor VII into a three-chain molecule that is inactive in coagulation.[80]

Common Coagulation Pathway

The activation of factor X to Xa begins the common coagulation pathway, so called because it is common to the intrinsic and extrinsic pathways. Equal amounts of factor Xa are generated by activation through either pathway.[73] Factor Xa binds to the platelet phospholipid surface and is thus prevented from diffusing away. On binding of factor Xa, a multimolecular complex known as the *prothrombinase complex* (see Fig. 48-1) is formed in the common pathway. The complex is Xa-Va-Ca^{2+}-platelet phospholipid. Factor V requires modification to factor Va by thrombin (factor IIa) to be active in this complex (Rxn 16).[53]

The prothrombinase complex converts prothrombin to thrombin (Rxn 17), a strong serine protease, in a two-step process. In the first step, peptide bonds in prothrombin are cleaved, which produces prethrombin 2 and either prothrombin fragment 1.2 or fragment 1.2.3 (PF1.2 or PF1.2.3). Laboratory tests for these fragments are important in assessing thrombotic risk (Chap. 51) and monitoring anticoagulant therapy. In the second step, a peptide bond is cleaved in prethrombin 2, releasing fully active thrombin that contains two chains, A and B, connected by a disulfide (S–S) bond. The common pathway reactions are completed with thrombin activation of fibrinogen to fibrin through a series of steps that stabilize the fibrin clot.

Coagulation Pathways Linking the Extrinsic, Intrinsic, and Common Pathways

The interaction and interdependence of the three coagulation pathways was not realized in older theories.[95] Some of these interactions have only been demonstrated *in vitro*

and remain to be confirmed *in vivo*. The more recently identified pathways are called "alternate" or "crossover" pathways. A major alternate pathway that has been demonstrated *in vitro* and is believed to occur *in vivo* is the extrinsic pathway activation of the intrinsic pathway. In this pathway, the tissue factor:factor VIIa- (TF:VIIa) − Ca^{2+} complex activates factor IX, thus bypassing the contact activation phase of coagulation (see Fig. 48-1).[56,59] If this pathway is confirmed *in vivo*, it could be the key to explaining the lack of bleeding associated with hereditary deficiencies of the contact factors XII, prekallikrein, and HMWK, and the lack of bleeding in some cases of factor XI deficiency.

In another alternate pathway, the intrinsic system factors XIIa and XIIf have been reported to activate the TF:VII complex in the extrinsic system.[81,119] Factor IXa and kallikrein of the intrinsic system also activate TF:VII in plasma that has been exposed to glass or other surfaces.[2,60,83,95] Factor Xa and thrombin in the common pathway provide a feedback mechanism to activate additional TF:VII. In yet another alternate pathway, thrombin in the common pathway has been demonstrated to activate the intrinsic pathway factor XI *in vitro*, thus bypassing the other contact factors in forming a fibrin clot.[27]

Figure 48-1 shows the traditional intrinsic, extrinsic, and common pathways along with the alternate coagulation pathways. It also shows the interaction of hemostasis with the kinin, complement, and fibrinolytic systems as well as platelets. As it has in the past, the model of the coagulation system can and probably will continue to change as new information becomes available.

Final Clot Formation and Stabilization

The action of thrombin on fibrinogen begins the final steps of coagulation (Rxn 18). Fibrinogen is a glycoprotein with the formula $(A\alpha, B\beta, \gamma)_2$. This means that fibrinogen is composed of three pairs of nonidentical but intricately interwoven polypeptide chains including two $A\alpha$ chains, two $B\beta$ chains, and two γ chains. The fibrinogen molecule is a dimer that is linked by disulfide bonds near the terminal ends. Both the $A\alpha$ and $B\beta$ chain pairs have small fibrinopeptides in their terminal region known as fibrinopeptides A and B (16 and 14 amino acids, respectively) for a total of four fibrinopeptides (two A and two B).

CONVERSION OF FIBRINOGEN TO FIBRIN

The conversion of fibrinogen to fibrin involves three steps (see Fig. 48-1).

The Enzymatic Step. First, there is cleavage of the two A and two B fibrinopeptides from the fibrinogen molecule by the enzymatic cleavage of thrombin. The γ chains remain intact and are not hydrolyzed during the formation of fibrin. Once the A and B fibrinopeptides are released, the molecule is referred to as a *soluble fibrin monomer* (Rxn 18a), which is essential for the second step, polymerization of fibrin. Fibrinopeptide A is released first and is required for fibrin polymerization; then fibrinopeptide B is released which makes the contact between the fibrin monomer units stronger.

The Polymerization Step. Fibrinopeptides A and B are negatively charged, and their release results in a fibrin monomer with a significantly decreased electronegativity, thus greatly reducing the intermolecular repulsive forces between the fibrin monomers. Thus, given the correct environment, including *p*H and ionic concentration, the fibrin monomers aggregate spontaneously by forming weak (primarily hydrogen) bonds between the fibrin monomers (Rxn 18b). First, they aggregate side to side (laterally) after fibrinopeptide A release, then end to end after fibrinopeptide B release. This results in an unstable clot (or gel) which can be dissolved *in vitro* in 5 M urea or weak acids such as 1% monochloracetic acid.

The Stabilization Step. The third step provides for formation of insoluble fibrin by clot stabilization. This requires thrombin, factor XIIIa, and Ca^{2+}. Thrombin activates factor XIII (Rxn 19), which then functions as a transamidinase, crosslinking adjacent fibrin monomers through formation of stabilizing covalent bonds. Both α and γ chains are involved in the formation of the stabilized fibrin clot (Rxn 20). Insoluble fibrin is more resistant to fibrinolysis than soluble fibrin. When plasmin lyses insoluble fibrin, characteristic stable fibrin degradation products (FDP) are formed (*e.g.*, the D–D dimer) which are not found when plasmin lyses soluble fibrin or fibrinogen. The stabilized clot is insoluble in 5 M urea and weak acid. Laboratory tests may be performed with these reagents to screen for factor XIII deficiency.

The Thrombin Feedback Mechanism

In addition to thrombin's role in the conversion of fibrinogen to fibrin (Rxns 18 and 18a) and fibrin stabilization, thrombin (factor IIa) has many roles in hemostasis. Most importantly, it acts to control and balance the hemostatic mechanism by providing feedback mechanisms to achieve control of the coagulation process (*i.e.*, to prevent excessive bleeding and clotting). Thrombin acts as both an activator and an inhibitor of coagulation.

THROMBIN'S ROLE AS COAGULATION ACTIVATOR

In vivo, thrombin activates coagulation factors I, V, VIII, XIII, and possibly XI.[27] It is said to be autocatalytic; that is, once it is generated, thrombin enhances the rate of prothrombinase complex production and is thus, to some extent, self-perpetuating. This activity is thought to relate to the enhancing effects of thrombin on factors V and VIII (Rxns 12 and 16). Thrombin also induces platelet aggregation.

THROMBIN'S ROLE AS COAGULATION INHIBITOR

Thrombin controls coagulation by acting also as an inhibitor to prevent excessive clotting. In high concentrations, thrombin has the opposite effect on factors V and VIII—it

can destroy them. The mechanism for this action is unclear. When bound to thrombomodulin on the endothelial cell surface, thrombin activates protein C, a potent anticoagulant (see Naturally Occurring Inhibitors of Coagulation, Proteins C and S).

THE FIBRINOLYTIC SYSTEM
Physiologic Fibrinolysis

Many similarities exist between the coagulation and fibrinolytic systems. Just as there are checks and balances in the formation of a clot, there are similar mechanisms for dissolution of the clot to promote wound healing. Fibrinolysis is the body's defense against occlusion of blood vessels. On the other hand, it is also important that bleeding does not recur because of premature lysing of the clot.

Activation of Plasminogen to Plasmin and Its Roles in Normal and Abnormal Fibrinolysis

Fibrinolysis is dependent on conversion of the zymogen plasminogen to the enzyme plasmin. Plasmin is not normally present in plasma. Plasmin's main physiologic role is the lysis (destruction) of fibrin. Plasminogen is a single-chain glycoprotein that is synthesized in the liver and has a molecular weight of 90,000. It is stored and transported in eosinophils and increased concentrations are found in association with inflammation.

Fibrin tends to adsorb plasminogen, which is normally present in plasma. Therefore, plasminogen is automatically incorporated into the fibrin clot. Once inside a fibrin clot, plasminogen is converted to plasmin by specific plasminogen activators (Fig. 48-3) and the slow destruction of the fibrin clot begins. Thus, conditions that initiate fibrin formation also initiate plasmin formation, which limits the coagulation process while leaving time for tissue repair. Any plasmin that escapes the clot is capable of destroying coagulation factors I, V, and VIII. Therefore, plasma contains antiplasmins capable of destroying the enzymatic activity of plasmin.

Destruction of coagulation factors by plasmin occurs in pathologic coagulation processes (*e.g.*, liver disease and some carcinomas). In such cases, the amount of plasmin in the plasma builds up because it exceeds the capacity of plasma antiplasmins to destroy it (see Fig. 48-3). Since fibrinogen is a single molecule, it is much more vulnerable to the action of plasmin than are fibrin monomers that are covalently bonded to one another in a clot. Since free plasmin in the plasma is destroyed by antiplasmins as rapidly as it is formed, these reactions do not normally occur. The two most rapidly acting antiplasmins are α_2-antiplasmin and α_2-macroglobulin (see Naturally Occurring Inhibitors of Fibrinolysis).

Activation of plasminogen to plasmin may occur through substances normally present in the plasma. Such activation is referred to as "intrinsic activation." Extrinsic activation occurs by substances that enter the plasma from an outside source (see Fig. 48-3).

ACTIVATION OF THE FIBRINOLYTIC SYSTEM

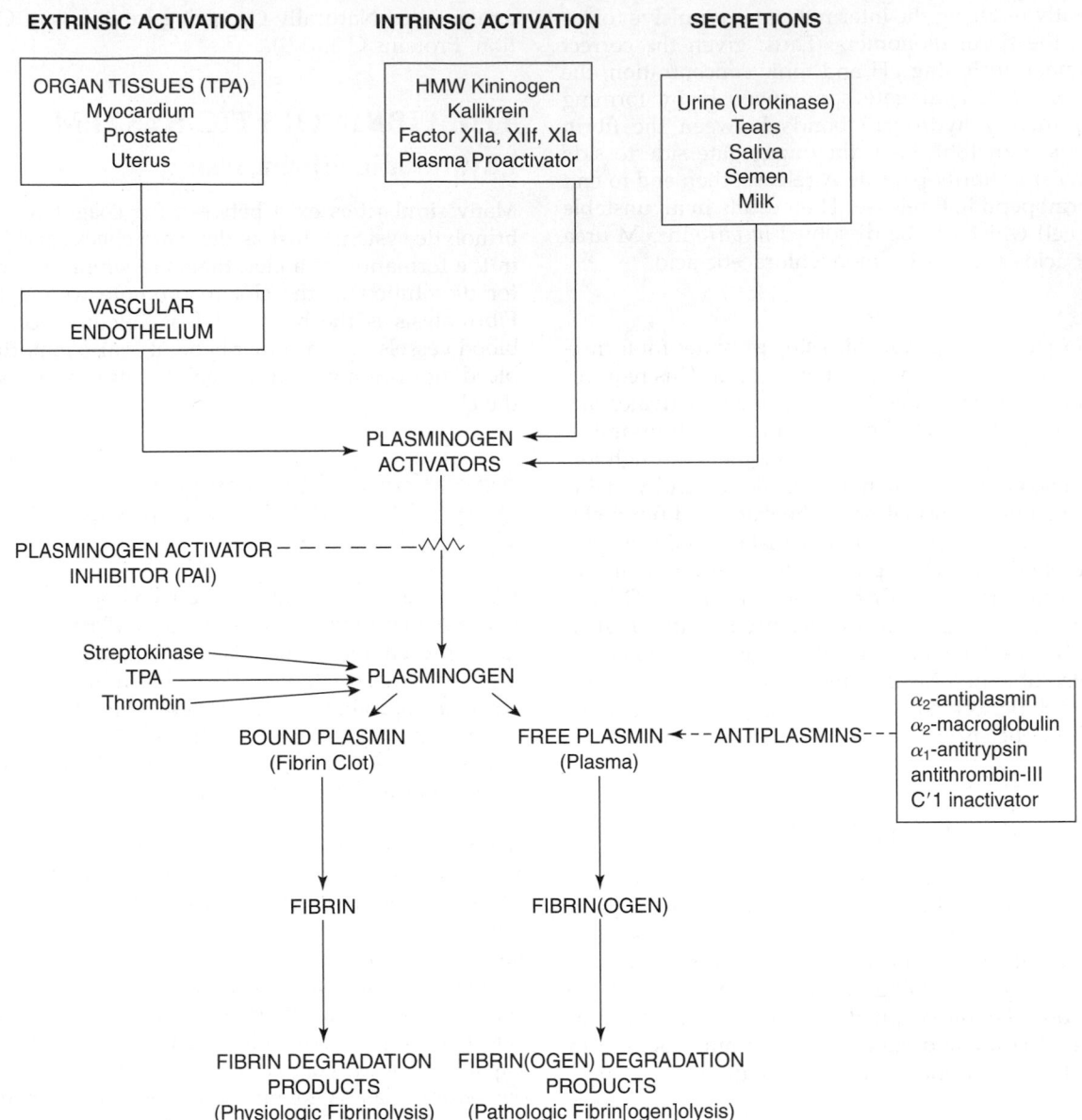

FIGURE 48-3. The fibrinolytic system may be activated by plasminogen activators from secretions, extrinsic sources such as tissue plasminogen activators (TPA) in organs and vascular endothelium, or by intrinsic sources. These plasminogen activators convert plasminogen to plasmin. Thrombin also activates plasminogen. Urokinase, streptokinase, or TPA administered therapeutically in thrombotic disorders act in the same way. Plasmin promotes fibrinolysis. Antiplasmins control (inhibit and neutralize) excess plasmin in the plasma, thus preventing excessive and premature (pathologic) fibrin(ogen)olysis. Plasminogen activator inhibitor (PAI) also inhibits fibrinolysis at a different step in the pathway.

INTRINSIC PLASMINOGEN ACTIVATION

Factors XIIa, XIIf, XIa, kallikrein, HMWK, and a specific plasma protein (proactivator) can activate plasminogen to plasmin intrinsically by contact activation through one or more pathways.[46] The plasma proactivator is activated by kallikrein during contact activation of coagulation.

EXTRINSIC PLASMINOGEN ACTIVATION

The extrinsic plasminogen activation pathway involves plasminogen activators present in organ tissues (see Fig. 48-3). Tissue plasminogen activators (TPA) have also been found in endothelial cells in the form of proteases,[113] particularly in the veins.[107]

Plasminogen activators are also present in body fluids (see Fig. 48-3). These activators may keep the secretory passages functioning properly.[64]

EXOGENOUS PLASMINOGEN ACTIVATION

To treat the abnormal formation of a thrombus, urokinase, a trypsin-like protease purified from urine, may be administered to a patient to activate plasminogen (see Fig. 48-3) to plasmin and induce fibrinolysis.[114] Streptokinase, a bacterial enzyme,[106] and tissue plasminogen activator (TPA)[78] are other therapeutic agents used to activate plasminogen to plasmin (Chap. 54). TPA is released *in vivo* following endothelial cell damage and can be manufactured *in vitro* through recombinant DNA techniques.

Fibrin(ogen) Degradation by Plasmin

In the process of fibrinogen or fibrin degradation by plasmin, specific fragments are produced called *fibrin(ogen) degradation products* (FDP) or *fibrin(ogen) split products* (FSP). Plasmin degrades both fibrinogen and fibrin. This results in the appearance of essentially the same fragments for fibrinogen and fibrin degradation, although the Aα and Bβ chains may remain intact in fibrinogen fragments.[105] These degradation products are removed by the liver, kidney, and reticuloendothelial system.

Figure 48-4 shows the sequence of reactions in the degradation of fibrin by plasmin and the four principal products, fragments X, Y, D (D–D dimer), and E. Note that plasmin acts on specific sites of each fragment to create smaller fragments throughout the reaction sequence. Fragments X and Y are referred to as *early* degradation products; fragments D and E are *late* degradation products.

Fragment X is the first and largest fragment formed (MW 250,000). Fragment X is the result of plasmin cleavage of the terminal portions of the alpha chains from a fibrin polymer, leaving isolated fibrin strands. Fragment

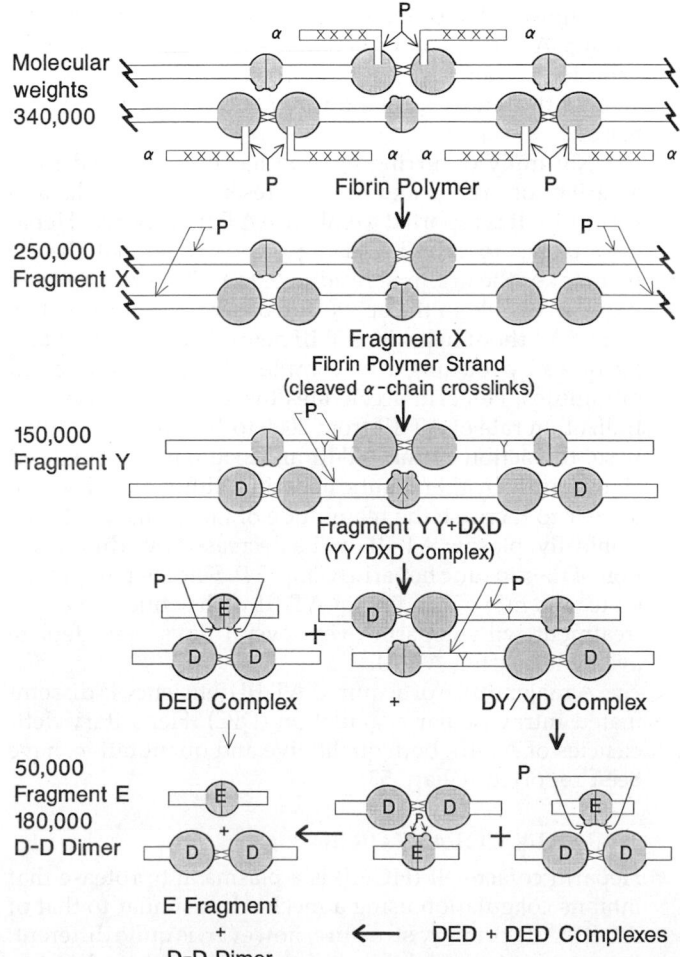

FIGURE 48-4. Degradation of fibrin by plasmin. P indicates sites where plasmin cleaves fibrin polymers, fibrin strands, and various complexes. (From Thompson AR, Harker LA: Manual of Hemostasis and Thrombosis, p 38. Philadelphia, FA Davis, 1983, with permission.)

X is then cleaved by plasmin (P) to form two fragments called Y (YY)[55] and an intermediate complex, DXD (see Fig. 48-4). This complex is further cleaved into intermediate complexes DED and DY/YD until finally, fragments E and D (D–D dimer) are formed. A single fragment D has a molecular weight of approximately 90,000, and that of the D–D dimer is approximately 180,000.[55]

It is now thought that the presence of the D–D dimer is a specific indicator of *in vivo* lysis of fibrin rather than fibrinogen. In the past, laboratory tests for FDP were incapable of distinguishing fibrin degradation products from fibrinogen degradation products.[26] Now, tests specific for the D–D dimer (Chap. 50) permit verification of *in vivo* fibrinolysis, because the presence of the D–D dimer is indicative only of fibrin (not fibrinogen) degradation products.[32]

Pathologic Effects of Fibrin Degradation Products

The FDP are significant because they can severely impair the hemostatic process and are presumably a major cause of hemorrhage in intravascular coagulation and fibrinogenolysis. The FDP demonstrate antithrombin activity, interfere with polymerization of the fibrin monomer, and interfere with platelet activity. Most FDP also form incoagulable or slowly coagulable complexes with fibrin monomers or fibrinogen. The early and larger fragments X and Y, along with the intermediate FDP, appear to be the most important in exerting anticoagulant effects. Most FDP inhibit coagulation, but fragment Y is the most potent of them. Fragments Y and D inhibit fibrin polymerization.[4] Fragment E is a powerful inhibitor of thrombin.[4] All four fragments, but particularly low-molecular-weight FDP,[100] have an affinity for coating platelet membranes and therefore cause a clinically significant platelet dysfunction by inhibiting aggregation.

Fibrin monomers are not normally present in the plasma. However, fibrin monomers complexed with FDP may be found in pathologic fibrinolytic states (*e.g.*, disseminated intravascular coagulation). Fibrin monomers and fragments X and Y form soluble complexes with fibrinogen. These soluble complexes will dissociate in the presence of protamine sulfate and ethanol to form gels or precipitates (a process referred to as paracoagulation). These reactions are the basis of two tests for detection of fibrin monomers in the plasma (ethanol gelation and protamine sulfate tests; Chap. 50).

INHIBITORS OF COAGULATION AND FIBRINOLYSIS

A regulatory system must exist within the body to control coagulation and fibrinolysis. This system includes both naturally occurring biochemical inhibitors and physiologic control mechanisms. The counterforces of the naturally occurring biochemical coagulation and fibrinolytic inhibitors are necessary to achieve a balance between activated clotting factors and fibrinolytic enzymes.[3] Some inhibitors quickly neutralize activated factors in the circulation, thus localizing coagulation to the sites where it is required, whereas others perform a similar function that limits fibrinolysis. Table 48-6 summarizes the features of the well-characterized inhibitors of coagulation and fibrinolysis.

Naturally Occurring Inhibitors of Coagulation

ANTITHROMBIN III

Antithrombin III (AT-III), also known as heparin cofactor I, is an important coagulation inhibitor found in plasma. It is a glycoprotein synthesized in the liver and has a half-life of approximately 2.7 days. AT-III inhibits most serine proteases including thrombin, XIIa, XIa, Xa, and IXa by forming complexes with these activated factors, thereby neutralizing them and preventing their action on other zymogens (see Fig. 53-1).[118] Factor VIIa is the only serine protease that AT-III does not significantly inhibit. AT-III also has an inhibitory effect on plasmin and kallikrein. Thus, AT-III plays a vital role in monitoring the coagulation, fibrinolytic, kallikrein-kinin, and complement systems. If these four systems are allowed to function without inhibition because of decreased levels of AT-III, the result can be severe, even fatal (Fig. 48-5).

A heparin-like substance known as hepa*ran* sulfate is normally present *in vivo* on cell surfaces including endothelium and platelets. It is an acidic mucopolysaccharide that may act as an anticoagulant similar to the action of commercially prepared heparin. A small amount of plasma AT-III binds to heparan sulfate on the vascular endothelial cell surface and protects uninjured vessels against thrombus formation by neutralizing serine proteases.

Naturally occurring hepa*rin* has been isolated from a variety of organs and also is present in mast cells and basophils. It is reported to enhance AT-III activity.[87] Heparin attaches to AT-III, causing a conformational change that makes the arginine residue of the AT-III reactive site more accessible to the active site of serine proteases (Fig. 48-6).[3,9] Without heparin, AT-III neutralizes thrombin and factor Xa by forming a 1:1 complex slowly over a period of minutes. Heparin accelerates the serine protease neutralization rate of AT-III from 2000 to 10,000 times.[54] Likewise, the action of the AT-III anticoagulant is enhanced significantly by therapeutic heparin,[94] although it does not appear to increase the magnitude of factor inactivation.[87] Ironically, plasma AT-III can be decreased by administration of therapeutic heparin (Chap. 54). Since heparin accelerates the rate of binding of AT-III with serine proteases, treatment with heparin over several days may deplete available plasma AT-III.

A major cause of acquired AT-III deficiency is disseminated intravascular coagulation (DIC). Hereditary deficiencies of AT-III, both qualitative and quantitative, have been reported (Chap. 53).[61]

HEPARIN COFACTOR II

Heparin cofactor II (HCFII) is a plasma antiprotease that inhibits coagulation using a mechanism similar to that of AT-III.[108] Its primary structure, however, is quite different. It is primarily an inhibitor of thrombin, although it has

TABLE 48-6
Naturally Occurring Inhibitors of Coagulation and Fibrinolysis

Inhibitor	Molecular Weight (daltons × 10³)	Plasma Concentration (mg/dL)	Rate of Inhibition	Rate Accelerated by Heparin?	System Inhibited	Function Inhibited
Antithrombin III	58	21–30	Slow	Yes	Coagulation	Thrombin, XIIa, XIa, Xa, IXa, and kallikrein
					Fibrinolytic	Plasmin and kallikrein
Heparin cofactor II	66	9	Slow	Yes	Coagulation only	Primarily thrombin
α_2-Macroglobulin	725	130–325	Variable	No	Coagulation	Thrombin and kallikrein
					Fibrinolytic	Plasmin and kallikrein
α_1-Antitrypsin	40–50	245–335	Slow	No	Coagulation	Potent inhibitor of XIa; weak inhibitor of thrombin
					Fibrinolytic	Plasmin
C′1 inactivator	105–135	14–30	Slow	No	Coagulation	XIIa, XIIf, XIa, and kallikrein
					Fibrinolytic	Plasmin
					Complement	C1 Esterase
Protein C–S system	62 (C)	0.2–0.6	Slow	No	Coagulation	Va and VIIIa
	71 (S)	1.5 (free)*			Fibrinolysis (enhanced)	May *enhance* fibrinolysis by inactivating plasminogen activator inhibitors (PAI)
Protein C inhibitor	67	0.5	?	Yes	Coagulation (enhanced)	Activated protein C
					Coagulation (inhibited)	Xa, thrombin, kallikrein
Plasminogen activator inhibitor-1 (PAI-1)	45–50	Trace†	Variable	No	Coagulation Fibrinolytic	Thrombin TPA‡, urokinase, activated protein C, plasmin
Tissue factor pathway inhibitor (TFPI)	30–40	0.01	Slow	Yes	Coagulation only	TF:VIIa, Xa
α_2-antiplasmin	65–70	5–7	Rapid	No	Fibrinolytic only	Principal inhibitor of plasmin; inhibits TPA‡; inactivates urokinase

*Protein S exists in plasma in both a free, active form and an inactive form bound to complement.
†PAI-1 plasma concentration (geometric mean) has been reported as 24 ng/mL.[45]
‡tPA = tissue plasminogen activators (see Fig. 48-3).

less affinity for thrombin and reacts more slowly with thrombin than AT-III. HCFII is activated by heparin and other mucopolysaccharides, particularly dermatan sulfate. Unlike AT-III, it does *not* inhibit plasmin. Hereditary deficiency of HCFII has been reported in a few families, but it does not always cause thrombosis.[88]

α_2-MACROGLOBULIN

α_2-Macroglobulin is a large, naturally occurring plasma glycoprotein.[41] This inhibitor binds with various proteo-lytic enzymes including thrombin, however its rate of thrombin inhibition is slower than that of AT-III. α_2-Macroglobulin does not completely inhibit its target enzymes.[75] This is because after binding with an enzyme, α_2-macroglobulin undergoes a conformational change that physically entraps an enyzme so that it may not bind with its substrate, but its active catalytic site remains intact. For example, thrombin bound to α_2-macroglobulin may still activate small amounts of factors V and VIII. In addition, α_2-macroglobulin seems to protect its bound enzymes against other circulating inhibitors.

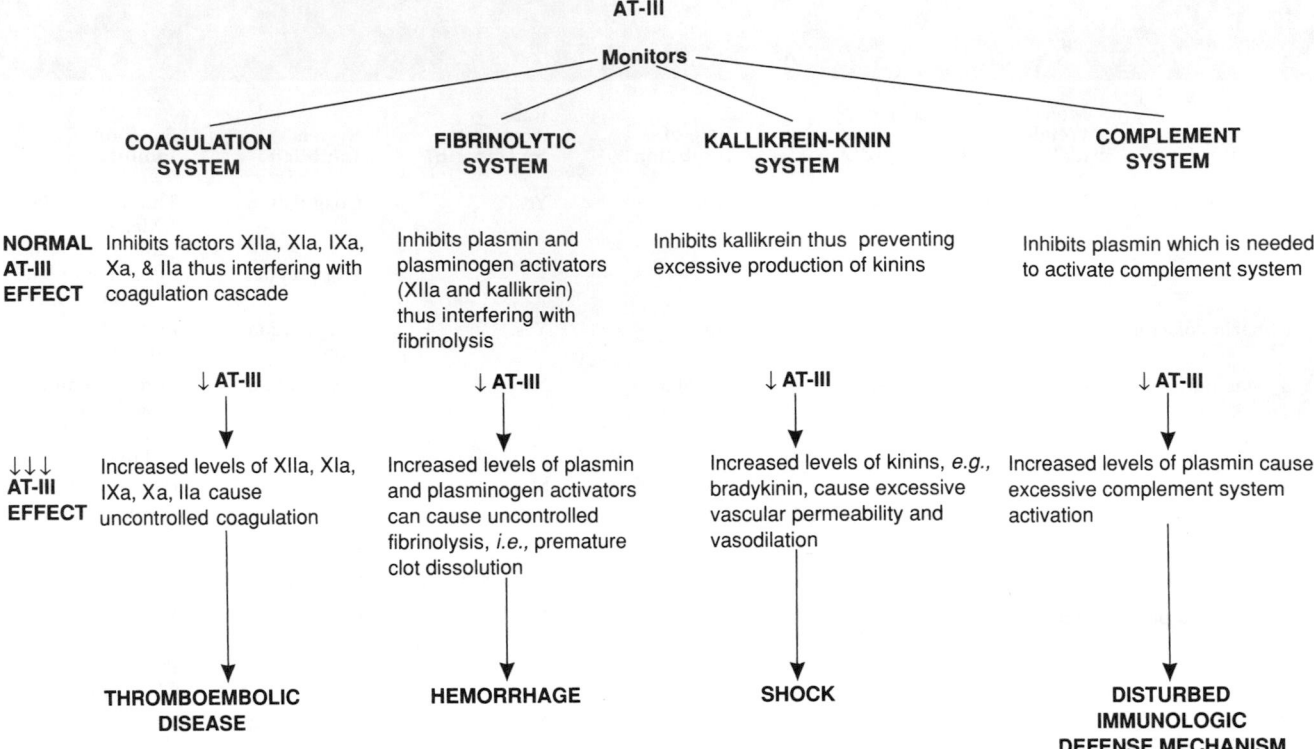

FIGURE 48-5. Antithrombin III (AT-III) is important in controlling four physiologic systems. Thus, if there is a decrease in the concentration of AT-III, serious clinical abnormalities can result.

α_2-Macroglobulin also inhibits kallikrein and fibrinolysis (see later). Two families have been reported with decreased α_2-macroglobulin levels equivalent to 20% to 40% of the normal levels in pooled plasma. Nevertheless, these persons were asymptomatic.[7,102]

α_1-ANTITRYPSIN

α_1-Antitrypsin (also known as α_1-antiprotease) is an α globulin[74] that is a potent inhibitor of factor XIa.[36] It may also inactivate thrombin at a slow rate, although this is still uncertain.[28] It is a weak inhibitor of trypsin (a substance that activates factor XII) and of the fibrinolytic system (discussed later).[28]

Hereditary deficiencies have been found in conjunction with liver cirrhosis (because of its production by the liver) and pulmonary disease such as emphysema (because α_1-antitrypsin is important to normal pulmonary function). Hereditary deficiencies have not been associated with thrombotic disorders.

C'1 INACTIVATOR (C1 ESTERASE INHIBITOR)

The C'1 inactivator is a glycoprotein[62] that was initially identified in the complement system as an inhibitor of C1 esterase, the first component of the complement system which is composed of the proteins C1q, C1r, and C1s (see Fig. 19-1). It is now known that the coagulation, fibrinolytic, kinin, and complement systems are all affected by this inhibitor. In the coagulation system, C'1 inactivator is the major inhibitor of the contact system. It inhibits factors XIIa, XIIf, and XIa. It accounts for 95% of the factor XIIa inhibitory capacity. In the kinin system, it accounts for 50% of the inhibitory capacity for kallikrein.

PROTEINS C AND S

Protein C and its cofactor protein S are vitamin K–dependent glycoproteins. Activated protein C complexed with protein S is a potent inhibitor of coagulation as it

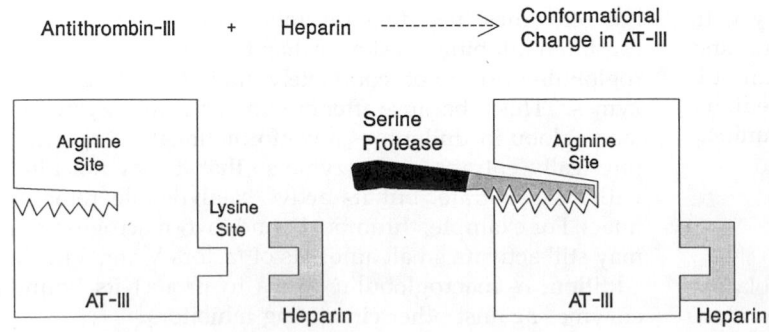

FIGURE 48-6. Antithrombin III (AT-III) inhibits serine proteases by binding them in an arginine site that is not easily accessible. If heparin is available, it binds to AT-III at a lysine site, causing a conformational change in AT-III that makes the arginine site more accessible to bind and inhibit serine proteases. With heparin, AT-III can inhibit serine proteases instantaneously.

destroys factors Va and VIIIa.[24] Protein C exists free in the plasma, but protein S exists in both an active free form and an inactive complement-bound form. Protein C activation, which occurs on the endothelial cell surface, requires calcium and thrombin bound to an endothelial cell surface receptor known as thrombomodulin (see Fig. 53-1).[23] There is disagreement about the continued ability of thrombin, once bound to thrombomodulin, to convert fibrinogen to fibrin, activate factor V, or stimulate platelet aggregation.[24a,59a]

There are four steps involved in the activation of protein C. First, it is believed that thrombomodulin forms a 1:1 complex with thrombin on the endothelial cell surface. Next, protein C binds to the thrombin–thrombomodulin complex by means of Ca^{2+} bridges and is slowly activated by proteolytic cleavage releasing a peptide (C activation peptide). Then protein S binds to the complex on the endothelial surface (see Fig. 53-1).[22] Finally, activated protein C, in the presence of protein S, proteolytically degrades factors Va and VIIIa.[57] In addition to regulation of clotting, the protein C–S complex may *enhance* fibrinolysis[58] by neutralizing plasminogen activator inhibitors (PAI; see Fig. 48-3 and Table 48-6).

Deficiency of either protein C or S results in serious thromboembolic disorders (Chap. 53). Protein C deficiencies are clinically similar to AT-III deficiencies[11] in that thromboembolic episodes present before 30 years of age.[12] A newly discovered entity referred to as activated protein C resistance explains more than half of the cases of hereditary thrombosis.[16a]

PROTEIN C INHIBITOR

A protein C inhibitor has been reported.[104,110] It is a heparin-activated serine protease that inhibits activated protein C, factor Xa, and thrombin. It does not affect plasmin or the plasminogen activator urokinase (see Fig. 48-3).[35] Deficiency of this inhibitor may cause a combined factor V and VIII deficiency since activated protein C destroys factors Va and VIIIa.

TISSUE FACTOR PATHWAY INHIBITOR (TFPI)

TFPI is a single polypeptide chain protein that is synthesized by endothelial and other cells. During coagulation, TFPI forms a complex with factor Xa (TFPI:Xa) that inhibits factor Xa and the tissue factor:factor VIIa (TF:VIIa) complex.[20,70,77,112] TFPI is a unique inhibitor since it is bivalent, that is, a single molecule has inhibitory sites for two factors. It is also unique in that the binding of factor Xa is apparently required for inhibition of TF:VIIa. Since factor Xa is a product of TF:VIIa generation, the requirement of factor Xa for TF:VIIa inhibition is referred to as a negative feedback control of coagulation. In contrast, other negative feedbacks in coagulation require an inactivating enzyme (activated protein C [discussed earlier]) rather than an inhibitor.

TFPI generally inhibits factor Xa at about the same rate as AT-III. Heparin induces TFPI normally pooled in the vasculature to move into the plasma, causing a several-fold rise in the plasma TFPI concentration and enhanced factor Xa inhibition.[49] Normal plasma does not contain a significant amount of the TFPI:Xa complex, therefore low levels of factor VIIa exist in plasma with a half-life of 1 to 2 hours without inhibition by TFPI.[69] No TFPI-deficient humans have been identified.

Naturally Occurring Inhibitors of Fibrinolysis

Fibrinolysis must be controlled to maintain a delicate balance between wound healing and clot dissolution. Excessive fibrinolysis is controlled by two naturally occurring inhibitors including (1) plasminogen activator inhibitor-1 (PAI-1), which inhibits tissue plasminogen activators (TPA) (see Fig. 48-3); and (2) antiplasmins (a group of inhibitors) which inactivate formed plasmin in the plasma. Excess plasmin is bound first by α_2-antiplasmin then, following its saturation, by α_2-macroglobulin. Finally, when α_2-macroglobulin is saturated, α_1-antitrypsin binds plasmin. Other antiplasmins also exist (see Table 48-6).

PLASMINOGEN ACTIVATOR INHIBITOR-1 (PAI-1)

An inhibitor of TPA (see Fig. 48-3) and urokinase called PAI-1 has been found in the plasma, in platelets,[21] and in many tissues including endothelium.[109] PAI-1 is a single-chain glycoprotein that is released from its storage site in platelet α granules upon platelet aggregation. It is also released in response to thrombin formation.[29] It forms a 1:1 complex with both TPA and urokinase, thus inhibiting fibrinolysis and contributing to the stabilization of fibrin.

PAI-1 can also inhibit plasmin, activated protein C, and thrombin. Congenital deficiency of PAI-1 causes a hemorrhagic disorder as a result of unopposed fibrinolysis. On the other hand, PAI-1 is itself inhibited by factor XIa produced during contact activation. This may provide some explanation for the role of contact activation in inducing fibrinolysis.

α_2-ANTIPLASMIN

α_2-Antiplasmin is an α_2-glycoprotein and a serine protease inhibitor.[115] It acts as a principal inhibitor of fibrinolysis by binding in a 1:1 irreversible complex to any plasmin that is free in the plasma,[66] thus neutralizing plasmin. This prevents plasmin from binding to fibrin and prevents plasmin's premature and uncontrolled digestion of fibrin, fibrinogen, and factors V and VIII by plasmin. It also permits a slow and orderly dissolution of the clot and adequate time for repair of damaged tissues.[66]

The complex formed between plasmin and α_2-antiplasmin is similar to the thrombin–AT-III complex. Both inhibitors bind to the active serine site of their respective enzyme targets, thus inactivating the serine protease and preventing its enzymatic action on its usual substrates. In addition, α_2-antiplasmin is crosslinked to fibrin by factor XIIIa, which assists in its inhibitory mechanism.[35]

Like other serine protease inhibitors, α_2-antiplasmin has been shown to inhibit many serine proteases,[67,91] including plasmin. Nevertheless, its physiologic role in inhibiting any other than plasmin appears negligible. The conversion of plasminogen to plasmin is also suppressed by α_2-antiplasmin through inhibition of tissue plasminogen activator.[82]

Studies have shown that α_2-antiplasmin is the most important naturally occurring inhibitor of fibrinolysis,[71] as it is the first to bind with plasmin in the plasma. *In vitro*, α_2-antiplasmin can decrease the normal binding rate of plasminogen to fibrin 30 times more effectively than a synthetic fibrinolytic inhibitor called epsilon-aminocaproic acid (EACA),[68] which is used to treat bleeding disorders,[85] particularly urinary tract bleeding, by inhibiting plasminogen activation.

Hereditary deficiencies of α_2-antiplasmin have been associated with a severe hemorrhagic tendency. In pathologic conditions involving excessive clotting (*e.g.,* diffuse or disseminated intravascular coagulation [DIC]) or excessive fibrinolysis (Chap. 52), the α_2-antiplasmin levels may be depleted secondary to increased concentrations of plasmin.

α_2-MACROGLOBULIN

α_2-Macroglobulin is a large, naturally occurring plasma glycoprotein that inhibits components in both the fibrinolytic and the coagulation systems (see Table 48-6). It rapidly inhibits plasmin after α_2-antiplasmin depletion, however, it does not totally eliminate plasmin's function in fibrinolysis.

α_1-ANTITRYPSIN

α_1-Antitrypsin (also known as α_1-protease) is the least significant of the three naturally occurring fibrinolytic system inhibitors. It inactivates plasmin slowly and does not bind plasmin until both α_2-antiplasmin and α_2-macroglobulin are saturated.[14,28,75]

OTHER FIBRINOLYTIC INHIBITORS

Antithrombin-III also functions to inhibit fibrinolysis by inhibiting plasmin and kallikrein. The C'1 inactivator also inhibits plasmin.[34]

Physiologic Coagulation Control Mechanisms

Physiologic control mechanisms work together with biochemical control mechanisms to maintain blood fluidity. These mechanisms include the nonthrombogenic characteristics of the vascular endothelium, the inhibiting processes at the site of clot formation, and hepatic and other clearance mechanisms for coagulation components.

VASCULAR ENDOTHELIUM MAINTENANCE OF NONTHROMBOGENICITY

The glycoprotein content and arrangement in the endothelial cell membrane favors blood fluidity and inhibits thrombus formation. Endothelial cells secrete many substances that are antithrombotic or fibrinolytic (see Table 47-2).

INHIBITING PROCESSES AT THE SITE OF CLOT FORMATION

Rapid blood flow through the vessels is important to prevent excessive propagation of a thrombus and dilute any excess procoagulants or profibrinolytic components at sites of injury.

Fibrin itself restricts the active coagulants to the interior of the fibrin clot. The platelets and endothelium also restrict coagulation to the site of injury.

HEPATIC AND OTHER CLEARANCE MECHANISMS FOR COAGULATION COMPONENTS

The hepatic clearance of soluble components such as plasminogen activators and activated serine proteases, including factors IXa, Xa, and VIIa,[19] prevents them from circulating in the venous system.[101] Consequently, liver impairment by conditions such as cirrhosis or hepatitis may cause systemic fibrinolysis or thrombosis.

Finely particulate procoagulants such as soluble fibrin components[47] and early FDP[13] may be removed in the pulmonary vascular bed. Peripheral blood leukocytes and tissue macrophages may also participate in the clearance of coagulation components.[96]

CHAPTER SUMMARY

The mechanism of hemostasis begins with injury to the endothelium, which triggers the release of components by platelets, the endothelium, and other tissues. These components interact with others in the plasma. The interdependent coagulation pathways and fibrinolysis (see Fig. 48-1) each exist to control hemotasis (*i.e.,* prevent excessive bleeding or clotting).

The *extrinsic coagulation pathway* is now considered of primary importance in initiation of *in vivo* clot formation. It is initiated when tissue factor (TF) is exposed on damaged endothelium and binds with plasma factor VII, forming the TF:VII complex. This complex may be activated to TF:VIIa by (1) factors XIIa, XIIf, and IXa from the intrinsic system; (2) kallikrein from the kinin system; and (3) Xa from the common pathway. On the other hand, TF:VIIa can activate factor IX in the intrinsic system. The TF:VIIa–Ca^{2+} complex activates factor X.

The *intrinsic coagulation pathway* begins with the contact phase of coagulation. However, factor XII and contact activation probably do not play a major role in *in vivo* coagulation. Nevertheless, the intrinsic system factors XI, IX, and VIII are important as deficiencies in these factors can all cause hemorrhagic disorders. The last reaction in this pathway is factor XIa or TF:VIIa activation of factor IX. Factor IXa binds with the cofactor VIIIa and Ca^{2+} and phospholipid to activate factor X.

Factor X is the first factor in the *common pathway* which ends in the formation of a stable fibrin clot. Factors Xa, Va, and Ca^{2+} form the prothrombinase complex on the platelet phospholipid surface, which is responsible for activation of prothrombin (factor II) to *thrombin* (factor IIa). Thrombin can accelerate or inhibit coagulation. It converts fibrinogen to fibrin. Factor XIIIa stabilizes the fibrin clot.

Fibrinolysis is the breakdown of fibrin by plasmin (see Fig. 48-3) contained within the fibrin clot. Fibrin(ogen) degradation results in the formation of fibrin(ogen) degradation products (FDP) (see Fig. 48-4).

Endothelial cells regulate coagulation by providing (1) tissue plasminogen activator (TPA) (see Fig. 48-3) that initiates fibrinolysis; (2) a site for AT-III adherence, allowing for its inhibitory effects on thrombin and other serine proteases (see Fig. 48-5); and (3) thrombomodulin, a receptor protein that binds thrombin, allowing for activation of protein C which binds with its cofactor, protein S. The protein C–S complex inhibits coagulation and enhances fibrinolysis (see Table 48-6).

In normal plasma, there are a number of naturally occurring inhibitors of coagulation and fibrinolysis (see Table 48-6). The principal inhibitor of fibrinolysis is α_2-antiplasmin.

Review Questions

48-1. The coagulation factors that are vitamin K dependent are

A. I, V, VIII, and XIII.
B. II, VII, IX, and X.
C. XII, XI, prekallikrein, and HMWK.
D. II, VII, IX, and XI.

48-2. The coagulation factors known as the contact group include

A. II, VII, IX, and X.
B. XII, XI, HMWK, and prekallikrein.
C. I, V, VIII, and XIII.
D. I, II, III, and IV.

48-3. The "early" split products of fibrin(ogen) degradation by plasmin are

A. X and Y.
B. X and D.
C. Y and D.
D. D and E.

48-4. The role of factor XIIIa in hemostasis is to

A. initiate the intrinsic coagulation pathway.
B. enhance the rate of prothrombinase production.
C. stabilize the fibrin clot.
D. initiate fibrinolysis.

For the following questions choose from these answers:
A. 1 and 3
B. 2 and 4
C. 1, 2, and 3
D. 4 only
E. all of the above

48-5. The coagulation factors that can activate factor VII include

1. XIIf.
2. Xa.
3. IXa.
4. kallikrein.

48-6. Thrombin has many roles in hemostasis including

1. activation of factor XIII.
2. activation of protein C.
3. conversion of fibrinogen to fibrin.
4. both enhancing and inhibiting coagulation.

48-7. Naturally occurring inhibitors of coagulation include

1. AT-III.
2. the protein C–S complex.
3. C'1 inactivator.
4. heparin cofactor II.

48-8. Antithrombin III inhibits

1. factors IIa, IXa, and Xa.
2. plasmin.
3. factors XIa and XIIa.
4. kallikrein.

48-9. Plasmin and thus fibrinolysis are inhibited by

1. α_2-macroglobulin.
2. α_1-antitrypsin.
3. α_2-antiplasmin.
4. the protein C–S system.

References

1. Aballi AJ, DeLamerens S: Coagulation changes in the neonatal period and in early infancy. Pediatr Clin North Am 9:785, 1962; Pediatrics 42:685, 1968
2. Altman R, Hemker HC: Contact activation in the extrinsic blood clotting system. Thromb Diath Haemorrh 18:525, 1967
3. Aoki N: Natural inhibitors of fibrinolysis. Prog Cardiovasc Dis 21:267, 1979
4. Arnesen H: The effect of products D and E on the thrombin induced conversion of fibrinogen to fibrin. Scand J Haematol 12:166, 1974
5. Bajaj SP, Butkowski RJ, Mann KG: Prothrombin fragments: Ca²⁺ binding and activation kinetics. J Biol Chem 250:2150, 1975
6. Bennett NB, Ogston CM, McAndrew GM: The thyroid and fibrinolysis. Br Med J 4:147, 1967
7. Bergqvist D, Nilsson IM: Hereditary α_2-macroglobulin deficiency. Scand J Haematol 23:433, 1979
8. Bithell TC: Blood coagulation. In Lee GR, Bithell TC, Foerster J et al (eds): Wintrobe's Clinical Hematology, 9th ed, p 566. Philadelphia, Lea & Febiger, 1993
9. Bjork I, Jackson CM, Jornvall H et al: The active site of antithrombin. J Biol Chem 257:2406, 1982
10. Brakman P, Albrechtsen OK, Astrup T: Blood coagulation, fibrinolysis, and contraceptive hormones. JAMA 199:69, 1967
11. Broekmans AW, Veltkamp JJ, Bertina RM: Congenital protein C deficiency and venous thromboembolism. N Engl J Med 309:340, 1983
12. Broekmans AW, Bertina RM, Loeliger EA et al: Protein C and the development of skin necrosis during anticoagulant therapy. Thromb Haemost 49:251, 1983
13. Budzynski AZ, Marder VJ: Degradation pathway of fibrinogen by plasmin. Thromb Haemost 38:793, 1977
14. Collen D, Wiman B: Fast-acting plasmin inhibitor in human plasma. Blood 51:563, 1978
15. Coopland A, Alkjaersig N, Fletcher AP: Reduction in plasma factor XIII (fibrin stabilizing factor) concentration during pregnancy. J Lab Clin Med 73:144, 1969
16. Crowell EB Jr, Clatanoff DV, Kiekhofer W: The effect of oral contraceptives on factor VIII levels. J Lab Clin Med 77:551, 1971
16a. Dahlbeck B, Carlsson M, Svensson PJ: Familial thrombophilia due to a previously unrecognized mechanism characterized by poor anticoagulant response to activated protein C: Prediction of a cofactor to activated protein C. Proc Natl Acad Sci 90:1004, 1993
17. Davie EW, Ratnoff OD: Waterfall sequence for intrinsic blood clotting. Science 145:1310, 1964
18. Davie EW, Fujikawa K, Kurachi K et al: The role of serine proteases in the blood coagulation cascade. Adv Enzymol 48:277, 1979
19. Deykin D, Cochios F, DeCamp G et al: Hepatic removal of activated factor X by the perfused rabbit liver. Am J Physiol 214: 414, 1968
20. Eaton D, Rodriquez H, Vehar G: Proteolytic processing of

human factor VIII. Correlation of specific cleavages by thrombin, factor Xa and activated protein C with activation and inactivation of factor VIII coagulant activity. Biochem 25:505, 1986

21. Erickson LA, Hekman CM, Loskutoff DJ: The primary plasminogen activator inhibitors in endothelial cells, platelets, serum, and plasma are immunologically related. Proc Natl Acad Sci USA 82:8710, 1985

22. Esmon CT: Protein C: Biochemistry, physiology, and clinical implications. Blood 62:1155, 1983

23. Esmon CT, Owen WG: Identification of an endothelial cell cofactor for thrombin-catalyzed activation of protein C. Proc Natl Acad Sci USA 78:2249, 1981

24. Esmon CT, Stenflo J, Suttie JW et al: A new vitamin K-dependent protein: A phospholipid-binding zymogen of a serine esterase. J Biol Chem 251:3052, 1976

24a. Esmon NL, Carroll RC, Esmon CT: Thrombomodulin blocks the ability of thrombin to activate platelets. J Biol Chem 258:12238, 1983

25. Fujikawa K, Davie EW: Human factor XII (Hageman factor). Methods Enzymol 80:198, 1981

26. Gaffney PJ, Perry MJ: Unreliability of current serum fibrin degradation product (FDP) assays. Thromb Haemost 53:301, 1985

27. Gailani D, Broze GJ Jr: Effects of glycosaminoglycans on factor XI activation by thrombin. Blood Coagul Fibrinolysis 4:15, 1993

28. Gans H, Tan BH: α_1-Antitrypsin, an inhibitor for thrombin and plasmin. Clin Chim Acta 17:111, 1967

29. Gelehrter TD, Sznycer-Laszuk R: Thrombin induction of plasminogen activator-inhibitor in cultured human endothelial cells. J Clin Invest 77:165, 1986

30. Gjonnaess H, Fagerhol MK: Studies on coagulation and fibrinolysis in pregnancy. Acta Obstet Gynecol Scand 54:363, 1975

31. Gotze O: Proteases of the properdin system. In Reich E et al (eds): Proteases and Biological Control: Cold Spring Harbor Symposium, p 255. Cold Spring Harbor NY, Cold Spring Harbor Laboratory, 1975

32. Greenberg CS, Devine DV, McCrae KM: Measurement of plasma fibrin D-dimer levels with the use of a monoclonal antibody coupled to latex beads. Am J Clin Pathol 87:94, 1987

33. Guccione MA et al: Reactions of ^{14}C-ADP and ^{14}C-ATP with washed platelets from rabbits. Blood 37:542, 1971

34. Harpel PC: C'1 inactivator inhibition by plasmin. J Clin Invest 49:568, 1970

35. Harpel PC: Blood proteolytic enzyme inhibitors: Their role in modulating blood coagulation and fibrinolytic enzyme pathways. In Colman RW, Hirsh J, Marder VJ et al (eds): Hemostasis and Thrombosis, 2nd ed, p 219. Philadelphia, JB Lippincott, 1987

35a. Hassouna HI: Laboratory evaluation of hemostatic disorders. Hematol Oncol Clin North Am 7(6):1161, 1993

36. Heck LW, Kaplan AP: Substrates of Hageman factor. I. Isolation and characterization of human factor XI and inhibition of the activated enzyme by α_1-antitrypsin. J Exp Med 140:1615, 1974

37. Hemker HC, Veltkamp JJ, Loeliger EA: Kinetic aspects of the interaction of blood clotting enzymes. III. Demonstration of an inhibitor of prothrombin conversion in vitamin K deficiency. Thromb Diath Haemorrh 19:346, 1968

38. Hoak JC, Wilson WR, Warner ED et al: Effects of triiodothyronine-induced hypermetabolism on factor VIII and fibrinogen in man. J Clin Invest 48:768, 1969

39. Hultin MB, Nemerson Y: Activation of factor X by factors IXa and VIII: A specific assay for factor IXa in the presence of thrombin-activated factor VIII. Blood 52:928, 1978

40. Iatridis SG, Ferguson JH: Effect of surface and Hageman factor on the endogenous or spontaneous activation of the fibrinolytic system. Thromb Diath Haemorrh 6:411, 1961

41. Jones JM, Creeth JM, Kekwick RA: Thiol reduction of human α_2-macroglobulin. Biochem J 127:187, 1972

42. Kasper CK, Hoag MS, Aggeler PM et al: Blood clotting factors in pregnancy: Factor VIII concentrations in normal and AHF-deficient women. Obstet Gynecol 24:242, 1964

43. Kato H, Nagasawa S, Iwanaga S: HMW and LMW kininogens. Methods Enzymol 80:172, 1981

44. Kerbiriou DM, Griffith JH: Human high-molecular-weight kininogen. J Biol Chem 254:12020, 1979

45. Kruithof EKO, Gudinchet A, Bachmann F: Plasminogen activator inhibitor 1 and plasminogen activator inhibitor 2 in various disease states. Thromb Haemost 59:7, 1988

46. Laake K, Vennerod AM: Factor XII-induced fibrinolysis: Studies on the separation of prekallikrein, plasminogen proactivator, and factor XI in human plasma. Thromb Res 4:285, 1974

47. Lewis JH, Szeto ILF: Clearance of infused fibrin. Fed Proc 24:840, 1965

48. Libre EP, Cowan DH, Watkins SP Jr et al: Relationships between spleen, platelets and factor VIII levels. Blood 31:358, 1968

49. Lindahl AK, Sandset PM, Abidgaard U: The present status of tissue factor pathway inhibitor. Blood Coag Fibrinol 3:439, 1992

50. Loeliger EA, van der Esch B, Mattern MJ et al: The biological disappearance rate of prothrombin, factors VII, IX, and X from plasma in hypothyroidism, hyperthyroidism, and during fever. Thromb Diath Haemorrh 10:267, 1964

51. Lombardi R, Mannucci PM, Seghatchian MJ et al: Alterations of factor VIII von Willebrand factor in clinical conditions associated with an increase in its plasma concentration. Br J Haematol 49:61, 1981

52. MacFarlane RG: The basis of the cascade hypothesis of blood clotting. Thromb Diath Haemorrh 15:591, 1966

53. Mann KG, Nesheim ME, Hibbard LS et al: The role of factor V in the assembly of the prothrombinase complex. Ann NY Acad Sci 370:378, 1981

54. Marciniak E: Thrombin-induced proteolysis of human antithrombin III: An outstanding contribution of heparin. Br J Haematol 48:325, 1981

55. Marder VJ, Budzynski AZ: Data for defining fibrinogen and its plasmic degradation products. Thromb Diath Haemorrh 33:199, 1975

56. Marlar RA, Griffin JH: Alternative pathways of thromboplastin-dependent activation of human factor X in plasma. Ann NY Acad Sci 370:325, 1981

57. Marlar RA, Kleiss AJ, Griffin JH: Human protein C: Inactivation of factors V and VIII in plasma by the activated molecule. Ann NY Acad Sci 370:303, 1981

58. Marlar RA, Kleiss AJ, Griffin JH: Mechanism of action of human activated protein C, a thrombin dependent anticoagulant enzyme. Blood 59:1067, 1982

59. Marlar RA, Kleiss AJ, Griffin JH: An alternative extrinsic pathway of human blood coagulation. Blood 60:1353, 1982

59a. Maruyama I, Salem HH, Ishii H et al: Human thrombomodulin is not an efficient inhibitor of the procoagulant activity of thrombin. J Clin Invest 75:987, 1985

60. Masys DR, Baja JSP, Rapaport SI: Activation of human factor VII by factor IXa and factor Xa. Blood 60:1143, 1982

61. Matsuo O: Incidence of thrombosis in inherited antithrombin III deficiency. Thromb Res 24:509, 1981

62. McConnell DJ: Inhibitors of kallikrein in human plasma. J Clin Invest 51:1611, 1972

63. McKusick VA: Mendelian Inheritance in Man: Catalogs of Autosomal Dominant, Autosomal Recessive and X-linked

Phenotypes, 9th ed. Baltimore, Johns Hopkins University Press, 1990

64. McNicol GP, Fletcher AP, Alkjaersig N et al: Impairment of hemostasis in the urinary tract: The role of urokinase. J Lab Clin Med 58:34, 1961

65. Morawitz P: Die Chemie der Blutgerinnung. Ergebn Physiol Biol Chem Exp Pharmakol 4:307, 1905. Available in the English translation as: The Chemistry of Blood Coagulation, translated by Hartman RC, Guenther PF. Springfield, IL, Charles C Thomas, 1958

66. Moroi M, Aoki N: Isolation and characterization of α_2-plasmin inhibitor from human plasma: A novel proteinase inhibitor which inhibits activator-induced clot lysis. J Biol Chem 251:5956, 1976

67. Moroi M, Aoki N: Inhibition of proteases in coagulation, kinin-forming and complement systems by α_2-plasmin inhibitor. J Biochem 82:969, 1977

68. Moroi M, Aoki N: Inhibition of plasminogen binding to fibrin by α_2-plasmin inhibitor. Thromb Res 10:851, 1977

69. Morrison SA, Jesty J: Tissue factor-dependent activation of tritium-labeled factor IX and factor X in human plasma. Blood 63:1338, 1984

70. Morrissey JH, Macik BG, Neuenschwander PF et al: Quantitation of activated factor VII levels in plasma using a tissue factor mutant selectively deficient in promoting factor VII activation. Blood 81:734, 1993

71. Mullertz S, Clemmensen I: The primary inhibitor of plasmin in human plasma. Biochem J 159:545, 1976

72. Nelsestuen GL, Suttie JW: The purification and properties of an abnormal prothrombin protein produced by dicumarol-treated cows: A comparison to normal prothrombin. J Biol Chem 247:8176, 1972

73. Nemerson Y, Bach R: Tissue factor revisited. Prog Hemost Thromb 6:237, 1982

74. Ogston D, Bennett B: Naturally occurring inhibitors of coagulation. In Ogston D, Bennett B (eds): Haemostasis: Biochemistry, Physiology and Pathology, p 202. London, John Wiley & Sons, 1977

75. Ogston D, Bennett B: Biochemistry of naturally occurring inhibitors of the fibrinolytic enzyme system. In Ogston D, Bennett B (eds): Haemostasis: Biochemistry, Physiology and Pathology, p 230. London, John Wiley & Sons, 1977

76. Østerud B, Laake K, Prydz H: The activation of human factor IX. Thromb Haemost 33:533, 1975

77. Parkinson JF, Garcia JG, Bang NU: Decreased thrombin affinity of cell-surface thrombomodulin following treatment of cultured endothelial cells with beta-D-xyloside. Biochem Biophys Res Commun 169:177, 1990

78. Pennica D, Holmes WE, Kohr WH et al: Cloning and expression of human tissue-type plasminogen activator cDNA in *E. coli*. Nature 301:214, 1983

79. Phillips LL, Rosano L, Skrodelis V: Changes in factor XI (plasma thromboplastin antecedent) levels during pregnancy. Am J Obstet Gynecol 116:1114, 1973

80. Radcliff RD, Nemerson Y: Mechanism of activation of bovine factor VII: Products of cleavage by factor Xa. J Biol Chem 251:4797, 1976

81. Radcliff R, Bagdasarian A, Colman R et al: Activation of bovine factor VII by Hageman factor fragments. Blood 50:611, 1977

82. Ranby M, Bergsdorf N, Nilsson T: Enzymatic properties of the one- and two-chain form of tissue plasminogen activator. Thromb Res 27:175, 1982

83. Rao LV, Rapaport SI: Activation of factor VII bound to tissue factor: A key early step in the tissue factor pathway of blood coagulation. Proc Natl Acad Sci USA 85:6687, 1988

84. Rapaport SI, Schiffman S, Patch MJ et al: The importance of activation of antihemophilic globulin and proaccelerin

by traces of thrombin in the generation of intrinsic pro-thrombinase activity. Blood 21:221, 1963; Scand J Clin Lab Invest Suppl 84:88, 1965

85. Reid WO, Hodge SM, Cerutti ER: The use of EACA in preventing or reducing haemorrhages in the haemophiliac. Thromb Diath Haemorrh 18:179, 1967

86. Rizza CR: Effect of exercise on the level of antihaemophilic globulin in human blood. J Physiol 156:128, 1961

87. Rosenberg RD: Heparin, antithrombin, and abnormal clotting. Annu Rev Med 29:367, 1978

88. Rosenberg RD: The heparin-antithrombin system: A natural anticoagulant mechanism. In Colman RW, Hirsh J, Marder VJ et al (eds): Hemostasis and Thrombosis. Philadelphia, JB Lippincott, 1987

89. Rosse WF: Complement. In Williams WJ, Beutler E, Erslev AJ et al (eds): Hematology, 2nd ed, p 87. New York, McGraw-Hill, 1977

90. Royle NJ, Nigli M, Cool D et al: Structural gene encoding human factor XII isolated at 5q 33-qter. Somat Cell Mol Genet 14:217, 1988

91. Saito H, Goldsmith GH, Moroi M et al: Inhibitory spectrum of α_2-plasmin inhibitor. Proc Natl Acad Sci USA 76:2013, 1979

92. Scott CF, Colman RW: Fibrinogen blocks the autoactivation and thrombin-mediated activation of factor XI on dextran sulfate. Proc Natl Acad Sci USA 89:11189, 1992

93. Scriver CR, Beaudet AL, Sly WS et al (eds): The Metabolic and Molecular Basis of Inherited Disease, p 2107. New York, McGraw-Hill, 1989

94. Seegers WH, Warner ED, Brinkhous KM et al: Heparin and the antithrombic activity of plasma. Science 96:300, 1942

95. Seligsohn U, Østerud B, Brown SE et al: Activation of human factor VII in plasma and in purified systems: Roles of activated factor IX, kallikrein, and activated factor XII. J Clin Invest 64:1056, 1979

96. Sherman LA, Lee J: Specific binding of soluble fibrin to macrophages. J Exp Med 145:76, 1977

97. Shore PA et al: Release of blood platelet serotonin by reserpine and lack of effect on bleeding time. J Pharmacol Exp Ther 117:232, 1956

98. Silverberg M, Nicoll JE, Kaplan AP: The mechanism by which the light chain of cleaved HMW-kininogen augments the activation of prekallikrein, factor XI and Hageman factor. Thromb Res 20:173, 1980

99. Simone JV, Abildgaard CF, Schulman I: Blood coagulation in thyroid dysfunction. N Engl J Med 273:1057, 1965

100. Solum NO, Rigollot C, Budzynski AZ et al: A quantitative evaluation of the inhibition of platelet aggregation by low molecular weight degradation products of fibrinogen. Br J Haematol 24:419, 1973

101. Spaet TH: Hemostatic homeostasis. Blood 28:112, 1966

102. Stenbjerg S: Inherited α_2 macroglobulin deficiency. Thromb Res 22:491, 1981

103. Stenflo J: Vitamin K, prothrombin and δ-carboxyglutamic acid. N Engl J Med 296:624, 1977

104. Suzuki K, Nishioka J, Kusumoto H: Mechanism of inhibition of activated protein C inhibitor. J Biochem 85:187, 1984

105. Thompson AR, Harker LA: Manual of Hemostasis and Thrombosis, 3rd ed, p 38. Philadelphia, FA Davis, 1983

106. Tillett WS, Garner RL: The fibrinolytic activity of hemolytic streptococci. J Exp Med 58:485, 1933

107. Todd AS: The histological localization of fibrinolysin activator. J Pathol Bacteriol 78:281, 1959

108. Tollefsen DM, Majerus DW, Blank MK: Heparin cofactor II. Purification and properties of a heparin-dependent inhibitor of thrombin in human plasma. J Biol Chem 257:2162, 1982

109. vanMourik JA, Lawrence DA, Loskutoff DJ: Purification of

an inhibitor of plasminogen activator (antiactivator) synthesized by endothelial cells. J Biol Chem 259:14914, 1984

110. Walker FJ: Regulation of activated protein C by a new protein. J Biol Chem 255:5521, 1980

110a. Walsh PN: Factor XI: A renaissance. Sem Hematol 29(3):189, 1992

111. Walsh PR, Biggs R: The role of platelets in intrinsic factor Xa formation. Br J Haematol 22:743, 1972

112. Warn-Cramer BJ, Maki SL, Zivelin A et al: Partial purification and characterization of extrinsic pathway inhibitor (the factor Xa-dependent plasma inhibitor of factor VIIa/tissue factor). Thromb Res 48:11, 1987

113. Wiggins RC, Loskutoff DJ, Cochrane CG et al: Activation of rabbit Hageman factor by homogenates of cultured rabbit endothelial cells. J Clin Invest 65:197, 1980

114. Williams JRB: The fibrinolytic activity of urine. Br J Exp Pathol 32:530, 1951

115. Wiman B, Collen D: Purification and characterization of human antiplasmin, the fast-acting plasmin inhibitor in plasma. Eur J Biochem 78:19, 1977

116. Witte S et al: Mikroskopische Befunde uber die Blutstillung bei Serotoninausschaltung. Thromb Haemost 5:505, 1961

117. Wright IS: The nomenclature of blood clotting factors. Thromb Diath Haemorrh 7:381, 1962

118. Yin ET, Wessler S, Stoll PJ: Biological properties of the naturally occurring plasma inhibitor to activated factor X. J Biol Chem 246:3703, 1971

119. Zur M, Radcliffe RD, Oberdick J et al: The dual role of factor VII in blood coagulation. Initiation and inhibition of a proteolytic system by a zymogen. J Biol Chem 257:5623, 1982

120. Zur M, Nemerson Y: The esterase activity of coagulation factor VII: Evidence for intrinsic activity of the zymogen. J Biol Chem 253:2203, 1977

CHAPTER 49

Routine and Special Laboratory Evaluation of Coagulation

Cheryl S. Cook

Objectives

1. List and describe the commonly performed tests for routine evaluation of coagulation.
2. Discuss the principles, methodologies, and interpretations of routine coagulation test results.
3. Describe some of the specialized tests currently being used to identify specific abnormalities of coagulation.
4. Recognize some of the advantages as well as potential problems in performing various coagulation procedures.

For centuries, man has been intrigued by the process of blood coagulation and has strived to perfect accurate and precise methods for evaluating the complex process. Since William Henson's discovery in the late 1700s that blood in ligated veins of a living animal clotted much more slowly than blood that has been shed from the body,[115] investigators have been avidly experimenting with ways to measure the blood's capacity to clot.[85,108]

In 1905, knowledge of coagulation took a significant step forward when Paul Morawitz, a young German scientist, published a comprehensive explanation of the chemistry of coagulation.[89] His observations that coagula-

tion did not occur when plasma was placed in containers with "nonwettable" surfaces, such as paraffin-lined tubes, but did so rapidly when placed in contact with "wettable" surfaces such as glass tubes, led to the development of methods for the measurement of coagulation.[5] Among the first researchers to expand on the theory of Morawitz were Drs. Roger Lee and Paul White.[81] Modifying the numerous procedures described in the literature in the early 1900s, these investigators developed a procedure known as the Lee and White whole blood clotting time (L-W). Today, more sensitive and precise procedures have replaced this test in most institutions. It was not until the mid-1930s that the next breakthrough in coagulation testing came about. At this time, Dr. Armand Quick[112] described a procedure called the prothrombin time (PT) test. With minor modifications, this test has become a routine coagulation procedure for evaluating the extrinsic coagulation system. In the 1950s, studies of blood from hemophiliacs, whose blood yielded normal prothrombin times despite its inability to clot normally, led to the development of the partial thromboplastin time (PTT) test.[72,74,132] Although procedural modifications have since been made, this test is still one of the best available for evaluating the intrinsic coagulation system.[62,73]

Separating the coagulation process into the extrinsic and intrinsic systems evolved from observations made in the laboratory (Fig. 47-4).[26] The extrinsic system requires the addition of a tissue extract to the plasma to induce coagulation. Damaged tissue will stimulate the extrinsic system by releasing a lipoprotein substance commonly referred to as tissue factor. This lipoprotein, in conjunction with factor VII, activates factor X in the common pathway and leads to the production of a fibrin clot. The extrinsic and common pathways include factors I, II, V, VII, and X. The intrinsic system is stimulated *in vitro* by activating blood or plasma with negatively charged surfaces in the presence of phospholipid supplied by platelets or other reagents. The intrinsic and common pathways include all factors except VII and XIII. Initially, the intrinsic pathway was thought to be the dominant one, with the extrinsic pathway having auxiliary status.[135] Recent studies have implicated the extrinsic system as dominant (Chap. 47). Refer to Figure 47-4 for diagrams of these pathways.

REFERENCE RANGES

Although approximate reference ranges will be given for each of the tests discussed in this chapter, it must be stressed that reference ranges in hemostasis are significantly affected by patient populations, methodology, reagent systems, instrument systems, and combinations thereof.[120] Refer to Chapters 44 and 58 for details on establishing reference ranges.

TESTING METHODOLOGIES

Traditionally, coagulation studies have been performed using the detection of clot formation (fibrin) as an endpoint. In recent years, technologic advances have increased the scope of special coagulation testing. The development of monoclonal antibodies has made highly specific antisera available for immunologic testing, and synthetic substrates have made it possible to view coagulation from an enzymatic perspective. In addition, new instruments and methods have been developed to keep pace with the expanding knowledge of hemostasis.

Fibrin Endpoint

Fibrin endpoint methodologies depend on detection of a fibrin clot as it is formed through proteolytic cleavage of fibrinogen. Methods for clot detection commonly used are the manual tilt-tube, electromechanical (fibrin strand), and optical density (turbidity) techniques. (See Chap. 58 for a detailed discussion of the instruments used in hemostasis.) Optical systems measure the rate of change of light absorbance, thus making the results potentially more reproducible than those of manual or electromechanical methods. Coagulation times will differ significantly depending on the instrument, reagent, and instrument–reagent combination being used. Thus, it is imperative that each laboratory establish the reactivity of its instrument–reagent combination or system to the various factors and its own reference ranges for each determination.

Immunologic Methods

Immunologic assays are gaining importance because of the recent discovery that there are inherited variants of coagulation proteins that have normal antigenic properties but lack functional activity. Such a protein is termed *crossreactive material* (CRM), and plasma containing such a protein is called CRM+. It is important to identify these variants in order to understand the pathophysiology of coagulation disorders.[64] Several immunologic techniques are available; the more commonly used procedures will be described very briefly below.[39,41,65,141] Refer to immunology texts for greater detail.

OUCHTERLONY DOUBLE DIFFUSION

The Ouchterlony technique is based on the principle that when antigen and the antibody specific to that antigen are placed in separate wells cut in agar they will diffuse toward each other in a radial manner and precipitate as immune complexes when they meet. The resultant precipitate can be seen as a transverse line (straight or curved) between the two wells. This method is not quantitative but will establish whether two antigens are serologically identical or different.

RADIAL IMMUNODIFFUSION

In radial immunodiffusion (RID) studies, specific antibody is incorporated into agar, and antigen is placed in wells cut in the agar. As the antigen diffuses, it precipitates with the antibody, forming a halo around the well. A linear relation exists between the square of the diameter of the ring and the concentration of antigen in the well.

LAURELL ROCKET ELECTROPHORESIS

In Laurell rocket electrophoresis, agarose containing antibody specific for the antigen to be measured is poured on a glass plate. Antigen is placed in wells cut on one side of the plate, and direct electrical current is applied. As the antigen migrates and contacts antibody molecules, a rocket-shaped precipitate is formed (Fig. 49-1). The area of the rocket or, more commonly, its height is proportional to the antigen concentration.[16,78,79]

CROSSED IMMUNOELECTROPHORESIS

Crossed immunoelectrophoresis (CIE) is a two-dimensional method. In the first dimension, plasma is electrophoresed through plain agarose to separate the antigens. Agar containing antibody specific to the antigen being measured is then poured on the plate, and a second electrophoresis is performed at right angles to the first. As the antigen–antibody complexes form, they create bell-shaped precipitin lines. Abnormalities can be detected by abnormal migration patterns or abnormally shaped precipitin areas (Fig. 49-2).

RADIOIMMUNOASSAY

In a radioimmunoassay (RIA), a known concentration of radiolabeled antigen and the unknown concentration of unlabeled antigen in a test sample compete for binding sites on a known and limited amount of antibody. For

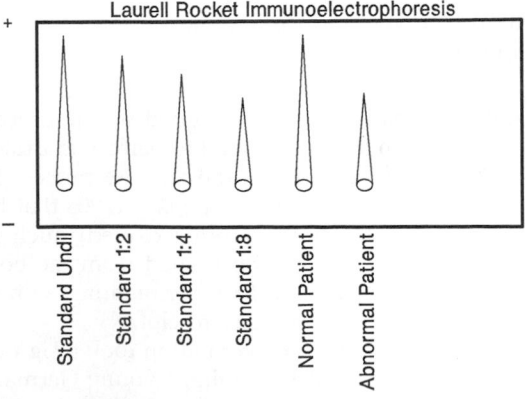

FIGURE 49-1. Laurell rocket electrophoresis. Height of "rocket" is proportional to antigen concentration.

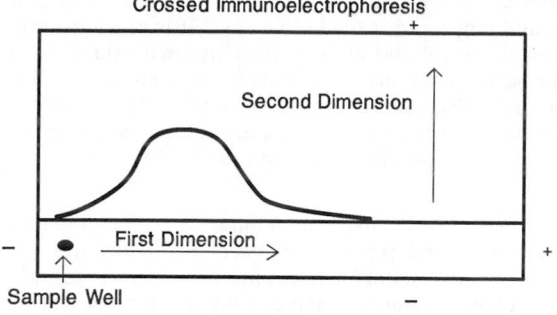

FIGURE 49-2. Precipitin lines formed during crossed immunoelectrophoresis.

example, there may be sufficient antibody to bind 50% of the labeled antigen. The greater the amount of unlabeled antigen in the test sample, the less amount of labeled antigen will be bound. The bound antigen is separated from the free antigen, and the ratio of radioactivity associated with the bound antigen to the free antigen is determined.[148]

ENZYME-LINKED IMMUNOSORBENT ASSAY

An enzyme-linked immunosorbent assay (ELISA) is an adaptation of RIA. Either the antigen or the antibody is immobilized on a solid support. In the latter case, an antigen-specific antibody is immobilized and known antigen is linked to an enzyme such as alkaline phosphatase or peroxidase. The labeled antigen competes with unlabeled antigen in the test sample for the bound antibody sites. Free antigen is washed away and a substrate for the enzyme label is then added. Color formed by cleavage of the substrate is read spectrophotometrically. The amount of color is directly proportional to the concentration of labeled antigen being measured. The ratio of labeled to unlabeled antigen can then be determined.[101,126]

Synthetic Substrates

Synthetic substrates are small peptide chains consisting of amino acid sequences that mimic the natural substrate of an enzyme. An indicator group, either a chromophore or a fluorophore, is attached to the synthetic substrate, which is cleaved by the enzyme that has specificity for that substrate (Chap. 58). Synthetic substrate assays allow coagulation testing to be approached as a series of enzymatic reactions in an accurate and sensitive manner. A sound knowledge of enzyme kinetics is necessary for optimal use of synthetic substrate assays. Endpoint or initial rate analysis may be performed, and many assays have been adapted for use on automated instrumentation.[38,51]

ROUTINE TESTS FOR THE INTRINSIC AND COMMON PATHWAYS

PLASMA RECALCIFICATION TIME

A modification of the whole blood clotting time is the recalcification time of plasma, using citrated plasma (instead of whole blood), $CaCl_2$, glass or siliconized tubes,

and either platelet-rich plasma (PRP), platelet-poor plasma (PPP), or both.[70] This test is based on the fact that except for calcium, normal PRP contains all the components of the coagulation mechanism necessary for generating a fibrin clot. Removal of red cells makes the clot easier to see. The time required for blood to clot after Ca^{2+} is added is a general measure of the intrinsic and common pathways. By using a parallel test on PPP, screening for a platelet function defect may also be accomplished. Reference ranges for PRP and PPP are 100 to 150 seconds and 130 to 240 seconds, respectively. Platelet-rich plasma should clot at least 20 seconds faster than platelet-poor plasma.[55]

The principal disadvantages of the plasma recalcification time are the difficulty in standardizing the number of platelets in the PRP and the length of time necessary to perform the test. Moreover, the test is insensitive to moderate factor deficiencies. In addition, errors in collection technique can significantly affect the results, as will the amount of glass contact. It is important that the same size tube always be used for testing and that the specimens be tilted uniformly. Because the procedure cannot be standardized, it is important to keep as many variables constant as possible. The sensitivity of this test is somewhat improved by diluting the plasma. This accomplishes three things: (1) it adjusts the PRP closer to the actual *in vivo* platelet count; (2) it increases the sensitivity of the test system to factor deficiencies; and (3) it dilutes the natural inhibitors to coagulation that are present. A normal control should be run with each test.

ACTIVATED CLOTTING TIME

By the mid-1960s, the lack of sensitivity and precision of earlier tests including the plasma recalcification test led researchers to look for better methods of monitoring heparin therapy (Chap. 54). Although by 1964, the PTT test was recognized to be sensitive to heparin, the test had not yet gained widespread acceptance as the heparin-monitoring procedure. Devising a new procedure based loosely on the now obsolete Lee-White test, Dr. Paul Hattersley developed the activated clotting time (ACT) test.[49,50] The ACT uses diatomaceous earth (diatomite) as an activator of the contact factors and requires the blood to be kept warmed to a constant 37°C by taking a special incubator to the patient's bedside.

Principle. Whole blood contains all the components necessary to produce a clot when removed from the veins and put into a glass tube. By adding an activator and keeping the blood at a constant 37°C, a reliable and rapid screen of the intrinsic and common pathways is achieved.

Reagents and Equipment

Two evacuated tubes containing 12 mg of diatomite.
A portable heat block
Thermometer
2 stopwatches

Procedure. The two tubes containing diatomite are brought to 37°C in a heat block at the patient's bedside. Using good venipuncture technique, at least 2 mL of blood is drawn into a tube and discarded. The tourniquet is removed, and the first tube with diatomite is attached to the needle. When blood starts to flow into the tube, the first stopwatch is started. The tube is filled, mixed, and placed in the heat block. The procedure is repeated with the second tube, and the second stopwatch is started. After 60 seconds, the first tube is observed by tilting it at 5-second intervals until a clot is formed, at which time the second tube is observed using the same procedure. The appropriate stopwatch is stopped at the first appearance of a clot in each tube. The duplicates should agree within 10 seconds. The average time is reported.[49]

Reference Range. The reference range is 75 to 120 seconds. The target range during heparin therapy is 140 to 185 seconds.

Interpretation. Prolongation of the ACT is indicative of one or more factor defects in the intrinsic or common pathways or the presence of a circulating anticoagulant such as heparin.

Comments. Temperature control is critical: all testing must be maintained at 37°C. The primary use of the ACT is during procedures requiring extracorporeal circulation, in which frequent testing and rapid turnaround time are required.[53] In fact, the ACT has enjoyed considerable popularity of late as a "point-of-care" test (*i.e.*, a test performed at the patient's bedside).[97] Another recent use of the ACT is in monitoring therapy with hirudin (a direct thrombin inhibitor derived from leaches).[17]

Other than the duplicate testing, there is no suitable method of quality control for this procedure.

PARTIAL THROMBOPLASTIN TIME

Several researchers observed that blood samples from classic hemophiliacs have a prolonged clotting time, but that when tissue thromboplastin is added, the plasma clots just as normal plasma does.[74] Expanded studies showed that thromboplastins, which are lipoproteins (protein + phospholipid), may be classified as complete or partial (only phospholipid). From these conclusions, investigators developed the partial thromboplastin time (PTT). This test is more sensitive to abnormalities in the early stages than were previous tests of the intrinsic system. An important refinement of the PTT was the addition of negatively charged activators to the system, resulting in significantly shorter clotting times.[87] This modification is now used exclusively. It is the test of choice to screen for factor deficiencies of the intrinsic and common pathways and also for monitoring heparin therapy. It also is the basis for assays of factors of the intrinsic system.

The PTT reagent consists of two components: a platelet substitute (phospholipid), prepared from brain or plant phospholipids, and an activator. Kaolin, Celite, micronized silica, or ellagic acid are used as activators, depending on the manufacturer.

Principle. The PTT measures all factors except VII and XIII. Maximum activation of the contact factors is accomplished by addition of the activator. Phospholipid is supplied to substitute for platelet factor 3 (PF3). From this point, the PTT is essentially the same as a recalcification time of plasma.

Specimen Requirements and Reagents. Citrated platelet-poor plasma should be collected according to the guidelines in Chapter 2. Reagents include phospholipid with activators (PTT reagent) and 0.025 M $CaCl_2$ (or as recommended by reagent manufacturer).[93]

Controls. Commercial lyophilized controls are available in normal, midrange, and extended ranges.[66] It is recommended that a normal control and at least one abnormal control be used.[94] In-house preparations of pooled/frozen plasma may be used as controls. Each laboratory must specify when controls are to be tested, what the satisfactory control limits are, and if duplicates are run, how closely the values should agree.

Equipment. For the manual method, 12 × 75 mm glass tubes, a heat block, and pipettes are needed. For the fibrin strand method, an instrument for electromechanical fibrin strand detection and appropriate cups and pipettes, as recommended by the manufacturer, are required. For the photo-optical method, the specialized instrument and appropriate accessories as listed by the manufacturer, are needed.

Procedure. Platelet-poor plasma (0.1 mL) is added to 0.1 mL of PTT reagent and incubated at 37°C for the period of time specified by the reagent manufacturer (approximately 3–5 minutes). After incubation, 0.1 mL of warmed $CaCl_2$ is added, and the time for clotting to occur is recorded.

Reporting, Reference Range and Interpretation. The PTT is reported in seconds, to the nearest tenth, along with the reference range.[94]

Reference ranges differ according to the reagent, method, and instrument used. The reference ranges may extend from a lower limit of 20 seconds to an upper limit of 45 seconds.

When properly performed, the PTT is an excellent screening test for the intrinsic and common coagulation pathway factors. Most commercial reagents will demonstrate a prolonged PTT if any factor measured by the PTT is less than 40% to 50% of normal. A prolonged PTT in the absence of heparin indicates a factor deficiency, an acquired circulating anticoagulant such as the lupus inhibitor, or an antibody to a specific factor such as factor VIII.

Comments. Sources of error in the PTT may be grouped into three categories: sample collection and preparation, reagent preparation, and instrumentation. Improper collection and processing of specimens may significantly affect the results. The anticoagulant volume should be adjusted for individuals with hematocrits greater than 0.55 L/L to avoid error caused by an incorrect anticoagulant-to-plasma ratio. Specimens with hematocrits greater than 0.55 L/L will have anticoagulant excess in the collection tube. The extra sodium citrate in the collection tube chelates the calcium in the PTT test system and may result in spuriously abnormal results. Sodium citrate volume should be adjusted in the collection tube to keep the recommended citrate–plasma volume correct.[94] Theoretically specimens with hematocrits less than 0.20 L/L need more anticoagulant in the collection tube to compensate for the increased plasma volume of the specimen. In practice, however, low hematocrits do not seem to cause problems with spurious results. Correction for citrate volume is not required for these specimens.[94] Hemolysis may cause a falsely shortened PTT. Platelets in the plasma sample may cause erratic results or falsely shorten the PTT. Unexpected heparin contamination (*e.g.*, from heparin locks) can falsely lengthen the PTT.

Reagents may be affected by improper storage, water impurities, or incorrect dilution. Reagent systems should be tested for sensitivity to factor deficiencies by performing the PTT on serial dilutions of plasma.

A failing light source, fluctuations in temperature, loss of calibration of tubing, or contamination will cause instrument error. A good quality control program should reveal any instrumental or reagent-related error. Refer to Chapter 58 for a discussion of instruments and quality control.

ROUTINE TESTS FOR THE EXTRINSIC AND COMMON PATHWAYS

PROTHROMBIN TIME

Early experiments by the French physiologist de Bainville[3] showed that blood could be made to clot quickly by adding tissue factors. The discovery that oxalate and citrate inhibit coagulation[119] led to the assumption that clotting was dependent on calcium.

The one-stage prothrombin time (PT), as described by Dr. Armand Quick in 1935,[112] was believed to be an indirect measure of prothrombin in plasma, dependent on the presence of fibrinogen. Subsequent discoveries of factors V, VII, and X showed that the PT is a reflection of the activities of several factors.[102,111] Thus, the PT used in the modern laboratory screens for deficiencies of factors I, II, V, VII, and X.

Although the PT is no longer considered a measure of prothrombin itself, it is still the test of choice for monitoring anticoagulant therapy by vitamin K antagonists (Chap. 54).[83,84,134,142] Three of the five factors measured by the PT (II, VII, X) are sensitive to and depressed by these anticoagulants.[109] Only factor IX, the other factor depressed by vitamin K antagonists, is not detected by the PT.

Principle. When tissue extract or thromboplastin[103] is added to PPP along with calcium, it reacts with factor VIIa to convert factor X to Xa. Factor Xa, along with factor Va, phospholipid, and Ca^{2+} converts prothrombin to thrombin. Thrombin subsequently converts fibrinogen to fibrin. The time from the addition of thromboplastin/$CaCl_2$ to the formation of a clot is reported.[55,56]

Specimen Requirements, Reagents and Equipment. Citrated platelet-poor plasma is collected according to the guidelines in Chapter 2. Thromboplastin/$CaCl_2$ (PT reagent) and controls (see discussion under PTT controls) are needed. Equipment is the same as that used for the PTT.

Procedure and Reference Range. Aliquots of control and patient plasma are warmed according to the method being used. The thromboplastin reagent is warmed by incubating it at 37°C for 3 to 5 minutes, and 0.2 mL of PT reagent is added to 0.1 mL of plasma (patient or control). The clotting time is recorded to the nearest tenth of a second.

Normal values differ with the reagent and method. These values may range from 10 to 12 seconds in some photo-optical systems and from 12 to 14 seconds using manual methods.

Reporting. Prothrombin times may be reported in several ways: (1) patient time (in seconds) with the reference range[94]; (2) patient time with the control time (in seconds); (3) prothrombin ratio (the PT of the patient divided by the mean of the reference range and multiplied by 100—rarely used in the United States); (4) percent activity (outdated and not recommended); and (5) the International Normalized Ratio (INR), which has been proposed as the standard method of reporting.[54,80,95] The INR is discussed in Chapter 54.

Interpretation and Comments. Prolongation of the PT indicates an abnormality of one or more common or extrinsic coagulation factors. This abnormality may be inherited or acquired. Prolongation may also occur with factor inhibitors. Using most commercial reagents, the PT is sensitive to factor deficiencies of less than 40% to 50% of normal.

Reporting of percent activity is no longer recommended because the dilution curve used to determine percent activity dilutes all factors, not just those affected by anticoagulant therapy, and is therefore an inaccurate representation of therapy. The most common method of reporting in the United States at the present time is patient time in seconds along with the reference range. The INR is gaining popularity in an effort to standardize PT reporting.[91] Portable instruments capable of determining PT and calculating the INR are available.[147] The sources of error in this test are similar to those discussed for the PTT.

OTHER TESTS

Two other laboratory determinations related to the extrinsic and common pathways are the Stypven time and prothrombin–proconvertin time.[71] Neither test has enjoyed widespread popularity. The reader is referred to textbooks dedicated to hemostasis and the indicated references for details on these rarely performed tests.[68,96,104]

OTHER ROUTINE TESTS

FIBRINOGEN

Many methods for the measurement of fibrinogen have been described. Five are most commonly performed.

1. Precipitation or denaturation methods,[44,60,128] in which heat, salt, or another agent is used to denature fibrinogen to an insoluble state. The suspended fibrinogen precipitate may be measured turbidimetrically, or the precipitated fibrinogen may be isolated and measured by colorimetric or ultraviolet protein quantitation. These methods generally are semiquantitative and are subject to many technical problems.
2. Turbidimetric or fibrin clot density procedures[28] are based on photo-optical measurement of the change in turbidity of plasma as fibrinogen is converted to fibrin by thrombin. The kinetics of this conversion have been used to measure the fibrinogen concentration.[58,141] Turbidimetric procedures are the basis for some automated fibrinogen methods that have been introduced.[130,149] Modifications of the original procedure have improved sensitivity at lower fibrinogen levels and have eliminated heparin interference.[122,123,130]
3. Coagulable protein assays are performed by clotting the plasma sample using thrombin or $CaCl_2$, isolating the fibrin clot, and then measuring the fibrin by weight, chemically, or by ultraviolet absorbance.[60,114,128] Ancrod, a thrombin-like enzyme that is specific for fibrinogen and not influenced by heparin, also has been used to clot plasma.[32] The coagulable protein assay is considered the reference procedure for fibrinogen measurement. The principal disadvantage of this type of assay is the time required to perform the test.[128]
4. Immunologic assays utilize antibodies to fibrinogen in assays such as radial immunodiffusion,[14,19,24] kinetic latex agglutinometry,[2] measurement of turbidity,[32] or

rocket immunoelectrophoresis. Immunologic assays are time consuming and they measure fibrin(ogen) degradation products. However, because immunologic assays measure dysfunctional as well as functional fibrinogen, performing an immunologic fibrinogen assay along with a functional fibrinogen assay is a useful tool in detecting dysfibrinogenemia (nonfunctional fibrinogen).

5. The modified thrombin clotting time is the most widely performed clinical fibrinogen assay[69] and its discussion follows. This assay was first described by Clauss in 1957.[21,131] The clotting time of diluted plasma to which a high concentration of thrombin has been added is inversely proportional to the fibrinogen concentration. This procedure is relatively insensitive to heparin and fibrin(ogen) degradation products.[63,90,128] A thrombokinetic procedure in which the maximal rate of change in optical density is measured during the modified thrombin time has been described.[92]

It is vital to realize that there may be discrepancies in the fibrinogen concentration as measured by the various methods described above on the same specimen. A dysfibrinogenemia will generally result in a low fibrinogen level as measured by the modified thrombin clotting time,[10] whereas immunologic techniques (or other techniques that do not depend on the formation of a clot) will yield normal or above-normal results in the same specimen.

MODIFIED THROMBIN CLOTTING TIME ASSAY FOR FIBRINOGEN

Procedure and Reference Range. A high concentration of thrombin is added to diluted, citrated, platelet-poor plasma to convert fibrinogen to fibrin. The clotting time is inversely proportional to the fibrinogen concentration. Quantitation is achieved through the use of standards with known concentrations of fibrinogen.[61,94]

Each laboratory must establish its own reference range. The range should be approximately 170 to 410 mg/dL.

Comments. Improper specimen collection with the wrong blood-to-anticoagulant ratio or lack of correction of citrate volume for a low or high hematocrit may cause erroneous results.

A higher dilution of the test plasma must be made if the clotting time is too short. A lesser dilution of plasma is necessary for very long clotting times; however, a dilution of less than a 1:3 (*e.g.*, 1:2) should not be tested. Appropriate dilution factors must be used in calculating results.

Fibrinogen degradation products at a concentration of greater than 100 μg/mL may affect the thrombin clotting time. High levels of the larger degradation products may interfere at lower fibrinogen concentrations.

Heparin concentrations greater than 1 U/mL may result in falsely low fibrinogen concentration measurements. Care must be taken to avoid obtaining specimens through heparinized lines.

If the patient is receiving fibrinolytic therapy, either ε-aminocaproic acid (EACA) or soybean trypsin inhibitor should be added to the collection tube to prevent *in vitro* clot lysis.

Hemolysis or lipemia may interfere with photo-optical measurements. Manual, semiautomated, or automated endpoint detection devices may be used, but each will result in a different endpoint.[94] The thrombin reagent (100 NIH units/mL) is unstable. (See comments under Thrombin Clotting Time.)

Known normal and abnormal controls should be run every 20 samples or every shift. Duplicates should agree within 0.5 seconds. A new standard curve must be established for each new lot of reagents. Only the linear portion of the calibration curve should be used to interpret plasma fibrinogen levels.

PLATELET COUNT

A platelet count is an important parameter in the routine evaluation of hemostasis. This count, usually performed by automated instrument (Chap. 42) but occasionally manually, may provide valuable information regarding the patient's hemostatic picture.

SPECIAL TESTS FOR COAGULATION PROTEINS OR SYSTEMS

Historic Tests for Coagulation Abnormalities

The *two-stage prothrombin time*[144,145] is of historic interest, as it was the first method to measure the prothrombin concentration indirectly in plasma.[15,125] This test is rarely used today, as it has been replaced by other methods such as factor assays for prothrombin using synthetic substrates or prothrombin depleted plasma.

The *prothrombin consumption test* is a prothrombin time (PT) study performed on serum from blood that has been allowed to clot for 60 minutes.[110] Severe deficiencies of factors V, VIII, IX, X, XI, or XII, as well as platelet deficiencies or abnormalities, will slow the rate of prothrombin conversion.[129] The test is unique in that the PT on normal serum will be long (usually greater than 20–25 seconds). This test has largely been replaced by more sensitive and specific assays.

The *thromboplastin generation test* (TGT) was based on the observation that barium sulfate or aluminum hydroxide will adsorb to certain coagulation factors.[36,52] If $BaSO_4$ or $Al(OH)_3$ is added to normal plasma, factors II, VII, IX, and X will be adsorbed and thus can be removed by centrifugation. Likewise, if blood is allowed to clot, the remaining serum will not contain fibrinogen, factor II, the labile factors V and VIII, or XIII. Therefore, if normal adsorbed plasma, normal serum, platelets, and $CaCl_2$ are mixed, the mixture cannot form a clot until prothrombin (factor II) is supplied by the addition of normal plasma. The assay was devised to identify deficiencies of specific factors.[7,105] The TGT is labor intensive and takes a significant amount of time to perform. It is not performed in most hemostasis laboratories today.

The TGT reagents (*i.e.*, normal adsorbed plasma and normal serum) can be used, however, in either the PT or the PTT systems (sometimes referred to as mixing studies or substitution studies). For example, if the patient has a normal PT and prolonged PTT, factors I, II, V, VII, and X are assumed to be normal. If the patient's PTT is corrected by addition of normal adsorbed plasma (containing factors I, V, VIII, XI, XII, and XIII) but not by addition of normal serum, factor VIII is presumed to be abnormal. If the patient's PTT is corrected by normal serum (containing factors IV, VII, IX, X, XI, and XII) but not by adsorbed plasma, factor IX probably is abnormal. The third possibility is for both serum and adsorbed plasma to correct the PTT. In this case, factors XI or XII may be abnormal. See Table 49-1 for a summary of the use of substitution studies in conjunction with other coagulation determinations to define factor deficiencies. Substitution or mixing studies are being replaced by factor assays in a number of institutions.

Current Tests for Coagulation Abnormalities

THROMBIN CLOTTING TIME

Principle. Addition of thrombin to plasma bypasses all coagulation reactions except polymerization of fibrinogen. The thrombin clotting time (TCT) measures the conversion of fibrinogen to fibrin and is not influenced by deficiencies of the other coagulation factors.[75] Dysfibrinogenemia, hypofibrinogenemia, fibrin split products, immunologic antithrombins, and the presence of abnormal globulins will prolong the TCT. The thrombin clotting time also is very sensitive to heparin and may be used to monitor heparin therapy.[64,107,113]

Procedure and Reference Range. A standardized thrombin solution is added to citrated platelet-poor plasma. The clotting time is a measure of the rate of conversion of fibrinogen to fibrin.

Depending on the thrombin concentration selected, reported reference ranges vary widely, *e.g.*, 8 to 9 seconds,[107] 15 to 20 seconds,[15] less than 24 seconds,[137] and 20 to 25 seconds.[113]

Comments. Platelets contain platelet factor 4, which is a heparin-neutralizing substance. Therefore, the specimen must be obtained and handled carefully to avoid platelet disruption. The plasma tested must be platelet free.

TCT should not be performed on heparinized plasma samples that have been frozen.[107]

Thrombin is highly unstable. To preserve its activity, it is diluted to 100 NIH units/mL with a solution of equal parts 0.15 M NaCl and glycerol. Aliquots are then frozen. Just prior to use, an aliquot of the stock thrombin is thawed and diluted with 0.15 M NaCl to give a control value established by each laboratory. Thrombin activity decreases after 20 minutes at 37°C.

Protamine can be added to determine if the thrombin time is prolonged because of heparin or other antithrombin activity, because protamine neutralizes heparin.[107]

Some procedures utilize a thrombin–CaCl$_2$ reagent. Calcium ions enhance the rate of polymerization of fibrin monomers.[75]

Plastic or siliconized glass should be used to pipette thrombin, because it will adhere to glass surfaces.[15]

A normal control sample must be run. Control and patient plasmas are tested in duplicate (duplicates should agree within 1.5–2.0 seconds). Each laboratory must establish its own control values based on the type of thrombin, reagents, and equipment used.

HIGH DOSE THROMBIN TIME

High dose thrombin time (HiTT), a highly modified version of the thrombin time, was developed by International Technidyne Corporation (Edison, NJ) and has become a popular method for monitoring high doses of heparin, such as those given to patients undergoing cardiopulmonary bypass.[143] In such cases, the activated clotting time (ACT) becomes unreliable because it is affected by factors such as hemodilution, hyperthermia, and by dysfunctional factors. The thrombin time described earlier correlates well with low doses of heparin but becomes unreliable at high doses (*i.e.*, >1.5 U/mL). In addition, there have been reports that the HiTT is superior to the ACT and PTT for monitoring patients receiving aprotinin, a powerful antifibrinolytic given to cardiopulmonary patients to decrease bleeding.

The reagent for the HiTT is a combination of a high concentration of lyophilized thrombin (10 U/mL), reptilase snake venom (see later), protamine, and calcium. This combination will provide full clotting of fibrinogen in the presence of fibrin(ogen) degradation products and heparin. The reagent is reconstituted with water and warmed to 37°C before 1.5 mL of blood is added. The time necessary for fibrin clot formation is recorded using

TABLE 49-1
Use of Substitution Studies in Conjunction with PT, PTT, and Thrombin Time to Define Factor Defects

Deficiency	PT*	APTT†	Thrombin Time‡	Substitution Studies		
				Normal Plasma§	Adsorbed Plasma‖	Aged Serum¶
I	Abn	Abn	Abn	C	C	NC
II	Abn	Abn	Nor	C	NC	NC
V	Abn	Abn	Nor	C	C	NC
VII	Abn	Nor	Nor	C	NC	C
VIII	Nor	Abn	Nor	C	C	NC
IX	Nor	Abn	Nor	C	NC	C
X	Abn	Abn	Nor	C	NC	C
XI or XII	Nor	Abn	Nor	C	C	C
Heparin	Abn	Abn	Abn	NC	NC	NC

*Screens extrinsic pathway (I, II, V, VII, and X).
†Screens intrinsic pathway (I, II, V, VIII, IX, X, XI, and XII).
‡Identifies presence of heparin and fibrinogen abnormalities.
§Contains all factors.
‖Contains I, V, VIII, XI, XII, and XIII.
¶Contains VII, IX, X, XI, and XII.
Abn = abnormal; Nor = normal; C = corrected; NC = not corrected.

an automated clot timing device (Hemochron). Comments on the thrombin time (given earlier) also apply to this test. Reference ranges vary and should be established by each laboratory. It should be noted that this test is *not* sensitive to heparin levels below 1.5 U/mL.

REPTILASE TIME

Principle. Reptilase is a thrombin-like enzyme isolated from the reptile *Bothrops atrox*. Reptilase cleaves fibrinopeptides from the alpha chain of fibrinogen, whereas thrombin releases fibrinopeptides from both the alpha and the beta chains. Fibrin monomers formed by the action of reptilase polymerize only end to end, whereas monomers formed by thrombin polymerize both side to side and end to end. The reptilase time is not influenced by heparin or immunologic antithrombins. Fibrin(ogen) split products will prolong the reptilase time to a lesser degree than the thrombin time,[76] whereas dysfibrinogenemia will more greatly affect the reptilase time. Therefore, if both the reptilase and the thrombin time tests are performed, the cause of the prolonged thrombin time can be identified more easily[40] (Table 49-2).

Procedure and Reference Range. Reptilase is added to citrated platelet-poor plasma. The time necessary for clot formation is proportional to the amount and quality of fibrinogen present. The reference range is approximately 18 to 20 seconds.

Comments. Platelet-poor plasma is required because, like thrombin, reptilase is capable of aggregating platelets. If thrombin is present in the specimen, it may interfere with reptilase. This problem can be eliminated by adding heparin, which will inhibit thrombin but not reptilase. After reconstitution with water, reptilase is stable for 6 hours at 37°C and for 5 days at 4°C. Clotting may be observed with either manual or automated techniques. A normal plasma control is run in the same manner as for the test plasma. Reptilase times should be determined in duplicate for each specimen.

INHIBITOR STUDIES

SCREENING TESTS

Principle. Coagulation testing abnormalities may be caused by either a factor deficiency or an inhibitor. The inhibitor's action may be (1) confined to a specific factor (*e.g.*, factor VIII inhibitor); (2) nonspecific (*e.g.*, lupus anticoagulant which is anti-phospholipid); or (3) global, affecting several factors simultaneously (*e.g.*, heparin). Correction studies with normal plasma are performed to differentiate a factor deficiency from an inhibitor (Table 49-3).[42,43]

Procedure and Reference Range. Patient plasma is mixed with normal plasma, which will correct the abnormality caused by a factor deficiency. If the abnormality is secondary to the presence of an inhibitor, it will not be corrected.[27,116] Testing is performed both immediately on mixing and after incubation for 2 hours at 37°C. Testing after incubation will reveal the time and temperature dependency of the inhibitor.

Depending on the type of test system used, the reference range for the PT or PTT will differ. Each laboratory must establish its own reference range.

Comments. The specimen should be centrifuged immediately to prevent interference from platelets. The normal control plasma is treated in the same manner as the patient specimen. For the control, fresh pooled normal plasma or healthy donor plasma is mixed 1:1 with Owren's veronal buffer and is incubated at 37°C. Additional controls may include undiluted patient plasma and undiluted pooled normal plasma that are treated in the same way as the patient mixture. Depending on the system to be tested, PT or PTT reagents will be necessary.

The interpretation of this test is based on the correction, if any, of the abnormal test time (Table 49-3). If the abnormality is attributable to a factor deficiency, the addition of one part normal plasma will correct the abnormal test time close to the normal range. If the abnormality is secondary to an immediate-acting inhibitor (*e.g.*, factor IX inhibitor, heparin), the addition of normal plasma will not correct the abnormal test time. If, however, the inhibitor is time or temperature dependent (*e.g.*, factor VIII inhibitor) an immediate correction will be noted, but on incubation, the test time will become prolonged if the inhibitor titer is high enough. Lupus anticoagulants generally are immediate acting but may be time dependent.[138] Equivocal results may be obtained in borderline or mild abnormalities.[82] If an inhibitor is indicated, a more sensitive and specific test should be performed to identify and quantify it.

INHIBITOR IDENTIFICATION AND QUANTITATION

As a special type of circulating anticoagulant or inhibitor, the lupus anticoagulant is an antibody which reacts with complexes of phospholipid and one or more cofactors (*e.g.*, prothrombin or β_2-glycoprotein). Although the inhibitor was first identified in patients with systemic lupus erythematosus (SLE), it has since been found in a wide variety of autoimmune conditions, and not all patients with SLE have the inhibitor.

Laboratory methods to screen for the lupus anticoagulant include tissue thromboplastin inhibition test (TTIT), dilute Russell's viper venom time (dRVVT), platelet neu-

---

TABLE 49-2
Comparison of Thrombin Times and Reptilase Times in Various Conditions

	Thrombin Time	Reptilase Time
Heparin therapy	Prolonged	Normal
Fibrin split products	Greatly prolonged	Prolonged
Hypofibrinogenemia	Prolonged	Prolonged
Dysfibrinogenemia	Prolonged	Greatly prolonged
Immunologic antithrombins	Prolonged	Normal

TABLE 49-3
Interpretation in Correction Studies Using Normal Plasma

	Immediate Testing	Testing After 2-Hour Incubation at 37°C
Factor Deficiency	Correction	Correction
Inhibitor		
Immediate acting (*e.g.*, heparin, factor IX inhibitor, most lupus anticoagulants)	No correction	No correction
Time dependent (*e.g.*, factor VIII inhibitor)	Correction	No correction

tralization test, agarose plasma gel test, and the textarin-to-ecarin ratio. In an attempt to find an assay that does not depend on clotting, an ELISA method using cardiolipin phospholipid in the immobile phase has been developed.[47] However, it was soon discovered that patients with the lupus anticoagulant are a heterogeneous group in that not all tests would necessarily be positive for any one patient. This implies that there may be several subgroups of antiphospholipid antibodies including the anti-cardiolipin antibodies. Specific factor inhibitors, such as factor VIII inhibitor, may be quantitated by the agarose inhibitor plasma gel technique or, more commonly, the Bethesda inhibitor assay.

TISSUE THROMBOPLASTIN INHIBITION TEST

The TTIT is a modified clotting test.[124] Citrated plasma is incubated at 37°C with dilute thromboplastin. CaCl₂ is added, and the clotting time is measured. The results are expressed as a ratio of the clotting time (in seconds) of the patient sample to that of the control sample. The TTIT is considered normal if this ratio is 1:1 or less; borderline if 1:2 to 1:3; and abnormal if it is greater than 1:3. Despite its popularity, the TTIT is neither sensitive nor specific.[139]

DILUTE RUSSELL'S VIPER VENOM TIME

The dRVVT[33] is a modification of the TTIT test using a reagent that will directly activate factor X and not be affected by several factor deficiencies (*e.g.*, factors XII, XI, VIII, or VII).

The reagent consists of dilute Russell's viper venom (approximately 1:2000 dilution), calcium, and phospholipid. Equal volumes of warmed reagent and platelet-poor citrated plasma are mixed and the time necessary for clot formation is measured. Results are reported as a ratio of the patient's clotting time to that of a normal control. Normally, the ratio should be less than 1.2. A deficiency of factors II, V, or X can be ruled out if a mixture of patient and normal plasma does not correct the ratio.

PLATELET NEUTRALIZATION PROCEDURE

In the platelet neutralization procedure, freeze-thawed platelets are added to the test plasma, and an PTT is performed. The platelets serve as an additional source of phospholipid and "neutralize" lupus anticoagulant. A significant shortening of the abnormal PTT is indicative of lupus anticoagulant.[139]

AGAROSE PLASMA GEL TECHNIQUE

Agarose containing fresh normal plasma is poured on a plate. Patient and control plasmas are placed in wells cut into the agar and allowed to diffuse into the gel. After incubation, the plate is flooded with CaCl₂ solution. The agarose will turn cloudy or opaque as fibrin is formed in the agarose. In the presence of an inhibitor, a clear area or zone of inhibition will be seen surrounding the well containing that plasma.[9,136]

TEXTARIN-TO-ECARIN RATIO

Triplett and associates[140] have recently proposed the use of two snake venoms as a sensitive and specific confirmatory test for the lupus anticoagulant. Textarin from the Australian eastern brown snake activates prothrombin in the presence of phospholipid, factor V, and calcium ions. Ecarin, a protein fraction of *Echis carinatus* venom, activates prothrombin in the absence of any cofactors. Therefore, in the presence of the lupus anticoagulant, the textarin time is prolonged and the ecarin time is unaffected. Test results are reported as a ratio of T/E. Normally, this ratio should be below 1.3. This test has since been evaluated by others and found to be highly sensitive for lupus anticoagulant.[35]

BETHESDA INHIBITOR ASSAY

Factor VIII inhibitor can be quantitated by mixing test plasma with a known amount of factor VIII and incubating the mixture for 2 hours at 37°C. After incubation, the amount of residual factor VIII is measured by specific factor assay (see following). By comparing the factor VIII activity in the patient incubation mixture with that in the control mixture, the amount of inhibitor present in the former can be calculated. The result is expressed in Bethesda units; one Bethesda unit of inhibitor is defined as the amount that will inactivate 50% of the factor VIII activity present.[67]

FACTOR ASSAYS

Currently, a variety of methods are in use for the measurement of factor activity, including one-stage clotting methods,[46,74] two-stage clotting methods,[8] fluorometric methods,[88] and colorimetric methods.[31,127] The fluorometric and colorimetric methodologies are based on the principles that govern synthetic substrates. The one-stage clotting method is widely used because of its simplicity.[6]

ONE-STAGE CLOTTING ASSAYS

Principle. One-stage factor assays are based on a simple modification of the PT or PTT. Assays for factors II, V, VII, and X generally are based on the PT, whereas assays for factors VIII, IX, XI, and XII are based on the PTT.

Procedure and Reference Range. The clotting time of a substrate plasma known to be deficient in the factor to be assayed is shortened or "corrected" by adding diluted factor-containing plasma. By using various dilutions of a known normal plasma or standard, a curve is constructed (Figs. 49-3 and 49-4). Unknown sample values are derived by using an appropriate dilution and converting the clotting time to factor activity from the standard curve.

The reference range for most factors is 50% to 150% of normal activity.

Comments. Because of the length of this procedure, the citrated platelet-poor plasma obtained from the patient and subsequent dilutions should be kept on slush ice. Plasma should be tested within 1 to 2 hours and dilutions within 30 minutes. Frozen plasma may be used provided the standard liquid reference plasma has likewise been frozen.

Normal reference plasma and factor-deficient plasma may be obtained commercially in lyophilized form. Care should be taken to ensure the accuracy of the stated values.

Known controls should be run simultaneously with the unknown samples. Other quality control measures should parallel those used in PT or PTT testing.

Only the linear portion of the calibration curve should be used. The curve may become flat at the most extreme dilutions if sensitivity is lost. Only a high-quality standard with an accurate value and a high-quality substrate should be used. The following is an example of the calculations for normal and abnormal plasmas using the curve shown in Figure 49-4.

	Dilution*	Clotting Time (seconds)	% Activity From Curve	% Activity Corrected for Dilution
Normal subject	1:10	46	74	74
	1:20	52.5	37	74
Factor-deficient	1:10	68	10	10
Patient	1:20	78	5	10

*Assume 1:10 dilution defines 100% of normal factor assay.

FACTOR VIII IMMUNOLOGIC ASSAYS

In addition to the functional factor assays discussed above, immunologic methods have been developed. Perhaps the coagulation protein most widely studied using immunologic methods is factor VIII-related antigen (factor VIIIC:Ag), which will measure both normal and abnormal factor VIII. The methodologies employed in quantitative immunologic assay of this factor include the Laurell rocket technique or rocket electroimmunodiffusion (EID),[78,150] the immunoradiometric assay (IRMA),[24,106,118] and the ELISA.[126] Crossed immunoelectrophoresis and SDS-polyacrylamide gel methods[59,117] are used to characterize qualitative abnormalities of the molecule. The Laurell rocket technique is the most convenient and popular method for the routine laboratory.[12]

RISTOCETIN COFACTOR

In addition to determining the antigenic level of factor VIIIC:Ag, it is highly recommended that the functional properties of the von Willebrand factor (vWF, VIII/vWF,

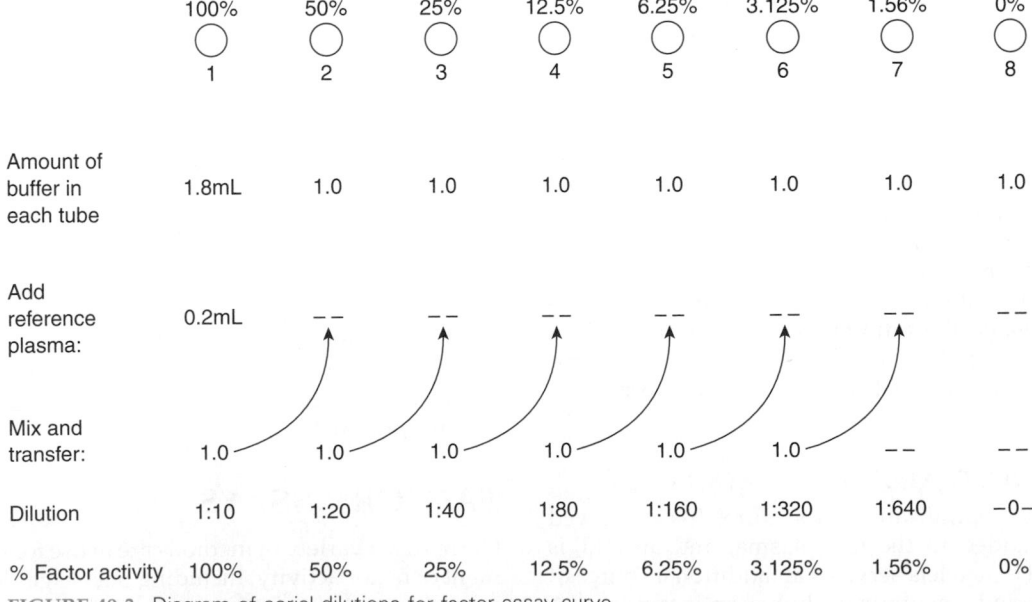

For 8 point factor assay curve, set up eight 12 x 75 tubes and label as indicated:

	100%	50%	25%	12.5%	6.25%	3.125%	1.56%	0%
	1	2	3	4	5	6	7	8
Amount of buffer in each tube	1.8mL	1.0	1.0	1.0	1.0	1.0	1.0	1.0
Add reference plasma:	0.2mL	--	--	--	--	--	--	--
Mix and transfer:	1.0	1.0	1.0	1.0	1.0	1.0	--	--
Dilution	1:10	1:20	1:40	1:80	1:160	1:320	1:640	-0-
% Factor activity	100%	50%	25%	12.5%	6.25%	3.125%	1.56%	0%

FIGURE 49-3. Diagram of serial dilutions for factor assay curve.

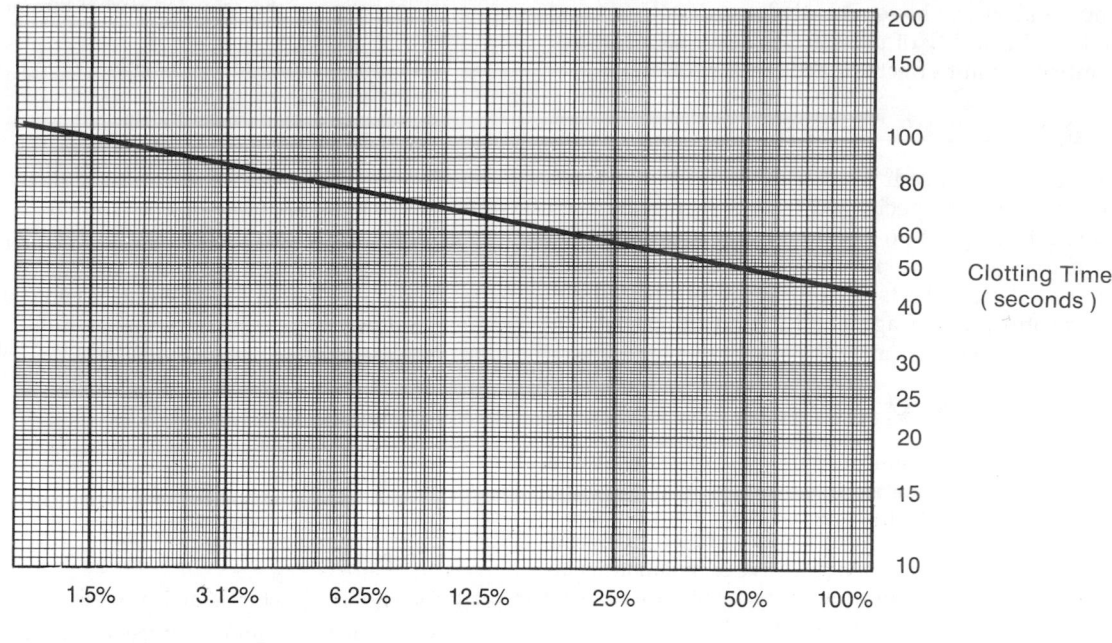

FIGURE 49-4. Sample factor activity curve based on dilutions of normal or standard plasma.

vWF:Ag, vWF:RCoF [ristocetin cofactor]; see Table 52-1) be assayed.[11,57] The vWF:RCoF assay is described in Chapter 56.

FLETCHER FACTOR

Fletcher factor (prekallikrein) participates in the contact phase of the intrinsic system (see Fig. 48-1) and was first described by Hathaway and associates in 1965.[48] Laboratory detection of prekallikrein deficiency is initially made by a simple screening test in which the prolonged PTT is corrected by additional incubation with an activator such as Celite or kaolin.[48] Partial thromboplastins containing ellagic acid as an activator *do not* usually detect this deficiency.[29] Fletcher factor deficiency is confirmed by a quantitative assay using a modified PTT technique and factor-deficient substrate or a synthetic substrate.[34]

REGULATORY PROTEIN ASSAYS

ANTITHROMBIN III

Antithrombin III (AT-III), which together with heparin will inactivate many activated serine proteases, may be assayed by either immunologic or functional methods. Immunologic assays commonly used include RIA,[18] RID,[86] and Laurell rocket immunoelectrophoresis.[78] Immunologic methods do not distinguish free-circulating AT-III from that which is complexed and inactive. The results are expressed in milligrams per deciliter. Normal plasma contains between 20 and 50 mg/dL of AT-III, depending on the assay.

Functional assays for AT-III activity may be performed by a clotting technique[20] or by employing synthetic substrates.[1,99] Functional assays are based on the fact that AT-III inhibits activated serine proteases. Exogenous heparin is added to the plasma to accelerate the action of AT-III. Thrombin or factor Xa is added in excess to the plasma. The amount of thrombin or factor Xa not inactivated by AT-III is quantitated by a clotting time or color formation (spectrophotometric). Functional values are expressed as a percentage of normal. Reference values should be established by each laboratory but should lie between 80% and 120% of normal activity.

PROTEIN C

Protein C plays a role in the fibrinolytic and coagulation systems as a regulatory protein and may be assayed immunologically and functionally.[45] Immunologic methods for protein C measurement involve the Laurell rocket immunoelectrophoresis technique,[44] RIA techniques,[30] or ELISA methodology.[13,146] Normal plasma contains approximately 3 to 4 μg of protein C per milliliter. Only recently have functional assays become available.[22,37,100,121] A relatively simple automated clot-based method for assaying the functional activity of protein C has been described by Odegard and associates.[100]

PROTEIN S

Protein S, which functions as a cofactor for activated protein C, may likewise be measured immunologically or functionally. Protein S determinations are complicated by the fact that it circulates both as a free protein and in a reversible complex with C4b-binding protein.[25] Protein S levels have been measured by Laurell rocket immunoelectrophoresis.[22] The reference level is approximately 1 μg/

mL. Functional assays have recently been developed and are based on the ability of protein S to serve as a cofactor for the anticoagulant effects of activated protein C.[23]

OTHER SPECIAL TESTS

In addition to the procedures discussed in this chapter, there are many other specialized tests that may be used to evaluate the coagulation system. There are several tests often used to evaluate the fibrinolytic or degradation aspects of coagulation. Tests including protamine sulfate, D-dimer, prothrombin fragment 1.2, and others will be discussed in Chapters 50 and 51.

CHAPTER SUMMARY

In this chapter, the development of the procedures used routinely in coagulation testing is discussed. General procedures are described including their reference ranges, the significance of abnormal results, and potential sources of error. Utilizing these procedures, general screening for basic coagulation abnormalities may be performed. In addition, many of these tests are suitable for monitoring anticoagulant therapy.

This chapter also focuses on specialized procedures performed in the coagulation laboratory that play a vital role in the assessment of the patient with a bleeding disorder. The methodologies employed by these tests are diverse.

Case Study 49-1

A coagulation panel was ordered on a 64-year-old man before coronary bypass surgery. The surgeon was concerned about an abnormal PTT result. The patient had a negative history of any bleeding or bruising tendency and denied any family history of bleeding disorders. The laboratory parameters on this patient were as follows: WBC 7.8×10^9/L; RBC 6.92×10^{12}/L; Hb 20.4 g/dL; Hct 0.62 L/L; PLT 335×10^9/L; PT 11.2 seconds; INR 1.05; PTT 58.4 seconds.

1. In addition to the elevated PTT, other test parameters in this panel are abnormal. What are they?
2. What steps should be taken to evaluate the abnormal PTT?
3. In light of the abnormalities, what is the probable cause of the spurious abnormal PTT in this patient?

Case Study 49-2

A 35-year-old female was referred to a hematologist for the evaluation of an abnormal PTT. All other laboratory tests, including WBC, RBC, Hb, Hct, PLT, PT, fibrinogen, and bleeding time were all within reference ranges. The patient had a negative history for bleeding or bruising problems. The original PTT was 72.4 seconds; a repeat PTT was 69.8 seconds (done in different laboratory).

1. Is a spuriously abnormal PTT suggested here?
2. What test(s) should be done to evaluate this abnormality?
3. What additional test(s) could be used to evaluate this patient?

Review Questions

For questions 49-1 and 49-2, choose your answer from the following:

A. 1 and 3 are correct
B. 2 and 4 are correct
C. 1, 2 and 3 are correct
D. only 4 is correct
E. all are correct

49-1. Prolongation of the activated partial thromboplastin time test may suggest

1. improper blood-to-anticoagulant ratio in the original specimen.
2. presence of heparin in the specimen.
3. a lupus inhibitor.
4. a deficiency of factor VII or factor XIII.

49-2. The prothrombin time test

1. is the most frequently used test to monitor anticoagulant therapy with vitamin K antagonists.
2. is a good screen for the intrinsic and common pathways.
3. is performed on citrated platelet-poor plasma.
4. is reported as a percentage of factor activity.

49-3. The thrombin time test will be prolonged by all of the following **EXCEPT**

A. dysfibrinogenemia.
B. fibrin split products.
C. elevated fibrinogen levels.
D. heparin.

49-4. The one-stage factor assay is used to

A. quantitate the amount of factor VIII inhibitor present.
B. measure the presence of heparin.
C. quantitate the amount of one specific coagulation factor.
D. measure antithrombin III.

49-5. Coagulation inhibitors against specific factors are best detected by

A. platelet neutralization test.
B. dilute thromboplastin inhibition test.
C. mixing studies using adsorbed plasma and serum.
D. Bethesda inhibitor assay.

References

1. Abildgaard U, Lie M, Odegard OR: Antithrombin (heparin cofactor) assay with "new" chromogenic substrates (S-2238 and Chromozym TH). Thromb Res 11:549, 1977
2. Babson AL, Opper CA, Crane LJ: Kinetic latex agglutinometry I: A rapid quantitative immunologic assay for fibrinogen. Am J Clin Pathol 77:424, 1982
3. de Bainville HMD: Injection de mati⟨age⟩re c⟨ae⟩r⟨aae⟩brale dans les veines. Gaz Med Paris 2:524, 1834
4. Barbui T, Rodeghiero F, Dini E et al: Subunits A and S inheritance in four families with congenital factor XIII deficiency. Br J Haematol 38:267, 1978
5. Brandt J: Principles of Coagulation—1982: Symposium sponsored by General Diagnostics Corporation, Lexington, KY, 1982
6. Barrowcliffe TW, Ingram GIC, Kirkwood TBL et al: A survey of VIII:C assays in the United Kingdom. Clin Lab Haematol 3:186, 1981
7. Biggs R, Douglas AS: The thromboplastin generation test. J Clin Pathol 6:23, 1953
8. Biggs R, Eveling J, Richards G: The assay of antihaemophilic-globulin activity. Br J Haematol 1:20, 1955
9. Bird P: Coagulation in an agarose gel and its application to the detection and measurement of factor VIII antibodies. Br J Haematol 29:329, 1975
10. Bithell TC: Hereditary dysfibrinogenemia. Clin Chem 31:509, 1985
11. Bouma BN, Wiegerinck Y, Sixma JJ et al: Immunological characterization of purified anti-haemophilic factor A (factor VIII) which corrects abnormal platelet retention in von Willebrand's disease. Nature 236:104, 1972

12. Bowie EJW, Owen CA: Abnormalities of factor VIII. In Triplett DA (ed): Laboratory Evaluation of Coagulation, p 115. Chicago, American Society of Clinical Pathologists, 1982

13. Boyer C, Rothschild C, Wolf M et al: A new method for the estimation of protein C by ELISA. Thromb Res 36:579, 1984

14. Brittin GM, Rafinia H, Raval D et al: Evaluation of single radial immunodiffusion for quantitation of plasma fibrinogen. Am J Clin Pathol 57:89, 1972

15. Brown B: Hematology: Principles and Procedures, 4th ed, p 202. Philadelphia, Lea & Febiger, 1984

16. Cann JR: A phenomenological theory of rocket and crossed immunoelectrophoresis. Immunochemistry 12:473, 1975

17. Carteaux JP, Gast A, Tschopp TB: Activated clotting time as an appropriate test to compare heparin and direct thrombin inhibitors such as hirudin or RO 46-6240 in experimental arterial thrombosis. Circulation 9:1568, 1995

18. Chan V, Chan TK, Wong V et al: The determination of antithrombin III by radioimmunoassay and its clinical application. Br J Haematol 41:563, 1979

19. Chen T, Lai CH: Fibrinogen assay by an immunodiffusion plate. Tech Bull Reg Med Technol 39(10):231, 1969

20. Chockly M, Penner J: An improved clinical assay for antithrombin III (heparin cofactor). Am J Clin Pathol 74:213, 1980

21. Clauss A: Gerinnungsphysiologische Schnellmethode zur Bestimmung des Fibrinogens. Acta Haematol (Basel) 17:237, 1957

22. Comp PC, Nixon RR, Cooper MR et al: Familial protein S deficiency is associated with recurrent thrombosis. J Clin Invest 74:2082, 1984

23. Comp PC, Nixon RR, Esmon CT: Determination of functional levels of protein C, an antithrombic protein, using thrombin-thrombomodulin complex. Blood 63:15, 1984

24. Counts RB: A solid-phase immunoradiometric assay of factor VIII protein. Br J Haematol 31:429, 1975

25. Dahlback B, Stenflow J: High molecular weight complex in human plasma between vitamin K-dependent protein S and complement component C4-binding protein. Proc Natl Acad Sci USA 78:2512, 1981

26. Davie EW, Ratnoff OD: Waterfall sequence for intrinsic blood clotting. Science 145:1310, 1964

27. Deutsch E, Lechner K: Circulating anticoagulants. In Bang NU, Beller FK, Deutsch E et al (eds): Thrombosis and Bleeding Disorders: Theory and Methods, p 286. New York, Academic Press, 1971

28. Ellis BC, Stransky A: A quick and accurate method for the determination of fibrinogen in plasma. J Lab Clin Med 58:477, 1961

29. Entes K, LaDuca FM, Tourbaf KD: Fletcher factor deficiency, source of variations of the activated partial thromboplastin time test. Am J Clin Pathol 75:626, 1981

30. Epstein DJ, Bergum PW, Bajaj SP et al: Radioimmunoassays for protein C and factor X. Am J Clin Pathol 82:573, 1984

31. Eriksson E, Rosen S, Knos M et al: Chromogenic substrate methods for the determination of factor VIII C, endotoxin and plasminogen activator (abstract). Thromb Haemost 46:315, 1981

32. Exner T, Burridge J, Power P et al: An evaluation of currently available methods for plasma fibrinogen. Am J Clin Pathol 71:521, 1979

33. Exner T, Papadopoulos G, Koutts J: Use of a simplified dilute Russell's viper venom time (dRVVT) confirms the heterogeneity among "lupus anticoagulants." Blood Coag Fibrinol 1:259, 1990

34. Fisher CA, Schmaier AH, Addonizio VP et al: Assay of prekallikrein in human plasma: Comparison of amidolytic, esterolytic, coagulation, and immunochemical assays. Blood 59:963, 1982

35. Forastiero RR, Cerrato GS, Carreras LO: Evaluation of recently described test for detection of the lupus anticoagulant. Thromb Haemost 72:728, 1994

36. Forbes CD, Douglas AS: Thrombin and thromboplastin generation techniques. In Bang NU, Beller FK, Deutsch E et al (eds): Thrombosis and Bleeding Disorders: Theory and Methods, p 82. New York, Academic Press, 1971

37. Francis RB, Patch MJ: A functional assay for protein C in human plasma. Thromb Res 32:605, 1983

38. Friberger P: Chromogenic peptide substrates: Their use for the assay of factors in the fibrinolytic and plasma kallikrein-kinin systems. Scand J Clin Lab Invest 42(suppl 162), 1982

39. Fudenberg HH, Stites DP, Caldwell JL et al (eds): Basic and Clinical Immunology, 2nd ed, p 337. Los Altos, CA, Lange Medical Publications, 1978

40. Funk C, Gmur J, Herold R et al: Reptilase-R: A new reagent in blood coagulation. Br J Haematol 21:43, 1971

41. Garvey JS, Cremer NE, Sussdorf DH (eds): Methods in Immunology: A Laboratory Text for Instruction and Research, 3rd ed, p 301. Reading, MA, WA Benjamin, 1977

42. Giddings JC: Hereditary coagulation disorders: Laboratory techniques. In Thomson JM (ed): Blood Coagulation and Haemostasis: A Practical Guide, 2nd ed, p 117. Edinburgh, Churchill Livingstone, 1980

43. Giddings JC: The investigation of hereditary coagulation disorders. In Thomson JM (ed): Blood Coagulation and Haemostasis: A Practical Guide, 2nd ed, p 48. Edinburgh, Churchill Livingstone, 1980

44. Goodwin JF: An evaluation of turbidimetric techniques for estimation of plasma fibrinogen. Clin Chem 13:1057, 1967

45. Griffin JH, Evatt B, Zimmerman TS et al: Deficiency of protein C in congenital thrombotic disease. J Clin Invest 68:1370, 1981

46. Hardisty RM, Macpherson JC: A one-stage factor VIII (anti-haemophilic globulin) assay and its use on venous and capillary plasma. Thromb Diath Haemorrh 7:215, 1962

47. Harris EN, Gharavi AE, Boey ML: Anticardiolipin antibodies: Detection by radioimmunoassay and association with thrombosis in lupus erythematosus. Lancet 2:1211, 1983

48. Hathaway WE, Belhasen LP, Hathaway HS: Evidence for a new plasma thromboplastin factor: I. Case report, coagulation studies and physiochemical properties. Blood 26:521, 1965

49. Hattersley P: Activated coagulation time of whole blood. JAMA 196:436, 1966

50. Hattersley P: Progress report: The activated coagulation time of whole blood (ACT). Am J Clin Pathol 66:899, 1976

51. Hemker HC: Handbook of Synthetic Substrates for the Coagulation and Fibrinolytic System. Boston, Martinus Nijhoff, 1983

52. Hicks ND, Pitney WR: A rapid screening test for disorders of thromboplastin generation. Br J Haematol 3:227, 1957

53. Hill J: A simple method of heparin management during extracorporeal circulation. Ann Thorac Surg 17:129, 1974

54. Hirsh J, Poller L: The International Normalized Ratio. A guide to understanding and correcting its problems. Arch Intern Med 154(Feb 14):282, 1994

55. Hougie C: Recalcification time test and its modifications (partial thromboplastin time, activated partial thromboplastin time and expanded partial thromboplastin time). In Williams WJ, Beutler E, Erslev A et al (eds): Hematology, 3rd ed, p 1662. New York, McGraw-Hill, 1983

56. Hougie C: One stage prothrombin time. In Williams WJ, Beutler E, Erslev AJ et al (eds): Hematology, 3rd ed, p 1665. New York, McGraw-Hill, 1983

57. Howard MA, Firkin BG: Ristocetin—A new tool in the investigation of platelet aggregation. Thromb Diath Haemorrh 26:362, 1971

58. Howard MA, Sawers RJ, Firkin BG: Ristocetin: A means of differentiating von Willebrand's disease into two groups. Blood 41:687, 1973

59. Hoyer LW, Shainoff JR: Factor VIII-related protein circulates in normal human plasma as high molecular weight multimers. Blood 55:1056, 1980

60. Huseby RM, Bang NU: Fibrinogen. In Bang NU, Beller FK, Deutsch E et al (eds): Thrombosis and Bleeding Disorders: Theory and Methods, p 222. New York, Academic Press, 1971

61. Inada Y, Okamoto H, Kanai S et al: Faster determination of clottable fibrinogen in human plasma: An improved method and kinetic study. Clin Chem 24:351, 1978

62. Jackson CM, Nemerson Y: Blood coagulation. Ann Rev Biochem 49:765, 1980

63. Jespersen J, Sidelmann J: A study of the conditions and accuracy of the thrombin time assay of plasma fibrinogen. Acta Haematol (Basel) 67:2, 1982

64. Jim RTS: A study of the plasma thrombin time. J Lab Clin Med 50:45, 1957

65. Jolgren VR, Triplett DA: Immunologic methods in the coagulation laboratory. ASCP Check Sample, Thrombosis and Hemostasis, TH 80-4 (TH-10). Chicago, American Society of Clinical Pathologists, 1980

66. Kahan J: Regional quality control of coagulation assay procedures. Thromb Diath Haemorrh 32:79, 1974

67. Kasper CK, Aledort LM, Counts RB et al: A more uniform measurement of factor VIII inhibitors. Thromb Diath Haemorrh 34:869, 1975

68. Keyser JW: Control of anticoagulant therapy by Thrombotest method. Br Med J 2:1514, 1963

69. Koepke JA, Gilmer PR, Filip DJ et al: Studies of fibrinogen measurement in the CAP survey program. Am J Clin Pathol 63:984, 1975

70. Korsan-Bengsten K: Routine tests as measures of the total intrinsic blood clotting potential. Scand J Haematol 8:359, 1971

71. Korsan-Bengsten K: Comparison of Thrombotest and simplastin A (a modified P&P test) in the detection of prolonged clotting times of whole blood and plasma during anticoagulant therapy. Scand J Haematol 8:369, 1971

72. Laki K, Lorand L: On the solubility of fibrin clots. Science 108:280, 1948

73. Langdell RD: Coagulation and hemostasis. In Davidsohn I, Henry JB (ed): Clinical Diagnosis by Laboratory Methods, 15th ed, p 414. New York, WB Saunders, 1974

74. Langdell RD, Wagner RH, Brinkhous KM: Effect of antihemophilic factor on one-stage clotting tests: A presumptive test for hemophilia and a simple one-stage antihemophilic factor assay procedure. J Lab Clin Med 41:637, 1953

75. Latallo ZS: Thrombin clotting assays. In Bang NU, Beller FK, Deutsch E et al (eds): Thrombosis and Bleeding Disorders: Theory and Methods, p 183. New York, Academic Press, 1971

76. Latallo ZS, Teisseyre E: Evaluation of Reptilase R and thrombin clotting time in the presence of fibrinogen degradation products and heparin. Scand J Haematol 13:261, 1971

77. Laurell CB: Antigen-antibody crossed electrophoresis. Ann Biochem 10:358, 1965

78. Laurell CB: Quantitative estimation of proteins by electrophoresis in agarose gel containing antibodies. Ann Biochem 15:45, 1966

79. Laurell CB: Electroimmunoassay. Scand J Clin Lab Invest 29(suppl 124):21, 1972

80. Le DT, Weibert RT, Sevilla BK et al: The International Normalized Ratio (INR) for monitoring Warfarin therapy: Reliability and relation to other monitoring methods. Ann Intern Med 120(7);552, 1994

81. Lee RI, White PD: A clinical study of the coagulation time of blood. Am J Med Sci 145:495, 1913

82. Lenahan JG, Smith K: Hemostasis, 18th ed. Durham, NC, Organon Teknika, 1986

83. Loeliger EA: Reliability of laboratory tests for the control of oral anticoagulation. Thromb Diath Haemorrh 32:483, 1974

84. Loeliger EA, van den Besselaar AMHP: Introduction. In van den Besselaar AMHP, Gralnick HR, Lewis SM (eds): Thromboplastin Calibration and Oral Anticoagulant Control, p 1. The Hague, Martinus Nijhoff, 1984

85. MacFarlane RG: The theory of blood coagulation. In Biggs R (ed): Human Blood Coagulation, Haemostasis and Thrombosis, 2nd ed, p 1. Oxford, Blackwell Scientific, 1976

86. Mancini G, Carbonara AO, Heremans JF: Immunochemical quantitation of antigens by single radial immunodiffusion. Immunochem 2:235, 1965

87. Marlar RA, Bayer PJ, Endres-Brooks JL et al: Comparison of the sensitivity of commercial PTT reagents in the detection of mild coagulopathies. Am J Clin Pathol 82:436, 1984

88. Mitchell GA, Abdullahad CM, Ruiz JA et al: Fluorogenic substrate assays for factors VIII and IX: Introduction of a new solid phase fluorescent detection method. Thromb Res 21:573, 1981

89. Morawitz P: Die Chemie der Blutgerinnung. Ergebn Physiol Biol Chem Exp Pharmakol 4:307, 1905

90. Morse EE, Panek S, Menga R: Automated fibrinogen determination. Am J Clin Pathol 55:671, 1971

91. Morse EE, Panek S, Pisciotto P et al: Reemergence of the international normalized ratio for the standardization of prothrombin time. Ann Clin Lab Sci 23:184, 1993

92. Natelson EA, Dooley DF: Rapid determination of fibrinogen by thrombokinetics. Am J Clin Pathol 61:828, 1974

93. National Committee for Clinical Laboratory Standards: Activated Partial Thromboplastin Time Test (APTT); Tentative Guideline, vol 12(23). Villanova, PA, NCCLS, 1992

94. National Committee for Clinical Laboratory Standards (NCCLS): Collection, Transport and Preparation of Blood Specimens for Coagulation Testing and Performance of Coagulation Assays, 2nd ed. H21-A2 vol 11(23). Villanova, PA, NCCLS, 1991

95. National Committee for Clinical Laboratory Standards: One-Stage Prothrombin Time Test (PT); Tentative Guideline, vol 12(22). Villanova, PA, NCCLS, 1992

96. National Committee for Clinical Laboratory Standards: Procedure for the Determination of Fibrinogen in Plasma, vol 14(2):3–7. Villanova, PA, NCCLS, 1994

97. Noureddin SN: Research review: Use of activated clotting times to monitor heparin therapy in coronary patients. Am J Crit Care 4:272, 1995

98. Nussbaum M, Morse B: Plasma fibrin stabilizing factor activity in various diseases. Blood 23:669, 1964

99. Odegard OR, Lie M, Abildgaard U: Heparin cofactor activity measured with an amidolytic method. Thromb Res 6:287, 1975

100. Odegard OR, Try K, Abildgaard U: Protein C: A simplified-automated activity assay. Thromb Res 42:257, 1986

101. O'Sullivan MJ, Bridges JW, Marks V: Enzyme immunoassay: A review. Ann Clin Biochem 16:221, 1979

102. Owren PA: The prothrombin activating complex and its clinical significance. In Report of 3rd International Congress of Hematology, p 379. New York, Grune & Stratton, 1950

103. Owren PA: Standardization of thromboplastin reagents and control plasmas. Haematologia (Budapest) 8:441, 1974

104. Owren PA, Aas K: The control of Dicumarol therapy and the quantitative determination of prothrombin and proconvertin. Scand J Clin Lab Invest 3:201, 1951

105. Owen CA, Thompson JH: Soybean phosphatides in pro-

thrombin-consumption and thromboplastin-generation tests: Their use in recognizing "thrombasthenic hemophilia." Am J Clin Pathol 33:197, 1960

106. Peake IR, Bloom AL: The use of an immunoradiometric assay for factor VIII related antigen in the study of atypical von Willebrand's disease. Thromb Res 10:27, 1977

107. Penner JA: Experience with a thrombin clotting time assay for measuring heparin activity. Am J Clin Pathol 61:645, 1974

108. Platt WR: Laboratory diagnosis of coagulation defects. In: Color Atlas and Textbook of Hematology, p 222. Philadelphia, JB Lippincott, 1969

109. Poller L, Thomson JM, Alderson MR: The British system for anticoagulant control and Thrombotest. J Clin Pathol 24:143, 1971

110. Quick AJ, Favre-Gilly J: The prothrombin consumption test: Its clinical and theoretic implications. Blood 4:1281, 1949

111. Quick AJ, Hussey CV, Geppert M: Prothrombin: Analytical and clinical aspects. Comparison of the one- and two-stage methods. Am J Med Sci 1:517, 1963

112. Quick AJ, Stanley-Brown M, Bancroft W: Study of coagulation defects in hemophilia and jaundice. Am J Med Sci 190:501, 1935

113. Rapaport SI, Ames SB: Clotting factor assays on plasma from patients receiving intramuscular injections of subcutaneous heparin. Am J Med Sci 234:678, 1957

114. Ratnoff OD, Menzie AB: A new method for the determination of fibrinogen in small samples of plasma. J Lab Clin Med 37:316, 1951

115. Ratnoff OD, Saito H: Surface mediated reactions. Curr Top Hematol 2:1, 1979

116. Rodman NF Jr, Barrow EM, Graham JB: Diagnosis and control of the hemophilioid states with the partial thromboplastin time (PTT) test. Am J Clin Pathol 29:525, 1958

117. Ruggeri ZM, Zimmerman TS: Variant von Willebrand's disease: Characterization of two subtypes by analysis of multimeric composition of factor VIII/von Willebrand factor in plasma and platelets. J Clin Invest 65:1318, 1980

118. Ruggeri ZM, Mannucci PM, Jeffcoate SL et al: Immunoradiometric assay of factor VIII related antigen with observations in 32 patients with von Willebrand's disease. Br J Haematol 33:221, 1976

119. Sabbatini L: Le calcium-ion dans le coagulation du sang. C R Soc Biol (Paris) 54:716, 1902

120. Sabo MG: Coagulation instrumentation and reagent systems. In Triplett DA (ed): Laboratory Evaluation of Coagulation, p 315. Chicago, American Society of Clinical Pathologists, 1982

121. Sala N, Owen WG, Collen D: A functional assay of protein C in human plasma. Blood 63:671, 1984

122. Saleem A, Fretz K, Krieg AF: Comparison of three methods for plasma fibrinogen. Ann Clin Lab Sci 6:65, 1976

123. Saleem A, Krieg AF, Fretz K: Improved micromethod for plasma fibrinogen unaffected by heparin therapy. Am J Clin Pathol 63:426, 1975

124. Schleider MA, Nachman RL, Jaffe EA et al: A clinical study of the lupus anticoagulant. Blood 48:499, 1976

125. Schroer H: Assay for prothrombin. In Bang NU, Beller FK, Deutsch E et al (eds): Thrombosis and Bleeding Disorders: Theory and Methods, p 175. New York, Academic Press, 1971

126. Schuurs AH: Enzyme-immunoassay. A powerful analytical tool. J Immunol 1:229, 1980

127. Seghatchian MJ, Miller-Andersson M: A colorimetric evaluation of factor VIII:C potency. Med Lab Sci 35:347, 1978

128. Shaw ST: Assays for fibrinogen and its derivatives. CRC Crit Rev Clin Lab Sci 8:145, 1977

129. Shulman NR: Prothrombin consumption tests. In Bang NU, Beller FK, Deutsch E et al (eds): Thrombosis and Bleeding Disorders: Theory and Methods, p 79. New York, Academic Press, 1971

130. Siefring GE, Riabov DK, Wehrly JA: Development and analytical performance of a functional assay for fibrinogen on the DuPont aca analyzer. Clin Chem 29:614, 1983

131. Tan V, Doyle CJ, Budzynski AZ: Comparison of kinetic fibrinogen assay with the vonClauss method and the clot recovery method in plasma of patients with conditions affecting fibrinogen coagulability. Am J Clin Pathol 104:455, 1995

132. Telfer TP, Denson KWE, Wright DR: A "new" coagulation defect. Br J Haematol 2:308, 1956

133. Thomas JE, Peake IR, Giddings JC et al: The application of a monoclonal antibody to factor VIII related antigen (VIII R:Ag) in immunoradiometric assays for factor VIII. Thromb Haemost 53:143, 1985

134. Thomson JM: Laboratory control of anticoagulant therapy. In Thomson JM (ed): Blood Coagulation and Haemostasis: A Practical Guide, p 279. Oxford, Churchill Livingstone, 1980

135. Triplett DA: The extrinsic system. Clin Lab Med 4:221, 1984

136. Triplett DA, Cassidy PG: The use of plasma-agarose gels in the coagulation laboratory. ASCP Check Sample. Thrombosis and Hemostasis, TH 85-3, (TH-39), vol 7(3). Chicago, American Society of Clinical Pathologists, 1985

137. Triplett DA, Harms CS: Procedures for the Coagulation Laboratory, p 20. Chicago, American Society of Clinical Pathologists, 1981

138. Triplett DA, Brandt JT, Maas RL: The laboratory heterogeneity of lupus anticoagulants. Arch Pathol Lab Med 109:946, 1985

139. Triplett DA, Brandt JT, Kaczor D et al: Laboratory diagnosis of lupus inhibitors: A comparison of the tissue thromboplastin inhibition procedure with a new platelet neutralization procedure. Am J Clin Pathol 79:678, 1983

140. Triplett DA, Stocker KF, Unger GA et al: The Textarin/Ecarin ratio: A confirmatory test for lupus anticoagulant. Thromb Haemost 70:925, 1993

141. Unanue ER, Benacerraf B: Textbook of Immunology, 2nd ed, p 56. Baltimore, Williams & Wilkins, 1984

142. van den Besselaar AMHP: Standardization of the prothrombin time in oral anticoagulant control. Haemostasis 15:271, 1985

143. Wang J-S, Lin C-Y, Karp RB: Comparison of high-dose thrombin time with activated clotting time for monitoring of anticoagulant effects of heparin in cardiac surgical patients. Anesth Analg 79:9, 1994

144. Ware AG, Seegers WH: Two-stage procedure for the quantitative determination of prothrombin concentration. Am J Clin Pathol 19:471, 1949

145. Warner ED, Brinkhous KM, Smith HP: A quantitative study on blood clotting: Prothrombin fluctuations under experimental conditions. Am J Physiol 114:667, 1936

146. Weber K, Osborn M: The reliability of molecular weight determinations by dodecyl sulfate polyacrylamide gel electrophoresis. J Biol Chem 244:4406, 1969

147. White RH, Becker DM, Gunther-Maker MG: Outpatient use of a portable international normalized ratio/prothrombin time monitor. South Med 87:206, 1994

148. Yalow RS, Berson SA: Immunoassay of endogenous plasma insulin in man. J Clin Invest 39:1157, 1960

149. Zacharski LR, Rosenstein R: Comparison of the reaction-rate and clot-density methods for determination of plasma fibrinogen. Am J Clin Pathol 68:45, 1977

150. Zimmerman TS, Hoyer LW, Dickson L et al: Determination of the von Willebrand's disease antigen (factor VIII related antigen) in plasma by quantitative immunoelectrophoresis. J Lab Clin Med 86:152, 1975

CHAPTER 50

Laboratory Evaluation of Fibrinolysis

Gordon E. Ens

Determination of Lysis Time
Historic Aspects
Euglobulin Clot Lysis

Determination of Lysis Products
Historic Aspects
Protamine Sulfate Dilution Test
Ethanol Gelation Test
Hemagglutination Test for Soluble Fibrin Monomers

Latex FDP Assay
D-Dimer Assay

Determination of Proteins Involved in Lysis
Plasminogen Assay
Tissue Plasminogen Activator
Plasminogen Activator Inhibitor-1
Alpha₂-Antiplasmin
Venous Occlusion Test

Case Study 50-1

Objectives

1. Discuss the advantages and disadvantages of the euglobulin clot lysis test.
2. Describe a screening test that detects both fibrin and fibrinogen degradation products.
3. Describe at least two laboratory tests designed to determine the presence of fibrin degradation products.
4. Compare and contrast the tests for activity of plasminogen, TPA, PAI, and α_2-antiplasmin.
5. List at least two precautions that must be taken when collecting specimens for most fibrinolytic system assays.

Laboratory evaluation of fibrinolysis has been evolving for the past 30 years. It began with a simple assay, the whole-blood clot lysis test (WBCLT), and has progressed to specific assays for many of the individual components involved in fibrinolysis.

In this chapter some assays commonly used for the evaluation of the fibrinolytic mechanism are discussed, including principles, expected results, and technical difficulties associated with their performance. The reader should already have a clear understanding of the fibrinolytic mechanism and is referred to Chapter 48 for a detailed discussion.

DETERMINATION OF LYSIS TIME

Historic Aspects

The WBCLT is significant from a historic perspective, even though it has been replaced by more sophisticated methods, which will be discussed later in this chapter. The WBCLT is based on the fact that whole blood will clot spontaneously when collected in a glass tube without anticoagulant. This clot should remain intact for approximately 48 hours at 37°C; significant clot lysis or dissolution prior to 48 hours is indicative of excessive systemic fibrinolysis. This test detects only grossly increased activity.[7]

Modifications of the WBCLT include the dilute whole-blood clot lysis time and the plasma clot lysis test, which are said to be more sensitive assays. They are based on the principle that dilution of blood or plasma with a buffer will decrease the activity of inhibitors to plasmin(ogen), thus leaving plasminogen activator or plasmin free to lyse the fibrin clot.[11]

The WBCLT, as well as its modifications, necessitate considerable experience for the reliable detection of lytic activity in the blood. Because of the technical difficulties, as well as the poor correlation of the results with clinical conditions, these tests are not routinely performed in the clinical laboratory.

Euglobulin Clot Lysis

The euglobulin clot lysis time (ECLT) avoids the problems of most plasmin(ogen) inhibitors in the assay system. The result is a more rapid and sensitive assay of lytic activity.

PRINCIPLE

Euglobulins are proteins that precipitate when plasma is diluted with water and acidified. They include plasminogen, plasmin, fibrinogen, and plasminogen activators. Most of the inhibitors of fibrinolysis (antiplasmin and antiplasminogen activators) remain in the supernatant fluid and therefore can be removed from the test system. Plasminogen activator inhibitor-1 (PAI-1) is only partially removed.[5]

PROCEDURE AND QUALITY CONTROL

The patient's citrated, platelet-poor plasma is diluted with water, acidified, and refrigerated. Euglobulins will precipitate, whereas inhibitors of fibrinolysis remain in the supernate, which is carefully decanted and discarded. The precipitate is then redissolved and clotted with thrombin. If the plasminogen in the euglobulin fraction is converted to plasmin, it will lyse the fibrin clot. The time needed for complete lysis at 37°C is recorded as the euglobulin lysis time.

Parallel testing of a presumed normal specimen can serve as a crude quality control measure. Strict adherence to a standardized procedure is necessary.

REFERENCE RANGE

The time required for complete clot lysis should be 1 to 2 hours.[4] In one recent study of 25 ambulatory normals, onset of clot lysis varied from 1.25 to 12 hours with a mean of 3.78 ± 2.45 (1 SD).[12] Lysis in less than 1 hour is usually indicative of increased fibrinolytic activity. Prolonged lysis times are indicative of decreased fibrinolytic activity frequently observed in association with elevated PAI-1 levels. The level of calcium ions in the system and the age of the patient may significantly affect the ECLT.[13,20]

COMMENTS

Blood collection is important in that lysis is enhanced if the tourniquet is left on for more than 1 minute and false-positive results may occur. In addition, laboratories should standardize the anticoagulant to be used, since reference ranges may vary depending on the anticoagulant (*e.g.*, citrate enhances lysis). The sample must be tested within 1 hour of collection or frozen immediately and stored at −70°C until assayed.

The procedure will detect increased fibrinolysis as a result of surgery, obstetric complications, various medical problems, and disseminated intravascular coagulation. This test does not detect fibrin(ogen) split products (X, Y, D, E).

The ECLT is performed by many specialized coagulation laboratories but has little application in the routine clinical laboratory because of the associated technical problems.

If the plasma fibrinogen concentration is less than 80 mg/dL, or if a significant concentration of fibrin(ogen) degradation products (FDP) is present, a poor clot will form, resulting in a false shortening of the lysis time, hence a false-positive result. In the case of greatly reduced plasminogen concentration, as in some cases of disseminated intravascular coagulation, there is insufficient plasminogen in the euglobulin fraction for activation and hence a false-negative (*i.e.*, normal appearing) result.[26]

Excessive agitation of the tube containing the clot may result in an erroneous endpoint.

DETERMINATION OF LYSIS PRODUCTS

The degradation of either fibrin or fibrinogen by plasmin results in fragments of protein referred to synonymously as either fibrin(ogen) degradation (or split) products (FDP or FSP).

Historic Aspects

For many years, the tanned red-cell hemagglutination inhibition (TRCHI) test was the standard against which all other quantitative assays of FDP were measured.[24] Although the TRCHI is still used in research laboratories, its usefulness in the routine clinical laboratory is limited because of its complexity.

The assay is based on the fact that rabbit-derived antihuman fibrinogen antisera, when mixed with the patient's serum, will combine with FDP. After incubation, formalin-fixed, fibrinogen-coated, human group O red cells (tanned RBC) are added to the mixture. These tanned RBC will then react with the residual antihuman fibrinogen antisera (antisera that has not combined with FDP). The mixture is evaluated for inhibition of red cell agglutination. The less tanned RBC agglutinate, the greater levels of serum FDP. Normally, there should be less than 12 μg of fibrinogen-like antigen per milliliter of plasma.

The staphylococcal clumping test[17] is of little use today even though it is a sensitive assay for detecting the presence of FDP X and Y (early breakdown products; Chap. 48), soluble fibrin monomers, and fibrinogen. To perform the test, whole blood is collected and allowed to clot, thus removing all fibrinogen. The remaining serum is diluted and then mixed with a suspension of *Staphylococcus aureus* strain Newman D2C (coagulase negative) in a microtiter plate. High-molecular-weight split products X and Y as well as monomers will complex with the bacteria, resulting in macroscopic agglutination. The highest dilution of patient serum that induces agglutination is determined. The sensitivity of the bacterial suspension is quantitated using a fibrinogen standard plasma and the final result is reported in fibrinogen equivalents per milliliter. Normally, there should be 0 to 8 μg of fibrinogen equivalents/mL of serum.

Protamine Sulfate Dilution Test

The purpose of this test is to detect fibrin monomers and the early FDP X and Y, which are present in plasma only in certain pathologic conditions. The action of thrombin on fibrinogen results in the formation of fibrin monomers that spontaneously polymerize to form a fibrin mesh. When FDP are present in large amounts, they may interfere with this polymerization reaction. The result is soluble (nonpolymerized) fibrin monomers. Primary (larger) degradation products X and Y also tend to polymerize but are inhibited from doing so by complexing with fibrinogen, as well as with the secondary (smaller) degradation products D and E.[17]

PRINCIPLE

When protamine sulfate is added to plasma, it displaces the secondary (smaller) degradation products from fibrin monomers and primary (larger) FDP, which will then polymerize spontaneously. This phenomenon is referred to as *paracoagulation*.[21]

PROCEDURE, QUALITY CONTROL AND REFERENCE RANGE

The assay is performed by adding patient's plasma to protamine sulfate in various dilutions. At the end of 30 minutes, the dilutions are examined for gel formation, which indicates polymerization of fibrin monomers and early FDP. The gel is somewhat difficult to detect, and reading of the results requires some experience.

There is no adequate quality control procedure for this method. Positive and negative controls should be run along with the patient sample. A positive control may be obtained from patients with known fibrinolytic activity. Strict adherence to procedure is essential.

Normally, no gel formation is seen.

COMMENTS

If fibrinogen is present in high concentrations, an amorphous precipitate will develop. This should not be mistaken for a positive reaction.[25]

Because this test is insensitive to fibrinogen and its degradation products, it readily distinguishes between primary and secondary fibrinolysis. Primary fibrinolysis (degradation of fibrinogen) results in a negative reaction, whereas secondary fibrinolysis (degradation of fibrin) yields a positive reaction.

A positive result may be expected in disseminated intravascular coagulation, pulmonary embolism, and during thrombolytic therapy, as well as in any other clinical conditions accompanied by degradation of fibrin clots. This reaction can be completely inhibited by high levels of plasmin, often found in patients with pulmonary embolism.[28]

False-positive reactions may be seen in healthy women immediately before and during menstruation and in patients with advanced cirrhosis or metastatic cancer.[15]

Generally speaking, this test is of limited value unless frequently performed, because experience in interpretation is of prime importance.

Ethanol Gelation Test

The ethanol gel test is said to be less sensitive but more specific than the protamine sulfate dilution test in detecting soluble fibrin monomers and polymers in plasma.[7]

PRINCIPLE

In the presence of a 50% solution of ethanol, any soluble fibrin monomer complexes present will dissociate, resulting in polymerization of the monomers and subsequent gel formation.[6] This is the same paracoagulation reaction involved in the protamine sulfate test.

PROCEDURE, REFERENCE RANGE AND COMMENTS

The test is performed by adding a 50% solution of ethanol to platelet-poor plasma and observing for gel formation. There should be no gel formation under normal conditions.

This test has been used in conjunction with, or substituted for, the protamine sulfate dilution test; however, it suffers from similar interpretation problems.

Hemagglutination Test for Soluble Fibrin Monomers

A European group developed this test, with claims of greater sensitivity and specificity than the two paracoagulation tests just described.

PRINCIPLE

The test reagent consists of erythrocytes coated with fibrin monomers. If soluble fibrin complexes are present in the test plasma, they will react with the fibrin monomers on the red cells and cause the red cells to agglutinate.

PROCEDURE, REFERENCE RANGE AND COMMENTS

Platelet-poor citrated plasma is incubated with coated red cells at 37°C for 10 minutes. The suspension is then placed on a ring slide and rocked for 6 minutes. It is then observed for agglutination. The strength of the agglutination will depend on the concentration of soluble fibrin monomers. Normally, there should be no agglutination of red cells.

Positive and negative controls must be run with the patient specimen. Timing and temperature are critical to the test. The test is not generally affected by the presence of FDP or heparin.

Latex FDP Assay

Because of the need for a convenient, rapid, and sensitive assay for fibrin degradation products, the latex FDP test was developed.

PRINCIPLE

Latex particles coated with antibody against either fibrin(ogen) fragments D and E or human fibrinogen are mixed with patient serum. Macroscopic agglutination of the latex particles indicates the presence of degradation products of either fibrinogen or fibrin.

SPECIMEN REQUIREMENTS

Certain precautions are required during blood collection. First, because trace amounts of fibrinogen will cause false-positive reactions, it is essential that the sample be thoroughly clotted with thrombin. Second, if heparin is present in the sample (e.g., from intravenous heparin infusion), a snake venom preparation (reptilase) must be added to ensure complete clotting.[7] Also, plasma from patients having excessive fibrinolytic activity may develop FDP in vitro after the specimen has been collected. Therefore, a plasmin inhibitor should be added to the collection tube to ensure the measurement of in vivo and not in vitro split products. Tubes containing thrombin and a plasmin inhibitor with or without venom, are commercially available.

PROCEDURE AND QUALITY CONTROL

The patient's serum in various dilutions is mixed with the latex particles, and the highest dilution in which macroscopic agglutination is present represents the titer of FDP. Depending on which manufacturer's kit is used, the sensitivity of the latex particles may be to degradation products D and E or to high-molecular-weight fragments X and Y.

Positive and negative controls should be run along with the patient specimens. These controls may be supplied by the manufacturer of the kit. If not, a positive control can be made by diluting normal plasma, which contains fibrinogen. A normal serum sample will serve as a negative control. The activity of the latex particles should be checked with dilutions of fibrinogen or plasma.

COMMENTS

Comparisons of these assays have been performed.[8,29,30] Positive results have been reported in disseminated intravascular coagulation, pulmonary embolism, deep vein thrombosis, acute myocardial infarction, abruptio placentae, preeclampsia, eclampsia, fetal death in utero, postpartum hemorrhage, malignant neoplasms, ovarian tumor, polycystic disease, renal failure, hydronephrosis, lupus nephritis, proliferative glomerulonephritis, renal transplantation, cirrhosis, after surgical complications, during thrombolytic therapy, and in healthy normal women during menstruation. Fluctuating levels have been observed during normal pregnancy.

False-positive results have been observed in samples that have not been clotted properly (e.g., heparin contamination or dysfibrinogenemia) or from patients with circulating rheumatoid factor. Also, if the latex–serum mixture is not read at the prescribed time, a false-positive reaction may result, because prolonged exposure to air will cause evaporation and apparent agglutination.

D-Dimer Assay

A more recent development in the evaluation of fibrinolytic activity is the D-dimer (D-D) assay, which measures a specific fragment arising from the degradation of cross-linked fibrin (D-dimer) and not fragments X, Y, D, or E. Because it measures fibrinolysis and not fibrinogenolysis, the presence of D-dimers is specific evidence of a physiologic response to intravascular fibrin formation[9] as opposed to primary fibrinolysis (*i.e.*, lysis in the absence of fibrin formation).

SPECIMEN REQUIREMENTS AND PROCEDURE

This assay may be performed on fresh citrated, heparinized, or EDTA plasma specimens as well as serum.

There are basically two methods to assay the D-dimer: enzyme immunoassay and latex bead. The enzyme immunoassay is useful when levels of D-dimer are low and a very sensitive assay is required. It does, however, require a special technique and is expensive and time consuming. A busy clinical laboratory has need for a rapid, simple, yet specific method. For this reason, the latex bead method has gained popularity despite the fact that it is not as sensitive as the enzyme immunoassay.

This method utilizes latex beads coated with monoclonal antibody specific for D-dimer but not to fibrinogen degradation products or early degradation products X and Y. The plasma or serum in various dilutions is mixed with a suspension of sensitized latex beads, and the highest dilution of plasma or serum that causes macroscopic agglutination of these beads is determined.

Under normal circumstances, levels of D-dimer should be less than 200 ng/mL.

COMMENTS

Positive results may be seen in patients with DIC, pulmonary and cerebral embolism, phlebitis, thrombosis, prethrombotic risk, and sickle cell disease, and after surgical procedures and during clot dissolution secondary to thrombolytic therapy.[3] The presence of rheumatoid factor, a heterologous antibody, may cause a false-positive reaction.[22] There is new evidence to suggest the usefulness of the D-dimer assay as a screening test for the diagnosis of venous thrombosis.[14,16,18,27]

Fresh citrated, heparinized, or EDTA plasma specimens may be used as well as serum. It should be noted, however, that D-dimer levels are somewhat lower in serum than in plasma[29]; this needs to be taken into consideration when interpreting test results.

DETERMINATION OF PROTEINS INVOLVED IN LYSIS

Since the fibrinolytic system shows circadian variation and responds to exercise, blood samples to be evaluated for fibrinolytic system components, including venous occlusion, should be obtained at a standardized time. The preferable time is early morning following an overnight fast and at least a 15-minute rest. Specimens should be processed immediately after phlebotomy, centrifuged to be platelet-free and if not evaluated immediately, placed into plastic vials and frozen at −70°C.

Plasminogen Assay

Over the years, many methods have been developed to assay plasminogen, among them are the fibrin plate assay[2] and the caseinolytic method.[1] These have been replaced by other methodologies having wider acceptance and application. Plasminogen should be assayed by both immunologic and functional assays in order to detect nonfunctional molecules. If only one assay is performed, it should be the functional assay.

Immunologic assays of plasminogen by radial immunodiffusion (RID)[10] and its modification[23] are available commercially. In these tests, the patient's plasma is added and allowed to diffuse from a well cut into an agarose matrix containing plasminogen antibody. The interaction of patient's plasminogen with the antibody results in an immunoprecipitation reaction, the diameter of which is measured and compared to that caused by control plasma. Although the test is simple to perform, 48 hours are required to obtain results. Also, it measures only the concentration of the plasminogen molecule immunologically, not taking into account its functional capabilities.

Functional assays are all based on the same principle: an excess of plasminogen activator, such as streptokinase, is added to a plasma sample. The resultant plasminogen–streptokinase complex generates plasmin activity that will react with a synthetic (chromogenic) substrate. The result is a color change proportional to the plasminogen level of the plasma. These assays are commercially available.

The problems inherent to the synthetic substrate procedure are (1) a spectrophotometer is required; (2) technique is critical: the timing of specific reactions as well as the narrow temperature range in which the assays are performed must be accurately monitored; and (3) icteric or hemolyzed plasma will interfere with the spectrophotometric measurement.

Tissue Plasminogen Activator

Tissue plasminogen activator (TPA) is a major player in the fibrinolytic system. Recombinant forms have been used therapeutically to dissolve clots in the vascular system. The TPA antigen can be measured immunologically or its activity can be determined.

TPA antigen levels are determined using an ELISA sandwich technique. The test sample (patient, control, or standard) is added to a microtest well coated with anti-TPA IgG and allowed to incubate for a specific time. During incubation, TPA binds to the immobilized anti-TPA antibodies, which are labeled with peroxidase. The wells are washed to remove unbound conjugate after which a color-linked peroxidase substrate is added. The amount of yellow color developed is directly proportional to the amount of TPA present in the sample. Several kits are available commercially. Each laboratory should evaluate any kits carefully as the quality of antibodies is of critical importance.

A fraction of circulating TPA may be inaccessible to the antibody (cryptic). EDTA or detergents are helpful in exposing these antigens so they will bind.

Reference ranges for immunologic assays range from 0.9 to 10.5 ng/mL.

Activity levels of TPA are determined indirectly by activating plasminogen in the presence of a fibrin-related stimulator (*e.g.*, soluble fibrin monomers) and measuring the plasmin generated. Reference values need to be established by each laboratory, since they vary widely. PAI inhibition of TPA can be a cause of analytical error. Many procedures call for the acidification of the sample to inhibit PAI–TPA binding.

Plasminogen Activator Inhibitor-1

Plasminogen activator inhibitor-1 (PAI-1) is synthesized by endothelial cells, hepatocytes, and megakaryocytes (platelets). By and large, platelet PAI is inactive. Increased levels of PAI are associated with thrombotic disorders. PAI is measured by a two-stage, indirect enzyme assay (Fig. 50-1). A standard amount of tissue plasminogen activator (TPA) is added to the plasma sample and incubated for a specific time. This allows TPA to complex with PAI. Plasmin inhibitors, such as α_2-antiplasmin, are removed by acidification. The unbound TPA (residual) is quantitated by adding the sample to a mixture of PAI-deficient plasma containing plasminogen and a chromogenic substrate and then measuring the color change caused by the generation of plasmin. The amount of color generated is inversely proportional to the amount of PAI in the specimen.

This test is not specific for PAI since other anti-TPAs exist; however, PAI is fast acting and placing a time limit on the incubation yields results reflecting PAI concentrations.

A variety of immunoassays are also available in kit form; however, they will not give any information on function nor are there adequate standards available. Every laboratory must establish its own reference ranges because those reported in the literature vary widely.

Alpha₂-Antiplasmin

The functional levels of α_2-antiplasmin, the primary plasmin inhibitor in plasma, are determined by an amidolytic method using a synthetic chromogenic substrate. Test plasma containing α_2-antiplasmin is incubated with a known amount of excess plasmin forming an antiplasmin–plasmin complex. The unbound plasmin then catalyzes the release of p-nitraniline (pNA) from a chromogenic substrate. The release of pNA is measured by either an endpoint or kinetic method. The amount of pNA generated is inversely proportional to the amount of α_2-antiplasmin in the specimen.

Venous Occlusion Test

The venous occlusion test provides an evaluation of the fibrinolytic system before and after a standardized amount of venous stasis.

A baseline sample is obtained by a nontraumatic venipuncture without use of a tourniquet. A blood pressure cuff is then applied at a pressure midway between systolic and diastolic pressure for a period of 10 minutes. (There is some indication that 20 minutes is preferable.) A second venipuncture is performed with the cuff still in place.

PAI $\xrightarrow{\text{TPA}}$ PAI:TPA + residual TPA

PLASMINOGEN $\xrightarrow[\text{(residual)}]{\text{TPA}}$ PLASMIN

PLASMIN + CHROMOGENIC SUBSTRATE $\longrightarrow$ COLOR

FIGURE 50-1. Reactions on which the activity assay for PAI is based.

Stasis normally results in the release of tissue plasminogen activator and plasminogen activator inhibitor-1 from endothelial cells. The response to stasis may be quantitated by assaying components of the fibrinolytic system. Normally, the release of TPA is greater than that of PAI, resulting in a decrease in euglobulin lysis time and a three- to fourfold increase in TPA concentration when compared to baseline. This increase in TPA post venous occlusion varies with sex (higher in men), increases with age, and is higher in obese subjects and in those with increased serum lipids.[31] Prolonged euglobulin lysis times indicate decreased TPA release from the endothelium or increased circulating PAI. Elevated PAI is not specific for thromboembolic disease, but rather has been observed in several clinical conditions including trauma, diabetes, extracorporeal circulation, and malignancy.[19]

CHAPTER SUMMARY

The laboratory assays described in this chapter measure various components of the fibrinolytic system. They are divided into three major categories: measurement of the time for lysis to occur, detection of products of lysis of fibrinogen and fibrin or of fibrin only, and measurement of specific reactants in the fibrinolytic system including plasminogen, its major activator (TPA) and inactivator (PAI-1), as well as antiplasmins. Only those tests most commonly employed in routine hemostasis laboratories have been discussed.

Most of the tests described are available commercially in kit form. The most important requirement for any of these tests is that they measure *in vivo* and not *in vitro* lysis and that platelets do not interfere. To accomplish this, the instructions pertaining to specimen collection, preparation, and assay must be strictly followed. If carefully performed, these assays will aid in the diagnosis and monitoring of events associated with the activation of the fibrinolytic system.

Case Study 50-1

A 35-year-old man was admitted through the emergency department with an anterior-wall myocardial infarction. It was determined that he was a candidate for clot dissolution with thrombolytic therapy (streptokinase). A coagulation profile was performed before and 2 hours after induction of the therapy. It was later determined in the cardiac catheterization laboratory that the clot was not effectively lysed. The patient was subsequently treated by conventional therapy using anticoagulants. Coagulation results were as follows:

	Pre-Therapy	Post-Therapy
PT (9–13 sec)	12.2 sec	17.0 sec
PTT (24–37 sec)	28 sec	55 sec
Fibrinogen (150–400 mg/dL)	300 mg/dL	32 mg/dL
FDP (latex) (<10 μg/mL)	<10 μg/mL	>160 μg/mL
D-dimer (<200 ng/mL)	<200 ng/mL	300 ng/mL
Plasminogen (68%–150%)	70%	22%

1. Explain the elevated FDP level.
2. Explain the decreased plasminogen level.
3. Why is the D-dimer level not elevated in proportion to the greatly elevated FDP level?

Review Questions

50-1. The euglobulin clot lysis test is shorter and more sensitive than previous tests of clot lysis because _____ are removed from the test system.

    A. plasminogen and plasminogen activators
    B. antiplasmin and antiplasminogen activators
    C. plasmin and plasmin activators
    D. fibrinogen and plasminogen activator inhibitor

50-2. A false-negative result for euglobulin clot lysis may occur if

    A. plasma fibrinogen levels are less than 80 mg/dL.
    B. significant amounts of FDP are present.
    C. the tourniquet is left on for several minutes during blood collection.
    D. the patient has disseminated intravascular coagulation.

50-3. The blood collection tube for any assay of fibrin(ogen) degradation products should contain

    A. thrombin, reptilase, and a plasmin inhibitor.
    B. reptilase and a plasmin activator.
    C. EDTA and a plasminogen activator inhibitor.
    D. antiplasmins and a trypsin inhibitor.

50-4. The presence of _____ the plasma is strong evidence that fibrin has been formed and is being lysed.

    A. X-Y
    B. D-E
    C. D-D
    E. E-E

50-5. A problem with the use of assays based on synthetic chromogenic substrates is

    A. poor sensitivity.
    B. a very narrow temperature range.
    C. poor specificity.
    D. high complexity since kits are not yet available.

50-6. Prolonged venous stasis will normally result in

    A. prolonged euglobulin clot lysis.
    B. release of plasminogen by endothelial cells.
    C. a greater release of endothelial cell TPA than of PAI.
    D. all of the above

References

1. Alkjaersig N, Fletcher AP, Sherry S: The mechanism of clot dissolution by plasmin. J Clin Invest 38:1086, 1959
2. Bang NU, Beller FK, Deutsch E et al: Thrombosis and Bleeding Disorders: Theory and Methods. New York, Academic Press, 1971
3. Berberian L, Cercek B, Laramee P et al: The serum level of D-dimer, a degradation product of crosslinked fibrin is elevated following intravenous streptokinase but not following conventional management in acute myocardial infarction (abstract). Proceedings of the 35th Annual Scientific Sessions of the American College of Cardiology, 1986
4. Blix S: Studies on the fibrinolytic system in the euglobulin fraction of human plasma. Scand J Clin Lab Invest 13(suppl):3, 1961
5. Bockenstedt PL: Laboratory methods in hemostasis. In Loscalzo J, Schafer AI (eds): Thrombosis and Hemorrhage, p 455. Boston, Blackwell Scientific Publications, 1994
6. Breen FA, Tullis JL: Ethanol gelation: A rapid screening test for intravascular coagulation. Ann Intern Med 69:1197, 1968
7. Brittin GM: Fibrinolysis. Chicago, American Society of Clinical Pathologists Commission on Continuing Education, 1972
8. Drewinko B, Surgeon J, Cobb P et al: Comparative sensitivity of different methods to detect and quantify circulating fibrinogen/fibrin split products. Am J Clin Pathol 84:58, 1985
9. Elms MJ, Bunce IH, Bundesen PG: Measurement of crosslinked fibrin degradation products: An immunoassay using monoclonal antibodies. Thromb Haemost 50:591, 1983
10. Fahey JL, McKelvey EM et al: Quantitative determination of serum immunoglobulins in antibody-agar plates. J Immunol 94:84, 1965
11. Fearnley GR, Balmforth G, Fearnley E: Evidence of diurnal fibrinolytic rhythm with a simple method for measuring natural fibrinolysis. Clin Sci 16:645, 1957
12. Glassman A, Abram M, Baxter G et al: Euglobulin lysis times: An update. Ann Clin Lab Sci 23:329, 1993
13. Gleerup G, Winther K: The effect of ageing on platelet function and fibrinolytic activity. Angiology 46:715, 1995
14. Goldhaber SZ: Epidemiology of pulmonary embolism and deep vein thrombosis. In Bloom AL, Forbes CD, Thomas DP et al (eds): Haemostasis and Thrombosis, vol 2, p 1327. New York, Churchill Livingstone, 1994
15. Gurewich V, Hutchinson E: Detection of intravascular coagulation by a serial-dilution protamine sulfate test. Ann Intern Med 75:895, 1971
16. Hathaway WE, Goodnight SH: Disorders of Hemostasis and Thrombosis, a Clinical Guide, p 323. New York, McGraw Hill, 1993
17. Hawiger J, Niewiarowski S, Gurewich V et al: Measurement of fibrinogen and fibrin degradation products in serum by staphylococcal clumping test. J Lab Clin Med 75:93, 1970
18. Heaton D, Billings J, Hickton C: Assessment of D-dimer assay for the diagnosis of deep vein thrombosis. J Lab Clin Med 110:588, 1987
19. Jensen R, Ens G: Coagulation Questions and Comments: Clin Hemostasis Rev 8(6):17, 1994
20. Kojima Y, Urano T, Kojima K et al: The significant enhancement of fibrinolysis by calcium ion in a cell free system: The shortening of euglobulin clot lysis time by calcium ion. Thromb Haemost 72:113, 1994
21. Kopec M, Kowalski E, Stachurashi J: Studies on paracoagulation: Role of antithrombin VI. Thromb Diath Haemorrh 5:285, 1961
22. Lane DA, Preston FE, Van Ross ME: Characterization of serum fibrinogen and fibrin fragments produced during disseminated intravascular coagulation. Br J Haematol 40:609, 1978
23. Mancini G, Carbonara AO, Heremans JF: Immunochemical quantitation of antigens by single radial immunodiffusion. Immunochem 2:235, 1965
24. Merskey C, Kleiner GJ, Johnson AJ: Quantitative estimation of split products of fibrinogen in human serum: Relation to diagnosis and treatment. Blood 28:1, 1966
25. Niewiarowski S, Gurewich V: Laboratory identification of intravascular coagulation: The serial dilution protamine sulfate test for the detection of fibrin monomer and fibrin degradation products. J Lab Clin Med 77:665, 1971
26. Penner JA: Blood Coagulation Laboratory Manual. Ann Arbor, University of Michigan Medical Center, 1977
27. Rowbotham B, Carol P, Whitaker A, Bunce I, Cobcroft R: Measurement of crosslinked fibrin derivatives—Use in the diagnosis of venous thrombosis. Thrombosis and Haemostasis 57:59, 1987
28. Sanfelippo M, Stevens D, Koenig R: Protamine sulfate test for fibrin monomers. Am J Clin Pathol 56:166, 1971
29. Smith L, Kitchens C: Experience with a commercially avail-

able kit for determining concentration of serum fibrin degradation products. Lab Med 14:554, 1983

30. Sorenson P, Galluzzo T, Tsao C: Evaluation of new latex FDP assay. Lab Med 13:688, 1982

31. Stegnar M, Pentek M: Fibrinolytic response to venous occlusion in healthy subjects: Relationship to age, gender, body weight, blood lipids and insulin. Thromb Res 69:81, 1993

32. Whitaker A, Elms M, Masci P et al: Measurement of cross-linked fibrin derivatives in plasma: An immunoassay using monoclonal antibodies. J Clin Pathol 37:882, 1984

CHAPTER 51

Markers of Thrombotic Activity

Gordon E. Ens

Definition and Diagnostic Applications

Thrombin–Antithrombin Complex

Prothrombin Fragment 1.2

Fibrinopeptide A

D-Dimer

Objectives

1. Define the term *markers of thrombosis*.
2. Describe why each of the following is considered to be an indicator of thrombosis when increased: thrombin–antithrombin (TAT), prothrombin fragment 1.2 (PF1.2), and fibrinopeptide A (FPA).
3. Describe at least one assay system used to detect markers of thrombosis.

DEFINITION AND DIAGNOSTIC APPLICATIONS

Evidence or markers of thrombosis range from enzyme–substrate complexes that reflect the body's attempts to regulate or inhibit coagulation to small fragments of peptides that are released as part of the process whereby coagulation factors are activated. Molecular markers are specific markers of activation of coagulation and fibrinolysis. Their measurement provides an ultrasensitive means of detecting minute changes in components of hemostasis.[14] Furthermore, they provide specific and pertinent data for the early diagnosis and management of disorders caused by excessive or inappropriate coagulation.[8,10]

Laboratory evaluation of thrombotic disorders and of molecular markers of thrombosis has recently undergone substantial development. Paramount to this development have been advances in understanding of the biochemistry of coagulation and fibrinolysis and technologic advances that permit the measurement of minute quantities of circulating products of hemostatic activation.[2] The assay systems most frequently used to measure molecular markers are competitive radioimmunoassay (RIA) procedures and enzyme-linked immunosorbent assays (ELISA) (Fig. 51-1). See Chapter 49 for a discussion of these two assay systems.

Biochemical markers in the blood are generated prior to thrombin becoming biologically available. These markers of thrombosis have three basic diagnostic applications: (1) the diagnosis of spontaneous thrombosis, (2) the prognosis and follow-up of thrombotic disease, and (3) the monitoring of anticoagulant therapy. Ideally, laboratory determinations of thrombosis markers should identify the pathologic process in the hemostatic mechanism as well as be inexpensive, reproducible, and easy to perform.[13]

Under normal conditions, all individuals demonstrate measurable quantities of thrombosis markers; these levels typically increase as part of the normal aging process. Marked elevations have been observed in persons with deep venous thrombosis, pulmonary emboli, disseminated intravascular coagulation, and other thromboembolic phenomena.[2] Because of their short half-lives, enzyme inhibitor complexes and activation peptides (protein fragments released as a result of factor activation) can be demonstrated in blood only as long as the thrombotic process is ongoing. Assays for activation peptides and inhibitor complexes provide physiologic evidence of *in vivo* processes and do not require the *in vitro* activation step necessary in many conventional assays. Additionally, very small samples are required for molecular marker studies. Marker testing frequently requires special anticoagulants for collection in addition to rapid sample processing.

This chapter will address three determinations for thrombosis markers that are beginning to be offered by routine hemostasis laboratories, particularly now that commercial kits are becoming increasingly available.

THROMBIN–ANTITHROMBIN COMPLEX

Upon activation of coagulation, antithrombin complexes with factors XIa, IXa, Xa, and IIa (Fig. 53-1). This reaction is reversible initially but becomes irreversible following the formation of a covalent bond between antithrombin and the serine protease. The antithrombin molecule is cleaved, which simultaneously modifies its structure. Then the thrombin–antithrombin (TAT) complex combines with vitronectin (complement S protein) in the blood to form a ternary complex, which is rapidly removed from circulation by an unidentified hepatic receptor.[17]

Principle. The TAT complex assay is considered a direct way to measure the hypercoagulable state, since the conversion of prothrombin to thrombin by an increase in factor Xa activity is one of the initial steps in hemostatic activation.

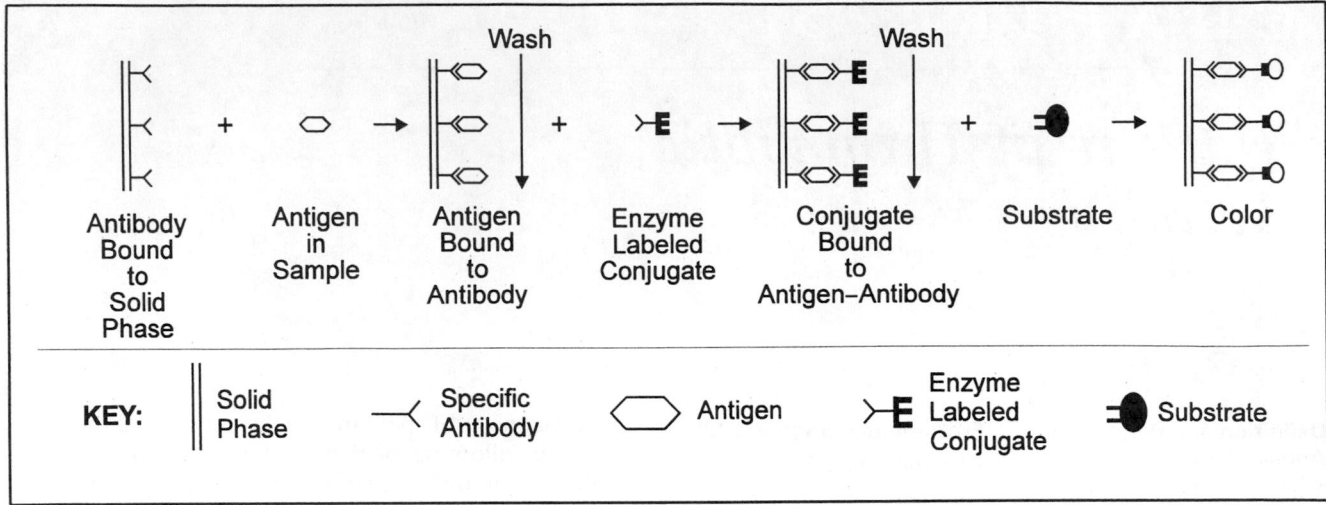

FIGURE 51-1. Enzyme-linked immunosorbent assay (ELISA).

Specimen Requirements. Testing for TAT is performed on plasma samples collected into trisodium citrate anticoagulant avoiding any trauma that might activate coagulation and falsely elevate TAT levels. After centrifuging, platelet-poor plasma is stable for 4 hours at 20° to 25°C, for 8 hours at 2° to 4°C, and for at least 30 days at −80°C.

Procedure and Reference Range. TAT levels can be determined immunologically by either radioimmunoassay or ELISA using monoclonal antibodies raised against the thrombin–antithrombin complex.

Reference ranges are less than 20 ng/mL.

Comments. TAT has an extremely short half-life (a few minutes); therefore, elevated levels are an indication of ongoing thrombin generation resulting in the consumption of antithrombin III (AT-III). The assay may be useful in monitoring a thrombotic episode, with decreasing levels indicating resolution of the thrombotic incident.

Disadvantages of the use of TAT in surgical patients and other patients in acute distress include the fact that levels may be elevated secondary to inflammation and microvascular thrombosis. However, levels below a certain threshold may suggest a protective mechanism in these patients.

PROTHROMBIN FRAGMENT 1.2

The prothrombin fragment 1.2 (PF1.2 or PF 1+2) is a polypeptide released from prothrombin when prothrombin is activated to thrombin through cleavage by the prothrombinase complex. The prothrombinase complex consists of activated factors X and V, calcium and phospholipid. PF1.2 has been used to assess thrombotic risk and monitor anticoagulant therapy.[6,7,12]

Specimen Requirements. Assays for PF1.2 are performed on plasma samples collected into heparin anticoagulant and should be centrifuged to obtain platelet-poor plasma within 1 hour of venipuncture. Samples are stable for up to 4 hours at 20° to 25°C and for at least 6 months at −80°C.

Procedure and Reference Range. Both polyclonal and monoclonal antibodies have been developed that are specific for the PF1.2 fragment even in the presence of large concentrations of prothrombin. These antibodies can be utilized to determine PF1.2 levels by either two-stage ELISA or RIA methodologies. Several commercial assays are available. Reference values are less than 3 ng/mL; however, this can vary between methods and laboratories.

Comments. PF1.2 is elevated in almost all patients with inherited antithrombin deficiency most likely because of the increased concentration of factor Xa observed in these patients. In some studies, PF1.2 is two times higher in antithrombin-deficient patients than healthy subjects. Patients with inherited thrombophilia and cancer also have elevated PF1.2 levels.[1,13]

PF1.2 levels were observed to increase with age in a study of approximately 200 males between ages 42 and 80 years.[6] PF1.2 also appears to be useful in monitoring the lowest dose of warfarin needed to protect against a thrombotic event. Circulating PF1.2, unlike thrombin, has a relatively long half-life of approximately 90 minutes.

FIBRINOPEPTIDE A

Principle. Circulating inhibitors normally neutralize activated coagulation factors. However, when free thrombin is allowed to circulate the fibrinogen molecule is degraded and fibrinopeptide A (FPA) and fibrinopeptide B are released. FPA is a small (molecular weight approximately 1500 daltons) polypeptide cleavage product and does not have any known independent function. It is specific for the action of thrombin on fibrinogen and the more stable of the two fibrinopeptides. Nevertheless, FPA has an *in vivo* half-life of only 3 to 5 minutes.[12] Fibrinopeptide B, on the other hand, forms at a slower rate during clot formation and is the product of the action of thrombin on fibrinogen as well as the action of plasmin on fibrin.[15]

Specimen Requirements. Strict sampling technique is essential in the accurate measurement of FPA. Samples for FPA testing are collected into a special anticoagulant containing trisodium citrate, heparin, and protease specific inhibitors. This combination of additives is designed to inhibit any possible *in vitro* coagulation reactions. The venipuncture must be rapid and the sample centrifuged immediately. If clotting is activated during sampling, falsely elevated FPA levels may be obtained. Fibrinogen is precipitated out by treating the plasma with bentonite; the specimen is then centrifuged and the supernate removed for testing. The removal of fibrinogen is critical since anti-FPA antibodies will react with fibrinogen as well. The sample is stable for 2 hours at $-2°$ to $4°C$ prior to bentonite treatment and at least 30 days at $-80°C$.

Procedure and Reference Range. FPA levels can be determined immunologically by modified ELISA or RIA procedures using anti-FPA antibodies. Commercial kits are available.

Reference ranges are generally considered to be 3 ng/mL or less; however, every laboratory must establish its own reference range, since there is considerable interlaboratory variability.[16]

Comments. Elevations of FPA have been observed in patients with disseminated intravascular coagulation, inflammatory processes, peripheral vascular disease, arterial thrombosis, venous thrombosis, and malignancy.

Studies of patients with peripheral vascular disease and bypass grafts showed serial declines in FPA levels following arterial bypass surgery.[4] These results suggest that FPA levels may be useful for estimating the severity of disease, degree of graft healing and patency (lack of obstructions causing poor blood flow), and the success of therapeutic intervention.

In a study of 70 healthy pregnant women, FPA levels rose significantly during delivery and remained elevated for 3 hours postpartum. Levels returned to prelabor values by 24 hours. FPA appears to be a sensitive indicator of clotting activation in this group of patients as well.[9]

Early coronary thrombosis in patients with acute transmural infarction results in marked elevation of FPA. Following the acute period, values then decline consistently. If initial elevations of FPA represent accelerated thrombosis with pathogenic importance, the detection of the marker may be useful in the selection of patients who are good candidates for thrombolytic therapy. FPA may also be useful in identifying those patients at risk for recurrent coronary thrombosis.[5]

D-DIMER

Fibrin clot formation is the end result of the action of thrombin on fibrinogen. Soluble fibrin monomers are polymerized into a fibrin fiber network that is further stabilized by the cross-linking action of factor XIIIa. Activation of the fibrinolytic system results in the generation of plasmin, which degrades the cross-linked fibrin thus producing D-dimer and other breakdown products. D-dimer is one of the most common molecular markers employed to evaluate hemostatic activation. D-dimer has gained in popularity because of its high sensitivity, relatively long half-life, and ease of detection. The D-dimer assay can aid in the diagnosis of rare primary fibrinolysis and distinguish between breakdown products of fibrin *versus* fibrinogen.[14] Since the D-dimer measurement is specific for fibrin derivatives, the assay is sensitive in patients with disseminated intravascular coagulation, liver disease, acute leukemia, and deep venous thrombosis.[3] See Chapter 50 for further discussion of this laboratory determination.

CHAPTER SUMMARY

This chapter has addressed markers of thrombosis that are currently available to clinical laboratories. Substantial investigation has been directed towards developing a better understanding of the changes that take place in the hemostatic mechanism prior to the clinical expression of thrombotic events. Continued studies relating the biochemical and molecular changes in the balance of naturally occurring anticoagulants and procoagulants to the clinical status of the patient will further enhance the diagnosis and management of venous and arterial thrombotic disorders.

Review Questions

51-1. A thrombosis marker that has proved to be useful for monitoring anticoagulant (warfarin) therapy is

A. thrombin–antithrombin (TAT).
B. prothrombin fragment 1.2 (PF1.2).
C. fibrinopeptide A (FPA).
D. D-dimer (D-D).

51-2. A thrombosis marker that has shown high sensitivity for disseminated intravascular coagulation (DIC) is

A. thrombin–antithrombin (TAT).
B. prothrombin fragment 1.2 (PF1.2).
C. fibrinopeptide A (FPA).
D. D-dimer (D-D).

51-3. Many markers of thrombosis reflect coagulation as it is occurring *in vivo* because of their

A. high affinity for coagulation factors.
B. stability.
C. neutralizing capability.
D. short half-life.

51-4. A common source of error for many laboratory determinations of thrombosis markers is

A. poor specimen collection.
B. lack of antibody specificity.
C. inadequate sample size.
D. presence of cross-reactive material.

51-5. A disadvantage of the thrombin–antithrombin (TAT) complex as a detector of thrombosis is that its levels may also be increased secondary to

A. malignancy.
B. bleeding.
C. inflammation.
D. pregnancy.

51-6. The age group that would be expected to have the highest levels of thrombosis markers is

A. newborn.
B. children.
C. adults.
D. elderly.

References

1. Bauer KA: Inherited hypercoagulable states. In Hoffman R, Benz EJ Jr, Shattil SJ et al (eds): Hematology, Basic Principles and Practice, 2nd ed, p 1781. New York, Churchill Livingstone, 1995
2. Bauer KA, Weitz JI: Laboratory markers of coagulation and fibrinolysis. In Colman RW, Hirsh J, Marder VJ et al (eds): Hemostasis and Thrombosis, Basic Principles and Clinical Practice, 3rd ed, p 1232. Philadelphia, JB Lippincott Company, 1994
3. Bounameaux H, Schneider PA, Reber G et al: Measurement of plasma D-dimer for diagnosis of deep venous thrombosis. Am J Clin Pathol 91:82, 1989
4. Donaldson MC, Matthews ET, Hadjimichael J et al: Markers of thrombotic activity in arterial disease. Arch Surg 122:897, 1987

5. Eisenberg PR, Sherman L, Schectman K et al: Fibrinopeptide A: A marker of acute coronary thrombosis. Circulation 71:912, 1985

6. Elias A, Bonfils S, Daoud-Elias M et al: Influence of long term oral anticoagulants upon prothrombin fragment 1+2, thrombin-antithromin III complex and D-dimer levels in patients affected by deep vein thrombosis. Thromb Haemost 69:302, 1993

7. Estivals M, Pelzer H, Sie P et al: Prothrombin fragment 1+2, thrombin-antithrombin III complexes and D-dimers in acute deep vein thrombosis: Effects of heparin treatment. Br J Haematol 78:421, 1991

8. Fareed J: Molecular markers of hemostatic activation. In Bick RL (ed): Clinics in Laboratory Medicine, part II, p 235. Philadelphia, WB Saunders Company, 1995

9. Gerbasi FR, Bottom S, Abdelmonem F et al: Changes in hemostasis activity during delivery and the immediate postpartum period. Am J Obstet Gynecol 162:1158, 1990

10. Hathaway WE, Goodnight SH Jr: Laboratory measurements of hemostasis and thrombosis. In: Disorders of Hemostasis and Thrombosis, p 21. New York, McGraw-Hill, 1993

11. Hathaway WE, Goodnight SH Jr: Thrombosis and cancer. In: Disorders of Hemostasis and Thrombosis, p 394. New York, McGraw-Hill, 1993

12. Horellou MH, Conard J, Samama MM: Laboratory tests for the diagnosis of venous thromboembolism. In Hull R, Pineo GF (eds): Disorders of Thrombosis, p 272. Philadelphia, WB Saunders, 1996

13. Jensen R, Ens G: Markers of thrombin activation. Clin Hemostasis Rev 8(9):1, 1994

14. Jensen R, Ens G: Diagnostic application of thrombotic markers. Clin Hemostasis Rev 5(7):1, 1991

15. Saito H: Normal hemostatic mechanisms. In Ratnoff OD, Forbes CD (eds): Disorders of Hemostasis, p 18. Philadelphia, WB Saunders, 1991

16. Owen J: The utility of fibrinopeptide assays. Thromb Haemost 62:807, 1989

17. Sheffield WP, Wu YI, Blajchman M: Antithrombin: Structure and function. In High KA, Roberts HR (eds): Molecular Basis of Thrombosis and Hemostasis. New York, Marcel Dekker, 1995

CHAPTER 52

Hemorrhagic Disorders of Coagulation and Fibrinolysis

Margaret C. Schmidt

Objectives

1. Describe the basic differences between inherited and acquired coagulation disorders.
2. Explain what is meant by the "contact phase" of coagulation.
3. Compare and contrast the clinical and laboratory effects of deficiencies in the four contact factors.
4. Compare and contrast the hemophilias A, B, and C, including their genetics, nomenclature, clinical effects, therapeutic modalities, and laboratory testing protocols.
5. List the von Willebrand disease variants (types) in the order of their frequency and indicate the laboratory test confirmation pattern for each variant (type).
6. Describe each of the inherited extrinsic and common pathway disorders, including the clinical effect and laboratory test results of each.
7. Cite an example of a circulating anticoagulant; describe its theory of origin, clinical effect, and the typical laboratory test results that demonstrate its presence.
8. Discuss how liver disease impairs the coagulation system and how laboratory tests reveal those disturbances.
9. Profile disseminated intravascular coagulation to include its etiology, clinical effects, and laboratory test results.

The disorders of hemostasis are complex. For purposes of clarity, this chapter classifies them into two major etiologic groups: inherited and acquired. Inherited disorders vary in severity but usually affect one hemostatic component. Acquired syndromes may also differ in severity as well as complexity and characteristically involve multiple hemostatic components or pathways. The section describing inherited disorders is arranged to follow the reactive sequence of events in the intrinsic, extrinsic, and common coagulation pathways as well as fibrin stabilization processes (Chaps. 47 and 48). The acquired disorders that are discussed are diverse but represent syndromes frequently encountered in clinical practice.

INHERITED DISORDERS OF COAGULATION

Intrinsic Pathway Disorders

The purpose of the intrinsic pathway is to bring about the *in vitro* activation of factor X to Xa. Three proteins in the plasma, collectively termed the *contact phase* of coagulation, begin the intrinsic pathway. In this context, "contact" refers to the contact between plasma hemostatic components and artificial surfaces after which a chain of reactions ensues. The product of the contact phase is the activation of factor XI (XIa), which carries the intrinsic pathway forward (Chap. 48).

Factor XII (Hageman), prekallikrein (Fletcher), and high-molecular-weight kininogen (HMWK) are the three contact proteins, whereas factor XI (plasma thromboplastin antecedent or PTA) is their substrate and may also be referred to as a contact factor. All are synthesized by the liver. Since the contact phase is an *in vitro* phenomenon, patients deficient in either factor XII, prekallikrein, or HMWK generally are hemostatically competent and asymptomatic. These same three proteins represent biochemical connections of intrinsic coagulation to *in vivo* surface-mediated defense reactions such as stimulation of neutrophils.[14] In the absence of these contact factors, fibrin can be generated by other means. The intrinsic system is markedly slowed by a defective contact phase only when tested *in vitro*. C1 inhibitor is also considered a contact factor whose deficiency does not produce coagulation disturbances; rather, its absence is associated with pulmonary disease in the form of hereditary angioedema.[14]

The roles of the four contact proteins are interdependent, and their structures are related (Fig. 52-1). Prekallikrein and factor XI circulate complexed to HMWK. In the absence of HMWK, activation of prekallikrein and factor XI does not occur.[14] The role of the catalytic cofactor HMWK is to configure these substrates so that their reactive sites are available for factor XIIa.

Factor XII, prekallikrein, and HMWK have roles in the fibrinolytic system, in the activation of factor VII, and in the body's response to systemic infectious agents.[26] These roles probably dominate *in vivo*.

FACTOR XII (HAGEMAN FACTOR) DEFICIENCY

Factor XII deficiency is an autosomal recessive trait that can be expressed in homozygous or heterozygous forms. The homozygote, possessing two abnormal alleles, has no factor XII; heterozygotes demonstrate variance in their factor XII plasma concentrations.[14]

Clinical Findings. Patients homozygous for factor XII deficiency do not suffer from a bleeding disorder. In fact, they may be vulnerable to excessive clotting (thromboses). It is noteworthy that the index patient (the first to be described with this disorder), Hageman, succumbed to pulmonary embolism.[14]

Laboratory Findings and Therapy. Laboratory findings are normal except for determinations involving the intrinsic system such as a prolonged partial thromboplastin time (PTT). The PTT is corrected with both adsorbed plasma and aged serum (Chap. 49). Factor XII assays will confirm the deficiency. Generally, no therapy is necessary for this disorder, since the coagulation abnormality is only an *in vitro* phenomenon.

PREKALLIKREIN (FLETCHER FACTOR) DEFICIENCY

Fletcher factor deficiency is believed to be transmitted as an autosomal recessive trait. As in Hageman factor

deficiency, prekallikrein-deficient patients generally do not demonstrate clinical bleeding and may be vulnerable to thrombotic events. Seventy-five percent of Fletcher factor is bound to HMWK in circulation; 25% is free in plasma.[14]

The laboratory findings are similar to those in factor XII deficiency. However, the PTT results will shorten if the plasma is incubated with a surface-activating substance such as kaolin.[25]

HIGH-MOLECULAR-WEIGHT KININOGEN (WILLIAMS, FITZGERALD, FLAUJEAC FACTOR) DEFICIENCY

High-molecular weight kininogen (HMWK), normally facilitates contact activation of factor XII and prekallikrein. Its absence results in poor contact-phase reactions, a deficiency of kinin formation (active forms derived from kininogen), and defective fibrinolysis reactions.[12]

The autosomal recessive HMWK defect does not produce clinical bleeding. The PTT results typically are mildly prolonged; other tests are within reference ranges.

FACTOR XI DEFICIENCY (HEMOPHILIA C; ROSENTHAL SYNDROME)

Once factor XII is activated during contact-phase reactions, the active form (XIIa), in the presence of HMWK, enzymatically cleaves factor XI (PTA) to XIa. This reaction takes place on a phospholipid-rich surface, such as a cell membrane.

Factor XIa behaves as a serine protease and can cleave more factor XII to XIIa to amplify the contact reactions. The other substrate for factor XIa in the intrinsic system is factor IX.

Originally described in 1953, factor XI deficiency represents the first inherited disorder in the intrinsic cascade to which a clinical bleeding syndrome is attributed. The defect is thought to be a result of decreased synthesis of the protein rather than production of an abnormal molecule and is controlled by an incompletely recessive autosomal dominant trait found largely in Jewish populations.[7]

Clinical Findings. The disorder produces a mild bleeding syndrome that responds well to therapy. Most factor XI-deficient patients are symptomatically "silent" until stressed by trauma or surgery. The clinical syndrome may include episodes of epistaxis (nosebleeds), hematuria, and menorrhagia. Surgery or trauma produces exaggerated bleeding. The same patient may differ in the degree of bleeding response from one event to another.

Laboratory Findings and Therapy. Deficiencies of factor XI produce prolonged PTT values that are corrected by both adsorbed plasma and aged serum. Factor assay reveals the specific factor deficiency and activity levels. Factor XIa increases in concentration when exposed to glass or after storage at 4°C. This fact can interfere with laboratory testing for the factor if the test sample is not handled properly. One-stage prothrombin time (PT) values and bleeding time results are not affected. A two-

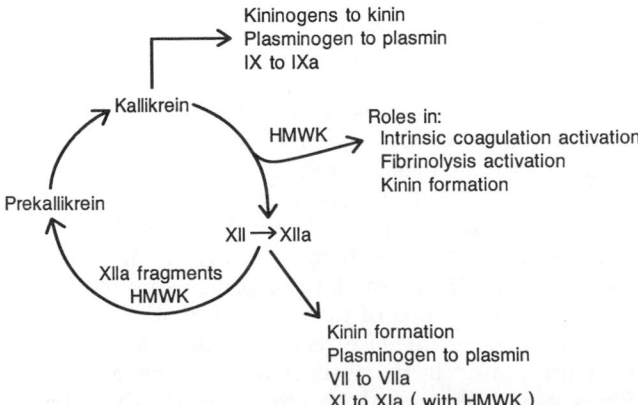

FIGURE 52-1. Interdependence of factors of contact activation phase of coagulation.

stage test utilizing a fluorogenic substrate to detect the presence of factor XIa has been described.[29]

No single specific blood component exists to treat factor XI deficiency. Fresh frozen plasma to maintain concentrations of 20% to 30% of normal activity will protect the patient.[7]

FACTOR X ACTIVATION PHASE DISORDERS

The activation of factor X may be considered the final reaction occurring in both intrinsic and extrinsic pathways, or conversely, it may be viewed as the first reaction of the "common" pathway. Once activated, factor Xa begins another series of reactions termed the common pathway leading to formation of fibrin. Factors VIII:C and IXa in the intrinsic pathway and the tissue factor–factor VIIa complex in the extrinsic pathway, in conjunction with lipid and Ca^{2+}, are required for the activation of factor X. Deficiencies of the factors necessary for the activation of factor X by way of the intrinsic pathway (VIII:C and IXa) cause serious bleeding disorders and occur frequently. Factor VII deficiency is rare.

FACTOR VIII:C DEFICIENCY (HEMOPHILIA A; CLASSIC HEMOPHILIA)

Classic hemophilia is recorded in antiquity. It is sometimes referred to as the "royal disease," because Queen Victoria of England was a carrier, and the condition eventually spread through Europe's royal families. It was first described scientifically in 1803. Much of the current knowledge about hemophilia A has evolved in the last 40 years.

Today, 85% of diagnosed congenital bleeding disorders are hemophilia A or factor VIII:C deficiency. Exact incidence figures are difficult to find, but best estimates cite 20 cases per 100,000 population.[7]

Hemophilia A is a sex-linked disorder transmitted on an X chromosome by carrier women to their sons. Carrier women produce clinically normal daughters who *may* carry the chromosomal defect. Sons of affected men are unaffected, but their daughters are obligatory carriers. One third of new cases occur spontaneously through mutations or variability in the expression of the X chromosome, causing skipped generations.

Factor VIII/vWF (or factor VIII complex) is a macromolecular complex circulating in plasma that consists of two distinct but related components (VIII:C and vWF). These two components have been characterized experimentally by their genetic, functional, and immunologic properties. Although there are a number of potential sites of factor VIII synthesis, the major production site appears to be the liver.[45,61] Table 52-1 presents the terms applied to this complex molecule. Figure 52-2 depicts the formation of the factor VIII/vWF complex and the pattern of inheritance of the two components.

The functional role of factor VIII:C is as cofactor to factor IXa for the activation of factor X to Xa. Thrombin is required to modify the structure of factor VIII:C in order for it to fulfill its role in accelerating the proteolytic action of factor IXa on factor X.

TABLE 52-1
Nomenclature for Factor VIII and von Willebrand Factor

VIII/vWF	The entire molecule as it circulates in the plasma. Composed of VIII:C and vWF protein portions noncovalently bound.
vWF	Glycoprotein responsible for binding to endothelium and supporting normal platelet adhesion and function; the carrier protein for VIII:C.
vWF:Ag	von Willebrand factor antigen as measured by immunoassay.
VIII:C	Intrinsic system cofactor to factor IXa (with Ca^{2+}) in the conversion of factor X to Xa. Tested by a clotting assay.
VIIIC:Ag	Antigenic property of procoagulant VIII:C as tested by immunoassay.
vWF:RCoF	Ristocetin (an antibiotic no longer used therapeutically) cofactor activity, which induces binding of vWF to platelets; reaction may be measured by aggregometry.
vWF B:Co	Botrocetin (a snake venom) cofactor activity, which detects vWF by inducing binding of vWF to platelets.
vW AgII	von Willebrand antigen II, a large propolypeptide of vWF released by platelets and endothelial cells along with vWF.

(From Montgomery RR, Coller BS: von Willebrand disease. In Colman RW, Hirsh J, Marder VJ, Salzman EW (eds): Hemostasis and Thrombosis: Basic Principles and Practice, 3rd ed, p 134. Philadelphia, PA, JB Lippincott, 1994.)

Clinical Findings. A bleeding diathesis arises from decreased or defective factor VIII:C. The severity of the disorder is tied to the degree of deficiency. Most severely affected patients possess less than 1% activity of factor VIII:C; moderately affected patients have 2% to 5% activity; and mildly affected patients generally have more than 5% activity. Clinical bleeding necessitating medical intervention occurs most frequently in severely afflicted hemophiliacs. Patients who maintain factor activity levels above 6% may remain clinically silent until traumatized or subjected to surgical procedures without prophylactic preparation. A patient's factor activity level remains fairly constant throughout life.

Typical bleeding episodes result from trauma but may be spontaneous in the most severe cases. Bleeding into soft tissues (hematomas) or joints (hemarthroses), epistaxis, hematuria, gastrointestinal or intracranial hemorrhages, and postoperative bleeding constitute the majority of hemorrhagic events in the hemophiliac. Repeated hemarthroses can cripple and deform over time. The joints of the knee, hip, elbow, ankle, and shoulder are most vulnerable. Taking analgesics such as aspirin during these events is contraindicated, because the drug inhibits platelet function.

Laboratory Findings. The screening test to detect factor VIII:C deficiency is the PTT. Prolonged PTT results that are corrected by fresh adsorbed plasma but not by serum

Factor VIII/vWF Complex Formation

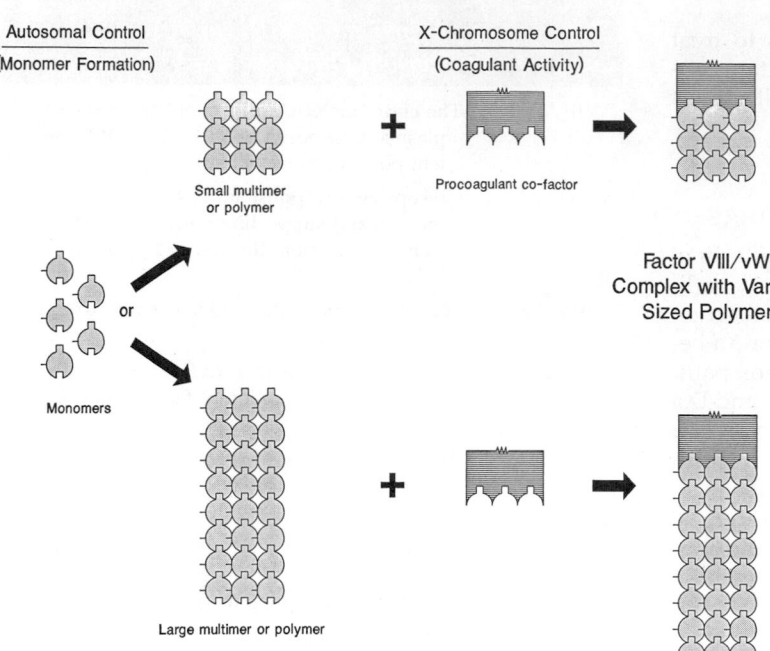

FIGURE 52-2. Factor VIII/vWF complex is composed of (a) procoagulant protein that is coded for by an X-linked gene (*at right*) and (b) a multimer that functions in platelet adhesion and whose synthesis is controlled by an autosomal gene (*at left*). For proper platelet adhesion, larger multimer complexes are necessary.

and results of factor VIII:C assays identify the deficiency and characterize the activity levels. Obligatory carriers have been detected by combined factor VIII:C and VIII:CAg assays. Genotypic detection of an abnormal VIII:C molecule is available through analysis of areas within or close to the VIII or XI gene.[27,33,44,47]

Therapy. The therapy for hemophilia A involves many issues. Replacement of factor VIII:C by infusion of concentrate products is done when the goal is to arrest bleeding. Simple estimation of dosage assumes that each unit of VIII:C (amount of factor VIII:C in 1 mL of normal plasma) infused per kilogram of body weight will invoke a 2% increase in the VIII:C level in plasma.[36] The VIII:C assay (not the PTT) should be used to monitor successful therapy.[57] Factor VIII:C levels of 30% will stop most bleeding into joints or muscles. Deeper joint bleeding and hematomas mandate 50% activity levels. Gastrointestinal bleeding, dental extractions, and surgery necessitate 80% to 100% activity levels.[7] The half-life of factor VIII in plasma is between 8 and 12 hours.

The decision to administer prophylactic (preventive) infusions depends on less well defined criteria: cost, availability, setting, age, status of joints, frequency of bleeding episodes, risk of hepatitis or AIDS, and the psychologic adjustment of the patient and family members. In milder cases, pharmacologic agents such as 1-desamino-8-D-arginine-vasopressin (DDAVP) may be substituted for donor products. This synthetic analog of the antidiuretic hormone 8-arginine vasopressin increases plasma factor VIII:C by causing its release from endogenous stores. Intravenous administration of DDAVP to mild hemophiliac patients may raise plasma levels of factor VIII:C threefold to sixfold. Baseline plasma levels of factor VIII:C must be sufficient so that an increase invoked by DDAVP will protect the patient.

Human factor VIII concentrates are variably treated by manufacturers to inactivate viruses and yield predictable products for dosage calculation. The cost per unit of factor VIII:C in these products is determined by the manufacturing and purification processes used. Hepatitis B virus (HBV) transmission has occurred even with the viricidal treatments employed with these products. HBV vaccinations are recommended for hemophilia patients. Human immunodeficiency virus (HIV) infection in hemophiliacs has been virtually eliminated by heat treatment of the concentrate products.[9] Recombinant products are now available which bypass the virus hazard (Recombinate or Kogenate). Persons with blood group A or B erythrocytes may have a hemolytic reaction to large doses of concentrates owing to exposure to anti-A or anti-B antibodies in the products. Group O cells should be used for transfusion when necessary.[53]

Inhibitors of (antibodies to) factor VIII:C have been recognized in patients with hemophilia A, in post-partum patients, in various immune disorders, and spontaneously in patients with no underlying disorder.[21] Inhibitors occur in 5% to 10% of hemophilia A patients, with the majority occurring in severe cases (<3% factor VIII:C).[5,31] These inhibitors appear without regard to the number of transfused products received or the type of product used. No linkage has been established between the major histocompatibility complex and the response to factor VIII:C. There is no method to determine who will develop antibodies and who will not. The antibodies are immunoglobulin G (IgG) with κ light chains, and γ_4 heavy chains.[54] These antibodies are characteristically found in patients who fail to respond to infusions of factor VIII:C products but who previously had responded well. A single patient may respond differently from infusion to infusion.[21]

Plasmapheresis may be employed to purge the antibody from plasma. Porcine factor VIII:C concentrates have been used because of the low cross-reactivity between human factor VIII:C antibodies and porcine factor VIII. Prothrombin complex concentrates present another option for patients with high titers of antibody. These concentrates bypass the need for factor VIII:C by providing factors II, VII, IX, and X, some of which may be activated. Use of these concentrates usually is reserved for life-threatening situations.

A modified PTT will detect weak inhibitors. In this procedure, a 4:1 patient-to-normal plasma mixture is incubated with a Kaolin-cephalin suspension for 2 hours at 37°C prior to recalcification.[17,37] The Bethesda inhibitor assay may be used to quantitate the inhibitor[32] (Chap. 49). The choice of therapy is dependent on the severity of the hemorrhage and the patient's previous response (titer) to infused concentrates.

FACTOR IX DEFICIENCY (HEMOPHILIA B; CHRISTMAS DISEASE)

In 1947, Pavlovsky demonstrated that *in vitro* mixing of plasmas from two "hemophilia" patients resulted in correction of the recalcification time of both plasmas.[43] At that time, all male patients exhibiting hemophilia symptoms were thought to have classic hemophilia; had that been the case, those results should not have been obtained. In 1952, other investigators found hemophilia patients who possessed factor VIII in their plasma but whose serum did not contain another substance that required vitamin K for synthesis and could be adsorbed to barium salts. The factor, now known as factor IX, was named plasma thromboplastin component (PTC) or Christmas factor for the surname of one index patient.

Clinical Findings. Factor IX deficiency (hemophilia B) is a sex-linked recessive trait and is expressed in mild, moderate, and severe forms. It generally is considered to be a milder form of hemophilia than factor VIII:C deficiency because clinically, these patients are not as prone to hemorrhages in the gastrointestinal tract, abdomen, central nervous system, or genitourinary tract. However, the severely factor IX–deficient patient is clinically indistinguishable from the factor VIII:C–deficient patient. Hemophilia B may occur as a result of synthesizing a dysfunctional factor IX molecule or decreased concentrations of the molecule.

Variants of the disease depend on the basis of the antigenic reactivity of factor IX:Ag. If the antigen reacts with specific antibody, the patient is termed cross-reactive material positive (CRM+); if the antigen is undetectable, the patient is termed CRM−; if the antigen reactivity is reduced but detectable, the patient is termed CRM[R] (reduced). Patients who are CRM+ have been the most extensively studied. No correlation exists between antigen presence and clotting activity (IX:C) of the factor IX molecule.[49] Carriers of hemophilia B have low procoagulant (IX:C) levels in plasma. Measurement of both IX:Ag and IX:C activity levels increases the accuracy of determining carrier status.[7]

Laboratory Findings. Moderate to severe factor IX:C deficiency is revealed by a prolonged PTT that is corrected with aged serum but not with adsorbed plasma. Mild cases can produce a PTT value within normal limits, yet

these patients may exhibit severe bleeding with trauma or surgery. The one-stage PT test using rabbit brain or lung thromboplastin will be within reference limits, but ox brain thromboplastin testing may reveal an abnormal result in a subgroup of these patients. Specific factor IX:C assay procedures are used for diagnosis and to assess activity levels during therapy. Severely affected patients may have activity levels below 1%. Moderately affected patients possess 1% to 5% of normal activity, and mild affliction is manifested as 6% to 49% activity.[50]

Therapy. Therapy involves either commercial concentrate products or human single-donor plasma units. Because of volume considerations, single plasma unit infusions may be unable to increase the activity to a level needed for hemostasis. One unit of factor IX activity is equal to the activity of factor IX in 1.0 mL of normal plasma. Calculations of dosage reveal that infusion of unrealistically large quantities of plasma would be necessary to bring factor IX activity levels to more than 20% of normal in most deficient patients. Commercial concentrates can achieve higher levels of activity in smaller infusion volumes but have the same infection risks discussed for factor VIII concentrates. Heparin is administered with these products to minimize the thrombotic risk, and the timing of the infusion is controlled over a short period. Concentrates are reserved for use in life-threatening situations. The promise of recombinant concentrates will eliminate the infection risk. Plasma exchanges with normal donor plasma have been performed to achieve greater than 50% activity levels and prevent cardiac overload.

Laboratory monitoring of the patient is achieved by factor IX:C assays before and after therapy. Factor IX:C activity levels of 20% to 30% will initially correct minor soft-tissue hemorrhages. Correction of hematuria, body cavity hemorrhage, central nervous system hemorrhage, or gastrointestinal bleeding requires activity levels greater than 50%. Dosage estimates are based on the premise that if one unit (activity of the factor in 1.0 mL of normal plasma) of factor IX:C is infused per kilogram of body weight, a 1% increase in the plasma level will occur.[7]

VON WILLEBRAND DISEASE

In 1926, Eric von Willebrand described the disorder that bears his name as an autosomal dominant trait that produces a prolonged bleeding time and evidence of vascular fragility.[62] Patients with this disease are vulnerable to bruising, epistaxis, menorrhagia, and hemorrhage from tooth extraction.

von Willebrand disease is now known to be an autosomal trait with either dominant or recessive inheritance. Both the factor VIII:C and the von Willebrand factor (vWF) of the factor VIII complex previously described (see Fig. 52-2) are involved. An important contribution by Zimmerman and associates in 1971 demonstrated that the vWF portion of the VIII complex (VIII/vWF) is reduced or absent in von Willebrand disease.[64] In that same year, it was demonstrated that platelets in von Willebrand plasma, in contrast to platelets in normal plasma, do not aggregate in the presence of an antibiotic called ristocetin.[8] The ristocetin effect is secondary to a lack of vWF (or factor vWF:RCoF) in the plasma,[16] since von Willebrand platelets react normally when placed in normal plasma.

Structural defects in the factor VIII complex in this disorder result in the production of a variety of vWF multimer combinations in plasma (see Fig. 52-2). Although decreased, the factor VIII:C component is nearly always present, as is vWF:Ag. Variation in the multimer sizes of vWF, and detectable presence of the vWF:Ag and vWF:RCoF in plasma is the basis for identifying variant types of this disease (Table 52-2).

von Willebrand disease is the most frequently inherited coagulopathy. True incidence figures are difficult to cite because many cases are clinically silent and thus undiscovered. No racial or ethnic prevalence is observed. Sometimes, the disorder is not manifested until adulthood when the patient is surgically or traumatically stressed. Cases of acquired von Willebrand disease have been reported[11,18,24,28,48] and generally are associated with autoimmune or lymphoproliferative disorders, in which abnormal antibodies are generated against the vWF. Treatment of the primary disease ameliorates the symptoms of acquired von Willebrand disease.

Clinical Findings. Bleeding appears to be more severe in children and decreases in severity with age. Muscular hematomas and hemarthroses are rare unless the patient inherits the autosomal recessive form of the disease. Type I and type II diseases (see Table 52-2)[51] are the most common forms of von Willebrand disease. In liver disease or pregnancy, levels of vWF are increased and clinical presentation will differ. Under these circumstances, patients with type I disease may have correction of the hemostatic defect; patients with type II disease will not.[1,42,58]

Laboratory Findings. Typical laboratory data include prolonged bleeding time, equivocal PTT results (depending on plasma levels of factor VIII:C), decreased activity of factor VIII:C, abnormal ristocetin-induced platelet agglutination or aggregation (vWF:RCoF), varying to absent levels of intermediate or large vWF multimers, and decreased quantities of vWF:Ag.

Therapy. Therapy is targeted at increasing levels of factor VIII:C in plasma and replacing functional vWF large multimers in circulation to shorten the bleeding time. Current therapy for von Willebrand disease employs the most conservative route, using DDAVP[38] whenever appropriate to avoid the risk of transfusion-transmitted disease. DDAVP may be administered intravenously and monitored by vWF:RCoF activity.[19] Concentrates of human material are used if tachyphylaxis occurs with DDAVP. Use of DDAVP requires attention to electrolyte balance, and concomitant administration of antifibrinolytic agents may be employed in some patients for oral surgery. Investigations are under way to administer DDAVP in intranasal mists for mucosal absorption.[35] If human material is required to control hemorrhage, cryoprecipitate or factor VIII concentrates containing sufficient quantities of intact large vWF multimers are the products of choice.[3]

Extrinsic and Common Pathway Disorders

In order for the extrinsic system to become operative, tissue damage and the release of tissue factor must occur. In the presence of Ca^{2+} and tissue factor, plasma factor VII is activated which, in turn, activates factor X to Xa.

TABLE 52-2
Classification of Types of von Willebrand Disease

Type	Mode of Inheritance	Effect	Results
I (Classic and most common)	Autosomal dominant	Variable; mild to moderate	Reduced vWF:Ag & vWF:RCoF; all multimers present; good response to DDAVP
IIA	Autosomal dominant	Variable	Reduced vWF:Ag and more severely reduced vWF:RCoF; loss of both intermediate & large multimers in plasma and platelets; poor response to DDAVP
IIB	Autosomal dominant	Variable	Mild reductions in vWF:Ag and variable effect on vWF:RCoF; lack of high MW multimers; platelet vWF multimers are intact in quantity & structure; thrombocytopenia especially after DDAVP
IIC	Autosomal recessive	Variable; moderate to severe	Rare; large multimers are absent in plasma; structure of complex multimers varies
III	Autosomal recessive	Severe	Heterozygotes are asymptomatic; homozygotes & doubly heterozygous patients lack vWF:Ag, vWF:RCoF, and all multimer sizes; VIII:C levels are low; no response to DDAVP
Platelet vW disease (pseudo vW disease)	Autosomal dominant	Variable	A platelet disorder; abnormal GPIb receptor on platelets; absent large vWF multimers which are bound to abnormal GP1b receptors; thrombocytopenia & large platelet forms on stained film; platelets aggregate with low concentrations of ristocetin; treat with transfusion of platelets

Note: The Subcommittee on von Willebrand Factor of the Scientific and Standardization Committee of the International Society on Thrombosis and Haemostasis has proposed a new phenotypic classification system for von Willebrand disorder subtypes.[51]
(From Montgomery RR, Coller BS: von Willebrand disease. In Colman RW, Hirsh J, Marder VJ, Salzman EW (eds): Hemostasis and Thrombosis: Basic Principles and Practice, 3rd ed, p 134. Philadelphia, PA, JB Lippincott, 1994.)

The intrinsic and extrinsic systems possess interrelated feedback loops. Examples include the ability of active factor XII (XIIf) fragments to amplify the activity of factor VII, the ability of factor IXa to activate factor VII, and the ability of factor VIIa to activate both factors IX and X (Chap. 48).

Factor Xa begins the common pathway. In combination with phospholipid, Ca^{2+}, and cofactor V, factor Xa will convert prothrombin (factor II) to thrombin (factor IIa), which in turn converts fibrinogen (factor I) to fibrin.

FACTOR VII DEFICIENCY

Factor VII deficiency is an autosomal recessive abnormality with intermediate expression. It is rare, occurring in approximately 1 in 500,000 individuals. Variants exist, labeled CRM+ and CRM[R] according to their antigenic reactivity. The behavior of this factor can vary in testing procedures depending on the tissue source of the thromboplastin used. Correlation between clinical bleeding tendency and activity levels in assays is poor.

Clinical Findings. Hemorrhage from mucous membranes and into soft tissues occurs most frequently in children. Adult heterozygotes usually tolerate surgery well but may be vulnerable to thrombotic events.

Laboratory Findings and Therapy. Diagnosis of factor VII deficiency is based on a family history and demonstrated prolongation of the one-stage PT, whereas the PTT and thrombin clotting time (TCT) results are within reference ranges. This is the only factor deficiency in which the PT is the single observed abnormality. Specific factor VII assay confirms the diagnosis; affected patients demonstrate 10% to 20% of normal activity. It should be noted that factor VII levels increase during pregnancy.

Donor plasma and serum components and commercial concentrates containing the prothrombin complex factors are used for replacement therapy.

FACTOR X (STUART-PROWER FACTOR) DEFICIENCY

Factor X was recognized as unique and given its numeral in 1959. The index patients' surnames (Stuart and Prower) are synonymous with factor X. Deficiency of this factor is inherited as an autosomal trait that is incompletely recessive but shows high penetrance. Immune variants (CRM+, CRM−, and CRM[R]) exist. This disorder is uncommon in the general population, although nine variants have been described.

Clinical Findings. The symptoms of factor X deficiency are highly variable. Patients may exhibit lifelong histories of bruising, soft-tissue bleeding, or postsurgical or posttrauma hemorrhages. All possible acquired causes, as well as the possibility of multiple factor deficiencies, must be eliminated in making the diagnosis.

Laboratory Findings and Therapy. The deficiency produces a prolonged PT and PTT and a prothrombin utilization abnormality. Specific factor X assay procedures are diagnostic. The PT is corrected by aged serum but not by adsorbed plasma.

Frozen plasma components or prothrombin complex concentrates (Konyne 80®) are used for therapy. Activity levels of 10% to 40% of normal are considered adequate for hemostasis.

FACTOR V DEFICIENCY (OWREN DISEASE; LABILE FACTOR DEFICIENCY)

Factor V deficiency was discovered in 1944 in Norway by Professor Owren. He demonstrated that adsorbed normal plasma, when added to his patient's plasma, corrected the prolonged PT. Other investigators subsequently described similar findings.

An autosomal recessive trait, factor V deficiency is demonstrated by homozygotes and is mild to silent in heterozygotes. Factor V also has been described as being deficient in conjunction with factor VIII:C (V–VIII deficiency) in another group of patients.[22,23,59] A variety of autoimmune disorders is known to produce mixtures of IgG and IgM antibodies to factor V, resulting in an acquired form of the disease.[20]

Clinical Findings. Factor V activity that is less than 10% of normal results in hemorrhagic diatheses. Clinical episodes are similar to those in the mild to moderate hemophilias. Deficiencies of platelet-borne factor V (platelet factor 1) may cause an abnormal bleeding time and seem to precipitate more clinical problems than decreases in plasma factor V levels do. It is suggested that activated platelet-borne factor V is the binding site for activated plasma factor X (Xa) and factor II (prothrombin).

Laboratory Findings and Therapy. Both the PT and the PTT are prolonged. If the PT is corrected with adsorbed normal plasma, evidence points to factor V deficiency. Platelet aggregation studies are normal. The possibility of combined (multiple) factor deficiencies must be eliminated. The specific factor V assay is considered diagnostic.

Therapy requires infusion of fresh frozen plasma, since factor V is labile in storage. Plasma activity levels of 25% to 30% of normal are sufficient in most cases to ensure hemostasis. Because of the apparent platelet involvement in this disorder, aspirin products should be avoided. The plasma supernatant fluid, removed after cryoprecipitates have formed in component preparations (cryo-free plasma), contains adequate levels of factor V when fresh and is used in some locations.

FACTOR II (PROTHROMBIN) DEFICIENCY

Factor II deficiency may be inherited as either a deficiency or a dysfunction and is rare in the general population. Hypoprothrombinemia is an autosomal recessive trait. Homozygotes have assayed levels of 2% to 25% of normal, whereas heterozygotes maintain levels of 50% or greater. Twenty-three variants of dysfunctional prothrombin molecules have been reported.[4,30,55,56]

Clinical Findings. Patients with less than 50% activity exhibit mild bleeding tendencies similar to those seen in mild hemophilia. Hemarthroses are rare. Medications containing aspirin may cause bleeding tendencies.

Laboratory Findings and Therapy. Laboratory values differ with activity levels of factor II. Both the PTT and one-stage PT are prolonged. The thrombin clotting time (TCT) procedure produces normal results. Diagnostic procedures include an assay for prothrombin activity and immune-based factor assays using antiprothrombin antisera.[55] Dysprothrombinemic patients will produce abnormal results in the activity (functional) assay but a normal immunologic (quantitative) assay. Care should be taken to rule out vitamin K deficiency, liver disease, and multifactor defects.

Therapy depends on which type of disorder is present and on its severity of expression. Fresh frozen plasma is the usual choice. Vitamin K–dependent protein concentrates (Konyne 80®) are also available but carry a risk of thrombosis.

FACTOR I (FIBRINOGEN) DEFICIENCY

A defect in fibrin formation may be the result of an inherited lack of fibrinogen (afibrinogenemia), an inherited deficiency of fibrinogen (hypofibrinogenemia), or an inherited production of a dysfunctional fibrinogen molecule (dysfibrinogenemia). The condition is rare. Afibrinogenemic patients have nearly undetectable amounts of fibrinogen; hypofibrinogenemic patients possess less than 100 mg/dL (reference range, 200–400 mg/dL), and in both cases, the molecular structure of fibrinogen is normal. Substitution of amino acids in fibrinogen's polypeptide chains produces a structural change (dysfibrinogenemia) that may result in (1) the inability to submit to proteolysis by thrombin, because the cleavage sites are inappropriate; (2) peculiar behavior during polymerization stages secondary to aberrant charge distribution across the molecule; (3) the addition of "dangling" (inappropriate) side groups that affect reactivity; or (4) the persistence of fetal fibrinogen into adulthood. Many variants involving these four possibilities have been described.[41] These patients demonstrate abnormal fibrinogen function but have normal levels when immunologic assays are performed.

All three forms of fibrinogen disorders are inherited as autosomal traits. Afibrinogenemia is recessive in expression and clinically severe. Hypofibrinogenemia and dysfibrinogenemia are phenotypically dominant, and bleeding episodes are less severe.

Afibrinogenemic patients' platelets appear to be affected because the bleeding time may be prolonged. Platelets have a surface receptor for fibrinogen, and fibrinogen apparently is necessary for platelet function *in vivo*.

A host of acquired disorders may reduce the plasma fibrinogen concentration. Examples include renal disease, hepatic disease, and "consumptive" disorders such as disseminated intravascular coagulation. The history and clinical features aid in the differentiation between inherited and acquired forms.

Clinical Findings. Hemorrhages in afibrinogenemia and hypofibrinogenemia differ in severity. With a complete lack of fibrinogen, spontaneous bleeding has occurred. Mucosal, intestinal, and intracranial sites are most commonly affected. Surgery and trauma present risks commensurate with the concentration of functional fibrinogen available, and poor wound healing has been observed.

Laboratory Findings. All laboratory tests that depend on fibrin formation will be prolonged in afibrinogenemia, whereas they may or may not be prolonged in hypofibrinogenemia. Thrombin and reptilase clotting times are sensitive to fibrinogen levels as well as function. Fibrinogen assays that do not depend on clot formation will differentiate decreased levels from abnormal function. Routine screening procedures such as the PTT and PT return variable results. Addition of reagent fibrinogen corrects these endpoints.

Postcoagulation Stabilization Defects

FACTOR XIII (FIBRIN-STABILIZING FACTOR) DEFICIENCY

Clinical Findings. A rare disorder, factor XIII deficiency is an autosomal recessive trait in which only homozygotes express the syndrome. The homozygous patient exhibits spontaneous bleeding and poor wound healing with unusual scar formation. General symptoms are similar to those of mild hemophilia. The syndrome is incompatible with pregnancy unless replacement therapy is provided throughout gestation. All such patients should avoid aspirin products.

Laboratory Findings and Therapy. Inadequate cross-linking of fibrin results in an unstable and friable clot with excessive red cell "fall out." Such unstable fibrin clots incubated in 5 M urea or 1% monochloroacetic acid dissolve rapidly. If adequate controls for excessive fibrinolysis are included, this test is relatively specific. The condition cannot be evaluated in the presence of heparin. Elaborate specific factor XIII assay procedures are available, and immunologic procedures exist.

Therapy is accomplished with infusion of donor plasma or commercial purified, lyophilized placental factor XIII.

ACQUIRED ABNORMALITIES OF COAGULATION AND FIBRINOLYSIS

Acquired Disorders

HEPATIC DISEASE

The liver is the principal site of synthesis of procoagulant and fibrinolytic proteins as well as coagulation inhibitory proteins. Liver disorders present two challenges: decreased synthesis of coagulation, lysis, and inhibitory proteins, and impaired clearance of activated hemostatic components.

The type of disorder differs in neonates and adults. Neonates display decreased levels of coagulation factors secondary to hepatic immaturity. They also lack sufficient levels of plasminogen and antithrombin III. In addition, neonates express a unique fetal fibrinogen that does not behave in the same manner as adult fibrinogen, and they have decreased levels of fibrinogen (hypodysfibrinogenemia). Decreased vitamin K–dependent factors in the neonate are discussed later in this chapter.

In adults, parenchymal liver diseases, such as cirrhosis and hepatitis, and diseases that infiltrate liver tissue, such as neoplasm, affect the synthetic capacity of the organ. Hemostatic changes often are subtle. Prolongation of the PT is considered a sign of worsening disease and may be caused by depression of vitamin K–dependent factor synthesis, poor dietary intake, or malabsorption of vitamin K. Fibrinolytic events and thrombocytopenia may also accompany liver disease.

Laboratory Findings and Therapy. Screening tests such as the PT, PTT, TCT, bleeding time, platelet count, fibrinogen levels, and fibrin split products determinations are used to monitor hemostatic status in liver disease.

Infusion of fresh plasma may bolster the circulating levels of procoagulants and minimize the hemorrhagic risk. Commercial prothrombin complex concentrates generally are not used in liver disease because of increased risk of thrombosis due to depressed levels of available inhibitory antithrombin III.

VITAMIN K DEFICIENCY

Vitamin K is a necessary cofactor for the conversion of terminal glutamic acid residues to γ-carboxyglutamic acid on factors II, VII, IX, and X as well as on protein C. This conversion takes place in the hepatocyte and is necessary for proper function. Vitamin K is produced by the normal flora of the gastrointestinal tract and absorbed. Deficiencies can occur if the normal flora is not present (because of broad-spectrum oral antibiotics), if absorption is decreased (obstructive jaundice), or if antagonistic drugs (coumarin family) are taken. Vitamin K may be a required dietary supplement for the neonate, because the supply through the placenta is minimal during gestation, and the gut is sterile for several days after birth. Less than 10% activity levels of prothrombin (factor II) in newborn plasma may result in hemorrhage. Premature infants are even more susceptible.

Breast-fed babies are more prone to vitamin K deficiency than are babies on prepared formulas, because maternal milk provides less of the vitamin than babies require. Breast milk also is sterile; therefore, seeding of the newborn gut with bacteria is further retarded. Injections of vitamin K administered to neonates help to overcome this temporary deficiency. Maternal drugs should be screened to ascertain that no antagonists to vitamin K are being ingested and transferred by way of milk to the baby. The one-stage PT is used to assess levels of vitamin K–dependent coagulation factors in the newborn when clinically indicated.

Therapeutic Anticoagulation

HEPARIN

Heparin is the intravenous anticoagulant most frequently used in clinical medicine. It is used extensively in specimen collection for laboratory studies and in preventing fibrin deposition on intravenous tubing devices residing in vessels. Heparin is an acid mucopolysaccharide that acts in conjunction with antithrombin III to inhibit most of the serine proteases in the coagulation pathways. It is metabolized by the liver and has a half-life of approximately 3 hours.

COUMARIN DRUGS (ORAL ANTICOAGULANTS)

The oral anticoagulants were discovered in Wisconsin during an investigation of hemorrhagic disease in cattle. The herds were consuming contaminated fodder containing spoiled sweet clover, which contains bishydroxycoumarin that caused the bleeding.

Warfarin is the most frequently used coumarin. It is water soluble and is administered orally. It is absorbed in the small bowel and circulates loosely bound to albumin in plasma. It can cross the placenta and appear in breast milk. Warfarin interferes with the carboxylation of the vitamin K–dependent plasma factors in the liver by interrupting the enzymatic phase of this reaction. This results in nonfunctional proteins circulating in plasma that are referred to as **p**roteins **i**nduced by **v**itamin **K** **a**ntagonist (PIVKA), or noncarboxylated K–dependent factors.

Circulating Anticoagulant (Inhibitory) Substances

Substances produced by the body that inhibit coagulation are termed *circulating anticoagulants*. Such products are considered pathologic and are produced in response to a variety of stimuli. The majority of these substances are immunoglobulins, and the existence of an antibody to each of the protein procoagulants has been demonstrated. Stimuli include infusion of blood or blood products, release of tumor substances into the circulation, and autoimmune disorders.

Inhibitory activity directed against factor VIII/vWF and factor IX has been discussed with the deficiency states. The laboratory results in the presence of such activity will mimic those seen in the hemophiliac states.

In 1960, an inhibitor was described in 5% to 10% of patients with systemic lupus erythematosus (SLE). Affected patients exhibited prolonged whole-blood clotting times and PTs.[46] A similar circulating anticoagulant activity has since been documented in patients who have drug-induced lupus and other immune disorders or malignant tumors, as well as in persons exhibiting no primary disease, thus rendering the term "lupus anticoagulant" a misnomer. The term *antiphospholipid antibody* may be more appropriate. Patients treated with phenothiazine, procainamide, hydralazine, quinidine, and long-term chlorpromazine are especially likely to produce these inhibitors.[2,10,13,63]

The lupus anticoagulant (LA) is more often associated with incidents of thrombosis than hemorrhage (Chap. 53). The LA has been documented in cases of acute viral infection in children and of HIV infection, and as an incidental medical discovery in patients with no underlying disorder. The antibody (anticoagulant) is IgG, IgM, or a combination in some patients, and is directed against *in vitro* procoagulant phospholipids in testing systems.

Other antiphospholipid immunoglobulins have been described against negatively charged phospholipids such as cardiolipin. Antiphospholipid activity interferes with many reactions in the coagulation pathways and reagent systems of phospholipid composition.

Patients exhibit a prolonged PTT, which remains prolonged when mixed with normal plasma. The sensitivity of the PTT to detect the presence of antiphospholipids depends on the makeup of the phospholipid reagent used. Detection of 80% to 90% of patients with antiphospholipid immunoglobulins is possible with commercially available products.[21] Rabbit brain phospholipid added to the PTT mixture has a sensitivity of 97% in detection of the LA.[21] The dilute Russell's viper venom time (dRVVT) test (Chap. 49), which is prolonged in the presence of LA, is also a sensitive phospholipid-dependent clotting test similar to the PTT.[39,60] An ELISA procedure employing human brain tissue as the antigen has been developed and is considered both sensitive and specific.[6] A comparison of sensitivities of various procedures to detect the LA has been published.[34] See Chapter 49 for a description of these and other tests for antiphospholipid immunoglobulins and Chapter 53 for a discussion of the thrombotic effects caused by these immunoglobulins.

Increased levels of fibrin(ogen) split (degradation) products (FSP or FDP), as seen in disseminated intravascular coagulation (DIC) and fibrinolytic disorders, exert an anticoagulant effect. The FSP interfere with the polymerization of fibrin strands and combine with procoagulant molecules in plasma to form complexes incapable of normal coagulant reactivity. If necessary, fibrin formation is controlled to limit the quantities of FSP produced. Laboratory procedures used to evaluate this process include latex D-dimer and FSP agglutination tests (Chap. 50), platelet counts, fibrinogen levels, PTT, and PT.[39]

Massive Transfusion Effects

Approximately 30% of patients who are transfused with large numbers of whole blood units have hemostatic problems. The leading defects are dilutional thrombocytopenia

and decreased levels of factors V and VIII. If extensive tissue damage and subsequent release of tissue factor have occurred, DIC may be precipitated, which will aggravate replacement therapy by consuming infused procoagulant material. Naturally occurring inhibitors will be consumed as well as procoagulants.[15]

Artificial Surface Effects

The demonstrated consequences of exposing blood to an artificial surface include the formation of thrombi and emboli, consumption of procoagulant proteins and platelets, alteration of the function of these proteins, and incitement of systemic syndromes (fever, vasoconstriction, and bronchial constriction).[52] When blood and an artificial surface meet, plasma proteins, especially fibrinogen, coat the exposed area (Fig. 52-3). Platelets may or may not attach, spread, and degranulate. Antifibrinogen antibodies do not react with layered fibrinogen, giving support to the theory that the deposited protein has changed its antigenic properties. The protein coat may change its composition over time, becoming less thrombogenic as it ages.

In the presence of complement, neutrophils and macrophages are attracted to protein-coated artificial surfaces and may assist in debriding the surface of both platelets and protein. Aggregates of leukocytes may form and be displaced into the circulation, forming microemboli as a result of complement activation.

The PTT, PT, platelet count, fibrinogen level, plasminogen level, antithrombin III assay, and FSP determinations may all be used to evaluate and monitor the effects of blood perfusing an artificial surface.

Disseminated Intravascular Coagulation

Disseminated intravascular coagulation (DIC) is a complication of other primary disorders. It results in consumption of coagulation proteins and platelets into thrombi, which are deposited locally or widely in the circulation. Coagulation and fibrinolytic processes occur simultaneously, and either one may dominate at a given time.

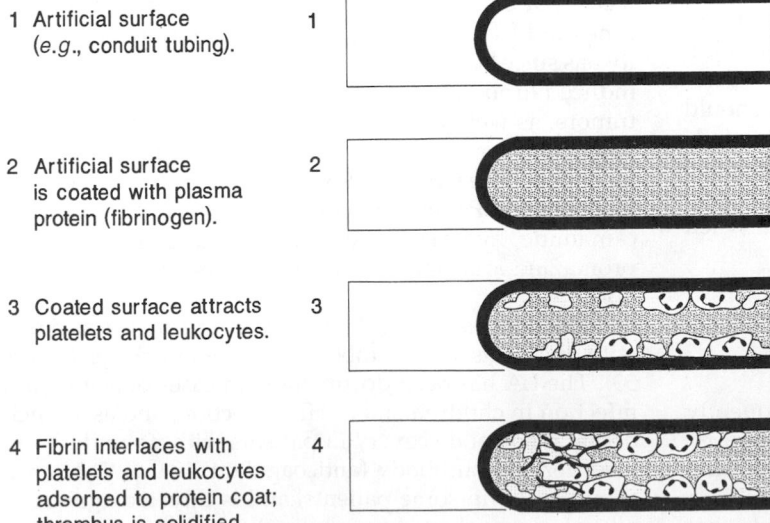

1 Artificial surface
   (e.g., conduit tubing).

2 Artificial surface
   is coated with plasma
   protein (fibrinogen).

3 Coated surface attracts
   platelets and leukocytes.

4 Fibrin interlaces with
   platelets and leukocytes
   adsorbed to protein coat;
   thrombus is solidified.

FIGURE 52-3. Interaction of blood components with artificial surface.

There is no age group or gender preference for DIC, and much variation occurs in its clinical presentation. The single common thread connecting all versions of DIC is the liberation of a thromboplastic substance that subsequently results in coagulation. Plasmin is activated by the contact phase reactions or by tissue activators released by damaged cells (see Fig. 48-3). The progress of DIC may be controlled by plasmin or thrombin at any given moment, which results in a dominant clinical exhibition of either lysis or thrombosis.

Damage to tissue and the resulting release of tissue substances brings about activation of coagulation. Endothelial cells may be damaged by bacterial toxins, hypoxic shock, acidosis, antigen–antibody reactions, overwhelming infections, and malignancies.[40] Thromboplastic substances also can be injected directly into the circulation through insect or snake bites or released along with plasminogen activators in obstetric complications, malignant diseases, and syndromes involving severe tissue trauma (burns, heat strokes, surgery, or crush injuries). Acute DIC develops in a matter of hours, and hemorrhage nearly always occurs; skin signs of purpura, gangrene, and bullae may appear.

Hemorrhage in chronic DIC is less frequent. Examples of conditions which can precipitate chronic DIC include neoplastic tumors, acute promyelocytic leukemia, liver disease, or retained dead fetus syndrome.

Laboratory evidence that DIC is in progress includes prolonged TCT, PT, and PTT; decreased platelet, fibrinogen, and AT-III levels; and elevated FSP. The D-dimer test (Chap. 50) is positive. Peripheral blood films may reveal erythrocyte fragments and decreased numbers of platelets. Hemoglobin and hematocrit values reflect the severity of hemorrhage.

Use of heparin in the treatment of DIC is controversial. Heparin may be of benefit if (1) thrombosis is damaging organ function; (2) reversal of the damage is possible; and (3) there are no contraindications to the use of heparin. It is most important to correct the disorder that invoked the DIC in the first place.

Replacement therapy with blood components may be necessary following acute DIC to control hemorrhaging. Fresh frozen plasma, platelet concentrates, and cryoprecipitate may be used. A complete profile of coagulation and lysis tests should be performed at clinically deter-

TABLE 52-3
Drug Interactions with Hemostatic Systems

Drug	Hemostatic Effect
Penicillin G (carbenicillin and ticarcillin)	Increases bleeding time; impairs platelet function, aggregation & interaction of vWF with platelets
DDAVP (1-desamino-8-D-arginine vasopressin)	Increases plasma levels of VIII:C by releasing endogenous stores of the protein; can shorten the PTT
Isoniazid (INH)	Can induce thrombocytopenia; increase bleeding time; stimulate production of inhibitors of factors I, V, and XIII after long-term exposure
Estrogen therapy (contraceptive/replacement)	Slight decrease in platelet numbers; has potential to provoke deep vein thrombosis; can degranulate platelets and shorten baseline coagulation tests
Aspirin products	Prolongs bleeding time; interferes with aggregation reactions
Dextran; high-molecular weight products	Increases bleeding time and impairs aggregation reactions; lowers circulating levels of vWF:Ag and vWF
Cephalosporins	Prolongs the PT; can provoke a thrombocytopenia or a thrombocytosis
Phenothiazines	Can invoke a lupus anticoagulant syndrome; prolongs the PTT and possibly the PT
Cholestyramine	Impedes the pharmacologic effect of warfarin; can shorten the PT in patients receiving warfarin
Phenylbutazone	Impairs platelet function and enhances effect of warfarin; can prolong the bleeding time; may increase the PT in a patient on both drugs
Metronidazole	Enhances the effect of warfarin in a patient on both drugs; can prolong the PT
Barbiturates	Accelerates the clearance of warfarin from the body; can shorten the PT
Oral hypoglycemic agents and phenytoin	Slows the clearance of warfarin; can prolong the PT
Procainamide	Known to stimulate lupus anticoagulant syndrome; interferes with contact phase reactants in coagulation
Streptomycin	Known to stimulate formation of inhibitors to factor V; can prolong the PT and possibly the PTT
Penicillin, sulfonamides, phenytoin	Known to stimulate formation of inhibitors to factor VIII; may prolong the PTT
Pentoxifylline	Decreases fibrinogen levels and platelet aggregation; may prolong PT
Quinidine, hydralazine, long-term chlorpromazine	May induce a lupus anticoagulant syndrome
Ciprofloxacin	Known to have induced an acquired von Willebrand syndrome

mined intervals to assess this syndrome during management.

Primary Fibrino(geno)lysis

Primary fibrino(geno)lysis syndrome in a pure form is rare. The disease is a result of the release of excessive amounts of plasminogen activators into the circulation either from damaged or malignant cells (as in prostatic carcinoma), or by introduction of plasminogen-activating substances (tissue plasminogen activator, streptokinase, urokinase) in thrombolytic therapy. These activators convert plasminogen into plasmin *in the absence of fibrin formation*. Plasmin is nonspecific in its action and will cleave fibrinogen, as well as factors V and VIII. As fibrinogen is broken down, FSP accumulate, which have an anticoagulant effect. The net result is the inability of the blood to clot and a bleeding disorder.

It is important to distinguish the primary process from secondary lysis, which occurs in DIC. The laboratory evidence for fibrino(geno)lysis is similar to that demonstrated in DIC. Nearly all coagulation tests are abnormal in both syndromes. Four tools may be applied to distinguish the two syndromes: (1) the euglobulin clot lysis time will be markedly shortened in primary fibrino(geno)lysis (PF) but normal to only slightly shortened in DIC; (2) the platelet count remains greater than $100 \times 10^9/L$ in PF, whereas it frequently drops below this level in DIC; (3) antithrombin III assays will demonstrate decreased levels in DIC and normal levels in PF; and (4) the D-dimer test, which is specific for the degradation of fibrin, will be positive in DIC and negative in PF.

In the absence of any evidence of thrombosis (DIC), antifibrinolytic drugs may be used to treat the primary lytic condition. These drugs include natural antiplasmins, bovine parotid extract (aprotinin), and synthetic lysine analogs epsilon-aminocaproic acid (EACA) or tranexamic acid. More frequently, DIC is assumed to be present and the patient managed accordingly. Prolonged cardiopulmonary bypass pump time in surgery and acute trauma to and hypoxia of tissues have precipitated the primary fibrinolytic state. Such cases are brief and self-limited. Prostatic carcinoma has produced a long-term lytic syndrome that necessitates therapy.

Drug Interactions with Coagulation Systems

Table 52-3 presents an abbreviated list of drugs with their known effects on hemostatic mechanisms. Drugs may directly enhance, retard, or inhibit coagulation reactions or indirectly stimulate the formation of inhibitory substances that neutralize reactants. Many of these drugs are in common use, and it therefore behooves the coagulation laboratory to be aware of their potential influence on testing systems and the possibility of within-patient variation during therapy with these agents.

CHAPTER SUMMARY

Coagulation disorders are categorized by mode of acquisition into inherited or acquired types. Inherited disorders may be further divided by site of biochemical disturbance within the intrinsic, extrinsic, common, or fibrin stabilization pathways. Most inherited disorders involve only one procoagulant defect. Multiple factor deficiencies and inhibitory substances may coexist in the acquired syndromes. The roles and effects of exogenous substances such as vitamins, drugs, transfusions, and introduction of artificial substances into the circulation have been considered.

The patient's history, demographic category, and clinical status are codeterminants in the interpretation and value of laboratory data in hemostatic disorders.

Case Study 52-1

A 12-year-old white male was seen for evaluation of frequent epistaxis and ecchymoses. Pertinent history revealed hematuria at 3 years of age without evidence of renal disease. Microhematuria was a consistent feature on urinalysis reports. Adenoidectomy at 5 years of age resulted in exaggerated hemorrhage that necessitated packing of the nasal passages. A knee injury at 7 years of age required hospitalization to manage the hemarthrosis. Loss of primary teeth resulted in exaggerated bleeding. To date, the patient has not received any tranfused components as therapy. He is an only child; no other positive history exists in the family.

The laboratory data (with reference ranges) were as follows: PTT 68 seconds (22–36 seconds); correction of PTT with adsorbed normal plasma was obtained; PT 10.5 seconds (10.3–12.5 seconds; ISI 2.0); Simplate bleeding time 17 minutes (3–9.5 minutes); PLT $289 \times 10^9/L$ (150–450 $\times 10^9/L$); factor VIIIC:Ag assay 11% (54%–195%); von Willebrand factor antigen (vWF:Ag) 30% (50%–150%); vWF multimer pattern, only small multimers present; von Willebrand ristocetin cofactor (vWF:RCoF) 5% (50%–150%).

1. What common denominator is evident in this patient's history? Of what significance is the family history?
2. This patient was diagnosed with von Willebrand disease. What laboratory data support this diagnosis?
3. What is the significance of the results of the vWF multimer pattern in this case? What is the type classification of this patient's disorder?
4. If DDAVP therapy is not effective, why is concentrated commercially prepared material such as "Humate P®" a superior source for replacement for this patient?

Review Questions

52-1. The category of coagulation disorders most likely to involve a deficiency in or defect of more than one procoagulant protein is

   A. inherited disorders.
   B. acquired disorders.
   C. post-coagulation stabilization defects.
   D. fibrinogen disorders.

52-2. A prolonged one-stage PT result in the presence of within-range results for all other screening coagulation tests would indicate a deficiency in

   A. platelet function.
   B. factor VIII.
   C. factor X.
   D. factor VII.

52-3. The method of choice to monitor successful DDAVP therapy in von Willebrand disease is the

   A. vWF:RCoF activity assay.
   B. PTT.
   C. vWF:Ag immunoassay.
   D. bleeding time.

52-4. A patient who has suffered a thrombotic event has a prolonged PTT which does not correct with normal plasma, a borderline PT, and a prolonged dilute Russell's viper venom time (dRVVT). These findings are consistent with

    A. increased amounts of circulating fibrin split products.
    B. dysfibrinogenemia.
    C. the presence of a lupus anticoagulant.
    D. contact phase coagulation disorders.

52-5. An inherited deficiency state that can generate a within-range PTT but a prolonged PT with ox brain thromboplastin reagent is factor

    A. VIII:C deficiency.
    B. IX deficiency.
    C. VII deficiency.
    D. X deficiency.

52-6. The most clinically serious form of von Willebrand disease

    A. is expressed by heterozygotes.
    B. reveals acceptable levels of all multimer sizes.
    C. responds well to DDAVP.
    D. reveals a lack of vWF:Ag, vWF:RCoF, and all multimers.

References

1. Baillod P, Gaucher C, Affolter B, et al: New variant of type II von Willebrand's disease with structural abnormality of plasma von Willebrand factor in a patient with very mild bleeding history. Am J Hematol 49(1):21, 1995
2. Bell WR, Boss GR, Wolfson JS: Circulating anticoagulant in the procainamide-induced lupus syndrome. Arch Intern Med 137:1471, 1977
3. Berntorp E: Plasma product treatment in various types of von Willebrand's disease. Haemostasis 24(5):289, 1994
4. Bezeaud A, Guillin MC, Olmeda F et al: Prothrombin Madrid: A new familial abnormality of prothrombin. Thromb Res 16:47, 1979
5. Biggs R: Complications of treatment. In Biggs R, Macfarlane RG (eds): Treatment of Hemophilia A and B and von Willebrand's Disease, p 181. London, Blackwell, 1978
6. Branch DW, Rote NS, Scott JR: The demonstration of lupus anticoagulant by an enzyme-linked immunoadsorbent assay. Clin Immunol Immunopathol 39:298, 1986
7. Brettler DB, Levine PH: Clinical manifestations and therapy of inherited coagulation factor deficiencies. In Colman RW, Hirsh J, Marder VJ, Salzman EW (eds): Hemostasis and Thrombosis: Basic Principles and Clinical Practice, 3rd ed. p 169. Philadelphia, JB Lippincott, 1994
8. Castaman G, Lattuada A, Mannucci PM, Rodeghiero F: Characterization of two cases of acquired von Willebrand syndrome with ciprofloxacin: Evidence for heightened proteolysis of von Willebrand factor. Am J Hematol 49(1):83, 1995
9. Centers for Disease Control: Safety of therapeutic products used for hemophilia patients. MMWR 29:441, 1988
10. Canoso RT, Hutton RA: A chlorpromazine-induced inhibitor of blood coagulation. Am J Hematol 2:183, 1977
11. Coccia MR, Barnes HV: Hypothyroidism and acquired vWD. J Adolesc Health 12:152, 1991
12. Colman RW: Formation of human plasma kinin. N Engl J Med 291:509, 1974
13. Davi S, Furie BC, Willey R: Circulating inhibitors of blood coagulation associated with procainamide-lupus erythematosus. Am J Hematol 4:401, 1978
14. DeLaCadena RA, Wachtfogel YT, Colman RW: Contact activation pathway: Inflammation and coagulation. In Colman RW, Hirsh J, Marder VJ, Salzman EW (eds): Hemostasis and Thrombosis: Basic Principles and Clinical Practice, 3rd ed, p 219. Philadelphia, JB Lippincott, 1994
15. Edmunds LH, Salzman EW: Hemostatic problems, transfusion therapy, and cardiopulmonary bypass in surgical patients. In Colman RW, Hirsh J, Marder VJ, Salzman EW (eds): Hemostasis and Thrombosis: Basic Principles and Clinical Practice, 3rd ed, p 956. Philadelphia, JB Lippincott, 1994
16. Ermens AA, deWild PJ, Vader HL, van der Graaf F: Four agglutination assays evaluated for measurement of von Willebrand factor (ristocetin cofactor activity). Clin Chem 41(4):510, 1995
17. Ewing NP, Kaspar CK: In vitro detection of mild inhibitors to factor VIII in hemophilia. Am J Clin Pathol 77:749, 1982
18. Facon T, Caron C, Cortin P et al: Acquired type II vWD associated with adrenal cortical carcinoma. Br J Haematol 80:488, 1992
19. Favaloro EJ, Dean M, Grispo L, Exner T, Koutts J: von Willebrand's disease: Use of collagen binding assay provides potential improvement to laboratory monitoring of desmopressin (DDAVP) therapy. Am J Hematol 45(3):205, 1994
20. Feinstein DI: Acquired inhibitors of factor V. Thromb Haemost 39:663, 1978
21. Feinstein DI: Immune coagulation disorders. In Colman RW, Hirsh J, Marder VJ, Salzman EW (eds): Hemostasis and Thrombosis: Basic Principles and Clinical Practice, 3rd ed, p 881. Philadelphia, JB Lippincott, 1994
22. Giddings JC, Seligsohn U, Bloom AL: Immunological studies in combined factor V and factor VIII deficiency. Br J Haematol 37:257, 1977
23. Girolami A, Violante M, Cella G et al: Combined deficiency of factor V and Factor VIII: A report of another case. Blut 32:415, 1976
24. Handin RI, Moloney WC: Antibody induced von Willebrand's disease. Blood 44:933, 1974; 48:393, 1976
25. Hathaway WE, Belhanson LP, Hathaway HS: Evidence for a new plasma thromboplastin factor: Case report, coagulation studies, and physiochemical properties. Blood 26:521, 1965
26. Hirsh EF, Magajima T, Oshima G et al: Kinin-system responses in sepsis after trauma in man. J Surg Res 17:147, 1974
27. Hoyer LW: Immunologic studies of antihemophilic factor (AHF, Factor VIII). IV. Radioimmunoassay of AHF antigen. J Lab Clin Med 80:822, 1972
28. Ingram GIC, Kingston PJ, Leslie J et al: Four cases of acquired von Willebrand's syndrome. Br J Haematol 21:189, 1971
29. Iwanga S, Kato H, Maruyama I et al: Fluorogenic peptide substrates for proteases in blood coagulation, kallikrein-kinin, and fibrinolysis systems: Substrate for plasmin and factor XIa. Thromb Haemost 42:49, 1979
30. Josso F, Rio Y, Beguin S: A new variant of human prothrombin: Prothrombin Metz, demonstration in a family showing double heterozygosity for congenital hypoprothrombinemia and dysprothrombinemia. Haemostasis 12:309, 1982
31. Kaspar CK: Incidence and course of inhibitors among patients with classic hemophilia. Thromb Diath Haemorrh 30:264, 1973
32. Kaspar CK, Aledort LM, Counts RB et al: A more uniform measurement of factor VIII inhibitors. Thromb Diath Haemorrh 34:869, 1975
33. Klein HG, Aledort LM, Bouma BN et al: A cooperative study for the detection of the carrier state of classic hemophilia. N Engl J Med 296:959, 1977
34. Lesperance B, David M, Rarick J et al: Relative sensitivity of different tests in the detection of low titer lupus anticoagulants. Thromb Haemost 60:217, 1988
35. Lethagen S, Ragnarson Tennvall G: Self-treatment with desmopressin intranasal spray in patients with bleeding disor-

ders: Effect on bleeding symptoms and socioeconomic factors. Ann Hematol 66(5):257, 1993

36. Levine PH: Hemophilia and allied conditions. In Brain MC (ed): Current Therapy in Hematology/Oncology. New York, BC Decker, 1983

37. Lossing T, Kaspar CK, Feinstein DI: Detection of factor VIII inhibitors with the activated partial thromboplastin time. Blood 49:493, 1977

38. Lusher JM: Response to 1-deamino-8-D-arginine vasopressin in von Willebrand disease. Haemostasis 24(5):276, 1994

39. Macik BG, Berkowitz SD, Ortel TL et al: Duke University Medical Center Clinical Coagulation Manual. October, 1994

40. Marder VJ, Feinstein DI, Francis CW, Colman RW: Consumptive thrombohemorrhagic disorders. In Colman RW, Hirsh J, Marder VJ, Salzman EW (eds): Hemostasis and Thrombosis: Basic Principles and Clinical Practice, 3rd ed, p 1023. Philadelphia, JB Lippincott, 1994

41. McDonagh J, Carrell N, Lee MH: Dysfibrinogenemia and other disorders of fibrinogen structure and function. In Colman RW, Hirsh J, Marder VJ, Salzman EW (eds): Hemostasis and Thrombosis: Basic Principles and Clinical Practice, 3rd ed, p 314. Philadelphia, JB Lippincott, 1994

42. Montgomery RR, Coller BS: von Willebrand Disease. In Colman RW, Hirsh J, Marder VJ, Salzman EW (eds): Hemostasis and Thrombosis: Basic Principles and Clinical Practice, 3rd ed, p 134. Philadelphia, JB Lippincott, 1994

43. Pavlovsky A: Contribution to the pathogenesis of hemophilia. Blood 2:185, 1947

44. Peake I: Carrier detection and prenatal diagnosis of hemophilia: Present and future strategies. Res Clin Lab 20:177, 1990

45. Piovella F, Giddings JC, Peake IR et al: Synthesis of procoagulant antihemophilic factor *in vitro*. Lancet 2:888, 1978

46. Rapaport SI, Ames SB, Duvall BJ: A plasma coagulation defect in systemic lupus erythematosus arising from hypoprothrombinemia combined with antiprothrombinase activity. Blood 15:212, 1960

47. Ratnoff OD, Steinberg AG: Detection of the carrier state of classic hemophilia. Ann NY Acad Sci 240:95, 1975

48. Richard C, Cuadrado MA, Prieto M et al: Acquired vWD in multiple myeloma secondary to absorption of vWF by plasma cells. Am J Hematol 35:114, 1990

49. Roberts HR, Grizzle JE, McLester WD et al: Genetic variants of hemophilia B: Detection by means of a specific PTC inhibitor. J Clin Invest 47:360, 1968

50. Roberts HR, Jones MR: Hemophilia and related conditions—Congenital deficiencies of prothrombin (factor II), factor V, and factors VII to XII. In Williams WJ, Beutler E, Erslev AJ, Lichtman MA (eds): Hematology, 4th ed, p 1453. New York, McGraw-Hill, 1990

51. Sadler JE: A revised classification of von Willebrand disease. For the Subcommittee on von Willebrand Factor of the Scientific and Standardization Committee of the International Society on Thrombosis and Haemostasis. Thromb Haemost 71(4):520, 1994

52. Salzman EW, Merrill EW, Kent KC: Interaction of blood with artificial surfaces. In Colman RW, Hirsh J, Marder VJ, Salzman EW (eds): Hemostasis and Thrombosis: Basic Principes and Clinical Practice, 3rd ed, p 1469. Philadelphia, JB Lippincott, 1994

53. Seeler RA: Hemolysis due to anti-A and B in factor VIII preparations. Arch Intern Med 130:101, 1972.

54. Shapiro SS: Antibodies to blood coagulation factors. Clin Haematol 9:207, 1979

55. Shapiro SS, Martinez J, Holburn RR: Congenital dysprothrombinemia: An inherited structural disorder of human prothrombin. J Clin Invest 48:2251, 1969

56. Shapiro SS, McCord IS: Prothrombin. In Spaet TH (ed): Hemostasis and Thrombosis, vol 4, p 177. New York, Grune & Stratton, 1978

57. Shulman NR: Surgical care of patients with hereditary disorders of blood coagulation. In Ratnoff OD (ed): Treatment of Hemorrhagic Disorders. New York, Harper and Row, 1968

58. Slaughter TF, Parker JK, Greenberg CS: A rapid method for the diagnosis of von Willebrand's disease subtypes by the clinical laboratory. Arch Pathol Lab Med 119(2):148, 1995

59. Soff GA, Levin J: Familial multiple coagulation factor deficiencies. I. Review of the literature: Differentiation of single hereditary disorders associated with multiple factor deficiencies from coincidental concurrence of single factor deficiency states. Semin Thromb Hemost 7:112, 1981

60. Thiagarajan P, Pengo V, Shapiro SS: The use of the dilute Russell viper venom time for the diagnosis of lupus anticoagulants. Blood 68:869, 1986

61. Tuddenham EGD, Lazarchick J, Hoyer LW: Synthesis and release of factor VIII by cultured human endothelial cells. Br J Haematol 47:617, 1981

62. von Willebrand EA: Hereditare Pseudohamophili. Finska Lak Sallsk Handl 68:87, 1926

63. Zarrabi MH, Zucker S, Miller F et al: Immunologic and coagulation disorders in chlorpromazine-treated patients. Ann Intern Med 91:194, 1979

64. Zimmerman TS, Ratnoff OD, Powell AE: Immunologic differentiation of classic hemophilic (factor VIII deficiency) and von Willebrand's disease. J Clin Invest 50:244, 1971

Disorders Leading to Thrombosis

Gordon E. Ens

Objectives

1. Define the term *hypercoagulable*.
2. Describe three natural anticoagulant mechanisms that control thrombus formation.
3. Describe the clinical and laboratory findings for each of the following conditions: antithrombin III deficiency, protein C deficiency, protein S deficiency, activated protein C resistance, and fibrinolytic system disorders.
4. Describe at least three secondary (acquired) disorders that may lead to thrombosis, emphasizing the laboratory findings.

Disorders leading to thrombosis are those abnormalities that result in an increased tendency to develop thrombi and emboli, sometimes called the *hypercoagulable* or *thrombotic risk state*.[22,41] Patients typically present with laboratory abnormalities (including deficiencies of the antithrombin or protein C pathway) or with clinical conditions (such as the postoperative state or malignancy) that have been associated with an increased incidence of thrombosis or thromboembolic complications.[7]

Thrombotic disorders have many etiologies that usually are divided into two broad categories.[3] These include primary (inherited) disorders, whose numbers continue to increase as new factors are discovered, and secondary or acquired disorders, which are composed of a heterogeneous group of clinical conditions associated with an increased risk of thrombosis compared to the general population.

PATHOPHYSIOLOGY

Hemostasis is the complex process of inhibition of blood loss through the combined action of platelets, coagulation factors, and blood vessel integrity. A critical balance between clot activating, inhibiting, and lysing factors is essential. Thrombosis results when hemostasis occurs at an inappropriate time or place.

There are three natural anticoagulant mechanisms that control thrombus formation (Fig. 53-1).[23,40] The first, *antithrombin III (AT-III)*, a globulin serine protease inhibitor, neutralizes thrombin and the other activated serine proteases in the coagulation cascade. Heparin accelerates the formation of antithrombin–thrombin complexes and the neutralization of thrombin activity.[39]

The second mechanism is the *protein C pathway*.[16] Protein C, a vitamin K-dependent glycoprotein, is converted by thrombin to activated protein C (APC or PCa), a serine protease. The rate of activation is greatly increased by thrombomodulin, a cofactor found on endothelial cell surfaces.[17] The APC exerts its anticoagulant effect by inactivating factors Va and VIIIa, with protein S, another vitamin K-dependent protein, serving as a cofactor.[10] In addition, APC facilitates fibrinolysis by neutralizing plasminogen activator inhibitor-1 (PAI-1).[30] The recent discovery of activated protein C resistance (APCR) as a result of a mutation in the factor V gene has greatly improved the ability to identify thrombotic risk.[24,48]

The third mechanism is the *fibrinolytic system,* the activation of which produces the serine protease plasmin, which lyses the fibrin clot into fibrin degradation products. The generation of plasmin from plasminogen is the result of plasminogen activators, which are found in various tissues (*e.g.*, prostate, uterus, kidney). Tissue plasminogen activator (TPA) has a high affinity for fibrin, making it available for converting plasminogen to plasmin in the forming clot. TPA is probably the principal plasminogen activator in blood vessels. PAI-1, having a high affinity for TPA and α_2-antiplasmin (the primary inhibitor of plasmin) helps regulate the fibrinolytic system.[15]

PRIMARY DISORDERS LEADING TO THROMBOSIS

The primary thrombotic disorders are inherited conditions involving one or more components of the hemostatic system, generally a protein of the coagulation or fibrino-

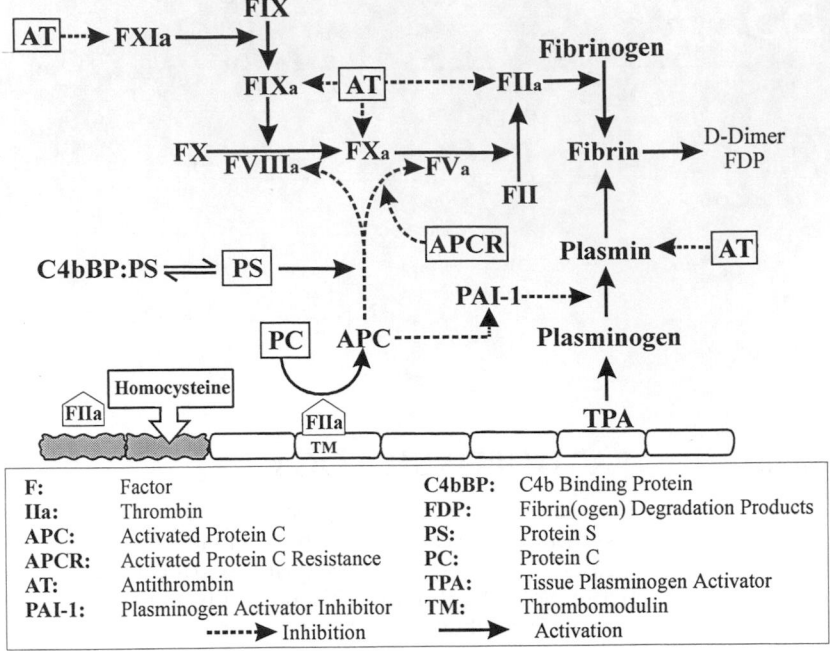

F:	Factor	C4bBP:	C4b Binding Protein
IIa:	Thrombin	FDP:	Fibrin(ogen) Degradation Products
APC:	Activated Protein C	PS:	Protein S
APCR:	Activated Protein C Resistance	PC:	Protein C
AT:	Antithrombin	TPA:	Tissue Plasminogen Activator
PAI-1:	Plasminogen Activator Inhibitor	TM:	Thrombomodulin
	------> Inhibition		——→ Activation

FIGURE 53-1. Interrelations among endothelial cells, protein C, protein S, antithrombin III, and coagulation scheme for regulation of thrombus formation.

lytic system rather than a platelet abnormality. The list of recognized primary disorders (Table 53-1) continues to grow.[14] Patients suffer recurrent thrombosis, often starting at an early age. Some patients are asymptomatic, the condition being discovered by laboratory testing as part of family studies. It is important to recognize that secondary risk factors such as malignancy, postoperative state, pregnancy, and lupus anticoagulant make these patients even more susceptible to thrombosis.

Antithrombin III Deficiency

Quantitative and qualitative defects of AT-III are the best defined and understood of the primary thrombotic disorders. As the principal inhibitor of thrombin in plasma, AT-III functions by complexing with and inhibiting thrombin and other activated serine proteases such as factors IXa, Xa, XIa, XIIa, and plasmin. The inhibition of thrombin and factor Xa are probably the most relevant interactions.[44] Heparin potentiates the action of AT-III *in vitro* and *in vivo*. A heparin-like substance (heparan sulfate) on the endothelial cell surface plays an important role in the *in vivo* regulation of thrombosis.[44]

TABLE 53-1
Primary Disorders of Thombosis

Antithrombin III deficiency

Protein C deficiency

Protein S deficiency

Activated protein C resistance

Fibrinolytic system disorders

Dysfibrinogenemia

Homocysteinuria

Congenital AT-III deficiency was first reported in 1965 in a family with recurrent venous thromboembolism and approximately 40% of normal plasma AT-III levels.[12] Since then, numerous families have been reported having partial deficiencies together with venous and arterial thrombotic disorders. The deficiency is more common than is generally realized, with the estimated incidence in the general population approaching 1 in 2000.[37] Two to five percent of patients hospitalized for deep venous thrombosis or pulmonary embolus have AT-III deficiency.[28] Typically, the defect is inherited as an autosomal dominant trait with males and females being affected equally.[34] Heterozygous persons have AT-III levels between 25% and 60% of normal. The homozygous state has not been reported.

CLINICAL AND LABORATORY FINDINGS

The most frequent clinical characteristics of AT-III deficiency are recurrent lower extremity thrombophlebitis and pulmonary embolism; however, thromboembolic events may also occur at other anatomic sites.[51] Thrombosis may be seen from the neonatal period to late in life, although the majority of affected persons manifest symptoms before the age of 35 years. At least 85% of AT-III–deficient individuals will have a thrombotic event by the age of 60.[18] Most thrombotic events are initiated by factors that may also cause thrombosis in persons *not* deficient in AT-III, especially surgery, trauma, pregnancy, oral contraceptive use, and infection.[51]

The deficiency is detected by measuring antigenic and functional levels of AT-III. Functional AT-III methods should be used to screen for the deficiency state, performing an immunologic measurement, if necessary, to confirm a molecular defect or decreased protein level. Radioimmunodiffusion or radioimmunoassay have been used to measure immunologic levels of the molecule, whereas functional activity is determined by measuring the ability of AT-III to inhibit thrombin. See Chapter 49 for details of these assays.

The reference range for functional AT-III in plasma is approximately 80% to 125% activity. Levels of 60% to 80% indicate a moderate thrombotic risk, and levels below 50% indicate significant risk. Serum rather than plasma levels of functional AT-III may be the preferred indicator of thrombotic risk, because serum reflects low plasma AT-III levels in addition to increased consumption of AT-III during the clotting process.[19] The reference range of serum AT-III is 70% to 125% activity.

EFFECTS OF TREATMENT ON LABORATORY RESULTS

Most patients with AT-III deficiency can be treated with heparin during the acute episodes, and with warfarin for maintenance therapy. Higher than the usual doses of heparin may be required for effective anticoagulation in patients with very low levels of AT-III.[38] Treatment with heparin may temporarily lower the AT-III level by 10% to 15% in patients with active thrombosis. Conversely, treatment with warfarin has been reported to raise AT-III levels, the mechanism being unknown.[29] Concentrates of AT-III are available and can be used to increase AT-III levels during acute episodes of thrombosis or periods of extreme thrombotic risk.

Protein C Deficiency

A more recently described cause of thrombotic disorders is a deficiency of another regulator of the hemostatic system, protein C.[45] A vitamin K–dependent glycoprotein, protein C is activated by the complex of thrombin–thrombomodulin on the endothelial cell surface. Activated protein C (APC) in the presence of protein S inactivates factors Va and VIIIa, important cofactors in the generation of a fibrin clot or thrombus.

Protein C was discovered in 1960; however, the initial report of a clinical deficiency was not made until 1981.[20] Two types of hereditary protein C deficiency have been reported. In type I, both the immunologic and activity levels are low, whereas in type II, only the activity is below normal. The incidence of type I protein C deficiency is about 5% in patients with venous thrombosis under 40 years of age. Protein C deficiency is inherited in an autosomal dominant or autosomal recessive manner. Homozygous deficiencies have been reported in infants with severe thrombosis who have almost no measurable plasma protein C.[43] The heterozygous state is associated with venous thrombotic disease and immunologic protein C levels of 40% to 50% of normal.[4]

CLINICAL AND LABORATORY FINDINGS

Individuals with protein C deficiency present at an early age with recurrent superficial or deep vein thrombophlebitis and frequent pulmonary emboli. Approximately 50% experience a thromboembolic episode before 30 years of age.

Protein C levels are measured in the laboratory by immunologic and functional assays. Normal ranges for both assays are approximately 70% to 125% of reference levels. Both assays should be performed to distinguish type I from type II deficiency. Because protein C is a vitamin K–dependent protein, levels will be low in patients receiving oral anticoagulant therapy. True deficiencies can be suggested in stabilized oral anticoagulated patients by measuring immunologic levels of other vitamin K–dependent factors and comparing them with the protein C immunologic level. Congenitally deficient individuals will have a disproportionately low level of protein C.

TREATMENT

Long-term warfarin therapy has been effective in management.[20,43] Warfarin-induced skin necrosis occurs in some patients during the initiation of such therapy, suggesting the advisability of the concomitant use of heparin during this time.[31] Protein C replacement therapy is currently being tested in clinical trials. Factor IX concentrates are rich in protein C and have been effective in a number of cases.[42]

Protein S Deficiency

Protein S, a vitamin K–dependent protein that functions as a cofactor for activated protein C, was first reported as a cause of thrombosis in 1984.[8] Protein S circulates in plasma in two forms. Approximately 50% is free protein S or the functional protein S that serves as a cofactor for activated protein C, while the other 50% protein S is bound to C4b-binding protein, an inhibitor in the complement pathway. The bound protein S is not functional.

CLINICAL AND LABORATORY FINDINGS

Heterozygous deficient individuals have recurrent venous thrombosis together with immunologic protein S levels of 30% to 60% of reference level activity. These persons are clinically similar to patients with heterozygous deficiencies of protein C and AT-III, having an increased tendency for recurrent venous thrombotic disorders that begin in early adulthood.[8]

Measurement of protein S by immunologic and functional methods is similar to that of protein C. Normal ranges are approximately 70% to 125% of reference level activity. Oral anticoagulant therapy will lower protein S levels, because protein S is vitamin K dependent. As in protein C, protein S deficiency may be inferred in stable oral anticoagulant patients by performing immunologic measurements of protein S and other vitamin K–dependent proteins and determining the ratio. Levels of C4b-binding protein can become elevated during inflammatory events and cause decreased levels of functional protein S.

TREATMENT

Oral anticoagulant therapy is the treatment of choice in those individuals with recurring venous thrombosis. Warfarin skin necrosis in protein S deficiency is similar to that seen in protein C deficiency.

Activated Protein C Resistance

Activated protein C resistance (APCR) is the most recently described genetic defect responsible for thromboembolic disease.[48] Activated protein C inhibits clot formation by selectively inactivating coagulation factors Va and VIIIa in the presence of cofactor protein S. A poor response to APC (*i.e.*, APCR) is caused by the presence of a molecular variant of factor V and has been shown to be the most frequent cause of venous thrombosis in hospitalized patients. It is due, 90% of the time, to a single point mutation in the factor V gene.[14]

CLINICAL AND LABORATORY FINDINGS

Clinical symptoms are similar to those for AT-III, protein C, and protein S deficiencies. APCR is reported to be found in 3% to 5% of the general population and is responsible for 20% to 50% of thrombosis in patients. Heterozygous individuals are at 5 to 10 times greater risk of thrombosis whereas homozygotes are at 50 to 100 times greater risk.

APCR is measured by determining the ratio of two PTT assays, one with APC added, the other without. Typically, a ratio of less than 2.0 is indicative of APCR. The baseline PTT must be in the normal range for the assay to be valid. Heparinized samples can be assayed by removing heparin prior to testing, whereas the effect of oral anticoagulants can be neutralized by the addition of factor V–deficient plasma. The mutation in the factor V gene can be determined by DNA-based analysis.

Fibrinolytic System Disorders

PLASMINOGEN

Plasminogen, the inactive precursor of plasmin, circulates in the blood in close association with fibrinogen and is trapped in the forming fibrin clot. Plasminogen is activated by tissue or plasma activators. Regulation of the activation to form plasmin is a complex process involving tissue plasminogen activator release from the vessel wall, generation of plasminogen activator inhibitor-1 (PAI-1) following plasminogen activation by factor XIIa, and the inhibition of PAI-1 by activated protein C. Inhibitors such as α_2-antiplasmin rapidly inactivate free plasmin in circulating blood.

Congenital and acquired disorders of fibrinolytic system components can result in impaired clot lysis, leading to excessive thrombus formation. Quantitative and functional abnormalities of plasminogen have been reported in individuals with recurrent thrombosis.[2] Deficiencies in factor XII may result in reduced activation of endogenous tissue plasminogen activator.[11]

Functional and immunologic assays for plasminogen are available (Chap. 50). Typically, the functional levels are decreased more than immunologic levels, indicating a qualitative defect in the plasminogen molecule.

TISSUE PLASMINOGEN ACTIVATOR/ PLASMINOGEN ACTIVATOR INHIBITOR-1

Tissue plasminogen activator (TPA) and plasminogen activator inhibitor-1 (PAI-1) produced by endothelial cells are the principal proteins that regulate the conversion of plasminogen to plasmin. Elevated levels of TPA have been associated with thrombotic events, particularly myocardial infarction. PAI-1 is an acute phase reactant protein and plasma concentrations are directly related to triglyceride levels.[33] Functional and immunologic assays exist for both TPA and PAI-1 although they are not routinely performed in most hospital laboratories.

Dysfibrinogenemia

Congenital disorders with clinically significant functional abnormalities of fibrinogen (dysfibrinogenemia) have been reported in conjunction with increased thrombosis.[1,2,13] Acquired dysfibrinogenemia is occasionally seen in hepatic diseases. Fibrinogen binds to proteins involved in fibrinolysis. Abnormalities at these binding sites or the binding site for plasmin may impair the fibrinolytic mechanism and facilitate thrombosis. Dysfibrinogenemia may be suspected when immunologic fibrinogen levels are significantly higher than functional levels.

Homocysteinuria

A rare autosomal recessive disorder, homocysteinuria causes severe premature arteriosclerosis and is associated with a high incidence of arterial and venous thrombosis early in life. Other syndromes including genetic disorders and vitamin deficiencies can lead to elevated levels of plasma homocysteine.[46] The mechanism of action is uncertain; however, homocysteine possibly interferes with the expression of thrombomodulin on endothelial cell surfaces, interfering with protein C activation.[47]

SECONDARY DISORDERS OF THROMBOSIS

The secondary disorders of thrombosis (Table 53-2) consist of a variety of clinical conditions associated with a high degree of thromboembolic complications. The pathophysiology leading to thrombosis is not fully understood in all cases; however, various abnormalities of hemostasis have been observed. Understanding these associations is important in selecting the most appropriate therapy or in eliminating the underlying cause. Many disorders have more than one mechanism affecting normal hemostasis, making classification difficult.[35]

Antiphospholipid Syndrome

Antiphospholipid syndrome (APLS) refers to a clinical disorder associated with thrombosis in conjunction with a positive laboratory test for antibody against phospholipid.[26] Two unique types of antibodies exist, antiphospholipid antibodies (APA) and lupus anticoagulant (LA). APA are quantitated by their ability to bind to negatively charged phospholipids such as cardiolipin. LA is an immunoglobulin that binds to the phospholipid reagent in clotting assays,[9] such as the PTT, dilute Russell's viper venom test, kaolin clotting time, and platelet neutraliza-

TABLE 53-2
Secondary Disorders of Thrombosis

LUPUS ANTICOAGULANT

HEMOSTATIC PROTEIN ABNORMALITIES

    Postoperative state

    Malignancy

    Pregnancy

    Oral contraceptives and estrogen

    Other

        Nephrotic syndrome
        Coronary artery disease
        Stroke

PLATELET ABNORMALITIES

    Diabetes mellitus

    Hyperlipidemia

    Myeloproliferative disorders

    Heparin-induced thrombocytopenia (HIT)

BLOOD VESSEL AND FLOW ABNORMALITIES

    Artificial surfaces

    Damaged vessels

    Abnormal blood flow

tion procedure (Chap. 49). No single assay is superior for determining thrombotic risk. Because of the transient nature of the antibodies, positive tests should be repeated after 1 to 2 months. APLS has been associated with cerebrovascular and cardiovascular disorders in addition to thrombosis at numerous sites. Women with APLS are at increased risk of recurrent pregnancy loss, fetal growth retardation, and infertility.

Hemostatic Protein Abnormalities

Several clinical conditions discussed below, such as postoperative states, malignancies, and pregnancy, have been associated with increased thrombosis. Typical laboratory findings include reduced levels of the naturally occurring anticoagulants or reduced fibrinolytic activity. Increased levels of molecular markers of thrombin generation may also be observed (Chap. 51).

POSTOPERATIVE STATE/TRAUMA

The postoperative state, particularly following orthopedic and gynecologic surgery, is a complex example of secondary hypercoagulability. The hemostatic mechanism reacts to surgery and blunt trauma in a similar manner, being activated through the extrinsic pathway following release of tissue thromboplastin (tissue factor) from sites of soft tissue injury and bone fracture.[27] The frequency of deep venous thrombosis in patients after hip surgery or fracture not treated prophylactically, is reported to be as high as 50%. Patients with primary hypercoagulable states are at increased risk. Contributing risk factors include immobilization, advanced age, obesity, malignancy, oral contraceptive use, pregnancy, and an increase in platelet count frequently observed after surgical trauma.

MALIGNANCY

Increased thrombosis in malignancy frequently is related to the release of coagulation activating factors by the neoplastic cells. This relationship has been observed for years, beginning with Trousseau's report more than a century ago.[50] The incidence of thrombosis in cancer patients varies from approximately 5% to 15%.[36]

Treatment of thrombosis in cancer patients is difficult because of resistance to anticoagulation and the potential for bleeding complications from necrotic tumor sites. Typically, the hemostatic abnormalities are corrected by elimination of the malignancy. The use of certain chemotherapeutic agents, specifically L-asparaginase has been associated with an increase in thrombosis and decreases in AT-III, protein C, and protein S levels.

PREGNANCY

The coagulation system undergoes a number of changes during pregnancy including increased levels of fibrinogen, factor VIII, and von Willebrand factor and decreases in AT-III, protein S, and fibrinolytic activity. The presence of antiphospholipid antibodies (APA) and lupus anticoagulant (LA) has also been strongly associated with spontaneous abortion, preeclampsia, and fetal growth retardation.[52] The actual frequency of thrombosis during pregnancy may be underestimated owing to difficulty in diagnosis. Antepartum subclinical events may become evident in the postpartum period as thrombophlebitis, venous insufficiency, pulmonary hypertension, or postphlebitic syndrome. During the first month after delivery, the risk of phlebitis and thromboembolism is substantially increased. Thromboembolic risk during pregnancy increases with age, prolonged bed rest, parity, hypertension, obesity, and nonvaginal delivery.

ORAL CONTRACEPTIVE OR ESTROGEN USE

The use of oral contraceptives has historically been associated with increased risk of thrombosis.[6] Since their inception in the 1960s, the estrogen content in oral contraceptives has been decreased significantly with a concomitant decrease in thrombotic events. The association of estrogen use with thrombotic risk is still hotly debated. Observed changes in hemostatic factors include increases in fibrinogen, factor VII, factor VIII, platelet aggregation and blood viscosity, and decreases in AT-III and protein S levels. Interestingly, the use of postmenopausal estrogen does not appear to be significantly associated with thrombosis.[5]

OTHER CAUSES

Increased incidence of thrombosis has also been observed in patients with cardiac and neurologic disease. Patients with nephrotic syndrome have increased incidence of venous thromboembolism, possibly owing to decreased levels of AT-III and protein S.[25] Increasing age, immobilization, and obesity are also associated with increased rates of venous thrombosis.[5]

Platelet Abnormalities

Platelet abnormalities typically observed in secondary thrombotic disorders include elevated numbers; increased aggregation response to ADP, collagen, and epinephrine; and increased levels of β-thromboglobulin and platelet factor 4.

Heparin-induced thrombocytopenia (HIT) is an unexpected, rapid decline in platelet numbers that occurs in 5% to 10% of individuals receiving heparin. Life-threatening thrombosis occurs in a significant number of patients with HIT.[25]

Blood Vessel and Flow Abnormalities

ARTIFICIAL SURFACES

Situations in which circulating blood is exposed to artificial surfaces create a substantial risk of thrombosis. The more common situations are vascular grafts, prosthetic heart valves, and procedures involving hemodialysis or hemoperfusion. The foreign surface activates platelets, causing increased adhesion and aggregation that in turn activates the coagulation system.

DAMAGED ENDOTHELIUM

Normal endothelium maintains a balance in the pro- and anti-thrombotic processes.[32] A variety of disease states such as vasculitis, scleroderma, systemic lupus erythematosus, Kawasaki disease, chronic occlusive arterial disease, and Bechet disease may contribute to damaged blood vessels which create a thrombotic risk state.

ABNORMAL BLOOD FLOW

The role of venous stasis as first described by Virchow has been documented by studies that show the association between venous stasis and thrombosis. Venous stasis is associated with a number of risk factors described earlier. Mechanisms creating thrombotic risk are not fully elucidated but probably include reduced fibrinolysis and slow removal of activated clotting factors from the site of vascular injury.

CHAPTER SUMMARY

This chapter has addressed laboratory and clinical recognition of disorders leading to thrombosis, as well as the pathophysiology of the primary thrombotic states and some of the clinical conditions associated secondarily with thrombotic states. Significant progress has been made in our understanding of thrombosis and thrombotic risk; however, much remains to be discovered. As new tests are developed and become more widely available, the diagnosis of thrombotic disorders and management of affected patients will be easier.

Review Questions

53-1. Heparin accelerates the action of

   A. protein C.
   B. antithrombin III.
   C. protein S.
   D. plasmin.

53-2. Vitamin K is necessary for the production of functional

   A. protein C.
   B. antithrombin III.
   C. thrombomodulin.
   D. plasmin.

53-3. Protein C inactivates factors Va and VIIIa and facilitates

   A. antithrombin–thrombin complexes.
   B. serine protease inactivation.
   C. plasmin–antiplasmin binding.
   D. fibrinolysis.

53-4. Inhibition of fibrinolysis is accomplished by

   A. tissue plasminogen activator.
   B. plasminogen activator inhibitor-1.
   C. protein C.
   D. activated protein C.

53-5. Treatment with _____ has been reported to increase levels of antithrombin III.

   A. TPA
   B. heparin
   C. warfarin
   D. hirudin

53-6. Protein C deficiency can best be determined on a patient receiving oral anticoagulants by

   A. comparing immunologic protein C assays to similar assays of coagulation factors II, VII, IX, or X.
   B. performing both functional and immunologic assays of protein C.
   C. comparing levels of protein C with those of protein S.
   D. treating the patient with heparin prior to performing protein C assays.

53-7. The circulating protein S bound to C4b-binding protein is

   A. the only form of protein S in plasma.
   B. a cofactor for protein C.
   C. a cofactor for AT-III.
   D. not functionally active.

53-8. Activated protein C (APC) resistance can be measured in the laboratory by determining the ratio of two _____ assays with and without APC added.

   A. PT
   B. PTT
   C. thrombin time
   D. APC

53-9. Patients who have circulating lupus anticoagulant have antibodies against

   A. cell membranes.
   B. negatively charged phospholipids.
   C. phospholipid in clotting assay reagents.
   D. cardiolipin phospholipid.

53-10. Pregnancy has been associated with an increased risk of thrombosis due to

   A. increased levels of fibrinogen and factor VIII.
   B. decreases in antithrombin III and protein S.
   C. decreased fibrinolytic activity.
   D. all of the above.

References

1. Al-Mondhiry HAB, Bilezikian SB, Nossel HL: Fibrinogen "New York," an abnormal fibrinogen associated with thromboembolism: Functional evaluation. Blood 45:607, 1975

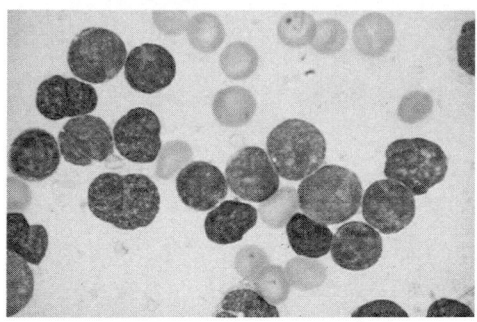

PLATE 36-1. L1 ALL. Homogeneous population of small cells with scanty cytoplasm. (1000×)

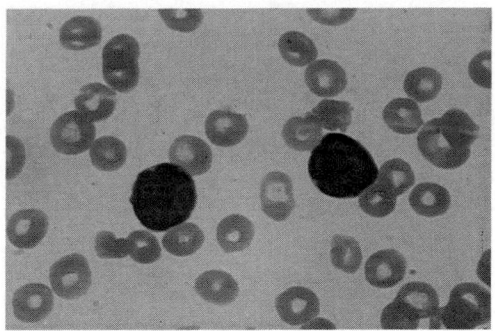

PLATE 36-2. L1 ALL. In contrast to Color Plate 36-1, this patient had a leukopenia. Both leukocytes in the field represent the typical L1 type lymphoblast: small, very high nuclear:cytoplasmic ratio and homogeneous morphology. (1000×)

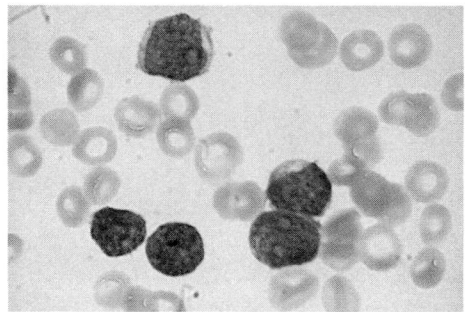

PLATE 36-3. L2 ALL. Heterogeneous population of large and small cells. Nucleoli are large; cytoplasm is moderately abundant. (1000×)

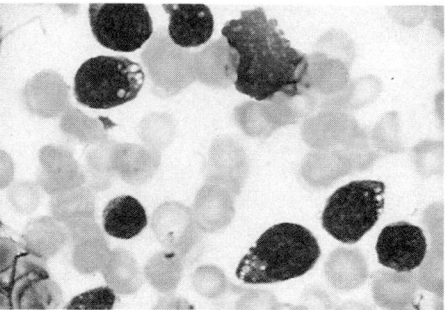

PLATE 36-4. L3 ALL. Primitive cells with abundant, very basophilic cytoplasm which is highly vacuolated. (1000×)

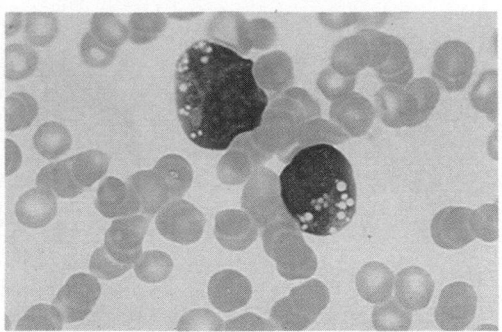

PLATE 36-5. L3 ALL. Another example showing the typical primitive, basophilic blasts containing numerous vacuoles in both cytoplasm and nucleus. (1000×)

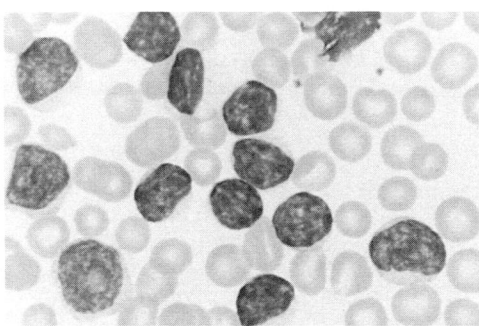

PLATE 37-1. Chronic lymphocytic leukemia. Note similarity of lymphocytes (monotonous picture). Also note smudge cell in upper part of field. (1250×)

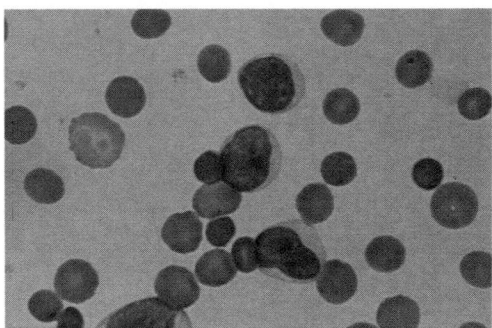

PLATE 37-2. Chronic lymphocytic leukemia (CLL) with evidence of autoimmune hemolytic anemia (note the presence of spherocytes). AIHA is not an unusual complication of CLL. (1000×)

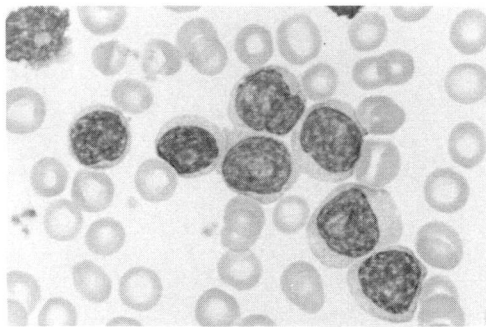

PLATE 37-3. Prolymphocytic leukemia. Note that nuclei of majority of lymphoid cells contain large vesicular nucleolus. (1250×)

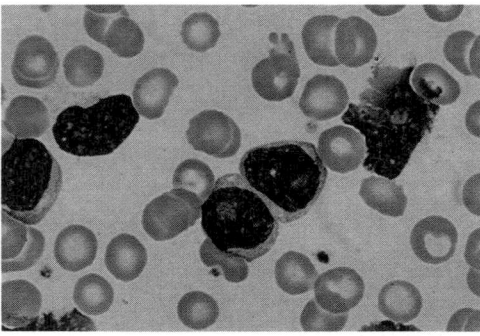

PLATE 37-4. Prolymphocytic leukemia (PLL). Note the large single nucleolus in the cells as well as in the smudge cell. (1250×)

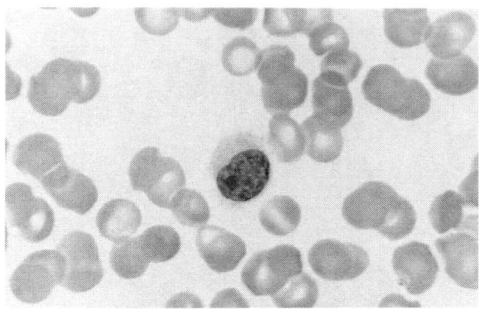

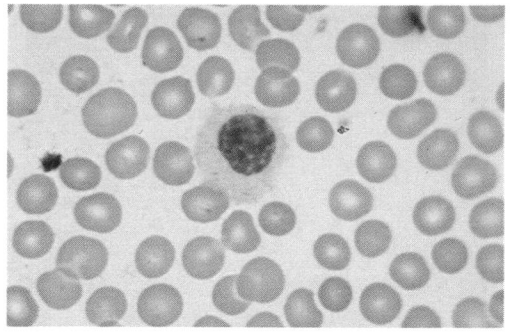

PLATE 37-5. Hairy cell leukemia. Presence of only one cell reflects the fact that the patient does not have an increased leukocyte count. Note hairlike projections of cytoplasm. (1250×)

PLATE 37-6. Hairy cell leukemia (HCL). Another example of these cells with hairlike cytoplasmic projections. (1000×)

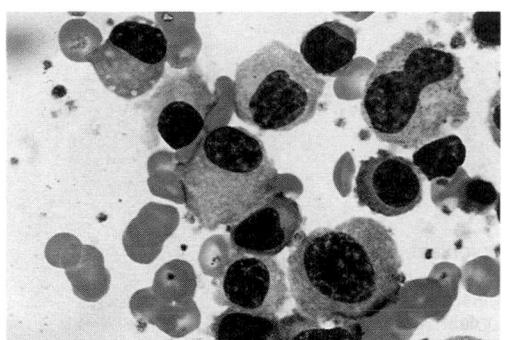

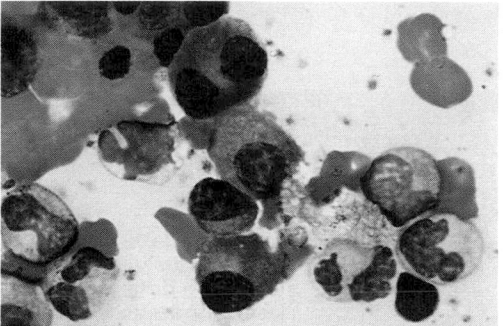

PLATE 39-1. Bone marrow fields from two patients with multiple myeloma. Note the marked difference in morphology of plasma cells in the two patients. (1000×)

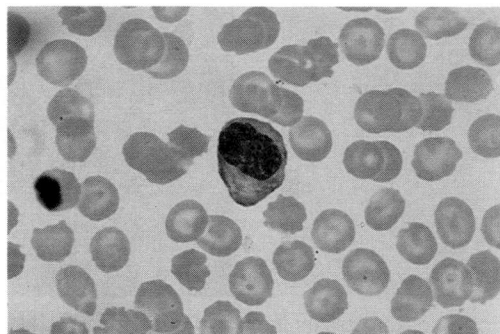

PLATE 39-2. Flame cell. Note pink areas in cytoplasm. (1000×)

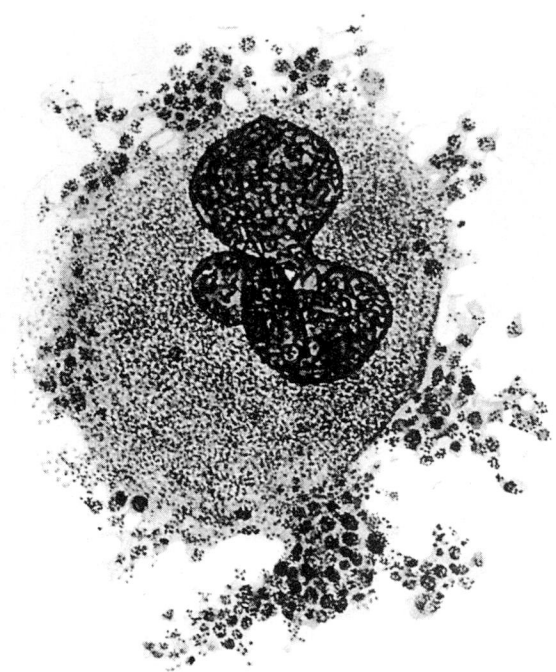

PLATE 55-7. Drawing of a platelet-producing megakaryocyte.*

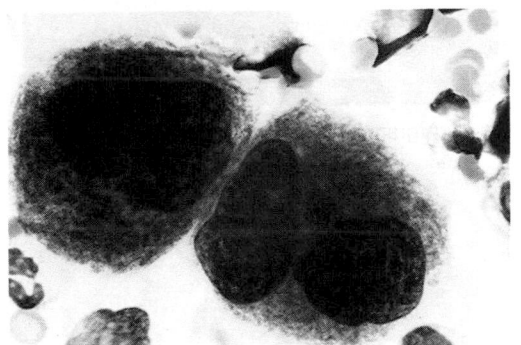

PLATE 55-8. Two mature megakaryocytes in normal marrow. The one to the left has visible platelet clusters within its cytoplasm.

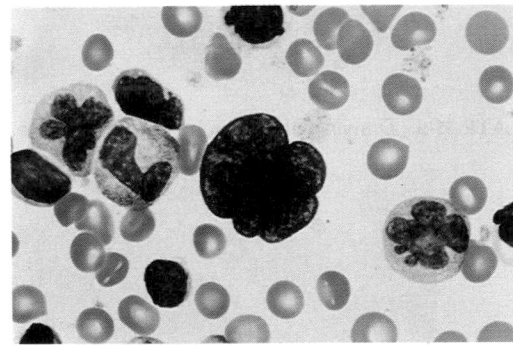

PLATE 55-9. A "naked" megakaryocyte nucleus remaining after platelets have been released into the venous sinus. This nuclear remnant will be phagocytized by macrophages. (1000×)

* From Diggs LW, Sturm D, Bell A: The Morphology of Human Blood Cells, 5th ed. Abbott Park, IL, Abbott Laboratories, 1985, with permission

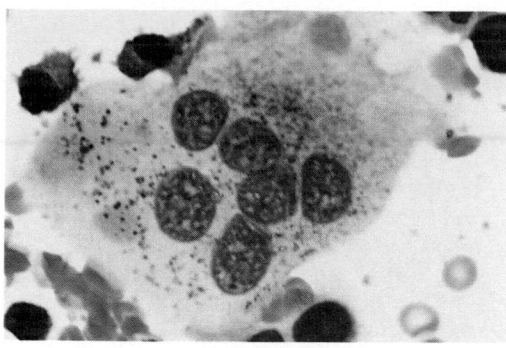

PLATE 55-10. Osteoclast. The "other giant cell" found in bone marrow that could be confused with megakaryocytes. See also Color Plates 27-4 and 27-6. (1000×)

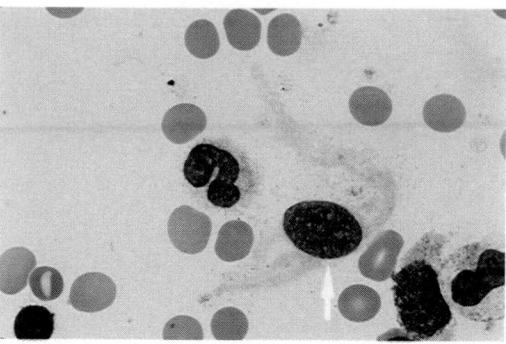

PLATE 55-11. Reticulo-endothelial cell. The *arrow* is pointing to the nucleus of the RE cell. The cytoplasm is frayed and can extend for quite a distance. (1000×)

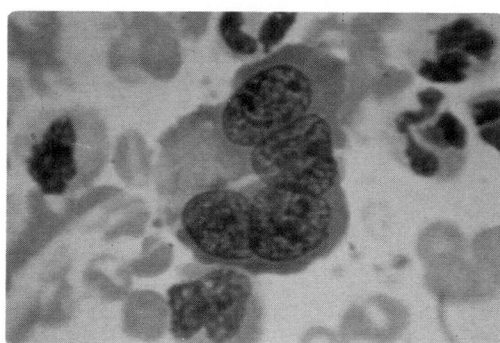

PLATE 55-12. Abnormal, giant multinucleated red cell precursor. Cells such as this might be found in bone marrow samples from individuals having the M6 acute myeloid leukemia, or who have received anti-DNA chemotherapy, or who have congenital dyserythropoietic anemia (CDA). This cell could be confused with a megakaryocyte. (1000×)

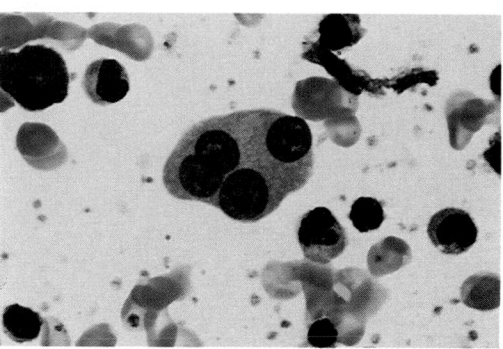

PLATE 55-13. Giant, multinucleated plasma cell that could be confused with a megakaryocyte. (1000×)

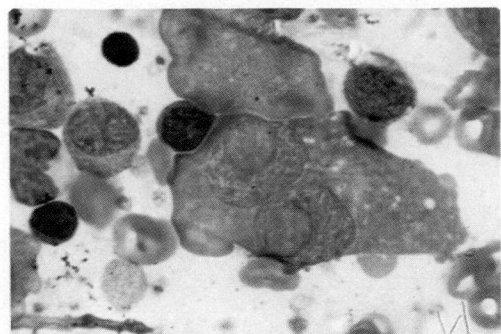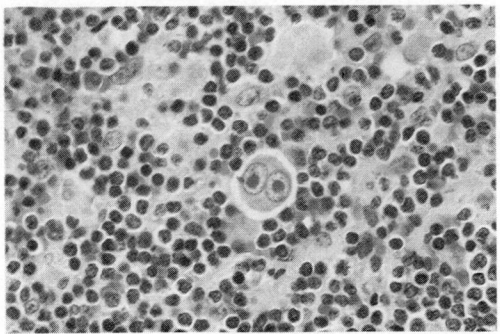

PLATE 55-14. Reed-Sternberg (RS) cell. (**A**) RS cell seen in bone marrow aspirate. Note the large nucleoli. (*Courtesy of the American Cancer Society of Hematology Slide Bank.*) (1000×). (**B**) RS cell seen in a bone marrow section. Note the large nucleoli that give the cell the appearance of an owl's face. The RS cell is sufficiently large in either aspirate or section material that it might be confused with a megakaryocyte. (400×)

2. Aoki N, Moroi M, Sakata Y et al: Abnormal plasminogen: A hereditary molecular abnormality found in a patient with recurrent thrombosis. J Clin Invest 61:1186, 1978

3. Bauer KA: Inherited hypercoagulable states. In Loscalzo J, Schafer AI (eds): Thrombosis and Hemorrhage, p 809. Cambridge, Blackwell Scientific Publications, 1994

4. Broekmans AW, Veltkamp JJ, Bertina RM: Congenital protein C deficiency and venous thromboembolism: A study of three Dutch families. N Engl J Med 309:340, 1983

5. Carter CJ: The natural history and epidemiology of venous thrombosis. Prog Cardiovasc Dis 36:423, 1994

6. Collaborative Group for the Study of Stroke in Young Women: Contraceptives and stroke in young women. JAMA 288:871, 1973

7. Collins GJ Jr, Ahr DJ, Rich NM et al: Detection and management of hypercoagulability. Am J Surg 132:767, 1976

8. Comp PC, Esmon CT: Recurrent venous thromboembolism in patients with a partial deficiency of protein S. N Engl J Med 311:1525, 1984

9. Comp PC: Congenital and acquired hypercoagulable states. In Hull R, Pineo GF (eds): Disorders of Thrombosis, p 339. Philadelphia, WB Saunders, 1996

10. Comp PC: Protein S: Clinical and laboratory aspects. In Green D (ed): Anticoagulants: Physiologic, Pathologic, and Pharmacologic, p 17. Boca Raton, CRC Press, 1994

11. Dyerberg H, Stoffersen E: Recurrent thrombosis in a patient with factor XII deficiency. Acta Hematol 63:278, 1980

12. Egeberg O: Inherited antithrombin deficiency causing thrombophilia. Thromb Diath Haemorrh 13:516, 1965

13. Egeberg O: Inherited fibrinogen abnormality causing thrombophilia. Thromb Diath Haemorrh 17:176, 1967

14. Ens GE: Cost-effective diagnosis of thrombotic disorders. Clin Hemost Rev 9(8):1, 1995

15. Ens GE, Jensen R: The fibrinolytic pathway. Clin Hemost Rev 8(6):1, 1994

16. Esmon CT: Clinical and physiological manifestations of the protein C anticoagulant pathway. In Green D (ed): Anticoagulants: Physiologic, Pathologic, and Pharmacologic, p 3. Boca Raton, CRC Press, 1994

17. Esmon CT: Protein-C: Biochemistry, physiology and clinical implications. Blood 62:1155, 1983

18. Filip DJ, Eckstein JD, Veltkamp JJ: Hereditary antithrombin III deficiency and thromboembolic disease. Am J Hematol 2:343, 1976

19. Gray AJ: Antithrombin III Check Sample: Thrombosis and Hemostasis, No. TH 80-5 (TH-11). Chicago, American Society of Clinical Pathologists, 1981

20. Griffin JH, Evatt B, Zimmerman TS et al: Deficiency of protein C in congenital thrombotic disease. J Clin Invest 68:1370, 1981

21. Griffin JH, Mosher DF, Zimmerman TS et al: Protein C, an antithrombotic protein, is reduced in hospitalized patients with intravascular coagulation. Blood 60:261, 1982

22. Hamstra RD: Personal communication, 1981

23. Hill RJ, Ens GE: The protein C pathway. Clin Hemost Rev 1:1, 1987

24. Jensen R: Activated protein C resistance. Clin Hemost Rev 9(6):1, 1995

25. Jensen RJ, Ens GE: Heparin induced thrombocytopenia with thrombosis. Clin Hemost Rev 8(4):1, 1994

26. Kitchens CS: Thrombophilia and thrombosis in unusual sites. In Colman RW, Hirsh J, Marder VJ et al (eds): Hemostasis and Thrombosis: Basic Principles and Clinical Practice, p 1255. Philadelphia, JB Lippincott, 1994

27. Lassen MR, Borris LC: Prevention in orthopedic surgery and trauma. In Hull R, Pineo GF (eds): Disorders of Thrombosis, p 209. Philadelphia, WB Saunders, 1996

28. Manco-Johnson MJ: Antithrombin III. In Green D (ed): Anticoagulants: Physiologic, Pathologic, and Pharmacologic, p 27. Boca Raton, CRC Press, 1994

29. Marciniak E, Farley CH, DeSimone PA: Familial thrombosis due to antithrombin III deficiency. Blood 43:219, 1974

30. Marlar RA, Kleiss AJ, Griffin JH: Mechanism of action of human activated protein C, a thrombin-dependent anticoagulant enzyme. Blood 59:1067, 1982

31. McGehee WG, Klotz TA, Epstein DJ et al: Coumarin necrosis associated with hereditary protein C deficiency. Ann Intern Med 101:59, 1984

32. Millenson MM, Bauer KA: Pathogenesis of venous thromboembolism. In Hull R, Pineo GF (eds): Disorders of Thrombosis, p 175. Philadelphia, WB Saunders, 1996

33. Nilsson IM, Krook H, Sternby NH et al: Severe thrombotic disease in a young man with bone marrow and skeletal changes and with a high content of an inhibitor in the fibrinolytic system. Acta Med Scand 169:323, 1961

34. Nossel HL, Yudelman I, Canfield et al: Measurement of fibrinopeptide A in human blood. J Clin Invest 54:43, 1974

35. Nucci MR, Bell WR: Acquired hypercoagulable states. In Loscalzo J, Schafer AI (eds): Thrombosis and Hemorrhage, p 835. Cambridge, Blackwell Scientific Publications, 1994

36. Rickles FR, Edwards RL: Activation of blood coagulation in cancer: Trousseau's syndrome revisited. Blood 62:14, 1983

37. Rosenberg RD: Actions and interactions of antithrombin and heparin. N Engl J Med 292:146, 1975

38. Rosenberg RD, Bauer KA: The heparin-antithrombin system: A natural anticoagulant mechanism. In Colman RW, Hirsh J, Marder VJ et al (eds): Hemostasis and Thrombosis: Basic Principles and Clinical Practice, p 837. Philadelphia, JB Lippincott, 1994

39. Rosenberg RD, Damus PS: The purification and mechanism of action of human antithrombin–heparin cofactor. J Biol Chem 248:6490, 1973

40. Rosenberg RD, Rosenberg JS: Natural anticoagulant mechanisms. J Clin Invest 74:1, 1984

41. Schafer AI: The hypercoagulable states. Ann Intern Med 102:814, 1985

42. Seghatchian MJ: Protein C in clinical factor IX concentrates. Lancet 1:1047, 1983

43. Seligsohn U, Berger A, Abend M et al: Homozygous protein C deficiency manifested by massive venous thrombosis in the newborn. N Engl J Med 310:559, 1984

44. Sheffield WP, Wu YI, Blajchman MA: Antithrombin: Structure and function. In High KA, Roberts HR (eds): Molecular Basis of Thrombosis and Hemostasis, p 355. New York, Marcel Dekker, 1995

45. Southern D, Ens GE: Normal hemostasis. In Rodak BF (ed): Diagnostic Hematology, p 465. Philadelphia, WB Saunders, 1995

46. Stampfer MJ, Malinow M, Willet WC et al: A prospective study of plasma homocyst(e)ine and risk of myocardial infarction in US physicians. JAMA 268:877, 1992

47. Stampfer MJ, Malinow MR: Can lowering homocysteine levels reduce cardiovascular risk? New Engl J Med 332(5):328, 1995

48. Svensson PJ, Dahlback B: Resistance to activated protein C as a basis for venous thrombosis. New Engl J Med 330:517, 1994

49. Teitel JM, Bauer KA, Lau HK et al: Studies of the prothrombin activation pathway utilizing radioimmunoassay for the F_2/F_{1+2} fragment and thrombin:antithrombin complex. Blood 59:1086, 1982

50. Trousseau A: Phelegmasia alba dolens. Clin Med Hotel Dieu Paris 3:94, 1865

51. Winter JH, Fenech A, Ridley W et al: Familial antithrombin III deficiency. Q J Med 51:373, 1982

52. Yasuda M, Takakuwa K, Tokunaga A et al: Prospective studies of the association between anticardiolipin antibody and outcome of pregnancy. Obstet Gynecol 86:555, 1995

CHAPTER 54

Laboratory Monitoring of Anticoagulant Therapy

Jamie E. Siegel and Powers Peterson

Heparin Therapy
Anticoagulant Activity
Administration
Laboratory Monitoring and
  Therapeutic Range

Oral Anticoagulants
Anticoagulant Activity
Administration
Laboratory Monitoring and
  Methods of Reporting
  Results

Antiplatelet Function Therapy
Anticoagulant Activity
Laboratory Monitoring

***In Vivo* Lysis of Thrombi**
Laboratory Monitoring

Case Study 54-1

Objectives

1. Describe how heparin, oral anticoagulants and platelet inhibitors decrease the coagulability of blood.
2. Discuss the differences between high and low molecular weight heparin.
3. Describe how the laboratory monitors the anticoagulant activity of heparin, oral anticoagulants and platelet inhibitors, respectively.
4. Describe how the international normalized ratio (INR) (1) is calculated and (2) is used to evaluate patient coagulation status.
5. Discuss the advantages and disadvantages of the international normalized ratio (INR).

Laboratory monitoring of anticoagulant therapy is imprecise but vital. The partial thromboplastin time (PTT) and the activated coagulation time (ACT) monitor heparin use, whereas the prothrombin time (PT) and the international normalized ratio (INR) monitor anticoagulants such as warfarin sodium. These assays provide an *estimate* of an anticoagulant drug's activity in protecting the patient from thrombus formation or hemorrhage. This chapter addresses the role of these laboratory tests in the clinical setting of thrombosis, the controversies surrounding monitoring drugs for anticoagulation, as well as the use of low molecular weight heparin (LMWH), antiplatelet agents, and thrombolytic therapy.

It is important to remember that the goal of anticoagulant therapy is to prevent or to treat thrombosis. Whether venous or arterial, thrombosis is the pathologic extension of normal hemostasis. The process leads to the formation of a solid mass from constituents of the blood within living, intact blood vessels or the heart. The resultant mass, known as a thrombus, is formed by a complex process involving the interaction of blood vessel walls, the formed elements of blood (RBC, WBC, platelets), and the plasma proteins that constitute the blood coagulation system.[4]

Approaches to the treatment of thrombosis differ because of the differences in the pathogenesis of arterial and venous thrombi. Treatment with anticoagulant drugs is more effective when intravascular fibrin formation is the predominant pathologic process (*e.g.*, deep vein thrombosis). Similar treatment may be of limited value when platelet aggregation is the principal factor in thrombus formation (*e.g.*, coronary artery thrombosis). Antiplatelet drugs may be appropriate for these patients. The objectives of therapy in deep venous thrombosis are to prevent propagation and embolization of the thrombus or thrombi and to minimize damage to the vein itself. Two treatments that have been used to slow the formation of fibrin are parenteral heparin and oral anticoagulants. An important therapeutic advance for treating arterial thrombosis caused by platelet emboli is drugs that inhibit normal platelet function. Agents such as aspirin, dipyridamole, and the newer platelet–receptor–GPIIb/IIIa antagonists impair platelet adhesion or aggregation. Plasminogen activators, which produce direct clot lysis *in vivo* are sometimes administered in acute life-threatening conditions such as massive occlusion of the coronary arteries, peripheral deep veins, or pulmonary arteries.

HEPARIN THERAPY

Heparin was the first agent administered as an anticoagulant.[14] Heparin is used to prevent the formation of thrombi in veins or to prevent the propagation of previously formed thrombi in veins or arteries. Currently, heparin is used to prevent or treat venous thromboembolism and to treat unstable angina and acute myocardial infarction. Heparin is also administered during and after coronary angioplasty and during cardiovascular surgery.[9]

Anticoagulant Activity

The commercial preparations of standard heparin are heterogeneous mixtures of glycosaminoglycans with molecular weights ranging from 5,000 to 30,000 daltons. The effects of heparin are mediated through its action on antithrombin III (AT-III). Heparin induces a conformational change in AT-III which creates a thousandfold enhancement of AT-III's natural activity against thrombin and activated factor X (Xa) (Fig. 53-1). Heparin enhances the effect of AT-III on thrombin by forming a complex with both AT-III and thrombin. On the other hand, the inactivation of Xa requires its binding to AT-III alone.[9,25] Low molecular weight heparin (LMWH) is produced from standard heparin by chemical or enzymatic depolymerization. Compared with standard heparin, LMWH has a decreased ability to inactivate thrombin because of its smaller molecular size and its inability to form a complex with AT-III and thrombin together. LMWH, however, inactivates Xa by binding to AT-III alone. Whereas standard heparin has an anti-Xa/antithrombin ratio of 1:1, LMWH has an anti-Xa/AT-III ratio of from 2:1 to 4:1. The activity ratio is determined by the molecular weight of the individual LMWH and, therefore, varies with different preparations of the drug. LMWH has a long plasma half-life, allowing once or twice-a-day administration when given subcutaneously. LMWH also has a more predictable response because of its lack of binding to heparin-binding proteins.

Heparin-induced thrombocytopenia (HIT) is a potentially lethal complication of heparin therapy. In this condition platelets are activated by heparin-dependent IgG antibodies against a complex of heparin and platelet factor 4 (a heparin-binding protein that is synthesized by platelets). Clinically this results in platelet aggregation and consumption leading to decreased platelet counts. Accepted clinical definitions of HIT are either (1) a decrease in the platelet count to less than 100×10^9/L during heparin treatment in patients who originally had normal platelet counts or (2) a decrease in the platelet count to less than 50% of baseline, even if the platelet count is greater than 100×10^9/L. HIT occurs in 2% to 5% of patients receiving therapeutic heparin.[15,36] Consequently, the platelet count is monitored daily in patients receiving intravenous (IV) heparin. If HIT develops, the appropriate initial response is to discontinue heparin immediately and to eliminate any possible hidden sources of heparin exposure such as heparin lines or heparin-coated catheters.[18] A further complication of heparin therapy is heparin-induced thrombocytopenia with thrombosis (HITT). The formation of thrombi is believed to be caused by the same heparin–platelet interactions described above. Although the incidence of HITT is less than the incidence of HIT, this clinical scenario is usually limb- or life-threatening.

Administration

Therapeutic anticoagulation is achieved with an initial heparin bolus followed by continuous intravenous (IV) infusion. Typically the bolus is administered as 5000 units (U) or as 80 U/kg. The infusion is started at 1300 U/h or as 18 U/kg/h.[13] "Therapeutic" levels of heparin as measured by the PTT must be achieved within 24 hours of hospitalization to prevent an increased risk of recurrent thrombosis. If oral anticoagulation is indicated, warfarin sodium is begun shortly after heparin treatment is initiated (see Oral Anticoagulants, Administration, following). Heparin anticoagulation should be continued for at least 5 days. During that period, the warfarin effects are also monitored. Heparin may need to be continued for a longer period in the clinical settings of massive pulmonary embolism or ileofemoral thrombosis.

If heparin must be administered in an outpatient setting for long-term management, it can be injected subcutaneously (10,000 to 20,000 U) every 12 hours. This situation may occur when a pregnant patient either develops a deep venous thrombosis or has a history of recurrent or life-threatening thromboses. The PTT levels are determined exactly 6 hours after a heparin injection. The goal is to have the patient's PTT level in the midlevel of the laboratory's previously determined therapeutic range. The dose of heparin is adjusted as needed.[6]

LMWH is administered by subcutaneous injection. It is given in a patient weight-based dosage for prophylaxis or treatment.

Laboratory Monitoring and Therapeutic Range

The first laboratory test used to monitor the effect of heparin was the Lee-White clotting time (LWCT), also known as the whole blood-clotting time (WBCT).[19] A prolonged LWCT occurs with increasing concentrations of heparin; however, there may be considerable scatter in the clotting times produced at any given concentration of heparin (poor reproducibility). Typical coefficients of variation range from 15% to 30%.[33] The LWCT also lacks sensitivity in that doubling the concentration of heparin may produce only a minimal change in the LWCT, whereas other assays often demonstrate a two- to threefold change. Finally, the test is time-consuming to perform and quality control is problematic at best.

Distinct differences in sensitivity to standard heparin preparations have been demonstrated for several laboratory assays, including the LWCT, ACT, PTT, PT and thrombin time (TT).[22] The effects of heparin on the recalcified TT results, as well as on PT and PTT results, are shown in Figure 54-1.

The PTT is a useful and sensitive assay for monitoring heparin therapy. Indeed, the College of American Pathologists survey data indicate that the PTT is the assay of choice.[1] The clinical goal is to attain an optimal dose (therapeutic range), one that prevents progression of thrombosis and simultaneously poses a minimum risk of hemorrhage.

It is recommended that each laboratory in which heparin therapy is monitored with the PTT determine its own therapeutic range, correlating PTT results to plasma heparin concentration (U/mL) so as to reflect the laboratory's specific reagents, instumentation and personnel.[20] Ideally, the laboratory should be able to demonstrate that the therapeutic PTT range is equivalent to a serum heparin level of 0.2 to 0.4 U/mL (as measured by protamine titration) or 0.3 to 0.7 U/mL anti-Xa activity.[9,16] Some phospholipid extracts as well as activators in current commercial reagents for the PTT may lack the sensitivity needed to

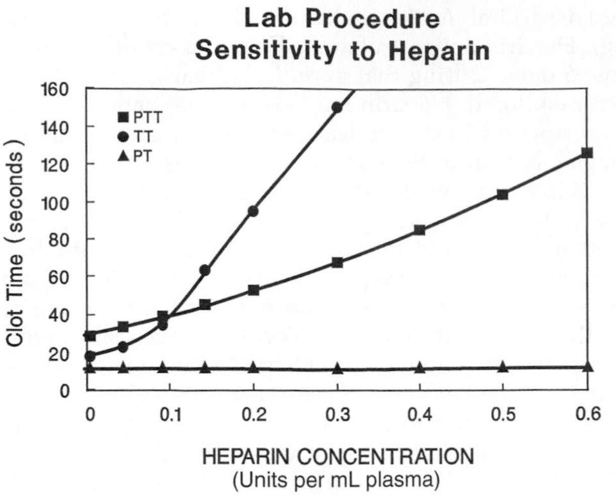

Lab Procedure
Sensitivity to Heparin

FIGURE 54-1. Sensitivity to heparin of various laboratory tests: Observe the sensitivity to small amounts achieved by recalcified thrombin time (TT). Note also that PT test is insensitive to therapeutic concentrations of heparin.

demonstrate the presence of small concentrations of heparin and so may fail to detect therapeutic levels adequately.[2,29] The *therapeutic range* was originally thought to be 1.5 to 2.5 times the patient's baseline PTT level. Although this therapeutic level (1.5 to 2.5 times baseline) was long a clinical standard, one report indicates a marked variability in the response (sensitivity) of the PTT reagents to the heparin preparations.[2] In other words, PTT results obtained on the same blood sample from a patient on a fixed dose of heparin may differ with different PTT reagents.[28] Therefore, the specific PTT thromboplastin reagent used by the laboratory must be noted when interpreting PTT results and calculating heparin dose(s). Attempts to standardize PTT reagents have not yet been successful.[23,24]

The PTT is sensitive over a heparin range of 0.1 to 1.0 U/mL. The relation becomes nonlinear above a heparin level of 1.0 U/mL. Therefore, the PTT cannot be used to monitor patients requiring very high doses of heparin, such as those undergoing angioplasty and coronary artery bypass surgery (Chap. 49). The recommended assay for monitoring serum heparin levels of 1 to 5 U/mL is the ACT.[9]

ORAL ANTICOAGULANTS

Warfarin, a derivative of 4-hydroxycoumarin, is the oral anticoagulant most commonly prescribed for venous thrombosis. Warfarin interferes with the metabolism of vitamin K. This vitamin is a required cofactor for the synthesis of coagulation factors II, VII, IX and X. Warfarin has no direct effect on clot lysis.

Anticoagulant Activity

Therapy with warfarin-type compounds prevents the liver from carboxylating the N-glutamyl residues of the prothrombin group factors (factors II, VII, IX and X). This results in lower plasma levels of these vitamin K-dependent factors. The nonfunctional proteins that are produced (previously referred to as *proteins induced by vitamin K antagonists* or PIVKA; now called des-γ-carboxy proteins) lack the calcium-binding properties that facilitate binding of coagulation factors to a phospholipid surface. Binding to a phospholipid surface is necessary for initiation of coagulation.[32]

The rate of reduction in the prothrombin group factors after administration of oral anticoagulants is related to the normal metabolic turnover (half-life) of each factor. Factor VII has the shortest plasma half-life and decreases first, 5 to 6 hours after initiation of warfarin therapy. Factor IX levels decrease within 28 to 40 hours, followed by factor X levels (half-life 40 to 50 hours). The last factor affected is factor II, the plasma half-life of which is 48 to 60 hours. Consequently, a stable anticoagulant effect is not attained until the patient has received warfarin for several days, even weeks. Laboratory monitoring, which consists of serial PT assays over the first weeks following initiation of warfarin therapy should reflect an understanding of the complex dynamics involved. In contrast to the immediate reversal of the anticoagulant activity of heparin by the injection of protamine sulfate, overcoming the interference of carboxylase activity produced by warfarin requires injection of vitamin K. Thereafter, 6 to 24 hours is required for vitamin K-dependent factors to return to normal plasma levels. If indicated, immediate reversal of the effects of oral anticoagulants may be achieved by transfusion of fresh frozen plasma.

The effects of warfarin are greatly affected by other drugs given concurrently. Agents that inhibit warfarin could result in thrombosis, whereas those that enhance its effects could lead to hemorrhage. Some of the drugs known to affect warfarin metabolism include various antibiotics, phenylbutazone, indomethacin, tolbutamide, salicylates, quinidine, barbiturates, diuretics, and oral contraceptive agents and other steroids. A complete listing of the many potential drug interactions can be found in other publications.[11,27] An abbreviated list is found in Chapter 52.

Administration

Oral anticoagulant therapy is usually initiated shortly after heparin: either immediately, after a therapeutic PTT level is achieved, or on the evening of the second day of heparin therapy. Warfarin is continued for at least 3 months for venous thromboembolic disease.

Laboratory Monitoring and Methods of Reporting Results

The laboratory test to monitor warfarin therapy has historically been the one-stage PT. The PT reflects the effects of warfarin on factors II, VII and X. (The PT does not measure depleted factor IX effects.) Standardization of the PT as a monitor of effective oral anticoagulant therapy was introduced in 1983 with the international normalized ratio (INR) system. This occurred after recognition that there were marked differences in the responsiveness of thromboplastin reagents to the vitamin K-dependent clotting factor levels. The thromboplastin reagents contain tissue factor, phospholipid and calcium. The active ingredient in the reagent is a lipoprotein (phospholipid–protein) extract derived from human or animal tissues. The PT result varies according to a particular thromboplastin reagent's "responsiveness" (sensitivity) to the effects of warfarin on factors II, VII and X. Thus, PT tests in different laboratories using different thromboplastin reagents may lead to different results even when the plasma warfarin concentration is the same. This could potentially cause the misinterpretation of a patient's anticoagulant status and consequently the risk of bleeding or thrombosis. To avoid this, reagent responsiveness is now determined by comparison with an internationally agreed on reference reagent: the World Health Organization (WHO) reference thromboplastin. All thromboplastin reagents distributed for laboratory use now have been calibrated against this reference preparation. The calibration number is known as the International Sensitivity Index (ISI). By design, the WHO reference thromboplastin has an ISI of 1.0. This ISI of 1.0 corresponds to appropriate responsiveness of the PT to the effects of warfarin. As the ISI increases, there is less responsiveness to the same (plasma) concentration of warfarin (*i.e.,* a decreased sensitivity of the PT to the effects of warfarin). This is shown in Figure 54-2.[5] For a patient receiving anticoagulants who has been stabilized and is receiving an unchanging dose of warfarin, the measured PT in seconds will decrease as the ISI of the individual thromboplastin reagent increases. For these reasons, laboratories should use a thromboplastin with a lower ISI (*i.e.,* less than 2.0).

The INR is the ratio of a patient's PT to the mean PT normal value determined using a given thromboplastin, and this ratio is raised to the power of the ISI. The formula is:[17]

$$INR = \left(\frac{PT_{patient}}{Geometric\ Mean\ PT_{normals}} \right)^{ISI}$$

where $PT_{patient}$ = patient PT in seconds for a given thromboplastin preparation; geometric mean $PT_{normals}$ = mean PT in seconds for healthy individuals using the same thromboplastin reagent; and ISI = international sensitivity index (provided by reagent manufacturer).

By using the INR, the degree of anticoagulation achieved by warfarin therapy may be compared regardless of thromboplastin used. Use of the INR allows PT results to be compared among clinical laboratories around the world, resulting in better patient management. It must be emphasized that the purpose of the INR is to monitor patients taking oral anticoagulants; it is not intended to be used for initial evaluation of the hemostatic system or thrombotic conditions.

Although the INR system is superior to reporting the PT in seconds alone or the PT ratio, problems with this system remain. If the INR is calculated on plasma from patients who are clinically stable and who have received warfarin for at least 6 weeks, it will evaluate the effects of factors II, X and VII. On the other hand, when a patient is *first* given warfarin, *only* its effects on factor VII influence the PT. Recall that the plasma half-life of factor VII is 6 hours, whereas the half-life of factor X is 40 to 50 hours and that of factor II is 48 to 60 hours. Therefore, the INR is unreliable early in treatment. Conservative clinical management would use the INR after the anticoagulated patient is stable, probably 2 to 3 weeks after initiation of warfarin. Other problems in using the INR include incorrect ISI values assigned to thromboplastin reagents, method and instrument variations and incorrectly calculated INR values.[11]

ANTIPLATELET FUNCTION THERAPY

Studies in the 1970s suggested that recurrent thrombotic episodes decreased when normal platelet function was curtailed by antiplatelet drugs. These drugs are now used in preventing arterial thrombosis, the pathologic counterpart of the beneficial role that normal platelets play in maintaining hemostasis.[7,29]

Anticoagulant Activity

Figure 54-3 demonstrates the effects of aspirin on normal platelet function. Under normal circumstances, when platelets are stimulated with a variety of agents (ADP, collagen, thrombin), arachidonic acid is made available by hydrolysis of membrane phospholipids. Subsequently, arachidonic acid is converted by cyclooxygenase to intermediate cyclic endoperoxides, which are precursors of thromboxane A_2. Thromboxane A_2 is a potent stimulant of platelet aggregation and is also a powerful vasoconstrictor. Aspirin, probably the most commonly prescribed inhibitor of platelet function, acts by irreversibly acetylating cyclooxygenase. Nonsteroidal anti-inflammatory

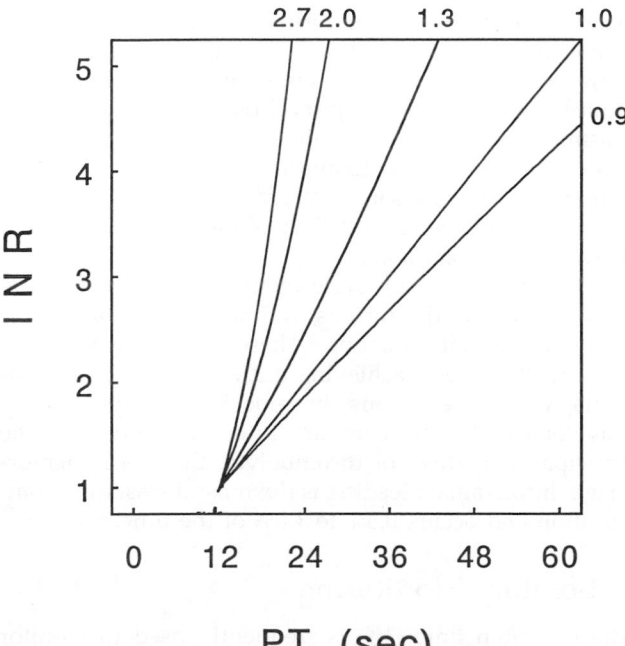

FIGURE 54-2. How thromboplastin reagent sensitivity affects the PT interval between INRs. ISI values are given at the end of each corresponding line. All lines intersect a theoretical mean normal clotting time of 12.0 sec. Notice that as the ISI increases, the time interval between INRs decreases.

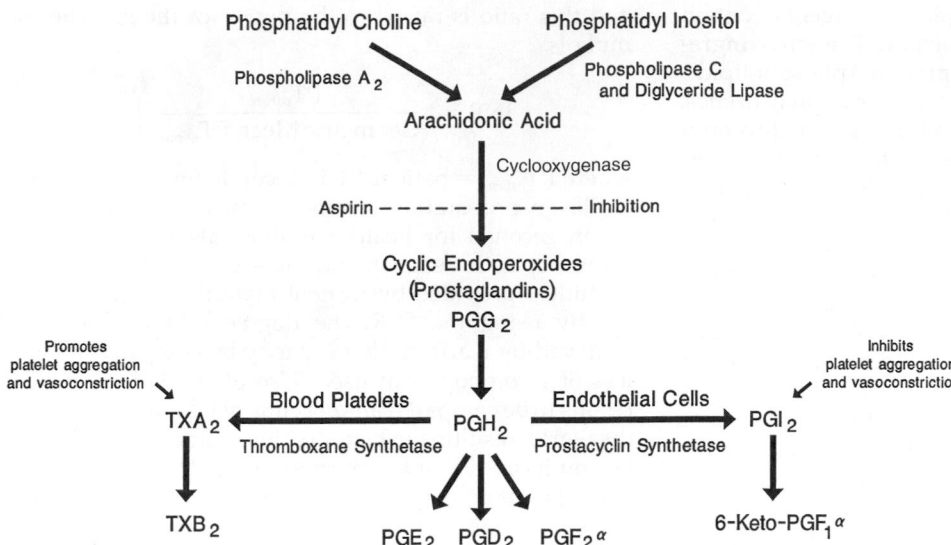

drugs (NSAIDs) also inhibit cyclo-oxygenase, but their effect on platelet function is reversible and short-lived.[26]

Ticlopidine™ is a newer antiplatelet agent that also irreversibly inhibits platelet aggregation by blocking the interaction between fibrinogen and platelet membrane glycoprotein receptor GPIIb/IIIa.[12] Platelet GPIIb/IIIa antagonists are being used to treat and prevent thrombotic complications in patients with cardiac disease. By inhibiting the GPIIb/IIIa receptor, these drugs mimic the defect present in the platelets of patients with Glanzmann's thrombasthenia (*i.e.*, the lack of GPIIb/IIIa; Chap. 57). This receptor mediates platelet aggregation but not adhesion. Other clinical applications are under evaluation.[3]

Laboratory Monitoring

Although antiplatelet drugs are reported to be effective in decreasing platelet adhesion or aggregation, their use usually requires no laboratory studies or assays for appropriate clinical management of the patient.[29] In some cases platelet aggregation assays, which monitor the platelet release reaction, may be useful. Ingestion of aspirin results in *in vitro* aggregation studies showing an absence of the second wave of aggregation in response to ADP and epinephrine. A reduced response to collagen and arachidonic acid also occurs.[20,31] See Chapter 56 for a further discussion of tests of platelet function.

IN VIVO LYSIS OF THROMBI

The previously discussed types of anticoagulant therapy have no effect on already formed (organized) thrombi. Fibrin deposits, both intravascular and extravascular, are removed through fibrinolysis, the enzymatic dissolution of insoluble fibrin polymer. This phenomenon is regulated by the plasminogen–plasmin system (Chap. 48), which can be enhanced by infusions of plasminogen activators. Agents in clinical use as plasminogen activators include streptokinase, urokinase, and tissue plasminogen activator (TPA).[21,34,35]

Plasmin that is formed after administration of plasminogen activators impairs hemostasis in two ways: (1) by direct lysis of fibrin in hemostatic clots and (2) by producing systemic fibrinolysis by cleaving fibrinogen as well as factors V and VIII. Resulting increases in fibrin degradation products (FDP) further enhance fibrinolysis because these fragments themselves act as direct thrombin inhibitors. In addition, the direct effect of plasmin on platelet membrane glycoproteins impairs platelet function.[8,21,27] Clinically, this condition is sometimes referred to as a *lytic state*.

Streptokinase and urokinase are administered by either systemic intravenous infusion or localized intra-arterial infusion. Streptokinase forms a 1:1 complex with plasminogen, which activates free plasminogen to plasmin. However, because it is a foreign antigen, it will usually stimulate an immune response. Urokinase directly cleaves plasminogen to form plasmin.[35] The clinical advantage of urokinase over streptokinase is that urokinase is less antigenic. The enzymatic activity of tissue plasminogen activator is enhanced by fibrin, making it a very sufficient activator of plasminogen.

Thrombolysis with these agents is used for the treatment of venous thrombosis, pulmonary embolism and acute myocardial infarction.[8] These plasminogen activators are effective in achieving early thrombolysis in patients with acute venous thrombosis, acute pulmonary embolism and acute coronary artery thrombosis.[27] The principal side effect of thrombolytic therapy is hemorrhage. Intracranial bleeding is the most devastating complication and occurs 0.3% to 1.0% of the time.[21]

Laboratory Monitoring

The thrombin time (TT) is frequently used to monitor fibrinolytic activity. The TT should be measured before thrombolytic therapy and 3 to 4 hours after starting therapy. A TT of 2 to 5 times baseline levels is desirable. Important "leading indicators" of an increased risk of hemorrhage include thrombocytopenias, low serum fibrinogen levels and increased levels of FDP measured by the D-dimer test (Chap. 50).[30]

CHAPTER SUMMARY

The correlation between hemorrhage and laboratory test results is imperfect. No single laboratory assay can predict the likelihood of clinical bleeding, nor is hemorrhage always associated with an abnormal test result. Judicious use of laboratory assays can enhance clinical management of the patient with a predisposition to thrombosis or an overt thrombotic state.

Case Study 54-1

A 28-year-old woman was admitted to the intensive care unit after a diagnosis was made of pulmonary embolism. Heparin (5000 U) was administered immediately by intravenous injection. Two hours later, the physician ordered a PTT. The laboratory reported a PTT of 40 seconds (reference range 25-36 seconds), and the physician called the laboratory to verify the results.
1. Identify any possible problems.
2. Identify possible solutions.

Review Questions

54-1. The laboratory test of choice for monitoring heparin therapy at a plasma concentration of 0.1 to 1.0 U/mL is the

A. prothrombin time.
B. partial thromboplastin time.
C. activated clotting time.
D. thrombin time.

54-2. The international sensitivity index (ISI) for thromboplastin reagents used in the clinical laboratory should be

A. less than 1.
B. less than 2.
C. greater than 2.
D. greater than 3.

54-3. The international normalized ratio (INR) is useful for

A. determining coagulation reference ranges.
B. monitoring heparin therapy.
C. monitoring thrombolytic therapy.
D. monitoring warfarin therapy.

54-4. The international normalized ratio (INR) is used to correct for differences in reagent preparations for the

A. prothrombin time.
B. partial thromboplastin time.
C. activated clotting time.
D. Lee-White clotting time.

54-5. If laboratory monitoring of antiplatelet function therapy is requested, the recommended test would probably be the

A. platelet count.
B. platelet aggregation assay.
C. Lee-White clotting time.
D. partial thromboplastin time.

54-6. Streptokinase, urokinase or tissue plasminogen activator is administered to patients to

A. inhibit cyclo-oxygenase.
B. inhibit the platelet GPIIb/IIIa receptor.
C. induce lysis of fibrin clots.
D. stimulate platelet aggregation.

54-7. Risk of hemorrhage may be detected by checking the

A. platelet count.
B. serum fibrinogen level.
C. D-dimer level.
D. all of the above.

References

1. Banez G, Triplett DA, Koepke JA: Laboratory monitoring of heparin therapy: The effect of different salts of heparin on the activated partial thromboplastin time: An analysis of the 1978 and 1979 CAP Hematology Survey. Am J Clin Pathol 74:569, 1980
2. Brandt JT, Triplett DA: Laboratory monitoring of heparin: Effects of reagent and instruments on the activated partial thromboplastin time. Am J Clin Pathol 76:530, 1981
3. Coller BS, Anderson K, Weisman HF: New antiplatelet agents: Platelet GPIIb/IIIa antagonists. Thromb Haemost 74:302, 1995
4. Cotran RS, Kumar V, Robbins RS: Pathologic Basis of Disease, 5th ed. Philadelphia, WB Saunders, 1994
5. Ebert RF: PTs, PRs, ISIs, and INRs: A primer on prothrombin time reporting. Clin Hemost Rev 7(11):1, (12)1, 1993
6. Ginsberg JS, Hirsh J: Use of antithrombotic agents during pregnancy. Chest 108:305S, 1995
7. Harker L: Hemostasis Manual, 2nd ed. Philadelphia, FA Davis, 1974
8. Hirsh J: Basis for the Therapeutic Range for Anticoagulant Therapy. Atlanta, Dade Company Thrombosis–Hemostasis Conference, 1984
9. Hirsh J, Raschke R, Warkentin TE et al: Heparin: Mechanisms of action, pharmacokinetics, dosing considerations, monitoring, efficacy, and safety. Chest 108:258S, 1995
10. Hirsh J, Levine MN: Low molecular weight heparin. Blood 79:1, 1992
11. Hirsh J, Dalen JE, Deykin D, Poller L, Bussey H: Oral anticoagulants: Mechanism of action, clinical effectiveness, and optimal therapeutic range. Chest 108:231S, 1995
12. Hirsh J, Dalen J, Fuster V et al: Aspirin and other platelet-active drugs. Chest 108:247S, 1995
13. Hyers TM, Hull RD, Weg JG: Antithrombotic therapy for venous thromboembolic disease. Chest 108:335S, 1995
14. Jorpes E: Heparin in the Treatment of Thrombosis: An Account of its Chemistry, Physiology and Application in Medicine, 2nd ed. New York, Oxford Press, 1946
15. King DJ, Kelton JG: Heparin-associated thrombocytopenia. Ann Intern Med 100:535, 1984
16. Kitchen S, Preston FE: The therapeutic range for heparin therapy: Relationship between six activated partial thromboplastin time reagents and two heparin assays. Thromb Haemost 75:734, 1996
17. Kovacs MJ, Weir K, Keeney M et al: Determining the mean normal prothrombin time (PT mn) for derivation of the International Normalized Ratio. Lab Hematol 1:23, 1995
18. Laster JL, Nichols WK, Silver D: Thrombocytopenia associated with heparin-coated catheters in patients with heparin-associated antiplatelet antibodies. Arch Intern Med 149:2285, 1989
19. Lee RI, White PD: A clinical study of the coagulation time of blood. Am J Med Sci 145:495, 1913
20. Lenahan J, Smith K: Hemostasis Manual, 18th ed. Durham NC, Organon Teknika, 1986
21. Levine MN, Goldhaber SZ, Gore JM et al: Hemorrhagic complications of thrombolytic therapy in the treatment of myocardial infarction and venous thromboembolism. Chest 108:291S, 1995

22. Palkuti H: Laboratory monitoring of anticoagulant therapy. J Med Technol 2:81, 1985

23. Ray M, Carroll P, Smith I et al: An attempt to standardize aPTT reagents used to monitor heparin therapy. Blood Coag Fibrin 3:743, 1992

24. Reed SV, Haddon ME, Denson KWE: An attempt to standardize the aPTT for heparin monitoring using the PT ISI/INR system of calibration. Results of a 13 centre study. Thromb Res 74:515, 1994

25. Rosenberg RD: Biochemistry of heparin antithrombin interactions, and the physiologic role of this natural anticoagulant mechanism. Am J Med 87(suppl 3B):2S, 1989

26. Shattil SJ, Bennett JS: Acquired qualitative platelet disorders due to diseases, drugs, and foods. In Beutler E, Lichtman MA, Coller BS, Kipps TJ (eds): Williams Hematology, 5th ed. New York, McGraw-Hill, 1995

27. Sherry S, Bell WR, Duckert FH et al: Thrombosis and Thrombolysis, 2nd ed. Somerville NJ, Hoechst-Rousel Pharmaceuticals, 1979

28. Shojania AM, Tetreault J, Turnbull G: The variations between heparin sensitivity of different lots of activated partial thromboplastin time reagent produced by the same manufacturer. Am J Clin Pathol 89:19, 1988

29. Thomson J: Blood Coagulation and Haemostasis, 2nd ed. New York, Churchill Livingstone, 1980

30. Tracy RP, Bovill EG: Fibrinolytic parameters and hemostatic monitoring: Identifying and predicting patients at risk for major hemorrhagic events. Am J Cardiol 69:52A, 1992

31. Triplett DA: Platelet Function: Laboratory Evaluation and Clinical Application. Chicago, American Society of Clinical Pathologists Press, 1978

32. Triplett DA: Anticoagulant therapy: Monitoring techniques. Lab Manage 20:32, 1982

33. Triplett DA: Laboratory Evaluation of Coagulation. Chicago, American Society of Clinical Pathologists Press, 1982

34. Triplett DA: Tissue plasminogen activator (t-PA). Thromb Hemost No. TH86-4(TH-46). Chicago, American Society of Clinical Pathologists Press, 1986

35. Verstraete M, Vermylen J, Schetz J: Biochemical changes noted during intermittent administration of streptokinase. Thromb Haemost 39:61, 1978

36. Warkentin TE, Levine MN, Hirsh J et al: Heparin-induced thrombocytopenia in patients treated with low-molecular-weight heparin or unfractionated heparin. N Engl J Med 332:1330, 1995

CHAPTER 55

The Megakaryocyte–Platelet System

Robert M. Rifkin

Objectives

1. Define the four stages of megakaryocytic maturation and describe the appearance of the nucleus and cytoplasm in each.
2. Explain the concept of endomitosis as it applies to megakaryocytic maturation.
3. List at least five normal or pathologic cells with which cells in the megakaryocytic series can be confused.
4. Describe the structure of the platelet plasma membrane and cytoskeleton.
5. State the life span and describe the turnover of platelets.
6. Describe the process of primary hemostasis including platelet adhesion, secretion, and aggregation.
7. Describe the interaction of platelets with the coagulation system.

The mysteries of platelet production and its regulation have recently begun to be unraveled. The megakaryocyte–platelet system is felt to be under the control of one or more thrombopoietins.[63] One such thrombopoietin has recently been isolated, purified, and cloned by several investigators.[25,67,114,135] This exciting discovery has allowed numerous studies to be performed to explore correlations between megakaryocytic structure, differentiation, and physiology.[145] A basic understanding of the megakaryocyte–platelet system is essential to appreciate the clinical significance of diseases which arise through states of platelet excess, deficiency, or dysfunction.

MEGAKARYOCYTE MATURATION AND STRUCTURE

A staging system to classify megakaryocyte maturation has been proposed based on light microscopic criteria.[148] It employs (1) nuclear-to-cytoplasmic ratio, (2) nuclear shape, (3) basophilia, and (4) cytoplasmic granularity (Table 55-1). The terms stage I, II, and III are often used with reference to the degree of maturity of megakaryocytes and correspond in general to the designations megakaroblast, promegakaryocyte, and granular megakaryocyte, respectively. Stage IV megakaryocytes represent mature megakaryocytes. The morphologically recognizable cells of the megakaryocytic line lack the capacity for self-renewal and are maintained by a continuous influx of precursor cells from the stem cell compartment.[135] The mature megakaryocyte is the cell that ultimately produces thrombocytes or platelets. This process is regulated in large part by the hormone thrombopoietin.[106]

Megakaryocytes and their precursors, the megakaryoblasts, at any stage of maturation normally are found only in small numbers in the bone marrow (1 to 4 per 1000 nucleated cells), and not in the peripheral blood. Megakaryocyte numbers are usually $6.1 \pm 0.7 \times 10^6$/kg body weight in man.[44,45] A few may also be found in the lungs. These cells constitute less than 1% of the nucleated cells within the bone marrow but are easily identified by their large size. A rough assessment of the number of megakaryocytes relative to the other marrow elements usually is sufficient for clinical purposes. Most of these cells in the marrow are in the third or fourth stage of maturation.

Stage I: The Megakaryoblast

The precise origin of platelets was initially puzzling, and they were at first felt to be little more than artifacts or precipitants on the peripheral blood film.[118] The modern view of platelets arising from the budding of megakaryocytes within the human bone marrow was originated at the turn of the century. James Wright provided evidence

TABLE 55-1
Maturation Stages of Megakaryocytes

Term	Size (μm)	Morphology
Megakaryoblast (Stage I)	>15	Lobed nucleus, basophilic cytoplasm
Basophilic megakaryocyte (Stage II)	>20	Horseshoe-shaped lobed nucleus, basophilic cytoplasm, azurophilic granules around centrosome
Granular megakaryocyte (Stage III)	>25–50	Large multilobed nucleus, acidophilic cytoplasm, numerous azurophilic granules
Mature megakaryocyte (Stage IV)	>25–50	Pyknotic nucleus, groups of 10–12 azurophilic granules

(From Williams N, Levine RF: The origin, development, and regulation of megakaryocytes. Br J Haematol 52:173, 1982.)

that platelets were derived from megakaryocytes within the bone marrow.[150,151] Since these initial observations, much work has been performed to better understand the life cycle of megakaryocytic cells and their offspring, platelets.

The primitive megakaryocyte arises from the transition of a multipotent progenitor cell (a primitive cell capable of producing erythrocytes, granulocytes, and megakaryocytes) to one that becomes lineage-restricted to megakaryocyte production. Commitment of a megakaryocytic precursor may be random, but the probability of commitment is dependent on the state of differentiation of the progenitor. Thus, the more primitive the progenitor is, the more likely it is to remain a mitotic cell.

The transition between multipotent progenitor and megakaryocyte-restricted progenitor involves the *mpl oncogene*, which is highly expressed in megakaryocytic progenitor cell lines and progenitor cells. Inhibition of *mpl* function *in vitro* decreases megakaryocytic differentiation of primitive progenitor cells.[130,134] A specific hormone, thrombopoietin, is responsible for the commitment of the megakaryoblast to differentiate further into more mature stages. The gene for thrombopoietin has recently been cloned using a variety of strategies giving rise to separate names for the same biologic activity. Megakaryocyte growth and differentiation factor (MGDF), thrombopoietin (TPO), and *mpl*-ligand all have the identical activities, and all represent thrombopoietin.

Megakaryocytic cells are unusual in that their nuclei are able to undergo multiple mitotic divisions without cytoplasmic division, generating giant multinucleated or polyploid cells. This is referred to as *endomitosis*. The multiple nuclei in these cells divide simultaneously and remain connected.[49] Thus, megakaryocytic cells, including the megakaryoblast, can have 1, 2, 4, 8, and even 16 or 32 nuclei. After the first nuclear division, megakaryo-

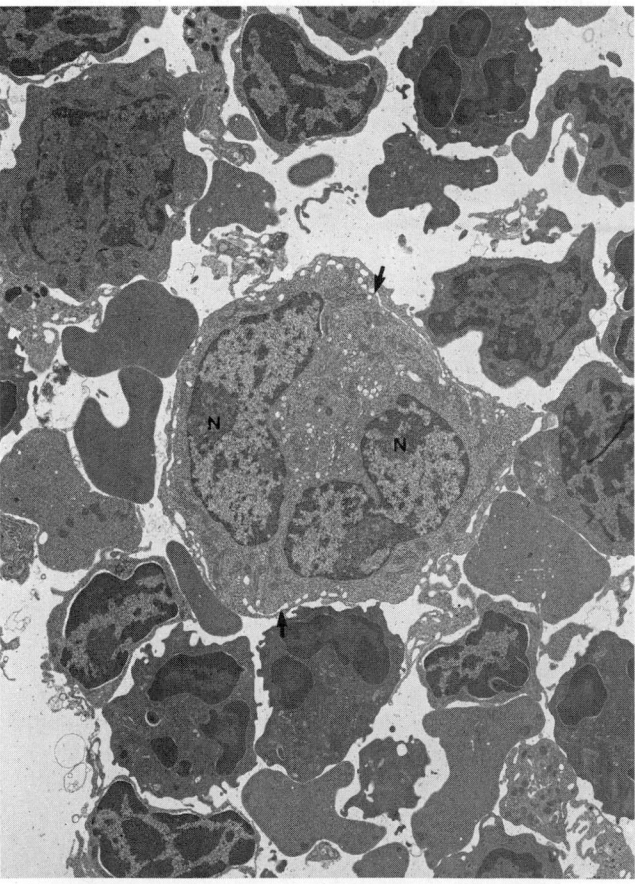

FIGURE 55-2. Immature mouse megakaryocyte. Some demarcation membranes are present at periphery (*arrow*). Nucleus (N) has two lobes, and Golgi complex along with some α-granules, mitochondria, and centrioles are present in cytoplasm (see also Fig. 55-7). ×4800. (With permission of photographer, Dr. P. E. Stenberg, Veterans Administration Medical Center, San Francisco.)

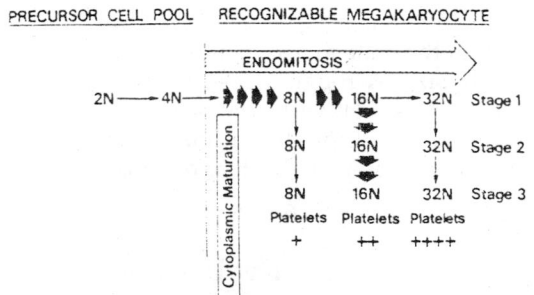

FIGURE 55-1. Theoretical model of megakaryocytopoiesis. The earliest recognizable cell is the 8N cell. The wide arrows indicate the major pathway of nuclear and cytoplasmic maturation. The relative platelet yield per megakaryocyte is indicated by the + signs. (Modified from Hirsh J, Doery JCG: Platelet function in health and disease. Prog Hematol 7:185, 1972.)

cytic cells always have an even number of nuclei (Fig. 55-1).

The megakaryoblast is the earliest recognizable stage of maturation. This cell displays blunt protrusions from its cytoplasmic membrane and contains a multitude of polyribosomes and clear vacuoles with diameters as large as 0.2 μm as seen by electron microscopy (Fig. 55-2). The central area of the megakaryoblast contains mitochondria and a primitive endoplasmic reticulum. The nucleus, which occupies most of the cell volume, has prominent nucleoli and distinct but barely marginated chromatin which is characteristic of immature cells (Fig. 55-3). The Golgi complex (vacuoles, lamellae, and vesicles) occupies the area surrounding the nucleus. Alpha-granules and centrioles are also found in the cytoplasm.

The megakaryoblast is identified by certain features using light microscopy on a Romanowsky-stained marrow specimen. First, it has a diameter of 15 to 50 μm. There may be a single, centrally located nucleus or multiple round and oval nuclei containing several nucleoli and distinct but fine delicate chromatin strands. The cytoplasm stains a diffuse blue, indicating absence of specific granules. The megakaryoblast is irregular in shape and has cytoplasmic tags extending into its external environment. These features are shown in Color Plates 55-1 and 55-2.

Stage II: The Promegakaryocyte

As the megakaryoblast matures to the promegakaryocyte stage, it increases in volume (see Fig. 55-3). Cell size ranges from 20 to 80 μm. The cell membrane retains its characteristic cytoplasmic tags, and the cytoplasm is rich in polyribosomes. The number of nuclear lobes begins to increase, but there is still only barely detectable margination of the chromatin around the nuclear membrane. Although the cell still appears somewhat immature, it is thought to be capable of protein synthesis, because, as seen by electron microscopy (Fig. 55-4), there is a more developed network of membranes within the cytoplasm. A network known as the *demarcating membrane system (DMS)* forms by invagination of the plasma membrane. Morphologic studies indicate that the outer cell membrane and the demarcating membranes have structural similarities. This suggests that the DMS functions as the future membrane system of the mature megakaryocyte's offspring, the platelet.[6,31,101,109,136,140] The development of the DMS also denotes individual platelet areas that finally result in the fragmentation of the mature megakaryocyte cytoplasm into platelets and other fragments.

The promegakaryocyte differs from the megakaryoblast in a number of ways when examined by light microscopy using a Romanowsky stain. These differences are illustrated in Color Plate 55-4. The promegakaryocyte is larger, and the nucleus has usually undergone one or two divisions. Bluish-stained granules (not present in the megakaryoblast) are apparent around the periphery of the nuclei. One promegakaryocyte variant has a distinct marginal zone with blunt cytoplasmic protrusions that stain a dark blue and often contain small colorless globules.

Stage III: The Granular Megakaryocyte

As viewed on Romanowsky-stained marrow by light microscopy, this cell is round and is expanded in volume,

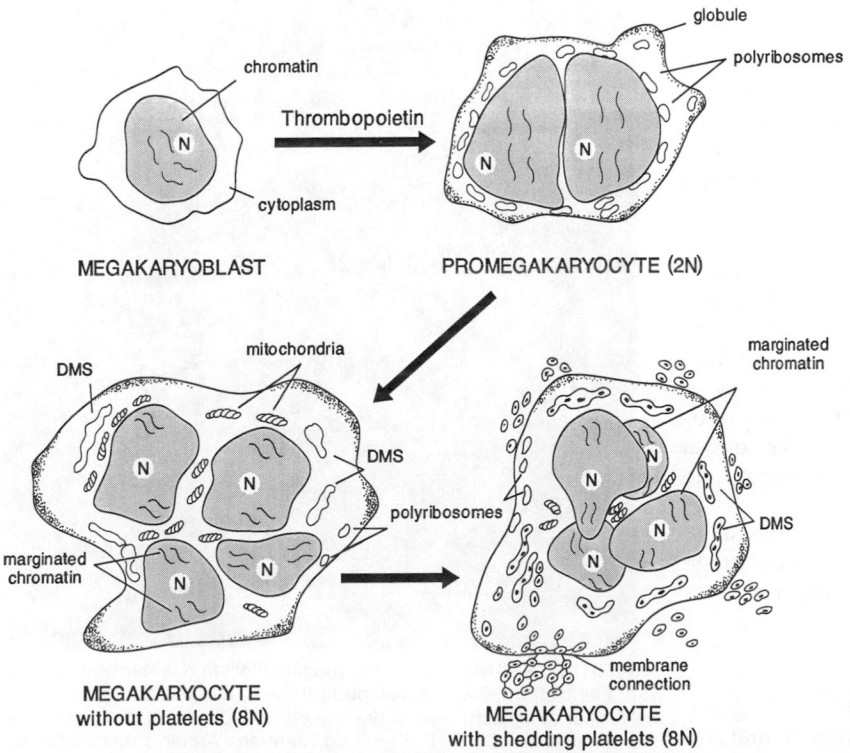

FIGURE 55-3. Diagrammatic representation of the morphologic maturation of the megakaryocyte system. DMS = demarcating membrane system; N = nucleus.

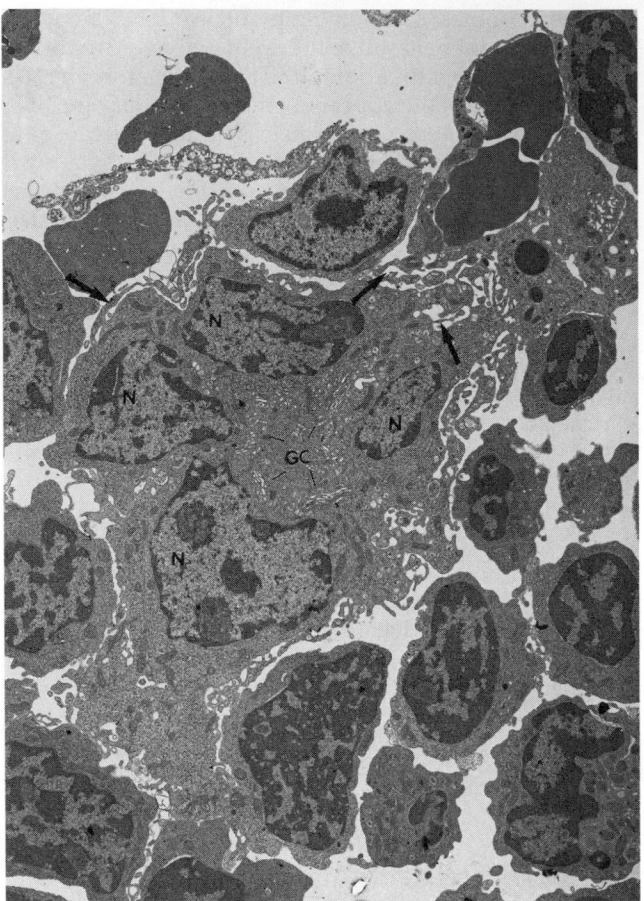

FIGURE 55-4. Maturing mouse megakaryocyte. Cell is more irregular in contour, and demarcation membranes (*arrows*) penetrate cytoplasm to greater extent than in immature cell. Also, nucleus (N) is more highly lobulated, and Golgi complex (GC) is enlarged. ×4800. (With permission of photographer, Dr. P. E. Stenberg, Veterans Administration Medical Center, San Francisco.)

with multiple nuclei and even peripheral margins. The abundant cytoplasm contains numerous small, rather uniformly distributed granules with a reddish-blue hue. The chromatin pattern is linear and coarse, with distinct spaces between the strands (see Color Plates 55-4 and 55-5).

As the megakaryocyte matures, it begins to contain all of the structural constituents of a thrombocyte; however, the organizational arrangement of these constituents and their number differ from that of a platelet when viewed by electron microscopy. The megakaryocyte cytoplasm is devoid of specific organelles other than polyribosomes and numerous mitochondria located in the central area of the cell (see Fig. 55-3). There is also an incomplete endoplasmic reticular system.

The granular megakaryocyte is known as the stage that does not ordinarily produce platelets. However, stage III megakaryocytes with at least four nuclei can produce platelets.[93]

Stage IV: The Mature Megakaryocyte

The mature megakaryocyte is the fourth stage of maturation. It is a very large cell, many times the size of the mature granulocyte, with a decreased nuclear-to-cytoplasmic ratio compared with the immature stages of development. By light microscopy on Romanowsky-stained marrow, the mature megakaryocyte nucleus is multilobed and polyploid (having more than two sets of homologous chromosomes in the cell, with 23 chromosomes per set) with ranges from 4N to 16N when not stressed to produce more platelets[64,93] (Fig. 55-3). For example, a four-lobed nucleus is termed 8N because it has eight single sets (four paired sets) of chromosomes. Ploidy levels can be as high as 32N or even 64N under abnormal conditions. In the cytoplasm, there are aggregations of granular material in masses that are separated by relatively clear areas that represent the DMS or vesicles. These aggregates of granular cytoplasm may be seen near the periphery of the cell (see Color Plates 55-6 through 55-8). Platelets may be seen adhering to the cell membrane as they begin to break away from the mature megakaryocyte.

On electron microscopy, the mature megakaryocyte periphery is seen to contain predominantly polyribosomes,[94] with occasional mitochondria. The remainder of the cytoplasm contains the extensive DMS (Fig. 55-5), which creates the future platelet fields. Each future platelet contains mitochondria and cytoplasmic granules.

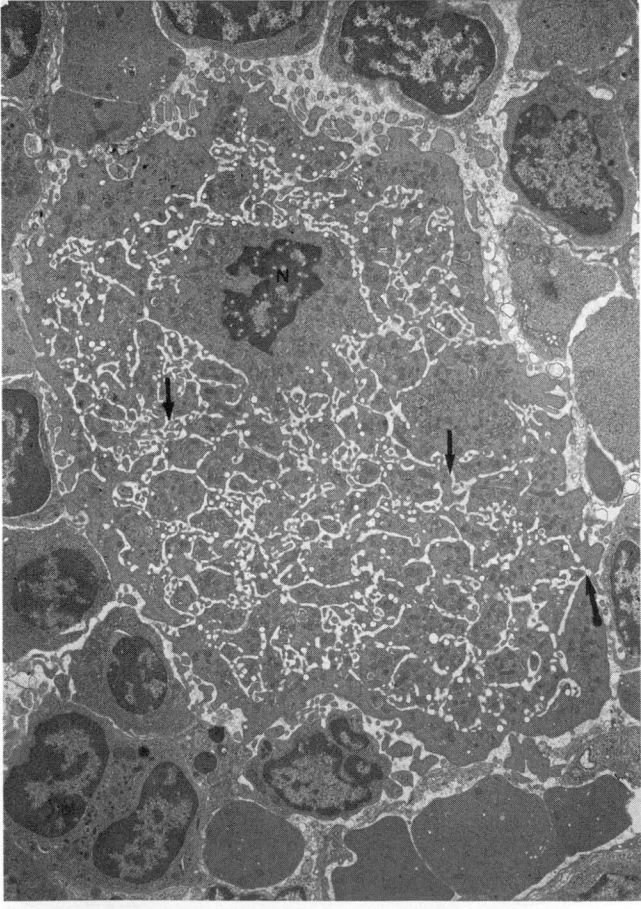

FIGURE 55-5. Mature mouse megakaryocyte. Demarcation membrane system is well developed (*arrows*), and nucleus is pyknotic. Nuclear:cytoplasm ratio is decreased. ×4800. (With permission of photographer, Dr. P. E. Stenberg, Veterans Administration Medical Center, San Francisco.)

Difficulties in the Identification of Maturation Stages and Cells in the Megakaryocytic Series

In differentiating the maturation stages of the megakaryocytic cells, emphasis should be placed on the cytoplasmic appearance. This is in contrast to emphasizing the number of nuclei or the chromatin structure, as is the rule in evaluating other hematologic cells. The reason is that occasionally, a megakaryocytic cell with only one or two nuclei can form platelets.

Granular and mature megakaryocytes are usually identified easily by their large size in comparison with other bone marrow cells and their 4N or greater ploidy. However, it should be recognized that there are other cell types in the marrow, both normal and pathologic, with which the megakaryoblast, promegakaryocyte, and granular and mature megakaryocyte can be confused. These include (1) the normal osteoclast, (2) the osteoblast, (3) the reticulum cell, (4) the abnormal multinucleated erythroblast, (5) the multinucleated plasma cell, (6) various tumor cells, and (7) Reed-Sternberg cells. (See Color Plates 55-10 through 55-14).

Platelet Formation and Shedding

A number of explanations have been offered for the initiation of platelet formation within the mature megakaryocyte.[7,97,101] Megakaryocytes normally develop close to the venous sinusoids so that platelet shedding is facilitated. Most likely, platelet formation begins with megakaryocyte development of long cytoplasmic processes within the extravascular marrow space. Such "proplatelet" processes penetrate the sinusoidal membrane through the endothelial cell body, rather than through pre-formed fenestrae (openings) as previously proposed.[100] These processes extend into the venous sinuses, frequently as a cluster that originates from a single megakaryocyte. Granular segments the size of platelets form between demarcation membranes within the proplatelet processes, and individual platelets are produced from fragmentation of these processes. The cytoplasmic fragments then undergo further dissolution within the sinus from which individual platelets evolve.[5,102] Mean platelet volume and megakaryocyte size can be predicted from a computerized fragmentation model.[122]

It has been estimated that each megakaryocyte can shed 1000 to 5000 platelets.[44,45] Once the megakaryocyte has released all of its platelet progeny, it is presumed that its nuclei (see Color Plate 55-9) and remaining cytoplasm are phagocytized by neighboring macrophages.

Megakaryocytic Microtubules and Microfilaments

Within the megakaryoblast and maturing megakaryocyte, there are a series of *microtubules* that converge on centrioles adjacent to the nucleus. The microtubules function as the mitotic spindle.[107] In contrast, within the mature megakaryocyte, the microtubule system is dispersed throughout the cell in a random fashion. This system is less developed than the one seen in the circulating platelet.

In contrast, the *microfilaments* in the immature megakaryocyte are abundant and disorganized. In the mature megakaryocyte, they become organized forming a pattern of microfilaments similar to that seen in the platelet. These microfilaments contain a significant amount of the contractile protein thrombosthenin (actomyosin), which comprises 15% to 20% of all proteins in the platelets.[13,81] Thrombosthenin is composed of actin and myosin and may be involved in maintaining the discoid shape of the platelet and in regulating changes in the platelet shape after activation.[10,11,99] When exposed to platelet-aggregating stimuli, the peripheral rim of microfilaments is reorganized to create a tight central formation. This facilitates the expulsion of megakaryocytic constituents such as serotonin and platelet-specific proteins.[31]

PLATELET STRUCTURE

The circulating platelet is a minute fragment of megakaryocyte cytoplasm measuring from 1 to 4 μm in diameter and from 0.5 to 1.0 μm in thickness.[45] Although quite small with an average platelet volume of 5 to 7 fL, the circulating thrombocyte is a complex structure. By light microscopy, the platelets appear as dense blue to purple particles with granules that stain with graded intensity during Romanowsky stain preparation.

The detailed anatomy of the platelet is best seen by electron microscopy and can be subdivided into four major areas: (1) *plasma membrane*, which consists of the platelet's outer membrane and related structures; (2) *submembrane area*, which links the membrane and the inner cell body; (3) *cytoskeleton (sol-gel zone)*, which constitutes the matrix or muscle and skeletal portion of the platelet; and (4) *organelles*, which consist of granules, dense bodies, lysosomes, and mitochondria (Fig. 55-6). These organelles serve as the metabolic center to influence platelet function in response to exogenous stimuli such as coagulation, infection, and the presence of foreign bodies.[142]

Plasma Membrane

The plasma membrane is approximately 7.5 nm in thickness and has a trilaminar unit structure (Fig. 55-7). It also has a surface coat or *glycocalyx* (see Fig. 55-6). Under homeostatic conditions, platelets circulate in the blood as discoid-shaped cells. The membrane and glycocalyx are relatively smooth and contain porelike indentations that open communication channels into the platelet cytoplasm, providing a distinct connection between the inside of the platelet and its surroundings. The glycocalyx is thicker and denser than that of most blood cells, ranging in thickness from 10 to 50 nm.[142] A number of glycoproteins are incorporated in this outer layer (Ia, Ib, Ic, IIa, IIb, III, IV, V, and IX), which play important roles in platelet adhesion and aggregation.[35,86,95] The glycocalyx also provides a surface to which some coagulation factors may adhere. These include factors I, V, VIII, X, XI, XII, and XIII. All of these are adsorbed selectively onto the platelet to facilitate assembly of the prothrombinase com-

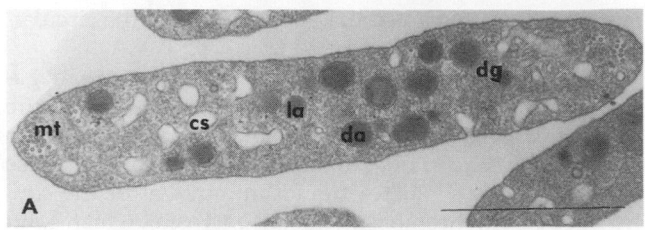

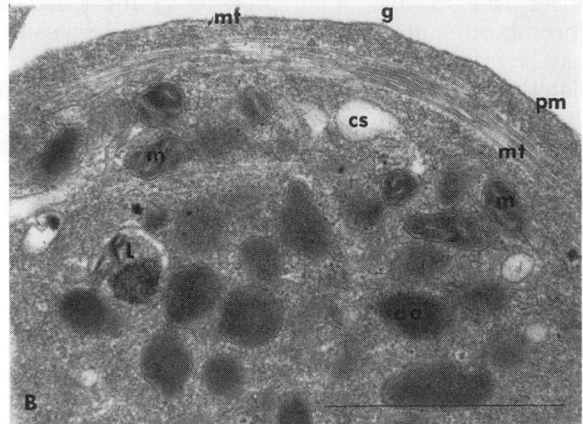

FIGURE 55-6. Transmission electron micrograph of normal human platelets in cross-section (*A*) and transverse section (*B*). Surface coat (glycocalyx, g) external to trilamellar plasma membrane (pm) is seen as a faint electron-semidense coating. (Cationic dye, such as ruthenium red, is necessary to see this structure fully.) Microtubular system (mt) is shown in both cross-section and transverse section at periphery of platelet. Microfilaments (mf) are randomly arranged throughout. Light α-granules (la), dark α-granules (da), and dense granules (dg) are present in the cytoplasm along with mitochondria (m) and lysosomal bodies (L). External canalicular system (cs) is seen as large empty spaces. Bar = 1 mm. (With permission of photographer, Dr. M. Richardson, Department of Pathology, McMaster University, Ontario, Canada.)

plex consisting of factors Va, Xa, and calcium. This complex then acts on prothrombin to convert it to thrombin (Chap. 48).

Underlying the glycocalyx is the plasma membrane, which serves as the physical and chemical barrier between the intracellular and extracellular constituents of the platelet. Within this membrane is the sodium/potassium ATPase ionic pump, which maintains a transmembrane ionic gradient.[146] The phospholipid constituents (phosphatidylserine, phosphatidylcholine, and phosphatidylinositol) and other fatty acid pools required for fatty acid metabolism are also located within this layer.[1,110] Finally, platelet factor VIII (von Willebrand factor), an important constituent for the acceleration of blood coagulation and for platelet adhesion, is also located in the lipoprotein-rich plasma membrane.

Submembrane Area

The submembrane area underlies the plasma membrane. This region is identified as a specific area because the organelles within the inner matrix of unaltered platelets never come in contact with the internal side of the platelet cell wall, but appear instead to be separated from it by the submembrane area (Fig. 55-7). This platelet region also contains an organized system of filaments, which are physically comparable to the microfilaments and submicrofilaments of the microtubule system.[139] They are dis-

tinct from the circumferential microfilaments and peripheral to them. They are usually obscured by the density of the cytoskeletal matrix but can be made visible by special techniques.[153] These structures are thought to prevent contact between organelles and the cell membrane by their physical presence. The submembrane filaments may also contribute to the regulation of the normal platelet discoid shape, act as a base for pseudopod formation, and interact with other contractile proteins to modulate platelet adhesion and clot retraction after activation.

Platelet Cytoskeleton (Sol-Gel Zone)

The platelet cytoskeleton underlies the submembrane area. The sol-gel zone represents the matrix of the platelet cytoplasm and consists of a circumferential microtubule system and randomly arranged microfilaments that form an intraplatelet matrix, both of which contribute to support of the platelet discoid shape. The microfilaments provide the contractile force after activation that directs the organelles toward the center of the cell with control and direction from the microtubules. The platelet cytoskeleton serves as a stabilizing component to regulate the arrangement of the internal organelles and microtubular system within the resting platelet body.[8] The cytoskeleton also facilitates communication between the organelles and the platelet's external surroundings. Cross-section microscopic examination of unstimulated platelets reveals the circumferential microtubules, which extend around the platelet perimeter (Fig. 55-7). Spaces in between the individual series of tubules contain submembrane filaments, which integrate one tubular system with another. In its position directly under the cell membrane,

TRANSVERSE SECTION

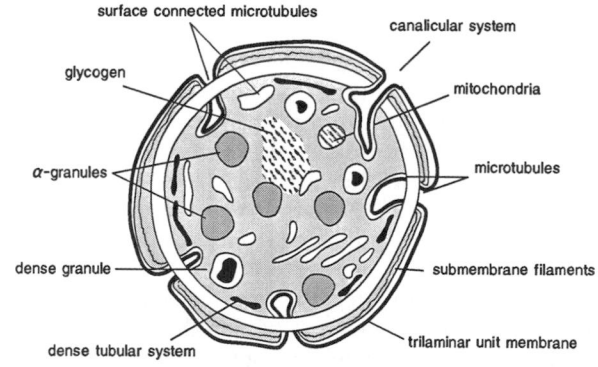

CROSS SECTION

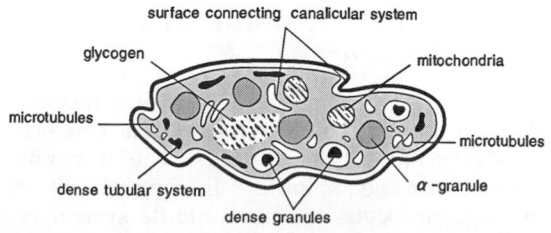

FIGURE 55-7. Diagrammatic representation of morphology of the platelet as viewed in transverse and cross-section.

this microtubular system probably contributes significantly to the cytoskeletal support system. When platelets are stimulated and lose their discoid form, the circumferential band of microtubules disappears, but on re-establishment of the discoid shape of the platelets, such as by treatment with cooling or biochemical agents (*e.g.*, prostaglandin I_2 or tannic acid) the microtubules reappear.[32,137,147]

It has been suggested that the microtubule system plays an important role in the contractile response of platelets to stimulation.[36,87,138] However, the microtubule system is not required for contraction. Instead, it most likely acts as a governor and influences the extent of the platelet contractile response.[137,152]

The microfilaments of a stimulated platelet can be identified readily and are projected outward, causing the formation of platelet pseudopodia. However, identification of microfilaments and their assembly within the cytoplasm of nonstimulated, discoid-shaped platelets is difficult. Platelet filaments are approximately 5 nm in diameter and contain two proteins, actin and myosin. This suggests that the microfilaments (unlike microtubules) within the platelet cytoskeletal system are necessary for the contractile process.[38] It also has been demonstrated that after secretion of platelet constituents in response to marked stimulation, platelets are able to recover their discoid form. When the stimulus is slight, aggregated platelets recover their discoid shape even more rapidly.[115] These observations suggest that microfilaments function in an organized and reversible manner.

An α-actinin and actin-binding protein has also been found in the platelet. This material is a transmembrane protein, linking the outer membrane to the microfilaments in the cytoskeletal area. This intracellular network may help to explain how the inner microfilaments influence platelet contraction by modulating the cytoskeleton of the outer layers of the platelet.[98] Thus, both circumferential and radial extensions of the microfilaments oriented in opposing directions may function as the platelet muscular system, which is able to facilitate, simultaneously, a centralized contraction of the platelet's granules and a reorganization of the platelet's shape in response to various stimuli.

Organelles

Organelles constitute the major portion of the platelet cytoplasm. These structures include dense bodies, α-granules, peroxisomes, lysosomes, and mitochondria. See Table 55-2 for a more complete list of platelet granule contents.

DENSE BODIES

The dense bodies (or dense granules) are 250 to 350 nm in diameter and are classified as dense because of their appearance by electron microscopy. They contain ADP and ATP (adenosine di- and triphosphate), GDP and GTP (guanosine di- and triphosphate), calcium, magnesium, and serotonin.[27,73,146,149] The nucleotide ADP is probably the most important component secreted from the dense granules after platelet stimulation. When ADP is released, it binds to specific receptors and initiates platelet aggrega-

TABLE 55-2
Platelet Granule Contents

DENSE BODIES

ADP, ATP

GDP, GTP

Calcium

Magnesium

Serotonin

α-GRANULES

Platelet-specific proteins
  Platelet factor 4 (PF4)
  β-Thromboglobulin family (platelet basic protein, low-affinity platelet factor 4, β-thromboglobulin, and β-thromboglobulin-F)

Multimerin

Adhesive glycoproteins
  Fibrinogen
  von Willebrand factor
  Fibronectin
  Thrombospondin
  Vitronectin

Coagulation factors
  Factor V
  Factor XI
  Protein S

Mitogenic factors
  Platelet-derived growth factor (PDGF)
  Transforming growth factor-β
  Endothelial cell growth factor
  Epidermal growth factor (EGF)

Fibrinolytic inhibitors
  α_2-Plasmin inhibitor
  Plasminogen activator inhibitor-1

Membrane-associated proteins
  P-selectin
  GMP 33
  24-kD GTP binding protein
  GP IV (CD36)
  Osteonectin

(Data from references 50, 56, 72, 76, 112, and 145.)

tion (Fig. 55-8). However, this is a short-lived effect, because ADP is rapidly degraded to adenosine which, in turn, inhibits platelet function by enhancing cyclic-AMP levels.

The importance of the minute amounts of calcium and magnesium ions released from the dense granules after platelet stimulation is not well understood. It is possible that the calcium concentration at the platelet surface or within the microtubule system is high and therefore influences the platelet microenvironment. Such a mechanism is thought to be important in the activation of membrane phospholipases, which are calcium dependent and influence the subsequent liberation of arachidonic acid, the precursor of a number of metabolites required for platelet function (see below).

ALPHA GRANULES

The α-granule is spherical and somewhat larger than the dense body, with an overall diameter of 300 to 500 nm. The predominant constituents released from these granules are coagulation factors and proteins such as platelet-

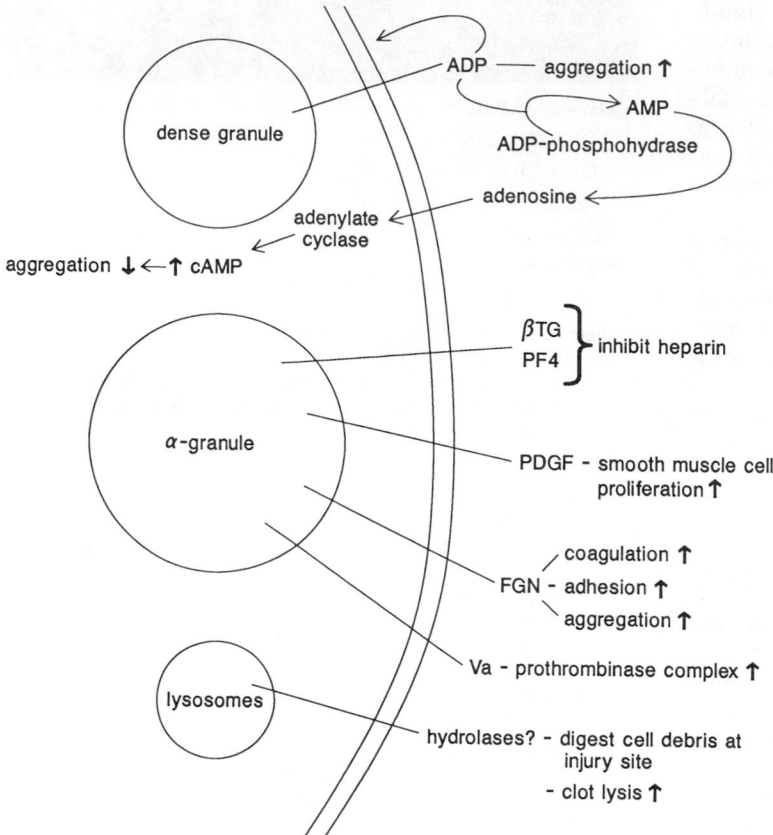

FIGURE 55-8. Release products of platelets and their effects. FGN = fibrinogen.

derived growth factor (PDGF) and thrombospondin, a glycoprotein apparently involved in platelet aggregation. Two other platelet-specific proteins are also released: platelet factor 4 (PF4) and β-thromboglobulin (βTG), both of which bind heparin (see Fig. 55-8).[14,104] It has been postulated that after platelet stimulation, PF4 binds endogenously released heparin and therefore neutralizes heparin's ability to inhibit coagulation. Finally, the α-granule also contains homologues of plasma proteins including glycoproteins IIb and IIIa, which serve as the receptors for fibrinogen and von Willebrand factor when complexed together.

The α-granule also contains fibrinogen and factor V (see Fig. 55-8). These two constituents are released after platelet stimulation and bind to the platelet surface at specific receptor sites. The binding of fibrinogen and factor V to the platelet surface provides a base for the binding and assembly of other coagulant factors, including prothrombin and factor Xa; and, the subsequent formation of the prothrombinase complex consisting of factors Va and Xa with calcium, which together stimulate activation of prothrombin on the platelet phospholipid surface. Fibrinogen acts as a bridge between ADP-stimulated platelets. It is likely that the release of fibrinogen from platelets within a hemostatic plug, rather than its recruitment from the plasma, better facilitates stabilization of the platelet plug. It is also possible that assembly of the fibrin matrix on the outer membrane of the platelet, in association with the contractile protein inside the platelet, acts synergistically to facilitate platelet-induced clot retraction, which is necessary for wound healing and vessel wall repair. Since platelets lack a nucleus and therefore have finite

metabolic capabilities, it is likely that the factor V or Va released from platelet α-granules is not synthesized by the platelet. Most likely, these proteins are acquired by platelet absorption from the plasma or through pinocytosis by the megakaryocytes, because these proteins have been identified in both megakaryocytes and platelets.[96,100]

The relative importance of platelet-associated *versus* plasma coagulation proteins is not entirely clear. The sequestration of coagulation factors within α-granules allows for high local concentrations of these proteins when platelets are stimulated. This property of activated platelets was formerly referred to as platelet factor 3 activity, a term which has largely been abandoned. It was not a discrete molecular species like PF4, but rather a catalytic ability of activated platelet membrane phospholipid to increase the reaction efficiency of the coagulation mechanism.

The most important cationic protein released from platelets is the mitogenic platelet-derived growth factor (PDGF). During platelet–vessel wall interactions after injury, PDGF is released from α-granules and stimulates smooth-muscle cell growth and proliferation.[103] For a number of years, it was thought that the hyperplastic response to vessel wall injury was mediated by PDGF. However, more recent studies suggest that endothelial cells and other blood cells also can release PDGF, indicating that PDGF is not specific to platelets.

LYSOSOMES

Lysosomes are platelet vesicles that contain a number of acid hydrolases including elastase, collagenase, cathepsins, heparinase, and enzymes that degrade polysaccharides (see Fig. 55-8). These hydrolases are obtained from fractions of platelets rich in both mitochondria and light α-granules.[133] The significance of their release is unclear; however, when platelets undergo secretion, lysosomal contents are more slowly and incompletely released than are the contents of the dense bodies and α-granules. Lysosomes may digest materials that the platelet endocytoses. However, platelets have limited ability to phagocytize any constituent. It is also possible that lysosome acid hydrolases may contribute to vascular damage at the site of platelet thrombus formation.[85]

Platelet Membrane System

The platelet membrane system has two components, the *open canalicular system* and the *dense tubular system*. The presence of an intracellular canalicular system that opens to the platelet's external environment is made evident by the presence of indented pores on the platelet surface and by cross-sections illustrating interconnecting tubules reaching from the outer membrane to the intercytosol components of the cell (see Figs. 55-6 and 55-7).[141] This is also known as the *surface-connected open canalicular system*, which may serve as a delivery route for substances ingested by the platelet, as well as the route of extrusion of substances released from the stimulated platelet. This canalicular system represents an extensive internal store of plasma membrane, and a storage site for platelet membrane glycoproteins. These canalicular systems remain readily visible and clear throughout the sequences of platelet shape change, contraction, adhesion, and aggregation.[143,144]

Channels of the dense tubular system are randomly dispersed in the platelet cytosol and appear to be close to the circumferential band of microtubules.[9] This suggests that the dense tubular system has an important role in influencing the microtubules supporting the discoid platelet shape. This role seems likely because there is no evidence of any communication between the open canalicular and the dense tubular systems. The dense tubular system can sequester ionized calcium and release it when platelets are activated. Platelets pump calcium out of the cytosol through the dense tubules, thus influencing the metabolic activity in the platelet. The dense tubular system also contains specific peroxidase activity important for prostaglandin synthetase activity and is likely to be the site of platelet prostaglandin synthesis.[16,37]

THROMBOKINETICS—PLATELET LIFE SPAN AND TURNOVER RATE

Under healthy steady-state conditions, the rate of platelet release from megakaryocytes is equivalent to the rate of platelet removal from the circulation. This net rate of production is expressed as *platelet turnover*, which has been estimated to be 35,000 ± 4300 platelets/mL/day.[45] Unlike erythrocytes, which circulate for approximately 120 days, platelets circulate for a short time. When platelet life span is studied using normal platelets injected into thrombocytopenic recipients, the life span ranges from 5 to 10 days and is, in part, dependent on the total number of platelets injected. In studies of "normal" recipients, the platelet life span ranged from 2 to 9 days.[2,47,48] These estimates, unfortunately, are influenced by the method of life span calculation.[79] Most investigators have used radiolabels such as indium 111 and chromium 51 and have analyzed the radiolabel recovery curves by various statistical approaches.[46]

Although the platelet life span is relatively short, the range in the general population is great. The significance of this wide range is unclear. However, it has been suggested that the circulating platelets can be divided into two major populations, young and old.[57,111] Young platelets are hemostatically more effective. As they circulate, presumably they interact with minuscule stimuli throughout the cardiovascular system and collide randomly with one another, as a result of which glycoproteins on their surfaces are destroyed. Hence, the old platelet is hemostatically less effective. The subsequent sequestration of old platelets from the circulation is also a matter of speculation; it may be attributable to a sufficiently altered membrane to render the platelet "foreign" to its surroundings, which results in sequestration by the reticuloendothelial system. In addition, at least 30% of the total circulating platelet population is normally sequestered in the spleen.[111] This platelet pool exchanges freely with the circulation. The significance of splenic sequestration is unclear, particularly because after splenectomy, platelet survival remains normal, and there is no apparent loss of hemostatic function.

PLATELET FUNCTION AND PRIMARY HEMOSTASIS

Platelets interact with injured vascular wall structures, plasma proteins, and other circulating blood cells, all of which are fundamental in the regulation of hemostasis and the pathogenesis of thrombosis.[76] When platelets are stimulated by way of these interactions, they release biologically active substances, which can interact with the vessel wall cells, including the endothelium, and influence plasma coagulation and the circulating cells that modulate hemostasis. In this section primary hemostasis will be discussed, including platelet adhesion, the platelet release reaction or secretion, and platelet aggregation.

Platelet Adhesion

Platelets do not adhere to the intact endothelial cell surface of blood vessels under normal conditions. However, they do adhere to detached endothelial cells, the subendothelium, media, and adventitia. Collagen, fibronectin, thrombospondin, laminin, vitronectin, and tissue factor are all hemostatically active following injury.[12,23,24,116,123] The degree of platelet response to such injury is, in part, influenced by the extent and depth of vessel wall injury (Fig. 55-9).

Stimuli that cause endothelial cell desquamation only (minor injury) expose platelets to the basement membrane, onto which they will adhere and spread. Under these conditions, the platelets do not release their constituents nor promote aggregation.[70] When the vessel is more

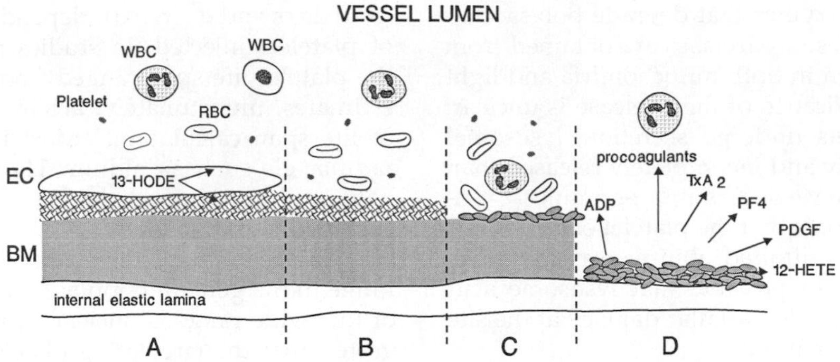

FIGURE 55-9. Platelet adhesion to the vessel wall. Avidity of platelet adhesion is dependent on degree of injury. (*A*) With an intact endothelium (EC), there is no adhesion, which is regulated, in part, by 13-HODE inside EC. (*B*) With selective removal of EC and exposure of basement membrane (BM) lying immediately below, there is little platelet adhesion, also presumed to be attributable, in part, to the presence of 13-HODE. (*C*) With exposure of deeper BM tissue, platelets adhere to the BM but do not release their constituents. (*D*) When the vessel wall is severely injured, platelets adhere to the damaged site, and platelet aggregates form in response to constituents released from adherent platelets.

severely injured (*e.g.*, rupture of an atherosclerotic plaque) resulting in exposure of the deeper structures of the vessel, platelets not only adhere to that surface but also undergo the release reaction, facilitating platelet aggregation and activating blood coagulation on their surfaces (see Fig. 55-8).[4,132]

The differences in these platelet responses are likely to be attributable to differences in the vessel wall components to which the platelets are exposed.[121] For example, smooth muscle cells and endothelial cells both synthesize collagen but of different types. Collagen types I and III, which are synthesized by smooth muscle cells, are located in the deeper regions of the vessel wall and promote platelet adhesion and facilitate aggregation and release.[3,4,108,120,132] Collagen types IV and V, which are synthesized by endothelial cells, are located immediately below the endothelium and promote platelet adhesion but do not cause platelet aggregation except under specific conditions.[4,24,53,105,132]

Platelet adhesion to some collagens requires the plasma protein von Willebrand factor (vWF), which acts as a link between the specific platelet membrane glycoprotein Ib/IX receptor complex (GP Ib/IX) and the subendothelial cell connective tissue.[22] High shear rates cause conformational changes in the vWF and/or platelet GP Ib.[124,126] Very high shear rates cause platelets to aggregate by a mechanism that involves vWF binding to GP Ib/IX followed by activation of GP IIb-IIIa. It is felt that platelets contribute significantly more to arterial thrombi than to venous thrombi, perhaps as a result of the differences in the shear rates in the different vascular beds.[41]

More recently, it has been demonstrated that 13-hydroxyoctadecadienoic acid (13-HODE) is a potent inhibitor of platelet adhesion as well as aggregation and thromboxane A$_2$ production.[19,20] 13-HODE is synthesized by endothelial cells. It is then released into the vascular tissues immediately underlying the endothelium thereby inhibiting platelet adhesion to that surface. This indicates that even the basement membrane is not initially thrombogenic (prone to producing a clot).[17] However, since other studies have not been able to confirm the effect of 13-HODE on platelet adhesion, its precise role remains unclear (Fig. 55-9). Platelet adhesion is also known to be affected by the age of the individual, the hematocrit, the speed of blood flow, the size of the vessel, and the shear rate (the forces tending to pull the platelet from a vessel wall).[26]

In order to understand the clinical relevance of platelet adhesion, it is helpful to consider two disease processes that arise from defects in the adhesion of platelets to the vascular endothelium. Bernard-Soulier syndrome is a rare autosomal recessive disorder that can cause serious platelet-related bleeding complications. The homozygous state is characterized by a prolonged bleeding time, thrombocytopenia, and giant platelets on the peripheral film. The GP Ib receptor is known to be virtually absent in this condition and GP IX is sometimes absent.[28]

Von Willebrand disease, in contrast to Bernard-Soulier syndrome, is an autosomal disorder with either dominant or recessive inheritance (see Table 52-2). The disease is caused by one of several qualitative or quantitative abnormalities in vWF glycoprotein.[22,54] In contrast to Bernard-Soulier syndrome, the adhesion defect of von Willebrand disease is due to an abnormality of plasma vWF rather than an intrinsic platelet defect. Thus, the therapy for this disease involves the transfusion of a source of normal protein (*i.e.*, cryoprecipitate) rather than platelets. However, platelet adhesion remains defective in both of these conditions.

Other plasma proteins likewise influence the interaction of platelets with artificial surfaces.[33,34,74,125] For example, when certain materials such as prosthetic valves or vessel wall grafts are implanted in the body, the surfaces rapidly become coated with plasma proteins such as albumin and fibrinogen (see Fig. 52-3). Thus, the biocompatibility of a prosthetic surface is influenced not only by its inherent physical properties but also by the effects of various plasma proteins bound to it, which in turn, influence platelet adhesion.

Platelet Release Reaction—Secretion

The two morphologically distinct platelet α-granules and dense bodies, as well as lysosomes, contain an abundance of constituents. These constituents influence platelet function, vessel wall tonicity, and coagulation.[21,50,51,52,56] A number of biologic materials, such as collagen, thrombin, epinephrine, thromboxane A_2 (TxA$_2$), and other arachidonic acid metabolites, cause platelets to release their granular contents. With relatively weak stimuli, only the contents of the α-granules are released, but with increased stimuli from higher concentrations of these agents, the contents of the dense bodies also are released.[61,80,91,92] Constituents released from the α-granules also contribute to platelet aggregation and activate the coagulation system by mechanisms currently under investigation.

The importance of the α-granules is made evident by the abnormal platelet function in patients with gray platelet syndrome (so named because the platelets appear ghostlike and pale on the peripheral blood film).[36] In this syndrome, the dense bodies and lysosomes are normal, but there is a deficiency of α-granules and their contents which results in a lifelong bleeding tendency.

On adhesion and subsequent platelet release, the cationic protein PDGF is released from the α-granules and influences smooth muscle cell proliferation and vessel wall hyperplasia after platelet–vessel wall interactions.[103]

Platelet Aggregation

Platelet aggregation is induced by a variety of stimuli including ADP, thrombin, thromboxane A_2 (TxA$_2$), collagen, and epinephrine (Fig. 55-10). The aggregation reaction is preceded by a change in platelet shape, which is mediated by the direction of the microtubular system and contraction of the microfilament system within the platelet. This response is also characterized morphologically by pseudopod formation that is attributable in part to the outward projection of the microfilaments. There appear to be at least three independent mediators of platelet aggregation: ADP, thrombin, and TxA$_2$.

ADP is released from the dense granules in response to collagen, epinephrine, or TxA$_2$ stimulation. It then acts on a specific receptor site and causes secondary, irreversible platelet aggregation. It may also recruit more platelets to participate in the thrombotic response at the site of injury.[50,56] The mechanism for ADP-induced aggregation appears to be dependent on the presence of a specific platelet glycoprotein receptor known as GP IIb-IIIa. The ADP-induced aggregation causes a change in the conformation of the GP IIb-IIIa complex on the platelet surface that allows binding of fibrinogen to the complex.

In the rare hereditary platelet disorder of Glanzmann thrombasthenia, the GP IIb-IIIa receptor is absent or mutated (Chap. 57). Thrombasthenic platelets do not aggregate with ADP, thrombin, collagen, epinephrine, or arachidonic acid as normal platelets do. Thus, the critical role of the platelet GP IIb-IIIa complex in mediating platelet aggregation was appreciated. It was anticipated and proven to be the case that mutations in this complex would cause thrombasthenia.[58] When thrombin and collagen are used together, however, thrombasthenic platelets undergo the release reaction.[87]

Thrombin induces platelet aggregation by at least three mechanisms. First, thrombin stimulates platelets to release ADP, mediating ADP-induced secondary irreversible aggregation.[50] Second, thrombin activates the platelet membrane phospholipases, initiating the formation of TxA$_2$.[65] Third, thrombin can induce platelet aggregation independently of the first two mechanisms.[92]

Thromboxane A_2, an arachidonic acid metabolite (Fig. 55-11), also induces platelet aggregation. When the platelet is activated by any of a number of stimuli (thrombin, endotoxin, and epinephrine), membrane phospholipases are activated, which in turn, liberate arachidonic acid from the platelet phospholipid stores. The free arachidonic acid is then oxidized in the cyclooxygenase pathway

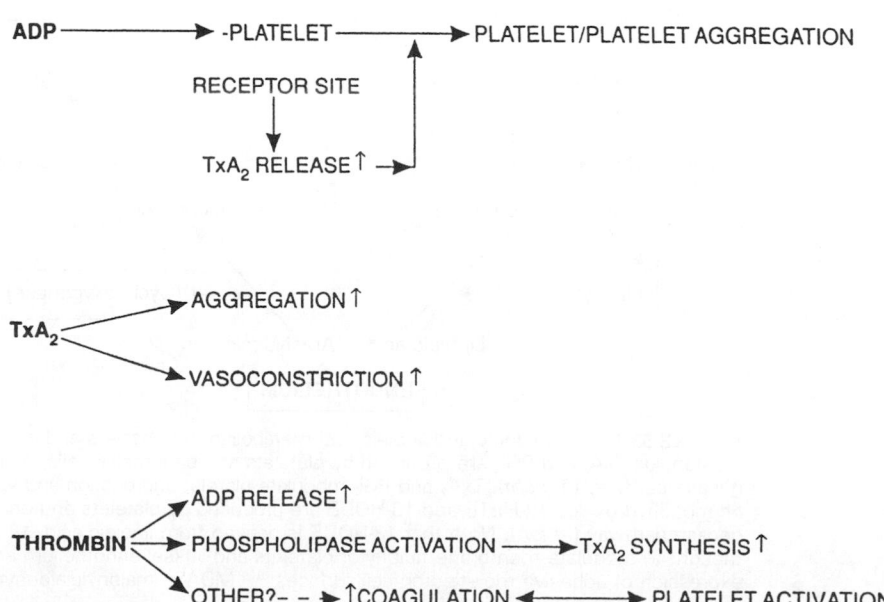

FIGURE 55-10. Schematic representation of platelet aggregation induced by *in vitro* and *in vivo* ADP, TxA$_2$, and thrombin stimulation.

to the unstable endoperoxides PGG$_2$ and PGH$_2$ by a reaction that utilizes molecular oxygen and is catalyzed by the enzyme cyclooxygenase (see Fig. 55-11). This is a step that is inhibited in an irreversible fashion by aspirin which acetylates cyclooxygenase. Interestingly, arachidonate metabolism in platelets is also altered in patients with myeloproliferative disorders, and may explain their bleeding tendency.[88] The endoperoxides are subsequently converted into TxA$_2$ (the principal metabolite) by the enzyme thromboxane synthetase and then by the peroxidases into a number of other prostaglandins (PGD$_2$, PGE$_2$, and PGF$_2$). TxA$_2$ promotes platelet aggregation directly and may also act synergistically with ADP and other stimuli (thrombin and collagen) to augment the platelet release reaction.[60] The endoperoxides PGG$_2$ and PGH$_2$ also are thought to induce platelet aggregation.[82] TxA$_2$ is also a potent vasoconstrictor and thus can assist hemostasis and coagulation indirectly.[39]

The same stimuli that activate arachidonic acid metabolism in the platelet also activate arachidonic acid metabolism in the vascular endothelium. As a result, endothelial cells metabolize arachidonic acid, through the cyclooxygenase pathway, into prostacyclin or PGI$_2$. This substance increases cyclic-AMP levels in platelets and in so doing inhibits platelet aggregation. The PGI$_2$ also causes vasodilation (see Fig. 55-10). These observations have led to the hypothesis that the relative amounts of TxA$_2$ and PGI$_2$ released from platelets and endothelial cells, respectively, with their opposing effects, modulate the hemostatic response at a site of vessel wall injury, thus ensuring adequate but not excessive coagulation activity.[78]

Free arachidonic acid also is metabolized in the platelet by the cytosol-located enzyme lipoxygenase into 12-hydroxy-eicosatetraenoic acid (12-HETE), which appears to be important for platelet adhesion (see Fig. 55-11). Studies of the role of lipoxygenase metabolites in platelet adhesion and aggregation have demonstrated that when TxA$_2$-mediated platelet aggregation is inhibited completely, and the platelets still are able to synthesize 12-HETE, the platelets adhere normally, if not better.[18] Conversely, when 12-HETE production is inhibited and platelet adhesion is impaired, the platelets still are able to synthesize TxA$_2$ and aggregate normally.

The hemorrhagic defect seen in a patient with primary thrombocythemia has also been associated with a lipoxygenase deficiency and decreased adhesion, even though the patient's platelets aggregated normally.[18,29] These studies indicate that platelet adhesion is modu-

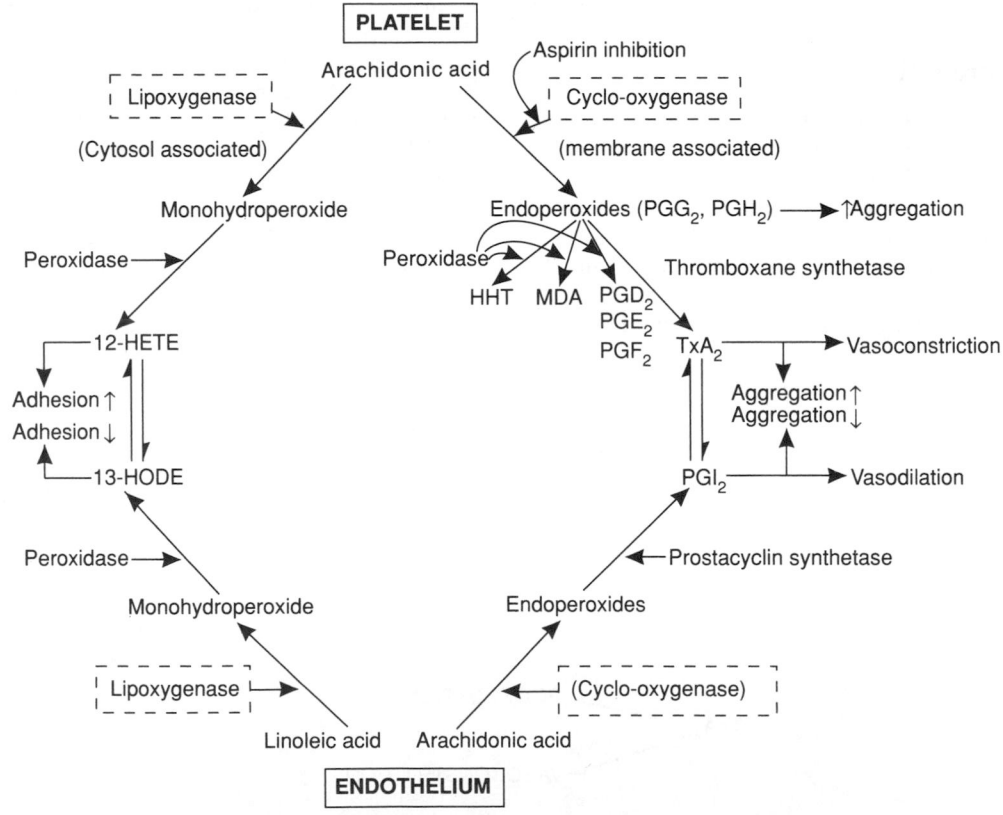

FIGURE 55-11. Arachidonic and linoleic acid metabolism by platelets and endothelium. Antagonistic prostanoids TxA$_2$ and PGI$_2$ are produced by platelets and endothelial cells, respectively, in the cyclooxygenase pathway (*at right*). TxA$_2$ and PGI$_2$ modulate platelet aggregation and vasoconstriction. Antagonistic monohydroxides 12-HETE and 13-HODE are produced by platelets and endothelial cells in the lipoxygenase pathway (*at left*). Note that 13-HODE is derived from linoleic acid. 12-HETE and 13-HODE are thought to modulate membrane fluidity of platelets and vessel endothelium and in so doing influence expression of adhesive moieties on cell surfaces.[19,20] MDA = malonyldialdehyde; HHT = 17-hydroxyheptadecatetraenoic acid.

lated, in part, by mechanisms regulated by lipoxygenase-derived arachidonic acid metabolites independent of the platelet aggregation phenomenon.

Platelet Regulation of Coagulation Reactions

In addition to their important role in primary hemostasis, platelets are one of the principal sites for plasma coagulation reactions. Platelets participate not only in the initiation of blood coagulation but also in thrombin generation in plasma.[112,119] Activated platelets provide a plasma membrane surface on which several clotting factors can bind in order to generate coagulation factor complexes. The Xase complex (factors IXa, VIIIa, and X) and the prothrombinase complex (factors Xa, Va, calcium)[42,131] both assemble on the platelet surface (Fig. 55-12).[62,83] The activated platelet surface accelerates two important reactions involving these complexes several thousand-fold by increasing the proximity and concentrations of reactants and providing the appropriate phospholipid moieties needed for both reactions. As previously noted, this property of activated platelets was formerly referred to as platelet factor 3 activity.

The participation of platelets in the activation of prothrombin by the prothrombinase complex on the platelet surface has been well defined. The assembly of the prothrombinase complex does not appear to require the presence of prothrombin.[83] Binding of prothrombin to the prothrombinase complex is calcium dependent.[71,117] The relative rate of conversion of prothrombin to thrombin by the prothrombinase complex on the platelet surface is 300,000 times the rate achieved by factor Xa alone.[84]

Stimulated platelets also are associated with a number of clotting factors including fibrinogen, factor Va, factor VIII (VIII:vWF), factor XI, and factor XII.[15,40,56,59,66,68,75,89,113,127,152] As a result of these activities, the coagulation reactions are further facilitated leading to fibrin clot formation.

Binding of VIII:vWF to platelets by a specific protein receptor is a prerequisite for *in vitro* platelet aggregation induced by ristocetin, which is used routinely to evaluate platelet function.[54,55] This interaction is similar to that in-

volved in the adherence of platelets to the subendothelium *in vivo*. It is unknown if the von Willebrand factor also serves as the platelet receptor site for the subsequent binding of the coagulant portion of factor VIII, which is required for intrinsic system activation of factor X.

The vitamin K–dependent clotting factors (II, VII, IX, and X) also interact with platelets. Although factors II, IX, and X can bind to negatively charged phospholipids, their ability to bind with high affinity to platelets in the absence of factor V has not been demonstrated.[77,84] It appears that factors IIa (thrombin) and Xa are the only vitamin K–dependent factors that can bind specifically to platelets.[77,117] Specific receptor sites for thrombin have been identified. The platelet-bound cofactor Va appears to be the receptor site for factor Xa as shown above (see Fig. 55-12). Preliminary studies also suggest that factors VII and VIIa bind to platelets, facilitating their delivery to the site of hemostatic plug formation.[90]

In plasma, the activation of factor X by factor IXa and cofactor VIIIa is dependent on the availability of platelet coagulant phospholipids.[72,84,128] This phospholipid reduces the concentration of factor X required to enable its activation by factors VIIIa and IXa.[128]

When platelets are activated *in vitro* with suboptimal concentrations of collagen or thrombin, there is an increase in both the rate and the amount of thrombin generated compared to using gel-filtered, unstimulated platelets as a surface for the activation of prothrombin to thrombin by factor Xa.[154] Platelet activation with either collagen or thrombin causes the appearance of phosphatidylserine on the platelet surface.[154] Phosphatidylserine increases the interaction of factor V/Va and prothrombin with platelets.[30,42] During this platelet activation, the surface changes initially favor the binding and activation of factor X in preference to the other coagulant factors.[69] However, it is unlikely that surface phosphatidylserine by itself accounts for the ability of activated platelets to enhance the conversion of prothrombin to thrombin by factor Xa. Possibly, intact activated platelets provide a second component that facilitates the receptor-site binding of factor Xa more efficiently than the binding of factor Xa to phospholipids alone.[14,129]

Platelets release other granular constituents that indirectly influence thrombin generation. In particular, PF4

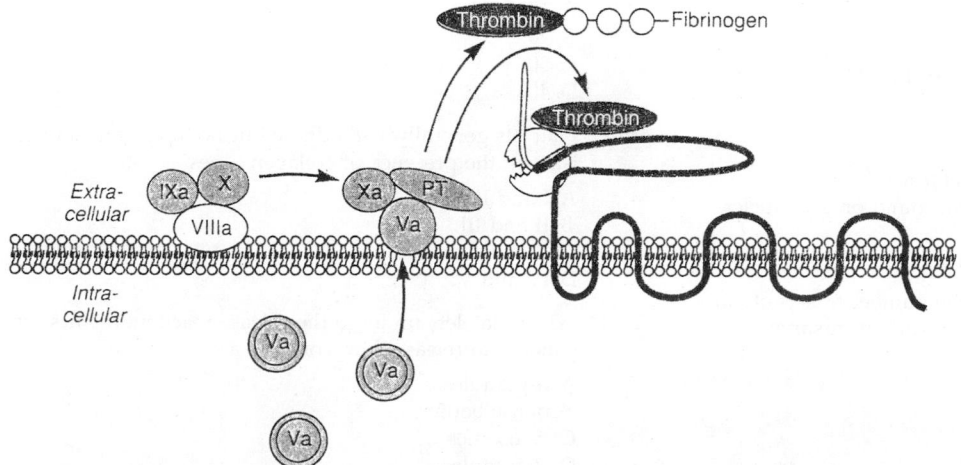

FIGURE 55-12. The role of the platelet in accelerating plasma coagulation reactions. The assembly of the "Xase" and the "prothrombinase" complexes both require phospholipid, which is supplied by the platelet membrane. Factor VIIIa, derived from plasma, binds to platelet membrane phospholipids and then binds factors IXa and X. Factor Xa generated from the complex then assembles with calcium and factor Va to form the prothrombinase complex. Factor Va is derived from plasma and platelet granules. Thrombin generated from the complex can bind to the platelet thrombin receptor or other cells, or generate fibrin from fibrinogen.

is released, which has specific anti-heparin–like activity, thus promoting coagulation.[14,104] On the contrary, vessel wall–derived glycosaminoglycans, such as heparin sulfate and dermatan sulfate, inhibit thrombin generation and act as regulators of the events at the site of injury.[43,104] Therefore, the effects of these constituents released from the vessel wall may be neutralized by PF4, thus blocking their potential anticoagulant activity at the site of injury.

CHAPTER SUMMARY

Circulating platelets are derived from megakaryocytes within the bone marrow. Under the influence of thrombopoietin (TPO), undifferentiated stem cells become committed to the megakaryocytic cell line through four stages: (1) the megakaryoblast, (2) the basophilic megakaryocyte, (3) the granular megakaryocyte, and, (4) the mature megakaryocyte. As the megakaryoblast matures, the demarcating membrane system (DMS) begins to form and develop making identification and formation of platelets possible. Ultimately, maturation proceeds to a point where the extensive DMS functions to create proplatelets which are shed from the mature megakaryocyte into the endothelial sinuses of the bone marrow to form individual platelets that are released into the circulation.

In the circulation, platelets perform a number of functions in both hemostasis and thrombosis. Platelets interact with injured vessel wall structures, plasma proteins, and other circulating blood cells. These interactions are fundamental to the regulation of hemostasis and to the pathogenesis of thrombosis. Adherence of platelets to the injured vessel wall provides a physical barrier to further blood loss. When platelets are stimulated by damage to the vessel wall, they release biologically active substances. Primary hemostasis including platelet adhesion, platelet secretion, and platelet aggregation all modulate hemostasis.

Specific constituents released from adhering platelets influence vessel wall tone (the vasoconstrictor TxA_2), vessel wall repair (PDGF), and coagulation. Coagulation influence is achieved by the platelet in furnishing a phospholipid surface on which the assembly of the Xase and prothrombinase complexes occurs, thus facilitating the catalysis of prothrombin to thrombin, leading to the formation of a stable platelet–fibrin clot.

Review Questions

55-1. Another name for thrombopoietin is

   A. interleukin 1.
   B. *mpl*-ligand.
   C. platelet-derived growth factor (PDGF).
   D. plateletpoietin.

55-2. The megakaryoblast

   A. has a diameter of 100 to 150 μm.
   B. may have a single or several round or oval nuclei.
   C. has cytoplasmic granules.
   D. shape is round and regular.

55-3. Under abnormal conditions, the number of sets of chromosomes in the nuclei of the mature megakaryocyte may range from

   A. 1 to 4.
   B. 4 to 16.
   C. 16 to 32.
   D. 32 to 64.

55-4. Cells that might be confused with the megakaryocyte include

   A. osteoclasts.
   B. reticulum cells.
   C. Reed-Sternberg cells.
   D. all of the above.

55-5. A normal megakaryocyte can produce _____ platelets.

   A. 50 to 100
   B. 100 to 500
   C. 1000 to 5000
   D. 10,000 to 50,000

55-6. The platelet glycocalyx

   A. is found immediately below the plasma membrane.
   B. is thinner than that seen in other cells.
   C. provides a surface to which coagulation factors can adhere.
   D. contains thrombosthenin.

55-7. The platelet's circumferential microtubule system

   A. disappears upon platelet stimulation.
   B. is required for platelet contraction.
   C. is responsible for pseudopod formation.
   D. all of the above.

55-8. Platelet stores of ADP and ATP are found in

   A. dense bodies.
   B. α-granules.
   C. peroxisomes.
   D. lysosomes.

55-9. Platelet factor 4 (PF4) is stored in

   A. dense bodies.
   B. α-granules.
   C. peroxisomes.
   D. lysosomes.

55-10. The platelet's dense tubular system is believed to

   A. provide an increased absorptive surface for the platelet.
   B. provide a route for extrusion of substances released by the platelet.
   C. act as a storage site for platelet glycoproteins.
   D. be the site for platelet prostaglandin synthesis.

55-11. Approximately _____% of platelets are normally sequestered by the spleen.

   A. 10
   B. 20
   C. 30
   D. 40

55-12. Platelets generally will adhere but not aggregate and release in the presence of collagen types

   A. I and II.
   B. II and III.
   C. III and IV.
   D. IV and V.

55-13. When platelets undergo the release reaction, the first organelles to release their contents are

   A. α-granules.
   B. dense bodies.
   C. lysosomes.
   D. β-granules.

For the following questions, use this format to answer:
A. 1 and 3 are correct
B. 2 and 4 are correct
C. 1, 2, and 3 are correct
D. only 4 is correct
E. all are correct

55-14. Platelets promote coagulation by

1. providing a phospholipid surface for binding coagulation factors.
2. releasing platelet factor 4 (PF4).
3. increasing the rate of thrombin formation.
4. providing receptor sites for thrombin.

55-15. The demarcating membrane system in the promegakaryocyte

1. surrounds developing platelets.
2. separates the megakaryocyte nuclei from the cytoplasm.
3. consists of invaginating plasma membrane.
4. has no known function.

References

1. Andersson LP, Brown JE: Interaction of factor VIII–von Willebrand factor with phospholipid vesicles. Biochem J 200:161, 1981
2. Aster RH, Jandl JH: Platelet sequestration in man. 1: Methods. J Clin Invest 43:843, 1964
3. Balleisen L, Gay S, Marx R et al: Comparative investigations on the influence of human bovine collagens type I, II, III on the aggregation of human platelets. Klin Wochenschr 53:903, 1975
4. Barnes MJ, Bailey AJ, Gordon JL et al: Platelet aggregation by basement membrane-associated collagens. Thromb Res 18:375, 1980
5. Becker RP, DeBruyn PP: The transmural passage of blood cells into myeloid sinusoids and the entry of platelets into sinusoidal circulation. A scanning electron microscope investigation. Am J Anat 145:183, 1988
6. Behnke O: Electron microscope study of the megakaryocyte of the rat bone marrow. J Ultrastruct Res 24:412, 1968
7. Behnke O: An electron microscope study of the megakaryocyte. II: Some aspects of platelet release and microtubules. J Ultrastruct Res 26:111, 1969
8. Behnke O: Microtubules in disc-shaped blood cells. Int Rev Exp Pathol 9:1, 1970
9. Behnke O: The morphology of blood platelet membrane systems. Sem Haematol 3:3, 1970
10. Behnke O, Emmersen J: Structural identification of thrombosthenin in rat megakaryocytes. Scand J Haematol 9:130, 1972
11. Behnke O, Kristensen B, Nielson L: Electron microscopic observations on actinoid and myosinoid filaments in blood platelets. J Ultrastruct Res 37:351, 1971
12. Bensusan HB, Koh TL, Henry KG et al: Evidence that fibronectin is the collagen receptor on platelet membranes. Proc Natl Acad Sci USA 75:5864, 1978
13. Bettex-Galland M, Luscher E: Thrombosthenin, the contractile protein from blood platelets and its relation to other contractile proteins. Adv Protein Chem 20:1, 1965
14. Bevers EM, Comforius P, van Rijn JLM et al: Generation of prothrombin converting activity at the outer surface of platelets. Eur J Biochem 122:429, 1982
15. Breederveld K, Giddings JC, tenCate JW et al: The localization of factor V within normal human platelets and a demonstration of a platelet-factor V antigen in congenital factor V deficiency. Br J Haematol 29:405, 1975
16. Breton-Gorius J, Guichard J: Ultrastructural localization of peroxidase activity in human platelets and megakaryocytes. Am J Pathol 66:277, 1972
17. Buchanan MR, Richardson M, Vallee E: Basement membrane underlying the vascular endothelium is not thrombogenic. Clin Invest Med 8(suppl B):B27, 1985
18. Buchanan MR, Butt RW, Markham B et al: Effects of aspirin and salicylate on platelet function. Prostaglandins Leukotrienes Med 21:157, 1986
19. Buchanan MR, Haas TA, Lagarde M et al: 13-Hydroxyoctadecadienoic acid is the vessel wall chemorepellant factor, LOX. J Biol Chem 260:16056, 1985
20. Buchanan MR, Butt RW, Magas J et al: Endothelial cells produce a lipoxygenase derived chemorepellant which influences platelet/endothelial cell interactions: Effect of aspirin and salicylate. Thromb Haemost 53:306, 1985
21. Buckingham S, Maynert EW: The release of 5-hydroxytryptamine, potassium and amino acids from platelets. J Pharmacol Exp Ther 143:332, 1964
22. Caen JP, Michel H, Tobelem G et al: Adhesion and aggregation of human platelets to rabbit subendothelium. A new approach for investigation: Specific antibodies. Experientia 33:91, 1976
23. Cazenave JP, Blondowska D, Richardson M et al: Quantitative radio-isotopic measurement and scanning electron microscopic study of platelet adherence to a collagen coated surface and to subendothelium with a rotating probe device. J Lab Clin Med 93:60, 1979
24. Cazenave JP, Packham MA, Kinlough-Rathbone RL et al: Platelet adherence to the vessel wall and to collagen coated surfaces. Adv Exp Med Biol 102:31, 1978
25. Chang MS, McNinch J, Basu R et al: Cloning and characterization of the human megakaryocyte growth and differentiation factor (MGDF) gene. J Biol Chem 270:511, 1995
26. Coller BS: Platelets in cardiovascular thrombosis and thrombolysis. In Foggard HA, Haley E, Jennings RB et al (eds): The Heart and Cardiovascular System, 2nd ed, pp 219–274. New York, Raven, 1991
27. Davis RB, White JG: Localization of 5 hydroxytryptamine in blood platelets: A radioautographic and ultrastructural study. Br J Haematol 15:93, 1968
28. Degos L, Tobelem G, Lethielluex P et al: Molecular defect in platelets from patients with Bernard-Soulier syndrome. Blood 50:899, 1977
29. Dutilh CE, Haddeman E, Don JA et al: The role of arachidonic lipo-oxygenase and fatty acids during irreversible blood platelet aggregation *in vitro*. Prostaglandins Med 6:111, 1981
30. Esmon CT: The subunit structure of thrombin activated factor V: Isolation of factor V, separation of subunits and reconstitution of biological activity. J Biol Chem 254:964, 1979
31. Fedorko M: The functional capacity of guinea pig megakaryocytes. 1: Uptake of 3H-serotonin by megakaryocytes and their physiology and morphologic response to stimuli for the platelet release reaction. Lab Invest 36:310, 1977
32. Fedorko M, Levine R: Tannic acid effect on membrane of cell surface origin in guinea pig megakaryocytes and platelets. J Histochem Cytochem 24:601, 1976
33. Feuerstein IA, Brophy JM, Brash JL: Platelet transport and adhesion to reconstituted collagen and artificial surfaces. Trans Am Soc Artif Intern Organs 21:427, 1975
34. Friedman LI, Liem H, Grabowski EF et al: Inconsequentiality of surface properties for initial platelet adhesion. Trans Am Soc Artif Intern Organs 16:63, 1970
35. George JN: Studies on platelet plasma membranes. IV:

Quantitative analysis of platelet membrane glycoproteins by ^{125}I-diazotized diiodosulfanilic acid labeling and SDS-polyacrylamide gel electrophoresis. J Lab Clin Med 92:430, 1978

36. Gerrard JM, Philips DR, Rao GHR et al: Biochemical studies of two patients with the gray platelet syndrome. J Clin Invest 66:102, 1980

37. Gerrard JM, White JG, Rao GHR: Towards localization of platelet prostaglandin production in the platelet dense tubular system. Am J Pathol 83:283, 1976

38. Gerrard JM, White JG: The structure and formation of platelets with emphasis on their contractile nature. In Ioachim HL (ed): Pathobiology Annual, p 31. New York, Appleton-Century-Crofts, 1976

39. Gibson BES, Buchanan MR, Barr RD et al: Primary thrombocythemia in childhood: Symptomatic episodes and their relationship to thromboxane A2, 6-keto-PGE1 and 12 hydroxy-eicosatetraenoic acid production: A case report. Prostaglandins Leukotrienes Med 26:221, 1987

40. Giddings JC, Shearn SAM, Bloom AL: Platelet associated coagulation factors: Immunochemical detection and the effects of calcium. Br J Haematol 39:569, 1978

41. Goldsmith HC, Turritto VT: Rheologic aspects of thrombosis and hemostasis: Basic principles and application. Thromb Haemost 55:415, 1986

42. Guinto ER, Esmon CT: Formation of a calcium-binding site on bovine activated factor V following reconstitution of the isolated subunits. J Biol Chem 257:1038, 1982

43. Handin RI, Cohen HJ: Purification and binding properties of platelet factor 4. J Biol Chem 251:4273, 1976

44. Harker LA: Megakaryocyte quantitation. J Clin Invest 47:458, 1968

45. Harker LA, Finch CA: Thrombokinetics in man. J Clin Invest 48:963, 1969

46. Harker LA: Platelet survival time: Its measurement and use. Prog Hemost Thromb 4:321, 1978

47. Heaton WA, Davis HH, Welch MJ et al: Indium-III: A new radionuclide label for studying human platelet kinetics. Br J Haematol 42:613, 1979

48. Hirsch ED, Favre-Gilly J, Dameshek W: Thrombopathic thrombocytopenia: Successful transfusion of blood platelets. Blood 5:568, 1950

49. Hoffman R: Regulation of megakaryocytopoiesis. Blood 74:1196, 1989

50. Holmsen H, Day HJ: The selectivity of the thrombin-induced platelet release reaction: Subcellular localization of released and retained substances. J Lab Clin Med 75:840, 1970

51. Holmsen H, Day HJ, Storm E: Adenine nucleotide metabolism of blood platelets. VI: Subcellular localization of nucleotide pools with different functions in the platelet release reaction. Biochim Biophys Acta 186:254, 1969

52. Hovig T: The ultrastructure of rabbit blood platelet aggregates. Thromb Diath Haemorrh 8:455, 1962

53. Howard BV, Macarak EJ, Gunson D et al: Characterization of the collagen synthesized by endothelial cells in culture. Proc Natl Acad Sci USA 73:2361, 1976

54. Kao KJ, Pizzo SV, McKee PA: Demonstration and characterization of specific binding sites for factor VIII/von Willebrand factor on human platelets. J Clin Invest 63:656, 1979

55. Kao KJ, Pizzo SV, McKee PA: Platelet receptors for factor VIII/von Willebrand protein: Functional correlation of receptor occupancy and ristocetin-induced platelet aggregation. Proc Natl Acad Sci USA 76:5317, 1979

56. Kaplan KL, Broekman MJ, Chernoff A et al: Platelet alpha-granule proteins: Studies on release and subcellular localization. Blood 53:604, 1979

57. Karpatkin S: Heterogeneity of human platelets. Metabolic and kinetic evidence suggestive of young and old platelets. J Clin Invest 47:1073, 1969

58. Kato A, Yamamoto K, Miyazaki S et al: Molecular basis for Glanzmann thrombasthenia (GT) in a compound heterozygote with glycoprotein IIb gene defects: A proposal for classification of GT based on the biosynthetic pathway of glycoprotein IIb-IIIa complex. Blood 79:3212, 1992

59. Keenan JP, Solum NO: Quantitative studies on the release of platelet fibrinogen by thrombin. Br J Haematol 23:461, 1972

60. Kinlough-Rathbone RL, Packham MA, Mustard JF: Synergism between platelet-aggregating agents: The role of the arachidonate pathway. Thromb Res 11:567, 1977

61. Kinlough-Rathbone RL, Reimers JJ, Mustard JF: Sodium arachidonate can induce platelet shape change and aggregation which are independent of the release reaction. Science 192:1011, 1976

62. Lajmanovich A, Hudry-Clergeon G, Freyssinet J-M et al: Human factor VIII procoagulant activity and phospholipid interaction. Biochim Biophys Acta 678:132, 1981

63. Levin J, Evatt BL: Humoral control of thrombopoiesis. Blood Cells 5:105, 1979

64. Levin J, Levin FC, Penington DG et al: Measurement of ploidy distribution in megakaryocyte colonies obtained from culture: With studies of the effects of thrombocytopenia. Blood 57:284, 1981

65. Lewis N, Majerus PW: Lipid metabolism in human platelets. II: De novo phospholipid synthesis and the effect of thrombin on the pattern of synthesis. J Clin Invest 48:2114, 1969

66. Lipscomb MS, Walsh PN: Human platelet factor XI: Localization in platelet membranes of factor XI-like activity and its functional distinction from plasma factor XI. J Clin Invest 63:1006, 1979

67. Lok S, Kaushansky K, Holly RD et al: Cloning and expression of murine thrombopoietin cDNA and stimulation of platelet production *in vivo*. Nature 369:565, 1994

68. Lopaciuk S, Lovette KM, McDonagh J et al: Subcellular distribution of fibrinogen and factor XIII in human platelets. Thromb Res 8:453, 1976

69. Luscher EF: Ein fibrinstabilisierender Faktor aus Thrombocyten. Schweiz Med Wochenschr 87:1220, 1957

70. Madri JA, Dreyer B, Pitlick FA et al: The collagenase components of the subendothelium: Correlation of structure and function. Lab Invest 43:303, 1980

71. Mann KG, Prendergast FG, Bloom JW: The metal ion and phospholipid interactions of the vitamin-K dependent factors. In Mann KG, Taylor FB Jr (eds): The Regulation of Coagulation, p 3. New York, Elsevier, 1980

72. Marcus AJ, Zucker-Franklin D, Safier LB et al: Studies on human platelet granules and membranes. J Clin Invest 45:14, 1966

73. Martin JH, Carson FL, Race GJ: Calcium containing platelet granules. J Cell Biol 60:775, 1976

74. Mason RG, Mohammad SF, Chuang HY et al: The adhesion of platelets to subendothelium, collagen and artificial surfaces. Semin Thromb Hemost 3:98, 1976

75. McDonagh J, Kiesselbach TH, Wagner RH: Factor XIII and antiplasmin activity in human platelets. Am J Physiol 216:508, 1969

76. Miale JB: Hemostasis and blood coagulation. In Miale JB (ed): Laboratory Medicine Hematology, 6th ed, p 772. St Louis, CV Mosby, 1982

77. Miletich JP, Jackson CM, Majerus PW: Properties of the factor Xa binding site on human platelets. J Biol Chem 253:6908, 1978

78. Moncada S, Vane JR: Arachidonic acid metabolites and the interactions between platelets and blood-vessel walls. N Engl J Med 300:1142, 1979

79. Murphy EA, Robinson GA, Rowsell HC et al: The pattern of platelet disappearance. Blood 30:26, 1967

80. Mustard JF, Perry DW, Kinlough-Rathbone RL et al: Factors responsible for ADP-induced release reaction of human platelets. Am J Physiol 228:1757, 1975

81. Nachman RL, Marcus A, Safier L: Platelet thrombosthenin: Subcellular localization and function. J Clin Invest 46:1380, 1967

82. Needleman P, Whitaker MO, Wyche A et al: Manipulation of platelet aggregation by prostaglandins and their fatty acid precursors: Pharmacological basis for a therapeutic approach. Prostaglandins 19:165, 1980

83. Nesheim ME, Eid S, Mann KG: Assembly of the prothrombinase complex in the absence of prothrombin. J Biol Chem 256:9874, 1981

84. Nesheim ME, Taswell JB, Mann KG: The contribution of bovine factor V and factor Va to the activity of prothrombinase. J Biol Chem 254:10952, 1979

85. Nieuwenhuis HK, van Osterhaut JJG, Rosenmuller E et al: Studies with a monoclonal antibody against activated platelets. Evidence that a secreted 53,000 molecular weight lysosome-like granule protein is exposed on the surface of activated platelets in the circulation. Blood 70:838, 1987

86. Nurden AT, Caen JP: Specific roles for platelet surface glycoproteins in platelet function. Nature 255:720, 1975

87. O'Brien JR, Woodhouse MA: Platelets: Their size, shape and stickiness *in vitro:* Degranulation and propinquity. Exp Biol Med 3:90, 1968

88. Okuma M, Uchina H: Altered arachidonate metabolism by platelets in patients with myeloproliferative disorders. Blood 13:1258, 1979

89. Osterud B, Rapaport SI, Lavine KK: Factor V activity of platelets: Evidence for an activated factor V molecule and for a platelet activator. Blood 49:819, 1977

90. Ozge-Anwar AH, Ofosu FA, Blajchman MA: Evidence that intact human platelets provide factor VII-like activity for the activation of factor X by the extrinsic coagulation pathway. Thromb Haemost 54:176, 1985

91. Packham MA: Stages in the interaction of platelets with collagen. Thromb Haemost 36:269, 1976

92. Packham MA, Kinlough-Rathbone RL, Reimers H-J et al: Mechanisms of platelet aggregation independent of adenosine diphosphate. In Silver MJ, Smith JB, Kocsis JJ (eds): Prostaglandins in Hematology, p 247. New York, Spectrum Publishing, 1977

93. Paulus JM: DNA metabolism and the development of organelles in guinea pig megakaryocytes: A combined ultrastructural, autoradiographic and cytophotometric study. Blood 35:298, 1970

94. Paulus JM: Platelet size in man. Blood 46:321, 1975

95. Phillips DR, Agin PP: Platelet plasma membrane glycoproteins. Evidence for the presence of nonequivalent disulfide bonds using nonreduced–reduced two-dimensional gel electrophoresis. J Biol Chem 252:2121, 1977

96. Piovella F, Ascaari E, Sofar GM et al: Immunofluorescent detection of factor VIII-related antigen in human platelets and megakaryocytes. Haemostasis 3:288, 1974

97. Pisciotta A, Stefanini M, Dameshek W: Studies on platelets. X: Morphologic characteristics of megakaryocytes by phase contrast microscopy in normal patients and in patients with idiopathic thrombocytopenia purpura. Blood 8:703, 1953

98. Pollard TD: Functional implications of the biochemical and structural properties of cytoplasmic contractile proteins. In Inoise S, Stephens RF (eds): Molecules and Cell Movement, p 259. New York, Raven Press, 1978

99. Puszkin E, Maldonado R, Spaet TH et al: Platelet myosin: Localization of the rod myosin fragment and effect of its antibodies on platelet function. J Biol Chem 252:4371, 1977

100. Rabellino EM, Nachman RL, Williams N et al: Human megakaryocytes. 1: Characterization of the membrane and cytoplasmic components of isolated marrow megakaryocytes. J Exp Med 149:1273, 1979

101. Rak K: Effect of vincristine on platelet production in mice. Br J Haematol 22:617, 1972

102. Rodley JM, Scurfield G: The mechanism of platelet release. Blood 56:996, 1980

103. Ross R, Glomset J, Kariya B et al: A platelet-dependent serum factor that stimulates the proliferation of arterial smooth muscle cells *in vitro.* Proc Natl Acad Sci USA 71:1207, 1974

104. Rucinski B, Niewiarowski S, James P et al: Antiheparin proteins secreted by human platelets: Purification, characterization and radioimmunoassays. Blood 53:47, 1979

105. Sage H, Crouch E, Bornstein P: Collagen synthesis by bovine aortic endothelial cells in culture. Biochemistry 18:5433, 1979

106. de Sauvage FJ, Hass PE, Spencer SD et al: Stimulation of megakaryocytopoiesis and thrombopoiesis by the c-*mpl* ligand. Nature 369:533, 1994

107. Schulz H, Schiller K: Microtubuli and Filamente in prospektiven Plattachenfeldern der Megakaryocyten. Z Zellforsch 87:309, 1968

108. Scott DM, Horwood R, Grant ME et al: Characterization of the major collagen species present in porcine aorta and the synthesis of their precursors by smooth muscle cells in culture. Connect Tissue Res 5:7, 1977

109. Shaklai M, Tavassoli M: Demarcation membrane system in rat megakaryocytes and the mechanism of platelet formation: A membrane reorganization process. J Ultrastruct Res 62:270, 1978

110. Shick PK, Kurica KB, Chacko GK: Location of phosphatidylethanolamine and phosphatidylserine in human platelet plasma membrane. J Clin Invest 57:1221, 1976

111. Shulman NR, Watkins JP, Hscoitz SB et al: Evidence that the spleen retains the youngest and hemostatically most effective platelets. Trans Assoc Am Phys 81:312, 1968

112. Sixma JJ: Platelet coagulant activities. Thromb Haemost 40:163, 1978

113. Slot JW, Bouma BN, Montgomery R et al: Platelet factor VIII-related antigen: Immunofluorescent localization. Thromb Res 13:871, 1978

114. Sohoma Y, Akahori H, Seki N et al: Molecular cloning and chromosomal localization of the human thrombopoietin gene. FEBS Lett 353:57, 1994

115. Steiner M, Ikeda Y: Quantitative assessment of polymerized and depolymerized platelet microtubules: Changes caused by aggregating agents. J Clin Invest 63:443, 1979

116. Stemerman MB, Spaet TH: The subendothelium and thrombogenesis. Bull NY Acad Med 48:289, 1972

117. Stenflo J, Dahlback B: Activation of prothrombin by factor Xa on the surface of platelets. In Mann KG, Taylor FB (eds): The Regulation of Coagulation, p 225. New York, Elsevier, 1980

118. Tobb-Smith AHT: Why the platelets were discovered. Br J Haematol 13:618, 1967

119. Tracy PB, Paterson JM, Nesheim ME et al: Interaction of coagulation factor V and factor Va with platelets. J Biol Chem 254:10354, 1979

120. Trelstad RL: Human aorta collagens: Evidence for three distinct species. Biochem Biophys Res Commun 57:717, 1974

121. Trelstad RL: Special state of the fibril end: Site of growth, point of cell surface attachment, and possible site for platelet interaction. In Gastpar H (ed): Collagen-Platelet Interactions, p 153. New York, Schattauer Verlag, 1978

122. Trowbridge EA: Platelet production: A computer-based biological interpretation. Thromb Res 31:329, 1983

123. Tschopp TB, Baumgartner HR, Silbergauer K et al: Platelet adhesion and platelet thrombus formation on subendothelium of human arteries and veins exposed to flowing blood *in vitro*: A comparison with rabbit aorta. Haemostasis 8:19, 1979

124. Turritto VT, Baumgartner HR: Platelet interaction with subendothelium in flowing rabbit blood. Effect of blood shear rate. Microvasc Res 17:38, 1979

125. Turritto VT, Leonard EF: Platelet adhesion to a spinning disc. Trans Am Soc Artif Intern Organs 18:348, 1972

126. Turritto VT, Muggli R, Baumgartner HR: Platelet adhesion and thrombus formation on subendothelium, Epon, gelatin, and collagen under artificial flow conditions. Trans Am Soc Artif Intern Organs 24:568, 1978

127. Tuszynski GP, Bevacona SJ, Schmaier AH et al: Factor XI antigen and activity in platelets. Blood 59:1148, 1982

128. van Dieijen G, Tans G, Rosing J et al: The role of phospholipid and factor VIIIa in the activation of bovine factor X. Biochemistry 256:3433, 1981

129. van Zutphen H, Bevers EM, Hemker HC et al: Contribution of platelet factor V content to platelet factor 3 activity. Br J Haematol 45:119, 1980

130. Vigon I, Marnon JP, Cocaoult L et al: Molecular cloning and characterization of *mpl*, the human homologue of the *v-mpl* oncogene. Identification of a member of the hematopoietic growth factor superfamily. Proc Natl Acad Sci USA 89:5640, 1992

131. Walsh PN, Biggs R: The role of platelets in intrinsic factor Xa formation. Br J Haematol 22:743, 1972

132. Wang CL, Miyata T, Weksler B et al: Collagen induced platelet aggregation and release: Critical size and structural requirements of collagen. Biochim Biophys Acta 544:468, 1978

133. Weiss HJ, deWitte L, Kaplan KL et al: Heterogeneity in storage pool deficiency: Studies in granule-bound substances in 18 patients including variants deficient in α-granules, platelet factor 4, β-thromboglobulin and platelet-derived growth factor. Blood 54:1296, 1979

134. Wendling F, Methia N, Louache F et al: Antisense oligodeoxynucleotides to mpl protooncogene specifically inhibit megakaryocytic differentiation. Blood 82:1395, 1993

135. Wendling F, Maraskovsky E, Debili N et al: cMpl ligand is a humoral regulator of megakaryocytopoiesis. Nature 369:571, 1994

136. White JG: Effects of colchicine and vinca alkaloids on human platelets. I: Influence on platelet microtubules and contractile function. Am J Pathol 53:281, 1968

137. White JG: Effects of colchicine and vinca alkaloids on human platelets. II: Changes in the dense tubular system and formation of an unusual inclusion in incubated cells. Am J Pathol 53:447, 1968

138. White JG: Fine structural alterations induced in platelets by adenosine diphosphate. Blood 31:604, 1968

139. White JG: The submembrane filaments of blood platelets. Am J Pathol 56:267, 1969

140. White JG: Effects of colchicine and vinca alkaloids on human platelets. III: Influence on primary internal contraction and secondary aggregation. Am J Pathol 54:467, 1969

141. White JG: Platelet morphology. In Johnson SA (ed): The Circulating Platelet, p 45. New York, Academic Press, 1971

142. White JG: Ultrastructural physiology and cytochemistry of blood platelets. In Brinkhous KM, Shermer RW, Mostofi FK (eds): The Platelet, p 85. Baltimore, Williams & Wilkins, 1971

143. White JG: Identification of platelet secretion in the electron microscope. Sem Haematol 6:429, 1973

144. White JG: Electron microscopic studies of platelet secretion. Prog Hemost Thromb 2:49, 1974

145. White JG: Physiochemical dissection of platelet structural physiology. In Baldini MG, Ebbe S (eds): Platelets: Production, Function, Transfusion and Storage, p 235. New York, Grune & Stratton, 1974

146. White JG, Conrad WJ: The fine structure of freeze-fractured blood platelets. Am J Pathol 70:45, 1973

147. White JG, Krivet W: An ultrastructural basis for the shape changes induced by chilling. Blood 30:625, 1967

148. Williams N, Levine RF: The origin, development, and regulation of megakaryocytes. Br J Haematol 52:173, 1982

149. Wood JG: Electron microscopic localization of 5-hydroxytryptamine (5-HT). Texas Rep Biol Med 23:828, 1965

150. Wright JH: The histiogenesis of blood platelets. J Morphol 21:263, 1910

151. Wright JH: The origin and nature of blood platelets. Boston Med Surg J 154:643, 1906

152. Zucker MB, Broekman MJ, Kaplan KL: Factor VIII-related antigen in human blood platelets: Localization and release by thrombin and collagen. J Lab Clin Med 94:675, 1979

153. Zucker-Franklin D: The submembranous fibrils of human platelets. J Cell Biol 47:293, 1970

154. Zwaal RFA, Hemker HC: Blood cell membranes and haemostasis. Haemostasis 11:12, 1982

CHAPTER 56

Laboratory Evaluation of Platelets

John A. Koepke

Objectives

1. Describe a method for performing peripheral blood film platelet estimates and two methods for manual platelet counts; include sources of error.
2. List two principles used in automated platelet counting, state a major advantage of such automation, and list several causes of both falsely increased and decreased platelet counts.
3. Discuss the procedure for the bleeding time test, state its usual reference range, and list several variables that affect it.
4. State the principle of platelet aggregometry, list six agonists used to evaluate platelet function, and discuss the interpretation of aggregometry tracings.
5. Describe the defect in von Willebrand disease, and recommend and briefly define tests that are helpful in its diagnosis.

The laboratory investigation of a disorder of hemostasis may include the evaluation of platelet number and their function.[20] These two aspects are interrelated in that abnormalities of either or both will result in a hemostatic defect; however, tests of platelet function are usually indicated only if platelet numbers are adequate. Formerly, the quantitation of platelets was primarily performed using manual microscopy methods. However, accurate and precise instrumental methods are now being used. The laboratory evaluations of platelet function provide a measure of adhesion, aggregation, granule release, or clot retraction, either separately or in their sum. The evaluation of qualitative platelet abnormalities is more complex, and most of this chapter will be devoted to this subject. Although von Willebrand disease (vWD) is not a disorder of platelet function *per se*, the deficiency of plasma von

Willebrand factor (vWF) prevents normal platelet adhesion *in vivo* and *in vitro*. Key tests for vWD include platelet aggregometry and analysis of vWF; consequently, vWD is included in the discussion of platelet function testing.

PLATELET COUNTING

Platelets must be present in sufficient numbers to play their supportive role in hemostasis. When evaluating a bleeding problem that may be traceable to platelets, platelet counting is an important and logical first step. This may be done simply by estimating the number of platelets on a peripheral blood film or, preferably, by using automated counting methods. The commonly stated platelet reference range for adults is 140 to 440×10^9/L; for pediatric patients, it is somewhat higher.

Platelet Estimates From Peripheral Blood Films

The procedure for peripheral blood film platelet estimates is detailed in Chapter 24. A method for calculation of a platelet count estimation factor on blood films is shown in Table 24-4 in the section on manual differentials. There should be one platelet for every 10 to 40 erythrocytes in normal peripheral blood. Thus, an oil-immersion field containing 100 erythrocytes should normally have between 3 and 10 platelets, whereas a field containing 200 erythrocytes should have between 5 and 20 platelets. See Automated Platelet Counts, Quality Control later in this chapter for a more precise method (Miller disc) for platelet count estimates on peripheral blood films.

The review of the peripheral blood film is also helpful in detecting causes of artifactually low counts secondary to platelet clumping caused by anticoagulant-dependent platelet agglutinins or microclots from improperly collected specimens. Giant platelets seen in some congenital platelet function defects and certain myeloproliferative disorders can also be detected in this way.

Manual Platelet Counts

The most commonly employed methods of manual platelet counts use a 1:100 or 1:200 dilution of blood loaded into a Neubauer hemocytometer chamber. Two different methods are used to make the platelets visible. The Tocantins method using Rees-Ecker diluent employs a citrate–formaldehyde buffer with brilliant cresyl blue as a platelet stain for light microscopy.[19] This diluent fixes and preserves erythrocytes as well as platelets to prevent their disintegration.

The more popular phase-contrast microscopy method requires a phase microscope and 1% ammonium oxalate diluting fluid, which lyses erythrocytes and allows platelets to form pseudopods.[5] It is generally agreed that platelet identification is improved with the phase contrast method.[9]

Specimen Requirements. When possible, venous blood collected with EDTA anticoagulant is preferable; skin puncture capillary blood samples can yield artifactually low counts due to platelet adhesion to the edge of the wound. If venipuncture is not possible, skin puncture should be performed with a larger blade so that a deep wound with freely flowing blood is obtained, and the specimen should be collected immediately to avoid significant platelet adhesion to the wound.

A convenient capillary blood collection system (Unopette®; Becton Dickinson) is available commercially. A precalibrated capillary tube is used for the collection of a measured amount of blood which is transferred into a premeasured volume of diluting fluid, thus providing an accurate dilution of the blood specimen.

Reagents and Equipment. A Neubauer hemocytometer with a rigid coverglass, erythrocyte diluting pipettes (or the Unopette® platelet counting system), and a light microscope are required for the Rees-Ecker method. To make diluent for the Rees-Ecker method, combine 3.8 g of sodium citrate, 0.2 mL of neutral formaldehyde (38%), and 0.1 g of brilliant cresyl blue in approximately 50 mL of distilled water. Bring to 100 mL with distilled water and filter.

For the phase-contrast method, the diluent is filtered 1% ammonium oxalate in distilled water. This method requires a special thin, flat-bottom counting chamber and a phase microscope with a phase objective and a long working distance phase condenser (Chap. 4).

Procedure and Calculations. Depending on laboratory preference, platelets may be counted either in ⅕ of a mm² or 1 mm² in the center of the counting chamber (see Fig. 24-2). Both sides of the chamber should be charged and counted and the results averaged. In the Rees-Ecker method, platelets appear as small, highly refractile; round, oval, or elongated bodies that stain light blue and are about 1/10 the diameter of the surrounding erythrocytes. In the phase-contrast method, erythrocytes are lysed, leaving only platelets and leukocytes, which can be distinguished easily. See Chapter 24 for a detailed description of hemocytometer cell counts.

Platelets are preferably reported as the number per liter (SI) but may be reported per μL (equivalent to mm³). The number of platelets counted is multiplied by the dilution factor (100 or 200), by a chamber depth-correction factor (10) because the depth of the chamber is 0.1 mm, and by an area correction factor (1 or 5) depending on whether 1 mm² or ⅕ mm² was counted. For example, if 1 mm² is counted and the dilution is 1:100, the number of platelets counted is multiplied by 1000 ($100 \times 10 \times 1$) to find the number of platelets per mm³ or μL. Multiplying this result by 10^6 gives the result per liter (L).

Comments and Sources of Error. Standardization of the technique and quality control of the method are extremely important in manual platelet counting. Results should be checked periodically against peripheral blood estimates, automated counts, or both. The expected coefficient of variation is around 10% for the phase-contrast method and 16% to 25% for the Rees-Ecker method. The phase microscope must be checked periodically according to manufacturer's recommendations to ensure that the phase objective and annulus

condenser are aligned correctly (Chap. 4). Special care should be taken to keep the counting chambers free of dirt or debris that might be mistaken for platelets. The chamber should be checked microscopically with a coverslip in place for such dirt or debris before adding the diluted platelet suspension. Ethyl alcohol (95% v/v) and a lint-free cloth or lens paper are recommended for cleaning.

Platelet clumping or discrepancies between the two counts of 20% or more necessitate repeat counts. A fresh specimen may be necessary. When the platelet count is low, a lesser dilution of the specimen may need to be counted to improve precision. For very low counts (*i.e.*, less than 50×10^9/L), a 1:20 dilution should be made in a leukocyte diluting pipette and a new dilution factor (20) used in the calculation. This allows for more platelets to be counted with a resultant increased precision.

Automated Platelet Counts

Most modern hematology analyzers count platelets. These instruments employ either optical methods (detection of the degree of light scattering) or electronic methods (change in the electrical resistance or capacitance across a circuit) to detect particles as they stream through an aperture tube or flow cell (Chap. 42). These instruments sample whole blood, lyse erythrocytes, and discriminate between platelets and leukocytes on the basis of their size, light scatter, or both. Varying the suspending diluent or the threshold settings of the circuitry allows separate counting of blood cells of different sizes. A significant advantage of instrumental platelet counts is their precision. Depending on the particular instrument, the coefficient of variation for platelet counts is between 2% and 5%.

Quality Control and Sources of Error. The key to reliable automated platelet counts is good quality control. Hematology instruments which include platelet counting must be standardized against reference methods such as the phase contrast method or against another instrument that has been calibrated for platelet counting. Once an instrument has been standardized or calibrated, stabilized suspensions of whole blood, which are available from several suppliers, are used as daily controls. Controls may be run at the beginning of each batch of blood counts or may be interspersed between patient samples. Records of quality control data must be examined to detect any subtle instrument or reagent problems (Chap. 45).

Samples from each batch may be screened for accuracy by platelet estimates performed on the peripheral blood film. One method for such estimates is discussed in Chapter 24. Another useful method requires a Miller disc and allows for a reasonably accurate estimate of the platelet count. The latter method relies on a determination of the platelet-to-erythrocyte ratio and therefore also requires an accurate erythrocyte count.[13] Histograms of platelet populations provide another quality control tool (Chap. 42).

There are several sources of error in automated platelet counts. Falsely high counts may result from contamination of reagents with particles of dirt or microorganisms or carryover from a prior sample with a high platelet count. Particles that should not be counted but that register as platelets include such platelet artifacts as erythrocyte and leukocyte fragments (*e.g.*, in patients undergoing chemotherapy for leukemia), lyse-resistant erythrocytes, or erythrocyte inclusion bodies (in methods that lyse erythrocytes). Artifactually low counts may occur with giant platelets, platelet agglutinins, or platelet satellitism. Each of these sources of error can be eliminated with a good quality-control regimen, including careful review of histograms generated by automated instruments and review of the peripheral blood film.

EVALUATION OF PLATELET FUNCTION

Patients with normal numbers of platelets and a long history of easy bruising, nosebleeds, gingival bleeding, and prolonged bleeding following surgery or injury may have a congenital functional platelet defect. Congenital platelet abnormalities, while uncommon, require careful and complete studies for appropriate patient treatment. The initial screening test for functional platelet disorders and for von Willebrand disease is the skin bleeding time (Table 56-1). Note that in all cases in Table 56-1, the bleeding time test is prolonged. Additional testing is indicated in such cases (see Table 56-1) until a definitive diagnosis is found. A fibrinogen determination is performed to rule out afibrinogenemia, which may mimic these platelet disorders.[23]

The Bleeding Time Test

Platelet adhesion to the exposed subendothelial collagen of severed capillaries (or to glass beads *in vitro*) requires the presence of plasma von Willebrand factor (vWF), platelets capable of interacting with vWF (platelets with the glycoprotein Ib-IX receptor complex), and platelet capacity to aggregate. Although several tests have been proposed to measure these aspects of platelet function, the preferred test is the skin bleeding time. In this test, a superficial incision, usually on the skin of the forearm, is made in a standard fashion. The time for the bleeding to stop is an *in vivo* measure of the interaction of platelets with the severed blood capillaries in the skin. It is affected by many variables, which are discussed in the following paragraphs. The bleeding time is a very useful initial test to be performed in patients suspected of having a congenital platelet abnormality or von Willebrand disease (vWD; discussed later in this chapter).

Procedure and Reference Ranges.[17] Make certain that the patient's platelet count is above a safe level (greater than $100 \times 10^9/$L). The bleeding time should be performed at room temperature since cooler or warmer ambient temperatures can affect the test. Inform the patient of possible scarring, keloid formation, and the risk of infection. Generally, this test should not be performed on individuals who are unable to cooperate or may have a tendency to form keloids. The testing should only be performed by individuals well-trained in the procedure. To ensure consistency in test performance and results, the procedure should be reviewed periodically with all personnel who perform it.

With the arm supine and on a firm support (preferably close to the level of the heart), select a site on the lateral one third of the forearm, 2 to 3 cm below the antecubital crease, in an area without hair (shaving may be required), surface veins, scars, tattoos, bruises, skin infection or edema, moles, or other abnormalities. If a suitable area is not found on the forearm, a location on the medial aspect of the calf about 6 to 8 cm below the knee has been shown to be an acceptable alternative location.

Place a blood pressure cuff on the upper arm (or thigh), clean the test site with an alcohol swab, and then inflate the cuff to 40 mm Hg for 30 to 60 seconds before the incision is made. The cuff should be kept at 40 mm Hg during the entire procedure. Firmly place the device (commercially available template or disposable device) on the site previously selected, using as little pressure as possible. Make the incision (5 mm long and 1 mm deep) either perpendicular (vertical) or parallel (horizontal) to the antecubital crease. The direction of the incision is at the discretion of the laboratory director, but once selected the same procedure should be used consistently. A horizontal incision gives a somewhat longer bleeding time; the vertical incision apparently results in less scarring.

Start the stop watch. Wick (touch), but do not blot, the drops of blood from the edge of the incision by bringing the edge of a filter paper (*e.g.*, Whatman #1) close to the incision every 30 seconds. Take care not to touch the actual incision or dislodge the developing platelet plug. The bleeding time is the time elapsed from when the incision was made until blood ceases to stain the filter paper, rounded to the nearest 30 seconds. No additional information is gained by continuing to measure the bleeding time after 20 minutes, and the test should be stopped when that limit is reached. Upon test completion, remove the cuff and clean the area around the incision. Place a butterfly closure to oppose the edges of the incision; it can be removed 24 hours later.

The upper limit of normal for most methods varies up to 9.0 minutes. Generally, the bleeding time increases with advancing age. However, each laboratory should establish its own reference ranges which vary with age as well as methodology.

Variables Affecting the Bleeding Time. Anemia prolongs the bleeding time. Also, as expected, patients with thrombocytopenia (less than $100 \times 10^9/$L) have an inverse correlation between the bleeding time and their platelet count. It is well known that many

---

TABLE 56-1
Laboratory Diagnosis of Platelet Function Disorders

| | Aspirin Ingestion | Storage Pool Defects | Platelet Thrombocytopathy | | von Willebrand Disease | Afibrinogenemia* |
			Bernard-Soulier Syndrome	*Glanzmann Thrombasthenia*		
Bleeding time	P	P	P	P	P	P
Platelet count	N	N	N/↓	N	N/↓**	N
PTT	N	N	N	N	N/↑	↑
Fibrinogen	N	N	N	N	N	↓
ADP response	Abn	Abn	N	Abn	N	Abn
Ristocetin response	N	N	Abn	N	Abn	N

KEY: P, prolonged; N, normal; ↓, decreased; ↑, increased; Abn, abnormal.
*Afibrinogenemia is not a thrombocytopathy, but a plasma fibrinogen deficiency which may mimic platelet disorders.
**Platelet count in von Willebrand disease occasionally decreased.

drugs prolong the bleeding time, aspirin being the most common offender. But other nonsteroidal anti-inflammatory drugs, ticlopedine (a platelet aggregation inhibitor), and antibiotics such as penicillin and cephalothin are also associated with a prolongation of the bleeding time. The aspirin effect persists for up to 3 days following ingestion, but with the other drugs, shorter durations of their effects have been noted. Devices which make smaller incisions are required for pediatric patients. For neonates, an even smaller incision is used. In both of these patient groups, a pediatric blood pressure cuff which maintains a pressure of 20 mm Hg must be used.[2]

Interpretation. The bleeding time should be interpreted in conjunction with the patient's clinical history. In von Willebrand disease, the bleeding time is usually prolonged, making it a useful screening test. The test is also prolonged in a number of hereditary platelet defects (Chap. 57) including Glanzmann thrombasthenia, Bernard-Soulier syndrome, and congenital storage pool disease (*e.g.*, Hermansky-Pudlak syndrome). The bleeding time is also prolonged in thrombocytopenia, afibrinogenemia, severe hypofibrinogenemia, and some vascular disorders. As noted previously, aspirin or other medications may lengthen the bleeding time.

Patients with mild qualitative platelet disorders and a significant bleeding history may manifest variability in their bleeding times and occasionally will have a normal result. Sometimes it is necessary to perform several bleeding time tests before a firm diagnosis can be made. There is no evidence that the bleeding time has any predictive value when used as a preoperative screening test for patients who do not have a history or clinical signs of functional platelet abnormalities.[11] Two possible exceptions to this general rule are screening prior to neurosurgical and intraocular procedures.

Historical Tests of Platelet Function

Prior to the widespread availability of platelet aggregation studies, several tests were advanced as methods for determining platelet function. They are now noted primarily for their historical interest. In the *in vitro* glass bead retention test, blood is passed through a column of glass beads. Normal platelets that have access to normal vWF will adhere and aggregate to the beads, with a resulting decrease in the platelet count of the effluent blood.[4] The normal percentage of platelets retained in the glass bead column is approximately 70% or greater.

The *in vivo* platelet adhesiveness test involves serial platelet counts on blood exuding from a forearm incision. Normally, the platelet counts decrease because of platelet adhesion to the wound. These counts are compared with a venous blood platelet count as a control to calculate percent platelet adhesiveness.[3] This test is rarely performed today because the results are no better or more specific than those of the bleeding time test.

The once popular clot retraction test is another platelet function test that is seldom, if ever, performed today. Whole blood is allowed to clot in a clean glass tube at 37°C. The clot begins to shrink and retract from the walls of the tube after 1 hour. This retraction process is maximal at 24 hours, by which time the clot occupies about half of the original blood volume.[6] This process depends on normal numbers of contractile platelets, the presence of calcium and ATP, and a normal concentration of fibrinogen. The interaction of platelets with fibrinogen and fibrin must also be normal for clot retraction to occur.

Platelet Factor Assays

Platelets facilitate plasma coagulation by providing a lipid surface onto which certain clotting factors bind, thereby enhancing their reaction rates. This facilitative platelet capacity in clot formation is synonymous with platelet factor 3 (PF3). PF3 is a functional concept rather than a discrete molecular substance, as is usually implied by the word "factor." When platelets are incubated with kaolin and epinephrine, they are stimulated to provide PF3 activity. Thus, the clotting time of platelet-rich plasma (PRP) incubated with kaolin and epinephrine is considerably shorter than that of platelet-poor plasma (PPP). The test for PF3 availability compares the clotting time of the patient's PRP with that obtained from a group of normal individuals. PF3 availability is decreased in acquired or congenital defects of platelet secretion or release.

Platelet factor 4 (PF4) and β-thromboglobulin are heparin-binding proteins found in platelet α-granules.[10] As such, their levels *in vivo* are an indicator of the presence of ongoing platelet activation in a variety of disease states such as myocardial infarction, venous thrombosis, diabetes, inflammatory states, and myeloproliferative disorders. Alternatively, release of these proteins from aggregating platelets in PRP can be examined for patients suspected of having storage pool disease or a release defect. PF4 and β-thromboglobulin assays are considered research procedures. There are several commercial RIA kits available for PF4 and β-thromboglobulin measurement in either plasma or from α-granule release.

Platelet Aggregometry

Principle. Studies of platelet aggregation *in vitro* are now commonly performed to assist in the diagnosis of hereditary and acquired platelet disorders. Aggregating agents (so-called agonists) added to a stirred suspension of PRP induce a shape change and aggregation of platelets. As a result, the PRP changes from a turbid suspension to one that transmits more light as the aggregates are formed. The process of platelet aggregation is monitored with a platelet aggregometer (Fig. 56-1) that measures and records a change in light transmission.

There have been several significant advances in aggregometry techniques. One is the impedance aggregometry system, which requires aliquots of undiluted, anticoagulated whole blood instead of PRP specimens. As with the PRP method, several platelet agonists are added in individual tests to the whole blood, and platelet aggregation is evaluated. Instead of using a change in light transmission, aggregation is monitored by the continuous increase in electrical impedance between two electrodes as platelets adhere and aggregate on the electrodes in a stirred, anticoagulated whole blood sample. A major advantage of whole blood aggregometry is the avoidance of PRP preparation, which can be problematic. Avoiding this step also significantly reduces the technical time required for testing. Whole blood aggregometry is believed by some to more closely approximate *in vivo* platelet reactivity than PRP aggregometry.

In another modification called lumi-aggregometry, platelet aggregation is monitored by the luciferase–luciferin reaction which, when ATP is released from the aggregating platelets, causes the luciferin to produce measurable light. This is the same chemical reaction that lights up fireflies.

In the following sections, details of aggregometry using PRP are given to illustrate the basic techniques and interpretations of aggregometry curves. The manufacturer's directions for platelet ag-

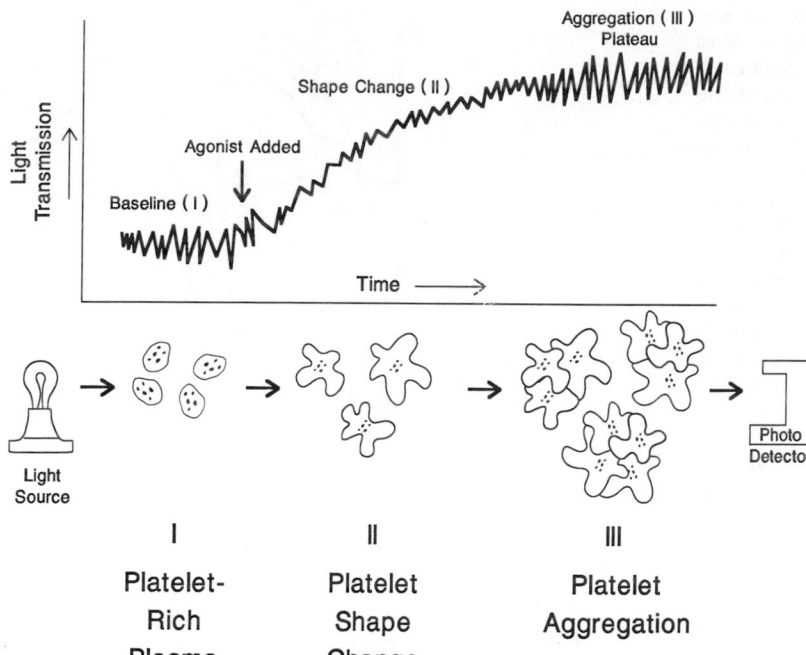

FIGURE 56-1. Principles of platelet aggregometry. (Modified from Penner JA: Manual of Blood Coagulation: Blood Coagulation Course. East Lansing, MI, Michigan State University College of Human Medicine, 1982, with permission.)

gregometry procedures must be carefully followed to generate valid information (see also Chap. 58).

Patient and Specimen Requirements. Preferably, the patient and the normal control individual should be fasting. Otherwise, they should have had a relatively fat-free meal to eliminate optical problems caused by lipemic plasma. Also, the patient should not be taking aspirin, nonsteroidal anti-inflammatory drugs, or other drugs known to interfere with platelet aggregation. Venous blood is drawn from the patient and from a normal individual into plastic syringes. Nine parts of blood are added immediately to a plastic test tube containing one part 3.2% trisodium citrate. PRP is obtained from both patient and control specimens by centrifuging at room temperature at 200 × g for 10 minutes. The supernatant PRP is carefully withdrawn (avoiding the aspiration of any erythrocytes), transferred to another plastic tube, stoppered, and kept at room temperature until testing. To ensure platelet viability, testing must be completed within 3 hours of specimen collection.

Platelet-poor plasma (PPP) is obtained from both specimens by additional centrifugation of the remaining PRP and red cells in the tubes at 2500 to 3000 × g for 30 minutes. The PPPs should also be kept at room temperature until use.[18] As a consequence of processing the PRP, platelets sometimes exhibit a "platelet shock" phenomenon and will be poorly responsive or even nonresponsive to ADP, collagen, and epinephrine for as long as 30 minutes. If a poor response is obtained with any of these reagents, the test should be repeated 30 minutes later. This problem may also be avoided by either waiting 30 minutes before initiating testing or by performing tests with these agents well into the testing session after recording the results with other agonists, such as ristocetin.

Platelet Agonists or Aggregating Agents. The platelet agonists used in the aggregometry procedure include ADP, epinephrine, collagen, thrombin, arachidonic acid, and ristocetin. Note that when aggregometry is performed using ristocetin, the test is referred to as ristocetin-induced platelet aggregation (RIPA) to differentiate it from another test that requires ristocetin, called the ristocetin cofactor (vWF:RCoF) activity assay. RIPA is a qualitative test used to determine the minimum concentration of ristocetin required to aggregate

platelets, whereas the vWF:RCoF assay (discussed later) is a quantitative test designed to evaluate the ability of plasma von Willebrand factor (vWF) to aggregate platelets in a fixed concentration of ristocetin.

There are many acceptable methods of maintaining stock solutions of aggregating agents. Stock concentrations and the volumes of aggregating agents added should be modified to suit the cuvette volumes of a particular aggregometer model. Follow the manufacturer's instructions for preparation and storage of aggregating agents.

Procedure

1. Perform platelet counts on patient and control PRP; adjust the platelet counts to between 200 and 300 × 10⁹/L by diluting with aliquots of PPP. Keep samples stoppered at room temperature.
2. Warm 0.5-mL aliquots of PRP in appropriate cuvettes to 37°C for several minutes as needed for testing.
3. Adjust the 100% transmittance of the platelet aggregometer using patient PPP.
4. Place warmed PRP samples in the aggregometer and adjust the baseline reading after at least 1 minute.
5. After stirring PRP for 2 minutes with small magnetic stir bars, forcefully add the appropriate volume of aggregating agent to ensure adequate mixing.
6. Record the aggregation curve for 3 to 5 minutes or until no further change is noted.
7. Repeat steps 2 through 6 for each aggregating agent with patient and control PRP.

Comments. Specimens for platelet aggregation studies should not come in contact with any type of glassware. Glass will prematurely activate platelets and thus result in a less-than-optimal response to aggregating agents. Nor should such specimens be refrigerated, as platelets kept cold do not respond optimally to aggregating agents. While awaiting testing, platelets are viable longer if they are kept at room temperature; however, aggregation occurs best at 37°C. Temperature monitoring should be done with a tube of plasma in the instrument heating block to determine the optimal warming time for samples.

Because stirring affects reagent mixing and platelet aggregate collisions, it has a significant effect on platelet aggregation. Most aggregation instruments rotate the stir bars at 1200 rpm. Multichannel instruments are synchronized to ensure comparability. Instruments should be checked periodically with a strobe light to determine the actual stirring rate. Stir bar characteristics can also be a source of variability; if two bars are used, they should be identical.

Extremes of hematocrit will affect the concentration of citrate anticoagulant in the plasma. If the hematocrit is low, the plasma concentration of citrate is relatively low, but if the hematocrit is high, plasma citrate levels will be high, *i.e.*, the decreased plasma volume is over-anticoagulated. Low levels of calcium are necessary for platelet aggregation; therefore, if a sample is over-anticoagulated with citrate (which could bind all or most of the calcium), it will appear less responsive and will require higher agonist concentrations to produce a response.[14]

The issue of pH is complex. The pH optima of the various aggregating agents are different: ADP and epinephrine responses are optimal between pH 7.7 and 8.0, whereas ristocetin responses are optimal at pH 7.3 but decline sharply above pH 7.7. Collagen has a broad optimal range, between 7.0 and 8.0. A pH of 7.7 is therefore a reasonable compromise. Unfortunately, PRP has weak buffering capacity, and CO_2 will diffuse out, causing a rise in PRP pH. Such a rise increases the chelation of calcium by citrate, and the responsiveness to aggregating agents declines as discussed above. Stoppering PRP tubes will retard the CO_2 loss, as will keeping the PRP under an oil layer or in a 5% CO_2-filled chamber. Attention to and monitoring of these pH effects will improve test reliability.

Interpretation of Aggregometry Tracings. Typical aggregation response curves are shown in Figure 56-2. At low concentrations of ADP or epinephrine, an initial (primary) response is seen, followed by platelet disaggregation and a return of the reading to baseline. At optimal reagent concentrations, two aggregation waves are seen; the primary response is followed by a brief plateau, and then a much larger secondary response occurs during which platelets aggregate irreversibly (Fig. 56-3). At higher concentrations of ADP and epinephrine, the stimulus is strong enough to obliterate the primary response, and a single wave of aggregation is seen. For the majority of normal samples, there is an optimal concentration of these two aggregating agents that results in a biphasic response. This concentration should be sought and used in testing to increase the sensitivity of the procedure to subtle defects in platelet secretion or storage pools, where there is an absence of the secondary aggregation wave. Using a concentration of ADP or epinephrine that is too high will cause a single large primary wave to be seen, leading to a mistaken interpretation of normality.

Because of the many variables that affect platelet aggregation (discussed previously), the optimal concentrations of ADP and epinephrine that give this important two-wave response may differ from laboratory to laboratory. It is also important to note that approximately 30% of the normal population does not respond to epinephrine, presumably because of a lack of surface membrane receptors responsible for platelet sensitivity to epinephrine. Another 30% of normal subjects have only a single wave of aggregation in response to ADP regardless of concentration.

Collagen produces a single wave of aggregation after a lag phase. The factors responsible for this response are the polymerization of acid-soluble collagen to the fibrillar form in plasma, adhesion of platelets to the collagen fibril, platelet release of ADP, and the response of other platelets to released ADP. An abnormal response can be secondary to Glanzmann thrombasthenia or to a defect in platelet release or storage pool ADP. As is the case with ADP and epinephrine, using a collagen concentration that is too high can camouflage a subtle release or storage pool defect. Only thrombasthenic platelets will not respond to excessively high concentrations of collagen. Thus, to increase the sensitivity of collagen aggregation, each laboratory should determine and use the lowest concentration

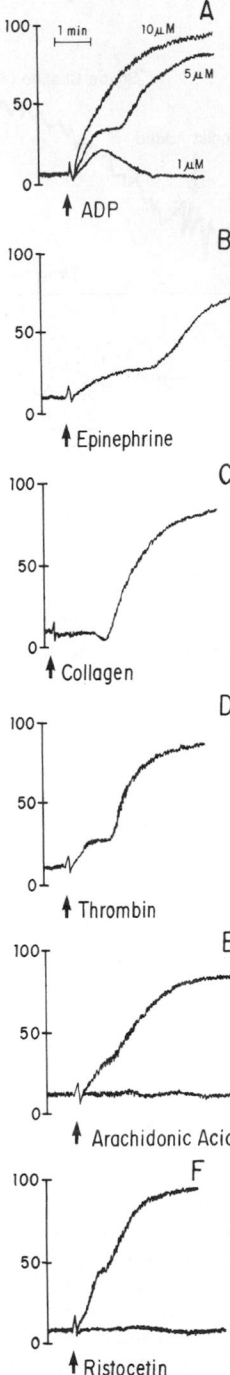

FIGURE 56-2. Typical platelet aggregation responses to various platelet agonists. The horizontal axis is time in minutes (usually 0 to 3–5 minutes) and the vertical axis is percent transmittance. The arrow indicates the addition of the particular agonist. (A) Dose response to ADP. There is only a primary wave to 1 μM ADP, followed by disaggregation, but a single large wave with 10 μM ADP, and the optimal two-wave response with 5 μM ADP. (B) Normal response to 10 μM epinephrine. Note subtle, shallow primary wave. (C) Normal response to collagen 5 μg/mL; note lag phase preceding single-wave response. (D) Normal response to thrombin 0.3 units/mL. (E) Responses to 1.0 mM arachidonic acid. Upper curve is normal; lower curve is an absent response in patient who had taken aspirin the day before. (F) Responses to ristocetin 1.5 mg/mL. Lower curve is an absent response from patient with severe von Willebrand disease; upper curve is a normal response. Note slight shoulder of primary wave occasionally seen with this agent.

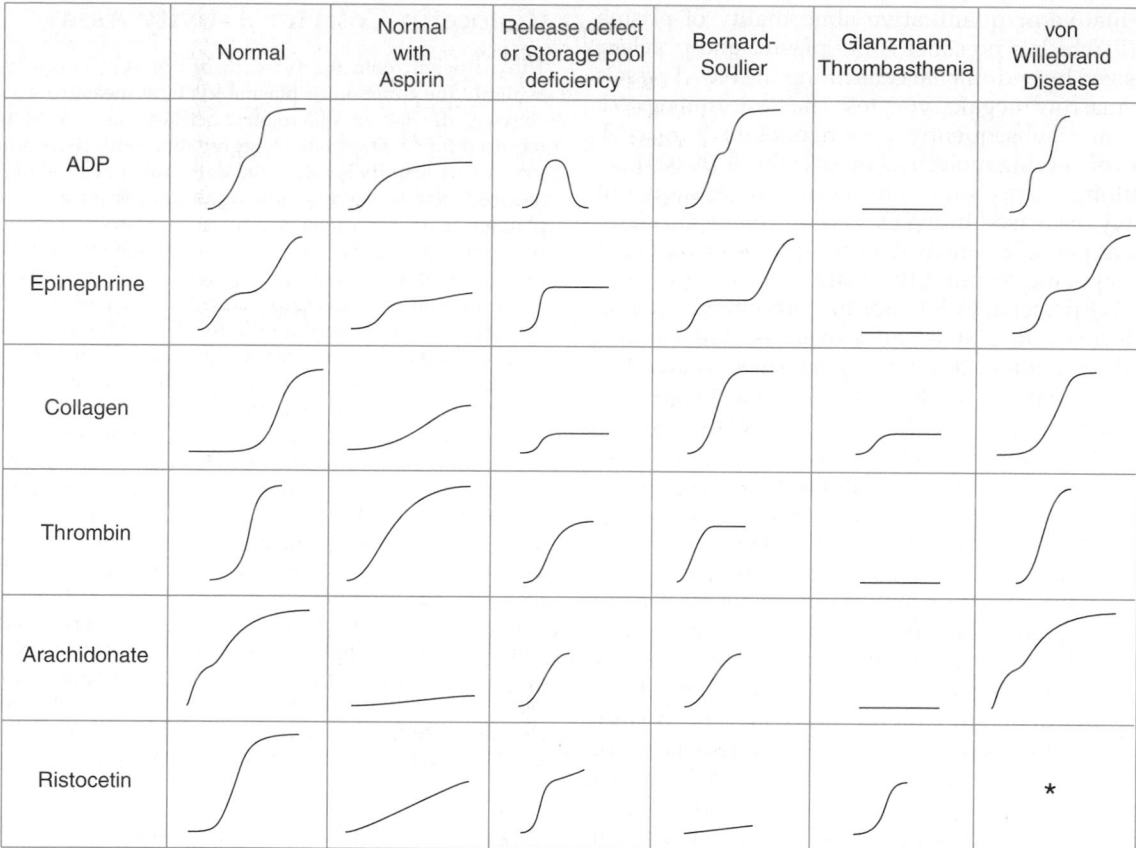

	Normal	Normal with Aspirin	Release defect or Storage pool deficiency	Bernard-Soulier	Glanzmann Thrombasthenia	von Willebrand Disease
ADP						
Epinephrine						
Collagen						
Thrombin						
Arachidonate						
Ristocetin						*

FIGURE 56-3. Typical platelet aggregation responses in various inherited and acquired (aspirin) platelet disorders. Agonist order is similar to that found in Fig. 56-2.* Responses of patients with von Willebrand disease subtypes differ according to the subtype (see text for details).

of collagen that still stimulates aggregation in a large number of normals. This concentration should be verified when lots or suppliers of collagen change.

Thrombin and ristocetin aggregation curves may also yield a two-wave response, depending on the concentration of the agonist. It is helpful to test both patient and control PRP at several concentrations of each agent before drawing conclusions. For example, the normal platelets from some individuals with normal levels of vWF will respond to ristocetin 1.0 mg/mL, whereas platelets from other normal subjects require a concentration of 1.5 mg/mL. Reliance on only one concentration of aggregating agent can lead to mistaken conclusions and further expensive and time-consuming workups. Additional comments on ristocetin aggregation responses are found in the following section on the diagnosis of von Willebrand disease.

Arachidonic acid typically produces a two-wave response. Abnormal responses are most commonly a perfect flat line and are easy to detect. The most common cause of an abnormal response is aspirin. Thrombasthenia, decreased thromboxane A_2 production, or a problem with the platelet cyclo-oxygenase enzyme are rare causes of an abnormal response. Other medications discussed in the bleeding time section also cause an abnormal response to arachidonic acid.

Interpretation of platelet aggregation tests first involves comparison of the patient's curves with the corresponding curves of a normal control. Minor differences (up to 25%) in the slope (rate) of aggregation and in the extent (plateau) of aggregation are not significant. In distinguishing normal from abnormal, however, it is not sufficient to compare a single control with the patient. One must keep in mind the many variables in the aggregation response and appreciate the variability of the curves of a large number of normal individuals. Thus, the interpretation of aggregometry is somewhat subjective and is best left to one who does interpretations frequently and appreciates the variability of normal responses. A file of normal

results and plotting of the upper and lower limits of a large number of normal controls is helpful. But this does not diminish the value of the daily normal control, which is a check on reagent stability, a guide to agent concentration adjustments, and a check on platelet viability during the testing session.

EVALUATION OF PLATELETS IN THE DIAGNOSIS OF VON WILLEBRAND DISEASE

There are an increasing number of platelet function disorders being discovered, primarily owing to increasingly sophisticated laboratory testing methods such as platelet aggregometry. Although not a primary platelet disorder, von Willebrand disease (vWD; Chap. 52) is another disease that may be diagnosed by an abnormal *in vitro* platelet aggregation test called the ristocetin cofactor activity assay. Another helpful test for diagnosing vWD is an assay of the von Willebrand factor antigen. Both of these assays are discussed in this section, following a brief review of vWD.

von Willebrand disease is thought to be the most common inherited bleeding disorder. Historically, vWD was thought to be a combined defect of factor VIII molecules and platelets. However, it is now known that in vWD, the von Willebrand factor (vWF) portion of the factor VIII molecule (now symbolized as VIII/vWF) is defective, but the platelets themselves *are normal*. vWD is actually a family of bleeding disorders characterized by a qualitative or quantitative abnormality of plasma vWF. vWF, which is present in both plasma and platelets, is synthesized by endothelial cells lining the blood vessels and bone marrow megakaryocytes. The basic unit of vWF dimerizes and subsequently polymerizes to form vWF multimers of varying molecular mass (1,000 to 20,000 kD). These multimers are required for normal hemostasis, but are variably decreased in vWD. vWF normally circulates in plasma as part of a noncovalent complex with the factor VIII procoagulant, forming the VIII/vWF complex.

The vWF defect in vWD leads to a prolonged bleeding time, a decrease in platelet adhesiveness, and reduced glass bead retention (a test rarely performed today). The qualitative or quantitative defect in vWF may be detected by using platelet aggregometry.[22] In vWD, platelet aggregation is abnormal in response to the ristocetin aggregating agent because this *in vitro* response requires the presence of vWF (which is lacking in vWD) and a platelet vWF receptor complex (glycoprotein Ib-IX).

The bleeding time is a useful screening test since almost all cases of vWD have abnormally prolonged bleeding times. If the bleeding time or initial clinical findings indicate the possibility of vWD, more definitive tests are needed to subcategorize the type of vWD, since therapy may differ depending on the vWD subtype. A large number of vWD subtypes have been identified and more continue to be discovered, but five of them make up the majority of cases (Table 56-2 and see Table 52-2; Chap. 52). These subtypes are differentiated on the basis of a panel of tests measuring several aspects of the double-protein VIII/vWF complex.[8] These tests include quantitation of factor VIIIC:Ag (Chap. 49) and vWF antigen by immunologic assays; ristocetin-induced platelet aggregation (RIPA; discussed earlier); ristocetin cofactor activity, in which plasma vWF function is evaluated using aggregometry (discussion follows); and plasma vWF multimers by electrophoresis.

Ristocetin Cofactor Activity Assay

The ristocetin cofactor (vWF:RCoF) activity assay is used to evaluate the function of plasma vWF by measuring vWF:RCoF activity, the factor VIII-related activity (*i.e.*, vWF) in plasma required for *in vitro* platelet aggregation with ristocetin. Percent vWF:RCoF activity is measured as the rate or extent of ristocetin-induced platelet aggregation/agglutination of a suspension of platelets in a series of plasma dilutions. Ristocetin is an antibiotic which was noted to cause platelet agglutination and thrombocytopenia in some patients. It was discovered that the degree of agglutination was inversely related to the patient's vWF:RCoF activity, *i.e.*, the lower the vWF:RCoF activity, the less platelets will agglutinate. This serendipitous discovery led to a useful test for the diagnosis of vWD. Needless to say, the drug was withdrawn for use as an antibiotic.

In this assay, a standard percent activity curve is first prepared by making dilutions of a reference plasma or a normal pooled plasma which has been calibrated against a reference preparation of vWF. These plasma dilutions are added to a suspension of washed or gel-filtered normal platelets in the presence of a fixed concentration of ristocetin (usually 1 mg/mL), and the degree of resultant platelet aggregation is measured using platelet aggregometry. Fixed or even lyophilized platelets can also be used since the platelets do not have to be metabolically active.[1] The test is repeated with the patient and control plasmas, and the percent vWF:RCoF activity is determined using the curve prepared from the standard plasmas. Details of testing can be found in the related NCCLS proposed guideline.[15]

von Willebrand Factor Assay

There are a number of assays for vWF:Ag that have differing sensitivities to sample preparation and high-molecular-weight vWF multimers.[7] One commonly used method is the Laurell rocket immunoelectrophoretic procedure. In this method, anti-vWF antibodies are incorporated into an agarose gel slab. Dilutions of normal reference plasma and patient plasma are placed into wells that have been cut into the gel. The well contents (and the agarose gel) are electrophoresed and migrate toward the

---

TABLE 56-2
Simplified Classification of von Willebrand Disease

Test	Type I	Type IIA	Type IIB	Type IIC	Type III
Bleeding time	P/N	P	P	P	P
Factor VIIIC:Ag	↓	N/↓	N/↓	N/↓	↓↓
RIPA	N/↓	↓↓	↑	↓↓	↓↓
vWF:RCoF	↓	↓↓	↓↓	↓↓	↓↓/A
vWF:Ag	↓	N/↓	N/↓	Abn dbl peak	↓↓/A
PLASMA					
wVF multimers					
High MW	N/↓	A	A	A	V/A
Intermed MW	N/↓	A	N	A	V/A
Low MW	N/↓	N*	N*	N**	V/A

KEY: P, prolonged; N, normal; ↑, increased; ↓, decreased; ↓↓, markedly decreased; A, absent; V, variable; Abn dbl peak, abnormal double peak on immunoassay; VIIIC:Ag, factor VIII coagulant portion; RIPA, ristocetin-induced platelet aggregation; vWF:RCoF, ristocetin cofactor activity assay; vWF:Ag, von Willebrand factor antigen assay; MW, molecular weight.
*Triplet multimer structure.
**Doublet multimer structure.

anode. An antigen–antibody reaction occurs which forms a rocket-shaped precipitin band when the gel is stained with Coomasie blue dye. The height of the rocket is proportional to the concentration of vWF in the well. The heights of the diluted standards are plotted on semilogarithmic paper and the patient's sample heights are read from this graph. Details of this method can be found in the related NCCLS proposed guideline.[16]

Patients with severe vWD can have a marked reduction in vWF (vWF:Ag). However, the concentration of vWF can vary, particularly in patients with mild forms of vWD, who sometimes have normal levels of vWF. Therefore if vWD is suspected, the test should be repeated at weekly or monthly intervals when normal levels are obtained for such individuals. In patients with factor VIII deficiency (hemophilia A), vWF levels are normal or even increased, apparently due to concomitant hepatic disease. vWF concentrations are also increased in pregnancy, with estrogen therapy, in inflammatory states, and after strenuous exercise. vWF levels (and factor VIIIC:Ag) are moderately low in preterm infants, then rise above the normal adult level at term; for this reason, the diagnosis of vWD may be missed in the newborn period.[21] Interestingly, vWF levels are somewhat lower in individuals with blood type O.

Since there are many vWF multimeric forms, vWF multimer structural analysis is sometimes useful in the differentiation of the various types of vWD. For instance, in type I, all forms of multimers are seen, but in other types of vWD, the largest multimers are absent in the plasma. Conversely, vWF multimers may be abnormal in plasma but normal in platelets. The methods of testing for multimers include either SDS-agarose gel electrophoresis or crossed immunoelectrophoresis. Details of testing are beyond the scope of this chapter. The place of multimer analysis in the diagnosis of vWD and related disorders and also the interpretation of the various determinations in vWD are summarized elsewhere.[12]

CHAPTER SUMMARY

Platelets must be present in the peripheral blood in sufficient numbers to be effective in their hemostatic role. Both manual and automated methods exist to enumerate platelets. Manual methods include blood film estimates, the Tocantins method using Rees-Ecker diluent and light microscopy, and the phase microscopy method. Platelet function may be evaluated provided platelet numbers are adequate. The most popular platelet function screening test is the skin bleeding time test, in which abnormalities simply indicate some type of platelet function problem. More specific tests include platelet factor assays such as PF3 availability, in which the ability of platelets to provide their surfaces for coagulation activities is evaluated. Platelet aggregometry is helpful in the diagnosis of a number of hereditary and acquired platelet function disorders, as well as the most common inherited bleeding disorder, von Willebrand disease (vWD), which is caused by abnormal plasma von Willebrand factor (vWF). Aggregometry involves the addition of various platelet agonists including ADP, epinephrine, collagen, thrombin, arachidonic acid, and ristocetin to observe platelet aggregation patterns indicative of various abnormalities. The ristocetin cofactor activity and vWF:Ag assays can also be used to assist in the diagnosis of vWD and other abnormalities.

Review Questions

56-1. An oil-immersion field containing 100 erythrocytes should normally have between _____ platelets.

A. 1 and 3
B. 3 and 10
C. 5 and 20
D. 20 and 40

56-2. The manual counting of platelets is best performed using a special thin, flat-bottom hemocytometer and

A. electron microscopy.
B. fluorescence microscopy.
C. light microscopy.
D. phase microscopy.

56-3. Falsely elevated automated platelet counts may result from

A. platelet satellitism.
B. platelet agglutinins.
C. exceptionally large platelets.
D. erythrocyte inclusion bodies.

56-4. The reference range for the skin bleeding time test is approximately a maximum of

A. 3 minutes.
B. 5 minutes.
C. 9 minutes.
D. 20 minutes.

56-5. When performing platelet aggregometry, it is NOT acceptable to

A. keep the platelet specimen at room temperature.
B. perform the test 5 hours after specimen collection.
C. use a whole blood specimen in some aggregometry systems.
D. perform the aggregation tests at 37°C.

56-6. The most common cause of an abnormal platelet aggregation response to arachidonic acid is

A. recent aspirin ingestion.
B. a defective cyclo-oxygenase enzyme.
C. Glanzmann thrombasthenia.
D. decreased thromboxane A_2 production.

56-7. The aggregation agent for platelet aggregometry most valuable in the diagnosis of von Willebrand disease is

A. arachidonic acid.
B. ADP.
C. ristocetin.
D. thrombin.

56-8. A manual platelet count was performed on a standard phase platelet counting chamber using a 1:200 specimen dilution. A 1-mm^2 area was counted, and 40 platelets were counted. The calculated platelet count is

A. 50×10^9/L.
B. 8000×10^9/L.
C. 80×10^9/L.
D. 8×10^9/L.

References

1. Allain JP, Cooper HA, Wagner RM et al: Platelets fixed with paraformaldehyde: A new reagent for assay for von Willebrand factor and platelet aggregating factor. J Lab Clin Med 85:318, 1975
2. Andrew M, Castle V, Mitchell L et al: Modified bleeding time in the infant. Am J Hemat 30:190, 1989
3. Borchgrevink CF: A method for measuring platelet adhesiveness *in vivo*. Acta Med Scand 168:157, 1960
4. Bowie EJW, Owen CA: The value of measuring platelet "adhesiveness" in the diagnosis of bleeding diseases. Am J Clin Pathol 60:302, 1973
5. Brecher G, Cronkite EP: Morphology and enumeration of human blood platelets. J Appl Physiol 3:356, 1950

6. Budtz-Olsen OE: Clot Retraction. London, Blackwell Scientific, 1951

7. Favalaro EJ, Facey D, Grispo L: Laboratory assessment of von Willebrand factor. Am J Clin Pathol 104:264, 1995

8. Hoyer LW: The factor VIII complex: Structure and function. Blood 58:1, 1981

9. International Committee for Standardization in Haematology: Selected method for visual platelet counting. Labmedica 5 (Aug/Sept):31, 1988

10. Kaplan KL, Nossel HL, Drillings M et al: Radioimmunoassay of platelet factor 4 and beta-thromboglobulin: Development of application to studies of platelet release in relation to fibrinopeptide A generation. Br J Haematol 39:129,1978

11. Lind SE: The bleeding time does not predict surgical bleeding. Blood 77:2547, 1991

12. Miller JL: von Willebrand disease. Hematol Oncol Clin North Am 4(1):107, 1990

13. Mogadam L: Application of the Miller's disc for the estimation and quality control of the platelet count. Lab Med 11:131, 1980

14. Muller MR, Salat A, Pulaki S et al: Influence of hematocrit and platelet count on impedance and reactivity of whole blood for electrical aggregometry. J Pharmacol Toxicol Methods 34:17, 1995

15. National Committee for Clinical Laboratory Standards: Assay for Ristocetin Cofactor. Proposed Guideline Document H41-P. Villanova, PA, NCCLS, 1993

16. National Committee for Clinical Laboratory Standards: Determination of von Willebrand Factor Antigen. Proposed Guideline Document HR49-P. Villanova, PA, NCCLS, 1993

17. National Committee for Clinical Laboratory Standards: Performance of the Bleeding Time Test. Proposed Guideline Document H45-P. Wayne, PA, NCCLS, 1995

18. Silver WP, Keller MP, Teel R et al: Effects of donor characteristics and platelet *in vitro* time and temperature on platelet aggregometry. J Vasc Surg 17:726, 1993

19. Tocantins LM: Technical methods for the study of blood platelets. Arch Pathol 23:850, 1937

20. Triplett DA (ed): Platelet Function: Laboratory Evaluation and Clinical Application. Chicago, American Society of Clinical Pathologists, 1978

21. Weinger RS, Cecalupo AJ, Olson JD et al: Neonatal von Willebrand's disease: Diagnostic difficulty at birth. Am J Dis Child 134:793, 1980

22. Weiss HJ, Hoyer LW, Rickles FR et al: Quantitative assay of a plasma factor deficient in von Willebrand's disease that is necessary for platelet aggregation: Relationship to factor VIII procoagulant activity and antigen content. J Clin Invest 52:2708, 1973

23. Yardumian DA, Mackie IJ, Machin SJ: Laboratory investigation of platelet function: A review of methodology. J Clin Pathol 39:701, 1986

CHAPTER 57

Quantitative and Qualitative Disorders of Platelets

Gerald L. Davis

Objectives

1. Describe the type of bleeding associated with platelet disorders.
2. Define thrombocytopenia, thrombocytosis, thrombocythemia, and thrombocytopathy and give examples of each.
3. Identify inherited and acquired causes of thrombocytopenia.
4. Compare and contrast hemolytic uremic syndrome, thrombotic thrombocytopenic purpura, and disseminated intravascular coagulation.
5. Compare the laboratory findings and clinical presentations of May-Hegglin, Bernard-Soulier, and Wiskott-Aldrich syndromes.
6. List three mechanisms by which drugs can induce thrombocytopenia.
7. Describe the differences between reactive and malignant (myeloproliferative) thrombocytoses.
8. List the glycoproteins that make up the von Willebrand factor receptor.
9. Describe the expected laboratory findings in von Willebrand disease, including platelet adhesion, platelet aggregation with ristocetin, and plasma levels of factor VIII coagulation activity.
10. List the glycoproteins associated with the fibrinogen receptor and describe the laboratory findings in Glanzmann's thrombasthenia.
11. Define storage pool defect and give an example, including the expected laboratory results.
12. Describe the effects of aspirin on the platelet release reaction.

The ability of platelets to aggregate and form a platelet plug is central to the maintenance of normal hemostasis. For effective platelet plug formation platelets must be present in adequate numbers and have normal function. The normal reference range for platelet counts (for neonates to adults) is usually stated as being 140 to 440 × 10^9/L.[14] Hemostatic disorders associated with platelet counts less than the reference range are classified as thrombocytopenias. The terms *thrombocytosis* and *thrombocythemia* both refer to conditions in which the circulating platelet count is greater than normal. Thrombocytosis is used when the increased platelet count is transitory and the total megakaryocyte mass is normal to only slightly increased. Thrombocythemia is a myeloproliferative disorder caused by a clonal neoplasm in which the increase in platelet count is persistent and the total megakaryocyte mass is greatly increased.[15] Classifications of the quantitative platelet disorders are presented in Tables 57-1 and 57-2. Regardless of the platelet count, the platelets must function normally for effective hemostasis. Conditions involving abnormal platelet function are classified as thrombocytopathies. Hemostatic disorders involving quantitative or qualitative platelet abnormalities can be either inherited or acquired. In some cases, such as Bernard-Soulier syndrome, thrombocytopenia and thrombocytopathy occur together.

The clinical presentations for thrombocytopenia and thrombocytopathy are the same. If platelets are deficient in either number or function, small vessel hemorrhage can occur. The clinical signs of small vessel bleeding include petechiae, purpura, and ecchymoses. Mucous membrane bleeding (wet purpura), gingival bleeding, menorrhagia, gastrointestinal or urinary bleeding and epistaxis are also associated with small vessel bleeding, but usually indicate a more serious hemostatic problem. Hemorrhage into the central nervous system (CNS) is the most serious site of spontaneous bleeding because it can cause severe disability or even death.

QUANTITATIVE PLATELET DISORDERS: THROMBOCYTOPENIA

Thrombocytopenia is defined as a platelet count of less than 140 × 10^9/L[14] and occurs whenever the rate of platelet production is insufficient to meet the need.[14] Such conditions occur whenever the rate of production is decreased

TABLE 57-1
Classification of Thrombocytopenia

DECREASED PRODUCTION

Megakaryocyte hypoproliferation
  Aplastic anemia
  Drug toxicity
  Alcohol toxicity
  Viral infection
  Congenital states

Ineffective thrombopoiesis
  Megaloblastic anemia
  Paroxysmal nocturnal hemoglobinuria (PNH)
  Thrombopoietin deficiency
  Ethanol abuse without malnutrition
  Severe iron-deficiency anemia
  Viral infection

Marrow replacement
  Leukemia
  Plasma-cell dyscrasia
  Metastatic carcinoma
  Myelofibrosis
  Lymphoma
  Granulomatous infections

INCREASED LOSS OR DESTRUCTION

Nonimmunologic
  Loss
    Severe hemorrhage
    Extensive transfusion
  Consumption
    Diffuse intravascular coagulation (DIC)
    Thrombotic thrombocytopenic purpura (TTP)
    Hemolytic uremic syndrome (HUS)
    Foreign surfaces
    Thermal injury
    Sepsis without DIC

Immunologic
  Isoimmune
    Neonatal purpura
    Post-transfusion purpura
    Refractory to platelet transfusions
  Autoimmune
    Immune thrombocytopenic purpura (ITP)
    Disease associated
  Drug induced
  Viral infection

SPLENIC SEQUESTRATION

---

or the rate of platelet loss is increased. Insufficient production can result from decreased stimulation by thrombopoietin, decreased number of megakaryocytes, or ineffective thrombopoiesis. An escalation in platelet loss from the circulation can occur when there is an increase in destruction (immunologic disorders), platelet consumption (thrombosis, DIC), hemorrhage, or sequestration (splenic, liver, bone marrow).

The severity of bleeding is related to the degree of thrombocytopenia. When platelet counts are less than $100 \times 10^9/L$, the prolongation of the bleeding time is inversely proportional to the platelet count.[52] If platelet function is normal, patients with platelet counts above $50 \times 10^9/L$ will have no hemorrhagic symptoms unless subjected to trauma or surgery. Platelet counts of less than $50 \times 10^9/L$ are referred to as severe thrombocytopenia, and spontaneous bleeding can occur when the

platelet count is less than $20 \times 10^9/L$. The number of red blood cells has an effect on the risk of hemorrhage. Among patients of similar platelet count, the anemic patient is at greater risk of bleeding.[6] In nonthrombocytopenic animals, the bleeding time varies inversely with the hematocrit.[18]

If platelet function is normal, the template bleeding time is usually within the reference range of 3 to 9 minutes when platelet counts are greater than $100 \times 10^9/L$.[72] When the count falls below this, the degree to which the bleeding time is prolonged is inversely proportional to the decrease in the platelet count.[52] If the platelets are large, as in May-Hegglin anomaly, the automated platelet counts need to be confirmed by manual techniques, since both aperture-impedance and light-scatter instruments tend to undercount platelets by 30% to 50% when giant platelets are present.[22]

Clot retraction is usually abnormal when the platelet count is below $60 \times 10^9/L$.[34] If platelet function is normal, platelet aggregation studies should be normal. Technical problems may occur with thrombocytopenic patients because such studies require platelet-rich plasma (PRP), which is difficult to obtain owing to the lack of platelets.

Inherited Megakaryocytic Hypoplasia

Inherited/neonatal megakaryocytic hypoplasia conditions are rare but must always be considered when the platelet count is low, especially if no platelet antibodies can be demonstrated. Fanconi anemia (FA), thrombocytopenia with absent radius (TAR), trisomy syndromes, and amegakaryocytic thrombocytopenia (AMT) are examples

TABLE 57-2
Classification of Thrombocytosis

PRIMARY–CHRONIC MYELOPROLIFERATIVE DISORDERS

Essential thrombocythemia

Polycythemia vera

Chronic granulocytic leukemia

Myelofibrosis with myeloid metaplasia

REACTIVE

Physiologic

Iron deficiency anemia

Rapid blood regeneration
  Acute blood loss
  Hemolytic anemia
  Rebound

Postoperative

Infections and inflammatory diseases
  Chronic disorders
    Tuberculosis
    Ulcerative colitis
    Sprue
    Rheumatoid arthritis
    Osteomyelitis
  Acute infections

Neoplasms
  Carcinoma
  Hodgkin disease

of inherited thrombocytopenias related to megakaryocytic hypoplasia.

Fanconi anemia and TAR are both inherited syndromes with autosomal-recessive transmission that are characterized by marked hypomegakaryocytic thrombocytopenia, skeletal deformities, and sexual and mental retardation. Although similar in clinical presentation, these two conditions differ in several ways. In FA the most notable skeletal abnormalities include absent or hypoplastic thumbs and short stature, whereas in TAR the bilateral deformities or absence of the forearm bones are notable. In FA the thrombocytopenia develops during childhood, becomes symptomatic between 18 months and 10 years, and is usually accompanied by a decrease in erythrocytes and leukocytes. Neonates with TAR present at birth with severe thrombocytopenia and normal erythrocyte and leukocyte counts.[42] The hematopoietic defect in FA exists at the stem cell level and involves early progenitors of all cell lines, whereas the defect in TAR appears to affect only the megakaryocyte progenitor cells.

Up to 90% of the neonates with TAR die in the first year of life, with hemorrhage being the most common cause of death.[32] If these patients survive the first 4 months of their life, there is a good chance that the platelet count will be close to normal by 5 to 6 years of age.[42] Mental retardation, which occurs in about 7% of the TAR neonates, is associated with intracranial hemorrhage.[82] Using ultrasound, absent radii can be detected in the fetus as early as 18 weeks, and thrombocytopenia can be confirmed by performing a platelet count on a fetal blood sample. If indicated, platelets can be transfused into the umbilical vein to reduce the risk of *in utero* hemorrhage as well as immediately after delivery.[122]

The cause of thrombocytopenia in TAR is not known. It has been suggested that it could be due to a maturational defect or arrest in the committed stem cells.[32] An immune-mediated defect has also been proposed, but failure of immunoglobulin and steroid administration to correct the thrombocytopenia suggests otherwise.[42]

AMT, a rare disorder, differs from TAR in that the thrombocytopenia persists and the patient deteriorates. In some cases there is complete failure of the marrow which affects all hemopoietic cell lines.

Acquired Megakaryocytic Hypoplasia

APLASTIC ANEMIA

Generalized bone marrow suppression leading to a decrease in all cell types is characteristic of aplastic anemia (Chap. 11). Acquired aplastic anemia may be the consequence of toxic chemical or physical agents. Ionizing radiation and chemotherapeutic agents produce a dose-dependent suppression of cells at the stem cell level. Viral infections have also been implicated in bone marrow hypoplasia.

Some drugs, such as chlorothiazide (a diuretic), cisplatin and carboplatin (anticancer drugs), and anagrelide (an anti-platelet function agent), appear to directly suppress megakaryocyte production. The mechanism by which these drugs and related compounds induce throm-bocytopenia appears to be related to drug toxicity rather than an immunologic response.[27,114]

MYELOPHTHISIC THROMBOCYTOPENIA

Myelophthisic thrombocytopenia refers to the crowding out of megakaryocytic precursors by space-occupying lesions in the marrow. Invasion of the marrow by nonmegakaryocytic tissues occurs in many conditions such as myelofibrosis, metastatic tumor, leukemia, Hodgkin and non-Hodgkin lymphomas, microangiopathic hemolytic anemia, and osteopetrosis (lack of a marrow cavity). Patients with infantile osteopetrosis have a deficiency of all hemopoietic elements and usually die from bleeding or infection.[111]

PROLONGED HYPOXIA

Extensive hypoxia has been reported to produce hypomegakaryocytic thrombocytopenia by reducing the pool of committed megakaryocyte progenitor cells by means of a greatly expanded erythroid progenitor pool.[106] It is also possible that the abnormal megakaryocytopoiesis is due to an acquired stem cell defect induced by the prolonged hypoxia.[107]

Inherited Ineffective Thrombopoiesis

Ineffective thrombopoiesis is characterized by a normal to increased number of megakaryocytes in the bone marrow, normal platelet life span, and decreased platelet count. In some conditions, such as the Wiskott-Aldrich syndrome, both ineffective thrombopoiesis and shortened platelet life span occur together and contribute to thrombocytopenia. In ineffective thrombopoiesis, up to 90% of the platelets are destroyed before they are released into the circulation.

MAY-HEGGLIN ANOMALY

May-Hegglin anomaly (Chap. 26) is a rare autosomal-dominant anomaly that is characterized by Döhle bodies within leukocytes, a variable degree of thrombocytopenia, and giant platelets. The degree of thrombocytopenia ranges from 20 to 120 $\times$ 10^9/L with a mean platelet volume (MPV) of 15 to 20 fL; platelet function is normal.[49] Bleeding is seldom a problem. Thrombocytopenia in these patients is usually attributed to ineffective thrombocytosis; however, the finding of increased levels of platelet-associated immunoglobulin G (IgG) in four members of the same family suggests a possible immune mechanism of platelet destruction.[22]

BERNARD-SOULIER SYNDROME AND WISKOTT-ALDRICH SYNDROME

Bernard-Soulier syndrome (BSS) and Wiskott-Aldrich syndrome (WAS) are two inherited disorders also associated with ineffective thrombopoiesis. BSS causes a platelet adhesion defect that leads to bleeding problems in affected individuals. WAS is an immunodeficiency syndrome characterized by severe thrombocytopenia and excessively small platelets that leads to bleeding. See Qualitative Platelet Disorders/Inherited for details on BSS and WAS.

PARIS-TROUSSEAU SYNDROME

Paris-Trousseau syndrome is a recently reported congenital thrombocytopenia with a mild hemorrhagic tendency that occurred in a woman and her child. Thrombocytopenia due to ineffective thrombopoiesis was indicated by the increased number of bone marrow megakaryocytes (a large percentage of which were micromegakaryocytes) and the normal platelet life span. Fifteen percent of the platelets in the peripheral blood showed giant α-granules resulting from the fusion of α-granules. This condition has been attributed to a deletion of the distal part of one chromosome 11 at 11q23.[20]

Acquired Ineffective Thrombopoiesis

Mild thrombocytopenia is a common finding in alcoholics. Ethanol suppresses thrombopoiesis at the level of the maturing megakaryocyte and decreases the platelet life span.[113] Even though alcohol suppresses both platelet production and platelet function, clinically significant hemorrhage is rare. Platelet counts usually start to increase after 2 to 5 days of abstinence from alcohol.

A deficiency of either vitamin B_{12} or folate results in an impairment of DNA synthesis (Chap. 12). A lack of DNA synthesis causes dyspoiesis and megaloblastic transformation of the red cell, myelocyte, and platelet precursors. The degree of ineffective thrombopoiesis and the morphologic appearance and size of the megakaryocytes are variable. Due to the short life span of platelets (10 days) compared to erythrocytes (RBC) (120 days), vitamin B_{12}–deficient patients may present with mild thrombocytopenia before the RBC megaloblastic changes are evident. The platelets in vitamin B_{12} deficiency appear to be normal in function.

Paroxysmal nocturnal hemoglobinuria (PNH) is an acquired mutational disorder (Chap. 18). Thrombocytopenia, which may be the initial manifestation of PNH, appears to be due to a defect that affects the hematopoietic stem cell.[17] Cells produced by the PNH hematopoietic stem cells have enhanced susceptibility to complement binding and lysis. These cells lack two membrane proteins that normally inhibit the binding and lytic action of complement. Even though the platelets in PNH, like the RBC, have an increased susceptibility to the lytic action of complement, they have a normal life span. The thrombocytopenia in PNH is due primarily to ineffective thrombopoiesis.[17]

Ineffective thrombopoiesis has also been linked to viral infections. Invasion of megakaryocytes by viral agents directly affects platelet production. The viruses can impair megakaryocytopoiesis by either interacting at the cell surface or through viral entry and intracellular replication.[75] Hepatitis B and C, herpes simplex, HIV, and Colorado tick fever are but a few of the viruses known to invade megakaryocytes.[2,35,97,101]

Nonimmune Platelet Destruction

Even with normal megakaryocyte production of platelets, thrombocytopenia can occur if platelets are lost or destroyed within the circulation. Platelet destruction may be either nonimmune or immune. Nonimmune platelet destruction may be subdivided into platelet consumption by either fibrin clots or platelet thrombi and a variety of miscellaneous conditions.

PLATELET CONSUMPTION

Thrombocytopenia can result from either acute or chronic activation of the coagulation system and the generation of thrombin. Disseminated intravascular coagulation (DIC; Chap. 52), hemolytic uremic syndrome (HUS; Chap. 18), and thrombotic thrombocytopenic purpura (TTP) are three major conditions characterized by nonimmune thrombocytopenia due to increased platelet consumption and shortened platelet life span.

It is important to distinguish between HUS, TTP, and DIC, since therapy for the different conditions will vary. Whereas DIC occurs in all age groups, TTP occurs primarily in adults, with more females being affected than males. HUS occurs most often in children less than 8 years of age. HUS occasionally occurs in adults with predisposing conditions associated with endothelial cell damage.[60]

Pathophysiology. Both HUS and TTP have a common pathomechanism involving endothelial cell damage which causes platelet thrombi to form. Endothelial cell injury can be caused by viral infections such as those reported in HIV patients,[29] hypertension, hypoxia, and immune complexes. Using a Western blot assay to detect autoantibodies to cryptic endothelial antigens that are normally hidden but exposed when the cell in injured, Koenig and coworkers presented evidence of endothelial cell damage in 13 of 14 TTP patients and 4 of 5 patients with HUS.[71] It has also been shown that activated leukocytes release elastase, which stimulates secretion of the very large vWF multimers from the endothelium in TTP patients.[40] The role of endothelial cell damage as the main pathogenesis of TTP is supported by the finding that the endothelial cell markers, tissue plasminogen activator (TPA) and thrombomodulin (TM), are increased at the onset of the syndrome. Recovery correlates with plasma TPA and TM levels.[121]

In the early stages of HUS, thrombi formation is primarily intraglomerular with renal dysfunction, proteinuria, and hematuria being prominent features. In TTP, the thrombus formation is diffuse and affects many organs. Several theories have been proposed on the etiology of these conditions but none completely explains the mechanism or the variability of the disease process. It has been suggested that TTP is really several diseases with common symptoms. Increased levels of the very large multimers of von Willebrand factor (vWF) accumulate in the patient's plasma for unknown reasons.[88] As the severity of TTP progresses these very large multimers disappear and the platelet count decreases. It is suggested that these very large multimers bind to the platelet membrane and promote intravascular formation of platelet thrombi.[88]

Most of the vWF in the circulation is produced by the endothelial cells. The endothelial cells of both normal and TTP patients release vWF that is made up of large to very large multimers that have molecular weights ranging into the millions. In normal individuals the plasma is believed to contain a substance that reduces these large multimers to the smaller size multimers found in normal plasma. A deficiency of this multimer-reducing substance would result in increased levels of the very large multimers. When patients are treated with fresh frozen plasma, the concentration of the very large multimers decreases and the patient improves. It is possible that the transfused plasma contains the reducing substance that is deficient in the TTP patient.[87]

Clinical Presentation. In children, vomiting and bloody diarrhea associated with verotoxin-producing *Escherichia coli* or *Shigella* infection frequently occurs before development of HUS. In some patients, a brief febrile disease may be the antecedent symptom. The patient may appear pale and jaundiced depending on the severity of the intravascular hemolytic anemia. Purpura and bleeding from the mucous membranes are usually present and platelet thrombi in the kidneys leads to renal failure. Hemolytic uremic syndrome is seen most frequently in children under 8 years of age and is a major cause of renal failure. In children less than 2 years of age the mortality rate is high. In older children the prognosis is generally excellent. Duration of oliguria, blood urea levels, and hypertension are important factors affecting therapy and survival.[31] HUS also occurs in adults but is much less common than in children. In adults HUS is usually secondary to conditions such as pregnancy, HIV infection, malignant hypertension, and organ transplantation.[84] Some families may possess an inherited predisposition to HUS.[61]

TTP is frequently associated with a preceding viral infection, pregnancy, or drug use. It is diagnosed most frequently in patients between the ages of 10 and 50, with a peak incidence in the fourth decade of life. Women are affected twice as often as men.[11] Fever, pallor, petechiae, neurologic manifestations, and renal disease are the chief clinical features. Neurologic manifestations, which are remittent and subject to sudden change, include headache, delirium, seizures, and coma. The neurologic problems, visual disturbance, and abdominal pain are associated with ischemia related to microvascular platelet thrombi.

Laboratory Findings. Laboratory findings in TTP, HUS, and DIC are similar and reflect the degree of hemolysis. Marked poikilocytosis, schistocytosis, and increased red cell distribution width (RDW) are indicators of red cell damage. Increased lactate dehydrogenase (especially LD isoenzyme LD-2), indirect bilirubin, and decreased haptoglobin values are associated with intravascular hemolysis.

In TTP both the anemia and thrombocytopenia are severe, with hemoglobin levels usually less than 10 g/dL, frequently less than 6 g/dL, and platelet counts less than 20×10^9/L. In HUS the anemia and thrombocytopenia are usually milder. The degree of anemia and thrombocytopenia in DIC depends on the severity of the condition.

Indicators of impaired renal function are present in HUS. BUN, creatinine, serum potassium, proteinuria, and microscopic hematuria are all increased. These variables are usually normal or only moderately elevated in TTP. Burr cells are present in the peripheral blood in HUS, but not in TTP or DIC.

Most coagulation tests such as the prothrombin time, activated partial thromboplastin time, and levels of coagulation factors, D-dimers, and fibrin split products are usually normal in TTP and HUS, but abnormal in DIC. Very large multimers of vWF are present in TTP except during crisis when their disappearance is associated with platelet agglutination and the development of thrombocytopenia.[88]

Treatment. Early diagnosis of TTP/HUS is of major importance in the treatment of these disorders. Before 1970 TTP was close to 100% fatal. With the introduction of plasma infusion and exchange the mortality rate is now less than 10%.[11] Although mild cases of TTP can be treated with either fresh frozen plasma or prednisone alone, most cases will require plasma exchanges. The patient must receive fresh frozen plasma every day until recovered; the patient also should be followed for early detection of relapse. Anti-platelet drugs such as aspirin and dipyridamole have proved to be ineffective in treating TTP.[11] Treatment with corticosteroids and intravenous injections of immunoglobulin has been unsuccessful, which suggests a nonimmune mechanism as the cause of the disease.[25,104] In addition to plasma infusions or plasma exchanges, therapy for HUS includes the use of dialysis and antihypertensive, antithrombotic, and anti-platelet drugs.[60]

An increase in the platelet count and a decrease in LD suggest a positive response to therapy. Platelet transfusions are to be avoided in patients with TTP because they can cause rapid clinical deterioration and life-threatening hemorrhaging. See Table 18-1 for a summary comparison of TTP, HUS, and DIC.

MISCELLANEOUS NONIMMUNE PLATELET DESTRUCTION

Dilutional Loss. Severe thrombocytopenia is a common occurrence following massive blood transfusions. It is generally accepted that the degree of thrombocytopenia is directly proportional to the number of units transfused.[5] However, a recent retrospective study failed to find a correlation between the number of transfused units and the severity of thrombocytopenia.[53] The number of functional platelets in blood that have been stored for more than a few days is close to zero. Thus, patients requiring extensive transfusions develop thrombocytopenia by three mechanisms: acute blood loss, platelet consumption, and dilution of their own platelet pool.

Artificial Surfaces. Platelet contact with artificial surfaces such as cardiovascular prosthetic devices, artificial organs,[3] prosthetic vascular grafts,[119] and dialysis membranes is associated with both quantitative and qualitative changes in platelet function. In dialysis patients the severity of the thrombocytopenia depends on the type and geometry of the material used in the dialysis membrane.[119] In cardiac bypass patients the development of thrombocytopenia has been associated with transfusion of blood collected by intraoperative and postoperative salvage systems.[112]

Drugs. Drug-induced platelet clumping can result in a thrombocytopenia. Ristocetin, an agonist that is used in platelet aggregation studies, was first used as an antibiotic until it was discovered that it caused thrombocytopenia by inducing *in vivo* platelet aggregation.[41] Heparin has also been implicated as causing platelet aggregation and concomitant thrombocytopenia.[69]

Infections. Sepsis-induced thrombocytopenia can result from the direct interaction between the organism and platelets, resulting in lysis or phagocytosis by the reticuloendothelial system. In a study of patients in an intensive care unit, sepsis was found to be an independent risk factor for thrombocytopenia. Thrombocytopenia was associated with longer hospital stay and increased mortality.[10]

Immune Platelet Destruction

In patients with normal platelet production, the most common cause of thrombocytopenia is due to immune mechanisms that result in platelet injury and removal from the circulation. These mechanisms involve the binding of platelet-associated immunoglobulin (PAIg). Antigenic determinants associated with immune platelet destruction include the human platelet antigens (HPA) such as HPA-1a (Pl[A1]), the major histocompatibility complexes (HLA), and the ABH(O) blood group system. The binding of IgM and IgA is associated with removal of platelets by the liver, whereas splenic sequestration and destruction is associated with IgG. The platelet count has been shown to be inversely correlated with the levels of PAIg, especially IgM.[92]

Immune thrombocytopenias can be caused by alloantibodies (isoimmune), autoantibodies (autoimmune), or drug-induced immune complexes and conditions secondary to autoimmune disorders such as systemic lupus erythematosus (SLE). Immune disorders affecting platelets are analogous to immune disorders that affect RBC. In autoimmune hemolytic anemia, destruction of the RBC is due to the binding of autoantibodies and removal of RBC by either the spleen or the liver. By a similar mechanism, binding of autoantibodies to platelets results in increased destruction of platelets. Neonatal alloimmune thrombocytopenia purpura (NATP) is analogous to Rh disease in the newborn, because thrombocytopenia in the fetus is due to maternal antibodies binding to the fetus' platelets. Post-transfusion purpura (PTP) is equivalent to a hemolytic transfusion reaction.

The direct antiglobulin test (DAT; formerly known as the Coombs' test) detects surface-bound RBC antibodies and is positive with immunohemolytic anemia. Similarly, tests for platelet surface-bound immunoglobulin are elevated in ITP. In addition, the amount of surface-bound immunoglobulin does not correlate with the degree of thrombocytopenia.[43]

ISOIMMUNE THROMBOCYTOPENIA

Alloantigens, also referred to as isoantigens, are substances that induce the production of alloantibodies when they are infused into individuals of the same species who lack the specific alloantigen. Infusion of platelets with alloantigens into a patient who lacks the antigen can induce an immunologic response. Some platelet-specific alloantigens are more immunogenic than others. The platelet-specific alloantigen HPA-1a is the most antigenic of the platelet alloantigens and is associated with most instances of NATP and PTP.

In Caucasians, approximately 3% of the population lack HPA-1a, whereas 100% of the Asian population tested to date have HPA-1a but lack other alloantigen that are found in Caucasians.[68] The frequency of occurrence of the platelet-specific alloantigens varies with race. The occurrence of the platelet-specific alloantigens in Caucasian Europeans and Americans is similar.

There is much confusion regarding the nomenclature of platelet-specific alloantigens. Originally the alloantigens were named based on the name of the patient in whom the alloantiserum was derived. This practice has resulted in several names for the same antigen. To standardize nomenclature, von Dem Borne and Decary proposed a system whereby the antigens are identified by a human platelet alloantigen (HPA) number.[120] The HPA numbers and the corresponding serologic designation of the antigen along with the location of the antigen may be found elsewhere. Based on molecular studies, HPA-1a, HPA-4a, HPA-6a, HPA-7a, and HPA-8a are probably five different names for the same alloantigen.[94]

Post-transfusion (Isoimmune) Purpura (PTP). PTP is a rare complication characterized by sudden, profound, and self-limited thrombocytopenia (less than $20 \times 10^9/$L). Bleeding occurs 2 to 12 days after the transfusion of products containing platelet antigens, with the time of recovery ranging from 5 to 60 days. Most cases have been reported in women who lacked the platelet-specific alloantigen HPA-1a (Pl[A1], Zw[a]) and who had been sensitized by pregnancy or transfusions. This alloantigen is located on platelet membrane glycoprotein IIIa and is present in 98% of the Caucasian population.[120] The antibody produced shows Pl[A1] specificity and fixes complement in some cases, although not in others.[46] The mechanism responsible for the destruction of the patient's Pl[A1]-negative platelets is unknown. After recovery, transfusion with blood containing the antigen does not always re-stimulate antibody production or cause thrombocytopenia, but recurrences have been reported years after the initial episode. Plasmapheresis appears to be most effective in resolving bleeding complications, with an increase in the platelet count within 48 hours following treatment.[21]

Neonatal Alloimmune Thrombocytopenia Purpura (NATP). NATP is analogous to hemolytic disease of the newborn (HDN), except that the fetal platelet is the target of the maternal IgG instead of the red cell. NATP is caused by transplacental passage of maternal IgG antibodies directed against fetal platelet antigens inherited from the father and absent on the mother's platelets. NATP also differs from HDN in that approximately 50% of the time it is evident in the first pregnancy. This suggests that sensitization to the platelet antigen by previous pregnancies or transfusions is not required.[45]

The infants may have a severe generalized petechial rash or purpura or may appear normal at birth and develop symptoms of thrombocytopenia within 2 or 3 days. Usually, all hematologic variables are normal except the platelet count, which can be $30 \times 10^9/L$ or less. Neonates with platelet counts less than $50 \times 10^9/L$ are a major concern, since the maternal antibodies are still present in the neonate's circulation and can promote continued destruction of the platelets.[74] Hyperbilirubinemia may be a problem due to excessive skin hemorrhage and frequently requires phototherapy.[73] Anti-HPA-1a has been implicated in 78% of NATP cases and 19% have been due to anti-HPA-5a. In Asian countries where close to 100% of the population has HPA-1a, no cases involving anti–HPA-1a have been reported. In these countries the presence of anti-HPA-4b appears to be of greater importance.[74]

Because maternal IgG antibodies can be transferred across the placenta and produce neonatal thrombocytopenia, it is important to differentiate alloimmune and autoimmune IgG antibodies to select the proper treatment. In suspected pregnancies, fetal platelet counts and platelet typing can be performed on specimens obtained by percutaneous umbilical blood sampling. If the fetus is determined to be at risk, platelet transfusions can be administered through the use of cordocentesis and delivery can be by cesarean section near term.[45] Intravenous immunoglobulin administration to the mother has been successful in elevating the fetal platelet count.[23] In neonates the treatment of choice is transfusion with either maternal platelets (washed with ABO-compatible plasma to reduce the likelihood of further transfer of maternal alloantibody to the infant) or antigen-negative platelets.[65]

Patients Refractory to Platelet Transfusion. The expression "refractory to platelet transfusion" means that infusion of platelets does not produce a sustained increase in platelet count. Patients who are refractory to platelet transfusion, such as those with aplastic anemia or acute leukemia who have received long-term platelet support, may have developed platelet alloimmunization which causes a rapid destruction of the transfused platelets. The alloantibodies produced in about two-thirds of the cases are directed against HLA antigens.

When ABO unmatched platelets are transfused, circulating immune complexes can be formed between the patient's soluble ABH antigens and the transfused antibodies, resulting in destruction of platelets by the innocent bystander mechanism. Destruction could also be through the binding of (1) circulating immune complexes to platelet Fc receptors or (2) complement component C3 to platelet membrane proteins.[54] Anti-HPA-1a and anti-HPA-1b in the plasma of bone marrow recipients can also cause refractoriness to platelet transfusions. It is suggested that all patients who are refractory to HLA-matched platelets be tested for platelet-specific antibodies.[37] Use of HLA-matched leukocyte-poor platelet concentrates may alleviate the problem for some recipients.[55] Use of high-dose intravenous immunoglobulin is effective in modulating platelet alloimmunization and increases the survival of transfused platelets. This therapy is recommended when patients with platelet alloimmunization have critical bleeding episodes or undergo surgical procedures.[24]

For life-threatening situations, two additional treatments are proposed: extensive platelet infusion and plasmapheresis.[70] Extensive platelet infusion temporarily reduces the level of offending alloantibody by adsorption, allowing the excess platelets to halt bleeding. Plasmapheresis reduces the alloantibody level prior to platelet transfusion.

PRIMARY AUTOIMMUNE THROMBOCYTOPENIA

Idiopathic or immune thrombocytopenic purpura (ITP) is a well-defined autoimmune disorder characterized by the destruction of antibody-coated platelets in the reticuloendothelial system and by normal to increased megakaryocytic production. The diagnosis of this relatively common hematologic problem is established by exclusion or ruling out other potential causes of thrombocytopenia.

The "I" in ITP can stand for either immune or idiopathic. Idiopathic means of unknown cause. Since ITP is known to be an autoimmune disorder, *immune* thrombocytopenia purpura is probably more descriptive. However, using the term *immune* does not separate these conditions from thrombocytopenias secondary to autoimmune disorders such as rheumatoid arthritis or systemic lupus erythematosus (SLE). Often the term *idiopathic* is more appropriate because the immune mechanism of the disorder is poorly defined. Clinically, idiopathic and immune are synonymous in reference to ITP.

ITP can be either acute or chronic based primarily on the duration of thrombocytopenia. Acute ITP is defined as ITP of less than 6 months, whereas chronic ITP persists for more than 6 months.

Pathophysiology. The association of acute ITP with a recent viral illness suggests that the immune system may be responding to viral antigens adsorbed onto the platelet surface or to immune complexes bound to the platelet.[16] The increased platelet-associated IgG (PA IgG) levels are consistent with either hypothesis.

Autoantibodies have been demonstrated in both acute and chronic ITP. Platelet membrane glycoproteins IIb-IIIa and Ib-IX are the principal targets of these autoantibodies. Significantly lower platelet counts have been reported in patients having antibodies to Ib-IX compared with patients having IIb-IIIa antibodies.[56] The binding of autoantibodies to platelets can cause (1) phagocytosis by the immune system by an Fc receptor mechanism and (2) activation of the complement pathway, which allows more efficient phagocytosis or *in vivo* cell lysis. Anti-platelet autoantibodies are able to bind to megakaryocytes in the bone marrow and to platelets in the peripheral blood.[93]

Decreased thrombocytosis associated with the binding of autoantibodies to megakaryocytes is debatable.

Splenectomy results in decreased levels of anti-platelet autoantibodies, which suggests a possible role of the spleen in antibody production. The spleen could release a product that stimulates antibody production, or it could be a site of antibody synthesis.[16] At the present time, the immunoregulatory defect that results in this autoimmune disorder is unknown.

Clinical Presentation. Acute ITP occurs primarily in young children 2 to 6 years of age. This self-limiting condition usually has a sudden onset and lasts less than 6 months. It is the most common cause of thrombocytopenia in children. It affects males and females equally, occurs most often in the winter and spring, and is frequently preceded by a viral infection 1 to 6 weeks prior to the appearance of bleeding.[30] Up to 90% of the children present with a transient bleeding episode and a platelet count less than 30×10^9/L. Children with a platelet count of less than 10×10^9/L can experience severe mucosal bleeding. Intracranial hemorrhage is a rare (<1%) complication of acute ITP and can be fatal.[58]

From 10% to 20% of the patients with acute ITP will develop chronic ITP based on the persistence of ITP for more than 6 months. These children are usually older (>7 years of age) and, like adult chronic ITP, more females than males are affected. There may be two different forms of childhood ITP.[58] Young children who show spontaneous remission have lower levels of autoantibodies whereas older children who go on to develop chronic ITP have elevated levels comparable to those found in adult chronic ITP.

The patient with chronic ITP is most often a young adult (age 20 to 40 years) who complains of hypermenorrhagia, easy bruising, petechiae, purpura, or prolonged bleeding (from superficial skin cuts) that has slowly increased in severity. Older patients are at the greatest risk of severe hemorrhage. Some patients are asymptomatic and only detected incidentally. In one case the diagnosis of chronic ITP was made after an alert phlebotomist observed that an abnormal number of petechiae appeared after the application of a tourniquet. Unlike acute ITP, there is usually no antecedent infection, platelet counts are usually higher (30 to 100×10^9/L), and remission is rare. In two recent large studies, the ratio of female to male patients was 2.2:1 and the age range at diagnosis was 14 to 78 years of age, with a median of 44 years and a peak incidence before age 30.[12,115] A possible explanation of the ratio of females to males might be the hemostatic challenge presented by the monthly menstrual cycle. In one study, 43% of the adult women presented with meno-metrorrhagia.[12]

Laboratory Findings. Decreased platelet counts, of less than 20×10^9/L in acute ITP and between 30 and 80×10^9/L in chronic ITP, are typical. In addition, there is an increased percentage of large platelets (MPV), and increased platelet distribution width (PDW). Platelet survival ranges from minutes to a few days. Bone marrow examination is of value primarily to rule out other causes of the thrombocytopenia. Bone marrow megakaryocytes are normal to increased in number. A prolonged bleeding time and abnormal clot retraction can be attributed to the thrombocytopenia and the binding of autoantibodies to glycoproteins IIb-IIIa. The large platelets represent young, metabolically active platelets and may explain why some patients with ITP have less bleeding than would be expected for the degree of thrombocytopenia.[52] Antibody bound to platelets is demonstrable in more than 90% of the cases of ITP. Coagulation tests such as the partial thromboplastin time (PTT) are usually normal. An increase in eosinophils and lymphocytes has been reported in some patients with acute ITP.[16]

Treatment. The goal of therapy is to raise the platelet count to a level that will maintain hemostasis. Therapy is indicated when there are signs of bleeding or the patient is at risk of hemorrhage.[58] Most cases of acute ITP can be treated successfully using corticosteroids. The fastest recovery from acute ITP has been accomplished using intravenous immunoglobulin. Anti-D antibody, interferon, and cyclosporin have also been used.[58]

Patients having chronic ITP with platelet counts of more than 50×10^9/L usually do not receive therapy unless there is a risk of hemorrhage. They are instructed to avoid all aspirin-containing drugs. Steroids or intravenous immunoglobulin are commonly used as the initial therapy. Splenectomy is the most effective treatment for patients who fail to respond to initial therapies.[12] Some cases of chronic ITP do not respond to splenectomy. Platelet transfusions are of minimal benefit since the infused platelets are rapidly destroyed.

The management of ITP in pregnancy requires special consideration, because maternal anti-platelet antibodies cross the placenta to the fetus, causing neonatal thrombocytopenia. Postnatal thrombocytopenia created by this mechanism usually is self-limited, with platelet counts returning to normal within 1 to 2 months.[99] Because of the risk of intracranial hemorrhage in severely thrombocytopenic infants due to trauma to the head associated with vaginal delivery, platelet counts on blood obtained from a fetal scalp vein are frequently performed when the mother's platelet count is less than 50×10^9/L. It has been recommended that delivery by cesarean should be performed when the fetal scalp vein platelet count is less than 50×10^9/L.[4]

SECONDARY AUTOIMMUNE THROMBOCYTOPENIA

Secondary autoimmune thrombocytopenia refers to thrombocytopenia that is secondary to another disease process. Examples include (1) lymphoproliferative disorders, such as chronic lymphocytic leukemia (CLL) and Hodgkin disease; (2) miscellaneous conditions, such as rheumatoid arthritis, SLE, and Crohn's disease; and (3) infectious diseases caused by bacterial infections, HIV, and a variety of other viruses.[66]

About 5% to 10% of patients with CLL and a smaller percentage of patients with other lymphoproliferative disorders develop immune thrombocytopenia.[59] Thrombocytopenia occurs frequently in SLE and is almost invariably autoimmune.[38] Patients with SLE are at a greater risk of thrombosis than hemorrhaging.[64] Splenomegaly is usual, and the bone marrow has a larger than normal number of megakaryocytes.

Immune thrombocytopenia appears to be a manifestation of acquired immunodeficiency syndrome (AIDS).[19] Bone marrow megakaryocytes are adequate to increased, PA IgG is increased, and patients are seropositive for antibodies to the causative retrovirus, human immunodeficiency virus (HIV).[1] Unexplained thrombocytopenia in otherwise healthy homosexual men may be an early manifestation of AIDS.[47]

DRUG-INDUCED IMMUNE THROMBOCYTOPENIA

A large number of cases of drug-induced immune thrombocytopenia are caused by a few drugs, notably quinidine, quinine, gold salts, sulfonamides and their derivatives, chloroquine, and rifampicin.[91] The diagnosis of drug-induced immune thrombocytopenia is based primarily on the clinical history of drug ingestion and the exclusion of other causes. The clinical history should document thrombocytopenia while the patient is receiving the drug and normalization of the platelet count after the drug is discontinued. Reproducible, sensitive, and specific *in vitro* tests for drug-induced thrombocytopenia are not widely available.

Pathophysiology. Drug-induced immune thrombocytopenias appear to be analogous to the drug-induced immune hemolytic anemias (Chap. 19). The antibody is directed against either a drug–platelet complex or a drug–plasma protein complex that then binds to the platelet.[85] Drug-induced synthesis of platelet autoantibody is a third possible mechanism, similar to that of methyldopa (Aldomet)–induced autoimmune hemolytic anemia, but there is no direct evidence for this. The drug can bind to the platelet membrane, with the antibody then attaching to the drug alone, or the drug may expose neoantigenic sites on the platelet membrane and the antibody then binds to these sites. The altered platelets are then removed from the circulation by the reticuloendothelial system. Drugs can also act as haptens, binding to a plasma protein and inducing production of antibodies that bind to the drug, forming an immune complex. The complexes settle on the platelets ("innocent bystanders"), which are then removed by the reticuloendothelial system.

Clinical and Laboratory Presentation. Most patients seek medical attention because of the sudden onset of petechiae, ecchymoses, blood-filled blisters in the mouth, and mucosal bleeding. The severity of the purpura may be disproportionate to the degree of thrombocytopenia, suggesting that the antibody also damages endothelium or induces a platelet-function defect.[85] Most patients experience spontaneous recovery, with the platelet count returning to normal limits 7 to 10 days after the drug is discontinued, although in some patients thrombocytopenia persists for 3 to 4 weeks. Laboratory results are similar to those described for other immune thrombocytopenias.

Treatment. The drug suspected of triggering the immune thrombocytopenia should be discontinued immediately. Corticosteroids may be administered because of their positive effects on vascular integrity.

PLATELET SEQUESTRATION

The spleen may be responsible for thrombocytopenia either by increased phagocytosis and destruction of damaged platelets or by increased sequestration of normal, undamaged platelets. Normally, 30% to 45% of the total circulating platelet pool is sequestered by the spleen from which it may be readily mobilized when needed.[8] In some conditions associated with splenomegaly, 50% to 90% of the platelets may be sequestered. The splenic pool consists of a larger proportion of megathrombocytes, which are younger and possibly more effective in hemostasis than the remainder of the circulating platelets.[62] Hypersplenism may be the chief mechanism of thrombocytopenia in Gaucher disease,[124] sarcoidosis,[33] and Felty syndrome.[9] Therapy usually is directed at correcting the primary disorder.

QUANTITATIVE PLATELET DISORDERS: THROMBOCYTOSIS

Thrombocytosis can be defined as an increase in platelets above 450×10^9/L. A large majority of patients with increased platelet counts are reacting to a stimulus (reactive thrombocytosis), *e.g.*, neoplasms and inflammatory conditions, iron deficiency, major trauma, post-splenectomy, post-surgery, epinephrine injection, or recovery from thrombocytopenia. In reactive thrombocytosis, the increase in platelet count is usually temporary, is less than 1000×10^9/L, and is not normally associated with any clinical problems. Nevertheless, reactive thrombocytosis 1 week after coronary bypass surgery has been implicated as an important risk factor for postoperative myocardial infarctions and venous thrombosis.[110]

The term *thrombocythemia* has been used to refer to the increased platelet counts associated with chronic myeloproliferative disorders (CMPD). The CMPD are a group of clonal disorders in which marked thrombocytosis is often found (Chap. 35). One in particular, essential thrombocythemia (ET) is characterized by increased megakaryocyte production with a persistent and massive elevation in platelet count.[36]

Clinical Presentation. Patients with reactive thrombocytosis generally do not have symptoms related to their increased platelet count. A small percentage may experience thrombosis, especially elderly patients.

Despite the elevated platelet count, up to 20% of patients with thrombocythemia related to a CMPD have a prolonged bleeding time. The severity of the bleeding problem does not correlate with the degree of abnormality in the platelet count. Paradoxically, some of these patients may present with both thrombosis and bleeding.

Laboratory Findings. In reactive thrombocytosis the platelet count is rarely above 1000×10^9/L and the increase is transitory, whereas ET is characterized by a

TABLE 57-3
Hereditary and Acquired Platelet Disorders

Hereditary	Acquired
Bernard-Soulier syndrome	Myeloproliferative disorders
Glanzmann thrombasthenia	Uremia
von Willebrand disease	Aspirin
Afibrinogenemia	Penicillin-type antibiotics
Gray platelet syndrome	Ethanol exposure
Wiskott-Aldrich syndrome	Dextran
Hermansky-Pudlak syndrome	C_{19} and C_{21} fatty acids
Chédiak-Higashi anomaly	Onions, garlic, etc.
Thrombocytopenia with absent radius (TAR)	Disseminated intravascular coagulation
Aspirin-like deficiency	Paraproteinemias
Cyclooxygenase deficiency	

platelet count greater than $1000 \times 10^9/L$, which is persistent. Platelet morphology, variation in platelet size, and platelet aggregation with epinephrine are typically abnormal in thrombocythemia of CMPD but normal in reactive thrombocytosis. Increases in megakaryocyte volume and leukocyte count are typical findings in thrombocythemia of CMPD compared to normal or decreased values in reactive thrombocytosis.

Reactive thrombocytosis is associated with increases in ESR, acute phase reactants (fibrinogen, VIIIC, vWF:Ag, C-reactive protein), and interleukin 6 (IL-6). In essential thrombocythemia these variables are usually normal or only slightly elevated. vWF:RCof and high molecular weight multimers are decreased in essential thrombocythemia.[83] Perez Encinas and coworkers[100] reported that the C-reactive protein levels in patients with essential

TABLE 57-4
Qualitative Platelet Abnormalities

Defects of Adhesion	Defects of Primary Aggregation	Defects of Release
Bernard-Soulier syndrome	Glanzmann thrombasthenia	Storage pool disease
Uremia	Afibrinogenemia	Gray platelet syndrome
Disseminated intravascular coagulation		Wiskott-Aldrich syndrome
Paraproteinemias		Hermansky-Pudlak syndrome
		Chédiak-Higashi anomaly
		Thrombocytopenia with absent radius (TAR)
		Uremia
		Aspirin
		Cyclooxygenase deficiency
		Ethanol

thrombocythemia were only twice the normal level as compared to a mean that was five times greater than normal in reactive thrombocytosis. The most potent stimulator for the hepatic synthesis of C-reactive protein is IL-6. IL-6, which also has thrombopoietic activity, is usually normal in chronic myeloproliferative diseases but increased in reactive thrombocytosis.[100]

Treatment. In reactive thrombocytosis the increased platelet count is usually temporary and requires no treatment. In ET the goal of therapy is to reduce the platelet count and to suppress the megakaryocytic proliferation. Drugs used include busulfan, hydroxyurea, recombinant interferon-α, and anagrelide.[76]

QUALITATIVE PLATELET DISORDERS: INHERITED

Thrombocytopathy is a term used to designate platelets that are qualitatively abnormal. The clinical picture of epistaxis, menorrhagia, easy bruising, and postoperative bleeding described for thrombocytopenia is also seen in cases of thrombocytopathy. Thrombocytopathies can be classified as either inherited or acquired (Table 57-3). These disorders can be due to either an intrinsic platelet defect or to an extrinsic defect. Extrinsic defects are frequently caused by the products of various diseases that inhibit platelet aggregation or adhesion. Most acquired intrinsic disorders are usually associated with drugs or myeloproliferative diseases (Table 57-4).

Adhesion Defects

Platelet adhesion refers to the sticking of platelets to any surface except that of another platelet. Disruption of the endothelial vascular lining exposes subendothelial components such as collagen and basement membrane. When normal platelets come in contact with these surfaces, they undergo a shape change, expose certain membrane-bound glycoproteins (GP), and adhere to the exposed foreign surface. The platelet membrane GP Ib-V-IX complex functions to bind to the von Willebrand factor (vWF) that is immobilized on the exposed subendothelium of damaged vessels. This coupling between the vWF and GP Ib-IX complex is required (GP V is not required) for platelet adhesion in small vessels.[95] In the smaller vessels, wall shear rates are much higher than in large arteries, therefore, platelet adhesion requires availability of GP Ib-IX and vWF. In the large arteries, GP Ib-V-IX and vWF are not required for platelet adhesion to the subendothelium.[78]

BERNARD-SOULIER SYNDROME (BSS)

In 1948, Bernard and Soulier first described a unique bleeding disorder.[13] To date, only a few additional cases have been reported. The condition is inherited as an autosomal recessive disorder, usually involving consanguinity. For some unexplained reason, the severity of the hemorrhagic problems, which usually are first observed during infancy or early childhood, tend to decrease with age. The severity of bleeding is usually greater than would be expected from the degree of thrombocytopenia. In two well-studied cases, the defect in this condition has been identified as a point mutation in codon 129 of the GP Ibα gene.[79]

Pathophysiology. Abnormal bleeding occurs because BSS platelets lack the vWF adhesion receptor GP Ib-V-IX that is necessary for the binding of vWF. The deficiency of this membrane receptor results in platelets that are unable to adhere to vWF. GP V appears to be a platelet substrata for thrombin, but this binding site is different from the platelet membrane thrombin receptor that has been cloned.

Laboratory Findings. Mild to moderate thrombocytopenia is a frequent but inconsistent finding. Some heterozygotes demonstrate thrombocytopenia and large platelets but have no symptoms. Platelet anisocytosis on a blood film is marked. The majority of the platelets are large (2.5–8 μm in diameter), with some of them being as big as lymphocytes.[81] The MPV of the giant platelets is about 12.5 fL compared to 7.5 ± 1.5 fL for normal platelets.[118] Other than size, the appearance of the large platelets generally is normal, although occasionally there is a central clustering of granules referred to as a *pseudonucleus*. The granular contents and the amount of vWF in these platelets are higher than in normal platelets.[57] In BSS, the platelet life span is shortened from the normal 10 days to 4.1 days.[118]

A bleeding time in excess of 20 minutes is a common finding. Clot retraction and platelet factor 3 (PF3) availability are normal. Platelet retention by glass bead columns is decreased. Ristocetin platelet agglutination studies are abnormal, and the addition of normal plasma, which contains vWF, does not correct the abnormal response. Both plasma and platelet factor VIII antigen levels are normal to increased.[57]

Platelet aggregation studies using ADP, epinephrine, and arachidonic acid produce normal results, but the results of aggregation studies with collagen and thrombin are variable. Platelet aggregation studies are difficult with BSS platelets, because it is hard to separate the large platelets from the red blood cells and lymphocytes, especially when using centrifugation for obtaining platelet-rich plasma. The influence of the large platelets may also affect the light scattering and size of the platelet aggregates, resulting in altered aggregation curves. The variable findings for the aggregation response to collagen and thrombin may be a consequence of these technical problems.

PLATELET-TYPE (PSEUDO) VON WILLEBRAND DISEASE

Platelet-type von Willebrand disease (vWD), also referred to as pseudo von Willebrand disease, is a form of thrombocytopathy that resembles type IIb vWD (Chap. 52). This autosomal-dominant bleeding disorder is due to a single point mutation that results in a single amino acid substitution at either residue 233 or 239 of GP Ibα.[108,117] The disease is characterized by abnormally enhanced binding of vWF to the platelet GP Ib-V-IX membrane receptor, which results in the loss of vWF from the plasma and removal of vWF-bound platelets from the circulation.

Clinical Presentation. Patients with platelet-type vWD present with mild bleeding typical of thrombocytopenia. In severe cases in which the factor VIII coagulation levels are decreased, deep wound bleeding and hemarthrosis can develop.

Laboratory Findings. The bleeding time is usually prolonged to a greater extent than would be predicted by the mild decrease in platelet count. The decrease in vWF and factor VIII coagulant activity is quite variable, resulting in variable PTT results.

Ristocetin platelet aggregation studies using the patient's own platelets show a hypersensitivity to aggregation typical of type IIb vWD. Control platelets (normal or formalin-fixed) show normal ristocetin aggregation. The hypersensitivity can also be demonstrated using normal plasma plus the patient's platelets. This information indicates that the patient's platelets are defective. Ristocetin aggregation is decreased when the patient's plasma plus normal platelets are used, which is reflective of the decreased vWF. Studies indicate that the decreased vWF is due primarily to the loss of the larger vWF multimers.[108] It is important to distinguish between type IIb vWD and platelet-type vWD, because the administration of vWF to platelet-type vWD patients will exacerbate their thrombocytopenia.

See Chapter 52 for a detailed discussion of true von Willebrand disease.

Aggregation Defects

Platelet aggregation is the sticking of platelets to platelets. Aggregation is a dynamic and metabolically active process that should not be confused with agglutination, which refers to platelet clumping and is not dependent on metabolic processes such as the release of ADP. Dead platelets, such as formalin-fixed or freeze-dried platelets used in the ristocetin test, will agglutinate, but they cannot aggregate. The ability of platelets to aggregate requires GP IIb and GP IIIa, which together form the fibrinogen receptor. This receptor, GP IIb-IIIa, as well as fibrinogen, are necessary for normal aggregation.

GLANZMANN THROMBASTHENIA

The autosomal recessive disorder known as Glanzmann thrombasthenia (GT), which has been associated with consanguinity, affects the two sexes equally. Only homozygotes have a clinically recognizable hemorrhagic disorder. GT appears to occur most frequently among Iraqi Jews, Jordanian Arabs, Indians, and French gypsies.[44,102] A number of point mutations have been demonstrated to cause GT.

Pathophysiology. Fibrinogen is a necessary cofactor for the aggregation of human platelets by ADP. When activated by agonists such as ADP or thrombin, the membrane-bound GP IIb-IIIa becomes available. Since fibrinogen binds rapidly to this complex, it is referred to as the fibrinogen receptor. However, other ligands such as fibrin, vWF, and vitronectin can compete for occupancy of the activated GP IIb-IIIa complex.[51] The exposure of the GP IIb-IIIa complex and binding to fibrinogen is required for normal platelet aggregation. GT is an example of a thrombocytopathy that is associated with a defect in the GP IIb-IIIa complex.

GT has been divided into type I and type II.[77] Type I is the more severe, with the platelets lacking GP IIb-IIIa as well as intraplatelet fibrinogen. Clot retraction is absent. In type II, platelets contain subnormal levels of fibrinogen, and the number of GP IIb-IIIa complexes is around 15% of normal. Clot retraction may be observable.

Clinical Presentation. The hemorrhagic symptoms of bruising, epistaxis, bleeding from mucous membranes, gastrointestinal bleeding, and menorrhagia are typical of platelet dysfunction. Ecchymoses frequently are seen at birth or early in life, but the severity of the hemorrhagic complications tends to decrease with age. In some individuals, the bleeding is severe enough to necessitate blood transfusions.

Laboratory Findings. The platelets are normal in number, size, and morphology and have a normal life span. However, they do not support clot retraction adequately, and PF3 availability is deficient. The bleeding time is usually markedly prolonged. When placed on a wettable surface such as a glass slide, the platelets fail to spread and form pseudopods; consequently, they will not form clumps on blood films made from capillary blood as normal platelets do. These platelets do not aggregate with ADP, epinephrine, collagen, or thrombin but will agglutinate on the addition of ristocetin.[78] The ability of the platelets to secrete the contents of their granules is not impaired. Normal amounts of platelet factor 4 (PF4), serotonin, and ADP secretion can be induced by exposure to thrombin.[123] Platelet retention in a glass bead column that requires both adhesion and aggregation is reduced markedly in most cases. Although adhesion to vascular subendothelium is usually normal, an adhesion defect associated with GT has been demonstrated. With few exceptions, the lack of clot retraction in the presence of a normal platelet count is diagnostic of GT.[44] Methods that are both sensitive and specific for thrombasthenia have been developed using monoclonal antibodies to detect deficiencies of the GP IIb-IIIa complex.

The platelet GP IIb-IIIa content is about 50% of normal in patients who are heterozygous for GT. However, these persons have normal clot retraction, aggregation studies, and bleeding times.

Treatment. Type I GT platelets lack the platelet-specific alloantigen HPA-1a (Pl^{A1}, Zw^a). Because 98% of the normal population has platelets that contain the HPA-1a antigen, platelet transfusions for the treatment of GT must be used with caution to reduce the chance of alloantibody formation. Multiply transfused patients with type I thrombasthenia may develop an IgG alloantibody to the GP IIb-IIIa complex. The addition of this antibody to normal platelets will cause them to exhibit the same laboratory abnormalities as GT platelets.

Other forms of treatment include the use of hormones in menorrhagia and oral iron supplements for the anemia associated with chronic bleeding. An allogeneic bone mar-row transplant was successful in correcting type I GT in a 4-year-old boy.[11a] Steroids have not proved to be beneficial.

Release Defects

Abnormal platelet release of ADP may be secondary to a lack of α- or δ (dense) granules. There may also be a deficient quantity of ADP stored within the granules, in which case, the condition is classified as a *storage pool disease.* A second type of release defect is characterized by impaired secretion of normal granule contents, which is sometimes referred to as *aspirin-like defect.* In both diseases the primary wave of aggregation usually is normal (Chap. 56). The secondary wave of aggregation, however, is abnormal because it is dependent on the release of endogenous ADP from the δ (dense) granules in response to exogenous ADP and epinephrine.

STORAGE POOL DISEASE

Platelet storage pool deficiencies (SPD) can involve defective or decreased α-granules, δ-granules, or both. This is a heterogeneous group of disorders. δ-granule deficiencies are much more common and are more likely to be associated with severe bleeding than are that α-granule deficiencies. Possible explanations for this are that α-granules are present in excess of need, the ratio being about 800 α-granules to 1 δ-granule, and that the contents of the δ-granules are more critical for platelet plug formation.

Gray Platelet Syndrome. Gray platelet syndrome is an example of an SPD in which α-granules are lacking. A Wright-stained blood film shows the platelets to be larger than normal and to be gray or blue-gray, in contrast to the lavender-purple granular appearance of normal platelets. The lack of normal α-granules has been demonstrated through electron micrographs of megakaryocytes. Tests for constituents of the α-granule, such as PF4, β-thromboglobulin, and fibrinogen, are abnormal. Decreases in PF3 also have been reported.[89] Tests for δ-granule contents (*e.g.*, uptake and storage of serotonin, ADP, and the ATP-to-ADP ratio) are normal. The dense tubular system (DTS), which is thought to be the storage site of calcium and cyclooxygenase, is abnormal in this syndrome and may be associated with abnormal release and variable aggregation findings.[90]

The gray platelet syndrome is rare, however, it appears to be autosomal-dominant.[89] A lifelong history of mild bleeding, easy bruising, moderate thrombocytopenia, and abnormal platelet morphology is characteristic. Platelet aggregations induced by ADP, epinephrine, and arachidonic acid are usually normal. Using thrombin and collagen the results are variable. These patients appear to be hemostatically normal, although serious bleeding has been reported in a few cases. In one case involving a 4-year-old girl, the bleeding was controlled with platelet infusions and antifibrinolytic therapy.[48]

Wiskott-Aldrich Syndrome (WAS). WAS is an immunodeficiency disorder characterized by small platelets and the triad of thrombocytopenia, recurrent infections, and eczema. It is X-linked, and affected boys rarely survive childhood because of the high risk of hemorrhage and infection. Females who carry the WAS gene are normal. The genetic defect has been mapped to the proximal portion of the short arm of the X chromosome (Xp11).[98]

The profound thrombocytopenia has been attributed to both rapid platelet turnover (shortened life span) and ineffective production.[96] The platelets are small, measuring about two-thirds of the normal size, with significantly reduced MPV, and they have abnormal cellular membranes because of the lack of a surface protein. This membrane defect also is present in the T lymphocytes.[96,103] Wiskott-Aldrich platelets have been reported to be lacking in storage pool nucleotides. In addition, decreases in the number of α-granules and mitochondria have been reported by several investigators, but these changes do not occur in all cases. Being qualitatively defective, the platelets are subject to rapid sequestration in the spleen. Splenectomy has been effective in increasing both the size and number of circulating platelets. An increase in the platelet-associated immunoglobulin G (PAIgG) has been reported to be elevated in these patients. Following splenectomy, PAIgG levels returned to normal, which suggests that the spleen plays a major role in this immunologically mediated condition.[28] Because of the associated risk of infection, splenectomy is not a universal treatment. Bone marrow transplantation may alleviate the symptoms. Infection, hemorrhage, and lymphoreticular malignancies are common causes of death.

Hermansky-Pudlack Syndrome. This syndrome is characterized by a triad of tyrosinase-positive oculocutaneous albinism, accumulation of ceroid-like pigment in macrophages, and a bleeding tendency associated with abnormal platelet function. This is an extremely rare autosomal recessive condition associated with a striking lack of δ (dense) granules. Numbers of α-granules are normal.

Chédiak-Higashi Anomaly. This syndrome is characterized by albinism, recurrent infections, hemorrhagic tendencies, and giant lysosomes in all granule-containing cells. Chapter 26 describes this disorder in detail. Although thrombocytopenia does occur, the prolongation of the bleeding time exceeds what would be expected on the basis of the platelet count, suggesting defective platelet function. The ratio of ATP to ADP in these platelets is consistent with a δ-granule deficiency.[105] The platelet response to ADP, epinephrine, collagen, arachidonic acid, and the calcium ionophore A231987, although variable, usually is deficient.[7] Typically, it is the secondary wave of aggregation that is abnormal or absent.

GRANULE-RELEASE DEFECTS

The clinical picture and laboratory findings in the heterogeneous group of granule-release defects (also known as aspirin-like defects) are similar to those for storage pool disease (SPD), except that the stored contents of the α- and δ-granules are normal. The absence of the secondary wave of aggregation with ADP and epinephrine and the abnormal collagen-induced platelet aggregation are at-

tributable to impaired release or secretion of ADP from the δ-granules.

Deficiencies of Platelet Prostaglandin Enzymes. These include defects in cyclooxygenase and abnormal thromboxane A_2 (TxA$_2$) activity. The abnormal platelet aggregation curve obtained by the addition of arachidonic acid to platelets deficient in cyclooxygenase is corrected by the addition of prostaglandin G_2. Only two families have been reported with TxA$_2$ deficiency, and little is known about the clinical and laboratory features. Prostaglandin G_2 does not correct the abnormal aggregation caused by deficient TxA$_2$ or impaired calcium mobilization.

Cyclooxygenase Deficiency. Patients with this deficiency have a mild bleeding disorder and treatment usually consists of avoiding anti-platelet drugs and controlling menorrhagia with hormonal therapy. Because thrombin will cause platelet release by way of a mechanism other than prostaglandin, the release of normal platelet contents in the presence of thrombin will differentiate this condition from an SPD.

QUALITATIVE PLATELET DISORDERS: ACQUIRED

Platelet function can be affected by many drugs, diets, and diseases. The effects may be biochemical, mechanical, or both.

Drugs

There is a long list of drugs reported to affect platelet function. Aspirin, the penicillins, and alcohol are the most frequently reported to cause clinical bleeding problems.[39] Aspirin and alcohol have a synergistic effect in increasing the bleeding time.

Patients taking aspirin have an abnormal secondary aggregation wave attributable to the inhibition of cyclooxygenase by irreversible acetylation of the enzyme's active site. Because platelets do not synthesize cyclooxygenase, the inhibitory effect lasts the life of the platelet (approximately 10 days). The prolongation of the bleeding time after aspirin ingestion is variable. Two hours after taking aspirin, most people show a 2- to 9-minute prolongation. About 10% to 15% of the population will have less than a 2-minute prolongation, and about 10% to 15% of the population will show greater than a 9-minute increase. The extent of prolongation of the bleeding time cannot be predicted by the bleeding time before aspirin ingestion. Marked prolongation of the bleeding time can be secondary to a variety of conditions, including vascular disorders, thrombocytopenia, vWF deficiency, and circulating anticoagulants. As in the SPD, the prolongation of the bleeding time is increased in proportion to the decrease in the ADP released from the δ-granules. Other drugs that similarly affect platelets are indomethacin, ibuprofen, and butazolidine. Collectively, this group of drugs is referred to as nonsteroidal anti-inflammatory agents.

Carbenicillin is the most potent of the penicillin group

of antibiotics capable of affecting platelet function. The mechanism of action is not clear, but it has been postulated that these drugs interact with glycoproteins on the surface of the platelet, causing a reduced response to most aggregating agents.

Prolonged exposure to alcohol, in addition to causing thrombocytopenia, impairs PF3 release and reduces secondary aggregation.[86] One possible mechanism is the direct impairment of prostaglandin synthesis by ethanol. Thromboxane A_2 release has been reported to be inhibited in alcoholic patients on hospital admission. During abstinence, the platelet count, bleeding time, and TxA_2 release return to normal.[86] The reduced platelet count and impaired platelet function may contribute to the increased incidence of gastrointestinal hemorrhage associated with excessive alcohol intake. Any drug, such as dipyridamole, that increases the platelet cAMP concentration will inhibit platelet function.

Finally, patients given significant amounts of intravenous dextran and related plasma expanders exhibit reduced platelet function. Because of the anti-platelet effect, dextrans are used as prophylaxis against deep venous thrombosis during surgery. The inhibitory effects of dextran probably result from the interaction between dextran and the platelet membrane or the reduced surface charge on the membrane due to the coating of the platelets by the plasma expanders.

Diet

Populations whose diet contains significant amounts of fish have decreased platelet function, as demonstrated in aggregation studies. It is believed that the C_{19} or C_{21} chain fatty acids or eicopentoic acids (omega-3 fatty acids) present in fish oils result in the replacement of arachidonic acid and production of inactive prostaglandin.[39] Another ethnic dietary component—an herb used in Szechwan cooking—decreases the platelet release reaction. Finally, onions, garlic, and related plants contain an extractable substance capable of inhibiting platelet aggregation.

A deficiency in vitamin B_{12} or folate may lead to a qualitative platelet defect, as well as to thrombocytopenia. Large amounts of vitamin E can also affect platelet lipids through peroxidation, with resulting defects in prostaglandin synthesis.

Diseases

Several diseases or conditions either produce abnormal platelets or produce substances that are responsible for inhibiting normal platelet function.

MYELOPROLIFERATIVE DISORDERS

Malignant myeloproliferative disorders frequently are associated with large, hypogranular platelets that can be defective in any or all functions (adhesion, aggregation, release, or contraction). These abnormalities reflect a fundamental defect in megakaryocyte maturation. A decrease in the epinephrine-induced secondary wave of aggregation is the most common aggregation defect. A decrease in the GP Ib-IX receptor has also been reported.

UREMIA

An increased blood urea nitrogen (BUN) is associated with qualitative platelet defects that can be corrected with dialysis. Various platelet defects have been described in conjunction with uremia, including decreased adhesion and aggregation and defective release. It is believed that these defects are a result of high concentrations of metabolites of urea such as guanidosuccinic acid and phenolic acids that inhibit platelet aggregation. Some patients with uremia also exhibit defective factor VIII / vWF complexes, especially the high molecular weight polymers necessary for adequate platelet adhesion.

DISSEMINATED INTRAVASCULAR COAGULATION

Disseminated intravascular coagulation (DIC) affects platelets in many ways in addition to overt destruction. Prematurely activated platelets may release granules, causing an acquired platelet SPD. In addition, the fibrin-(ogen) degradation products that circulate in DIC are believed to interact with platelet membranes and inhibit adhesion or aggregation.

IMMUNOGLOBULIN PRODUCTION

Antibody binding to platelets accelerates platelet destruction and inhibits platelet function. The reduced platelet aggregation using collagen, ADP, and epinephrine seen in SLE and immune thrombocytopenia purpura has been associated with increased levels of immunoglobulin. Specific antibodies such as anti–HPA-1a which binds to GP IIIa, can bind to membrane receptors and inhibit platelet function. Some antibodies can affect the uptake of substances into the platelet granules during megakaryocytopoiesis.[50]

CHAPTER SUMMARY

Platelets are an important element in preventing blood from escaping from vessels. Platelet defects can lead to bleeding, thrombosis, or both. Platelets can be abnormal in number (quantitative disorders) or function (qualitative disorders) and these abnormalities may be inherited or acquired. Quantitative disorders include decreased numbers (thrombocytopenia) or increased numbers (thrombocytosis or thrombocythemia). Thrombocytopenia may be caused by decreased production or increased loss or destruction whereas thrombocytosis may be reactive or part of a malignant myeloproliferative disorder. Qualitative disorders include the inability to adhere, to aggregate, or to release internal contents of granules. Inherited defects in platelet function may involve the platelet itself or a plasma protein that is necessary for platelet function. Acquired defects in platelet function are relatively common and may be related to drugs, diet, or disease.

Case Study 57-1

A 36-year-old black woman was admitted through the emergency room with chief complaints of headache, dizziness, lethargy, nausea, vomiting, and weakness. Three months earlier, she underwent a subtotal gastrectomy for adenocarcinoma of the stomach. She was placed on mitomycin therapy, a cancer chemotherapeutic drug. Diagnostic procedures indicated a recurrence of the carcinoma.

Laboratory testing revealed a moderately increased leukocyte count with a neutrophilia and a normocytic, normochromic anemia with marked anisocytosis and red cell fragmentation. There were 3 nucleated RBC per 100 leukocytes. Repeated manual platelet counts ranged from 10 to 50 $\times$ 10^9/L except for brief increases following platelet transfusions. The PTT and fibrinogen assays remained within normal limits throughout most of the patient's hospitalization. The PT was slightly prolonged (13–17 seconds; reference range was 10.5–13.0 seconds) until her death from respiratory failure on day 19. Urinalysis revealed increased protein, 60 to 100 RBC per high power field, and granular and hyaline casts. Serum chemistries showed increased LD, creatinine, and BUN and decreased haptoglobin.

1. Why was the patient's platelet count monitored by manual rather than automated methods?
2. What are the possible diagnoses and why?
3. What may have triggered the acute onset?
4. What other laboratory data may be of value in determining the pathogenesis of the thrombocytopenia?

Case Study 57-2

A 6-year-old boy had repeated nosebleeds and a tendency to bruise. This concerned his aunt, a clinical laboratory scientist. She examined a blood film made from a capillary skin puncture sample and noted that the platelet count appeared normal but that, contrary to expectation with a capillary puncture sample, his platelets were not clumped on the blood film. She persuaded her sister to take the boy to a physician. The patient's CBC was normal but his bleeding time exceeded 15 minutes. The PT, PTT, thrombin time (TT), and fibrinogen assay were all normal. Platelet aggregation studies revealed a total lack of response to ADP, a partial response to collagen, and a normal response to ristocetin.

1. What is a likely cause for the patient's bleeding history and what other laboratory tests might be helpful?
2. What is the basic defect in this condition?
3. What information was obtained by the original capillary puncture blood film?

Review Questions

57-1. Chronic ITP affects primarily

  A. neonates.
  B. young children.
  C. young adults.
  D. men.

57-2. After receiving 15 units of whole blood a patient's platelet count decreased to less than 20 $\times$ 10^9/L. The most probable explanation is

  A. decreased platelet life span.
  B. dilutional loss.
  C. antibodies to platelet-specific alloantigen HPA-1a.
  D. splenic sequestration.

57-3. When homologous platelets were infused into a patient, the platelet life span was normal, but when the patient's own platelets were infused the life span was markedly shortened. This observation suggests an

  A. intrinsic platelet defect.
  B. extrinsic platelet defect.
  C. immune mechanism.
  D. *in vivo* platelet aggregation.

57-4. A 2-year-old girl was admitted with a Hb of 10 g/dL, decreased RBC, and increased RDW. The platelet count was 17 $\times$ 10^9/L. Other laboratory results were within reference ranges. Except for a minor viral infection 6 weeks before, the patient had been in excellent health. These findings are typical of

  A. disseminated intravascular coagulation.
  B. hemolytic uremic syndrome.
  C. Bernard-Soulier syndrome.
  D. acute idiopathic thrombocytopenic purpura.

57-5. Neonatal alloimmune thrombocytopenia (NATP) is analogous to

  A. transfusion-induced thrombocytopenia.
  B. hemolytic disease of the newborn.
  C. ineffective thrombocytosis.
  D. inherited neonatal thrombocytopenia.

57-6. Reactive thrombocytosis is usually associated with

  A. a chronic myeloproliferative disorder.
  B. older adults.
  C. a temporary increase in platelet count.
  D. males more often than females.

57-7. The enzyme inhibited by aspirin is

  A. thromboxane synthetase.
  B. cyclooxygenase.
  C. lactate dehydrogenase.
  D. phospholipase.

57-8. The platelet membrane von Willebrand receptor is composed of

  A. platelet factor 3.
  B. GP V-Xa.
  C. GP Ib-V-IX.
  D. GP IIb-IIIa.

57-9. Pseudo (platelet-type) von Willebrand disease is characterized by

  A. a storage pool defect.
  B. defective platelet vWF.
  C. liver disease.
  D. enhanced binding of vWF to the platelet vWF receptor.

57-10. The platelets in Wiskott-Aldrich syndrome

  A. are about two-thirds normal size.
  B. fail to bind fibrinogen.
  C. fail to bind vWF.
  D. are unable to release their granule contents.

References

1. Abrams DI, Kiprov DD, Goedart JJ et al: Antibodies to human T-lymphotropic virus type III and development of the acquired immunodeficiency syndrome in homosexual men presenting with immune thrombocytopenia. Ann Intern Med 104:47, 1986
2. Abzug MJ, Levin MJ, Rotbart HA: Profile of enterovirus disease in the first two weeks of life. Pediatr Infect Dis J 12:820, 1993
3. Addonizio VP: Platelet function in cardiopulmonary bypass and artificial organs. Hematol Oncol Clin North Am 4:145, 1990
4. al Mofada SM, Osman ME, Kides E et al: Risk of thrombocytopenia in the infants of mothers with idiopathic thrombocytopenia. Am J Perinatol 11:423, 1994

5. American Association of Blood Banks Technical Manual, 9th ed, p 252. Washington DC, AABB, 1985

6. Anand A, Feffer SE: Hematocrit and bleeding time: An update. South Med J 87:299, 1994

7. Apitz-Castro R, Cruz MR, Ledezma E et al: The storage pool deficiency in platelets from humans with the Chédiak-Higashi syndrome: Study of six patients. Br J Haematol 59:471, 1985

8. Aster RH: Pooling of platelets in the spleen: Role in the pathogenesis of "hypersplenic" thrombocytopenia. J Clin Invest 45:645, 1955

9. Barnes CG, Turnbull AL, Vernon-Roberts B: Felty's syndrome: A clinical and pathologic survey of 21 patients and their response to treatment. Ann Rheum Dis 30:359, 1971

10. Baughman RP, Lower EE, Flessa HC et al: Thrombocytopenia in the intensive care unit. Chest 104:1243, 1993

11. Bell WR, Braine HG, Ness PM et al: Improved survival in thrombotic thrombocytopenic purpura–hemolytic uremic syndrome. Clinical experience in 108 patients. N Engl J Med 325:398, 1991

11a. Bellucci S, Devergie A, Gluckman E et al: Complete correction of Glanzmann's thrombasthenia by allogeneic bone marrow transplantation. Br J Haematol 59:635, 1985

12. Ben Yehuda D, Gillis S, Eldor A: Clinical and therapeutic experience in 712 Israeli patients with idiopathic thrombocytopenic purpura. Israeli ITP Study Group. Acta Haematol 91:1, 1994

13. Bernard J, Soulier JP: Sur une nouvelle variété de dystrophie thrombocytaire hémorrhagipare congénitale. Sem Hôp Paris 24:3217, 1948

14. Bithell TC: The diagnostic approach to the bleeding disorders. In Lee GR, Bithell TC, Foerster J et al (eds): Wintrobe's Clinical Hematology, 9th ed, p 1306. Philadelphia, Lea & Febiger, 1993

15. Bithell TC: Thrombocytosis. In Lee GR, Bithell TC, Foerster J et al (eds): Wintrobe's Clinical Hematology, 9th ed, p 1390. Philadelphia, Lea & Febiger, 1993

16. Bithell TC: Thrombocytopenia caused by immunologic platelet destruction: Idiopathic thrombocytopenic purpura (ITP), drug-induced thrombocytopenia, and miscellaneous forms. In Lee GR, Bithell TC, Foerster J et al (eds): Wintrobe's Clinical Hematology, 9th ed, p 1329. Philadelphia, Lea & Febiger, 1993

17. Blaas P, Weber S, Hansch GM et al: Paroxysmal nocturnal hemoglobinuria. Klin Wochenschr 68:247, 1990

18. Blajchman MA, Bordin JO, Bardossy L et al: The contribution of the haematocrit to thrombocytopenic bleeding in experimental animals. Br J Haematol 86:347, 1994

19. Blockmans D, Vermylen J: HIV-related thrombocytopenia. Acta Clin Belg 47:117, 1992

20. Breton-Gorius J, Favier R, Guichard J et al: A new congenital dysmegakaryopoietic thrombocytopenia (Paris-Trousseau) associated with giant platelet alpha-granules and chromosome 11 deletion at 11q23. Blood 85:1805, 1995

21. Budd JL, Wiegers SE, O'Hara JM: Relapsing post-transfusion purpura: A preventable disease. Am J Med 78:361, 1985

22. Burns ER: Platelet studies in the pathogenesis of thrombocytopenia in May-Hegglin anomaly. Am J Pediatr Hematol Oncol 13:431, 1991

23. Bussel J, Kaplan C, McFarland J: Recommendations for the evaluation and treatment of neonatal autoimmune and alloimmune thrombocytopenia. The Working Party on Neonatal Immune Thrombocytopenia of the Neonatal Hemostasis Subcommittee of the Scientific and Standardization Committee of the ISTH. Thromb Haemost 65:631, 1991

24. Chen SH, Liang DC, Lin M: Treatment of platelet alloimmunization with intravenous immunoglobulin in a child with aplastic anemia. Am J Hematol 49:165, 1995

25. Chintagumpala MM, Hurwitz RL, Moake JL et al: Chronic relapsing thrombotic thrombocytopenic purpura in infants with large von Willebrand factor multimers during remission. J Pediatr 120:49, 1992

26. Coller BS: Disorders of platelets. In Ratnoff OD, Forbes CD (eds): Disorders of Hemostasis, p 73. New York, Grune & Stratton, 1984

27. Comis RL: Cisplatin: The future. Semin Oncol 21(5 Suppl 12):109, 1994

28. Corash L, Shafer B, Blaese RM: Platelet-associated immunoglobulin, platelet size, and the effects of splenectomy in the Wiskott-Aldrich syndrome. Blood 65:1439, 1985

29. Cruccu V, Parisio E, Pedretti D et al: HIV-related thrombotic thrombocytopenic purpura (TTP) as first clinical manifestation of infection. Haematologica 79:277, 1994

30. Davis GL, Fritsma GA: Platelet disorders. In Corriveau DM, Fritsma GA (eds): Hemostasis and Thrombosis in the Clinical Laboratory, pp 304–342. Philadelphia, JB Lippincott, 1988

31. Dayal R, Agarwal S, Prasad R et al: A clinico-hematological profile of hemolytic-uremic syndrome. Southeast Asian J Trop Med Public Health 24(Suppl 1):280, 1993

32. de Alarcon PA, Graeve JA, Levine RF et al: Thrombocytopenia and absent radii syndrome: Defective megakaryocytopoiesis-thrombocytopoiesis. Am J Pediatr Hematol Oncol 13:77, 1991

33. Dickerman JD, Holbrook PR, Zinkham WH: Etiology and therapy of thrombocytopenia associated with sarcoidosis. J Pediatr 81:758, 1972

34. Didisheim P: Screening tests for bleeding disorders. Am J Clin Pathol 47:622, 1967

35. Dominguez A, Gamallo G, Garcia R et al: Pathophysiology of HIV related thrombocytopenia: An analysis of 41 patients. J Clin Pathol 47:999, 1994

36. el Kassar N, Hetet G, Li Y et al: Clonal analysis of haemopoietic cells in essential thrombocythaemia. Br J Haematol 90: 131, 1995

37. Evenson DA, Stroncek DF, Pulkrabek S et al: Posttransfusion purpura following bone marrow transplantation. Transfusion 35:688, 1995

38. Fabris F, Steffan A, Cordiano I et al: Specific antiplatelet autoantibodies in patients with antiphospholipid antibodies and thrombocytopenia. Eur J Haematol 53:232, 1994

39. Firkin BG: The Platelet and its Disorders. Boston, MTP Press, 1984

40. Galbusera M, Ruggenenti P, Noris M et al: Alpha 1-Antitrypsin therapy in a case of thrombotic thrombocytopenic purpura. Lancet 345:224, 1995

41. Gangarosa EJ, Johnson TR, Ramos HS: Ristocetin-induced thrombocytopenia: Site and mechanism of action. Arch Intern Med 105:83, 1960

42. George D, Bussel JB: Neonatal thrombocytopenia. Semin Thromb Hemost 21:276, 1995

43. George JN: Platelet IgG: Measurement, interpretation, and clinical significance. In Coller BS (ed): Progress in Hemostasis and Thrombosis, vol 10, pp 97–126. Philadelphia, WB Saunders, 1991

44. George JN, Reimann TA: Inherited disorders of the platelet membrane: Glanzmann's thrombasthenia and Bernard Soulier disease. In Colman RW, Hirsch J, Marder VJ et al (eds): Hemostasis and Thrombosis: Basic Principles and Clinical Practice, p 496. Philadelphia, JB Lippincott, 1982

45. Glassman AB, Shieh WJ: Neonatal alloimmune thrombocytopenia: Current considerations. Ann Clin Lab Sci 24:407, 1994

46. Gockerman JP, Shulman NR: Isoantibody specificity in posttransfusion purpura. Blood 41:817, 1973

47. Goldsweig HG, Grossman R, William D: Thrombocytopenia in homosexual men. Am J Hematol 21:243, 1986

48. Gootenberg JE, Buchanan GR, Holtkamp CA et al: Severe hemorrhage in a patient with gray platelet syndrome. J Pediatr 109:1017, 1986

49. Greinacher A, Mueller-Eckhardt C: Hereditary types of thrombocytopenia with giant platelets and inclusion bodies in the leukocytes. Blut 60:53, 1990

50. Handagama PJ, Shuman MA, Bainton DF: Incorporation of intravenously injected albumin, immunoglobulin G, and fibrinogen in guinea pig megakaryocyte granules. J Clin Invest 84:73, 1989

51. Hantgan RR, Nichols WL, Ruggeri ZM: von Willebrand factor competes with fibrin for occupancy of GPIIb:IIIa on thrombin-stimulated platelets. Blood 75:889, 1990

52. Harker LA, Slichter SJ: The bleeding time as a screening test for evaluation of platelet function. N Engl J Med 287:155, 1972

53. Harvey MP, Greenfield TP, Sugrue ME et al: Massive blood transfusion in a tertiary referral hospital. Clinical outcomes and haemostatic complications. Med J Aust 163:356, 1995

54. Heal JM, Masel D, Rowe JM et al: Circulating immune complexes involving the ABO system after platelet transfusion. Br J Haematol 85:566, 1993

55. Herzig RH, Herzig GP, Bull MI et al: Correction of poor platelet transfusion responses with leukocyte-poor HLA-matched platelet concentrates. Blood 46:743, 1975

56. Hou M, Stockelberg D, Kutti J et al: Antibodies against platelet GPIb/IX, GPIIb/IIIa, and other platelet antigens in chronic idiopathic thrombocytopenic purpura. Eur J Haematol 55:307, 1995

57. Howard MA, Montgomery DC, Hardisty RM: Factor VIII-related antigen in platelets. Thromb Res 4:617, 1974

58. Imbach P: Immune thrombocytopenia in children: The immune character of destructive thrombocytopenia and the treatment of bleeding. Semin Thromb Hemost 21:305, 1995

59. Kaden BR, Rosse WF, Hauch TW: Immune thrombocytopenia in lymphoproliferative diseases. Blood 53:545, 1979

60. Kanfer A: Hemolytic-uremic syndrome with renal thrombotic microangiopathy. Rev Prat 44:1205, 1994

61. Kaplan BS, Chesney RW, Brummond KN: Hemolytic uremic syndrome in families. N Engl J Med 292:1090, 1975

62. Karpatkin S: Heterogeneity of human platelets. VI: Correlation of platelet function with platelet volume. Blood 51:307, 1978

63. Kaushansky K: Thrombopoietin: The primary regulator of platelet production. Blood 86:419, 1995

64. Keeling DM, Isenberg DA: Haematological manifestations of systemic lupus erythematosus. Blood Rev 7:199, 1993

65. Kelton JG, Blanchette VS, Wilson WE et al: Neonatal thrombocytopenia due to passive immunization: Prenatal diagnosis and distinction between maternal platelet alloantibodies and autoantibodies. N Engl J Med 302:1401, 1980

66. Kelton JG: The serological investigation of patients with autoimmune thrombocytopenia. Thromb Haemost 74:228, 1995

67. Kieffer N, Phillips DR: Platelet membrane glycoproteins: Function in cellular interactions. Annu Rev Cell Biol 6:329, 1990

68. Kim HO, Jin Y, Kickler TS et al: Gene frequencies of the five major human platelet antigens in African American, white, and Korean populations. Transfusion 35:863, 1995

69. King DJ, Kelton JG: Heparin-associated thrombocytopenia. Ann Intern Med 100:535, 1984

70. Klein CA, Blajchman MA: Alloantibodies and platelet destruction. Semin Thromb Hemost 8:105, 1982

71. Koenig DW, Barley-Maloney L, Daniel TO: A Western blot assay detects autoantibodies to cryptic endothelial antigens in thrombotic microangiopathies. J Clin Immunol 13:204, 1993

72. Kumar R, Ansell J, Deykin D: Clinical trial of a new bleeding time device. Am J Clin Pathol 70:640, 1978

73. Kunicki T, Beardsley DS: The alloimmune thrombocytopenias: Neonatal alloimmune thrombocytopenic purpura and post-transfusion purpura. In Coller BS (ed): Progress in Hemostasis and Thrombosis, vol 9, pp 203–232. Philadelphia, WB Saunders, 1989

74. Kunicki TJ, Newman PJ: The molecular immunology of human platelet proteins. Blood 80:1386, 1992

75. Kunzi MS, Groopman JE: Identification of a novel human immunodeficiency virus strain cytopathic to megakaryocytic cells. Blood 81:3336, 1993

76. Kuramoto A: Diagnosis and treatment of essential thrombocythemia. Rinsho Ketsueki 36:480, 1995

77. Lee H, Nurden AT, Thomaidis A et al: Relationship between fibrinogen binding and the platelet glycoprotein deficiencies in Glanzmann's thrombasthenia type I and type II. Br J Haematol 48:47, 1981

78. Legrand YJ, Karniguiah A, Lefrancier P et al: Interaction of platelets with a nonpeptide derived from type III collagen. Blood 58:198a, 1981

79. Li C, Martin E, Roth GJ: The genetic defect in two well-studied cases of Bernard-Soulier syndrome: A point mutation in the fifth leucine-rich repeat of platelet glycoprotein Ibα. Blood 86:3805, 1995

80. López JA: The platelet glycoprotein Ib-IX complex. Blood Coag Fibrinolysis 5:97, 1994

81. Lusher JM, Barnhart MI: Congenital disorders affecting platelets. Semin Thromb Hemost 4:123, 1977

82. MacDonald MR, Schaefer GB, Olney AH et al: Hypoplasia of the cerebellar vermis and corpus callosum in thrombocytopenia with absent radius syndrome on MRI studies. Am J Med Genet 50:46, 1994

83. Messinezy M, Westwood N, Sawyer B et al: Primary thrombocythaemia: A composite approach to diagnosis. Clin Lab Haematol 16:139, 1994

84. Michelson AD: Thrombocytopenia associated with environmental exposure to polyurethane. Am J Hematol 38:145, 1991

85. Miescher PA: Drug-induced thrombocytopenia. Semin Hematol 10:311, 1973

86. Mikhailidis DP, Jenkins WJ, Barradas MA et al: Platelet function defects in chronic alcoholism. Br Med J 293:715, 1986

87. Moake JL, Chintagumpala M, Turner N et al: Solvent/detergent-treated plasma suppresses shear-induced platelet aggregation and prevents episodes of thrombotic thrombocytopenic purpura. Blood 84:490, 1994

88. Moake JL, McPherson PD: von Willebrand factor in thrombotic thrombocytopenic purpura and the hemolytic-uremic syndrome. Transfusion Med Rev 4:163, 1990

89. Mori K, Suzki S, Sugai K: Electron microscope and functional studies on platelets in gray platelet syndrome. Tohoku J Exp Med 143:261, 1984

90. Mori K, Suzki S, Sugai K et al: Morphological changes of platelets during the process of platelet aggregation in gray platelet syndrome. Tohoku J Exp Med 149:425, 1986

91. Moss RA: Drug induced immune thrombocytopenia. Am J Hematol 9:439, 1980

92. Movahed Shariat Panahi MR, Le Blanc S, Schober O et al: Study of platelet-associated immunoglobulins of IgG, IgM, IgA, and IgE classes and platelet kinetics in 33 patients with idiopathic thrombocytopenic purpura. Ann Hematol 69:121, 1994

93. Nagasawa T, Hasegawa Y, Komeno T et al: Simultaneous

measurements of megakaryocyte-associated IgG (MAIgG) and platelet-associated IgG (PAIgG) in chronic idiopathic thrombocytopenic purpura. Eur J Haematol 54:314, 1995

94. Newman PJ: Nomenclature of human platelet alloantigens: A problem with the HPA system? Blood 83:1447, 1994

95. Nurden A, Nurden P: A review of the role of platelet membrane glycoproteins in platelet-vessel wall interaction. Bailliere's Clin Hematol 6:653, 1993

96. Ochs HD, Slichter SJ, Harker LA et al: The Wiskott-Aldrich syndrome: Studies of lymphocytes, granulocytes and platelets. Blood 55:243, 1980

97. Patt YZ, Charnsangavej C, Yoffe B et al: Hepatic arterial infusion of floxuridine, leucovorin, doxorubicin, and cisplatin for hepatocellular carcinoma: Effects of hepatitis B and C viral infection on drug toxicity and patient survival. J Clin Oncol 12:1204, 1994

98. Peacocke M, Siminovitch KA: The Wiskott-Aldrich syndrome. Semin Dermatol 12:247, 1993

99. Pearson HA, McIntosh S: Neonatal thrombocytopenia. Clin Haematol 7:111, 1978

100. Perez Encinas MM, Bello Lopez JL, Perez Crespo S et al: C-reactive protein in differential diagnosis of primary thrombocytosis. Med Clin Barc 104:441, 1995

101. Philipp CS, Callaway C, Chu MC et al: Replication of Colorado tick fever virus within human hematopoietic progenitor cells. J Virol 67:2389, 1993

102. Reichert N, Seligsohn U, Ramot B: Clinical and genetic aspects of Glanzmann's thrombasthenia in Israel. Thromb Diath Haemorrh 34:806, 1975

103. Remold-O'Donnell, Rosen FS, Kenney DM: Defects in Wiskott-Aldrich syndrome blood cells. Blood 87:2621, 1996

104. Remuzzi G, Ruggenenti P: Plasma manipulation in hemolytic uremic syndrome and thrombotic thrombocytopenic purpura. Ann Med Interne Paris 143(Suppl 1):19, 1992

105. Rendu F, Breton-Gorius J, Lebret M et al: Evidence that abnormal platelet functions in human Chédiak-Higashi syndrome are the result of a lack of dense bodies. Am J Pathol 111:307, 1983

106. Rolovic Z, Basara N, Biljanovic Paunovic L et al: Megakaryocytopoiesis in experimentally induced chronic normobaric hypoxia. Exp Hematol 18:190, 1990

107. Rolovic Z, Basara N, Stojanovic N et al: Abnormal megakaryocytopoiesis in the Belgrade laboratory rat. Blood 77:456, 1991

108. Russell S, Roth GJ: Pseudo-von Willebrand disease: A mutation in the platelet glycoprotein Ib alpha gene associated with a hyperactive surface receptor. Blood 81:1787, 1993

109. Schafer AI: Essential thrombocythemia. In Coller BS (ed): Progress in Hemostasis and Thrombosis, vol 10, pp 69–96. Philadelphia, WB Saunders, 1991

110. Schmuziger M, Christenson JT, Maurice J et al: Reactive thrombocytosis after coronary bypass surgery. An important risk factor. Eur J Cardiothorac 9:393, 1995

111. Shapiro F: Osteopetrosis. Current clinical considerations. Clin Orthop 294:34, 1993

112. Sloand E, Alyono D, Yu M et al: Platelet from postop membrane glycoproteins and microvesicles in blood from postoperative salvage: A study in cardiac bypass patients. Transfusion 35:738, 1995

113. Smith CM 2d, Tobin JD Jr, Burris SM et al: Alcohol consumption in the guinea pig is associated with reduced megakaryocyte deformability and platelet size. J Lab Clin Med 120:699, 1992

114. Spencer CM, Brogden RN: Anagrelide. A review of its pharmacodynamic and pharmacokinetic properties, and therapeutic potential in the treatment of thrombocythaemia. Drugs 47:809, 1994

115. Stasi R, Stipa E, Masi M et al: Long-term observation of 208 adults with chronic idiopathic thrombocytopenic purpura. Am J Med 98:436, 1995

116. Stuart MJ, McKenna R: Diseases of coagulation: The platelet and vasculature. In Nathan DG, Oski FA (eds): Hematology of Infancy and Childhood, 2nd ed, p 123. Philadelphia, WB Saunders, 1981

117. Takahashi H, Murata M, Moriki T et al: Substitution of Val for Met at residue 239 of platelet glycoprotein Ib alpha in Japanese patients with platelet-type von Willebrand disease. Blood 85:727, 1995

118. Tomer A, Scharf RE, McMillan R et al: Bernard-Soulier syndrome: Quantitative characterization of megakaryocytes and platelets by flow cytometric and platelet kinetic measurements. Eur J Haematol 52:193, 1994

119. Verebeelen D, Jochmans K, Herman AG et al: Evaluation of platelets and hemostasis during hemodialysis with six different membranes. Nephron 59:567, 1991

120. Von dem Borne AE, Decary F: ICSH/ISBT working party on platelet serology. Nomenclature of platelet-specific antigens. Vox Sang 58:176, 1990

121. Wada H, Kaneko T, Ohiwa M et al: Increased levels of vascular endothelial cell markers in thrombotic thrombocytopenic purpura. Am J Hematol 44:101, 1993

122. Weinblatt M, Petrikovsky B, Bialer M et al: Prenatal evaluation and in utero platelet transfusion for thrombocytopenia absent radii syndrome. Prenat Diagn 14:892, 1994

123. White GC II, Workman EF, Lundblad RL: Thrombin binding to thrombasthenic platelets. J Lab Clin Med 91:76, 1978

124. Zimran A, Kay A, Gelbart T et al: Gaucher disease. Clinical, laboratory, radiologic, and genetic features of 53 patients. Medicine Baltimore 71:337, 1992

Instrumentation and Quality Control in Hemostasis

*Ruth Ann Henriksen and
Robert A. Van Dyne*

Objectives

1. Describe three ways to detect fibrin clot formation that are used in coagulation instrumentation.
2. Discuss the principles involved in currently used laboratory instrumentation including point-of-care testing.
3. Identify three parameters and associated variables that affect coagulation testing and quality control.
4. Describe how control values, reference ranges, and factor activity curves are obtained and used in the coagulation laboratory.
5. Explain the basis for synthetic substrate assays and some limitations of these assays.

In this chapter, practical considerations for obtaining consistent and reliable results in the clinical coagulation laboratory are presented. The development of instrumentation, beginning with manual techniques and extending to modern instruments controlled by microprocessors and designed for computer interfacing, is reviewed, along with considerations in selecting instrumentation. Because of the complex enzymatic nature of the coagulation process and the common use of the biologic phenomenon of fibrin clot formation as an endpoint in many coagulation tests, the results of these tests may have a larger coefficient of variation than do many tests in the clinical laboratory. Nevertheless, careful adherence to principles of quality control (QC) in instrument maintenance, specimen collection and handling, use of controls, preparation of standards, and selection of reagents will yield results that provide important information for patient diagnosis and treatment.

INSTRUMENTATION FOR TESTS OF HEMOSTASIS

Historical Development

The blood coagulation process and its associated disorders have been investigated for nearly two centuries. As early as 1911, the length of time required for a fibrin clot to form in glass tubes was used to study the characteristics of normal and hemophilic plasmas.[1] This manual technique for clotting time determination was used in the clinical laboratory for many years to identify patients with disorders of blood coagulation.[4,15,22,23] Later, the need to monitor anticoagulant therapy used in the treatment of thrombotic disorders brought additional demands for coagulation testing.

To increase the efficiency and precision of the determination of plasma clotting times, semiautomated instruments were introduced in the 1950s. Although these instruments generally required the manual addition of specimen and reagents, they provided an automatic clotting time determination. In general, the clotting time is inversely proportional to the rate of thrombin generation or fibrinopeptide A release from fibrinogen and is detected by a change in a physical property associated with conversion of the soluble fibrinogen molecule to insoluble polymerized fibrin.

During the 1970s, instruments were designed that automatically added reagents to a plasma sample and determined the clotting time. Such instrumentation now is used extensively and usually incorporates photo-optical sensing of fibrin clot formation. The 1990s have seen additional automation and data handling capabilities incorporated into instruments, which may also perform multiple coagulation tests.

Visual Detection of Fibrin Clot Formation

The use of glass tubes, a water bath for temperature regulation, a timing device, and visual observation for determination of clotting time continues to have limited application. Variables that must be controlled include the temperature, pipetter calibration, and the accuracy of the timing devices. It is difficult to control temperature in this method because the tube is repeatedly removed from the water bath to tilt it and check for clot formation (thus the name tilt tube method). However, the most difficult and least controllable aspect is the visual detection of the clotting endpoint. Nevertheless, with a little practice, it is possible to develop considerable skill with this method and to obtain much useful information.

Today, in most laboratories, manual methods have been replaced with more precise automated or semiautomated instruments. However, in situations in which plasma fibrinogen levels are severely decreased, it may be possible to detect an endpoint in the prothrombin time (PT) or partial thromboplastin time (PTT) tests visually by the tilt tube method when automated methods fail. The tilt tube method may also be used to perform the kaolin clotting time, in which a kaolin suspension which is not suitable for optical methods (see later) is the activator in the PTT test. This test is very sensitive to lupus-like anticoagulants, which cause a prolongation of the clotting time.[13,16,17] In addition, manual techniques may be useful in research laboratories whose experimental protocol does not adapt easily to available instrumentation. In smaller laboratories, manual techniques may serve as backup methods when instruments fail. When instruments are not available, manual procedures may be used to diagnose coagulation disorders and monitor anticoagulant therapy.

Electromechanical Detection of Fibrin Clot Formation

Principle of Operation. Electromechanical systems monitor the formation of polymerized fibrin. These instruments, which include the Fibrometer (Fig. 58-1) manufactured by BBL Microbiology Systems, Division of Becton Dickinson (Cockeysville, MD), or the ST4 (Fig. 58-2) from American Bioproducts Company (Parsippany, NJ), require the operator to add all the reagents to a reaction cup. Temperature control and a timing device for clot detection are part of the instruments. Timing is initiated either automatically through activation by the pipetter or by manually activating a timer. For the Fibrometer, clot formation is detected when a fibrin strand is formed between the moving and stationary electrodes and maintains electrical contact as the moving electrode rises out of the reaction mixture, thus causing the timer to stop. For the ST4, an iron ball oscillates in an alternating electromagnetic field. As fibrin polymerizes, the oscillations of the ball decrease. The instrument uses an algorithm based on these variations in oscillation to determine the clotting time.

Accuracy and Sensitivity. Although the timer for the Fibrometer is calibrated to the nearest 0.1 second, the mechanical nature of this instrument results in detection of clot formation at only 0.5-second intervals. With the software available on the ST4, precision of endpoint determination is improved to 0.1 second. Instruments that employ a mechanical clot detection system may

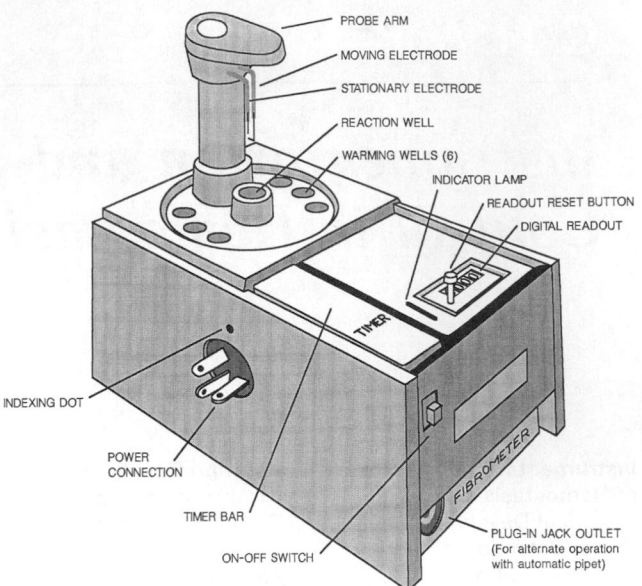

FIGURE 58-1. The Fibrometer, with essential features indicated. Instrument uses electromechanical principle for detection of fibrin clots. (Courtesy of BBL Microbiology Systems, Division of Becton Dickinson, Cockeysville, MD 21030.)

detect clot formation at somewhat lower fibrinogen levels (50 mg/dL) than optical instruments.

Sources of Error. For any electromechanical instrument, proper system operation requires accurate volume measurements to ensure proper mixing and clot detection. To meet the requirements of different test procedures, two types of probes are available for the Fibrometer, one for a 0.3-mL reaction volume and another for 0.4 mL. It is also important that the reaction cups be manufactured to exact specifications so that the cup has the correct diameter and may be seated properly in the reaction well.

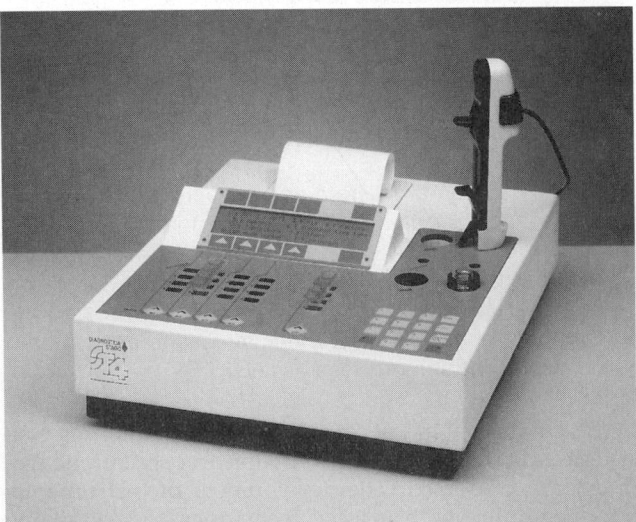

FIGURE 58-2. ST4 coagulation analyzer. The ST4 employs a magnetic-mechanical method for detecting fibrin clot formation. A software package allows storage and modification of instrument operating parameters and reference curves for a variety of clot-based assays. (Courtesy of American Bioproducts Company, Division of Diagnostica Stago, Parsippany, NJ 07054.)

For the ST4, mixing of the reagents and specimen is dependent on the size of the pipette tip used and the angle at which the reagent is pipetted into the reaction cuvette. Deviations in reagent delivery technique can significantly affect endpoint detection.

Because the electrodes on the Fibrometer probe are transferred to succeeding sample mixtures, it is important that activated coagulation factors not be transferred from one sample to the next, because such contamination will result in shortened clotting times. To prevent contamination, cleaning of the probes may be accomplished by dipping them into a dilute acid solution, such as 2% acetic acid, and rinsing with distilled water. This potential for contamination has been eliminated with the ST4 since no part of the instrument itself contacts the sample.

Comments. Use of semiautomated electromechanical instruments is less labor intensive than manual techniques, and operator-dependent variability is reduced considerably. The 1994 College of American Pathologists (CAP) survey shows that approximately 40% of all laboratories use a mechanical clot detection system for fibrinogen determinations.[11] These instruments continue to serve as a backup for photo-optical instruments, and because of differences in sensitivity, they frequently are used to recheck suspected aberrant results (*e.g.*, PT and PTT) obtained from optical instruments.

Software available on the ST4 allows for storage and modification of various testing parameters, reference curve data, reagent and control lot numbers, and for storage of data to check precision of replicate tests. The electromechanical instruments are relatively inexpensive and, therefore, may be well suited for use in research laboratories or where test volume is low.

Photo-optical Detection of Fibrin Clot Formation

Principle of Operation. Another method for detecting fibrin clot formation depends on the increase in light scattering associated with the conversion of soluble fibrinogen to the insoluble polymerized fibrin clot. In general, visible light passes through the reaction mixture and the transmitted light is detected by a photocell. As the fibrin clot forms, more light is scattered, and the amount of light transmitted decreases. The signal generated by the photocell is analyzed by algorithms that determine the point at which clot formation occurs in each sample. These instruments also have a timer to determine the interval between the addition of the final reagent, which initiates the clotting reaction, and the point of clot formation. Other features of photo-optical instrumentation depend on the level of complexity of the instrument.

Instruments. Semiautomated photo-optical instruments include the Electra 750 and 750A (Medical Laboratory Automation, Inc., Pleasantville, NY) and the AccuStasis 1000 and 2000 (Sigma Diagnostics, St. Louis, MO).

Instruments designated as automated will automatically add reagents to a sample supplied to the instrument in a disposable cuvette. These instruments include the Coag-A-Mate XM and RA4 (Organon Teknika Corp., Durham, NC), the MLA Electra series (Medical Laboratory Automation, Inc., Pleasantville, NY), the ACL series (Instrumentation Laboratory, Lexington, MA), the AccuStasis 5000 (Sigma Diagnostics, St. Louis, MO), and the Microsample Coagulation Analyzer 210 (Bio/Data Corp., Horsham, PA). These instruments generally feature control by microprocessors and data storage. Several may be interfaced with a computer for sample identification and test reporting. These instruments differ in flexibility for performing different tests, compatibility with single or duplicate testing, rate

of test throughput, sample volume required, and the option of operating with random access to different tests.

The newest automated coagulation instruments have enhanced hardware and software operating systems that provide direct specimen identification and sampling, perform complex serial dilutions on patient samples, and support extensive data management capabilities for patient results, calibration data, factor assay curves, reagent usage, and quality control. These instruments include the Multi-Channel Discrete Analyzer 180 (MDA 180, Organon Teknika Corp., Durham, NC) (Fig. 58-3), Electra 1600 (Medical Laboratory Automation, Inc., Pleasantville, NY), Microsample Coagulation Analyzer 310 (Bio/Data Corp., Horsham, PA), the Fibrintimer A (Behring Diagnostics Inc., Westwood, MA), and the STA (American Bioproducts, Parsippany, NJ) (Fig. 58-4).

Sources of Error. To allow for specimen variability and to avoid false endpoint detection secondary to the optical rippling that typically follows the addition of reagents to a sample, all instruments delay endpoint detection for a set time after reagent addition. During this "guard interval," a baseline is established for the transmitted light intensity of each sample. Therefore, a specimen with a clotting time shorter than the guard interval may be reported erroneously as having the maximum clotting time.

Photo-optical systems detect a rapid and substantial decrease in light transmission. Therefore, optical instruments may

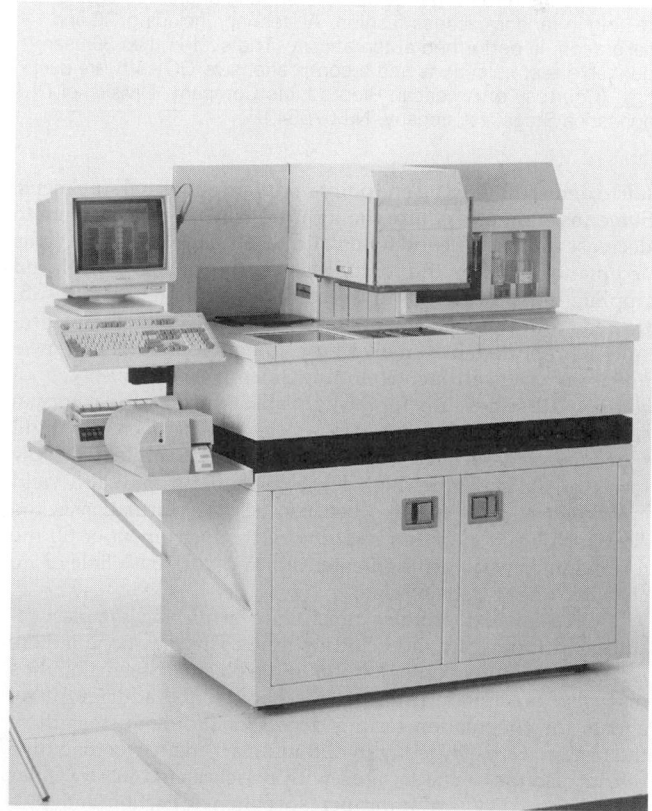

FIGURE 58-3. The MDA 180 system from Organon Teknika. This is a fully automated random access analyzer for clotting, chromogenic, and immunoassay procedures. Design includes positive displacement pumps for accurate delivery of plasma and reagents, closed tube sampling, and positive identification with automated bar code scanning and bidirectional LIS interface. The reagent tray can accommodate 30 reagents, thus providing random access for 12 assays. A modem link to technical and service groups provides support and easy interlaboratory QC program participation. (Courtesy of Organon Teknika Corporation, Durham, NC 27704.)

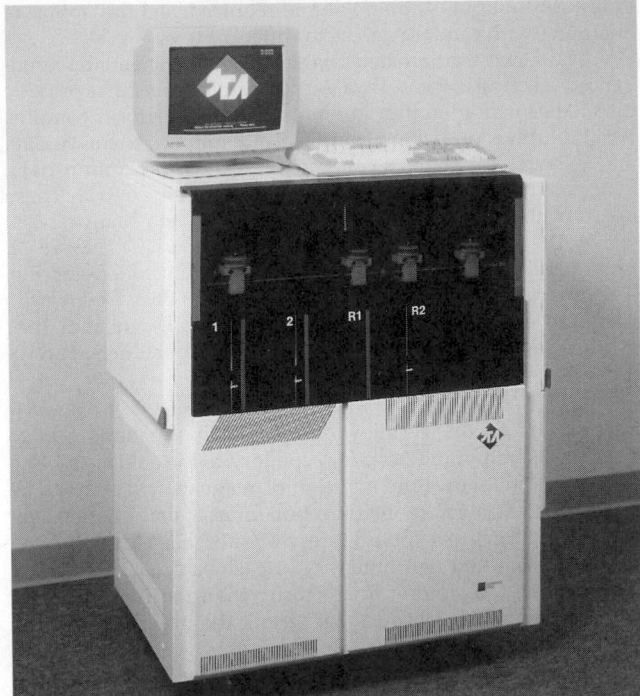

FIGURE 58-4. STA hemostasis system from American Bioproducts. This instrument performs both clotting and chromogenic testing in random access fashion. All testing, including QC and calibration, is performed automatically. The system has 80 user-definable test selections and a comprehensive QC software package. (Courtesy of American Bioproducts Company, Division of Diagnostica Stago, Parsippany, NJ 07054.)

fail to detect the clotting endpoint in certain abnormal specimens. Some instruments require the light transmission to continue to decrease for a full second for a valid result. This feature prevents acceptance of false endpoints that can be caused by delayed rippling in the sample. The 1-second observation period is subtracted from the instrument clock automatically before the results are reported. Extremely icteric, lipemic, or hemolyzed specimens may yield erroneous clotting times if an instrument cannot compensate sufficiently for the light absorbance by the abnormal specimen itself, which prevents detection of decreased light transmission associated with clot formation. Samples with low levels of fibrinogen or high levels of heparin may also yield erroneous results, perhaps because: (1) clot formation is too slow for detection of an endpoint by the instrument or (2) the formation of weak or fragmented fibrin occurs with little or no change in light transmission.

Occasionally, proteins precipitate in plasma samples, resulting in apparently short clotting times. This may occur if there is a large amount of cryoglobulin in the plasma. Macroglobulins may also precipitate from plasma because the addition of reagents for coagulation testing decreases the ionic strength of the test mixture. Difficulty in obtaining acceptable clotting time results also may be associated with disseminated intravascular coagulation (DIC) or improper specimen collection and processing. When any of these problems is present, the sample should be tested again using another method to ensure accurate results. Other possible sources of error in photo-optical instrument operation are discussed under Quality Control for Instrument Operation.

Comments. Reproducibility of clotting times determined by photo-optical instruments is expected to be 0.1 second. Photo-optical clot detection is the basis of most automated and semiau-

tomated instruments used in clinical laboratories today, and was the method used for more than 90% of PT and PTT results reported in the 1994 CAP survey.[11] As new instruments are introduced, improvements in optics permit more accurate detection of clot formation. Organon Teknika Corporation (Durham, NC) has incorporated multiple channels into the optics module of the MDA 180 so that it simultaneously monitors multiple reaction mixtures at 35 discrete light wavelengths over a spectral range of 405 to 710 nm. This allows the instrument to photo-optically detect clot formation at one wavelength while other wavelengths are used to inspect specimens for the presence of hemolysis, bilirubin, and lipemia.

Selecting an Instrument for the Laboratory

INSTRUMENT AND OPERATIONAL COSTS

A number of factors need to be considered in selecting a coagulation instrument. An initial consideration is the instrument cost. Manufacturers of coagulation reagents may make instruments available as part of a purchase agreement for reagents. Although such agreements are attractive because no capital equipment expenditure is required, it may be worthwhile to determine the cost of purchasing reagents and equipment separately.

Both the cost of the equipment and the labor cost for instrument operation should be considered in purchase decisions. Newer instruments that minimize the need for specimen handling and processing may offer considerable labor savings. However, in small laboratories performing only a few tests daily, it may not be possible to recover the cost of expensive instrumentation. Therefore, semiautomated equipment or smaller automated instruments may be a better choice. Additional considerations are the performance record of similar equipment, the cost and accessibility of repairs, and the cost of maintenance contracts.

Finally, the cost of disposables associated with instrument operation must be considered. Because the reaction cuvettes usually are unique to each instrument, it may be necessary to buy the cuvettes from the equipment manufacturer, allowing little possibility for competitive pricing. Reagent tubing may need to be replaced regularly. Other disposables are the reagent vessels, stir bars, pipette tips for handling reagents and specimens, waste containers, printer paper, and minor instrument parts.

MATCHING THE INSTRUMENT WITH LABORATORY NEEDS

It is important to consider what tests the laboratory wishes to perform and which of these can be done on a given instrument. Most instruments have a number of testing options which need to be matched to the needs of the laboratory. In some laboratories, it may be preferable to have two or more small instruments that can provide additional backup in case of equipment failure rather than one large instrument with more options than needed. Examination of current CAP survey reports[11] provides information about the reproducibility of results for different instrument–reagent systems for various tests and also indicates the extent to which a given instrument is being used in other clinical laboratories.

Other features to be considered are instrument flexibility for adding new tests, varying test parameters, throughput needed during peak testing periods, and compatibility with the reagents currently being used, or reagents from alternative vendors. Adaptability to the laboratory's desired testing pattern is also important. It may be helpful to be able to perform more than one test (*e.g.,* PT and PTT) in a single run rather than be limited to performing a single test on each batch of samples. Random access (*i.e.,* the ability to choose what tests are to be performed) to tests allows even more versatility. Laboratories that use single test results rather than duplicate testing should determine whether the instrument performs tests in one or both of these configurations. Decreasing the plasma volume required for testing may be particularly attractive to laboratories in which there is a need to minimize specimen volume. In addition, decreasing specimen size reduces the required reagent volume, which results in considerable cost savings. The instrument's software should be compatible with the laboratory data handling needs. Finally, to enhance laboratory efficiency, the instrument should be simple to operate and maintain.

QUALITY CONTROL FOR INSTRUMENT OPERATION

The quality control checks selected to monitor instrument operation will depend on the instrument and types of assays performed. Many modern automated instruments have internal system operation detection circuits. For temperature-regulated equipment including refrigerators, freezers, and water baths, the laboratory should regularly (at least daily or every shift) monitor and record temperatures. For instruments without a self-contained system for monitoring temperature, test and reagent wells may be filled with water and the temperature determined with a calibrated thermometer. In this method, thermometer bulbs must be small enough to be immersed in the liquid, and sufficient time must be allowed for equilibration. If these precautions are not observed, inaccurate and nonreproducible temperatures will be observed. Surface temperature probes may permit faster and more accurate monitoring.

Inconsistent reagent delivery may cause erratic problems in automated instruments. Although some newer instruments can monitor reagent delivery or reaction volume, older instruments generally do not. Being aware of potential problems such as crimped tubing, insufficient reagent stock, or other causes of erratic delivery is important. In the extreme case, these problems appear as a series of results with the maximum clotting time. Such an occurrence always demands further investigation.

Personnel also must know how to operate all instruments properly. Consider, for example, the selection of an incorrect testing mode. If PT testing is selected accidentally instead of PTT, the instrument may not be able to detect the error. In this situation, the wrong reagent volume may be dispensed to the reaction cuvettes, causing all specimen results to be erroneous. This scenario is a particular problem when it is necessary to change instrument settings continually because the same instrument is used for several tests.

Instrument operation manuals contain general guidelines for maintenance and QC. Some important variables are listed in Table 58-1. No program for monitoring and recording variables will detect all possible sources of error in a testing system, and there is no substitute for careful attention to system operation. Consider, for example, an acute failure in instrument temperature regulation. If this is not detected before the next scheduled temperature check, many inaccurate results could be reported. An alert operator will detect inconsistencies in patient or control results, or both, thus avoiding a larger problem that ultimately could affect patient care. The need for careful attention to changes in performance becomes even more critical as laboratories become increasingly computerized and results are reported with minimal review by personnel.

QUALITY CONTROL FOR HEMOSTASIS TESTING

Specimen Quality Control

Quality control in hemostasis begins with proper specimen collection, handling, and processing, as presented in Chapter 2. Table 58-1 lists specimen variables affecting coagulation test results. In some disease states, the delicate balance of the coagulation/anticoagulation pathways is disturbed so that the rate of thrombin generation during phlebotomy in the absence of anticoagulant is faster than normal. In these situations, it is very important

TABLE 58-1
Some Variables Affecting Coagulation Testing and Quality Control

INSTRUMENT
Temperature
Light source
Detector
Timer
Disposables
Reagent delivery

SPECIMEN
Collection system
Anticoagulant
Phlebotomy technique
Centrifugation
Delays in handling
Storage conditions

REAGENTS AND CONTROLS
Shipping conditions
Storage conditions
Reconstitution
Contamination
Deterioration
Lot changes

that the QC procedures associated with specimen collection be followed carefully.

Reagent Quality Control

In this section, the focus is on the quality control procedures for ensuring satisfactory reagents for performing routine coagulation tests: the PT, PTT, functional fibrinogen level, and thrombin time. See Chapter 49 for additional comments on the reagents.

Commercially available thromboplastin reagents for the PT are derived principally from bovine and rabbit brain or lung. Surface activators used in activated PTT reagents include kaolin, silica, diatomaceous earth (Celite), or ellagic acid,[6] all of which provide a surface for the activation of factor XII.

Test results are dependent on the specific reagents and instrumentation used.[7] Therefore, reference ranges and sensitivity to individual factor deficiencies will differ according to the test system used. (*System* is defined as any instrument–reagent combination.)

REAGENT SELECTION FOR PROTHROMBIN TIME AND PARTIAL THROMBOPLASTIN TIME TESTING

In selecting reagents for use in laboratory testing, several factors should be considered as outlined here.

Purpose of Testing. Although the PT and PTT may be used as routine screening tests for coagulation disorders, these tests may be used even more frequently to monitor anticoagulant therapy (Chap. 54). Therefore, reagent performance in producing reliable results for both types of testing must be considered.

Instrument–Reagent Compatibility. It is important that the reagents selected be compatible with available instrumentation. This may be readily achieved by selecting reagents and equipment marketed by the same vendor. However, this kind of package may be more costly and may not always best satisfy laboratory needs. CAP proficiency testing surveys are a useful indicator of the performance of various instrument–reagent combinations. These surveys can be used as indicators of the sensitivity of various systems in detecting abnormal survey samples. These surveys also report a laboratory's performance with respect to others using the same system, in addition to its performance relative to the total group of participants.

Reagent Cost. Cost must be considered in light of budgetary constraints. When more than one reagent will perform satisfactorily, a cost savings may be realized by requesting competitive bids from suppliers. A cost per test analysis is often helpful in evaluating the operational costs of an instrument. The cost per test analysis should also include the break-even volume of each test (*i.e.*, the minimum number of tests that must be performed within a specified time period to avoid a negative effect on the laboratory budget) to ensure that new assays provided by the instrument can be offered in a cost-effective manner.

Reproducibility. Reproducibility of the results obtained with a given reagent may be determined by the laboratory or from examination of the results obtained by many laboratories on survey samples. Examination of the data provided by various voluntary interlaboratory QC programs can be helpful in determining the reproducibility of quality control results between laboratories which can be an indicator of reagent lot-to-lot variability as well as instrument performance.

Reagent Sensitivity. In evaluating a reagent, the laboratory needs information regarding test system sensitivity to specific factor deficiencies, sensitivity of the PTT to therapeutic levels of heparin, and the expected results for the PT in patients receiving coumarin derivatives. Because of its possible association with an increased incidence of thrombosis, there is considerable interest in the sensitivity of PTT reagents to the lupus anticoagulant.

An important feature of a satisfactory reagent is its sensitivity to changes in coagulation factors of interest at the normal–abnormal interface. Adequate information regarding reagent sensitivity often is not available from the manufacturer or literature sources. To determine sensitivity to a specific coagulation factor, the concentration of the factor in question must be varied by mixing a factor-deficient plasma and the plasma reference pool obtained from 20 normal donors who are taking no medications and have no known illnesses. For example, this is achieved for coagulation factor VIII by mixing plasma severely deficient only in factor VIII (commercially available) with the reference pool (in which factor VIII is defined as 100%) in various proportions. The percentage of the plasma reference pool contained in each mixture corresponds to the percentage of factor VIII present. Using semilogarithmic graph paper, a plot of factor concentration in percent is made on the logarithmic scale against the PTT in seconds on the linear scale (Fig. 58-5). The straight line that best fits all points indicates reagent sensitivity. Using this graph, the percent of factor VIII at which the PTT becomes abnormal, according to the reference range established by the laboratory for this reagent, may be determined. To screen adequately for mild factor VIII deficiency, an abnormal PTT should be obtained at no less than 35% factor VIII if the population reference range has been determined correctly. If this criterion is not met, further investigation is required. This may include attention to proper handling of all plasma specimens and evaluation of alternative reagents or different lots of the same reagent.

As an example, the graph in Figure 58-5 indicates that for this instrument–reagent system, a 35% factor VIII level corresponds to a PTT of 32.5 seconds. Therefore, the upper limit of this laboratory's population reference range should be no higher than 32.0 seconds; otherwise, patients with a mild factor VIII deficiency would go unidentified using this system. Refer to Figure 58-5 for further details. It should be recognized that this determination of sensitivity assumes that the level of only a single factor is significantly decreased, in this case factor VIII. Sensitivities to other factors may be determined similarly. In situations in which multiple factor levels are slightly decreased but still technically within the normal range, an abnormal PT

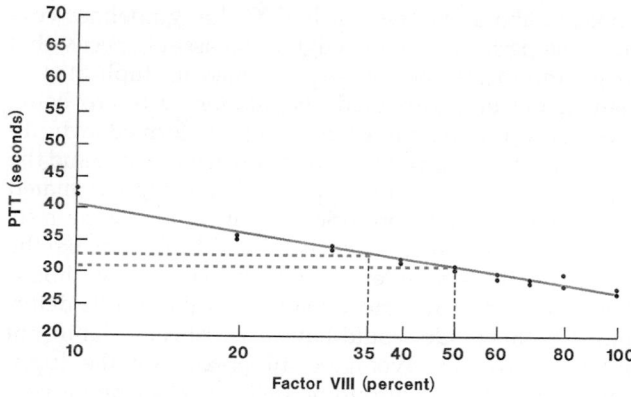

FIGURE 58-5. Sensitivity of PTT reagent to factor VIII level. The PTT was determined for plasma containing various concentrations of factor VIII. Plasma samples were mixtures prepared from a reference pool and plasma severely deficient in factor VIII. For this particular reagent and instrument combination, the graph indicates that 50% factor VIII activity corresponds to 30.5 seconds, whereas 35% factor VIII activity corresponds to 32.5 seconds. To detect deficiency conditions adequately, a reagent–instrument system should detect an abnormal PTT at a minimum of 35% factor activity. To achieve this goal, this laboratory should set its PTT upper limit to 31 to 32.0 seconds. This should correspond to the upper limit of the laboratory's population reference range for PTT. If the two limits are not almost identical, the population range may need to be determined again. Sensitivity of reagent to each intrinsic pathway factor should be checked using this technique. Every laboratory must determine its own sensitivity curve using its reagents and instrumentation. This graph is presented as an example from one laboratory. (Data supplied by Special Hematology Laboratory, Department of Pathology, University of Iowa Hospitals and Clinics, Iowa City, IA.)

or PTT may be observed.[9] This situation may be seen in patients in whom either a disease condition or therapeutic intervention causes a mild decrease in several factors.

Once a reagent has been selected, the laboratory should secure enough from a single lot to permit use for at least 1 year. Most reagents will have some lot-to-lot variability; as a result, reference ranges and sensitivities need to be checked for each new lot even though the reagent is obtained from the same manufacturer.[5,8,12,25]

REAGENT SELECTION FOR FIBRINOGEN DETERMINATION

As with the PT and PTT, the results of fibrinogen determination by the Clauss method[10] are somewhat dependent on the reagent and equipment manufacturer.[11] Therefore, the reference range for fibrinogen may be system dependent and the same instrument–reagent pair should be used to establish the reference range and to determine patient values. For fibrinogen assays, the fibrinogen standard used should be traceable to a primary standard for which the total clottable protein has been determined.

The laboratory selection of reagents depends on a combination of reagent cost and the equipment available. Fibrinogen may be determined by either semiautomated electromechanical detection of fibrin clot formation or by photo-optical instruments.[11] Generally, photo-optical instruments use the same methodology and reagents as the electromechanical ones. Alternative methods for evaluating fibrinogen are available on some instruments. The

ACL System (Instrumentation Laboratory, Lexington, MA) monitors fibrin polymerization in the PT test to determine the fibrinogen level. In this case, the PT reagent contains an antiheparin agent to prevent heparin in the undiluted plasma from interfering with the test.

SOURCES OF ERROR IN COAGULATION REAGENT USE

Once reagents are selected for the laboratory, it is important that they be shipped, stored, and reconstituted as appropriate and used in accordance with the manufacturer's recommendations. If these guidelines are not followed, erroneous test results may be obtained.

Several possible sources of error are associated with coagulation reagents. Deterioration will prolong clotting times. Evaporation from opened vials of reagent also must be avoided. If not attributable to a change in reagent lot number, short clotting times usually result from reagent contamination. Shipping or storage problems related to excessive exposure of reagents to either heat or cold, especially temperatures around 0°C, causing liquid reagents to freeze and later thaw, can cause deterioration of reagents.

Lyophilized reagents are far less susceptible to damage caused by excessive heat or cold. They must be reconstituted, using a volumetric pipette, with the volume of distilled or deionized water specified by the manufacturer. Erroneous clotting times may result from too little or too much diluent.

Expiration dates and stability guidelines for reconstituted reagents are provided by the manufacturers and must be heeded. The laboratory regulatory and licensing agencies do not approve of using reagents beyond their expiration dates. All manufacturers' reagents and controls are different and have different claims; copies of package literature should be filed with the procedures and posted with QC guidelines. Optimally, a laboratory should verify the time limitations for stability of reagents based on its own evaluation, with instrumentation, environment and usage conditions considered as important variables.

Problems may arise with changes in reagent lot. These changes can be expected and may necessitate reevaluation of the laboratory's control and population reference ranges when switching to a new reagent lot. The change in the control range may be more noticeable in abnormal than in normal control ranges. Therapeutic ranges for anticoagulation may also need to be reestablished with changes in reagent lot.

Control Materials

PROTHROMBIN TIME AND PARTIAL THROMBOPLASTIN TIME

A control plasma is intended only to monitor the performance of the testing system. A control is not a standard. Control values do not in any way define a reference range. Further, it should be remembered that the use of control plasmas in the laboratory does not detect problems associated with specimen collection, handling, processing, or storage. Most laboratories use commercially prepared and lyophilized plasmas as normal and abnormal controls to verify the performance of reagents and equipment.

Because these materials are intended only for use as coagulation controls, they are not a satisfactory substitute for normal human plasma in other procedures, such as factor and inhibitor assays or mixing studies.

Commercially available controls generally perform as specified by the manufacturer and provide both convenience and a method of monitoring precision to ensure reliable results. In many instances, reagent manufacturers will assist in interlaboratory comparison of results, which may be particularly helpful for smaller laboratories. If this type of interlaboratory comparison is not needed, a large volume of normal plasma may be obtained by the laboratory, aliquoted, and stored at −70°C for use as a control.

The CAP hematology inspection checklist suggests that controls for coagulation tests be run once each shift to verify system performance. A troubleshooting guide for unacceptable control results is given in Table 58-2. Besides monitoring the testing system, repeated performance of a given test on the same lot of control plasma permits determination of the standard deviation of the clotting time for the particular reagent and instrumentation being used. This information may be helpful in interpreting patient results, particularly those at the borderline between normal and abnormal. Long-term monitoring of the mean and standard deviation for control results may indicate subtle shifts or trends in the testing system attributable, for example, to one of the variables listed in Table 58-1. For additional quality control, some laboratories use data management systems that monitor changes in the population mean of the PT, PTT, and fibrinogen assays based on a moving average similar to the moving average programs associated with many automated blood cell counting instruments (Chap. 45).

Because of the nature of coagulation test systems, these tests generally do not have the precision of clinical chemistry tests. As a result, the National Committee for Clinical Laboratory Standards (NCCLS) guidelines covering the performance of coagulation assays specify that coagulation tests should be performed in duplicate.[19] If manual or semiautomated coagulation tests are being used, these tests are almost uniformly performed in duplicate. However, in an effort to decrease testing time and the expense of reagents and supplies when using automated equipment, some laboratories perform only single tests for routine procedures such as PT and PTT. To make the change to the single-test mode, the laboratory should demonstrate that not more than 1% of the results determined in this mode would have a statistically significant difference from the average result obtained in the duplicate mode. The use of on-line delta checks (comparison of current result with the most recently reported result for any given patient) also may assist the laboratory in detecting occasional aberrant test results that warrant verification.[18]

FIBRINOGEN AND THROMBIN TIME

Fibrinogen values usually are available for commercially prepared control plasmas supplied for PT and PTT testing. However, the laboratory may not obtain this stated result if the reagent and instrument system are not the same as those specified by the supplier of the control plasma.

Because the thrombin time test is very sensitive to small changes in thrombin concentration, the control clotting time obtained on a normal plasma prepared and handled similarly to patient plasma should be reported with the patient result. If the laboratory wishes to use a commercially prepared normal control plasma in this test, it must be established that the control plasma yields the same clotting time as fresh normal plasma. Some thrombin reagents available for automated instrument systems are stabilized sufficiently to enable laboratories to establish a population reference range for each lot of reagent, in which case, the reference range can be reported rather than the control plasma clotting time.

Establishing the Population Reference Range

Test results for the normal population (reference range) should be determined by each laboratory.[25] Commercial controls are not acceptable for use in determining reference ranges. A population reference range is established by testing plasma specimens from a group of at least 20 healthy individuals, without personal or family history of bleeding disorders, who are not currently receiving any anticoagulant treatment. These specimens should be obtained and processed in the same manner as patient specimens. The population reference range determined in this way provides an objective means of deciding whether patient specimen results are normal or abnormal. Further information on establishing population reference ranges is found in Chapter 44.

The sensitivity of the PTT reagent, particularly to factor VIII and IX levels, should also be considered (see earlier, Reagent Selection for Prothrombin Time and Partial Thromboplastin Time Testing) in arriving at the best

TABLE 58-2
Troubleshooting Unacceptable Prothrombin Time and Partial Thromboplastin Time Controls

Problem	Possible Cause*
Unacceptable normal and abnormal control results in only one test system (PT or PTT)	Test reagents
Unacceptable normal and abnormal control results in both PT and PTT	Instrumentation variables
Unacceptable results only on normal control in both PT and PTT	Normal control
Unacceptable results only on abnormal control in both PT and PTT	Abnormal control
Mixed pattern of longer and shorter results	Lot changes of reagents or controls; instrumentation variables

*See Table 58-1 for additional details.

estimate for the laboratory's population reference range. Once established, the reference range should not vary unless there is a change in the test system. System changes that might influence the reference range include changes in the sample collection system (*e.g.*, changing the concentration of sodium citrate used as an anticoagulant); changes in testing methodology (*e.g.*, from manual to automated); a change in instrumentation (another manufacturer or another model from the same manufacturer); a change in reagents or reagent lot number; and repair or replacement of instrument parts.

Reporting Results for Prothrombin Time and Partial Thromboplastin Time

The PT and PTT results are routinely reported to the nearest 0.1 second along with the population reference range. For the PT, another reporting method may be used to facilitate interlaboratory comparison and, more importantly, to assist physicians in prescribing more consistent oral anticoagulant therapy.[21] This method, the international normalized ratio (INR), is a calculated value comparing the patient PT result to the mean value for the reference range with a correction to normalize for the specific thromboplastin reagent that is used. The calculation and use of the INR are described in more detail in Chapter 54.

A corresponding standardization in reporting PTT results has not been achieved. It should be noted, however, that PTT reagents have variable sensitivities to heparin and that therapeutic ranges are reagent dependent.[5,7,8]

Reference (Activity) Curve Generation for Factor Assays

The fundamental point of reference in blood coagulation is a plasma pool obtained from 20 normal donors. Generation of factor assay reference curves (also called "standard" or "factor activity" curves) requires the use of either a reference pool collected from 20 normal donors or a commercial reference plasma with assayed factor concentrations.

For laboratories choosing to prepare and store their own reference pool, special care must be taken to ensure the quality of the pooled plasma and its stability during long-term storage. Samples from all 20 donors must be drawn within a short time (30–60 minutes) into the same anticoagulant used in routine sample collection. These samples are then processed rapidly by centrifugation to separate the plasma and cells, followed by high-speed recentrifugation of the pooled plasma to remove residual platelets. The platelet-free plasma is aliquoted quickly and frozen at −70°C. This procedure must be completed rapidly to prevent degradation of the labile coagulation factors. Obtaining a reference pool requires attention to detail and a commitment by both laboratory personnel and donors to the task at hand. For smaller laboratories, it may not be feasible to collect such a pool.

By definition, the level of coagulation factors and other coagulation-related proteins in the plasma reference pool is 100% of normal or 1 unit/mL. For fibrinogen, the concentration (mg/dL) is based on a determination of the clottable protein. Further information on the preparation and use of the reference or standard curve for factor assays may be found in Chapter 49. A sample reference curve is shown in Figure 49-4.

After the lyophilization of commercially available reference plasmas, it generally is not possible to recover all the factor activity. Therefore, the assay values for the lyophilized material are determined by repeated assay of the reconstituted material against a 20-donor plasma pool. A frozen reference plasma is commercially available with the stated values of about 100% for all coagulation proteins. Variability in handling both the reference plasma and patient specimens contributes to considerable variation in factor assay results, as may be seen in CAP coagulation survey results.

The commercial pooled reference plasma cannot be used to determine the population reference range or expected normal values for the PT or PTT. Rather, it is used specifically for establishing reference curves in assays for specific coagulation factors.

There are few primary reference materials available with known activity for coagulation proteins. One primary standard plasma with assay values for fibrinogen, factor VII, factor VIII, von Willebrand antigen, and ristocetin cofactor activity is available from the CAP (Northfield, IL). In the United States, this reference material serves as a standard for calibration of other reference plasmas and should assist in standardizing these assays.

Proficiency Testing

The use of single lots of plasma for interlaboratory comparison of coagulation test results assists individual laboratories in identifying and assessing their performance relative to that of other laboratories. Such interlaboratory comparison should increase the reliability of coagulation tests performed in all laboratories. Because the results obtained for PT and PTT are dependent on the instrument–reagent system used, results in CAP surveys are compared with those of other laboratories that use the same testing system. However, as new instruments and reagents are marketed, a particular instrument–reagent pair may not be used by enough laboratories to allow a statistically valid comparison of results. In general, clotting times are more dependent on the reagents used than on the instrumentation.

COAGULATION POINT-OF-CARE TESTING

Instrumentation

In recent years, coagulation instruments designed for point-of-care testing (POCT) have been developed. In critical-care situations, these instruments can provide rapid PT or PTT results with unprocessed (whole blood) samples, proving to be valuable as a real-time monitor of hemostasis.[2,3,20,24] This is particularly true when clotting conditions may be rapidly changing, such as during a surgical procedure or when a patient is receiving anticoagulant therapy. Point-of-care coagulation instrumentation includes the Thrombolytic Assessment System (TAS,

Cardiovascular Diagnostics, Inc., Raleigh, NC) and the CoaguChek System (Boehringer Mannheim Corp., Indianapolis, IN). Both of these instruments are portable and may be used with either whole blood or plasma specimens. Clot formation is determined by variations of the photo-optical method. The CoaguChek instrument employs a laser photometer which detects clot formation by detecting the cessation of blood flow by capillary action into a reagent chamber, where the reagent is rehydrated with either a thromboplastin (PT) or a chemical activator and soybean phosphatide (PTT). The TAS analyzer (Fig. 58-6) uses a disposable test card with a reaction chamber containing the reagents necessary for a particular test. A magnetic strip on the back of the test card provides the instrument with instructions concerning the type of test, card lot characteristics, and other test parameters. The test cards also contain paramagnetic particles which move under the influence of an electromagnet in the analyzer. When a drop (35 μL) of whole blood or plasma is added to the reaction chamber, the sample is drawn by capillary action to mix the particles, reconstituting the reagents. A photodetector observes a light change when a sample is added and automatically begins the test. The electromagnet turns on and off every second. The paramagnetic particles in the test mixture stand up when the magnet is on, causing more light to pass through the detector. When the magnet is off, the particles fall down, causing less light to be detected. Clot formation causes a cessation of this particle signal and a software algorithm is used to determine the clotting time in seconds.

Similar kinds of instrumentation are commonly used in performing the activated whole blood clotting time in cardiac surgery or intensive care units where heparin levels are monitored. These instruments generally require a special specimen collection tube containing a surface activator, which is filled and then inserted into the instrument which is temperature-controlled and times clot formation.

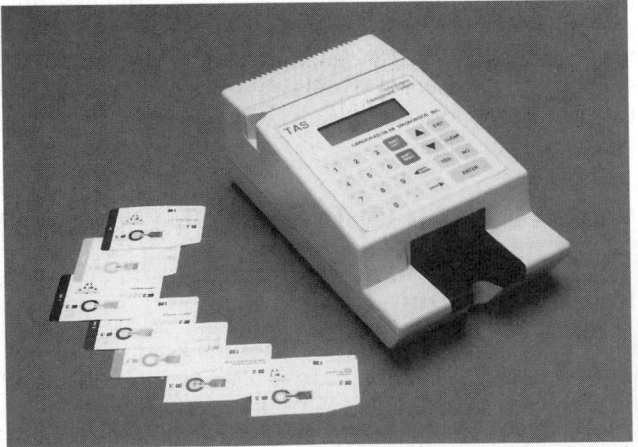

FIGURE 58-6. Thrombolytic Assessment System (TAS) point-of-care analyzer. This is a lightweight, portable instrument designed for *in vitro* diagnostic use in decentralized areas of the hospital. The TAS analyzer uses specifically developed test cards to detect the onset of clot formation or lysis in citrated whole blood or plasma samples. (Courtesy of Cardiovascular Diagnostics, Inc., Raleigh, NC 27604.)

Accuracy and Sensitivity. Point-of-care coagulation instruments have shown good correlation with traditional methods of clot detection. Studies reveal that the correlation of results with traditional methods is dependent on both reagents and instrumentation. The PT shows much better correlation with photo-optical–based systems than the PTT does. Because of the variability in reagents, instrumentation, and sample type (whole blood or plasma), laboratories must evaluate each new method in the same manner as traditional methodologies are evaluated. Good laboratory practice requires that each system used be validated with its own normal population range, heparin and coumarin therapy ranges, and sensitivity and specificity trials to ensure the accuracy of patient results. Point-of-care coagulation reagents also have lot-to-lot variability and, as a result, reference ranges and sensitivities need to be checked for each new lot, just as with traditional methods.

Sources of Error. The performance of the various POCT instruments is largely dependent on the type of specimen tested. The use of non-anticoagulated whole blood will, in many cases, severely affect the precision and accuracy of the test owing to the presence of high levels of tissue thromboplastin and activated factors in the sample.[2] Because many of these instruments are designed to use a variety of sample types (fingerstick whole blood, citrated whole blood, citrated plasma, or control plasma), performing a test using the wrong sample mode can lead to an inaccurate result.

The hematocrit can affect results as a consequence of the plasma-to-anticoagulant ratio as may be seen with other methods of clot detection. Hematocrits below 0.20 L/L and higher than 0.60 L/L can influence the rate at which the sample and reagent are mixed, especially when using a whole blood specimen. When hematocrits are outside these limits, tests should be performed using a plasma-based system with adjustment of the anticoagulant-to-blood ratio as required for the reagents used. The drop size of the sample used in the test can also affect the test result. In addition, the presence of hemolysis, bilirubin, or lipemia in moderate to large amounts may interfere with testing. Because temperature can affect movement of the sample, both the test cards and specimens should be tested only after warming them to room temperature.

Comments. Point-of-care testing will play an increasing part in patient care and is appropriate when rapidly reported results lead to therapeutic decisions. Coagulation point-of-care instruments are being designed for use by individuals without technical laboratory training. Therefore, the laboratory's challenge will be to ensure that quality control procedures are carefully followed. Documentation of QC procedures is required by several accrediting and regulatory bodies including the Clinical Laboratory Improvement Amendments of 1988 (CLIA '88), the Joint Commission on Accreditation of Healthcare Organizations (JCAHO),[14] and the College of American Pathologists (CAP).

AGGREGOMETRY QUALITY CONTROL

A platelet aggregometer measures the decrease in light scattering or the increase in light transmission as a function of time as platelets aggregate or clump in response to a stimulus added to platelet-rich plasma (PRP) (see Fig. 56-1). Several companies market instruments for measuring platelet aggregation, and manufacturer's recommendations for operation and maintenance should be followed. Proper operation requires correct function of the light source, photodetector, temperature regulation, the motor that operates the small magnetic specimen stir bars, and the recording device for data output. It is also possible to monitor platelet aggregation in whole blood by monitoring changes in electrical impedance.

Release of platelet granule contents is associated with normal platelet aggregation, and the release response may be assessed in parallel with aggregation with some commercially available instruments. Stimulation of platelets results in the release of both ATP and ADP from the dense granules. The release of ATP may be monitored with the addition of a firefly luciferase reagent to the PRP. In this reaction, ATP supplies energy for visible light production that is detected by a sensitive photocell. The ATP release and platelet aggregation may be detected simultaneously if two photocells are positioned at a 90-degree angle, one to measure the increase in light transmission as the stirred platelets aggregate and the other to measure light emission secondary to ATP release. By using a compound that fluoresces in the presence of ionized calcium, it is possible, in a similar manner, to determine the release of Ca^{2+} from platelets in response to various stimuli.

To interpret results of platelet aggregation studies properly, it is important that reproducible procedures be followed. Citrated PRP should be prepared by a standard reproducible centrifugation procedure (Chap. 56). The preservatives in commercial specimen collection tubes may affect platelet function, and for this reason caution should be exercised in the use of such tubes.

Reagents used in stimulating platelet aggregation need to be stored under conditions that will maintain maximum stability. Reagents in solution generally may be stored for 1 year at $-70°C$. Because of its susceptibility to oxidation, arachidonic acid is particularly difficult to handle. A concentrated solution of arachidonic acid prepared in dimethyl sulfoxide that has been purged with nitrogen is stable for several months at $-70°C$ when stored in polypropylene microcentrifuge tubes that have been swept with nitrogen before filling and closing.

Although maintaining the quality of reagents is the best assurance of satisfactory platelet aggregation results, a further QC measure may include performing aggregation studies on a normal specimen in parallel with the patient specimen. Because of individual variability in platelet aggregation responses and the frequent presence of aspirin or other antiplatelet drugs in either patient or control specimens, the occurrence of abnormal responses should be confirmed by repeat testing with particular attention to excluding all medication.

SYNTHETIC SUBSTRATES IN TESTS OF HEMOSTASIS

Basis for Coagulation Assays with Synthetic Substrates

Because the blood coagulation cascade consists of a series of enzymatic reactions catalyzed by serine proteases, the activity of these enzymes may be measured by methods similar to those used in the clinical chemistry laboratory. Application of synthetic substrate methods to coagulation testing presents new opportunities to test specific constit-

uents not testable with more conventional clotting tests. These constituents include coagulation inhibitors, plasminogen, individual clotting factors, and activation fragments derived from clotting factors. Substrates with various degrees of specificity for several activated coagulation factors are available. At this time, the principal drawback of the technology is the expense of the reagents and instrumentation.

Generally, these assays of enzymatic activity use a synthetic peptide substrate in which the free carboxyl group is blocked by a phenol derivative or substituted aniline. Enzymatic hydrolysis of an ester or anilide substrate results either in measurable fluorescence changes or in a change in light absorption. Figure 58-7 illustrates the spectral change resulting from hydrolysis by thrombin of a tripeptide-*p*-nitroanilide to yield *p*-nitroaniline and the tripeptide. The change in molar absorptivity per 1 cm at 405 nm (the wavelength at which the change in absorbance is measured to determine enzymatic activity; see Fig. 58-7 for explanation) is 10^4 (*i.e.*, when a 1.0 M solution of substrate is completely hydrolyzed, the absorbance at 405 nm increases by 10,000 for a sample path length of 1 cm). Because of this large change in molar

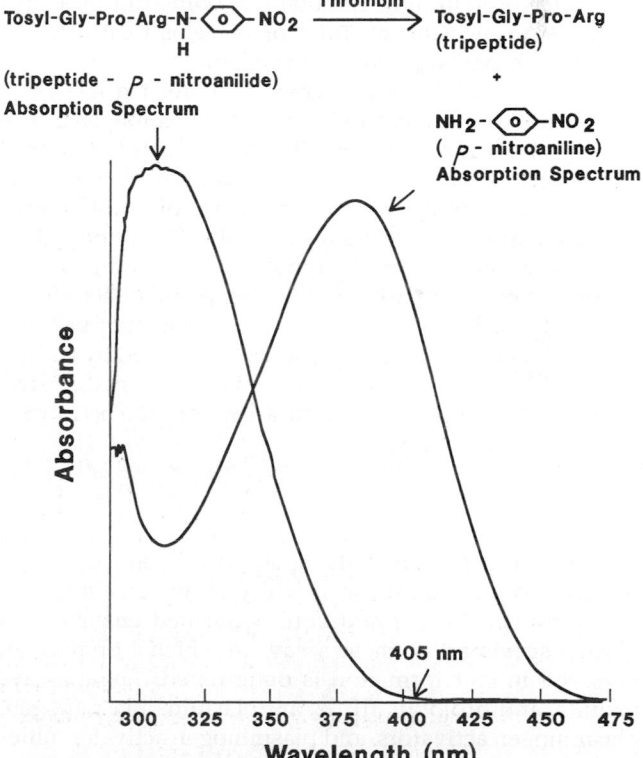

FIGURE 58-7. Spectral shift resulting from enzymatic hydrolysis of chromogenic substrate *p*-nitroanilide by coagulation enzyme thrombin. The spectrum of tripeptide-*p*-nitroanilide (Tos-Gly-Pro-Arg-*p*-nitroanilide) is shown before enzymatic hydrolysis. Wavelength of maximum absorbance for the *p*-nitroanilide is 316 nm. After hydrolysis by thrombin at pH 8.3, maximum absorption of the product *p*-nitroaniline occurs at 381 nm. Note that absorbance by substrate becomes negligible at approximately 405 nm, whereas the product has significant absorbance at 405 nm. Thus, by monitoring the change in absorbance at 405 nm, thrombin activity may be quantitatively measured with minimal interference from substrate absorbance.

absorptivity, assays with this type of substrate are sensitive to low levels of enzyme.

Instrumentation

Substrates with various degrees of specificity for several activated coagulation factors are available. Several of the available coagulation instruments (*i.e.*, ACL 3000 from Instrumentation Laboratory, Electra 900-1600C from Medical Laboratory Automation, Inc., or the MDA 180 from Organon Teknika Corporation) can perform synthetic substrate assays, and methods have also been developed in which assays of coagulation-related proteins are performed on clinical chemistry analyzers. Coagulation assays using synthetic substrates have been described for a number of centrifugal analyzers. Other automated kinetic analyzers also have been used for synthetic (chromogenic) substrate assays of coagulation proteins. DuPont has several assays available on their ACA instrument. In general, these analyzers provide automatic addition of a plasma specimen, reagents, and substrate to a reaction cuvette. The extent of substrate hydrolysis is then determined from the change in light absorbance or, in a few cases, a change in fluorescence. Through the use of a calibration curve, a quantitative measure of a particular protein may be obtained. Some ELISA assays designed to measure peptides or proteins related to the coagulation pathway are also available.

In a small laboratory where it is not feasible for a coagulation instrument to be used for chromogenic substrate testing, it may be possible to perform the desired assays on an available clinical chemistry instrument. It is not necessary that the equipment be fully automated, because many of these assays may also be performed on a visible-range spectrophotometer with a temperature-controlled cell compartment; the assays are either kinetic (substrate hydrolysis is followed as a function of time) or endpoint (the enzymatic reaction is stopped by adding acid before the absorbance change is determined). Alternatively, chromogenic substrate assays may be performed on a microplate reader.

Applications

Of the synthetic substrate assays available, the most widely accepted are those in which an enzyme inhibitor is determined by the addition of purified enzyme to a plasma specimen, or those assays in which a protein not involved in clot formation is determined. These assays include antithrombin III, α_2-antiplasmin, plasminogen, plasminogen activators, and plasminogen activator inhibitors. Quantitation of heparin and heparinoids (low-molecular-weight heparin) likewise is readily achieved by this type of assay.

Some special considerations arise with respect to coagulation factor assays. Some coagulation factors, such as factor VIII, do not catalyze a biochemical reaction but are instead cofactors for an enzymatic reaction. Therefore, factor VIII concentration cannot be measured *directly* using chromogenic substrates, and a coupled assay must be used. A coupled assay that is commercially available for factor VIII depends on the hydrolysis of a chromogenic

substrate by factor Xa generated in the presence of factor IXa and the cofactor, factor VIIIa, derived from the test sample. Knowledge of the design of these assays is also important for their proper interpretation. For example, chromogenic substrate assays may frequently use plasma samples at a higher dilution than are used in clot-based assays, and the presence of mild coagulation inhibitors thus may be masked.

The serine protease coagulation factors have limited biologic specificities, and the low-molecular-weight synthetic substrates may not discriminate among various enzymatic activities. To overcome this difficulty, a coupled assay needs to be designed. Specificity may be introduced by using specific activators or inhibitors and by careful selection of substrates and assay conditions to maximize the activity of the enzyme of interest. Because the specificity determinants for low-molecular-weight synthetic substrates are different from those of biologic substrates, it is particularly important that chromogenic substrate assays be carefully selected and interpreted when they are being used to evaluate congenital coagulation factor deficiency states or acquired deficiencies in response to coumarin therapy. Similar considerations pertain to the use of immunologic assays for the detection of deficiency states, since a cross-reactive protein may be present that reacts in the immunologic assay but lacks functional activity.

In selecting which hemostasis tests the laboratory should offer, it is important to consider not only the costs for labor and reagents and the availability of required instrumentation but more significantly, the need for a particular test in making clinical decisions. In general, tests will most frequently be needed to diagnose congenital or acquired deficiency states that may result in excessive bleeding or a tendency toward thrombosis and to monitor factor replacement or anticoagulant therapy.

CHAPTER SUMMARY

Testing in the clinical coagulation laboratory relies heavily on photo-optical instrumentation in which the change in light scattering associated with fibrin clot formation is detected as a decrease in visible light transmission through reaction mixtures containing the test plasma. In selecting instruments for purchase, laboratory needs should be matched with the available instrumentation, with consideration given to providing adequate backup during instrument failure. Careful and consistent adherence to QC procedures in specimen collection, handling, and processing, as well as in the performance of tests and maintenance of equipment, is essential to obtaining reliable results.

For the PT and PTT, the test results are system dependent, differing with both the instrumentation and the reagents used. Therefore, it is important for each laboratory to establish a population reference range using its own test systems to permit identification of coagulation abnormalities.

For coagulation factor assays, the primary standard is a reference plasma pool obtained from at least 20 donors within 30 to 60 minutes, processed quickly, and frozen. The enzymatic nature of the coagulation pathway makes factor assays sensitive to differences in the handling of the factor-deficient plasma, commercial standards, or the reference plasma pool, as well as specimens. As a consequence, large laboratory-to-laboratory variability in results is seen.

Coagulation point-of-care testing is receiving increased attention as a means of providing rapid results for therapeutic decisions. These tests generally use dry reagents that are rehydrated by the specimen. Clotting endpoint detection employs modified optical sensing systems.

As understanding of the biochemical features of the coagulation pathway has increased, enzymatic methods for detecting and quantitating proteins of the coagulation and fibrinolytic pathways have been developed that use synthetic substrates. Some caution, in terms of both assay specificity and utility for patient management, needs to be exercised in applying these assays in the clinical laboratory.

Case Study 58-1

An 8-year-old boy was seen in the emergency room for uncontrollable bleeding from a wound to the knee. The parents reported no known bleeding disorder in this child; however, they had heard of relatives who had had "bleeding problems." The clinician ordered a PTT to screen for factor VIII deficiency before deciding on any further, more expensive testing. The patient's PTT was 32.0 seconds, the PTT control value was 31.5 seconds, the commercial control range for PTT was 31.0 to 33.0 seconds, and the population reference range established for this laboratory was 22.0 to 29.0 seconds.
1. Of what significance is the control range and population reference range in the interpretation of the patient result?
2. Is there any indication for follow-up testing? If so, what might be recommended?

Case Study 58-2

In the coagulation laboratory, PT and PTT results on controls run at the beginning of the evening shift were within acceptable limits. During the next 2 hours, it was noticed that there was an excessive number of PT and PTT results that were shorter than the reference range. The short clotting times generally did not occur on the same patient (*i.e.*, if the PT for any patient was short, the PTT for that patient was within the reference range or *vice versa*). There were occasional discrepancies between duplicates. When specimens with discrepant duplicate results were retested, the results agreed with the longer clotting time of the discrepant pair. A physician called the laboratory and requested to speak with the supervisor because the PTT on a patient receiving heparin was reported as normal, and the physician believed this could not possibly be correct.
1. Is there cause for concern in this situation? Why or why not?
2. Did the controls at the beginning of the shift indicate any problem?
3. Do the erratic, discrepant results indicate any particular problem (*i.e.*, instrument, reagent, or specimen abnormalities)? Why or why not? Must all variables listed in Table 58-1 be reviewed as possible sources of the problem?
4. Should the physician be told that the specimen result is definitely correct because the controls were within acceptable limits prior to running that specimen? If not, what should be done?
5. Should the controls be repeated at this point?
6. Would a check of system precision be useful at this time? If so, how could this be performed? Should control material be used?
7. If the problem is not identified after reviewing all possibilities and erratic results persist, is it necessary to switch to a backup instrument if one is available? Should the manufacturer's technical service be contacted, or should the laboratory continue to investigate the problem on its own?
8. In any situation in which a problem is suspected, should the PT and PTT be performed in duplicate until the problem is resolved, even if the laboratory normally uses a single determination for these tests? Why or why not?

Review Questions

58-1. Electromechanical detection of fibrin clot formation is
    A. dependent on light scattering from the fibrin clot.
    B. the most commonly used method to detect fibrin clot formation in current instrumentation.
    C. dependent on the mechanical and electrical properties of the fibrin strand formed in coagulation.
    D. a complex method of clot detection, not used in modern laboratories.

58-2. Good quality control practices
    A. include reevaluation of the reference range when the PT or PTT reagent lot number changes.
    B. are not necessary with fully automated instrumentation.
    C. require that a control specimen be run with each PTT test.
    D. do not include consideration of how the specimen was obtained.

58-3. Point-of-care testing
    A. can be used for all coagulation tests usually performed by a hospital laboratory.
    B. may be a satisfactory method for routine monitoring of anticoagulant therapy.
    C. works best with refrigerated, non-anticoagulated whole blood samples.
    D. uses dry reagents, thus eliminating the need to reevaluate the sensitivity to anticoagulants when reagent lot numbers are changed.

References

1. Addis T: The pathogenesis of hereditary hemophilia. J Pathol Bacteriol 15:427, 1911
2. Ansell J, Tiarks C, Hirsh J et al: Measurement of activated partial thromboplastin time from a capillary (fingerstick) sample of whole blood. A new method for monitoring heparin therapy. Am J Clin Pathol 95:222, 1991
3. Belsey RE, Fischer PM, Baer DM: An evaluation of whole blood analyzer designed for use by individuals without formal laboratory training. J Fam Pract 33:266, 1991
4. Biggs R, Douglas AS: The thromboplastin generation test. J Clin Pathol 6:23, 1953
5. Bjornsson TD, Nash PV: Variability in heparin sensitivity of APTT reagents. Am J Clin Pathol 86:199, 1986
6. Bock PE, Srinivasan KR, Shore JD: Activation of intrinsic blood coagulation by ellagic acid: Insoluble ellagic acid-metal ion complexes are the activating species. Biochemistry 20:7258, 1981
7. Brandt JT, Triplett DA: Laboratory monitoring of heparin. Effect of reagents and instruments on the activated partial thromboplastin time. Am J Clin Pathol 76:530, 1981
8. Brill-Edwards P, Ginsberg JS, Johnston M, Hirsh J: Establishing a therapeutic range for heparin therapy. Anal Int Med 119:104, 1993
9. Burns ER, Goldberg SN, Wenz, B: Paradoxic effect of multiple mild coagulation factor deficiencies on the prothrombin time and activated partial thromboplastin time. Am J Clin Pathol 100:94, 1993
10. Clauss A: Gerinnungs physiologische schnell Methode zur Bestimmung des Fibrinogens. Acta Haematol 17:237, 1957
11. College of American Pathologists: Comprehensive Coagula-

tion Module 1994 Survey, Set C2G-2. Northfield, IL, CAP, 1994

12. Hirsch J, Dalen JE, Deykin D: Oral anticoagulants: Mechanism of action, clinical effectiveness and optimal therapeutic range. Chest 102:312, 1992

13. Jensen R, Ens GE: Advances in the diagnosis of lupus anticoagulant. Clin Hemost Rev 7:1, 1993

14. Joint Commission on Accreditation of Healthcare Organizations: 1995 Comprehensive Accreditation Manual for Hospitals, p 105. Oakbrook Terrace, IL, JCAHO, 1995

15. Langdell RD, Wagner RH, Brinkhous KM: Effect of antihemophilic factor on one-stage clotting tests: A presumptive test for hemophilia and a simple one-stage antihemophilic factor assay procedure. J Lab Clin Med 4:637, 1953

16. Lazarchick J, Kizer J: The laboratory diagnosis of lupus anticoagulants. Arch Pathol Lab Med 113:177, 1989

17. Lo SC, Oldmeadow MJ, Howard MA et al: Comparison of laboratory tests used for identification of the lupus anticoagulant. Am J Hematol 30:213, 1989

18. Morris MW, Brooker DW, Miller JL et al: Single versus duplicate prothrombin time assays. Lab Med 18:524, 1987

19. National Committee for Clinical Laboratory Standards: Collection, Transport, and Preparation of Blood Specimens for Coagulation Testing and Performance of Coagulation Assays. Approved guidelines. NCCLS Document H21-A. Villanova, PA, NCCLS, 1986

20. Oberhardt BJ, Dermott SC, Taylor M et al: Dry reagent technology for rapid, convenient measurements of blood coagulation and fibrinolysis. Clin Chem 37:520, 1991

21. Poller L: Progress in standardization in anticoagulation control. Hematol Rev 1:225, 1987

22. Proctor RR, Rapaport SI: The partial thromboplastin time with kaolin: A simple screening test for first stage plasma clotting factor deficiencies. Am J Clin Pathol 36:212, 1961

23. Quick AJ, Stanley-Brown M, Bancroft FW: A study of the coagulation defect in hemophilia and in jaundice. Am J Med Soc 190:501, 1935

24. Sane DC, Gresalfi NJ, Enney-O'Mara LA et al: Exploration of rapid bedside monitoring of coagulation and fibrinolysis parameters during thrombolytic therapy. Blood Coagul Fibrinolysis 3:47, 1992

25. Triplett DA, VanderSluys C: The importance of establishing the normal population range in coagulation testing. The Texan, Texas J Med Technol 3(4):8, 1986

APPENDIX A

Case Study Answers

CHAPTER 1

Case Study 1-1

1. Follow the steps in Table 1-5.
2. Cracked tubes should not be placed in an automated cell counter, as they may break in the instrument. If possible, the tube should be mixed thoroughly and the blood then transferred to an intact tube along with the patient label. If the tube is badly cracked, the specimen must be redrawn.

Case Study 1-2

1. Either the technologist is not using the fume hood properly, *i.e.*, with the closure at the proper level, or the hood is not functioning properly. If the hood is being used properly, it should be put out of service until someone can check its drawing and venting capabilities.

CHAPTER 2

Case Study 2-1

1. Since the Hb was falsely decreased, and there was no indication that the instrument was malfunctioning, phlebotomy error should be considered. The specimen volume was appropriate, but the lower test result suggests specimen dilution. This could be caused by excess tissue fluid in the specimen, owing to excessive squeezing at the puncture site. When questioned, the phlebotomist indicated that she had first performed two unsuccessful venipunctures before performing the capillary puncture. She was desperate to obtain a CBC specimen so that another phlebotomist would not have to travel to the patient's home. The finger puncture resulted in an inadequate flow of blood, so the phlebotomist resorted to forceful squeezing to obtain at least the minimum volume for the Microtainer, significantly diluting the specimen.
2. This situation could have been avoided by the phlebotomist's adhering to proper skin puncture technique. Warming the puncture site and performing the puncture properly using an adequately-sized puncture device should have resulted in an adequate flow of blood without resorting to excess squeezing. She should have been aware of the problems associated with poor technique and should not have submitted the specimen for testing.

Case Study 2-2

1. Again there is reason to suspect phlebotomy error. When questioned, the first phlebotomist admitted that he had only collected a single sodium citrate anticoagulated tube for PT testing and that he had had trouble entering the vein. The combination of the difficult venipuncture and failure to collect blood in a discard tube before filling the sodium citrate tube resulted in significant tissue thromboplastin contamination of the specimen. This served to activate coagulation prior to testing, resulting in the decreased PT result despite the patient's effective therapy.
2. This situation could be avoided by discontinuing the venipuncture procedure for coagulation testing specimens if a vein is not entered cleanly. All phlebotomists should be familiar with the procedural requirements for acceptable coagulation specimens. Also, the required discard tube could be submitted with the citrated specimen as an indication that appropriate technique was followed. Specimens without discard tubes could be rejected.

CHAPTER 3

Case Study 3-1

1. Since the total leukocyte count is significantly low, a buffy coat preparation would be most appropriate to look for the abnormal nucleated cells in question.
2. A leukocyte differential, red cell morphology, and platelet estimate are three determinations that cannot be done on a buffy coat preparation, because centrifugation will cause layering of cell types based on cell density. Therefore, platelets will be concentrated (they are least dense and layer on top of the buffy coat); there will be increased numbers of polychromatophilic red cells (which are less dense than mature red cells and layer just below the buffy coat); and the distribution of leukocyte types will not be totally random even after mixing owing to the fact that they also layer according to density (*e.g.*, neutrophils will layer at the bottom of the buffy coat).
3. When leukocytes are concentrated as they are in a buffy coat, the rare immature forms (*e.g.*, metamyelocyte and myelocyte) and fragments of megakaryocyte nuclei are more likely to be seen. In addition, since monocytes have a tendency to stick to one another, they may be concentrated in single areas on a buffy coat preparation.

Case Study 3-2

1. The stain pack should be checked to be sure it isn't outdated, the platen should be cleaned, and the tubing should be changed.
2. Precipitate on a blood film can sometimes be removed by dipping the slide in 30% ethanol (two to three quick dips).
3. Advantages of the platen-type stainer include reagent conservation, total automation (*i.e.*, the laboratorian can walk away), time savings, and the ability to insert stat specimen slides.

CHAPTER 4

Case Study 4-1

The technologist should check to see if the specimen is upside down. It should only take a minor adjustment, using the fine focus knob when changing from one objective to another. Most objective lenses are manufactured so that minimal refocusing is required when magnifications are changed.

Case Study 4-2

The technologist should always perform the basic steps for Koehler illumination at the beginning of any work using the microscope. Koehler illumination precisely focuses and centers the light path and spreads the light uniformly over the field of view ensuring optimal contrast and resolution of the specimen image.

Case Study 4-3

The technologist needs to align the annular ring in the condenser with the phase-changing ring in the objective. Exact centering is critical for obtaining the best contrast effect and therefore should be checked frequently. Even a slight decentering of the annular ring and the phase-changing ring can produce low contrast and a shadow effect that can cause an inaccurate, usually falsely decreased, platelet count.

Case Study 4-4

Air bubbles sometimes occur when lowering the objective into the oil or when contact is broken between the lens and the slide. Bubbles can sometimes be removed by "sweeping" the oil immersion objective from side to side. The technologist could also clean the slide and begin the oil immersion procedure again. Also, when applying oil to the slide, be careful not to introduce any air bubbles. For example, remove any air bubbles trapped in the nozzle of the oil dispenser.

CHAPTER 9

Case Study 9-1

1. The discrepancy in these results relates to the rule of three, which states that $3 \times Hb = Htc \pm 3$. In this sample, $3 \times 15 = 45$, which is not equal to 36 ± 3.
2. The four possible sources of this discrepancy are an elevated leukocyte count, a lipemic specimen, abnormal globulins in the specimen, or Hb S or Hb C.
3. To correct for an elevated leukocyte count, centrifuge the Hb mixture and determine Hb on the supernatant fluid; to correct for lipemia, add 0.02 mL of patient plasma to 5.0 mL of the cyanmethemoglobin reagent and use this as the patient blank. Abnormal globulins should not be a problem when using the recommended cyanmethemoglobin reagent. If using the original Drabkin's reagent (which is *not* recommended), correct for globulin presence by adding 0.1 g of potassium carbonate to 1 L of Drabkin's before use to keep the globulins in solution. If Hb S or Hb C is present, correct for the cells' resistance to hemolysis by diluting the hemoglobin mixture 1:2 with distilled water (1 part mixture to 1 part water), and multiplying the result by 2.

Case Study 9-2

1. No. The Hb and Hct are not normal for an adult female, because normally, the Hb does not exceed approximately 16.0 g/dL and the Hct does not exceed 0.46 L/L. These values are "falsely" elevated in this case by the extreme dehydration (fluid loss) associated with the burn.
2. The Hb and Hct are technically accurate and comply with the rule of three. However, there is a physiologic error inherent here, because this is a burn victim. Burn victims normally lose a significant amount of fluid at the burn sites, causing plasma volume to drop. This causes the temporary appearance of a high Hb and Hct. When fluids lost because of the burn are replaced in treatment, the Hb and Hct will fall sharply. In addition, erythrocytes damaged by the heat are expected to lyse, causing an even further decrease in the Hb and Hct (Chap. 18).

Case Study 9-3

1. (1) Adequate time may not have been allowed for conversion of the Hb to cyanmethemoglobin, causing the Hb to be falsely decreased; or (2) the technologist may not have centrifuged the Hct specimens long enough to achieve maximum packing time, thus causing falsely increased Hct values.

Case Study 9-4

1. Setting the rack of sedimentation rate tubes on top of the refrigerator could lead to: (1) a falsely decreased ESR because of the lower temperatures from air rushing out on opening the refrigerator or freezer; (2) a falsely increased ESR attributable to vibrations from opening and closing the refrigerator and freezer doors; or (3) a falsely increased ESR because of heat released from the refrigerator motor.

Case Study 9-5

1. A technologist could consistently read hematocrits higher than coworkers because of: (1) incorrect reading of the Hct scale on the reader wheel; (2) incorrect use of the reader wheel; or (3) including the buffy coat in the Hct reading when the leukocyte count is elevated.

Case Study 9-6

1. The RBC, Hb, and Hct are all suspect in this case, because they do not meet the criteria of the rule of three.
2. The most likely reason for the abnormal results is the markedly elevated WBC.
3. Because the abnormality seems to relate to the elevated WBC, one should investigate whether the Hb was erroneously determined *before*, or correctly determined *after* centrifugation of the mixture to remove the WBC. For the Hct, it should be verified that the buffy coat was not included. Any procedural errors should be corrected and the results rechecked, which will most likely correct the discrepancies. The RBC count is probably correct, because this value would be unaffected by a WBC count at this level.

Chapter 9 Exercises

$$MCV = \frac{28.2 \times 10}{3.20} = 88 \text{ fL} \qquad \text{9-1}$$

$$MCH = \frac{9.6 \times 10}{3.20} = 30.0 \text{ pg}$$

$$MCHC = \frac{9.6 \times 100}{28.2} = 34.0 \text{ g/dL}$$

$$RPI = \frac{14.3 \times \dfrac{0.282}{0.45}}{2.0} = 4.5$$

$$ARC = \frac{(14.3) \times (3.20 \times 10^{12}/L)}{100}$$

$$= 457.6 \times 10^9/L$$

$$CRC = 14.3 \times \frac{0.282}{0.45} = 9.0\%$$

$$\text{Retic (\%)} = \frac{20}{1000} \times 100 = 2.0\% \qquad \text{9-2}$$

CHAPTER 10

Case Study 10-1

1. The child is anemic, as indicated by a decreased RBC, Hb, and Hct.

2. Microcytic, hypochromic based on an MCV of $\dfrac{18 \times 10}{3.0} = 60$ fL and MCHC of $\dfrac{5.0 \times 100}{18} = 27.8$ g/dL.

3. Ineffective erythropoiesis, based on an RPI of $\dfrac{2.5 \times \dfrac{0.18}{0.45}}{2.5} = 0.4$.

4. Iron studies are needed to rule out or confirm the presence of iron deficiency anemia, the most common microcytic, hypochromic anemia. If iron deficiency is not present, other microcytic, hypochromic anemias need to be considered.

Case Study 10-2

1. The student is anemic, as indicated by a decreased RBC, Hb, and Hct. Her WBC and PLT are also decreased.

2. Normocytic, normochromic based on an MCV of $\dfrac{17 \times 10}{2.0} = 85$ fL and MCHC of $\dfrac{5.5 \times 100}{17} = 32.4$ g/dL.

3. Ineffective erythropoiesis based on an RPI of $\dfrac{0.5 \times \dfrac{0.17}{0.45}}{2.5} = 0.08$.

4. A normocytic, normochromic anemia with normal RBC morphology demonstrating ineffective erythropoiesis along with a decreased WBC and PLT suggests a hypoproliferative anemia. Bone marrow evaluation is needed to establish a definitive diagnosis.

Case Study 10-3

1. He is anemic, as indicated by a decreased RBC, Hb, and Hct.

2. Normocytic, normochromic based on an MCV of $\dfrac{16 \times 10}{1.7} = 94$ fL and MCHC of $\dfrac{5.2 \times 100}{16} = 32.5$ g/dL

3. Effective erythropoiesis based on an RPI of $\dfrac{22.0 \times \dfrac{0.16}{0.45}}{2.5} = 3.1$.

4. The presence of a normocytic, normochromic anemia and an effective bone marrow response indicates the presence of an anemia caused by hemolysis or blood loss. The blood film should be examined for schistocytes indicative of a hemolytic process. The direct antiglobulin test (DAT) would be helpful in determining whether the anemia is related to an immune process.

Case Study 10-4

1. He has erythrocytosis, as indicated by an increased RBC and Hct (male Hct reference range: 0.41—0.53 L/L). He also has a slight increase in WBC and PLT. All of this suggests polycythemia vera.

2. First the erythrocytosis should be classified as relative or absolute on the basis of a blood volume study and a red cell mass (RCM) determination. The differential diagnosis of absolute erythrocytosis often requires other complex laboratory testing including arterial oxygen saturation (sO_2), P_{50}, carboxyhemoglobin, and renal studies. See Chapter 35 for additional criteria for the diagnosis of polycythemia vera.

CHAPTER 11

Case Study 11-1

1. The results are typical of aplastic anemia based on the hypocellular bone marrow with mostly fat cells and the biopsy demonstrating less than 5% cellularity. Also the peripheral blood absolute granulocyte and platelet values and the reticulocyte count meet the criteria for severe aplastic anemia (see Table 11-1). The marrow in acute leukemia, megaloblastic anemia, and most myelodysplastic syndromes is hypercellular. The patient is not likely to have Fanconi anemia, because the disorder appeared at age 25.

2. Peripheral blood cell counts would be expected to begin to rise 2 to 4 weeks following successful engraftment. Reticulocyte counts should rise within a week.

3. The marrow aspirate results do *not* provide sufficient information for the physician to make the diagnosis. Therefore, the laboratory report of the marrow biopsy is critical to verify aplastic anemia. The aspirate alone may not give a true picture because of the sometimes focal nature of this condition.

4. Possible etiologies would include exposure to chemicals, drugs (both prescribed and over-the-counter), radiation, and recent infections, particularly viral (*e.g.*, viral hepatitis).

Case Study 11-2

1. Chromosomal (cytogenetic) abnormalities are seldom found in secondary acquired aplastic anemia but are commonly found in congenital aplastic anemia.

2. The disease in this case is inherited based on two facts: (1) at 10 years of age a chromosomal abnormality was found, and (2) 5 to 10 years of age is the typical presenting age for congenital aplastic anemia.

3. The most likely classification of this man's disease is congenital Fanconi anemia, a primary aplastic anemia and the only form of inherited aplastic anemia.

4. Cultured lymphocytes from patients with Fanconi anemia are uniquely hypersensitive to agents such as diepoxybutane which interfere with DNA synthesis.

5. Patients less than 10 years of age may have a normocellular marrow, but as they grow older, the marrow becomes progressively more hypocellular and eventually aplastic.

6. Progression to acute leukemia is common in patients with Fanconi anemia. This was suspected in this patient because of the slight increase in myeloblasts in the bone marrow, and because of the additional chromosomal abnormalities found on this admission.

CHAPTER 12

Case Study 12-1

1. The RBC, Hb, and Hct values are all decreased; the MCV and MCH are elevated. They indicate macrocytic anemia, the cause of which must be sought through additional tests, patient history, and physical examination. The increased MCV and MCH values are common, but not always found, in cases of megaloblastic anemia.

2. Serum B_{12} is markedly decreased since the approximate reference range is 100 to 700 pg/mL. Serum folate is within the approximate reference range of 3 to 16 ng/mL.

3. After administration of B_{12} alone, the Schilling test result indicates that the patient is not absorbing B_{12} since the 24-hour urine ^{57}Co-labeled B_{12} is less than 8%. After administration of labeled B_{12} with intrinsic factor (IF), the results indicate correction of the B_{12} absorption problem. Figure 12-6 shows the possible causes of the malabsorption, including pernicious anemia (PA) and inert IF among others.

4. IF-blocking antibodies bind with IF and block its B_{12} binding site, rendering IF unable to bind and protect B_{12} during its

transit through the GI tract. The positive result of the IF-blocking antibodies test indicates a strong possibility that the patient has PA because it is the immunologic test of choice for diagnosis of PA.

5. No. Oval macrocytes and hypersegmentation of the neutrophil nucleus do not differentiate between B_{12} and folate deficiency. Together they indicate the possibility of a megaloblastic anemia, but they do not allow identification of the specific cause. This morphology is not specific for megaloblastic anemia; nuclear hypersegmentation of neutrophils and oval macrocytes can also be found in the myelodysplastic syndromes. To be considered hypersegmented, a neutrophil should have at least six nuclear lobes.

6. Yes, the results are consistent with those for PA, including the decreased serum B_{12}, positive IF-blocking antibodies, Schilling test results, increased MCV, oval macrocytes, hypersegmented neutrophils, and the patient's age and diabetic condition.

Case Study 12-2

1. This patient needed vitamin B_{12} injections for the rest of his life because of his ileal resection. This surgery often leads to vitamin B_{12} malabsorption since vitamin B_{12} is normally absorbed in the ileum.

2. Yes, the patient could develop a megaloblastic anemia without vitamin B_{12} injections owing to the vitamin B_{12} malabsorption in the resected ileum. Of course, anemia would probably not be apparent for several years given a normal supply of B_{12} in the liver at the time of his surgery.

3. Yes, the RBC, Hb, and Hct values all indicate a slight anemia for an adult male. The anemia is normocytic based on the MCV of 82 fL.

4. Of the chemistry values given, the only abnormal values are the decreased serum ferritin and positive stool occult blood. They are not indicative of a megaloblastic anemia. However, decreasing serum ferritin is one of the first laboratory indicators of iron deficiency.

5. Yes, the increasingly microcytic erythrocyte size associated with a decreasing serum ferritin could cause an otherwise macrocytic MCV to become a normocytic MCV in this case. The decreased serum ferritin could indicate an iron deficiency which can mask a simultaneous megaloblastic anemia by causing a normal MCV since the MCV is an average value of all erythrocyte sizes.

6. Yes, the decreased serum ferritin and positive stool occult blood (which indicates gastrointestinal bleeding) are likely to be related to each other and to the peripheral blood values in this case. These values go hand-in-hand to indicate chronic blood loss and quite possibly a developing iron deficiency anemia since gastrointestinal bleeding is a common cause of iron deficiency anemia (Chap. 13).

7. Plasma total homocysteine and serum methylmalonic acid could both be recommended because they have been shown to be abnormal in the earliest stages of B_{12} deficiency, even when there are no hematologic abnormalities and the serum B_{12} is normal.

8. Yes, it does appear that the patient has been receiving his vitamin B_{12} injections regularly since his serum B_{12} and RBC folate are both normal.

CHAPTER 13
Case Study 13-1

1. From the patient's history, nutritional anemia might be expected. Because iron deficiency anemia is the most common form of anemia and occurs with high frequency in premeno-pausal women, it is the most likely cause for anemia in this case.

2. The CBC shows that the patient has microcytic (MCV 70 fL), hypochromic (MCHC 31.2 g/dL) erythrocytes. Morphologically, there is significant anisocytosis and poikilocytosis with hypochromia. These features rule out certain nutritional deficiencies that typically produce macrocytosis (e.g., folate deficiency) and further suggest iron deficiency anemia.

3. Yes, the chemistry findings do confirm the suspected diagnosis. The absence of ferritin indicates that iron stores are totally depleted. Serum iron is also extremely low, as is transferrin saturation. These features are indicative of iron deficiency.

4. The patient's reticulocyte count is expected to increase significantly in response to a therapeutic trial of ferrous sulfate. If reticulocytosis does not occur within 2 weeks of the beginning of therapy, the iron should be discontinued, and the patient should be reevaluated.

5. Most likely, a sound diagnosis of iron deficiency could have been made on the basis of the CBC results and the serum ferritin alone. If the diagnosis were incorrect, this would become obvious if the patient did not respond to iron therapy with an increase in her reticulocyte count within 1 to 2 weeks.

6. On initial diagnosis, a bone marrow examination is not appropriate, because the laboratory tests and patient history point to the most common type of anemia, iron deficiency, for which treatment is simple and patient response easily monitored without a bone marrow examination.

Case Study 13-2

1. Using the MCV, this anemia is classified as macrocytic. Considering the age of the patient, the dimorphic RBC, and the large number of ringed sideroblasts in the bone marrow, it is most likely an acquired sideroblastic anemia.

2. Yes, basophilic stippling on the peripheral blood film is a common finding in connection with ringed sideroblasts in the bone marrow.

3. The bone marrow study was performed because the anemia persisted with no response to treatment. The findings of ringed sideroblasts and dyserythropoiesis are consistent with a diagnosis of idiopathic acquired sideroblastic anemia (IASA), a myelodysplastic syndrome.

4. Cytogenetic (chromosomal) abnormalities frequently are seen in patients with IASA. Their presence confirms the neoplastic disorder, which in some cases, is difficult to unequivocally diagnose based on morphology alone. Cytogenetic studies were performed on this patient's bone marrow and a deletion of chromosome Y was documented. This abnormality, although not the most common one, is associated with myelodysplasias (see text).

CHAPTER 14
Case Study 14-1

1. The WBC is increased and the RBC and Hb are decreased. The neutrophils are probably increased and the lymphocytes decreased, depending on the established reference ranges. The most probable disorder indicated is sickle cell disease, owing to (1) the elongated red cells and target cells on the peripheral blood film, (2) the recurring chronic ulcers in the lower tibial region, and (3) the severity of the anemia.

2. A solubility test for sickling Hb should be performed as a quick method of screening for Hb S before further laboratory testing decisions are made.

3. If the solubility screening test is positive, cellulose acetate Hb electrophoresis (pH 8.4) should be performed next to confirm Hb S. If Hb S is present, it will migrate between Hb A_2 and Hb F (Fig. 14-3).

4. The elevated WBC count and neutrophilia are indicative of an infection, as is the fever. The most common infections associated with Hb S disease are pneumonia and *Salmonella* infections.

Case Study 14-2

1. The first laboratory procedure performed should be the solubility test as a screening measure. For Hb S, the results should be positive.
2. The Hbs that could be indicated on cellulose acetate electrophoresis include (1) in the Hb S position: Hb S, Hb D, Hb G, or Hb Q India; and (2) at or near the Hb A_2 position: Hb A_2, Hb C, Hb C-Harlem, Hb E, or Hb O-Arab.
3. To confirm the results on cellulose acetate, citrate agar electrophoresis at acid *p*H should be performed, which separates all of these Hbs. The resulting migration must be compared to those for known Hbs and the control (Fig. 14-3) to identify the abnormal variants.

CHAPTER 15

Case Study 15-1

1. The RBC count, Hb F, and Hb A_2 are all increased; the MCV and MCH are decreased, and the Hb and Hct are borderline-normal. These results suggest heterozygous β thalassemia (β^0/β or β^+/β). The increased Hb A_2 and Hb F exclude α-thalassemia. The lack of clinical findings in this 22-year-old patient exclude β thalassemia major, and most likely exclude thalassemia intermedia, since there is essentially no anemia. Thalassemia minima (silent carrier) is excluded because Hb electrophoresis is normal in this condition, and this patient's electrophoresis pattern is slightly abnormal.
2. The blood film evaluation for red cell morphology was expected to and did show the following: microcytosis, slight hypochromia, slight poikilocytosis with target cells, and basophilic stippling.
3. Heterozygous β thalassemia usually is not associated with any clinical disability, therefore, treatment is not necessary.
4. Affected persons have a normal life span.
5. The thalassemias follow simple Mendelian segregation. Assuming, for example, that both parents had the heterozygous genotype β^0/β, possible outcomes for offspring are: 25% chance of inheriting homozygous β-thalassemia (β^0/β^0); 50% chance of inheriting heterozygous β-thalassemia (β/β^0 or β^0/β); and 25% chance of being normal (β/β).

		Mother	
		β^0	β
Father	β^0	β^0/β^0	β^0/β
	β	β/β^0	β/β

Case Study 15-2

1. A hemoglobinopathy or thalassemia would be likely in this case because the disorder appears to be hereditary, and these abnormalities are common in Southeast Asians. Hemoglobin electrophoresis at alkaline *p*H on cellulose acetate is a reasonable test to perform, because this is an initial screening procedure that can be helpful in identifying many hemoglobinopathies and thalassemias.
2. Alpha thalassemia in Southeast Asians may be associated with a one- ($-\alpha/\alpha\alpha$), two- ($--/\alpha\alpha$ or $-\alpha/-\alpha$), three- ($--/-\alpha$), or four- ($--/--$) α-gene deletion. The four-gene deletion, Bart's hydrops fetalis, is ruled out since the patient is 17 years old. Little or no anemia is associated with one or two α-gene

deletions. Most likely, this patient has Hb H disease ($--/-\alpha$), since her anemia is moderate.
3. Because the mother has mild anemia, her genotype is most likely heterozygous α^0 thalassemia ($--/\alpha\alpha$). The father is not anemic, but the daughter is believed to have Hb H disease ($--/-\alpha$), so he may have heterozygous α^+ thalassemia ($-\alpha/\alpha\alpha$).
4. If this patient does in fact have Hb H disease, Hb H (2 to 40%) should appear on cellulose acetate electrophoresis (alkaline *p*H) along with Hb A and decreased A_2. A trace amount of Hb Bart's might also be seen.

Case Study 15-3

1. The abnormalities shown by electrophoresis include a decreased percentage of Hb A and the presence of Hb S. Alkali denaturation indicates an increase in Hb F (for adults, normal is less than 2%), and microchromatography indicates an increase in Hb A_2 (normal is 2.0% to 3.5%).
2. For the hemoglobinopathies listed, increased levels of Hb F are associated with sickle cell disease and Hb S–thalassemia, and may be associated with Hb SC, whereas increased A_2 usually occurs only in Hb S–thalassemia.
3. The most likely diagnosis is Hb S–β^+-thalassemia. β^+-thalassemia is indicated by the presence of 21% Hb A, which requires some production of β chains. Also a rare sickle cell is more indicative of Hb S–β^+- than Hb S–β^0- thalassemia.
4. The MCV of 84 fL and the severe anemia are not generally consistent with a diagnosis of Hb S–β^+-thalassemia. This disorder usually causes a decreased MCV, whereas 84 fL is within the reference range for adults. Perhaps this patient's usual MCV is near the high point of the reference range, and therefore the MCV is depressed for him as an individual. The MCH is decreased, which is typical of Hb S–β^+-thalassemia.
5. The most likely diagnosis would be Hb S–β^0-thalassemia. In β^0-thalassemia, no Hb A is produced because no β chains are produced.

CHAPTER 16

Case Study 16-1

1. Judging from the RBC morphology, the RDW is expected to be increased. The normal MCV represents the average cell volume of a mixture of small and large erythrocytes as seen on the blood film. The reticulocyte count should be elevated if the patient's bone marrow is able to respond to the anemia. The presence of moderate polychromasia suggests that the reticulocyte count is elevated.
2. The presence of schistocytes, microspherocytes, and echinocytes suggests hemolysis caused by mechanical damage. This patient's anemia was caused by both erythrocyte destruction by the prosthesis and blood loss in the lungs.
3. Red cell fragmentation caused by prosthetic valves can occur in the immediate postoperative period as a result of poor valve design or placement. Later, if the valve becomes infected, local clotting may occur. Deposition of fibrin strands in the area injures red cells as they pass through the vessels. Also the infection and clotting may cause the valve to function poorly, forcing red cells to pass through an irregular opening with more turbulence than is normal in the heart.
4. The prolonged PT and PTT, along with the decreased platelet count and the abnormal red cell morphology, suggest intravascular coagulation, though it may be local rather than disseminated in this case. The presence of fibrin split products or decreased fibrinogen would support the diagnosis, although the patient's liver disease may affect the reliability of those results. Chemistry laboratory results would probably show increased serum unconjugated bilirubin and LD, and decreased

serum haptoglobin. Urinalysis would probably reveal increased urobilinogen, free hemoglobin, and hemosiderin.

Case Study 16-2

1. The reddish tinge indicates the presence of increased free hemoglobin in the plasma and is strongly indicative of an intravascular hemolytic process.
2. The low Hb and Hct were most likely caused by acute intravascular hemolysis due to *Clostridium* septicemia. They do not match according to the rule of three. The Hb appears high compared to the Hct. This is caused by the fact that the cyanmethemoglobin reaction measures both intra- and extracellular Hb, *i.e*, both in the red cells and that which is free in the plasma from hemolysis, whereas the Hct must be calculated based only on intact red cells.
3. Additional studies to confirm the presence of a severe intravascular hemolysis would include serum haptoglobin (absent); hemopexin (decreased); plasma hemoglobin (increased); and urine hemoglobin and hemosiderin (both positive). Elevated levels of plasma unconjugated bilirubin, urine urobilinogen, and lactate dehydrogenase (LD) would also be present in this case, as well as in cases of increased extravascular hemolysis.

CHAPTER 17

Case Study 17-1

1. The peripheral blood film and other laboratory data indicate a nonimmune (DAT negative) spherocytic hemolytic anemia.
2. The laboratory data and family history suggest hereditary spherocytosis.
3. An osmotic fragility test is necessary for diagnosis, and results should reveal increased susceptibility of the patient's red cells to osmotic lysis.
4. The patient is suffering from aplastic crisis. The viral infection associated with influenza temporarily halted erythropoiesis while hemolysis continued.
5. The patient's mother and brother most likely suffer from the same disorder. Both should have increased numbers of microspherocytes on the peripheral blood film with mild anemia. Although it might be expensive and probably unnecessary to check, both most likely have an increased erythrocyte osmotic fragility.

Case Study 17-2

1. The ascorbate-cyanide test is positive because the brown color indicates that methemoglobin formed as a result of G6PD deficiency in the patient's specimen. This test is less specific but more sensitive than the G6PD fluorescent spot test. On the contrary, the demonstration of fluorescence on the fluorescent spot test probably indicates a false-normal G6PD caused by the suspected hemolytic episode. Hemolytic episodes cause increased levels of reticulocytes and some younger cells in circulation, which may temporarily elevate G6PD levels to the normal range in G6PD-deficient individuals.
2. The fluorescent spot test can be repeated using a centrifuged specimen from which the top quarter (1/4) of the erythrocyte population, which contains reticulocytes, has been removed. This procedure lessens the effect of higher levels of G6PD in reticulocytes and younger red cells and would be expected to yield no fluorescence in the G6PD fluorescent spot test, indicating a G6PD deficiency.
3. The RPI calculation is

$$\frac{22 \times \dfrac{0.19}{0.45}}{2.5} = 3.7$$

Since the general rule for adequate response to anemia is >3.0 (Chap. 10), it appears that the bone marrow in this case is mounting a good erythropoietic response to anemia.
4. A quantitative G6PD assay could be done to confirm or rule out G6PD deficiency.

CHAPTER 18

Case Study 18-1

1. For a 4-year-old boy, the RBC, Hb, and Hct are decreased. The MCV and MCHC are just slightly out of the reference range according to Table 9-1. The neutrophils appear slightly increased, probably as a result of the infection, and the lymphocytes appear decreased according to Table 24-3.
2. The variable red cell morphology may be caused by a combination of hemolysis (as indicated by schistocytes) and oncoming iron deficiency, both of which could produce the population of microcytic cells and the slight hypochromia. Iron deficiency may be the result of inadequate dietary intake, since the child's appetite has been poor, and he is at an age when iron requirements are increased because of growth.
3. Yes, the poikilocytes are significant in this case. It is not normal to see moderate burr cells in an acceptable area of blood film examination. And even a few schistocytes can be very significant in the diagnosis of a hemolytic disorder.
4. Hemolytic uremic syndrome (HUS) is particularly associated with the finding of burr cells. HUS is usually found in infants and young children.
5. There are a number of significant urinalysis and chemistry findings in HUS. Urinalysis generally demonstrates the presence of protein, WBC, RBC, and casts. The uremic portion of HUS usually causes measurements of blood urea nitrogen and creatinine to be markedly elevated, and serum unconjugated bilirubin may be elevated. The hemolytic portion of HUS causes plasma Hb to be increased, which causes an expected decrease in haptoglobin.
6. The expected results of coagulation and platelet function tests in HUS are generally within reference ranges. Therefore none would be recommended unless the diagnosis was unclear from other laboratory results, except perhaps a routine prothrombin time and partial thromboplastin time as a screen for coagulation competency.
7. If HUS is the correct diagnosis, the prognosis is good if the renal failure can be treated.
8. The finding of β-hemolytic *Streptococcus pyogenes* in the throat culture does relate to the HUS condition. Often in HUS there is an inciting event such as infection or trauma, which may have been the case for this child. Treating the infection might go a long way toward correcting both the renal damage and the hemolytic process.

Case Study 18-2

1. Yes, problems such as pre-eclampsia, a common complication of pregnancy, are known to cause microangiopathic hemolytic anemia (Table 18-2).
2. The burr cells and schistocytes indicate hemolysis.
3. Yes the elevated liver enzyme alanine aminotransferase does relate to the suggested diagnosis of pre-eclampsia, because it suggests that the patient may have developed the syndrome called hemolytic anemia with elevated liver enzymes and low platelet count (HELLP), which is a subset of severe preeclampsia. This patient's platelet count is borderline normal, but may be decreased as compared to her usual platelet count.
4. In TTP, the liver enzyme alanine aminotransferase should not be elevated as it is in the HELLP syndrome. Also in TTP, the signs and symptoms include cerebral manifestations such as

loss of consciousness and seizures. These are not found in the HELLP syndrome.

CHAPTER 19
Case Study 19-1

1. Yes. The Hb and Hct match according to the rule of three, because the Hb is 8.0 g/dL and $3 \times 8.0 = 24.0$. By definition, the Hct must fall within $24 \pm 3\%$, and it does at 22% or 0.22 L/L.
2. The most likely cause of the red urine is hemoglobin caused by sudden hemolysis. It can also be caused by intact red cells, myoglobin (muscle Hb), some drugs and dyes, and congenital erythropoietic porphyria (CEP; Chap. 7).
3. The combination of having had the flu and playing out in the snow might be significant.
4. Since ingestion of drugs or other toxic material was denied, the physician might consider paroxysmal cold hemoglobinuria (PCH), the disorder brought on by cold and viruses, and also hemoglobinopathies, other types of hemolytic anemias, and red cell metabolic defects.
5. Additional tests that could be recommended include each of the following, for which the results in this case are indicated: urinalysis revealed Hb; the DAT was positive with polyspecific sera and anticomplement sera; the antibody showed anti-P specificity; the blood film revealed rouleaux; serum haptoglobin was decreased; and the Donath-Landsteiner (D-L) test was positive.
6. None except a recommendation that the boy be kept out of cold temperatures. The boy's problem was diagnosed as PCH with hemolysis owing to the viral infection and cold exposure. This hemoglobinuria is self-limited, and the boy recovered spontaneously.

Case Study 19-2

1. No. The Hb and Hct do not match according to the rule of three, because the Hb is 13.5 g/dL and $3 \times 13.5 = 40.5$. By definition the Hct must fall within $40.5 \pm 3\%$ which, at 36% or 0.36 L/L, it does not. The laboratorian should not expect the Hb and Hct values to match because the indices indicate macrocytic and hyperchromic cells, whereas the rule of three applies only to normal cells.
2. No. The RBC and Hb do not match. In general the RBC $\times$ 3 = Hb, however in this case $3.2 \times 3 = 9.6$, which is significantly different from the Hb of 13.5 g/dL. The lack of correlation discussed in answer number 1 and in this answer might also be accounted for by the fact that the whole blood Hb measurement includes Hb inside the red cells *and* that which is free in the plasma, whereas the Hct measurement and RBC count are based only on intact red cells. Therefore, in severe intravascular hemolysis, the Hb reading will appear disproportionately high compared to the RBC count and the Hct.
3. All red cell indices are above the usual reference range, and the MCH is particularly suspicious because it is grossly abnormal. Also the RBC count is decreased in comparison to the Hb (see number 2 above). Such abnormalities are often indicative of cold agglutinins.
4. The laboratory scientist could observe the sample tube carefully for clumping of red cells on the walls of the tube at room temperature. This was done and small red cell clumps were noted. The patient indeed had a significant amount of cold agglutinins. Red cell clumps cause a false decrease in the RBC count and an elevated MCV (each clump is seen as one large cell by the automated cell counter). The Hct is lower than it should be; therefore, it must be performed manually.

The MCH and MCHC values are abnormal because of the agglutinating cells.
5. Yes, the WBC and Hb results are accurate as they are usually unaffected by cold agglutinins. All cells, single or clumped, are hemolyzed for the Hb reading.
6. The specimen should be warmed to 37°C for at least 15 minutes, mixed while warm, and sampled immediately in order to produce reliable results.

CHAPTER 20
Case Study 20-1

1. Yes, these results are all consistent with chronic blood loss (Table 20-2).
2. Iron deficiency anemia is the most common of the microcytic, hypochromic anemias. An elevated RDW is often associated with, but not specific for, iron deficiency.
3. Gastrointestinal (GI) bleeding is the most likely cause of anemia in adult men and postmenopausal women.
4. The stool occult blood test could be useful to confirm GI blood loss, in which the test is usually positive. Also serum ferritin may be useful to rule out a heterozygous, clinically mild or silent hemoglobin disorder, such as α-thalassemia minor or β-thalassemia trait (Chap. 15). Both of these disorders could also cause a low MCV, but a normal or increased serum ferritin, whereas serum ferritin is decreased in iron deficiency anemia.

Case Study 20-2

1. The results are consistent with acute blood loss, which results in a proportional loss of red cells and plasma. The Hb and Hct are expected to be normal in early acute blood loss. As intravenous solutions are given and the body compensates by drawing fluid from interstitial spaces, the blood becomes diluted to reflect the true degree of red cell loss.
2. The reticulocyte count would probably be normal at admission and rise dramatically over the next several days reaching a maximum of 15% (RPI greater than 3) in ten days.
3. It is important to calculate the RPI rather than using the uncorrected reticulocyte count when assessing recovery from acute blood loss, because under intense erythropoietic stress, the number of reticulocytes circulating may be markedly increased without a corresponding increase in bone marrow reticulocytes. An RPI greater than 3 indicates an adequate bone marrow response to anemia (Chaps. 9 and 10).

CHAPTER 22
Case Study 22-1

The rapidly elevated leukocyte count was probably caused by a shift of leukocytes from the marginated to the circulating pool. An increase occurring this rapidly indicates a physiologic response possibly caused by patient anxiety. An increase owing to neutrophils being recruited from the bone marrow storage pool as a result of tissue damage would not occur for approximately 4 to 5 hours.

Case Study 22-2

The new employee is probably using different criteria (*e.g.*, the nucleus must have no indentations to be called a band) for identification of band neutrophils. These criteria differ widely depending on the laboratory. The supervisor should review the criteria being used in this laboratory with the new employee and ensure that the he or she understands the criteria before reports are released.

CHAPTER 23

Case Study 23-1

1. The two cells most likely to be confused with the small lymphocyte are the microblast and the rubricyte. The arrangement of the nuclear chromatin is the single most helpful characteristic in the identification of the majority of cell types.
2. Normal lymphocytes, like the ones in this case, characteristically have dense blocks of heterochromatin located predominately in the central and peripheral areas of the nucleus. The nuclear chromatin of microblast cells may be delicate, giving a stippled appearance, or dense and structureless (hematogones), whereas the dense clumps of heterochromatin with pale or unstained areas of parachromatin of the rubricyte give a checkerboard appearance. The cytoplasm of the rubricyte has a mingling of blue (RNA) and pink (hemoglobin) to give a "muddy" appearance. In this case, the large volume of nucleus with scant, blue, nongranular cytoplasm is characteristic of either a small lymphocyte or a blast cell; however, the nuclear chromatin as described is not characteristic of a blast.
3. CD8 surface markers indicate that the cells are T cells belonging to the suppressor and/or cytotoxic subset.

Case Study 23-2

1. The cells are most likely B cells, but not CFU-L. The morphologic description of the cells and the presence of cell markers CD10 and CD19 are compatible with the pre-B cell (hematogone). TdT is sometimes positive for pre-B cells. The CFU-L (lymphoid stem cell) is characterized by the absence of cell markers CD10 and CD19 and by the presence of CD34 and *c-kit*. These characteristics are absent from the cells of this marrow. Cell markers for the T cell lineage (CD2, cytoplasmic CD3, and CD7) are absent.
2. The most likely cause for the presence of the pre-B cell in this patient's marrow is regeneration of the lymphoid population following bone marrow transplantation. These cells may be found in the bone marrow in several conditions, *e.g.*, in very young children, following bone marrow transplantation, in acute lymphoblastic leukemia in remission, and in iron deficiency anemia.

CHAPTER 24

Case Study 24-1

1. No. Tech number 3's results do not fall within the 95% confidence limits. According to Table 24-6, the 95% confidence limits for a 100-cell differential count for the observed automated value of 10% should be 4% to 18% monocytes. All other laboratory scientists' results are within the expected range.

Case Study 24-2

1. Assuming that the baby is closer to 12 hours old than 1 week old (Table 24-3), the relative and absolute lymphocyte counts are below the reference range; the relative and absolute monocyte counts are above the reference range. The smudge cells may indicate abnormally fragile lymphocytes.
2. Yes, the WBC count does need correction since there are more than 5 NRBC per 100 WBC. The calculation is:

$$\frac{30.0 \times 10^9/L}{8 + 100} \times 100 = 27.8 \times 10^9/L$$

3. In addition to all of the leukocyte percentages (totalling 100%), the differential report should include the number of smudge cells found, since smudge cells may indicate the presence of abnormal lymphocytes. The report should also include the number of NRBC per 100 WBC and the corrected WBC count, although NRBC are normal on a newborn's blood film. And finally, the report should include the number of megakaryocyte fragments found, although these are also normal on a newborn's blood film.

Chapter 24 Exercises

24-1. $(250 + 265)/2 = 257.5$ = Average no. cells counted

$$\frac{257.5 \times 20}{4 \times 0.1} \times 10^6/L = 12.9 \times 10^9/L$$

24-2. (A). Based on the peripheral blood findings, the leukocyte count estimate is $(70 \times 1.5 \times 10^9/L) = 105.0 \times 10^9/L$

(B). Based on Table 24-1, a 1:200 dilution should be made for manual WBC counting. An RBC Thoma pipette should be used.

(C). $(170 + 184)/2 = 177$ = Average no. cells counted

$$\frac{177 \times 200}{4 \times 0.1} \times 10^6/L = 88.5 \times 10^9/L$$

24-3. Yes, all differential counts that reveal more than five nucleated RBC per 100 WBC indicate the need for a WBC count correction.

$$\frac{20.0 \times 10^9/L \times 100}{20 + 100} = 16.7 \times 10^9/L$$

24-4. (A). $\dfrac{194 \times 10}{4 \times 0.1} \times 10^6/L = 4.9 \times 10^9/L$

(B). $\dfrac{383 \times 20}{4 \times 0.1} \times 10^6/L = 19.2 \times 10^9/L$

(C). $\dfrac{273 \times 10}{8 \times 0.1} \times 10^6/L = 3.4 \times 10^9/L$

(D). $\dfrac{207 \times 200}{8 \times 0.1} \times 10^6/L = 51.8 \times 10^9/L$

(E). $\dfrac{50 \times 32}{40 \times 0.2} \times 10^6/L = 0.2 \times 10^9/L$

24-5. $(0.08 \times 8.4 \times 10^9/L) = 0.7 \times 10^9/L$. This result is *not* within the usual reference range for an adult; it indicates eosinophilia. It *is* within the reference range for infants and small children (Table 24-3).

CHAPTER 25

Case Study 25-1

1. The findings that indicate CML include the markedly increased WBC count, severe left shift (including blast forms), and the presence of NRBC, which might indicate marrow replacement by leukemic cells. The findings that are unusual for CML are the lack of increased eosinophils and basophils and the lack of circulating immature forms of eosinophils and basophils. NOTE: The toxic neutrophil morphology cannot be used to diagnose *or* rule out CML, since patients with CML and a superimposed infection and those receiving chemotherapy may exhibit toxic morphology, such as toxic granulation in their neutrophils.
2. The toxic granulation is most likely real for two reasons: (1) only 60% of neutrophils are affected, and (2) the presence of Döhle bodies supports the toxic morphology.
3. There is an absolute monocytosis. Three percent multiplied by the total leukocyte count equals $3.18 \times 10^9/L$, an increased number of monocytes per liter (Table 24-3).

4. An NAP of 316 is increased and indicates reactive rather than malignant leukocytosis. The NAP is usually decreased in CML. Further investigation revealed that this patient had a brain abcess; the infection was subsequently controlled with antibiotics. It should be noted that occasionally a patient with CML may experience bacterial infections or other stressful conditions that cause the normal granulocytes to react with an increased amount of alkaline phosphatase. For example, a patient with CML and an NAP score of 2 contracted a bacterial infection. The patient's NAP score rose to 98, which is within the normal reference range.

Case Study 25-2

1. Probable diagnosis: sepsis; possible toxic shock syndrome. Cause of thrombocytopenia could be bone marrow depression, or possibly peripheral destruction of platelets. Cause of the left shift, a toxic reaction to foreign antigens.
2. A viral infection, possibly CMV, acquired through the transfusions.
3. The absolute lymphocyte count equals $(14.0 \times 10^9/L) \times 0.60 = 8.4 \times 10^9/L$.
4. Confirmation tests: CMV antibody titers and negative heterophil antibody test.

CHAPTER 26
Case Study 26-1

1. The most likely cause of the differential findings is the presence of Pelger-Huët anomaly.
2. These cells should be reported as mature neutrophils with a comment about the presence of Pelger-Huët cells.
3. It is important that these cells not be confused with immature granulocytic forms such as bands, metamyelocytes, and myelocytes whose presence might indicate an infectious process with a "shift to the left."

Case Study 26-2

1. Both red cells and platelets were being sequestered and possibly destroyed by the enlarged spleen.
2. Thrombocytopenia, abnormal platelet function, and liver dysfunction leading to a decrease in coagulation factors could all have contributed to the bleeding problem.
3. The increased bilirubin, increased liver enzymes, and the prolonged prothrombin time indicate liver dysfunction.

CHAPTER 28
Case Study 28-1

1. The optimum time for leukapheresis was on day 9 of mobilization therapy, when the patient's leukocyte count recovered from its lowest point. At this time, the most immature progenitors and pluripotent stem cells are mobilized into the peripheral circulation.
2. The leukapheresis product and after-antibody fractions should have about the same CD34+ purity. The initial numbers in this patient are very good. The eluate should be enriched, while the unadsorbed fraction from the column should have a greater volume and be depleted of CD34+ cells. The case study data correlate with theoretical expectations.
3. The patient was considered to engraft on day +11 (11 days following the transplant) according to the criteria (*i.e.*, when the absolute neutrophil count is higher than $0.5 \times 10^9/L$ for three consecutive days). This timely recovery occurred because the autograft was enriched with progenitors and stem cells.
4. The autograft was concentrated to a small volume with high CD34 purity. This purged the graft of occult tumor cells, which

provided one more safeguard in addition to high dose chemoradiotherapy.

Case Study 28-2

1. A T-cell depletion was performed because the father and son had a one-antigen mismatch in their HLA types; T-cell depletion minimizes GVHD. It would be rare if all six HLA-A, -B, and -DR loci of a father and son were identical since one set of alleles is inherited from each parent. The probability of such a match is higher among siblings.
2. No. Judging from the laboratory data, there was an apparent enrichment of CFU-GM colonies. Note that the decrease in BFU-E is not likely to be a problem because erythroid engraftment is seldom a concern.
3. (a) The limiting dilution assay (LDA) is a quantitative assay of cultured T cells, whereas flow cytometry using a fluorescence-activated cell sorter (FACS) separates a cell population using a monoclonal antibody-fluorescent conjugate. (b) The log depletion fell within the expected range of a successful depletion, between 1.0 and 3.0 in both assays (see data chart). (c) The results of both methods correlate very well because both accurately measure T cells.
4. Ineffective depletion of T cells produces severe graft-versus-host disease (GVHD). However, mild GVHD is desirable for the graft-versus-leukemia (GVL) effect, therefore the T-cell depletion method should not be so sensitive as to exceed a 3.0 log depletion.

CHAPTER 29
Case Study 29-1

1. Periodic acid-Schiff stain is used to demonstrate carbohydrate (*e.g.*, glycogen) present in cells—either in the granules (granular positivity) or free in the cytoplasm (diffuse or granular). Ordinarily, this is seen in cells of granulocytic, monocytic, and megakaryocytic lineage. Erythrocyte precursors normally do not stain, but in M6 erythroleukemia, intense cytoplasmic PAS positivity may be seen in erythroid precursors. Likewise, lymphocytes usually do not stain (or only stain very faintly). However, in acute lymphoblastic leukemia, the lymphoblasts are frequently strongly PAS positive with large granular or "chunky" positivity.
2. The diagnosis is most likely FAB M6—erythroleukemia that developed following a history of a dysmyelopoietic syndrome (Chap. 33). Sudan black B and peroxidase are negative in M6 erythroleukemia (as in this case) but positive in the myelocytic and monocytic leukemias (FAB M1—M5) (Table 34-1).

Case Study 29-2

1. Nonspecific esterase.
2. Monocytes.
3. Alpha-naphthyl butyrate.
4. The most likely diagnosis is acute monocytic leukemia (FAB M5).

CHAPTER 30
Case Study 30-1

1. The CSF cell count reference range for a child <1 year old is WBC 0 to $30 \times 10^6/L$ and RBC $0 \times 10^6/L$. Therefore, the WBC count is normal, but the RBC count is markedly elevated.
2. Not necessarily. The blasts could result from peripheral blood contamination from a traumatic tap. The RBC:WBC ratio in the peripheral blood must be compared with that in the CSF. If these two ratios are approximately equal or the ratio is higher in the CSF, it cannot be determined whether the patient actually has CNS disease, because a traumatic tap has oc-

curred. The peripheral blood RBC count was $2.5 \times 10^{12}/L$, which must be converted to the same power of 10 (10^9) for comparison with the WBC count, *i.e.*, $2500 \times 10^9/L$. The RBC:WBC ratios in the peripheral blood and CSF are calculated as follows:

$$\text{Peripheral blood: } \frac{\text{RBC}}{\text{WBC}} = \frac{2500 \times 10^9/L}{283 \times 10^9/L} = 8.8$$

$$\text{CSF: } \frac{\text{RBC}}{\text{WBC}} = \frac{5180 \times 10^6/L}{2 \times 10^6/L} = 2590$$

Because the ratio in the CSF is much higher than that in the blood, a traumatic tap did occur in this patient, and CNS disease cannot be diagnosed using this specimen.

3. Yes. ALL is the most common leukemia to infiltrate the CNS.

Case Study 30-2

1. No, particularly in immunocompromised patients; the appropriate cellular and humoral immune response to infections may not occur.
2. Absolutely. The cytocentrifuge will concentrate the organisms and thus increase the chances of detection on the slide.
3. The organism will stain with Wright stain as little purple oval bodies surrounded by a clear area (the capsule). The clear capsule may not be apparent unless the organism is intracellular.
4. India ink, fungal stains, fungal cultures, and serology for fungal antigens.

CHAPTER 31

Case Study 31-1

1. They are of T-cell origin. All the cell surface markers are consistent with this, but the gene rearrangement results are confirmatory. This information may be useful for treatment decisions.
2. Because of the high sensitivity of this molecular test, it allows the detection of low levels of malignant cells that may reflect minimal residual disease or early relapse. Furthermore, the observed rearranged fragments are unique markers of that patient's tumor and can indicate whether subsequent disease originated from the same or a different malignant clone of cells.
3. The translocations t(9;22) (known as Philadelphia chromosome), t(4;11), and t(1;19) are all indicators of a poor prognosis.

Case Study 31-2

1. It is caused by a single nucleotide base substitution. The sickle cell anemia mutation is easier to test for because all cases of sickle cell anemia are caused by the same mutation, whereas different cases of thalassemias are likely to be caused by different mutations, and thus analysis is more complicated.
2. The parents would not have to be tested using molecular methods. In the adult, much less expensive methods can be used, such as the solubility test for sickling hemoglobin or hemoglobin electrophoresis. If it were discovered that only one or neither parent was a carrier, then there would be no possibility of them together producing an affected child (*i.e.*, one with sickle cell anemia; homozygous SS state). However, if both parents were carriers (heterozygous AS state), and they wished to know whether this fetus had the disease, molecular methods would be necessary since a fetus produces very few β-chains (the hemoglobin chain that carries the Hb S defect) and thus very little Hb S is available in the fetus to detect using traditional laboratory methods. For all future pregnancies of two carrier parents, molecular methods would be necessary in each case to determine whether the fetus is homozygous Hb SS since two carrier Hb AS parents

have a 25% chance of having a Hb SS child (see Table 5-7 on genetic probabilities).

CHAPTER 33

Case Study 33-1

1. A dysmyelopoietic disorder seems likely because of the two cytopenias (RBC and WBC), the macrocytic RBC population with a dimorphic picture, and the marrow evidence of both dyserythropoiesis (megaloblastoid morphology and ringed sideroblasts) and dysmegakaryocytopoiesis (single round nuclei).
2. This patient was most likely classified as refractory anemia with ringed sideroblasts (RARS) because of the large number of ringed sideroblasts found in the marrow. Other DMPS subgroups may have ringed sideroblasts but they generally comprise less than 15% of the RBC precursors.

CHAPTER 34

Case Study 34-1

1. The most likely FAB classification is M5 (acute monocytic leukemia). Based on the description of the marrow, it appears to be M5a (predominance of monoblasts).
2. The abnormal cells appear to be monocytic in nature; therefore, the cells should be strongly positive for nonspecific α-naphthyl acetate esterase or α-naphthyl butyrate esterase.
3. Finding megaloblastoid RBC precursors in the marrow is not surprising because cytarabine (ara-C) inhibits DNA synthesis (Table 34-6).

Case Study 34-2

1. The most likely FAB classification is M0, acute myeloblastic leukemia with minimal differentiation.
2. Ultrastructural demonstration of peroxidase positivity within the blasts would substantiate the myeloid origin of these cells.
3. CD34 positivity has been associated with an adverse outcome, *i.e.*, difficulty in achieving remission and/or a shortened survival rate.

CHAPTER 35

Case Study 35-1

1. The sudden appearance of a marked basophilia is one of the signs of impending blast transformation. Other signs may be: (1) the appearance of dysplastic myelogenesis; (2) a sudden onset of thrombocytopenia coupled with an increase in the blast count; (3) an increase in the leukocyte and blast count and a decrease in the platelet count; and (4) appearance of lymphoblasts.
2. Color Plate 35-6 illustrates micromegakaryoblasts and micromegakaryocytes.
3. The final diagnosis is megakaryocytic blast transformation of CML. The prognosis is grave. Most treatment at this point is supportive only, with transfusions and antibiotics. Standard chemotherapy appears insufficient for treatment of nonlymphocytic blast transformation of any of the CMPD.

Case Study 35-2

1. The finding of Ph^{1-} cells is unusual in CML. Rather, cells from the malignant proliferating clone in most CML patients are Ph^{1+}. Because Ph^{1+} cells are usually paramount in the diagnosis of CML, one must speculate on the possibility that Ph^{1-} CMLs are truly dysmyelopoietic syndromes (DMPS) rather than CMPD.
2. Patients with CML often respond to standard chemotherapy and enter remission for a period of time. The fact that these four patients, whose cells were Ph^{1-}, did not respond to che-

motherapy suggests misdiagnosis. Note that the DMPS do *not* respond to conventional therapy for CMPD.

3. The prognosis is less favorable for Ph[1-] (8–15 months survival) than for Ph[1+] (40–42 months survival) patients. The possibility that these patients have a DMPS could be part of the explanation for the less favorable prognosis.

Case Study 35-3

1. The most likely diagnosis is polycythemia vera (PV). The patient's age is typical for a CMPD. The laboratory values indicate PV, because by definition, for the tentative diagnosis of PV in a female patient, the Hb should be greater than 15.5 g/dL, and the Hct should be greater than 0.47 L/L. This patient's Hb and Hct far exceed these criteria in their marked abnormality. The RBC count is also markedly increased over the diagnostic criterion of $>5.9 \times 10^{12}$/L. The MCV indicates a microcytic population of red cells, also typical of PV. Another key finding is the RCM of 43.6 mL/kg, which far exceeds the diagnostic criterion of >32 mL/kg for females. It is also common in PV to find a low-normal MCHC and leukocytosis, which this patient displayed, and a thrombocytosis, which was not quite definitive on her first blood count but was on the second.

2. Her itching eyes is one of the many possible symptoms in patients with PV. The purple color of her skin is a classic physical finding. Patients with PV may have a ruddy (reddish-purple) complexion, also known as "ruddy cyanosis."

3. Serum iron, serum B_{12}, and arterial O_2 saturation are useful in differentiating PV and absolute secondary erythrocytosis (secondary polycythemia; see Table 35-3). If these indicators are not definitive, a serum EPO measurement may help, because the value is usually decreased in PV, but normal or increased in secondary polycythemias. An LAP test could also be useful; however, it is probably the least reliable test because of its susceptibility to technical error in staining and interpretation.

4. Usually, the plasma volume is elevated in PV, whereas, this patient's was decreased at 30.9 mL/kg (reference range 40 to 50 mL/kg) for some unknown reason.

5. Treatment with ^{32}P and therapeutic phlebotomy were routine treatment regimens for PV patients in the early 1980s when this patient was treated. More recently, hydroxyurea provides an alternative to ^{32}P and may be the drug of choice for myelosuppression, because it has been reported to be less leukemogenic than other myelosuppressive drugs.

CHAPTER 36

Case Study 36-1

1. The blasts must have been small and homogeneous with scanty cytoplasm and indistinct nucleoli.

2. Anemia and thrombocytopenia were probably caused by marrow replacement by the abnormal cell population.

3. Yes. L1 ALL is most frequently seen in children 15 years of age or younger.

4. Pre-B ALL because immunologic marker studies showed a predominance of CD10, CD19, and HLA-DR. In addition, cytoplasmic μ was positive and sIg was negative.

Case Study 36-2

1. The cases have similar features: a high leukocyte count with a predominance of blasts along with anemia and thrombocytopenia. Cytochemical stains and immunologic markers show similar results although PAS reactivity is frequently not as positive in L2 as it is in L1 ALL. Morphologically, the blasts in this case showed more variability in size and the cytoplasm was more abundant. Nucleoli were also more visible. The patient was a young adult. These are features consistent with L2 ALL.

2. The CD34 surface marker, along with the other B cell markers, indicates the presence of cells in the earliest stage of B-cell development. CD34 is found on hematopoietic stem cells.

3. Children with ALL have a better prognosis than adults. Improved survival for patients with ALL has occurred with intrathecal chemotherapy and bone marrow transplantation.

CHAPTER 37

Case Study 37-1

1. Chronic lymphocytic leukemia (CLL), based on the severe lymphocytosis. The patient's age and gender, as well as the accompanying positive direct antiglobulin test (DAT) all correlate with a diagnosis of CLL.

2. Autoimmune hemolytic anemia.

3. Because the Hb and Hct are decreased, whereas the reticulocyte count and the serum bilirubin are increased.

4. The prednisone helps suppress the activity of the immune system, thus decreasing hemolysis. As long as the marrow is not replaced by lymphocytes and retains its ability to make erythroid precursors, the red cell destruction is compensated for by new production.

Case Study 37-2

1. Hairy cell leukemia, based on the morphology of the abnormal cells and the positive TRAP stains.

2. The bone marrows of hairy cell leukemia patients are often fibrotic.

3. The patient's enlarged spleen may have sequestered platelets peripherally and the abnormal bone marrow, which was packed with more than 90% hairy cells, accounted for decreased production of platelets.

4. Tartrate-resistant acid phosphatase. The TRAP stain is positive in hairy cells but negative in most other lymphoid cells.

CHAPTER 38

Case Study 38-1

1. No, it is not unusual for a patient with Hodgkin disease to have a normal Hb and Hct.

2. Yes, it is common to find a normal bone marrow aspirate but an abnormal biopsy core in Hodgkin disease. Particularly in stage IV disease, there is usually an associated fibrosis such that the neoplastic cells are retained in the biopsy but are not aspirated and therefore not found free in bone marrow films.

3. Chemotherapy may cause a decrease in RBC, granulocyte, and platelet counts.

4. No, a platelet count of 35×10^9/L is not cause for a platelet transfusion, unless there are signs of bleeding. Usually a platelet transfusion is indicated when the platelet count is $\leq 20 \times 10^9$/L, at which point there is a significant risk of spontaneous bleeding.

5. A relative increase in monocytes usually heralds a coming increase of peripheral blood granulocytes, usually 3 to 5 days prior to the granulocytosis.

CHAPTER 39

Case Study 39-1

1. The ESR, rouleaux, and plasma cells on the blood film and the increased serum total protein all indicated the need for further testing.

2. Multiple myeloma.

3. No. A 100-cell differential is not a statistically sound sample. Malignant cells frequently tend to cluster together and therefore distribution on a blood film may be poor.

Case Study 39-2

1. Monoclonal IgM is the most likely cause of this patient's problems. Clinical symptoms and the lack of bone lesions suggest Waldenström's macroglobulinemia.
2. The RBC, Hb, and Hct are low as a result of blood loss. The ESR is elevated owing to increased Ig. The PTT and PT are prolonged as a result of interaction of the M protein with coagulation factors. Platelets are coated with the abnormal protein, affecting their function in both aggregation studies and in the patient.
3. Monoclonal IgM may exhibit the properties of a cryoglobulin causing plasma or serum precipitates on exposure to cold. A greatly elevated MCV and unrealistic MCH and MCHC are clues that laboratory results may be erroneous. The platelet count and occasionally the WBC value can be spuriously elevated owing to inclusion of aggregates formed as a result of either cold- or pH-related precipitation of the M protein.

CHAPTER 42

Case Study 42-1

1. MCV = 105.1 fL; MCH = 54.5 pg; MCHC = 51.9 g/dL
2. The MCH and MCHC are incompatible with life; the MCV is "OK."
3. The RBC count and Hct parameters.
4. MCV = 94.8 fL; MCH = 33.3 pg; MCHC = 35.2 g/dL.
5. RBC agglutination disappeared with warming of the sample (37°C for approximately 10 minutes) before repeat testing. There are two choices when looking only at the numeric data: (1) the Hb is too high, owing to some interference or (2) the RBC and Hct are too low. Since an instrument problem was ruled out, the low RBC and Hct may be due to hemolysis or individual RBC not being counted because of cold agglutination. If hemolysis was the cause of the low RBC count, the same sample will not give different results after warming. The repeat results show increases in both RBC count and Hct, whereas the Hb remained the same. Warming of the sample has brought about separation of the agglutinated RBC for them to be analyzed individually when tested "warm."

Case Study 42-2

1. The Hb and Hct don't agree. The MCH and MCHC are unreasonable.
2. The plasma color and clarity can be observed for hemolysis or lipemia.
3. Ammonium oxalate dilution clears the sample of lyse resistant RBC for a correct WBC and differential analysis. Prior to this dilution, the lyse resistant RBC were being counted as WBC and were "seen" as lymphs. This shifted the relationship of the true cell counts by falsely increasing the lymphocyte count.
4. The plasma Hb reading was caused by lipemia.
5. The Hb value (12.2 g/dL in this case) must be adjusted for the interference caused by the lipemic plasma. If whole blood is 1.0 unit, then this patient has an Hct of 0.28 units and a plasma of 0.72 units. The plasma Hb interference is therefore equal to the plasma Hb reading (4.0 g/dL) times 0.72 which equals 2.88 (4.0 × 0.72 = 2.88). To correct the Hb for lipemia, the calculation is 12.2 − 2.88 = 9.32 g/dL. The corrected Hb of 9.3 g/dL is in agreement with the Hct value of 0.28 L/L.

Case Studies 42-1 and 42-2 each have extremely high MCH and MCHC values. This is caused in the first case by RBC analysis being falsely low and in the second case by Hb measurement being falsely high. Other parameter values and relationships give clues as to which red cell parameters have most likely been affected. The fastest check for RBC cold agglutination is to mix the whole blood sample well, then hold it still and observe the

blood coating the inside of the tube as it moves down the side of the tube. A grainy appearance may be observed rather than smooth draining of the red cells down the inside of the tube. The agglutination of RBC can also be seen on the blood film preparation. Spinning a microhematocrit will help identify a falsely lowered automated RBC count and Hct. It also permits observation of the plasma for evidence of hemolysis or lipemia. In Figure 42-21A, the RBC histogram shows a characteristically decreased red cell population in the normal size range because of cold agglutination and an increased second population of "larger" cells.

CHAPTER 43

Case Study 43-1

1. Thiazole orange will also stain DNA within red cells. Howell-Jolly bodies are made up of DNA; therefore, the presence of large numbers of Howell-Jolly bodies will result in a falsely increased automated reticulocyte count using thiazole orange.
2. Reticulocyte counts by flow cytometry are statistically superior for two reasons: (1) a significantly greater number of cells are examined in order to obtain the percent of reticulocytes (10,000 vs 1000); and (2) the distribution of reticulocytes on reticulocyte films is poor compared to their distribution in the flow cytometer.
3. An IRS is based on the difference in the intensity of fluorescence between early or prematurely released reticulocytes and those that are released after a specific time in the bone marrow.

Case Study 43-2

1. This test is usually performed to monitor HIV infections.
2. A problem in evaluating CD4+ counts by flow cytometry is the inability of many flow cytometers to generate an absolute cell count. Consequently, absolute CD4+ cell counts must rely on the percentage generated by the flow cytometer multiplied by a total lymphocyte count generated by a hematology analyzer. Instrument errors are compounded and comparison between laboratories is difficult.
3. All human material prepared for flow analysis should be prepared in a biohazard hood and the flow cytometer must be a closed system. The fluidics system must be rinsed with a disinfectant at least once daily. Centrifuges used for preparing specimens must be equipped to prevent aerosol leakage.

CHAPTER 45

Case Study 45-1

1. Too few data points are given in this case to identify either a shift or a trend; at least six successive points are needed. A shift and a trend are illustrated in Figure 45-2.
2. The platelet parameter is out of control since the 3rd, 4th, and 5th data points are beyond the acceptable (lower) limit.
3. Using fresh whole bloods as controls presents a problem in separating instrument problems from sample deterioration. The problem in this case is sample-related, not instrument-related. The sample developed platelet clumping over the first few hours of use as a control, and the dramatic decrease in platelet number reflects this sample change. It was identified by preparing and staining a blood film for microscopic examination. Platelet clumps were easily identified microscopically, which explained the decrease in platelet numbers. An advantage of using fresh whole blood as part of a control program is that it is exactly like (rather than similar to) the unknown samples being tested. Note: The slight increase in the WBC in this case may be related to some interference from the platelet clumps.

CHAPTER 47
Case Study 47-1

1. Dietary vitamin C (ascorbic acid) deficiency.
2. The disorder is scurvy. It affects the vascular system by preventing the formation of intact, stable collagen in blood vessels. Without vitamin C, there is also a deficiency of the cement substance that holds endothelial cells together. This causes capillary fragility and serious bleeding problems.
3. The best diagnostic approach is observation of the clinical response to vitamin C replacement therapy, which is usually rapid if vitamin C deficiency is the underlying disorder causing the bleeding abnormalities.
4. Administration of vitamin C usually brings the plasma level of vitamin C and the vascular integrity back to normal and rapidly eliminates the hemorrhagic manifestations in this disorder.

Case Study 47-2

1. The intrinsic coagulation system since the PTT is abnormal, but the PT is normal.
2. Coagulation factors XII, XI, prekallikrein (PK), high-molecular-weight kininogen (HMWK), IX, or VIII.
3. No, this is not surprising. The finding of an abnormal PTT does not necessarily mean that a patient has a bleeding abnormality. It is now recognized that patients with deficiencies in factor XII, PK, or HMWK do not have bleeding abnormalities, and only about half of those with a factor XI deficiency have a bleeding problem. Deficiencies of factors IX and VIII *are* both associated with bleeding disorders.
4. Factors XII, PK, or HMWK and possibly factor XI (see answer 3). This child was discovered to have a PK (Fletcher factor) deficiency.
5. Factor assays should be performed to determine the plasma levels of all the intrinsic pathway coagulation factors (see answer 2).
6. She would not be expected to have bleeding complications from a dental extraction; in fact, the procedure was performed without any bleeding problems.

CHAPTER 49
Case Study 49-1

1. The RBC, Hb, and Hct are significantly elevated.
2. The first step in the evaluation is redrawing the PTT specimen after making adjustments in the amount of sodium citrate used as anticoagulant in the collection tube and repeating the PTT on this specimen.
3. The probable cause is anticoagulant excess in the collection tube, caused by the unusually low plasma volume that resulted from the elevated red cell volume. The excess sodium citrate, a calcium chelator, interferes in the PTT test system, falsely prolonging the clotting time.

Case Study 49-2

1. No. Repeated results with a new specimen as well as all other test parameters being normal does not suggest a spurious abnormality.
2. An inhibitor study with pre- and post-incubation testing should be done.
3. If the inhibitor study was *positive*, a platelet neutralization test and an agarose plasma gel test could be done to confirm a possible Lupus inhibitor. Specific factor assays could be done to confirm normal factor levels. If the inhibitor study was *negative* for inhibitor, testing for von Willebrand's disease should be done, including a factor VIII assay, bleeding time, and ristocetin cofactor assay.

CHAPTER 50
Case Study 50-1

1. The FDP level is elevated because the streptokinase resulted in fibrin(ogen) lysis. This process generated many FDP (X, Y, D, and E). The latex particles in this particular test are sensitive to the latter two products (D and E).
2. The decreased plasminogen level is a result of the conversion of plasminogen to plasmin by streptokinase.
3. The D-dimer assay is not greatly elevated because the thrombolytic therapy did not lyse the clot. In order for this test to be positive, degradation products arising from cross-linked fibrin must be present. In this case, the streptokinase caused lysis of the fibrinogen in the plasma (which caused the greatly elevated FDP level) but was unsuccessful in lysing the clot.

CHAPTER 52
Case Study 52-1

1. This patient has demonstrated a continuous hemorrhagic pattern throughout his life. The family history is significant in that no known close relative is similarly afflicted; therefore, the possibility of an acquired syndrome could not be dismissed.
2. The laboratory data that support a diagnosis of von Willebrand disease include: the PTT and its subsequent correction with adsorbed normal plasma; the bleeding time results in the presence of platelet numbers within reference range; the PT within reference range eliminating the extrinsic and common coagulation pathways; the factor VIIIC:Ag assay level; the vWF:Ag assay; the vWF multimer pattern; and the ristocetin cofactor assay.
3. The presence of small-sized vWF multimers and the absence of intermediate- and large-sized vWF multimers is consistent with type IIA von Willebrand disease (Table 56-2).
4. Individuals affected by type IIA von Willebrand disease do not respond well to DDAVP as a therapeutic agent. Replacement of intermediate- and large-sized vWF multimers with correction of the bleeding time and an increase in the plasma level of VIIIC:Ag are best achieved by products containing the required vWF multimers and VIIIC:Ag.

CHAPTER 54
Case Study 54-1

1. The PTT should be prolonged considerably over the normal range because heparin acts immediately, and the test was requested only 2 hours after administration. Possible causes for the unexpected result are: (1) laboratory error; (2) a low level of AT-III, which is a cofactor for heparin; (3) an excessively high number of platelets that were activated during the PTT specimen collection and released platelet factor 4 (antiheparin); or (4) the presence of a drug that is inhibiting the effects of heparin (*e.g.*, digitalis, antihistamines).
2. Possible solutions: (1) eliminate discrepancies attributable to laboratory error by checking the procedures used for specimen collection and processing, checking quality control results, and reviewing reagents and instrumentation. Then repeat the PTT; (2) assuming no laboratory error, inquire about the possible existence of any underlying diseases or conditions that decrease the level of AT-III, such as cirrhosis, nephrotic syndrome, or, in this patient, the use of oral contraceptives. Suggest the determination of AT-III levels; and (3) review the patient's drug history, as the anticoagulant properties of heparin can be inhibited by synergistic effects of other drugs.

CHAPTER 57
Case Study 57-1

1. Platelet counts performed by automated particle counters may be spuriously increased in the presence of microcytic or fragmented erythrocytes. The first CBC performed on this patient revealed the problem because the automated platelet count was 48×10^9/L, but a phase platelet count was 25×10^9/L which correlated much better with the blood film platelet estimate.

2. The CBC results and red cell fragmentation are consistent with a microangiopathic hemolytic anemia (MAHA). The increased LD and decreased haptoglobin are characteristic of intravascular erythrocyte destruction associated with MAHA. MAHA may be associated with conditions such as disseminated intravascular coagulation (DIC), thrombotic thrombocytopenic purpura (TTP), or hemolytic uremic syndrome (HUS). In both HUS and TTP, platelets are consumed and deposited in the microvasculature without consumption of coagulation factors. Symptoms and data supporting renal disease are characteristic of these conditions. TTP is more common in women, and neurologic problems, including headaches, are frequently associated with TTP.

3. The acute onset of symptoms is probably related to several factors. Mitomycin has been implicated as the etiologic factor in a number of patients who developed concomitant fragmentation hemolysis, thrombocytopenia, and renal failure. In addition, this patient's symptoms may have been caused by the development of immune complexes, which have been demonstrated in patients with gastric carcinoma and TTP-like syndromes. One of the demonstrated immune complexes has been shown to react with tumor cells and a glycoprotein from autologous platelets (platelets from the same person in whom the immune complex was found), producing platelet aggregation.

4. Detection of circulating immune complexes or platelet-associated immunoglobulin (PAIg) may provide further information as to the pathogenesis of the thrombocytopenia.

Case Study 57-2

1. This is a typical example of Glanzmann's thrombasthenia. Other helpful laboratory tests include clot retraction and platelet retention on glass beads, both of which should be abnormal, and a vWF assay, which should be normal.

2. The basic defect is decreased or defective platelet membrane glycoproteins IIb and IIIa, without which the platelet cannot bind fibrinogen. This causes abnormal platelet function *in vivo* and *in vitro*.

3. A blood film taken from a capillary puncture has sometimes been referred to as the "poor man's aggregation test." The fact that the patient's platelets were normal in number but did not form small clumps (*i.e.*, the blood film looked like it had been taken from an EDTA sample rather than from a capillary puncture [fingerstick]) points to a platelet function abnormality.

CHAPTER 58
Case Study 58-1

1. The commercial control range for the PTTs in this laboratory has no bearing on the interpretation of the patient's test result except to ensure that the test system is functioning properly. The narrow range of 31.0 to 33.0 seconds for the control is used only to check for system performance and to determine shifts and trends in control results indicating a possible system failure (Table 58-2). Patient results must be compared with the laboratory's established PTT population reference range based on a sample of "healthy" subjects. In this laboratory, the patient's PTT of 32.0 seconds appears prolonged in comparison with the normal population, for which the upper limit of the reference range was 29.0 seconds.

2. Further testing is warranted because the PTT is prolonged. The tests to assist in diagnosis would most likely include a prothrombin time, thrombin time, and fibrinogen, with factor assays to follow, as indicated by other test results and the patient's history.

Case Study 58-2

1. The unexpected occurrence of erratic PT and PTT results should definitely raise suspicion, as this causes doubt about precision and accuracy. Further investigation is warranted.

2. The controls at the beginning of the shift indicated that the system was in control. Therefore, at the time, there was no cause for concern.

3. Erratic, discrepant results do not point specifically to a problem with the instrument, reagent, or specimens, which makes problem identification difficult. Therefore, all variables listed in Table 58-1 should be reviewed as possible problem sources. Possible instrument problems include malfunction of the light source, detector, clotting timer, electrical circuitry, or some combination. Incorrect reagent delivery is not a likely cause of the problem, because this error usually results in excessively long clotting times. Reagents do not appear to be a source of trouble in this case; however, it is good to be certain that they are being used in accordance with established guidelines for stability. Reagents should be in homogeneous suspension without large particles or aggregates. The erratic pattern of discrepant results most likely does not indicate a specimen-handling problem either, because the short results generally do not occur on the same patient. However, it would be good to verify that specimens are being drawn properly, delivered to the laboratory promptly, and processed and tested with minimal delay.

4. No. The physician should not be told that the specimen result is definitely correct. If the system problem has not yet been resolved, it would be best to review the procedure for obtaining and delivering coagulation specimens with the personnel involved and request another specimen for repeat testing. Until the source of the problem is known, repeat testing should be done on a backup instrument if available.

5. Yes. The controls should be repeated at this point to be certain they are still within acceptable limits.

6. Yes. A check of system precision would be useful. A series of 15 tests for the PT and PTT should be run on the same normal plasma to check for precision and reproducibility. It is unnecessary to use commercial control material, which is expensive, to check system precision when running each test 15 times. A normal plasma serves the same function.

7. If the problem is not detected and corrected, a backup instrument should be used, if available, until the malfunction can be evaluated by a service technician. Technical service definitely should be called. Alternatively, if after running the controls again and checking system precision, no problem with the instrument is found, the laboratory should continue to monitor the results carefully on this instrument with an increased use of controls to try to identify any pattern of discrepant results.

8. Yes, when a problem is suspected, all tests should be performed in duplicate (even if the laboratory normally performs only single tests) and the average result reported to assist in identifying the problem and verifying patient results. Duplicate testing should be continued until the problem is resolved.

Answers to Review Questions

Q	A		Q	A		Q	A		Q	A		Q	A		Q	A
1-1	B		8-1	D		13-1	C		19-6	C		27-5	D		35-3	A
1-2	C		8-2	D		13-2	C		19-7	D		27-6	A		35-4	D
1-3	A		8-3	C		13-3	B					27-7	B		35-5	B
1-4	A		8-4	A		13-4	D		20-1	D						
			8-5	C		13-5	B		20-2	A		28-1	D		36-1	B
2-1	C		8-6	H					20-3	C		28-2	C		36-2	C
2-2	B		8-7	A		14-1	A		20-4	B		28-3	A		36-3	C
2-3	A		8-8	G		14-2	B					28-4	B		36-4	D
			8-9	F		14-3	B		22-1	C		28-5	A		36-5	B
3-1	B		8-10	D		14-4	D		22-2	B					36-6	D
3-2	C		8-11	B		14-5	A		22-3	A		29-1	C		36-7	B
3-3	D		8-12	C		14-6	D		22-4	D		29-2	B		36-8	D
3-4	C		8-13	E		14-7	D		22-5	C		29-3	D			
3-5	D					14-8	C		22-6	A		29-4	A		37-1	A
3-6	C		9-1	B					22-7	C					37-2	B
			9-2	C		15-1	B					30-1	C		37-3	B
4-1	A		9-3	A		15-2	C		23-1	A		30-2	D		37-4	B
4-2	A		9-4	A		15-3	C		23-2	C		30-3	A			
4-3	B		9-5	B		15-4	D		23-3	B		30-4	A		38-1	A
4-4	C		9-6	B		15-5	D		23-4	B		30-5	D		38-2	C
4-5	A		9-7	E		15-6	A		23-5	E		30-6	B		38-3	D
						15-7	A		23-6	D					38-4	C
5-1	D					15-8	D		23-7	E		31-1	A		38-5	B
5-2	B		10-1	A		15-9	E					31-2	C		38-6	A
5-3	C		10-2	C					24-1	C		31-3	B		38-7	C
5-4	D		10-3	C		16-1	A		24-2	B						
5-5	B		10-4	B		16-2	D		24-3	B		32-1	B		39-1	D
5-6	B		10-5	A		16-3	B		24-4	C		32-2	C		39-2	A
5-7	A		10-6	D		16-4	B		24-5	C		32-3	A		39-3	C
5-8	D					16-5	C		24-6	D					39-4	C
						16-6	B					33-1	B			
6-1	A		11-1	B					25-1	D		33-2	C		40-1	C
6-2	B		11-2	D		17-1	C		25-2	B		33-3	A		40-2	D
6-3	B		11-3	C		17-2	A		25-3	A		33-4	D		40-3	B
6-4	D		11-4	D		17-3	E		25-4	C		33-5	C		40-4	A
6-5	A		11-5	C		17-4	D		25-5	C		33-6	E			
6-6	C		11-6	A					25-6	C		33-7	C		41-1	B
6-7	D		11-7	D		18-1	D					33-8	E		41-2	D
						18-2	C		26-1	D		33-9	D		41-3	A
7-1	C		12-1	B		18-3	A		26-2	B					41-4	C
7-2	A		12-2	C		18-4	B		26-3	B		34-1	C			
7-3	C		12-3	E		18-5	C		26-4	B		34-2	D		42-1	D
7-4	B		12-4	C					26-5	B		34-3	D		42-2	C
7-5	D		12-5	A		19-1	C					34-4	A		42-3	B
7-6	B		12-6	C		19-2	C		27-1	B		34-5	B		42-4	D
7-7	D		12-7	E		19-3	A		27-2	C					42-5	A
7-8	C		12-8	C		19-4	B		27-3	C		35-1	B		42-6	D
7-9	A		12-9	A		19-5	B		27-4	A		35-2	A		*(continued)*	

42-7	1.	B	44-1	C		47-1	D		50-3	A		53-7	D		55-14	E
	2.	C	44-2	B		47-2	B		50-4	C		53-8	B		55-15	A
	3.	A	44-3	D		47-3	B		50-5	B		53-9	C			
	4.	D	44-4	C		47-4	A		50-6	C		53-10	D		56-1	B
	5.	C	44-5	B		47-5	E								56-2	D
42-8	1.	D	44-6	B		47-6	B		51-1	B		54-1	B		56-3	D
	2.	A	44-7	A					51-2	D		54-2	B		56-4	C
	3.	E	44-8	E		48-1	B		51-3	D		54-3	D		56-5	B
	4.	B	44-9	C		48-2	B		51-4	A		54-4	A		56-6	A
	5.	D	44-10	A		48-3	A		51-5	C		54-5	B		56-7	C
	6.	B	44-11	C		48-4	C		51-6	D		54-6	C		56-8	C
	7.	E				48-5	E					54-7	D			
	8.	E				48-6	E								57-1	C
	9.	E	45-1	B		48-7	E		52-1	B		55-1	B		57-2	B
	10.	A	45-2	D		48-8	E		52-2	D		55-2	B		57-3	A
	11.	F	45-3	D		48-9	C		52-3	A		55-3	D		57-4	D
	12.	C	45-4	A					52-4	C		55-4	D		57-5	B
42-9	E		45-5	B					52-5	B		55-5	C		57-6	C
42-10	B					49-1	C		52-6	D		55-6	C		57-7	B
42-11	C					49-2	A					55-7	A		57-8	C
						49-3	C					55-8	A		57-9	D
43-1	A		46-1	A		49-4	C		53-1	B		55-9	B		57-10	A
43-2	C		46-2	D		49-5	D		53-2	A		55-10	D			
43-3	A		46-3	B					53-3	D		55-11	C		58-1	C
43-4	D		46-4	D					53-4	B		55-12	D		58-2	A
43-5	B		46-5	C		50-1	B		53-5	C		55-13	A		58-3	B
43-6	A		46-6	C		50-2	D		53-6	A						

APPENDIX C

Percent Transmittance— Absorbance Conversion Table

% T	0.00	0.25	0.50	0.75	% T	0.00	0.25	0.50	0.75	% T	0.00	0.25	0.50	0.75	% T	0.00	0.25	0.50	0.75
	ABSORBANCE*					ABSORBANCE*					ABSORBANCE*					ABSORBANCE*			
1	2.000	1.903	1.824	1.757	26	0.585	0.581	0.577	0.573	51	0.292	0.290	0.288	0.286	76	0.119	0.118	0.116	0.115
2	1.690	1.648	1.602	1.561	27	0.569	0.565	0.561	0.557	52	0.284	0.282	0.280	0.278	77	0.114	0.112	0.111	0.100
3	1.523	1.488	1.456	1.426	28	0.553	0.549	0.545	0.542	53	0.276	0.274	0.272	0.270	78	0.108	0.107	0.105	0.104
4	1.398	1.372	1.347	1.323	29	0.538	0.534	0.530	0.527	54	0.268	0.266	0.264	0.262	79	0.102	0.101	0.100	0.098
5	1.301	1.280	1.260	1.240	30	0.523	0.520	0.516	0.512	55	0.260	0.258	0.256	0.254	80	0.097	0.096	0.094	0.093
6	1.222	1.204	1.187	1.171	31	0.509	0.505	0.502	0.498	56	0.252	0.250	0.248	0.246	81	0.092	0.090	0.089	0.088
7	1.155	1.140	1.126	1.112	32	0.495	0.491	0.488	0.485	57	0.244	0.242	0.240	0.238	82	0.086	0.085	0.084	0.082
8	1.097	1.083	1.071	1.059	33	0.482	0.478	0.475	0.472	58	0.237	0.235	0.233	0.231	83	0.081	0.080	0.078	0.077
9	1.046	1.034	1.022	1.011	34	0.469	0.465	0.462	0.459	59	0.229	0.227	0.226	0.224	84	0.076	0.074	0.073	0.072
10	1.000	0.989	0.979	0.969	35	0.456	0.453	0.450	0.447	60	0.222	0.220	0.218	0.216	85	0.071	0.069	0.068	0.067
11	0.959	0.949	0.939	0.930	36	0.444	0.441	0.438	0.435	61	0.215	0.213	0.211	0.209	86	0.066	0.064	0.063	0.062
12	0.921	0.912	0.903	0.894	37	0.432	0.429	0.426	0.423	62	0.208	0.206	0.204	0.202	87	0.061	0.059	0.058	0.057
13	0.886	0.878	0.870	0.862	38	0.420	0.417	0.414	0.412	63	0.201	0.199	0.197	0.196	88	0.056	0.054	0.053	0.052
14	0.854	0.846	0.838	0.831	39	0.409	0.406	0.403	0.401	64	0.194	0.192	0.191	0.189	89	0.051	0.049	0.048	0.047
15	0.824	0.817	0.810	0.803	40	0.398	0.395	0.392	0.390	65	0.187	0.186	0.184	0.182	90	0.046	0.045	0.043	0.042
16	0.796	0.789	0.782	0.776	41	0.387	0.385	0.382	0.380	66	0.181	0.179	0.177	0.176	91	0.041	0.040	0.039	0.037
17	0.770	0.763	0.757	0.751	42	0.377	0.374	0.372	0.369	67	0.174	0.172	0.171	0.169	92	0.036	0.035	0.034	0.033
18	0.745	0.739	0.733	0.727	43	0.367	0.364	0.362	0.359	68	0.168	0.166	0.164	0.163	93	0.032	0.030	0.029	0.028
19	0.721	0.716	0.710	0.704	44	0.357	0.354	0.352	0.349	69	0.161	0.160	0.158	0.157	94	0.027	0.026	0.025	0.024
20	0.699	0.694	0.688	0.683	45	0.347	0.344	0.342	0.340	70	0.155	0.153	0.152	0.150	95	0.022	0.021	0.020	0.019
21	0.678	0.673	0.668	0.663	46	0.337	0.335	0.332	0.330	71	0.149	0.147	0.146	0.144	96	0.018	0.017	0.016	0.014
22	0.658	0.653	0.648	0.643	47	0.328	0.325	0.323	0.321	72	0.143	0.141	0.140	0.138	97	0.013	0.012	0.011	0.010
23	0.638	0.634	0.629	0.624	48	0.319	0.317	0.314	0.312	73	0.137	0.135	0.134	0.132	98	0.009	0.008	0.007	0.006
24	0.620	0.615	0.611	0.606	49	0.310	0.308	0.305	0.303	74	0.131	0.129	0.128	0.126	99	0.004	0.003	0.002	0.001
25	0.602	0.598	0.594	0.589	50	0.301	0.299	0.297	0.295	75	0.125	0.124	0.122	0.121	100	0.000	0.0000	0.0000	0.000

* Absorbance = $2 - \log \%\,T$

Relative Centrifugal Force Nomograph

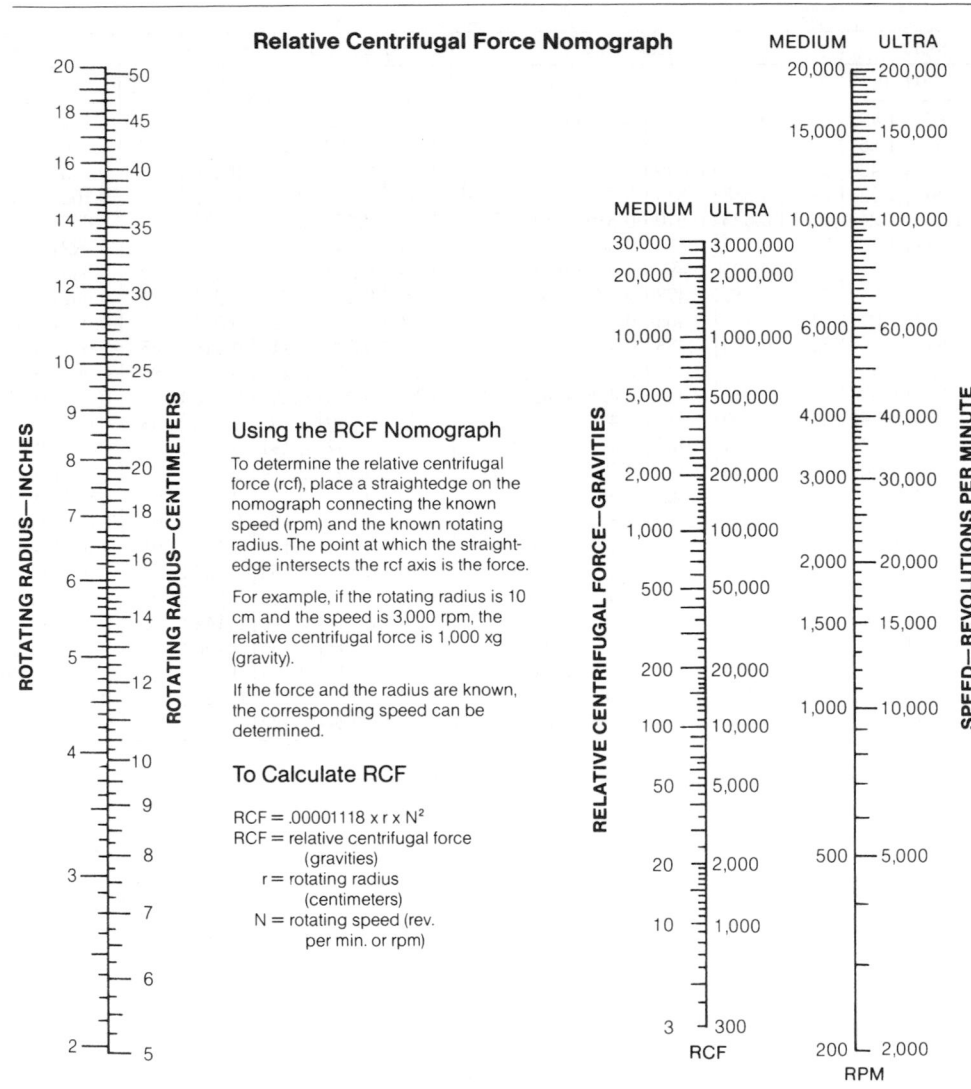

Relative Centrifugal Force Nomograph

Using the RCF Nomograph

To determine the relative centrifugal force (rcf), place a straightedge on the nomograph connecting the known speed (rpm) and the known rotating radius. The point at which the straightedge intersects the rcf axis is the force.

For example, if the rotating radius is 10 cm and the speed is 3,000 rpm, the relative centrifugal force is 1,000 xg (gravity).

If the force and the radius are known, the corresponding speed can be determined.

To Calculate RCF

$RCF = .00001118 \times r \times N^2$
RCF = relative centrifugal force (gravities)
   r = rotating radius (centimeters)
   N = rotating speed (rev. per min. or rpm)

ROTATING TIP RADIUS

The distance measured from the rotor axis to the tip of the liquid inside the tubes at the greatest horizontal distance from the rotor axis is the rotating tip radius.

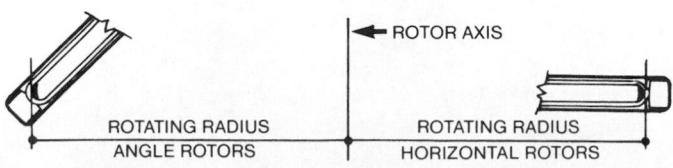

(Reprinted by permission from International Equipment Co., Damon Corporation)

Glossary

aberrations Optical lens defects (chromatic, spherical, and field curvature) that degrade the quality of an image seen when using a microscope.

abetalipoproteinemia A very rare hereditary disorder characterized by the absence of apolipoprotein B–containing lipoproteins. This results in decreased serum levels of low-density lipoproteins (LDL), very low density lipoproteins (VLDL), and chylomicrons. Also called hereditary acanthocytosis.

ablative therapy Treatment to destroy, as in the treatment of leukemia or tumor cells.

absorbance A measure of light absorbed (taken in and not reflected) by a solution.

acanthocyte (Gr. *acantho*: thorn or spike) A small, densely stained erythrocyte that is no longer disc-shaped and has a few irregularly spaced, pointed spicules or thornlike projections of various lengths and widths over its surface (Fig. 8-9).

acanthocytosis, hereditary See abetalipoproteinemia.

accuracy The closeness of a test result to the true value.

achlorhydria Absence of free hydrochloric acid in the stomach.

achylia gastrica An acquired atrophy of the stomach lining that causes reduced or total elimination of hydrochloric acid and intrinsic factor secretion from gastric parietal cells in the stomach.

acid-elution slide test A staining technique used to identify Hb F in erythrocytes. Also called the Kleihauer-Betke stain.

acidophilic Staining readily with the eosin (or acid) component of a Romanowsky stain. Literally, means "acid-lover."

acrocyanosis Blue-gray discoloration of finger tips and other extremities (see Raynaud's phenomenon).

actin A peripheral erythrocyte membrane protein composed of short filaments. It interacts with the protein spectrin, and both are thought to underlie the lipid bilayer on the cytoplasmic side, and to regulate membrane shape and deformability. Also called band 5.

acute In leukemia, refers to the presence of large numbers of primitive cells (blasts) in the blood and bone marrow.

acute phase reactant Long list of proteins that share in common an elevation in concentration as a response to stressful or inflammatory states associated with infection, trauma, surgery, and different degrees of tissue injury including necrosis.

Addison disease Hypoadrenalism in which there is a decrease in adrenal cortex production of cortisol that characteristically leads to anemia.

adenopathy Swelling of glands. Lymphadenopathy refers to swelling of lymph nodes.

adenosine diphosphate (ADP) A product, along with organic phosphate, of the hydrolysis of adenosine triphosphate (ATP), with the release of free energy; used in the laboratory as a platelet agonist. ADP can be readily rephosphorylated to ATP. ADP is one of many substances found in platelets.

adenosine triphosphate (ATP) The source of energy for erythrocytes (and all cells) that is generated in the Embden–Meyerhof pathway (EMP).

aerosol A liquid or solution that has been dispersed in the air as a fine mist or particles.

affinity Strength and avidity with which binding occurs. Antibodies have variable affinity for antigens as do antigen receptors for antibodies.

agglutination The aggregation of cells into random clusters or masses (Fig. 8-3) when exposed to various erythrocyte antibodies. The outline of each individual cell is not seen.

agnogenic From the Greek word meaning obscure; of unknown origin or etiology (see idiopathic).

agonist In the hemostasis laboratory, an agent that aggregates platelets, *e.g.*, ADP or thrombin.

albinism Partial or total absence of pigment in skin, hair, and eyes.

aleukemic leukemia A term used to describe the absence of leukemic cells in the peripheral blood of a patient with leukemia. Pancytopenia is also frequently seen in these individuals.

alkylating agent Synthetic compounds containing two or more end (alkyl) groups that combine readily with other molecules. They are used in the treatment of many types of malignancies to inhibit both cell division and the production of mutations and have a toxic effect on many types of normal and malignant cells.

alloantibody An antibody produced by one member of a species that will react with antigens of another member of the same species; also known as isoantibody.

alloantigen An antigen that is coded for at the same gene locus within a species. It will induce an immune response if transferred to another member of that species who lacks the antigen; also known as isoantigen.

allogeneic Derived from a genotypically nonidentical donor of the same species; antigenic interaction is expected.

allograft A tissue transplant from an allogeneic donor.

alloimmune Immunity found in a member of a species to antigens found in the same species (alloantigens), but not on the exposed member's cells; also known as isoimmune.

alopecia Loss of hair; baldness.

alpha (α) granule A spherical organelle in the platelet that releases a number of constituents, some derived from the plasma, and others synthesized by the megakaryocyte, that affect coagulation, platelets, smooth muscle cells, and vessel walls.

alveolar Anatomic term pertaining to small sac-like dilatations; plural: alveoli. Pulmonary alveoli are thin-membrane sacs in the lungs where gas exchange takes place.

amphoteric Capable of being negatively or positively charged and therefore acting both as an acid (proton donor) and as a base (proton acceptor). Hemoglobin and water are amphoteric.

amplification An increase in the number of copies or the detection of a target nucleic acid sequence.

amyloid A starch-like protein produced and deposited in tissues in certain disease states.

anaphylatoxin An agent produced during complement fixation on cells that serves as a mediator of inflammation by inducing mast cell degranulation and histamine release, thus producing an anaphylactic response.

anaphylaxis An exaggerated allergic reaction of an organism to a protein or foreign substance.

anemia A condition characterized by a decrease in circulating erythrocytes (destruction or loss exceeds production), or a hemoglobin level that is below the reference range.

aneuploid Having an abnormal number of chromosomes, either too many or too few.

aneurysm A weakened area in the wall of an artery that forms a saclike dilatation.

anion Negatively-charged monatomic or polyatomic ion, such as chlorine (Cl^-) or hydrogen carbonate (HCO_3^-), that migrates toward a positive electrode (anode).

anisochromia The term used to describe the variation in hemoglobin content when both hypochromic and normochromic erythrocytes are present on a peripheral blood film.

anisocytosis The term used to describe variation in an erythrocyte population size or diameter on a peripheral blood film.

Ann Arbor staging system A system for classifying Hodgkin disease based on the number of lymph node regions and/or organs that have been infiltrated by lymphocytes; essential for treatment and evaluation of treatment success.

anode Positively-charged electrode.

antecubital fossa The anatomic area corresponding to the bend of the elbow.

antenatal Prior to birth.

antibody A protein substance produced by lymphocytes, especially plasma cells, in response to foreign antigen stimulation. See immunoglobulin.

antibody, cold Harmless autoantibody reacting optimally at 0–4°C, including anti-I, anti-H, and anti-IH. However, there is a pathologic form of anti-I antibody (IgM) that leads to complement-mediated extravascular (principally hepatic) hemolysis. See cold agglutinin syndrome.

antibody, warm Autoantibodies that are usually IgG, but some are IgM or IgA and react optimally at 37°C. The IgG type do not bind complement and are often specific for Rh antigens. They cause extravascular (principally splenic) destruction of erythrocytes.

anticoagulant A chemical substance that inhibits blood coagulation. 1. Normal or abnormal plasma proteins that act as inhibitors of blood coagulation. 2. The chemical used to prevent blood coagulation in a whole blood specimen. 3. Chemicals administered therapeutically to patients to prevent blood coagulation.

anticoagulant, oral Refers to vitamin K antagonists, such as coumarin or warfarin, administered therapeutically by mouth to prevent blood coagulation.

anticoagulant therapy A pharmaceutical agent administered to a patient to inhibit the normal blood coagulation reaction. This therapy is commonly monitored with blood coagulation tests such as the prothrombin time or partial thromboplastin time.

antigen A substance that is capable of inducing an immune response which results in production of antibodies specific for the substance.

antihemophilic factor Factor VIII, a cofactor in the intrinsic coagulation pathway needed for factor IXa activation of factor X. See Table 52-1 for details on the many terms applied to this complex molecule.

antinuclear antibody (ANA) Autoantibodies directed against a variety of intracellular nuclear proteins. They are found in association with systemic rheumatic diseases including systemic lupus erythematosus. Both an immunofluorescent method and an indirect immunoenzyme antibody technique are now used to detect ANA. Also called antibody to nuclear antigen.

antiplasmins A group of substances that inactivate plasmin and thus inhibit fibrinolysis. The most important is α_2-antiplasmin.

α_2-antiplasmin A naturally occurring glycoprotein that is the first to bind with any plasmin that is free in the plasma, thus preventing excessive fibrinolysis.

antiseptic An agent or substance capable of preventing infection by inhibiting the growth of infectious agents without necessarily destroying them; applied particularly to agents used on living things including people. See disinfectant.

antithrombin III (AT-III) A naturally occurring inhibitor of coagulation that inhibits serine proteases including thrombin, XIIa, XIa, Xa, and IXa. It also inhibits fibrinolysis by inhibiting plasmin. Its action is enhanced significantly by therapeutic heparin (Fig. 48-6). Deficiencies are associated with thrombosis. Also called heparin cofactor I.

α_1-antitrypsin An α globulin that is a potent inhibitor of factor XIa. Also the least significant of the three major naturally occurring fibrinolytic system inhibitors. Also known as α_1-antiprotease.

anuria A lack of urine production.

aplastic Absence of all bone marrow cells in all three cell lines (leukocytes, erythrocytes, and platelets).

aplastic anemia An acquired or inherited disease in which there is a primary defect in the bone marrow causing a severe decrease in all bone marrow cells, replacement of the bone marrow by fat, and a peripheral blood pancytopenia.

aplastic crisis A transient failure of erythrocyte production most commonly caused by viral infection. It may occur in association with hemolytic conditions and lead to a rapid decrease in the hemoglobin level, a so-called "crisis."

apoferritin A protein that binds iron in plasma to form ferritin (see ferritin).

apoptosis See necrobiotic.

arthralgia Joint pain.

artifact An abnormal finding on a blood film that is not naturally occurring. It may be caused by poor staining quality, slow blood film drying, poor preparation technique, cell damage, or fat particles. Artifacts should NOT be reported.

ascites Accumulation of serous fluid in the abdominal cavity.

ascorbic acid Vitamin C.

aseptic Characterized by the absence of pathogenic organisms; sterile.

aspirate, bone marrow The fluid portion of the marrow obtained with a syringe; a suspension of blood, fat, and particles of developing hematopoietic cells.

ataxia Defective muscular coordination.

atheroma A deposit of yellowish fatty plaque on arterial walls occurring in atherosclerosis.

atherosclerosis A common form of arteriosclerosis in which deposits of yellowish plaques (atheromas) containing cholesterol and lipids are formed within the large and medium-sized arteries.

athymic An inherited condition characterized by the absence of the thymus gland; results in the inability to produce T lymphocytes.

atrophy Wasting away; decrease in size or volume of a cell, tissue, organ, or part.

Auer rod Azurophilic rod-like structure found in the cytoplasm of nonlymphoid blasts or progranulocytes which represents a fusion of primary lysosomal granules.

autoantibodies Antibodies that react with the host's own cell or tissue antigens produced in autoimmune diseases.

autograft A reinfusion of tissue from the same individual (from self).

autoimmune Abnormal immunity to one's own antigens caused by the reaction of one's own immune system against oneself.

autologous Derived from the same individual (self).

autosome Any of the chromosomes other than the sex (X and Y) chromosomes.

autosplenectomy Splenic infarction and fibrosis that causes the spleen to shrivel to practically nothing and become nonfunctional. This is particularly due to sickle occlusion in sickle cell anemia.

azo dye A synthetic dye with one or more N=N groups as its color group(s). Examples include fast garnet and fast blue.

azurophilic granules 1.The bluish-red or purple granules that first appear in the promyelocyte stage in the neutrophilic maturation sequence; also called primary granules. 2. Prominent reddish-purple granules occasionally seen in the cytoplasm of mature lymphocytes.

Babesia Protozoan organisms transmitted to humans by a tick bite. *Babesia* are found in erythrocytes as ringlike structures resembling the ring stages of malarial parasites. The rings may be round, oval, elongated, amoeboid, or pear-shaped, and are often tiny (Figs. 8-28, 8-31).

band 3 An erythrocyte membrane integral protein that acts as an inorganic anion (Cl^-—HCO_3^-) transport channel.

band neutrophil Immature form of segmented neutrophil with an elongated, curved, or sausage-shaped nucleus and numerous pinkish-tan granules in the cytoplasm; represents 0% to 11% of leukocytes in normal adult peripheral blood; also called stab or staff.

bandpass filter A filter that transmits a specific portion of the spectrum of light. All other parts of the spectrum are blocked or attenuated.

Barts hydrops fetalis A lethal syndrome resulting from homozygosity for α° thalassemia (—/—).

basal value The normal baseline value in any individual for any laboratory test.

base pair (bp) Two complementary nucleotides joined by hydrogen bonding.

base sequence The linear order of purine and pyrimidine bases in a DNA molecule.

basket cell A nuclear remnant that may be found on stained blood films made with the wedge technique. It differs from a smudge cell only in that the basket cell is more spread apart (greater diameter) and has a loosely woven appearance.

basopenia An absolute decrease in basophilic leukocyte numbers.

basophil Granulocytic leukocyte with large purple-black granules in the cytoplasm when stained with Wright stain; represents 0% to 1.6% of leukocytes in normal adult peripheral blood.

basophilia 1. The reaction of cellular material that has an affinity for basic dyes; with a Romanowsky stain, material that stains blue. 2. An absolute increase in the leukocyte basophil numbers.

basophilic Staining readily with the methylene blue (or basic) component of a Romanowsky stain. Literally, means "base-lover."

basophilic stippling The fine or coarse, deep blue to purple-staining inclusion that may appear in erythrocytes on a dried Wright-stained film (Figs. 8-22, 8-28). It appears homogeneously throughout the Hb portion of the erythrocyte. Stippling represents aggregates of ribosomes that appear during the drying and staining of films. It may be found in nucleated red blood cells or diffusely basophilic red blood cells.

battlement track A specific search pattern (Fig. 24-5) used to count leukocytes in the appropriate examination area of a blood film. Used to perform the leukocyte differential.

beam splitter A mirror or prism capable of splitting a light beam into two or more separate beams.

Beer's Law The absorbance of a homogeneous sample containing an absorbing substance is directly proportional to the concentration of the absorbing substance and to the thickness of the sample in the optical path.

Bence Jones protein Low-molecular-weight free light chains of immunoglobulin often found in the urine of patients with a monoclonal gammopathy (plasma cell disorder). The protein has a characteristic solubility pattern when the urine is heated.

benign Abnormal uncontrolled cell maturation with abnormal appearing cells that have abnormal organelle shape and structure. However, the abnormal cells are restricted to a localized area and usually surgically removable as opposed to malignant cells.

Bernard–Soulier syndrome (BSS) A hemorrhagic disorder (named after the two French investigators who first described it) characterized by giant platelets. The platelets in BSS lack an adhesion receptor consisting of glycoproteins Ib, V, and IX.

Bethesda unit The amount of factor VIII inhibitor that will inactivate 50% of the factor VIII in one mL of normal plasma.

bilineage The presence of two distinct leukemic cell populations based on immunophenotyping of surface markers.

bilirubin The breakdown product of heme (a component of hemoglobin) and its precursors.

bilirubinuria The presence of conjugated bilirubin in the urine.

biohazard Any item, body part, or substance that is capable of producing infectious disease. Examples include cultures, body fluids, tissues, organs, or anything (*e.g.*, needles) that is contaminated with the foregoing.

biphenotypic A leukemic cell population in which both myeloid and lymphoid markers are present on the same cell.

birefringence The quality of transmitting light unequally in different directions; double refraction.

blast (types I, II, and III) Myeloblasts with varying amounts of azurophilic granules. Type I has no granules; type II has less than 20 granules; and type III has more than 20 granules, a central nucleus, and a small Golgi apparatus.

blind loop syndrome A disorder resulting from alterations in the small intestine to which intestinal contents may gain access but not readily move away from. This causes bacterial overgrowth and results in malabsorption of vitamin B_{12}, steatorrhea, and anemia.

blister cell An erythrocyte poikilocyte with a vacuole-like area formed as the result of being caught on a fibrin strand (Fig. 8-12C). This vacuole ruptures to form the keratocyte.

blood film review An organized review of a stained blood film including evaluation of cell morphology and estimates of cell concentrations.

blot, dot A molecular technique in which nucleic acid samples are transferred (blotted) in an ordered array onto a membrane. The shape of the transfer area determines whether it's called a dot (circular) or slot (oblong) blot. The target nucleic acid sequence is detected by hybridization with specific probes.

Bohr effect The change in oxygen affinity of hemoglobin with a change in blood *p*H.

bone marrow architecture The microscopic structure of the marrow; the juxtaposition of the cellular and noncellular elements as seen in sectioned marrow.

brilliant cresyl blue inclusion body test A test for microscopic detection of hemoglobin (Hb) H that requires incubation of blood with brilliant cresyl blue stain, a redox dye that causes the precipitation of Hb H *in vitro*. Erythrocytes that are positive for Hb H contain small, irregularly-shaped bodies that are blue-green and have a pitted golf ball-like appearance (Fig. 14-9B).

burr cell An erythrocyte with irregularly-sized and unevenly-spaced spicules on its surface (Figs. 8-8B, 8-13). The number of burr cells varies from one microscopic field to another. A burr cell results from an acquired membrane abnormality in the presence of plasma chemical abnormalities typically related to anemia of renal insufficiency. Sometimes called an echinocyte.

burst-forming unit–erythroid (BFU-E) The earliest identified erythroid-committed cell in the bone marrow which is a precursor of the colony-forming unit–erythroid (CFU-E) progenitor. In bone marrow culture, colonies of BFU-E grow in clusters or "bursts."A few BFU-E are normally present in the bone marrow.

butterfly needle A needle and tubing attached to a plastic wing-shaped device, resembling a butterfly, between the needle and the tubing (Fig. 2-1). The tubing may be attached to a syringe, evacuated collection tube holder, or an intravenous fluid infusion set.

Cabot ring A thin ringlike structure in erythrocytes that stains reddish-blue to violet in Wright stain (Figs. 8-25, 8-28). It may be circular and appear at the cell periphery, or form a figure eight, incomplete rings, or other configurations. More than one ring may be present in a single cell.

calibration Any adjustments made to an instrument to correct the results recovered so that they match "truth." Truth is defined by standards or reference procedures.

carboxyhemoglobin A carbon monoxide (CO) derivative of hemoglobin (Hb) that normally represents less than 1% of the total Hb. Hb affinity for CO is more than 200 times stronger than that for O_2.

carboxyhemoglobinemia An acquired condition in which blood carboxyhemoglobin levels are elevated causing various symptoms. At carboxyhemoglobin levels of 50% to 70% of total Hb, an individual can be asphyxiated.

carcinogen Any agent or substance that has been reported to cause neoplasia (cancer).

cardiac output The volume of blood pumped by the heart per minute.

cardiolipin A phospholipid extracted from beef heart and an important component of tissue membranes.

cardiomegaly Increased size of the heart.

cathode Negatively-charged electrode.

cation Positively-charged monatomic or polyatomic ion such as potassium (K^+) or ammonium (NH_4^+) that migrates toward a negatively-charged electrode (cathode).

CD3 Cell surface marker that is the hallmark of the T-lymphocyte lineage.

CD34 Surface antigen that identifies a very early hematopoietic cell (probable stem cell).

cell-adhesion molecules (CAM) Molecules that serve as ligands or coreceptors for a number of different cell surface proteins allowing for adhesion of cells, *e.g.*, lymphocyte adhesion to endothelial cells in preparation for moving into the tissues. CAMs also provide special signals for cell development, homing, and recirculation of lymphocytes.

cellularity, bone marrow A comparison of the amount of hematopoietic tissue with the amount of fat in relation to the age of the patient; best judged from sectioned marrow. Reported as normocellular, hypercelluar, or hypocellular.

cerebrospinal fluid (CSF) A body fluid (normally clear and colorless) that circulates over the brain and around the spinal cord to protect them from sudden changes in pressure and provide a site for metabolic exchange of nutrients and waste.

cerebrovascular accident A sudden hemorrhage, embolism, or thrombus in the vessels of the brain that may lead to a stroke including dizziness, numbness, and even paralysis in some cases.

Charcot–Leyden crystals Hexagonal bipyramidal crystals sometimes found in secretions or exudates of patients with allergic asthma; formed from disintegration of eosinophils.

chelation Process related to the therapeutic administration of a chemical compound by which a metallic ion is sequestered and firmly bound into a ring within the chelating molecule. When used to treat lead intoxication, the chelated lead is excreted in the urine.

chemiluminescence Cold light or light produced as a result of a chemical reaction without the production of heat.

chemotaxis Response of phagocytic cells to chemical stimuli resulting in cellular movement toward the stimulus.

chemotherapy The treatment of a disease such as leukemia by use of chemical agents rather than other modalities such as radiation, surgery, or transplant.

chloride shift The normal movement of chloride (Cl^-) ions into the erythrocyte in exchange for bicarbonate (HCO_3^-) ions moving out of the erythrocyte to maintain electroneutrality. This results from hemoglobin's function in acid-base balance of the blood (Fig. 7-7).

choroid plexus Folds (villi) of the pia mater membrane that are highly vascular and are located in the third, fourth, and lateral ventricles of the brain.

chromatin The genetic material of the nucleus, primarily composed of DNA. There are two forms: heterochromatin, which stains well, is coiled, condensed, and clumped; and euchromatin, which appears as dispersed threads that often do not stain well. During mitosis, chromatin condenses and separates into chromosomes.

chromogenic Capable of generating color after reacting with an appropriate reagent.

chromosomal translocation The transfer of a part of one chromosome to a different chromosomal location.

chronic disease, anemia of (ACD) Anemia seen in chronic infections and inflammatory and malignant conditions but not related to bleeding, hemolysis, or marrow replacement by tumor.

chronic myeloproliferative disorders See myeloproliferative disorder, chronic.

C'1 inactivator A naturally occurring inhibitor of coagulation, fibrinolysis, and the complement and kinin systems (Table 48-6).

circadian A 24-hour period; circadian rhythm refers to the repetition of an activity or process at the same time every day.

c-kit ligand A hematopoietic growth factor that stimulates primitive hematopoietic progenitors. Also called stem cell factor.

CLIA'88 Clinical Laboratory Improvement Amendments of 1988; the regulations that describe laboratory standards that must be met to receive Medicare and Medicaid reimbursement. The "Final Rules" were published on February 28, 1992 in the Federal Register. There have been several updates since 1992.

clonal disorder A condition derived from an abnormality in a single bone marrow precursor cell that leads to a genetically identical abnormal group of cells.

clone To establish a strain of cells in culture (or *in vivo*) from a single cell.

clot retraction An *in vitro* phenomenon in which blood clot contraction can be observed after a few hours, leaving clear serum adjacent to the test tube walls. This is subjectively indicative of normal platelet function *in vivo* but requires verification using platelet function tests.

cluster designation (CD) A classification system for monoclonal *antibodies* specific for antigens on normal or neoplastic cells. Antibodies specific for similar antigens are clustered together under a single CD number.

cluster differentiation (CD) antigen An international classification system of numerically designated cell surface *antigens* that are detected by monoclonal antibodies and used for cell identification and differentiation.

coagulation The complex process that leads to the conversion of fibrinogen to fibrin to form a blood clot; also referred to as hemostasis. See hemostasis.

coagulation pathway, common The final series of reactions that leads to formation of a fibrin clot. The factors in this pathway include factor X, prothrombin, fibrinogen, factor XIII, and the cofactor V. It is activated by either the extrinsic or intrinsic coagulation pathway.

coagulation pathway, extrinsic A series of reactions that begins the process of forming a fibrin clot. It is initiated when tissue factor (TF) is exposed on damaged endothelium and forms a

Ca^{2+}-dependent complex with factor VII. The TF:VIIa-Ca^{2+} complex activates factor X in the common coagulation pathway. See Figure 48-1, tissue factor, and coagulation pathway, common.

coagulation pathway, intrinsic A series of reactions that begins the process of forming a fibrin clot. It is initiated *in vitro* when factor XII is exposed to the negatively-charged surface of a substance such as glass. It includes the contact factors (XII, XI, prekallikrein, and HMWK) and factors IX and VIII. Factor IXa combines with the factor VIII cofactor (VIIIa) and Ca^{2+} on the platelet phospholipid surface to activate factor X in the common coagulation pathway. See Figure 48-1, contact coagulation factor group, and coagulation pathway, common.

cobalamins A family of vitamins (including vitamin B_{12}) with a corrin ring containing cobalt at their center bound to four nitrogen atoms. The corrin nucleus contains four pyrrole rings and is similar to the porphyrin nucleus of heme. The corrin ring is attached to the nucleotide 5,6-dimethylbenzimidazole. See vitamin B_{12}.

codocyte (Gr. *kodon*: bell) See target cell.

codominant Exhibiting the full expression in a heterozygote of both alleles of a pair without either being influenced by the other, as in a person with blood group AB or one with sickle cell trait (Hb AS).

codon A group of three adjacent nucleotides on a strand of DNA that code for an amino acid.

cold agglutinin syndrome A disorder in which there is a pathologic form of anti-I antibody that leads to complement mediated hemolysis; these antibodies bind avidly to erythrocytes at 0–10°C, causing agglutination. Blood samples of these patients must be incubated 15 minutes at 37°C before performing a complete blood count.

colon The last part of the large intestine, which is attached at its end to the rectum.

colony A group of organisms (bacteria or cells) growing on nutrient media that are derived from a single organism (see clonal).

colony-forming unit–erythroid (CFU-E) Primitive cells in the bone marrow thought to be derived from erythroid precursors (burst-forming unit–erythoid). CFU-E are stimulated by erythropoietin to form colonies and committed to forming erythrocytes. May also be found in peripheral blood.

commitment In referring to developing cells, this term is used to depict the cell's inability to develop into anything other than a specific cell type or family.

complement Enzymatic proteins (C1–C9) that interact to mediate certain effects of the body's inflammatory response to tissue injury or exposure to foreign substances. The complement system also interacts with the coagulation, fibrinolytic, and kinin systems. Complement binding with antibodies on erythrocyte surfaces can cause extravascular or intravascular hemolysis (Fig. 19-1).

complement, alternate pathway A sequence of reactions involving complement that is activated by certain cells, particles, or microorganisms without the presence of antibodies.

complement, classic pathway A sequence of reactions involving complement that is activated when IgG or IgM antibodies complex with antigens on erythrocytes resulting in hemolysis (Fig. 19-1).

complementary nucleotides Nucleotides that can pair specifically with each other. In DNA adenine (A) pairs with thymine (T), and cytosine (C) pairs with guanine (G).

condenser Optical lens system that directs and focuses light from an illumination source onto a specimen positioned on a microscope stage.

congenital Describes any condition existing at, and usually before, birth; conditions present at birth whether hereditary or acquired.

congenital Heinz body hemolytic anemia Unstable Hb disease that results in denaturation and precipitation of globin chains and formation of Heinz bodies. An unstable Hb usually causes little or no clinical findings, but it may cause a severe hemolytic anemia. See hemoglobin, unstable.

consumption coagulopathy A condition in which there is excessive coagulation and all the coagulation factors are consumed at a faster rate than they can be replenished.

contact coagulation factor group A group of factors that is adsorbed by contact with a negatively-charged surface such as the subendothelium *in vivo*. It includes prekallikrein, HMWK, and factors XII and XI. This group initiates the intrinsic coagulation pathway, fibrinolysis, kinin formation, and activates the complement system (Fig. 48-1 and Table 48-4).

contamination Introduction of an extraneous substance (*e.g.*, chemical or infectious agent) thereby rendering the original material impure, unsuitable, or unhealthy.

continuous quality improvement (CQI) A program established to develop achievable goals that are then continuously monitored in an effort to document improving laboratory services.

Cooley's anemia See β thalassemia major.

Coombs' test See direct antiglobulin test.

Cooper and Cruickshank stain A seldom used stain for direct absolute basophil counts performed on a Fuchs-Rosenthal or Speirs-Levy hemocytometer.

Coplin jar A wide-mouthed glass or plastic jar with a screw cap and ridges on two sides of its inner surface to accommodate up to 10 slides for staining.

corrected reticulocyte count (CRC) A correction of the reticulocyte percentage to a normal hematocrit of 0.45 L/L to allow correction for the degree of patient anemia.

cortisol A hormone produced by the adrenal cortex that stimulates erythrocyte production.

coumarin See anticoagulant, oral.

coverslip A thin, clear sheet of glass that may be round, square, or rectangular that is placed over an object to be viewed with a microscope. Its purpose is to protect the object or change the refractive index of the object. Also known as a coverglass.

crenated Adjective used to describe cells with outlines that are notched or scalloped or "wrinkled." See echinocyte.

crescent cell See semilunar body.

cross-reactive material Hereditary variants of coagulation proteins that have normal antigenic properties but lack functional activity.

cryogen A substance capable of reducing the temperature to very low levels (freezing).

cryoglobulin An abnormal protein in the blood that precipitates in the cold and redissolves at body temperature.

culling The splenic process of removing senescent and abnormal erythrocytes.

Cushing disease Hyperadrenalism in which there is an increase in adrenal cortex production of the hormone cortisol which may lead to abnormally increased erythrocyte production.

cyanocobalamin Another name for vitamin B_{12}. See vitamin B_{12}.

cyanosis A bluish discoloration of the skin and mucous membranes; appears when blood levels of methemoglobin exceed 10% of the total hemoglobin and also in acrocyanosis.

cyclin Nuclear proteins that play a role in the progression of the cell cycle.

cyclooxygenase An oxygenating enzyme found in fatty acid metabolism for the synthesis of prostaglandins. Various prostaglandins have significant effects in both stimulating and inhibiting platelet aggregation. Aspirin will acetylate and cause the malfunction of cyclooxygenase; this inhibits platelet aggregation.

cytocentrifuge A device that uses centrifugal force to concentrate nucleated cells into a small area of a 3 × 1-inch glass slide.

cytochemistry The application of chemical reactions to cells to reveal their chemical composition.

cytogenetics The study of chromosomes, their structure, and function.

cytokine Any substance (also called a growth factor) synthesized and released by a cell (*e.g.*, T lymphocytes or epithelial cells) that affects or alters the function or activity of other types of cells. Cytokines promote proliferation and differentiation of cells. A complex network of cytokines facilitates communication among cells of the immune system. Lymphokines are cytokines produced by lymphocytes. Interleukins are cytokines (see interleukin). Many have been identified.

cytopenia Decrease in the number of any type of blood cell in the peripheral blood, *e.g.*, thrombocytopenia is a decrease in peripheral blood platelets.

cytosol Liquid medium of the cell cytoplasm without organelles and insoluble components.

dacryocyte Teardrop-shaped erythrocyte.

dactylitis See hand-foot syndrome.

darkfield A type of illumination for the microscope involving the blockage of direct light rays so that the object is illuminated with obliquely angled light. The result is a bright object on a black background.

DC Direct current generated from a low-voltage, low-frequency source used in automated hematology analyzers to count cells and determine their overall volume using the electrical impedance principle.

D-D dimer One of the late fibrin degradation products that result from plasmin dissolution of a fibrin clot (Fig. 48-4). A laboratory test for the D-D dimer provides a specific indicator of excessive *in vivo* fibrin formation and fibrinolysis which are common in diffuse intravascular coagulation (DIC).

deferoxamine A chelating agent that binds with iron to form a soluble complex. Used as an antidote for iron poisoning and in the treatment and prevention of iron overload in some β thalassemia conditions.

defibrination Removal of fibrin from whole blood. It may be an *in vitro* or *in vivo* (defibrination syndrome) process.

definitive Fixed or final form; as in definitive red cell precursors produced during hepatic hematopoiesis.

definitive flag An automated, instrument-generated message that appears when numeric data limits (that are determined and set by the user) are exceeded. These flags indicate patient values or other conditions that require follow-up action before release of a report. See suspect flag.

demarcating membrane system A platelet-specific diffuse membrane organelle that may mark the boundary of platelet fields in the maturing megakaryocyte.

demyelinate To destroy or remove the myelin (lipid) sheath surrounding the axons of many nerves.

denaturation The separation of the two strands of a double-stranded nucleic acid molecule by the loss of hydrogen bonding between complementary nucleotides.

dense body A spherical organelle in the platelet that releases a number of constituents including ADP, ATP, calcium, pyrophosphate, and serotonin among others. ADP initially stimulates platelet aggregation, but is later degraded to adenosine which inhibits platelet function. Also called dense granule.

dense tubular system A series of membranes in the platelet derived from smooth endoplasmic reticulum and closely apposed to the open canalicular system. It contains several structures and substances important to the activation of platelets, *e.g.*, prostaglandins.

deoxyribonucleic acid (DNA) The molecule that encodes and transmits the genetic information needed for cellular structure and function.

deoxyuridine (dU) suppression test A radioactive assay that requires bone marrow cells and detects deficient thymidylate synthesis caused by either vitamin B_{12} or folate deficiency.

Diamond-Blackfan anemia The inherited form of pure red cell aplasia. See pure red cell aplasia.

diapedesis Process by which leukocytes move from blood vessels into tissues by squeezing between junctions in the endothelial cells lining blood vessel walls.

diaphorase See NADH-methemoglobin reductase.

diastolic pressure The minimum pressure of the blood on the walls of the arteries that is measured when the ventricles of the heart are relaxed. The adult normal range is approximately 65 to 90 mm Hg.

diathesis Condition; disease or group of diseases.

differential lysis Controlled alterations of blood cells by reagent systems to enhance automated separation and counting of cell populations and subpopulations.

differentiation A generally irreversible process by which stem cells lose their ability to self-renew and gain the ability to carry out specialized functions. For example, granulation in the cytoplasm of a myeloblast is morphologic evidence that the cell has undergone differentiation and belongs to the granulocyte family.

diffusely basophilic red cell See polychromatophilic red cell (Fig. 8-28).

dimorphism Property of having or existing under two forms, such as an erythrocyte population on a blood film demonstrating both macrocytic and microcytic cells.

2,3-diphosphoglycerate (2,3-DPG) An organic phosphate produced in the Embden–Meyerhof pathway, specifically, in the Rapoport–Luebering shunt. When Hb binds 2,3-DPG, O_2 affinity decreases. Conversely, when plasma 2,3-DPG decreases, Hb 2,3-DPG is released, and the Hb affinity for O_2 increases.

Diphyllobothrium latum A large tapeworm that can be found in improperly cooked fish causing parasitic disease in humans. It interferes with vitamin B_{12} absorption by competing with intrinsic factor for binding B_{12}.

direct antiglobulin test (DAT) A test for the presence of antibodies that have attached to an erythrocyte surface *in vivo*. Previously called the Coombs' test.

disinfectant A substance capable of killing microorganisms or inhibiting their growth; applied particularly to agents used on inanimate objects, *e.g.*, surfaces, floors. See antiseptic.

dissociation curve, carbon dioxide (CO_2) A curve that reflects the relationship between blood CO_2 content and the pCO_2 for 0% HbO_2, nonoxygenated blood, and 97.5% HbO_2, oxygenated blood. The difference in these curves demonstrates a phenomenon known as the Haldane effect (Fig. 7-6). See Haldane effect.

dissociation curve, oxyhemoglobin An S-shaped (sigmoidal) curve representing the affinity of hemoglobin for oxygen. A shift to the left in this curve represents increased O_2 affinity; a shift to the right represents decreased O_2 affinity (Fig. 7-5).

diuretic Medication to increase urine output.

diurnal Daily; happening in the daytime.

diverticulitis, intestinal Inflammation of a diverticulum (see diverticulosis), especially in the colon.

diverticulosis, intestinal The presence of small pouches or sacs (diverticulum) formed by hernial protrusion of the mucous membrane lining through a defect in the muscular coat of the intestine in the absence of inflammation.

Donath–Landsteiner (D–L) autoantibody An IgG antibody that causes the autoimmune hemolytic disease paroxysmal cold hemoglobinuria (PCH), which is associated with hemolysis following the exposure of affected individuals to varying degrees of cold. See paroxysmal cold hemoglobinuria.

drepanocyte (Gr. *drepane*: sickle) See sickle cell.

dry tap The inability to aspirate marrow; usually due to fibrosis, hypercellular marrow, or poor technique.

duodenum The first part of the small intestine into which stomach contents are sent.

dyscrasia A general term for disease.

dyserythropoiesis Abnormal maturation of erythrocytes in the bone marrow causing abnormalities in appearance in the bone marrow and peripheral blood, *e.g.*, multinuclearity or megaloblastoid appearance, and sometimes abnormalities in function. Also known as megaloblastoid maturation. See megaloblastoid.

dyserythropoietic anemia, congenital (CDA) Hereditary anemias of abnormal nuclear development characterized by variable degrees of anemia and bone marrow erythrocyte precursor nuclear abnormalities such as multinuclearity and other bizarre changes, but normal serum vitamin B_{12} and folate levels.

dysfibrinogenemia A qualitative abnormality in the fibrinogen molecule (about 40 have been described), usually transmitted as an autosomal dominant trait, which may interfere with normal hemostasis. Some abnormalities may be asymptomatic, some may cause bleeding, and a few have been associated with thrombosis.

dysgranulopoiesis Abnormal maturation of granulocytes in the bone marrow causing abnormalities in appearance in the bone marrow and peripheral blood, *e.g.*, pseudo-Pelger–Huët or giant granules, and sometimes abnormalities in function.

dysmegakaryocytopoiesis Abnormal maturation of megakaryocytes in the bone marrow causing abnormalities in appearance in the bone marrow and peripheral blood, *e.g.*, mononuclear or dwarf-sized megakaryocytes, and sometimes abnormalities in function.

dysmyelopoietic syndrome (DMPS) A clonal proliferative disorder of the bone marrow characterized by dyspoiesis or dysplasias of bone marrow precursor cells and peripheral blood cytopenias. Blast forms in the bone marrow make up less than 30% of the bone marrow cells. Also called myelodysplastic syndrome, preleukemia, or preleukemic syndrome. Five have been classified (Tables 33-1 and 33-2).

dysplasia Developmental abnormalities in myeloid cell maturation causing unusual size and shape, organization, nuclear/cytoplasmic maturation asynchrony, and a shift in position of organelles. Such cells are likely to become neoplastic (malignant) without treatment.

ecchymosis A form of purpura in which blood escapes into large areas of skin or mucous membranes, but not into deep tissue. The area turns black and blue (bruise) and later, greenish brown or yellow (Fig. 47-6).

echinocyte (Gr. *echinos*: sea urchin) An erythrocyte that has evenly distributed, uniform-sized, blunt spicules or bumps on its surface (Figs. 8-8A, 8-13). Echinocytes may be seen on films made from anticoagulated blood that is several hours old, but such cells are artifacts. They are artifacts if practically every cell in the thin portion of the film is an echinocyte. This should not be reported. Also called a crenated cell.

eclampsia Convulsions and coma that may occur in pregnancy in association with preeclampsia, *i.e.*, hypertension, edema, and proteinuria. Preeclampsia is a common cause of microangiopathic hemolytic anemia.

ectopic Displaced. Abnormal location.

edema Presence of abnormally large amounts of fluid in the intercellular tissue spaces of the body.

EDTA (Ethylenediaminetetraacetic acid) A disodium or tripotassium salt which binds calcium ions and is commonly used as an anticoagulant in hematology testing.

effector cell A cell capable of accomplishing a specific task or function. For example, the plasma cell, which is capable of producing immunoglobulin, is an effector cell of B-cell lineage.

effusion The movement of fluid into a tissue or cavity.

Ehlers–Danlos syndrome A hereditary connective tissue defect in which the individual has hypermobile joints and hyperextensible skin that can be stretched much more than normal, but returns to normal on release.

electrical impedance An increase in the resistance to electric current flow caused by an object that is a poor conductor of electric current (*e.g.*, a cell).

electrophoresis The migration of charged particles, such as various hemoglobins, in an electrical field.

elliptocyte An erythrocyte that has an elliptical shape (Fig. 8-7). It may result from an inherited or acquired condition and its shape can range from egg-shaped or slightly oval to sausage-, rod-, or pencil-shaped.

elliptocytosis, hereditary A heterogeneous group of erythrocyte membrane skeletal disorders in which spectrin is structurally abnormal. Large numbers of elliptical erythrocytes are found on the peripheral blood film, and there are varying degrees of hemolysis.

embolus A particle made up of a blood clot, fat, gas bubbles, tumor cells, or other debris present in blood vessels that can cause blockage of blood flow (embolism). Plural, emboli.

Embden–Meyerhof pathway (EMP) The major source of erythrocyte energy through anaerobic conversion of glucose to lactate to produce ATP (Fig. 6-7).

encephalitis Inflammation of the brain.

end cell A fully mature cell with a finite life span.

endomitosis The replication of nuclear elements within an intact nuclear envelope without subsequent chromosomal movement or cytokinesis. Also referred to as endoduplication.

endothelial cells Squamous epithelial cells that line the blood vessels and prevent blood from leaving the vascular system. They do not promote coagulation or platelet activation; they facilitate blood flow.

engraftment In bone marrow transplantation, the result of successful transplantation of donor cells into recipient marrow.

enzymopathy A hereditary defect in or deficiency of an enzyme, *e.g.*, the erythrocyte enzymes G6PD or PK.

eosinopenia An absolute decrease in eosinophilic leukocyte numbers.

eosinophil Granulocytic leukocyte with large orange-pink granules in the cytoplasm when stained with Wright stain; represents 0% to 7% of leukocytes present in normal adult peripheral blood.

eosinophilia An absolute increase in eosinophilic leukocyte numbers.

eosinophilic Staining readily with eosin. See ''acidophilic.''

epigastric Located in the upper-middle portion of the abdomen, including the area over and in front of the stomach.

epistaxis Nosebleed.

ependyma The membrane that lines the ventricles of the brain and the central canal of the spinal cord.

epidermal Pertaining to the outermost layer of skin composed of squamous epithelium.

erythremia A clonal disorder that affects bone marrow production of erythrocytes only, causing an increase in the total red blood cell mass.

erythroblast General term for nucleated red blood cells.

erythroblastosis fetalis Another name for hemolytic disease of the newborn.

erythrocyte A mature red blood cell that contains no nucleus. Its chief function is to carry hemoglobin through the circulation to deliver oxygen to the tissues and to carry CO_2 away from tissues back to the lungs.

erythrocyte sedimentation rate (ESR) A measure of the degree of settling of erythrocytes in plasma in an anticoagulated whole-blood specimen during a specified period of time.

erythrocytosis A condition characterized by an increase in circulating erythrocytes and thus an increased red blood cell mass. There is also an increased hemoglobin content and hematocrit.

erythrocytosis, absolute primary A true increase in red blood cell mass caused by a chronic myeloproliferative disorder known as polycythemia vera. See polycythemia vera.

erythrocytosis, absolute secondary A true increase in red blood cell mass caused by either appropriate or inappropriate mechanisms. In an appropriate response, erythrocyte production is increased in response to tissue hypoxia caused by various conditions, *e.g.*, pulmonary disease or certain hemoglobinopathies. In an inappropriate response, erythrocyte production is increased owing to increased erythropoietin production caused by renal disease or extrarenal tumors that produce some substance that stimulates erythrocyte production.

erythrocytosis, relative A decrease in plasma volume causing an apparent, but not true, increase in red blood cell mass demonstrated by an increase in hematocrit; some causes include dehydration secondary to vomiting, diarrhea, burns, or the use of diuretics.

erythroderma Skin disorder characterized by reddening and exfoliation.

erythrokinetics The movement of erythrocytes from the time of generation to their destruction; the balance between erythrocyte production and destruction.

erythron The entire mass of mature and immature erythrocytes in both intravascular and extravascular locations.

erythrophagocytosis The consumption of erythrocytes by cells in the reticuloendothelial system.

erythropoiesis The process of producing erythrocytes.

erythropoiesis, ineffective A process in which an abnormally increased number of developing erythrocytes do not become normal circulating erythrocytes, but rather are destroyed in the bone marrow before maturation.

erythropoietin (EPO) A glycoprotein hormone secreted primarily by the kidneys that stimulates stem cells of the bone marrow to produce erythrocytes.

essential Fundamental, basic, or inherent; when referring to a disease, it implies a primary disease, *i.e.*, one not acquired from another condition.

etiology Origin.

euchromatin Finely granular, evenly-distributed nuclear chromatin characteristic of immature cells.

euglobulin Any globulin protein that is soluble in salt solution but not soluble in water.

examination area Refers to the monolayer of cells on a blood film where at least 50% of the cells are free (do not overlap). This area is considered best for examination of cellular morphology and estimation of cell numbers. The location depends on the type of preparation. On a wedge-type blood film, it is located just behind the feathered end. On a coverslip preparation, it is located in the middle of the blood film.

extramedullary Occurring outside of the bone marrow; extra = outside, medullary = bone marrow.

extravascular Outside the vessels; for example, in reticuloendothelial organs.

exudate An effusion resulting from trauma or inflammation. Characterized by high protein concentration and presence of cells.

eyepiece Optical lens that further magnifies the intermediate image formed by the objective lens of a microscope.

fagot cell Cell containing bundles of Auer rods.

Fanconi anemia A rare, inherited (autosomal recessive) form of aplastic anemia. It is accompanied by other abnormalities such as hypoplasia of the kidneys, skeletal abnormalities, and mental retardation. See aplastic anemia.

favism A severe, potentially fatal hemolytic condition caused by ingestion of fava beans that occurs in a few individuals whose erythrocytes are severely G6PD deficient; particularly associated with the G6PD Mediterranean variant.

Fc receptor (FcR) Cell surface molecules capable of binding the Fc fragment of immunoglobulin molecules.

feathered end Refers to the thin end of a wedge-type blood film preparation where the blood that was being pulled by the spreader slide runs out. Also known as the "tail end."

ferritin A substance composed of iron bound to a protein called apoferritin. Ferritin is the main iron storage form in the body and is found in the plasma and in cells. Serum ferritin reflects the body's tissue iron stores and is thus a good indicator of iron storage status.

ferrochelatase The last enzyme required in the synthesis of the heme molecule; it catalyzes the chelation of ferrous (Fe^{2+}) iron to protoporphyrin IX to form heme. Hereditary deficiency of this enzyme causes a disorder called protoporphyria.

fibrin The molecule that remains after the amino terminal peptides A and B have been removed from fibrinogen by the enzyme thrombin. This permits the formation of soluble fibrin monomers that polymerize spontaneously and are held together by weak noncovalent bonds. Then, in the presence of thrombin, factor XIIIa (activated fibrin stabilizing factor), and Ca^{2+}, fibrin is stabilized by formation of covalent bonds to form an insoluble blood clot. Normal lysis by plasmin slowly dissolves the clot as the tissues heal.

fibrin monomer The initial material remaining after thrombin cleavage of fibrinopeptides A and B from fibrinogen. Fibrin monomers polymerize to form polymers. See fibrin.

fibrinogen A high-molecular-weight plasma protein (coagulation factor I) that is hydrolyzed by thrombin to form fibrin in the final stage of fibrin clot formation.

fibrinogen coagulation factor group This group includes fibrinogen (factor I) and factors V, VIII, and XIII. These factors are the only ones that act as substrates for the fibrinolytic enzyme plasmin (*i.e.*, they are destroyed by plasmin) (Table 48-4).

fibrin(ogen) degradation products (FDP) Specific molecular fragments produced in the process of fibrinogen or fibrin degradation by plasmin within a clot. The four principal products are fragments X, Y, D (D-D dimer), and E. Also called fibrin(ogen) split products (FSP).

fibrin(ogen) split products (FSP) See fibrin(ogen) degradation products.

fibrinolysin See plasmin.

fibrinolysis The dissolving of a fibrin clot, usually accomplished by plasmin.

fibrinolytic system A series of reactions that slowly dissolves a blood clot through the degradation of fibrin by the glycoprotein plasmin (Fig. 48-4).

fibrinopeptide A (FPA) A small polypeptide molecule that is released when thrombin degrades fibrinogen.

fibrin stabilizing factor Coagulation factor XIII which is activated by thrombin (factor IIa) and acts on fibrin to stabilize the fibrin clot.

FITC Fluorescein-isothiocyanate. A fluorescent dye (fluorochrome) used in flow cytometry to assist in characterizing cell populations. See also fluorescence-activated cell sorter (FACS).

fixation Immersion of a tissue into a solution of one or more chemicals for the purpose of preserving the cells as closely as possible to their living state and to prevent cellular breakdown and autolysis. Fixation is required to preserve cells for staining and examination.

floating discriminators Adjusted gates (see gate) in hematology instruments that are controlled by computer algorithms. They are used to provide optimal separation of cell populations for automated identification and counting.

flow cytometer An instrument that characterizes cells and their internal contents by detection of various types of light scatter and fluorescence as the cells pass one at a time in front of a light beam (usually a laser; see laser).

fluorescence-activated cell sorter (FACS) Analytical instrument that separates and quantitates cells by fluorescent emissions of conjugated monoclonal antibody bound to cells.

fluorochrome A molecule capable of absorbing light energy and emitting photons of a longer wavelength as it releases excess energy.

folate A family of compounds derived from folic acid, also called pteroylglutamic acid. They are required for three reactions that lead to DNA synthesis. A diet restricted in folate for three to six months can lead to folate deficiency and megaloblastic anemia. Sources of food folate include green leafy vegetables, among others.

follicular cell Cell derived from the follicle or nodule in the cortex of the peripheral lymphatic organ such as a lymph node.

forward scatter The light diffracted by a cell in a direction axial to a laser light beam as the cell passes through that beam.

free erythrocyte protoporphyrin (FEP) Protoporphyrin within erythrocytes that is not bound with iron to form heme. It is increased in several situations including iron deficiency anemia and lead toxicity.

Fuchs-Rosenthal hemocytometer A special hemocytometer (Fig. 24-6) designed for counting larger volumes than the Neubauer hemocytometer. It is used for manual eosinophil and basophil counts to provide absolute cell count results that may be useful in certain diagnostic situations.

Gaisböck's syndrome Relative erythrocytosis associated with a condition seen in individuals experiencing anxiety and stress. Also called stress syndrome and spurious erythrocytosis.

gamete A germ cell (either ovum or spermatozoon) containing one-half the normal number of chromosomes. See haploid.

gammopathy Abnormal proliferation of antibody-producing cells that results in an increase in serum immunoglobulins.

gastritis Inflammation of the stomach.

gate A region that specifies the boundaries set for an instrument to analyze a specific cell population. By using one or more gates, that population may be analyzed without interference by other cell types.

gene rearrangement The physical reorganization of parts of the same gene or between different genes.

gene therapy A method of disease treatment in which a defective gene is replaced with a normal gene in order to provide the body with the functional protein product of the gene.

genome The complete genetic information of an organism.

genotype The entire genetic constitution of an individual including the nature of the individual alleles for a specific gene.

germinal matrix Consisting of primitive stem cells found in early stages of development.

Giemsa Name of a German bacteriologist who developed a blood stain known as the Giemsa stain that consists of methylene blue azures.

Glanzmann thrombasthenia A hemorrhagic condition (named after the first investigator who described it) characterized by ab-

normally functioning platelets and poor clot retraction. The platelets lack a surface receptor for fibrinogen consisting of glycoproteins IIb and IIIa (GP IIb-IIIa).

globin Varied sequences of amino acids called polypeptide chains that bind with heme to form hemoglobin. The chains are designated by the Greek letters α, β, γ, δ, ε, and ζ, depending on the amino acid sequence.

globin chain synthesis study A test to reveal the ratio of β to α (β/α) globin chains.

glucose-6-phosphate dehydrogenase (G6PD) An important erythrocyte enzyme in the hexose monophosphate shunt (HMS). It is the most commonly deficient enzyme of the HMS. G6PD converts glucose-6-phosphate (glucose-6-P) to 6-phosphogluconate (6-PG) allowing for the subsequent production of NADPH and reduced glutathione (GSH) (Figs. 6-7 and 17-4) . G6PD is required to protect hemoglobin against oxidation. G6PD is present in increased amounts in reticulocytes and is also found in leukocytes.

glucose-6-phosphate dehydrogenase (G6PD) deficiency An X-linked inherited hemolytic disorder caused by a deficiency in the G6PD enzyme.

glutathione Reduced glutathione (GSH) is the principal reducing agent in the erythrocyte and it is produced in the hexose monophosphate shunt (HMS). GSH is used to reduce oxidized sulfhydryl groups in hemoglobin (Hb) and other proteins. It protects enzymes and Hb against oxidation by detoxifying hydrogen peroxide and free radicals (Figs. 6-7 and 17-4). The reducing reaction, which depends on NADPH generated in the HMS, yields reduced sulfhydryl groups and oxidized glutathione (GSSG).

glycocalyx An outer coating of carbohydrate-rich molecules detected with the electron microscope on the free surface of platelets. It contains a variety of platelet glycoproteins and coagulation factors.

glycophorin A An erythrocyte membrane integral protein that bears some blood group antigens.

gout Recurrent attacks of inflammation in joints caused by deposits of urate crystals. Gout may be either hereditary or acquired. Accelerated purine metabolism may lead to gout.

G-protein A complex of three proteins located in the cell membrane that, when activated by means of receptor ligand binding, are capable of inducing certain cellular activities.

graft-versus-host (GVH) reaction Immunologic response of lymphocytes in a graft against the foreign antigens in the tissues of an immunocompromised host who is incapable of rejecting the foreign cells of the graft. In a bone marrow transplant, cytotoxic T lymphocytes in the bone marrow inoculum are responsible for the GVH reaction. Clinical manifestations involve mostly the skin, liver, lung, and gastrointestinal tract.

graft-versus-leukemia (GVL) effect The same immune response that elicits cytotoxic T lymphocytes causing GVHD is also toxic to and inhibits proliferation of tumor cells.

granulocyte A leukocyte containing distinct granules in the cytoplasm; includes neutrophils, eosinophils, and basophils.

granulocyte-colony stimulating factor (G-CSF) A specific peptide that stimulates granulocytic development.

granuloma A granular tumor or growth which is usually composed of lymphoid and epithelioid cells.

growth factor See cytokine and interleukin.

Haldane effect The shift in the CO_2 dissociation curve, which reflects the relationship between whole blood CO_2 content and the pCO_2 for 0% HbO_2 (nonoxygenated blood) and 97.5% HbO_2 (oxygenated blood). This shift reflects the increased affinity of 0% HbO_2 for CO_2 in the tissues, where pCO_2 is high, and the decreased affinity of 97.5% HbO_2 for CO_2 in the lungs where pCO_2 is low, and thus it is excreted by means of expired air.

half-moon cell See semilunar body.

Ham's acidified serum test A test to assist in the diagnosis of paroxysmal nocturnal hemoglobinuria (PNH). It is based on the fact that erythrocytes from patients with PNH have an abnormal sensitivity to complement-mediated lysis in acidified serum.

hand-foot syndrome A condition in sickle cell disease caused by decreased blood flow to the hands and feet resulting in swelling and pain. Also called dactylitis.

haploid The number of chromosomes in a gamete—usually one-half the adult number. In the human, this number is 23.

haploidentical Refers to an incomplete match of human leukocyte antigens (HLA-A, -B, or -DR) between donor and recipient. See human leukocyte antigen (HLA).

hapten A low molecular weight substance (less than 5000) that rarely stimulates antibody production. However, some drug haptens can stimulate antibody production, causing drug-induced immune hemolytic anemia.

haptoglobin A protein made by the liver that binds free hemoglobin in the plasma.

harbinger Something that comes before to give an indication of what follows.

harvest In bone marrow transplantation, the collection of bone marrow or peripheral blood nucleated cells to yield sufficient numbers of stem cells for engraftment.

heat of fusion Heat released at the point when a solution in the liquid state transforms to the solid state.

Heinz body A round refractile erythrocyte inclusion not visible on a Wright-stained film. It ranges in size from about 1 to 3 μm and is attached to the cell membrane (Fig. 8-26). It may appear singly or multiply. It is best identified by supravital staining with basic dyes such as crystal violet, methylene blue, or brilliant cresyl blue.

helmet cell An abnormal, fragmented erythrocyte shape that looks like a helmet or hat. Suggestive of a microangiopathic hemolytic anemia or traumatic hemolytic anemia.

hemangioma Benign tumor of the blood vessels; may be congenital or acquired erythrocyte and may cause microangiopathic hemolytic anemia.

hemarthrosis A leakage of blood into a joint cavity.

hematemesis Vomiting of blood.

hematocrit (Hct) Packed red blood cell volume determined from an anticoagulated blood sample; denotes the percentage of erythrocytes in a known volume of whole blood. Reference range for adults is generally between 0.36 L/L and 0.48 L/L (Table 9-1).

hematoidin Substance formed in tissues from the breakdown of hemoglobin; chemically similar to bilirubin.

hematology The study of the appearance, development, physiology, kinetics, and pathology of the formed elements in blood (erythrocytes, leukocytes, and platelets).

hematoma A collection of blood in an organ, body space, or tissue caused by a break in a blood vessel wall. The blood usually clots, and subcutaneous hematomas may appear purplish-black.

hematopoiesis The production of blood cells. Also known as hemopoiesis.

hematoxylin and eosin (H&E) stain The routine histologic stain for tissue sections; used to stain bone marrow trephine and particle sections.

hematuria Intact erythrocytes in the urine.

heme A compound formed from the chelation of an iron atom in the ferrous (Fe^{2+}) state with protoporphyrin IX, a reaction catalyzed by the ferrochelatase enzyme (Figs. 7-3 and 13-1). Heme combines with globin to form hemoglobin.

heme-heme interaction In hemoglobin (Hb), the increased affinity of other heme molecules for O_2 as each heme molecule binds O_2. The more O_2 bound by Hb, the greater its affinity for O_2.

hemiglobin Another name for methemoglobin.

hemochromatosis An inherited (idiopathic) or acquired (see hemosiderosis) disorder of iron metabolism characterized by the abnormal deposition of iron in the tissues of multiple organs such as the liver, pancreas, heart, and pituitary gland causing tissue damage and bronze skin pigmentation. Associated with an increase in the number of siderotic granules (approximately 20 per cell) and an increase in the size of the siderotic granules in erythrocytes.

hemoconcentration Concentration of blood components due to the loss of plasma from the blood.

hemocytometer An apparatus (Figs. 24-1, 24-2) used to perform manual leukocyte, erythrocyte (now rarely done), and platelet counts on highly abnormal peripheral blood specimens whose cells cannot be accurately counted by automated methods. Also used to count cells in body fluids.

hemodilution Dilution of blood components due to an increase of fluid in the blood from the interstitial spaces.

hemoglobin (Hb) Main constituent of the erythrocyte; a protein that serves as the vehicle for transport of O_2 and CO_2 and maintains blood pH. It is composed of 4 globin (polypeptide) chains and 4 heme molecules. 2,3-DPG is sometimes resident in Hb.

hemoglobin Barts Hb composed of four gamma chains (γ_4) which has an extraordinarily high oxygen affinity. A significantly reduced rate of α chain synthesis in fetal life results in an excess of γ chains that form Hb Barts.

hemoglobin CC crystal An intraerythrocytic hexagonal crystal of Hb C with blunt ends that stains darkly (Fig. 8-18). It is found in patients with homozygous C (Hb CC) disease. The remainder of the erythrocyte is relatively Hb free and colorless (Fig. 8-20). It is not observed in all patients with Hb CC and is not seen in Hb C trait (Hb AC).

hemoglobin Gower I and Gower II Normal hemoglobin variants with molecular structures $\zeta_2\varepsilon_2$ and $\alpha_2\varepsilon_2$, respectively; produced only in the first 3 months of fetal development.

hemoglobin H Hb composed of four beta chains (β_4).

hemoglobin H disease A moderately severe hemolytic condition resulting from the compound heterozygous state for α^0 and α^+ thalassemia ($-/-\alpha$).

hemoglobin H inclusion Intracellular hemoglobin (Hb) H that can be demonstrated in affected erythrocytes *in vitro* by their exposure to an oxidant, such as brilliant cresyl blue, which precipitates Hb H. The inclusions occur in multiples and cover the cell surface, producing a golf-ball-like appearance (Fig. 14-9B). See brilliant cresyl blue inclusion body test.

hemoglobin M Inherited methemoglobin variants, of which there are 5. The amino acid substitutions causing the hemoglobin Ms cause hemoglobin to enter the ferric state resulting in methemoglobin formation.

hemoglobinopathy Condition caused by one or more qualitative structural abnormalities of the globin polypeptide chains that result from alteration of the deoxyribonucleic acid (DNA) genetic code for those chains. Many hemoglobinopathies exist.

hemoglobin Portland A normal hemoglobin with molecular structure $\zeta_2\gamma_2$ produced only in the first 3 months of fetal development.

hemoglobin S An abnormal β-globin chain variant in which valine is substituted for glutamic acid in the sixth position. See sickle cell anemia and sickle cell trait.

hemoglobin SC crystal A dark-hued intraerythrocytic crystal of condensed hemoglobin that distorts the erythrocyte membrane (Fig. 8-19). It is found in Hb SC disease. The characteristic type of crystalline projection is often straight with parallel sides and one blunt, pointed, protruding end ("Washington monument" shape). Multiple crystals may also protrude in different directions as fingerlike projections from a common crystalline center (Fig. 8-20).

hemoglobin, unstable A hemoglobin characterized by reduced solubility and a tendency to precipitate, forming intracellular Heinz bodies that are rigid and incapable of traversing the splenic microcirculation, thus predisposing the erythrocytes to hemolysis, *e.g.,* Hb Köln.

hemoglobinuria The presence of free hemoglobin (not intact erythrocytes) in urine.

hemoglobin variants Abnormal forms of hemoglobin (Hb) that differ because of variable amino acid sequences or numbers in their globin chains. Variants are usually caused by amino acid substitutions in normal Hbs (Table 14-3). See Table 7-2 for comparison to normal Hbs. The variants are numerous, *e.g.,* Hbs C, D, H, and S.

hemolysis The destruction of erythrocytes, which results in a release of their intracellular contents.

hemolysis, extravascular The erythrocyte destruction that occurs when intact or fragmented cells are phagocytized in the reticuloendothelial system (RES) with subsequent release of hemoglobin into the macrophages.

hemolysis, intravascular The destruction of erythrocytes in the blood vessels without phagocytic cell involvement resulting in the release of hemoglobin directly into the plasma.

hemolytic anemia An anemia that develops when the rate of erythrocyte destruction is accelerated and the bone marrow is normal but is not capable of keeping up with the erythrocyte destruction.

hemolytic anemia, immune Acquired hemolytic anemia characterized by accelerated destruction of erythrocytes by antibodies. The resultant anemia is due to the function, or in some cases malfunction, of the body's immune system.

hemolytic disease of the newborn (HDN) An anemia caused by destruction of an infant's erythrocytes when a maternal antibody that is specific to an antigen on the infant's erythrocytes crosses the placenta. Antibodies to Rh, ABO, and Kell antigens, among others, can cause HDN. Also known as erythroblastosis fetalis.

hemolytic uremic syndrome (HUS) A syndrome of infants and young children that involves acute intravascular hemolysis and renal failure.

hemolyze To undergo hemolysis.

hemopexin A plasma protein capable of combining with free heme.

hemophilia A group of sex-linked inherited coagulation disorders in which the level of blood coagulation factor VIII (hemophilia A) or factor IX (hemophilia B) is decreased below the normal level.

hemoptysis Expectoration of blood secondary to hemorrhage in the larynx, trachea, bronchi, or lungs.

hemorrhage Escape of blood from the vessels into the surrounding tissue or into the environment. Acute hemorrhage refers to immediate and severe bleeding, whereas chronic hemorrhage refers to less blood volume lost more gradually.

hemosiderin An insoluble form of storage iron that is produced when apoferritin is unavailable to complex with iron to form ferritin. A complex of oxidized iron and protein.

hemosiderinuria The presence of hemosiderin, an insoluble form of storage iron, in urine.

hemosiderosis An acquired focal or general increase in tissue iron stores without associated tissue damage. It is often caused by long-term transfusions that are required in certain disorders and may eventually cause tissue damage (see hemochromatosis). Associated with an increased number of siderotic granules in erythrocytes.

hemostasis The arrest of bleeding by physiologic properties of vasoconstriction and coagulation or by surgical means. Normal hemostasis depends on the types of surrounding tissues, the integrity of the blood vessels, normal platelet number and function, and the presence of adequate amounts of functioning coagulation promoting and inhibiting proteins.

hemostasis, primary The vascular and platelet response to vessel injury.

hemostasis, secondary The coagulation system response to vessel injury that leads to formation of a fibrin clot.

heparan sulfate A substance found on the endothelial cell surface that enhances antithrombin III activity.

heparin A mucopolysaccharide that enhances the effects of antithrombin III. It is used as an anticoagulant for laboratory testing and as a therapeutic agent.

heparin cofactor I Another name for antithrombin III.

heparin cofactor II (HCFII) A plasma antiprotease that inhibits coagulation primarily by inhibition of thrombin.

hepatosplenomegaly Increased size of the liver and spleen.

hereditary erythroblast multinuclearity with positive acidified serum test (HEMPAS) Type II congenital dyserythropoietic anemia (CDA), which is the most common CDA type. Characterized by an abnormal erythrocyte sensitivity to acidified normal serum, which is similar to that seen in paroxysmal nocturnal hemoglobinuria (PNH). HEMPAS and PNH can be distinguished by the failure of HEMPAS erythrocytes to lyse in the sugar water screening test.

hereditary persistence of fetal hemoglobin (HPFH) A disorder characterized by persistence of fetal hemoglobin (Hb F) production into adult life, which is sometimes associated with extremely mild forms of thalassemia.

heterochromatin Coarse, granular, irregularly-distributed chromatin forming medium-sized to large aggregates or clumps in the nucleus of a cell; characteristic of mature cells.

heterogeneity Of unlike nature or characteristics.

heterozygous Possessing different alleles at a given locus for a particular genetic characteristic. Also, inheriting the expression of both a normal allele and a genetic abnormality, *e.g.,* sickle cell trait (Hb AS).

heterozygous, doubly Inheriting two phenotypically interacting but separate genetic abnormalities, *e.g.,* Hb S–β thalassemia.

hexose monophosphate shunt (HMS) A pathway associated with the Embden–Meyerhof pathway that helps prevent oxidative damage to the erythrocyte (Fig. 6-7). Also called the pentose phosphate pathway.

high endothelial venules (HEVs) Venules that are lined with specialized endothelium found in lymphoid organs.

high-molecular-weight kininogen (HMWK) See kinin system.

high penetrance A genetic term that indicates a large number of individuals having a genotype that exhibits a phenotype. Low penetrance implies a low number of people who have a genotype that exhibits a phenotype.

histochemistry The application of chemical processes to cut sections of tissue to reveal their chemical composition.

histocompatible In a bone marrow transplant, refers to tolerance between donor and recipient cells to enable successful transplant engraftment: donor and recipient HLA-A, -B, and -DR loci are identical; six of six antigens match. See human leukocyte antigen (HLA).

histogram On automated hematology instruments, a display of data with the Y axis usually being relative number (or concentration), whereas the X axis is a measured characteristic of a particle (*e.g.,* volume, density, or staining intensity).

HIT Heparin-induced thrombocytopenia.

Hodgkin disease One of two principal groups of lymphomas diagnosed by lymph node biopsy, which reveals a mixture of normal cells (which predominate) and malignant Reed–Sternberg cells.

homing The circulation and migration of particular cells to specific tissues; also called trafficking.

homocysteine A sulfur-containing amino acid that is present in plasma either bound to protein (70%) or in a free form, both of which can be measured together as total homocysteine. It is required for DNA synthesis and increased in both folate and vitamin B_{12} deficiency.

homocysteinemia An excess of homocysteine in the blood.

homocysteinuria The presence of homocysteine in the urine (reference range, negative).

homologous Having similar appearance, function, or structure. Homologous chromosomes are two chromosomes, one donated by each parent. They have the same genes.

homozygous Possessing identical alleles at a given locus for a particular genetic characteristic. Also, inheriting all abnormal alleles of a gene, *e.g.*, sickle cell disease (HB SS).

Howell–Jolly body Small, round fragments of the nucleus (resulting from karyorrhexis or nuclear disintegration) of a late nucleated red blood cell or metarubricyte that stain reddish-blue with Wright stain (Figs. 8-21, 8-28).

human leukocyte antigen (HLA) Histocompatibility antigens (glycoproteins) on the surface of circulating and tissue cells determined by a region on the short arm of chromosome 6. This region includes a complex of several genes designated HLA-A, -B, -C, -DP, -DQ, and -DR, which are used to determine compatibility of tissues or organs that are proposed to be used for transplant.

humoral antibodies Immunoglobulins circulating in the plasma, all of which are part of the immune system. See immunoglobulin.

hyaluronidase Enzyme which breaks down hyaluronic acid (the "cement" of tissues).

hybridization The process by which the nucleotides of complementary nucleic acid sequences interact to form double-stranded molecules.

hydrocytosis See stomatocytosis, hereditary.

hydrodynamic focusing The fluidic narrowing of a liquid (*e.g.*, blood sample) stream injected into the center of a fast-flowing stream of cell-free (sheath) fluid. If laminar flow characteristics are maintained, the sample fluid in the middle flows faster than the surrounding sheath fluid and is not diluted by the sheath fluid. This causes the particles to line up in a single-file passage as they progress through the capillary sensing zone (aperture) for counting and measurement of other particle characteristics.

hydrogen peroxide (H_2O_2) A highly toxic substance generated in small amounts during normal erythrocyte metabolism, and in larger amounts when an oxidant drug interacts with oxyhemoglobin.

hydroxyapatite $Ca_{10}(PO_4)_6(OH)_2$ found in bones and teeth and responsible for the rigidity of these structures.

hyperbilirubinemia Increased plasma or serum bilirubin. See bilirubin.

hyperchromic A descriptive (although seldom used) word for erythrocytes that lack central pallor even though they lie in a desirable area for morphologic observation. Such erythrocytes are associated with a high MCHC and are common in hemolytic anemias.

hypercoagulable Characterized by the inappropriate formation of fibrin clots within the vascular system.

hypercoagulation Uncontrolled thrombosis.

hyperplasia The abnormal multiplication or increase in the number of normal cells in normal arrangement in a tissue such as bone marrow.

hypersegmented neutrophil A mature neutrophil having 6 or more nuclear lobes.

hypertension, malignant A rapidly progressive form of high blood pressure associated with severe vascular damage.

hypoadrenalism See Addison disease.

hypochromic A descriptive word used for erythrocytes with decreased hemoglobin content; commonly found in many anemias including iron deficiency.

hypocoagulation Excessive bleeding.

hypofibrinogenemia An abnormally low concentration of fibrinogen in the blood. It may be acquired due to consumptive processes of coagulation or from impaired synthesis. It may be inherited as an autosomal recessive trait and is usually of no clinical significance.

hypogammaglobulinemia An immunologic deficiency of all gamma globulin (IgG) antibodies.

hypoplastic Decreased number of bone marrow cells in all three cell lines (leukocytes, erythrocytes, and platelets).

hyposthenuria A condition characterized by inability to form urine of a high specific gravity.

hypoxia Decreased oxygen availability to the tissues.

icteric Affected by jaundice; yellow. Yellow discoloration of plasma, skin, sclerae, and mucous membranes caused by bilirubin accumulation associated with liver disease.

idiopathic Of unknown etiology (cause). See agnogenic.

idiopathic acquired sideroblastic anemia (IASA) See refractory anemia with ringed sideroblasts.

idiosyncratic Characterized by abnormal susceptibility to some drug, protein, or other agent that is peculiar to the individual.

Ig superfamily A large number of immunoglobulin-like cell-surface molecules known to be important for recognition of other molecules, cell adhesion functions, and triggering of events at the cell surface.

ileum The section of the small intestine farthest from the stomach.

iliac crest, posterior The upper margin of the hipbone in the back; the preferred site for bone marrow specimen collections.

Imerslund syndrome A rare hereditary disorder that causes vitamin B_{12} malabsorption in homozygotes within the first two years of life causing megaloblastic anemia and proteinuria.

immature reticulocyte fraction (IRF) A new parameter referred to as the "left shifted" reticulocyte count that is measured by several flow cytometric reticulocyte counters. It is clinically useful in following chemotherapy, erythropoietin therapy, and marrow failure.

immune thrombocytopenic purpura (ITP) A condition where autoantibodies cause the destruction of circulating platelets; may be acute or chronic.

immunity, humoral Acquired immunity provided by circulating antibodies produced by B lymphocytes and plasma cells.

immunocytochemistry The use of monoclonal or polyclonal antibodies to identify specific antigens on or within cells for purposes of identifying the cell type.

immunoglobulin A protein with antibody activity produced by lymphocytes and plasma cells. There are 5 classes including IgG, IgM, IgA, IgD, and IgE. See antibody.

immunophenotyping Detection of the genetic phenotype of a cell by analyzing for the presence of specific antigens on or within the cell through the use of monoclonal antibodies.

immunosuppression Depression of the function of the immune system through the use of various agents; usually accomplished by destruction of cells of the immune system (lymphocytes and macrophages).

incompatibility, major ABO Recipient has antibodies against donor erythrocytes.

incompatibility, minor ABO Donor has antibodies against recipient erythrocytes.

indolent Causing little or no symptoms, *e.g.*, pain; slow growing. See insidious.

infarct An area of tissue cell death caused by obstruction of blood circulation, most commonly by a thrombus or embolus, and thus lack of tissue oxygenation.

inhibitor A substance, often an antibody, that interferes with the normal reactions in a test system or biological activity *in vivo*. In coagulation, an inhibitor may be directed toward a specific factor, toward a reaction (non-specific), or toward several factors simultaneously (global).

insidious Stealthy and deceitful; of gradual and subtle onset. When used in relation to the onset of a disease, the patient has had no symptoms or signs of disease. See indolent.

in situ hybridization (ISH) A molecular technique in which cells immobilized on microscope slides are exposed to probes specific for a certain target sequence. The intracellular presence and location of the target:probe hybrid are detected by microscopic examination. When the probes are tagged with fluorescent markers, the method is called FISH.

integral proteins Erythrocyte membrane proteins that are in contact with both the inner and outer surfaces of the membrane (Fig. 6-6). The principal ones are the glycoproteins designated glycophorin A and band 3 that span the lipid bilayer.

integrins A large family of cell surface adhesion molecules composed of $\alpha\beta$ heterodimeric protein.

intercurrent Breaking into and modifying the course of an already existing disease.

interleukin (IL) A large group of glycoproteins called hematopoietic growth factors that sustain the proliferation, differentiation, and survival of immature hematopoietic progenitor cells and influence the survival and function of mature cells.

international normalized ratio (INR) A number used to monitor patients taking oral anticoagulants. Using this number, clinicians may interpret the prothrombin time (PT) results among laboratories using different thromboplastin preparations with different sensitivities to the effects of anticoagulants. It is calculated as the ratio of a patient's PT to the mean PT normal value (from a laboratory's plasma reference pool) and this value raised to the power of the thromboplastin international sensitivity index (see ISI). The ISI is provided by the thromboplastin manufacturer.

international sensitivity index (ISI) A number that indicates the comparative slope of a thromboplastin reagent to the World Health Organization reference thromboplastin preparation. It is used to calculate the international normalized ratio (see INR) and provided by the manufacturer on the thromboplastin package insert.

intrathecal injection Injection of a substance through the theca (enclosing case or sheath) of the spinal canal into the subarachnoid space.

intravascular In the vessels.

intrinsic factor (IF) A protein secreted by the gastric parietal cells that forms a protective complex with vitamin B_{12} that is transported down the gastrointestinal tract to the ileum where B_{12} is released from IF and absorbed. It is also known as Castle's intrinsic factor, after its discoverer William Castle.

iodophor A preparation containing iodine that is capable of inhibiting the growth of microorganisms.

iron A major component of the hemoglobin molecule. Iron is chelated (in the ferrous [Fe^{2+}] form) to protoporphyrin IX, a reaction catalyzed by the enzyme ferrochelatase to form heme (Fig. 13-1).

iron deficiency anemia Anemia associated with a decreased hemoglobin level, MCV, and microcytic, hypochromic erythrocytes related to an absolute decrease of iron available to synthesize hemoglobin.

iron, serum Refers to ferric iron (Fe^{3+}) bound to serum transferrin.

isoantibody See alloantibody.

isoantigen See alloantigen.

isoelectric focusing A modified form of electrophoresis in which the support medium along which proteins migrate has a *p*H gradient or gradually increasing *p*H, *e.g.*, 3 to 10, such that proteins migrate in the electric field to the *p*H that is equal to their isoelectric point. There they have no more charge and cease to move. Used to assess abnormal hemoglobin variants.

isoelectric point (pI) The *p*H of the surrounding environment at which a protein has no net charge.

Jenner Name of a British physician who developed a type of Romanowsky stain. The Jenner stain differs from other Romanowsky stains in the ratio of methylene blue to eosin that is used.

kallikrein Activated form of prekallikrein; a form of kinin. See kinin system.

kaolin Fine white clay used in the manufacture of porcelain and also as an *in vitro* activator of coagulation factor XII. Named after the mountain in China where it was first mined.

karyorrhexis Rupture of the cell nucleus in which chromatin disintegrates into formless granules or spheres. The inability of chromosomes to reform into a nucleus after mitosis, resulting in disintegrated, structureless chromatin fragments.

karyotype The systematic display of all the chromosomes from a single cell lined up and numbered according to size, location of centromere, and banding patterns revealed by special stains. Humans are normally characterized by 22 pairs of autosomal chromosomes and a pair of sex chromosomes.

keratocyte (Gr. *keras*: horn) An erythrocyte poikilocyte with horns (Fig. 8-12D) that is the result of the rupturing of the vacuole of a blister cell. It should be reported as a schistocyte.

kernicterus Brain damage in infants afflicted with high levels of plasma bilirubin.

kinetics 1. In hematology, the dynamic forces that move cells into and out of different body compartments or tissues. 2. The rate at which a reaction proceeds.

kinin A peptide of low molecular weight composed of a series of amino acids.

kinin system In hemostasis, certain kinins are activated by the coagulation and fibrinolytic systems (Fig. 48-1). They include prekallikrein and its activated form kallikrein, kininogen (both low-molecular-weight [LMWK] and high-molecular-weight [HMWK] forms), and the kinins, *e.g.*, bradykinin. Prekallikrein and HMWK are important in the contact activation phase of the intrinsic coagulation pathway and in complement activation.

Kleihauer–Betke stain See acid-elution slide test.

Köhler illumination An illumination method that ensures optimum contrast and resolution of specimen details seen when using a microscope.

koilonychia Abnormal change of the fingernails sometimes associated with iron deficiency anemia (Fig. 13-2). The nails become thin and concave and have raised edges (spoon nails).

Kupffer cells Macrophages (phagocytic cells) in the liver that form part of the reticuloendothelial system and destroy severely abnormal erythrocytes.

lactate dehydrogenase (LD) An enzyme widely distributed in the tissues of the body that catalyzes the oxidation of lactate to pyruvate. Erythrocytes contain high concentrations of isoenzymes LD-1 and LD-2.

lactoferrin An iron-binding glycoprotein found in the secondary granules of the neutrophil that competes with bacteria for iron.

laminar flow The passage of two liquids through a channel in which the two liquids do not mix; used in hydrodynamic focusing. They travel in parallel or layered configuration with central layers flowing faster than outer layers.

laser Acronym for light **a**mplification by **s**timulated **e**mission of **r**adiation. A device that produces an intense, nondiverging, monochromatic beam of light. Used as the light source in many flow cytometers, in several instruments performing automated 5-part differentials, and in those counting reticulocytes.

latex An emulsion of finely divided particles of rubber or plastic.

lavage To wash out or irrigate an organ or space.

lead intoxication Clinical condition related to the chronic or acute ingestion of lead which is highly toxic. Toxic effects may involve many organs and the clinical manifestations parallel the blood lead levels.

Leishman Name of a British surgeon who developed a type of Romanowsky stain specifically for staining blood parasites. The Leishman stain differs from other Romanowsky stains in the ratio of methylene blue to eosin that is used.

leptocyte (Gr. *lepto*: thin) An erythrocyte that is thinner than normal with a colorless center. It has an increased surface area that is out of proportion to the volume and may be normocytic or microcytic. Microcytic leptocytes are formed because of a lack of hemoglobin, as seen in severe iron deficiency. Small leptocytes may be seen in thalassemia and hemoglobinopathies such as Hb C.

lethargy Feeling of drowsiness.

leukapheresis The removal of leukocytes from the peripheral circulation followed by reinfusion of the remainder of the blood components to the donor.

leukemia, acute lymphocytic (ALL) A clonal proliferative disorder of lymphoid precursor cells characterized by lack of cell maturation and differentiation. They include the FAB subtypes of L1, L2, and L3.

leukemia, acute nonlymphocytic (ANLL) A clonal proliferative disorder of erythroid, granulocytic, monocytic or megakaryocytic precursor cells characterized by lack of cell maturation and differentiation. Blast forms of these precursors make up at least 30% of the bone marrow cells. They include the FAB subtypes of MO, M1, M2, M3, M4, M5, M6, and M7. Also called acute granulocytic (AGL) and acute myeloid leukemia (AML).

leukemogen A drug or chemical that is capable of causing bone marrow depression, aplasia, and malignancy.

leukemoid Condition with an outward appearance of leukemia that is transient in nature. Usually characterized by very high leukocyte counts with a severe left shift.

leukocyte White blood cell; colorless nucleated cell that circulates in peripheral blood and functions as the body's main defense against infection.

leukocyte alkaline phosphatase (LAP) A phosphatase enzyme found in varying amounts in the cytoplasm of neutrophils and their precursors. Also called neutrophil alkaline phosphatase (NAP).

leukocyte differential count A procedure performed on a stained peripheral blood film during which 100 leukocytes are classified according to their type and observed for abnormalities, the leukocyte count is estimated, morphologic erythrocyte abnormalities are identified, and platelet number is estimated.

leukoerythroblastic Presence of immature neutrophils and nucleated red blood cells in the same blood film. Usually indicative of a space-occupying lesion in the bone marrow.

Levy counting chamber A type of hemocytometer. See hemocytometer.

ligand A molecule that binds to a specific receptor on the surface of or within a cell.

ligase An enzyme that connects pieces of DNA.

ligase chain reaction (LCR) A molecular technique in which a target sequence is amplified using primers that encompass the sequence and are then joined together by a ligase.

limiting dilution assay (LDA) Analytical method to determine the frequency of T-cell growth in increasing dilutions (decreasing cell concentrations) of the graft before and after T-cell depletion; log of T-cell depletion is calculated from this frequency.

lineage specificity Any substance, function, or activity that is peculiar to a particular cell line or cell family.

lipemia Excessive fat or lipids in the blood causing plasma to have a "milky" appearance.

low-molecular-weight kininogen (LMWK) See kinin system.

lumbar Part of the back between the thorax and the pelvis; loins.

lupus erythematosus cell See systemic lupus erythematosus.

lupus inhibitor An immunoglobulin (IgG, IgM, or both), first observed in the plasmas of patients with systemic lupus erythematosus, found with a variety of clinical conditions that interferes with the *in vitro* phospholipid-dependent tests of coagulation (*e.g.*, PTT, dilute Russell's viper venom test).

lymphadenopathy Disease of the lymph nodes that results in their swelling.

lymphocyte Leukocyte that has a deep purple, dense nucleus and bright sky-blue cytoplasm, usually containing no granules; represents 10% to 44% of leukocytes in normal adult peripheral blood.

lymphocyte transformation Process by which resting lymphocytes enter the cell cycle and begin the process of mitosis. Characterized by increasingly larger size and decreasing nuclear clumping.

lymphocyte, variant Lymphocyte responding to an antigenic stimulus; may represent 0% to 7.5% of leukocytes in normal adult peripheral blood; also called reactive, stimulated, or atypical lymphocyte or virocyte.

lymphokine Cytokine produced by lymphocytes. See cytokine.

lymphokinetics The process of lymphocyte multiplication, maturation, storage, and migration to tissues, including sites of infection or cell damage.

lymphoma A group of malignant diseases with abnormal lymph node enlargement causing abnormal histology. Peripheral blood abnormalities usually do not occur until advanced stages of the disease.

lymphoma, non-Hodgkin One of two principal groups of lymphomas (the other being Hodgkin disease) in which the lymph node cellular infiltrates are generally uniformly composed of similar-appearing neoplastic cells that are usually B lymphocytes.

lymphopoiesis Formation of lymphocytes.

lymphostasis Absent or reduced flow of fluid within the lymph ducts.

Lyon hypothesis A theory that one of the two X chromosomes in female's cells is inactivated at random during embryogenesis. Therefore, some cells have maternal X chromosome characteristics, whereas the remainder have paternal X chromosome characteristics. This is particularly important in explaining G6PD deficiency among women.

lysosome A membrane-bound granule in the cytoplasm of a cell that contains a variety of enzymes and other chemicals necessary for the degradation and digestion of phagocytosed foreign materials. Lysosomes are found in macrophages, granulocytes, and platelets.

lysozyme An anti-bacterial hydrolase enzyme found in both primary and secondary neutrophil granules and monocytes that catalyzes the hydrolysis of mucopolysaccharides or mucopeptides; also known as muramidase. It aids in phagocytosis by destroying the capsule of some bacteria.

M Symbol for molar, which denotes the strength of a solution.

macrocyte A macrocytic erythrocyte (see macrocytic). Macrocytes may occur with or without anemia.

macrocytic The descriptive term for erythrocytes that have a mean cell volume (MCV) exceeding 100 fL or a diameter exceeding 8.5 to 9.0 μm.

α_2-macroglobulin A naturally occurring glycoprotein that is the second to bind with any plasmin that is free in the plasma (following saturation of α_2-antiplasmin), thus preventing excessive fibrinolysis. It also inhibits components in the coagulation system.

macroglobulinemia Increase in an unusually high-molecular-weight globulin in the blood, often an immunoglobulin of the IgM class.

macroovalocyte See oval macrocyte.

macrophage A phagocytic cell found in the tissues; the tissue counterpart of the blood monocyte.

major histocompatibility complex (MHC) The chromosomal region that contains the genes that regulate immune functions.

malaise Discomfort, uneasiness.

malaria A disease caused by the protozoan *Plasmodium* (see Plasmodium) which invades erythrocytes. It is transmitted to man by the bite of the *Anopheles* mosquito.

malignant An abnormal uncontrolled process of cellular growth in which cells do not resemble their tissue of origin and multiply and spread rapidly (metastasize), destroying normal tissue. The cells' organelle structure and shape is abnormal, and the process is often irreversible and rapidly fatal.

MAPSS™ Multiple angle polarized-scatter separation; acronym of Abbott Laboratories' technology used in 5-part differential analysis.

march hemoglobinuria A condition in which hemoglobin is found in the urine and schistocytes are found on the blood film most likely due to mechanical damage to the cells in the feet of individuals on long walking expeditions.

marginated neutrophil pool (MNP) Term describing location of neutrophils while adhering to vessel walls; approximately one-half of the neutrophils in blood vessels are contained in this pool and are constantly exchanged with the circulating neutrophil pool.

mast cell Cell resembling and functionally similar to the basophil that is found throughout the connective tissues of the body.

mastectomy The surgical removal of a breast.

maturation The process of becoming fully developed and obtaining all the functional characteristics of a mature or end cell.

May–Grünwald Names of two German physicians who developed a type of Romanowsky stain. The May–Grünwald stain differs from other Romanowsky stains in the ratio of methylene blue to eosin that is used.

May–Hegglin anomaly A condition characterized by giant, poorly-functional platelets and large blue inclusions in all granulocytes. It was named after the two investigators who first described it.

mean corpuscular hemoglobin (MCH) The average weight of hemoglobin of a single erythrocyte in a given blood sample; expressed in picograms (pg).

mean corpuscular hemoglobin concentration (MCHC) The average concentration of hemoglobin in a single erythrocyte of a given blood sample; expressed in g/dL.

mean corpuscular volume (MCV) The average volume of a single erythrocyte in a given blood sample; expressed in femtoliters (fL).

megakaryocytic hypoplasia Condition characterized by fewer than normal numbers of megakaryocytes in the bone marrow.

megaloblast A very large erythrocyte precursor with characteristically fine nuclear chromatin at all stages of maturation. Early megaloblasts have an extremely basophilic cytoplasm. See megaloblast, orthochromic.

megaloblast, orthochromic A characteristic erythrocyte precursor in megaloblastic anemia. It has an abundant, mature-looking pink cytoplasm similar to that of an orthochromic normoblast, but its nucleus resembles that seen in a polychromatophilic normoblast, a less mature precursor. This is referred to as nuclear-cytoplasmic asynchrony.

megaloblastic anemias A large subgroup of anemias of abnormal nuclear development classically associated with very large, oval erythrocytes (macroovalocytes), an increased mean cell volume, and hypersegmented neutrophils and commonly caused by either vitamin B_{12} or folate deficiency.

megaloblastoid Literally means "resembling megaloblastic." A form of abnormal erythrocyte maturation commonly found in the myeloproliferative and dysmyelopoietic disorders. It is characterized by large (even giant) RBC precursors having an open chromatin pattern that is more coarse than that of megaloblastic maturation, making the parachromatin more prominent. The chromatin may be attached to the nuclear membrane in large clumps. Multinuclearity and abnormally-shaped nuclei may be present.

megathrombocyte Giant platelet.

melena Stool containing dark red or black blood. The black color is caused by the action of intestinal juices on blood that has escaped into the gastrointestinal tract from the vascular system.

memory lymphocyte A lymphocyte that has encountered specific antigen(s) and is programmed for recognition and action with the next encounter.

meninges The three membranes that cover the brain and spinal cord: the pia mater, dura mater, and arachnoid.

menorrhagia Excessive uterine bleeding occurring at the usual intervals of menstruation.

mesothelium Lining cells derived from the mesoderm that make up the surface of serous membranes.

metamyelocyte An immature neutrophil stage in which the round nucleus begins to flatten or indent and the cytoplasm is similar to the mature neutrophil; normally found only in the bone marrow.

metaplasia 1. Production of cells outside the normal location. When referring to myeloid cells (myeloid metaplasia), implies production of myeloid cells outside of the bone marrow. See extramedullary. 2. Controlled abnormal cell growth associated with adaptive substitution of cell types, *e.g.*, lung epithelial cell replacement in smoking.

metarubricyte The last nucleated red blood cell stage (Color Plates 6-1–6-3 and 6-6). It has a pale, blue-gray-violet polychromatophilic to pinkish cytoplasm and a dense nuclear chromatin pattern. The nucleus is pyknotic and extruded at this stage (Fig. 6-4); hemoglobin is the main cytoplasmic constituent.

metastasis The transfer of disease from one organ or part to another not directly connected with it as is typical of the cells of malignant tumors.

methemalbumin The product formed when free heme is oxidized in the plasma and bound to albumin.

methemalbuminemia The presence of methemalbumin in the plasma.

methemoglobin A hemoglobin derivative in which the ferrous iron (Fe^{2+}) has been oxidized to ferric iron (Fe^{3+}). It cannot function to transport O_2 or CO_2. It is normally reduced in the methemoglobin reduction pathway, a part of the Embden–Meyerhof pathway (Fig. 6-7).

methemoglobinemia The presence of elevated levels of methemoglobin in the plasma. Rarely this is an inherited disorder caused by deficiency of the NADH-methemoglobin reductase enzyme; more commonly it is acquired from exposure to various substances including certain drugs and foods. Clinical manifestations are few and generally mild.

methemoglobinuria The presence of methemoglobin in urine.

α-methyldopa A medication frequently prescribed for hypertension that may cause drug-induced immune hemolytic anemia.

methylmalonic acid (MMA) An organic compound that is found in the plasma as a result of catabolism of propionic acid and increased if vitamin B_{12} is deficient.

MHC class I molecule A transmembrane glycoprotein, composed of a large, heavy α chain and a smaller chain known as β_2-microglobulin, that is found on most nucleated cells.

MHC class II molecule A transmembrane heterodimer composed of an α and a β chain linked by noncovalent bonds and found primarily on B lymphocytes, monocytes and macrophages, dendritic cells, endothelial cells, and other cells subsequent to activation.

microangiopathic Pertaining to a disease of small blood vessels.

microangiopathic hemolytic anemia (MAHA) The characteristic anemia found in diseases of small blood vessels including DIC, TTP, HUS, and other disorders which cause hemolysis with characteristic erythrocyte fragments on the peripheral blood film.

microcyte A small erythrocyte with a reduced volume, normal or decreased hemoglobin content, and a reduced, normal, or increased diameter. "Microcytic" is the descriptive term.

microfilament The contractile fiber in platelets formed by actomyosin, about 5 to 7 nm in diameter.

microspherocytes Small, round erythrocytes (smaller than platelets) that result from thermal damage. Also called microspherules.

microtubule A cyclindrical structure, 20–27 nm in diameter, found in many types of cells. It is composed of protein subunits called tubulin. Microtubules serve as part of the cytoskeleton.

Miller disc An optical device for use in estimating peripheral blood film platelet counts.

mitogen A substance usually derived from plants that stimulates cells, especially lymphocytes, to undergo blastic transformation and mitosis. Examples include pokeweed mitogen (PWM), concanavalin-A (con-A), and phytohemagglutinin (PHA).

mitosis Division of a cell that forms two daughter cells with nuclear chromosomes identical to those of the original cell.

molecular probe A fragment of DNA or RNA used to detect a complementary nucleic acid within a cell by means of hybridization.

Monge's disease Chronic mountain sickness that is caused by a loss of tolerance for hypoxia in individuals exposed to high altitudes with low atmospheric pressure that results in decreased arterial oxygen content.

monoclonal Arising from a single precursor cell; relating to a single clone of cells. Most malignancies are monoclonal; they arise from a single parent cell that is transformed by a neoplastic event.

monoclonal antibody(mAb) A specific antibody of a single molecular species obtained from a hybridoma (*i.e.*, a single antibody-producing lymphocyte fused with a single myeloma cell) that is specific for a single antigen. The hybridoma is grown in culture and enables the production of unlimited quantities of the specific antibody.

monoclonal gammopathy A disease in which there is an increase in serum immunoglobulin produced by cells derived from one abnormal parent cell; thus, the immunoglobulin is structurally homogeneous.

monocyte Leukocyte with lobulated or horseshoe-shaped nucleus and abundant, pale gray-blue cytoplasm with fine, indistinct

granules; represents 2% to 10% of leukocytes in normal adult peripheral blood.

monomer A molecule that is the repeating unit of a string of identical molecules (polymer).

mononuclear phagocyte system (MPS) System of mononuclear phagocytic cells located throughout the body; includes mature and immature monocytes in the blood and bone marrow, and both free and fixed tissue macrophages; formerly called the reticuloendothelial system.

morphogenesis The alteration in appearance that a cell undergoes during any type of activity such as maturation.

mosaicism Refers to an organ or tissue that is made up of cells from two or more genetically distinct sources.

Moschcowitz syndrome Alternate name for thrombotic thrombocytopenic purpura (TTP).

multiple myeloma A malignant proliferation of plasma cells characterized by bone infiltration and the presence of abnormal monoclonal immunoglobulin in the serum. Also known as plasma cell myeloma.

muramidase See lysozyme.

mutation Any change in the base sequence of a genomic nucleic acid.

mycosis fungoides A rare form of cutaneous T-cell lymphoma characterized by skin lesions but no systemic involvement (see Sézary syndrome).

myeloblast A primitive cell of myeloid origin whose lineage is uncertain when based solely on light microscopy (it could be a precursor cell for granulocytes, monocytes, erythrocytes, or megakaryocytes). Special stains, surface markers, and electron microscopy indicate that the majority of these cells are neutrophil precursors.

myelocyte An immature neutrophil stage in which the nucleus remains round, the cytoplasm remains slightly blue and secondary granules begin to form in the cytoplasm. It is the most mature stage still undergoing mitosis and normally found only in the bone marrow.

myeloid cells Normal cells of the bone marrow including maturing leukocytes (except lymphocytes), erythrocytes, and platelets.

myeloid:erythroid (M:E) ratio A ratio of the percentage of developing myeloid (usually the granulocytes and their precursors) to the percentage of developing erythroid (erythrocyte) precursors. Derived from the bone marrow differential and reported in whole numbers. The expected ratio in adults ranges from 2:1 to 4:1.

myeloma A tumor composed of cells normally found in the bone.

myelomonocytic leukemia, chronic (CMML) A dysmyelopoietic syndrome characterized by 5 to 20% blasts in the bone marrow, less than 5% blasts in the peripheral blood, a prominent monocytic component in the bone marrow, and moderate dysgranulopoiesis (Table 33-2).

myeloperoxidase An enzyme located in the primary granules of the neutrophil that aids the cell in killing phagocytized bacteria.

myelophthisic Space-occupying lesion in the bone marrow caused by fibrous tissue, metastatic tumor, or leukemia. Usually accompanied by leukoerythroblastic reaction.

myelophthisic anemia Anemia secondary to bone marrow infiltration and replacement by abnormal cells (*e.g.*, leukemia).

myeloproliferative Disorder resulting in the abnormal proliferation of myeloid cells.

myeloproliferative disorder, chronic (CMPD) A clonal proliferative disorder of bone marrow precursor cells in which cells retain maturation and differentiation. No more than 5% blasts are found in the bone marrow in these disorders during the chronic phase of the disease.

myelosuppression Inhibition of hemopoiesis in the myeloid (bone marrow) tissues.

NADH–methemoglobin reductase An enzyme in the Embden–Meyerhof pathway, specifically in the methemoglobin reduction pathway, which reduces methemoglobin in the blood (Fig. 6-7). Also called diaphorase.

naive lymphocyte A lymphocyte that has not encountered an antigen.

NAP Neutrophil alkaline phosphatase. See leukocyte alkaline phosphatase.

necrobiotic Normal (programmed) cell death resulting from development. Also known as apoptosis (noun) or apoptotic (adj). Not to be confused with necrosis or necrotic.

necrosis Cell death resulting from abnormal and irreversible cell damage.

necrosis, skin Death of skin cells that frequently results in open sores; caused by a wide variety of agents from microbes to vascular blockage to toxins.

neoplasia Abnormal cell growth and appearance that can be benign (see benign) or malignant (see malignant).

Neubauer hemocytometer A standard device (Fig. 24-1) used to perform manual leukocyte, erythrocyte (now rarely done), and platelet counts. See hemocytometer.

neutrophil, segmented A leukocyte with a multilobed nucleus and a cytoplasm containing numerous light pinkish-tan granules when stained with Wright stain; represents 37% to 77% of leukocytes in normal adult peripheral blood; also known as seg, polymorphonuclear neutrophil (PMN), and poly.

normoblast Nucleated red blood cell.

normoblastic A descriptive word for normal erythrocyte precursor maturation.

normochromic A descriptive word used for erythrocytes with normal hemoglobin content.

normocytic A descriptive word used for normal-sized erythrocytes.

Northern blot See Southern blot.

nuclear–cytoplasmic asynchrony An abnormal relationship between the degree of maturation of the nucleus and the cytoplasm of an erythrocyte or leukocyte precursor. Erythrocyte precursors show a mature, pink cytoplasm surrounding an immature nucleus with fine, delicate chromatin.

nuclear:cytoplasmic (N:C) ratio The area of the cell which is nucleus in relation to the area which is cytoplasm; a high nuclear to cytoplasmic ratio (large amount of nucleus in proportion to amount of cytoplasm) usually denotes cellular immaturity.

nucleated red blood cell (NRBC) A maturing red blood cell that contains a nucleus and is normally found in the bone marrow, but may be found in the peripheral blood in many abnormal hematogic conditions. Also called a normoblast.

nucleoli Plural of nucleolus.

nucleolus (pl. nucleoli) A round, refractile body present in the nucleus of most cells. It is electron dense and more than one may be present in the early stages of a cell's maturation. It contains RNA, proteins, and small amounts of DNA. Nucleoli are involved in the production and distribution of RNA.

nucleoproteins A combination of protein (*e.g.*, histones) and nucleic acids (*e.g.*, DNA). Nuclear chromatin is generally made up of nucleoproteins.

nucleotide A purine (adenine or guanine) or pyrimidine (cytosine, thymine, or uracil) base containing a sugar (ribose or deoxyribose) and a phosphate moiety.

nucleotides, complementary Nucleotides that can pair specifically with each other. In DNA, adenine (A) pairs with thymine (T), and cytosine (C) pairs with guanine (G).

nucleus A round or oval mass of protoplasm within the cell that contains chromatin and sometimes nucleoli. The nucleus directs cell activity.

numerical aperture The performance rating of a lens for gathering light, for example an objective lens on a microscope.

objective Optical lens system that forms the magnified intermediate image of a specimen viewed on a microscope.

occlusion, venous Mechanical blockage of the return of venous blood from extremities to the heart.

occult blood A test using a fecal sample for the presence of blood that is not visible to the unaided eye.

oliguria Secretion of a diminished amount of urine compared to the fluid intake.

oncogene A mutated proto-oncogene capable of causing malignant (neoplastic) development.

open canalicular system (OCS) A membrane system that permeates normal platelets and connects to the open surface. The OCS absorbs large quantities of plasma proteins to help form the glycocalyx.

opsonization Process by which bacteria or foreign particles are coated by antibodies and/or complement to enhance phagocytosis by certain leukocytes.

organomegaly A general term to describe enlargement of one or more organs.

orthochromic normoblast See metarubricyte.

osmolarity The concentration of osmotically active particles in solution.

osmosis The passage of pure solvent from a solution of lesser to one of greater solute concentration when the two solutions are separated by a membrane which selectively prevents the passage of solute molecules but is permeable to the solvent.

osmotic fragility The capacity of erythrocytes to take up fluid in hypotonic solutions, *e.g.*, 0.35% NaCl. Spherocytes have increased osmotic fragility (*i.e.*, low tolerance for hypotonic fluid uptake), whereas target cells have decreased osmotic fragility (*i.e.*, increased tolerance for hypotonic fluid uptake).

osteolysis Destruction of bone, especially owing to the removal or loss of calcium.

o-toluidine dihydrochloride A chemical used in the counterstain for differentiation of heme from nonheme proteins when a band is migrating near the specimen application point on cellulose acetate hemoglobin electrophoresis. Heme stains purple; nonheme protein remains pink.

oval macrocyte A very large (macrocytic), oval erythrocyte. It usually has a markedly increased MCV (more than 125 fL) and strongly implicates megaloblastic erythropoiesis caused by vitamin B_{12} or folate deficiency. A nuclear maturation defect in the early nucleated red blood cells of the bone marrow leads to development of oval macrocytes (Fig. 8-4B). May be called a macro-ovalocyte.

ovalocyte An erythrocyte that has an oval or egg shape. It results from hereditary or acquired conditions.

overt Apparent, observable, not hidden.

oxyhemoglobin Hemoglobin that is carrying oxygen.

P_{50} The partial pressure of oxygen at which hemogobin is half saturated.

pancytopenia A decrease in all cellular constituents (leukocytes, erythrocytes, and platelets); may be seen, for example, in aplastic anemia.

panmyelosis Increased proliferation of all myeloid cells (erythrocytes, granulocytes, and platelets).

Pappenheimer bodies Small, irregular, dark-staining granules that appear near the periphery of a young erythrocyte in a blood film stained with Wright or supravital stain (Figs. 8-23, 8-28).

With Perls' Prussian blue stain (Chap. 29), these bodies stain positively, indicating their iron content (Color Plate 13-1). Also called siderotic granules.

parachromatin The nonstaining or clear areas between chromatin clumps in the nucleus of myeloid and lymphoid cells; becomes more prominent as cells mature.

paracoagulation The formation of gels or precipitates caused by the reaction between protamine sulfate or ethanol and fibrin monomers or fragments X and Y. This phenomenon is used in the laboratory to detect fibrin monomers that are not normally present in the plasma.

paraneoplastic Clinical symptoms and signs that are associated with a malignancy but not caused directly by the malignancy.

paraprotein An abnormal plasma protein produced by a clone of neoplastic plasma cells proliferating abnormally. It is often the abnormal immunoglobulin produced in a monoclonal gammopathy.

parasthesias A prickling, tingling, "pins and needles" sensation in the hands and feet; a symptom sometimes reported by patients with pernicious anemia.

paroxysmal cold hemoglobinuria (PCH) The rarest form of autoimmune hemolytic anemia (AIHA); it is caused by binding of the Donath–Landsteiner (D-L) autoantibody to erythrocytes following exposure to cold, which results in intravascular hemolysis and gross hemoglobinuria.

paroxysmal nocturnal hemoglobinuria (PNH) A rare acquired intracorpuscular defect of blood cells causing a hemolytic anemia. It is caused by a mutation in a single bone marrow precursor that results in an abnormal clone of bone marrow stem cells that produce abnormal blood cells.

partial thromboplastin time (PTT) A clinical laboratory test that measures the function of the intrinsic and common blood coagulation pathways and requires citrated platelet-poor plasma preincubated with a reagent containing a surface activator. Coagulation is initiated by addition of Ca^{2+}. Agents are added to the test reagent that expedite activation of contact coagulation factors decreasing the total time of the test. The PTT is commonly used to monitor heparin therapy.

pathognomonic Characteristic of a disease; a sign or symptom on which a diagnosis can be made.

pentose phosphate pathway (PPP) See hexose monophosphate shunt.

percent transmittance (%T) The amount of light that passes through a medium.

perfusion Supplying oxygen and nutrients to tissues and organs by way of circulating blood.

pericardium A membranous sac that surrounds the heart and great vessels attached to the heart. The inner layer is a serous membrane.

peripheral proteins Erythrocyte membrane proteins that are attached to the integral proteins on the inner (cytoplasmic) portion of the membrane (Fig. 17-1). They include, among others, three important erythrocyte skeletal proteins: α and β spectrin (also called bands 1 and 2, respectively) and actin (band 5).

peritoneum A serous, membranous sac that lines the abdominal and pelvic walls and encloses the gastrointestinal viscera.

pernicious anemia (PA) A form of megaloblastic anemia associated with vitamin B_{12} deficiency that results from a lack of intrinsic factor secretion in the stomach caused by an acquired atrophy of the stomach lining called achylia gastrica.

petechiae Purplish-red, pinpoint hemorrhagic spots (<3 mm in diameter) in the skin caused by loss of capillary ability to withstand normal blood pressure and trauma. Poor capillary integrity allows erythrocytes to leak out of capillary beds into tissue. Many petechiae close together can create purpura. Petechiae are more indicative of a vascular or platelet disorder than of coagulation or fibrinolytic defects.

phagocytosis Process by which certain leukocytes engulf and dispose of microorganisms and cellular debris.

phagosome Vacuole formed when a phagocytic cell completely surrounds a particle or microorganism.

phenotype The entire physical, biochemical, and physiologic makeup of an individual as determined both genetically and environmentally (as opposed to genotype); the physical and/or physiologic expression of the genotype.

pH gradient Having an increasing pH (*e.g.*, 3–10). See isoelectric focusing.

Philadelphia chromosome (Ph^1) An abnormal chromosome resulting from the translocation of chromosomal material between chromosomes 9 and 22, technically written as t(9q$^+$; 22q$^-$); found in over 95% of patients with chronic myelogenous leukemia. Its presence in patients with acute lymphoblastic leukemia is considered a poor prognostic sign.

phlebotomist A person who performs phlebotomies.

phlebotomy Any opening of a vein, usually associated with venipuncture, for the collection of a blood specimen.

phospholipid (PL) A substance found on the surface of platelets, where many coagulation reactions take place. PL and calcium on the platelet surface are essential for enzyme and substrate functions in the coagulation pathways.

photocutaneous lesion Skin abnormality found in people with some porphyrias. The increase in blood porphyrins causes an increase in skin absorbance of sunlight, which leads to the formation of these lesions.

photomultiplier tube (PMT) An electronic detector that is sensitive to weak optical (light) signals. It amplifies the weak signals and converts optical signals into electrical current.

phototherapy Exposure of an infant with hyperbilirubinemia to natural sunlight or fluorescent light to reduce the plasma bilirubin level.

phytohemagglutinin Lectin extracted from the red kidney bean capable of causing erythroctyes to agglutinate and T lymphocytes to proliferate.

pitting, splenic Removal of inclusion bodies from an erythrocyte by the macrophages of the spleen.

plasma The liquid portion of anticoagulated whole blood.

plasmacytoma Tumor composed of plasma cells. Typically, several are seen in bone marrow from patients with multiple myeloma.

plasmapheresis Process in which plasma is selectively collected. Blood is drawn and separated by centrifugation. Cells are then returned to the donor.

plasmin A serine protease and fibrinolytic enzyme formed upon the activation of plaminogen within a fibrin clot by plasminogen activators (Fig. 48-3). It is not normally found in the plasma because antiplasmins immediately degrade it. Plasmin plays multiple roles in hemostasis. Also called fibrinolysin.

plasminogen A single-chain glycoprotein zymogen that normally circulates in the plasma. It is the inert precursor of the enzyme plasmin. See plasminogen activator and plasmin.

plasminogen activator A substance released by damaged tissues that activates plasminogen to its active form, plasmin; also called tissue plasminogen activator (TPA).

platelet A fragment of megakaryocyte cytoplasm found in the peripheral blood (1 to 4 μm diameter). Viewed by light microscopy, it has a discoid shape, has no nucleus, and appears violet-purple with Romanowsky stain. It interacts with injured vessel wall structures, plasma proteins, and other circulating blood cells in the regulation of hemostasis and pathogenesis of thrombosis.

platelet-poor plasma (PPP) Plasma that has been centrifuged at sufficiently high relative centrifugal force to remove platelets.

platelet-rich plasma (PRP) Plasma that has been centrifuged at sufficiently low relative centrifugal force to allow platelets to remain in suspension.

plethoric Characterized by a ruddy or reddish complexion caused by overfullness of blood vessels.

pleura A serous, membranous sac that lines the thoracic cavity and encloses the lungs. Right and left pleura are separate and distinct.

pluripotent Capable of producing more than one cell line; see stem cell, pluripotent.

pneumothorax An accumulation of air (or gas) within the pleural cavity that is lined by the pleura.

pocketbook cells Folded erythrocytes characteristic of Hb SC disease (Fig. 14-8) .

poikilocyte An abnormal erythrocyte shape.

Plasmodium A protozoan parasite of which there are four species (*Plasmodium vivax, P. malariae, P. ovale,* and *P. falciparum*) that infect humans and invade erythrocytes. They are transmitted to man by the bite of the *Anopheles* mosquito and cause the disease called malaria.

polarize To confine the vibrations of light waves to one plane or one direction.

polychromasia A variation in the color of Romanowsky-stained erythrocytes on the peripheral blood film; cells appear bluish or gray due to the diffuse mixture of hemoglobin with retained basophilic substances.

polychromatophilia See polychromasia.

polychromatophilic normoblast See rubricyte.

polychromatophilic red cell A young red blood cell that no longer has a nucleus but still contains some RNA. Also called diffusely basophilic red cell (Fig. 8-28). The cell stains diffusely blue with Wright stain (Color Plate 9-1).

polyclonal Derived from different parent cells; relating to several clones of cells (in contrast to monoclonal).

polycythemia Literally, means an abnormal increased production of more than one cell line (*e.g.,* erythrocytes, granulocytes, and platelets). Derived from Greek words poly (many), cyte (cell), and emia (blood disesase). Sometimes used to refer to the condition polycythemia vera (see that entry).

polycythemia vera (PV) A chronic myeloproliferative disorder with an absolute increase in red blood cell mass resulting from a clonal, pluripotent stem cell disorder. Leukocytosis and thrombocytosis are common in PV.

polymerase An enzyme that facilitates the synthesis of a nucleic acid (DNA or RNA) sequence that is usually a copy of a template sequence.

polymerase chain reaction (PCR) A molecular technique of *in vitro* DNA synthesis in which many copies of a target DNA sequence are made (amplification) during a series of cycled reactions. RNA can serve as the target if its sequence is first converted into a complementary DNA copy in a method variation called reverse transcriptase-PCR (RT-PCR).

polymorphism A naturally occurring variation in the base sequence of genomic DNA between individuals of the same species.

polymorphonuclear neutrophil (PMN) See neutrophil, segmented.

porphyrias Acquired or inherited disorders caused by various enzyme deficiencies. This leads to the accumulation of porphyrin precursors or of one or more of the porphyrin(ogen)s in the bone marrow (erythropoietic porphyrias) or in the liver (hepatic porphyrias). Decreased hemoglobin production is the result. Some patients demonstrate neurologic abnormalities and pronounced skin sensitivity to sunlight.

porphyrin One of a group of iron-free or magnesium-free cyclic tetrapyrrole derivatives found in all vertebrate and plant cells. They form the basis of the respiratory pigments, *e.g.,* hemoglobin, which contains protoporphyrin IX.

precision The ability to reproduce a test result on the same sample.

preeclampsia See eclampsia.

preleukemia (preleukemic syndrome) See dysmyelopoietic syndrome.

priaprism Persistent and painful erection of the penis without sexual arousal.

primary lymphoid organs (PLO) Organs that supply the secondary lymphoid tissue with partially differentiated lymphocytes.

primer A short DNA sequence which, after binding to a complementary nucleic acid sequence, can initiate the synthetic activity of a polymerase.

probe A nucleic acid sequence used in molecular techniques to hybridize to its specific complementary target sequence. It usually has a discernable marker attached to it (often a radioisotope) that allows detection of the hybridization.

prodromal Pertaining to the initial stage of a disease in which symptoms indicate oncoming overt disease.

proficiency testing (PT) PT is comprised of samples with unstated quantities of analytes that are to be tested in the same manner as patient samples. The measured values are known by the provider. A laboratory's test results are compared to those of its peer group. Rules for testing and performance are set forth by CLIA'88.

prognosis Predicted outcome of a disease or condition; the chance that recovery will occur.

proliferation The process by which the number of organisms increases. Cells generally proliferate by means of mitosis.

promyelocyte The immature granulocyte stage in which primary granules begin to form; normally found only in the bone marrow; also called progranulocyte.

pronormoblast See rubriblast.

prophylactic Preventing disease; an agent acting as a preventive against disease.

propionic acid An acid normally produced by intestinal bacteria.

prorubricyte The second nucleated red blood cell stage found in the bone marrow (Color Plate 6-5) . The cytoplasm is basophilic with the Golgi apparatus usually visible as a light area near the nucleus. The nucleus is round; its chromatin is dark violet and definitely coarser and more clumped than that of the rubriblast. Parachromatin is slightly visible between the clumps of chromatin. Nucleoli are not usually visible.

prostacyclin (PGI$_2$) Substance released from endothelial cells that inhibits platelet aggregation.

protein C A vitamin K–dependent glycoprotein that is a potent anticoagulant. Optimal activation of protein C requires thrombomodulin, Ca^{2+}, and thrombin. Activated protein C complexed with its cofactor, protein S, inhibits factors Va and VIIIa. It may also enhance fibrinolysis (Table 48-6) . Deficiencies are associated with thrombosis.

protein S A vitamin K–dependent glycoprotein that acts as a cofactor with protein C (see protein C). Deficiencies are associated with thrombosis.

prothrombin A zymogen (factor II) that is converted to the serine protease thrombin (factor IIa) by the prothrombinase complex in the common coagulation pathway.

prothrombinase complex The complex of factor Xa, the nonenzymatic cofactor Va, and Ca^{2+} that form on the platelet phospholipid surface (Fig. 48-1) as part of the common coagulation pathway. It is responsible for prothrombin activation to thrombin.

prothrombin coagulation factor group Refers to the vitamin K–dependent coagulation factors II, VII, IX, and X, which are synthesized in the liver. Vitamin K is necessary to γ-carboxylate the enzyme precursors of these factors so that they may function in the coagulation process (Table 48-4).

prothrombin time (PT) A clinical laboratory test that measures the function of the extrinsic and common blood coagulation pathways and requires citrated platelet-poor plasma. Coagulation is initiated by the addition of thromboplastin (tissue factor) and Ca^{2+}. This test is commonly used to monitor therapy with coumarins and related drugs.

proto-oncogene A normal gene associated with control of cellular growth and proliferation. If mutated, a proto-oncogene may become an oncogene which is capable of causing malignancy.

protoporphyria A disorder caused by an inherited deficiency of the enzyme ferrochelatase which causes an abnormal accumulation of porphyrin precursors in the bone marrow. Patients demonstrate photocutaneous lesions and mild to severe hepatobiliary disease.

protoporphyrin IX, erythrocyte A porphyrin that is chelated with Fe^{2+} to form heme. This reaction is catalyzed by ferrochelatase (Fig. 13-1). See free erythrocyte protoporphyrin.

pruritic Itchy; making one want to scratch the skin to obtain relief.

Prussian blue stain A stain used to detect siderotic (iron) granules in erythrocytes. Also called Perls' Prussian blue stain.

pure red cell aplasia (PRCA) An acquired or inherited disease in which there is a primary defect in the bone marrow causing a severe decrease in maturing erythroid elements and severe anemia.

purpura A hemorrhage of blood into small areas of skin, mucous membranes, and other tissues (Fig. 47-6). These areas first appear red but later turn purple and finally brownish-yellow. The colors coincide with the conversion of heme to biliverdin. As the color fades, biliverdin is converted to bilirubin, which is removed from the area and processed in the liver. See petechiae and ecchymosis.

pyelonephritis Inflammation of the kidneys.

pyknotic Having a dense nuclear mass such as that seen in a metarubricyte just prior to nuclear extrusion.

pyogenic Producing pus.

pyropoikilocyte A tiny, round, fragmented erythrocyte shape also called a microspherocyte because of its extremely low MCV (Fig. 8-15B). It is associated with abnormal RBC heat sensitivity.

pyropoikilocytosis, hereditary A rare disorder characterized by severe hemolytic anemia with extreme anisocytosis and micropoikilocytosis.

pyruvate kinase (PK) An erythrocyte enzyme in the Embden–Meyerhof pathway (EMP) that catalyzes the formation of pyruvate from phosphoenol-pyruvate (PEP) and is accompanied by the transformation of adenosine diphosphate (ADP) to adenosine triphosphate (ATP) (Fig. 6-7). This is the most commonly deficient enzyme in the EMP. PK is also found in leukocytes and platelets.

pyruvate kinase (PK) deficiency A hereditary hemolytic erythrocyte disorder resulting from a deficiency of the PK enzyme.

5q⁻ syndrome A clonal proliferative disorder that is characterized by numerous small or medium-sized mononuclear or bilobed megakaryocytes in the bone marrow (Fig. 33-2), an acquired deletion of the long arm of chromosome 5 involving the region 5q15 to 5q31, and a macrocytic anemia. The disorder may progress to acute nonlymphocytic leukemia.

quality assurance Encompasses comprehensive concepts, including components of quality control, that are primarily quantitative and statistical, and those aspects of laboratory management that impart perceptions of credibility and medically useful results to the clinician.

quality control A laboratory program established ideally to reduce both systematic and random errors to zero through the use of quantitative data and statistical tools.

radio frequency (RF) A high-frequency alternating current provided by an electromagnetic probe used in some automated cell counters to determine cellular density and intracellular composition.

radioimmunoassay A laboratory method based on competition for a limited number of protein-binding sites (in the form of antibody to the test substance) between a known added amount of "tagged" or "radioactively labeled" test substance and unlabeled test substance found in the patient's serum. It is used to quantitate serum ferritin, hormones, and vitamins among other things.

random error A laboratory measurement error caused by chance and sampling errors. It affects the precision of a measurement method, introduces increased variability into an analysis, and cannot be detected by testing control specimens. Also called indeterminate error.

Rapoport–Luebering shunt A bypass pathway in the Embden–Meyerhof pathway that generates 2,3-diphosphoglycerate (2,3-DPG).

Raynaud's phenomenon A vascular disorder that causes acrocyanosis (blue-gray discoloration of extremities) and pain (especially in the tip of the nose, ear lobes, or fingertips) on exposure to cold temperatures. It is usually reversible.

recessive gene A gene that, in the presence of its dominant allele, does not express itself.

recirculation The movement of lymphocytes back and forth between the peripheral blood, lymph, and secondary lymphoid tissue.

recombinant human erythropoietin (r-HuEPO) A manufactured substance that is a highly effective treatment for the anemia of chronic renal disease.

red cell distribution width (RDW) A numeric quantitation made by electronic cell counters that is said to quantitate anisocytosis and identify minor populations of microcytic or macrocytic erythrocytes that are not apparent from the mean cell volume (MCV).

red cell mass (RCM) The total mass of erythrocytes in the circulation based on body weight and reported in mL/Kg. The RCM may be determined from blood volume studies using radioisotopic dilution techniques. It is important in the differentiation of absolute and relative polycythemia.

Reed–Sternberg cell A cell associated with Hodgkin disease found in affected lymph nodes. It is a large cell (4 to 8 times the size of a normal lymphocyte) that may contain multiple nuclei, two nuclei, or a single bilobed nucleus. The nucleoli are large and eosinophilic with a distinct halo, giving the cell an "owl-eyed" appearance.

reference method A method that is specific for an analyte and quantitates the true concentration of the analyte.

refractory anemia (RA) A dysmyelopoietic syndrome characterized by less than 5% blasts in the bone marrow, less than 5% blasts in the peripheral blood, and marked dyserythropoiesis (Table 33-2). Also a general term for an anemia that does not readily respond to treatment.

refractory anemia with excess blasts (RAEB) A dysmyelopoietic syndrome characterized by 5 to 20% blasts in the bone marrow, less than 5% blasts in the peripheral blood, and moderate dysgranulopoiesis (Table 33-2).

refractory anemia with excess blasts in transformation (RAEBIT) A dysmyelopoietic syndrome characterized by 20 to 30% blasts in the bone marrow, greater than 5% blasts in the peripheral blood, and some dysplasia of the myeloid cell lines (Table 33-2).

refractory anemia with ringed sideroblasts (RARS) An acquired form of sideroblastic anemia also called idiopathic acquired sideroblastic anemia (IASA). It is considered a dysmyelopoietic syndrome and characterized by ringed sideroblasts in the bone marrow.

remission Disappearance of symptoms and clinical (laboratory) evidence of disease.

reptilase A thrombin-like enzyme, obtained from the reptile *Bothrops atrox*, that is capable of cleaving fibrinopeptide A from the α chain of fibrinogen.

resistance A conductor's opposition to the flow of electric current.

resolution The ability of a lens to delineate detail in a specimen viewed on a microscope.

restriction endonuclease An enzyme that recognizes a specific short nucleotide sequence in double-stranded DNA and cleaves the double strands there or nearby.

reticulin A type of collagen that makes up reticular fibers.

reticulocyte An immature erythrocyte that has lost its nucleus. It retains mitochondria and other organelles and precipitated aggregates of ribonucleic acid (RNA) within its ribosomes. The RNA produces varying amounts of polychromasia on a Romanowsky-stained blood film.

reticulocyte maturation index (RMI) A number that is derived from the amount of RNA present in individual reticulocytes (quantitated by a flow cytometer) within an erythrocyte population. It reflects the overall maturity of the reticulocyte population (the more RNA, the younger the cell).

reticulocyte production index (RPI) A calculated value that provides a general indication of the rate of effective erythropoiesis in anemias; a further correction of the reticulocyte count for "shift" reticulocytes based on the hematocrit value.

reticulocytosis Increase in the number of peripheral blood reticulocytes.

reticuloendothelial system (RES) The aggregate of all the cells and tissues that comprise the cellular and immunologic defense mechanism of the body and destroy normal and abnormal erythrocytes. It includes the phagocytic cells of the spleen, liver, lymph nodes, bone marrow, and to a lesser extent, the lungs and other tissues. Formerly called the mononuclear phagocyte system (MPS).

retinitis pigmentosa A degenerative condition of the retina seen in abetalipoproteinemia.

retrovirus A family of RNA viruses characterized by the possession of reverse transcriptase in the virion.

ribonucleic acid (RNA) A nucleic acid similar to DNA except that it contains ribose instead of deoxyribose. There are several types, including messenger RNA, transfer RNA, and ribosomal RNA, each of which has a specific cellular function.

Romanowsky stain A stain used to differentiate blood cells and blood parasites; the components include methylene blue, eosin, and methylene blue azures. The stain is generally made by dissolving the dye in absolute methanol.

rouleaux A French term that means roll. An erythrocyte formation in the usual observation area in which erythrocytes are not separated from one another; rather, they appear in short or long stacks resembling coins or flat plates (Fig. 8-2). The entire outline of each cell is not visible.

rubriblast The earliest and largest erythrocyte precursor in the bone marrow (Color Plate 6-4). The nuclear/cytoplasmic ratio is high. The cytoplasm is basophilic (intense dark blue). The Golgi apparatus may be visible as a pale area next to the nucleus. The nucleus is usually round to slightly oval, has dispersed fine clumps of chromatin, and contains nucleoli. This cell may be confused with a myeloblast.

rubricyte A nucleated stage of erythrocyte maturation in which the nucleus is round and may be eccentric with very coarse and condensed chromatin (Color Plate 6-6). The cytoplasm has an opaque, violet-blue color called polychromasia. This cell may be confused with a lymphocyte.

Russell bodies Globular inclusions of immunoglobulin that may be present in plasma cells.

Rye classification The classification of Hodgkin's disease into four histologic groups based on the extent of lymphocyte infiltration and abundance of Reed–Sternberg cells detected by lymph node biopsy.

satellitism The clinging of one cellular element to the outer surface of another cellular element. Most frequently a phenomenon of platelets clinging to the outer surface of a phagocytic cell such as a neutrophil or monocyte.

scattergram A two-dimensional display of two cell characteristics produced by automated leukocyte differential counters. Each cell is represented by a dot based upon X- and Y-axis analytical measurements. When many cells are plotted, clusters develop that represent relative concentrations of cells with very similar characteristics. Other terms include cytogram and dot plot.

Schilling test A laboratory test to measure the body's ability to secrete viable intrinsic factor and absorb orally-administered free ^{57}Co-cyanocobalamin in the ileum. Normal absorption is reflected by a minimum level of urinary excretion of radiolabeled B_{12}.

Schilling test, food A laboratory test in which ^{57}Co-cyanocobalamin bound to egg yolk is given orally to test for the ability to absorb food-bound ^{57}Co-cyanocobalamin. This test is usually performed as a follow up if classic Schilling test results are normal in patients whose serum vitamin B_{12} is decreased. The food Schilling test is abnormal when there is malabsorption of food-bound vitamin B_{12} but normal absorption of free vitamin B_{12}.

schistocyte (Gr. *schistos*: cloven) An abnormal erythrocyte shape that results from passing through fibrin strands, altered vessels, or a damaged heart valve prosthesis causing the erythrocyte to cleave and fragment (Figs. 8-12A, B and 8-13).

schizocyte (Gr. *schizo*: split) See schistocyte.

scurvy See vitamin C deficiency.

secondary lymphoid tissue (SLT) Tissue that produces lymphocytes in response to antigen, *e.g.*, spleen, lymph nodes.

selectins A family of three protein adhesion molecules found on the cell surface, designated as E (endothelial cell), P (platelet), and L (leukocyte).

semilunar body A large, pale-pink staining ghost of an erythrocyte—the membrane remaining after the contents have been released (Fig. 8-16). It is as large as a leukocyte and always acquired. It is also called a half-moon cell or crescent cell and frequently is seen in malaria and other hemolytic conditions.

senescent Descriptive term for erythrocytes that have lived their normal 120-day life span, and therefore will be destroyed by phagocytic cells in the RES.

septicemia Systemic disease associated with the presence of microorganisms in the blood; blood poisoning.

serine protease An active enzyme derived from the action of an enzyme on a zymogen. It has an exposed, serine-rich, active enzyme site. Serine proteases selectively hydrolyze arginine- or lysine-containing peptide bonds of other zymogens, thus converting them to active enzymes. Coagulation factors II, VII, IX, X, XI, and XII, and protein C are all serine proteases.

serum The liquid portion obtained from coagulated blood.

Sézary syndrome A rare form of cutaneous T-cell lymphoma characterized by both skin lesions and systemic involvement.

shift reticulocyte A very large, diffusely basophilic cell (reticulocyte) that indicates premature release from the bone marrow during intense erythrocyte production. Also called a shift cell.

shift to the left Presence in the peripheral blood of immature stages of neutrophils that are normally found only in the bone marrow; an indication of a reactive or stressful condition.

shock A clinical syndrome in which peripheral blood flow is inadequate to return sufficient blood to the heart for normal function; caused by hemorrhage, infection, or heart failure.

sickle cell A thin and elongated erythrocyte with pointed ends that is well filled with hemoglobin (Hb) (Figs. 8-17 and 14-6). The sickle shape is caused by long rod-shaped polymers of Hb

S. Hb S crystals cause cells to become rigid, and they impede blood flow to tissues, resulting in tissue death, organ infarction, and pain. They are seen in sickle cell anemia (Hb SS) and sometimes in the sickle trait condition (Hb AS). Also called a drepanocyte.

sickle cell anemia Homozygous inheritance of the sickle hemoglobin gene (Hb SS) which causes a life-threatening disease. Also called sickle cell disease.

sickle cell crisis A painful condition that occurs in patients with Hb S, particularly in sickle cell anemia, caused by any situation that produces excessive deoxygenation of erythrocytes causing them to sickle (*e.g.*, infection, dehydration, and high altitude).

sickle cell trait Heterozygous inheritance of the sickle hemoglobin gene (Hb AS). The condition usually causes no symptoms, but affected individuals may experience painful sickle crises if they encounter situations that cause extreme tissue hypoxia.

sideroblast A nucleated red blood cell that contains iron (siderotic granules) not yet incorporated into hemoglobin. The iron is stainable with an iron stain such as Perls' Prussian blue.

sideroblast, ringed An abnormal nucleated red blood cell (NRBC) found in the bone marrow of patients with sideroblastic anemia and the dysmyelopoietic syndrome refractory anemia with ringed sideroblasts (RARS). It contains large iron granules that are deposited within mitochondria and situated in a ring or collar around the NRBC nucleus (Color Plates 29-10 and 33-2). If 5 or more iron granules in a given NRBC occupy at least 30% of the circumference of the nucleus, the NRBC is called a type III pathologic ringed sideroblast. The iron stains blue to blue-green with Prussian blue.

sideroblastic anemia Group of different anemias that can be inherited or acquired (Table 13-5) that all demonstrate defective iron utilization in the production of heme for hemoglobin and the presence of ringed sideroblasts in the bone marrow (Color Plates 29-10 and 33-2).

siderocyte A mature erythrocyte containing particles of iron (siderotic granules) not yet incorporated into hemoglobin. These particles are visualized by an iron stain such as Perls' Prussian blue (Fig. 8-24). They are also visible on a Wright-stained peripheral blood film as Pappenheimer bodies (Fig. 8-23).

siderotic granules Iron granules found in erythrocytes. See Pappenheimer bodies.

side scatter The light that is refracted and reflected from a cell in a direction that is angled from the laser light beam axis as the cell passes through that beam.

silent carrier An individual who carries an abnormal gene that causes no clinical abnormality, *e.g.*, one who has heterozygous α^+ thalassemia (-α/$\alpha\alpha$) has no clinical or hematologic abnormalities.

sinusoids Thin-walled, irregular vascular channels.

skin puncture A procedure in which the skin is punctured by a sharp device to obtain capillary blood specimens.

smudge cell A nuclear remnant from a damaged or disintegrating leukocyte. Usually appears as a round or oval purple smudge (hence the name). See basket cell.

sO₂ Arterial blood oxygen saturation.

sodium citrate An anticoagulant that binds calcium ions and is commonly used in hemostasis testing.

sol-gel zone A term for the grouping of the platelet microfilaments, microtubules, and aqueous cytoplasm.

Soret band The absorbance bands in the lower part of the visible light range between 400 and 430 nm where heme compounds have characteristic sharp, narrow, and pronounced absorption peaks, *e.g.*, for oxyhemoglobin the band is from 412 to 415 nm.

Southern blot A molecular technique in which DNA fragments separated by gel electrophoresis are transferred (blotted) to a membrane on which a specific DNA target sequence can be de-

tected by hybridization to a complementary probe. When RNA is analyzed, it is called a Northern blot.

spectrin A peripheral erythrocyte membrane protein composed of long, rod-shaped molecules (Fig. 17-1). Two types have been designated, α and β (also called bands 1 and 2, respectively). It interacts with the membrane protein actin. Both proteins are thought to underlie the lipid bilayer on the cytoplasmic side and to regulate membrane shape and deformability. Abnormal membrane spectrin has been linked to hereditary spherocytosis and elliptocytosis.

Speirs-Levy hemocytometer A special hemocytometer (Fig. 24-7) designed for counting larger volumes than the Neubauer hemocytometer. It is used for manual eosinophil and basophil counts to provide absolute cell count results.

spherocyte Abnormal round erythrocyte lacking central pallor, showing increased staining intensity, and having a smaller volume (MCV) than a normal erythrocyte (Fig. 8-6) and an increased MCHC and osmotic fragility. Presence on a blood film suggests a hemolytic anemia. Even rare spherocytes should be reported.

spherocytosis, hereditary A group of erythrocyte membrane skeletal disorders characterized by numerous spherocytes on the blood film and varying degrees of hemolysis.

spleen A large vascular, abdominal organ (part of the RES) that removes senescent and abnormal erythrocytes from the circulation.

spur cell An erythrocyte with sharp points similar to an acanthocyte. It is found in severe hemolytic anemia associated with cirrhosis and in metastatic liver disease.

standard, primary A stable material of precise analyte concentration and purity against which the analyte in other materials can be compared or measured; used in instrument calibration. In hematology, a primary standard exists for hemoglobin only, but it is not widely available.

standard, secondary A whole blood sample in which an analyte concentration is measured using reference methods.

stasis Literally, means "standing still." Refers to the cessation of circulation.

steatorrhea Fatty feces.

stem cell A primitive cell capable of self-renewal as well as differentiation along one of several cell lines.

stem cell, myeloid The precursor in the bone marrow from which all erythrocytes, platelets, and leukocytes (except lymphocytes) are derived.

stem cell, pluripotent (multipotent) Hematopoietic cell that differentiates into erythroid, myeloid, and lymphoid cellular elements.

stenosis Constriction or narrowing of a passage.

stippled red blood cell An erythrocyte containing basophilic stippling (see basophilic stippling).

stomatocyte (Gr. *stoma*: mouth) An abnormal erythrocyte with an elongated, slit-like, or "mouth-shaped" central pallor (Fig. 8-10) instead of the usual circular form. It may be hereditary, acquired, or an artifact. It is normal to find a few stomatocytes on a blood film, but an increased number is usually associated with alcoholism, cirrhosis, obstructive liver disease, and Rh null disease.

stomatocytosis, hereditary An erythrocyte membrane disorder in which stomatocytes result from altered membrane permeability to cations; also called hydrocytosis.

storage pool disease A heterogeneous group of platelet disorders characterized by defects in or lack of platelet α granules, dense granules (bodies), or both, that result in defective platelet release of storage granule contents. These intraplatelet granules normally contain and store a variety of substances involved in hemostasis.

stromal cell A cell that is part of the supporting matrix of an organ as opposed to a parenchymal cell that performs a specific function related to the organ (*e.g.*, connective tissue).

subleukemic Minimal morphologic and quantitative evidence of malignancy. Leukocyte count is normal and only a few abnormal cells can be found on the peripheral blood film.

substrate A chemical substance whose makeup is changed through the action of a specific enzyme, *e.g.*, hydrogen peroxide is the substrate of the enzyme peroxidase.

sugar water screening test A test to assist in the diagnosis of paroxysmal nocturnal hemoglobinuria (PNH). Whole blood is incubated at 37°C in a low ionic strength solution that promotes erythrocyte binding of complement components. Normal erythrocytes do not hemolyze under these conditions, but erythrocytes from patients with PNH do.

sulfhemoglobin A hemoglobin (Hb) derivative formed during the oxidative denaturation of Hb by the addition of a sulfur (S) atom to each heme molecule. It is not normally formed, but occurs on exposure to some drugs and is not reversible.

sulfhemoglobinemia An acquired and generally benign condition caused by excessive sulfhemoglobin in the blood in which the only significant effect is cyanosis.

supravital stain A substance used to stain unfixed cells in the living state to study vital and functional processes, *e.g.*, new methylene blue stain for visualization and enumeration of reticulocytes.

suspect flag In a multiparameter hematology instrument, a flag generated by a computer program that is designed to identify abnormal conditions in a blood sample. The sample patterns and limits that trigger these flags are set by the instrument manufacturer; they are not adjustable by the user. See definitive flag.

syngeneic Genetically identical, *e.g.*, identical twins.

synthetic substrate Small peptide chains consisting of amino acid sequences that mimic the natural substrate of an enzyme. It is often linked with a chromophore at the site where the proteolytic enzyme will cleave it, producing a detectable color reaction when clipped by that enzyme.

systematic error A laboratory measurement error caused by factors other than chance, *e.g.*, deteriorating reagents or loss of instrument calibration; usually detected by testing control specimens. Also called determinate error.

systemic lupus erythematosus (SLE) An autoimmune disease in which the patient's sera contains the LE factor, an antibody to nuclear DNA (antinuclear antibody [ANA]). SLE may be diagnosed by a test for ANA or an older manual method called the LE preparation that induces the formation of the characteristic LE cell, although neither test is specific for SLE. The LE cell is a neutrophil containing one or more large spherical inclusions of disintegrated nuclear material in the cytoplasm.

systolic pressure The maximum pressure of the blood on the walls of the arteries that results from the height of contraction of the left ventricle of the heart as it pumps blood to the aorta. The adult normal range is approximately 110 to 140 mm Hg.

tachyphylaxis Rapid and progressive decrease in response to an administered pharmacologic or physiologic substance.

target cell An abnormal erythrocyte having a central area of hemoglobin (Hb) surrounded by a relatively colorless ring and a peripheral ring of Hb (Fig. 8-11). It is also called a codocyte and a Mexican hat cell. It has a high surface-to-volume ratio and decreased osmotic fragility. This shape is always acquired.

target nucleic acid sequence The base sequence of interest for a particular molecular assay. For hybridization assays, it is the sequence for which a probe is specific. For amplification assays, it is the sequence that is amplified.

T-cell receptor (TCR) Disulfide-linked cell surface heterodimers α, β, γ, and δ.

TCR/CD3 signaling complex Definitive surface marker for T lymphocytes.

telangiectasias Thin, dilated vessels causing red to violet skin lesions that range from pinpoint size to 3 mm. They may bleed either spontaneously or from minor trauma (Fig. 47-5).

terminal deoxynucleotidyl transferase (TdT) An intranuclear DNA polymerase enzyme that can be detected in human thymocytes, primitive lymphoid precursors, and a few other cells in the bone marrow. It catalyzes the elongation of polynucleotide chains. Tests for TdT activity are used to identify the lymphoid nature of cells in the diagnosis of acute lymphocytic leukemia and lymphoblastic lymphomas. TdT is also known as DNA nucleotidyl transferase.

α thalassemia A disorder with various forms that results from a decrease in the number of α chains produced. It is caused by a deletion or mutation affecting one, two, three, or all four α-globin genes (Tables 15-3 and 15-4).

α thalassemia minor A form of α thalassemia that has two genotypic forms: heterozygous α^0 thalassemia ($—/\alpha\alpha$) and homozygous α^+ thalassemia ($-\alpha/-\alpha$). Both result in a decrease in α chain synthesis. Neither condition produces clinical disease, but hematologic abnormalities are found. Also known as α thalassemia trait.

β thalassemia Conditions in which there is a reduced synthesis of β chains. They are classified according to clinical severity and include, in order from most to least severe, β thalassemia major, β thalassemia intermedia, β thalassemia minor, and β thalassemia minima (Tables 15-5, 15-6, and 15-7).

β thalassemia intermedia A clinical phenotype of intermediate severity between the trait (β thalassemia minor) and the disease (β thalassemia major), in which significant anemia occurs but chronic transfusion therapy is not absolutely required.

β thalassemia major A clinical phenotype caused by two thalassemic β genes, associated with a severe, transfusion-dependent hemolytic anemia. Also known as Cooley's anemia.

β thalassemia minima The "silent carrier" state of heterozygous β thalassemia which causes no detectable clinical or hematologic abnormalities.

β thalassemia minor A clinical phenotype caused by inheritance of a single β-thalassemia allele. It is rarely associated with any clinical disability and produces little or no anemia, although peripheral blood erythrocyte morphology is abnormal.

thermal amplitude The temperature range in which antibodies bind to erythrocytes.

Thoma pipet A glass pipet (Fig. 24-3) used to make dilutions ranging from 1 part in 10 (1:10) to 1 part in 1000 (1:1000) for manual cell counting.

threshold A point of beginning. With respect to cell counts, refers to the size of voltage pulse above which the pulse will not be counted, or below which the pulse will be counted. Both lower and upper thresholds can be set.

thrombin A serine protease coagulation factor (factor IIa) derived from the zymogen prothrombin. Thrombin converts fibrinogen to fibrin. It plays multiple roles in both activation and inhibition of coagulation.

thrombocythemia Increase in the number of circulating platelets related to one of the chronic myeloproliferative disorders.

thrombocytopathy Condition accompanied by poor platelet function.

thrombocytopenia A decrease in the number of peripheral blood platelets.

thrombocytosis An increase in the number of peripheral blood platelets.

thromboembolic conditions Those in which a blood vessel is obstructed with thrombotic material, which is then carried to another vessel causing another obstruction.

thromboembolism An embolus made up of a blood clot.

thrombolytic Dissolving or splitting up a thrombus (blood clot).

thrombomodulin A protein found on the surface of endothelial cells that acts as a cofactor in the activation of protein C, a potent anticoagulant. See protein C.

thrombophilia Increased production of thrombi.

thrombophlebitis Presence of a fibrin clot (thrombus) within a vein (usually in the lower extremities), which is frequently accompanied by an inflammatory response.

thromboplastin reagent A phospholipid/tissue factor preparation that binds factor VII, resulting in a complex that can activate both factor X and factor IX in the presence of calcium ions.

thrombopoietin The hormone responsible for stimulating megakaryocyte progenitors to differentiate into more mature states.

thrombosis The formation, development, or presence of a thrombus.

thrombotic thrombocytopenic purpura (TTP) An acquired condition that affects primarily young adults and is characterized by nonimmune thrombocytopenia owing to increased platelet consumption and a shortened platelet life span. TTP often causes a microangiopathic hemolytic anemia. Also called Moschkovitz syndrome.

thrombus An aggregation of blood factors, primarily platelets and fibrin with entrapment of cellular elements, frequently causing vascular obstruction at the point of its formation.

tinnitus A ringing sound in the ear.

tissue factor (TF) A high-molecular-weight lipoprotein found in most organs and in large blood vessels. When the vessel endothelium is damaged, tissue factor is exposed and binds with factor VII to form the tissue factor:VII (TF:VII) complex that, upon activation and complexing with Ca^{2+}, activates factor X in the common coagulation pathway. Also called factor III and tissue thromboplastin.

tissue factor pathway inhibitor (TFPI) A protein that binds and inhibits factor Xa and subsequently (on the same molecule) binds and inhibits the tissue factor-factor VIIa (TF:VIIa) complex, thus inhibiting coagulation.

tissue thromboplastin A substance contained in tissues that activates coagulation. See tissue factor.

T lymphocyte (T cell) Thymic-dependent subpopulation of lymphocytes responsible for cell-mediated immunity including effector, helper, suppressor, secretor, and memory functions.

tonicity Osmotic tension in the plasma.

total iron binding capacity (TIBC), serum A measurement of the maximum concentration of iron that can be bound by serum proteins, primarily transferrin.

total quality management (TQM) A program of coordination and cooperation among hospital departments and clinicians to ensure quality patient care.

totipotent Having the capacity to differentiate along any cell line. Pluripotent is sometimes used synonymously.

totipotent stem cell The most primitive hematopoietic progenitor that is capable of developing along any of the cell lines that are inherently possible.

tourniquet A device placed around an extremity that impedes venous or arterial flow.

trafficking See homing.

transcobalamins (TC) The plasma vitamin B_{12}–binding proteins called TC I, II, and III. The most important is TC II which transports some B_{12} to storage sites and is necessary for transport of cobalamin through cell membranes.

transferrin A plasma protein that binds and transports iron.

transferrin receptor, serum Cell membrane protein that facilitates intake of the iron-transferrin complex into nucleated red blood cells. A small number of these receptors circulates, and this number is believed to parallel the density of receptors in cells. Both the number of cell receptors and the quantity circulating in plasma are increased in iron deficiency anemia.

transferrin saturation Calculated value obtained from the serum iron and TIBC, both in $\mu g/dL$, as follows:

$$\text{transferrin saturation (\%)} = \frac{100 \times \text{serium iron}}{\text{TIBC}}$$

transmittance See percent transmittance (%T).

transmural Extending through the wall of an organ or cavity.

transudate An effusion formed by mechanical factors such as osmotic or hydrostatic pressure.

trephine biopsy, bone marrow A solid core of bone and marrow tissue obtained by using a needle with a sharp cutting edge.

Türk cell Variant or atypical lymphocyte, also called a plasmacytoid lymphocyte (Color Plate 25-2).

Türk's solution A diluent for leukocyte counting that lyses erythrocytes without destroying leukocytes. Türk's solution enhances leukocyte nuclear definition.

Unopette system (Becton Dickinson, Rutherford, NJ) A series of reservoirs containing premeasured diluent and pipets that automatically measure the appropriate amount of sample required for diluting blood specimens in preparation for manual counting. Various reservoirs are available for leukocyte, platelet, and eosinophil counts as well as a complete blood count from a skin puncture specimen and for measurement of erythrocyte osmotic fragility.

unstable hemoglobin disease See congenital Heinz body hemolytic anemia.

upregulate To influence the synthesis of a molecule resulting in its increase. The opposite is downregulate.

urobilinogen A derivative of bilirubin formed by the action of intestinal bacteria.

vasoconstriction Narrowing or constriction of a blood vessel that leads to reduced blood flow.

vasoocclusive crisis A painful condition that occurs in sickle cell disease when rigid sickle cells increase blood viscosity and block blood vessels, which can cause organ failure.

vector A plasmid (extrachromosomal DNA found in bacteria) or phage (bacterial virus) that can be used to introduce foreign DNA into host cells.

venipuncture A procedure in which a vein is entered, usually with a needle, for the withdrawal of blood or the introduction of fluids.

ventricle A cavity or chamber within an organ, *e.g.*, ventricles of the heart or brain.

vertigo Feeling of being off balance or dizzy, caused by disorders of the inner ear.

villi Small vascular protrusions from the surface of a membrane (*e.g.*, choroid plexus).

viscoelastic Properties of viscosity and elasticity; viscosity being the property of a substance that is dependent on the friction of component molecules as they slide by one another and elasticity being resilience or the ability to stretch, compress, or distort its shape and then return to its original shape.

vitamin B_{12} An organic compound that is composed of a cobalt-containing corrin ring attached to 5,6-dimethylbenzimidazole, a structure similar to riboflavin. It is required for normal DNA synthesis and normal erythrocyte maturation. Dietary sources include meat, fish, eggs, and milk. Normal body stores of B_{12} are adequate for several years if no more is ingested. B_{12} deficiency causes megaloblastic anemia. Also called cyanocobalamin. See cobalamins.

vitamin C deficiency The dietary deficiency of vitamin C (ascorbic acid) that may result in serious bleeding problems and anemia because vitamin C is needed to form the intact structure of vascular collagen.

vitamin K A fat soluble vitamin required for production of the vitamin K–dependent coagulation factors II, VII, IX, and X. See prothrombin coagulation factor group. It is normally ingested in the diet and is also manufactured by the gut flora. There is no substantial storage of vitamin K in the body.

vitamin K coagulation factor group See prothrombin coagulation factor group.

vitronectin A serum and extracellular multifunctional glycoprotein. It inhibits complement-mediated cytolysis, is involved in cell adhesion, and is capable of binding heparin and thrombin. Also known as complement S protein. This glycoprotein must be distinguished from protein S, another cofactor in the hemostatic system.

von Willebrand disease (vWD) A family of bleeding disorders transmitted as an autosomal dominant trait in which the von Willebrand factor portion of the factor VIII molecule is defective. Most vWD classification types (Table 56-2) are characterized by decreased levels of factor VIIIC:Ag, decreased von Willebrand factor antigen (vWF:Ag), a prolonged bleeding time, and impaired ristocetin-induced platelet aggregation (RIPA).

von Willebrand factor (vWF) A protein that is part of the factor VIII molecule (Fig. 48-2) and is required for normal platelet adhesion and function.

Waldenström's macroglobulinemia Monoclonal proliferation of lymphocytes and plasma cells in the bone marrow synthesizing immunoglobulin of the IgM class.

"Washington monument" projections See Hb SC crystals.

wedge blood film Blood film made by spreading a drop of blood over a glass slide by pulling the blood behind a "spreader" slide until the blood runs out; synonymous with spreader-slide blood film or push blood film.

WIC, WOC WIC is the white [cell] impedance counting method and WOC is the white [cell] optical counting method. Acronyms for the technology of Abbott Laboratories' leukocyte counting methods.

xanthochromia Term used to describe cerebrospinal fluid having a yellow color. See cerebrospinal fluid.

xenogeneic Belonging to another species.

yolk sac In the embryo, a sac of extraembryonic endoderm with some nutritional function in lower animals. In humans, the first blood cells are formed here.

zeta potential Amount of repulsion among erythrocytes as a result of their like negative charges from integral proteins on the membrane.

zinc protoporphyrin (ZPP) A form of protoporphyrin that forms when iron is deficient or cannot be properly coupled with protoporphyrin. ZPP can be measured by a hematofluorometer method.

zymogen An inactive enzyme precursor with no biologic activity that is converted to an enzyme by the action of another enzyme, an acid, or some other means. In coagulation, they include factors II, VII, IX, X, XI, XII, XIII, and prekallikrein.

Common Abbreviations

ACD Anemia of chronic disease
ADP Adenosine diphosphate
AGL Acute granulocytic leukemia
AIHA Autoimmune hemolytic anemia
ALL Acute lymphocytic leukemia
AML Acute myeloid leukemia
ANA Antinuclear antibody
ANLL Acute nonlymphocytic leukemia
AT-III Antithrombin III
ATP Adenosine triphosphate
BCB Brilliant cresyl blue inclusion body test
BFU-E Burst-forming unit—erythroid
CC crystal Hemoglobin CC crystal
CDA Dyserythropoietic anemia, congenital
CFU–E Colony-forming unit—erythroid
CLIA'88 Clinical Laboratory Improvement Amendments of 1988
CLL Chronic lymphocytic leukemia
CLLD Chronic lymphoproliferative leukemic disorders
CMML Chronic myelomonocytic leukemia
CMPD Chronic myeloproliferative disorder
CRC Corrected reticulocyte count
CSF Cerebrospinal fluid
DAT Direct antiglobulin test
DIC Disseminated intravascular coagulation
DMPS Dysmyelopoietic syndrome
2,3-DPG 2,3-diphosphoglycerate
EDTA Ethylenediaminetetraacetic acid
EPO Erythropoietin
ESR Erythrocyte sedimentation rate
FACS Fluorescence-activated cell sorter
FCM Flow cytometry
FDP Fibrin(ogen) degradation products
FEP Free erythrocyte protoporphyrin
FITC Fluorescein-isothiocyanate
FPA Fibrinopeptide A
FSP Fibrin(ogen) split products
G6PD Glucose-6-phosphate dehydrogenase
GSH Reduced glutathione
GSSG Oxidized glutathione
GVHD Graft-versus-host reaction
GVL effect Graft-versus-leukemia effect
Hb Hemoglobin
HCFII Heparin cofactor II
HCL Hairy-cell leukemia
Hct Hematocrit
HDN Hemolytic disease of the newborn
HEMPAS Hereditary erythroblast multinuclearity with positive acidified serum test
Hi Hemiglobin
HIT Heparin-induced thrombocytopenia
HLA Human leukocyte antigen
HLA-DR Human leukocyte antigen
HMWK High-molecular-weight kininogen
HMS Hexose monophosphate shunt
HPFH Hereditary persistence of fetal hemoglobin
HUS Hemolytic uremic syndrome
IASA Idiopathic acquired sideroblastic anemia
IF Intrinsic factor
IgG Immunoglobulin G
IgM Immunoglobulin M
IL Interleukins

IRF Immature reticulocyte fraction
ITP Immune thrombocytopenic purpura
LAP Leukocyte alkaline phosphatase
LD Lactate dehydrogenase
LE Lupus erythematosus
LMWK Low-molecular-weight kininogen
M Molar
mAb Monoclonal antibody
MAHA Microangiopathic hemolytic anemia
MAPSS™ Multiple angle polarized-scatter separation
MCH Mean corpuscular hemoglobin
MCHC Mean corpuscular hemoglobin concentration
MCV Mean corpuscular volume
MDS Myelodysplastic syndrome
M:E ratio Myeloid:erythroid ratio
MHC Major histocompatibility complex
MMA Methylmalonic acid
MNP Marginated neutrophil pool
MPS Mononuclear phagocyte system
NAP Neutrophil alkaline phosphatase
NHL Non-Hodgkin lymphoma
NRBC Nucleated red blood cell
PA Pernicious anemia
PAIg Platelet-associated immunoglobulin
PCH Paroxysmal cold hemoglobinuria
PCV Packed cell volume; see hematocrit
PGI$_2$ Prostacyclin
pI Isoelectric point
PK Pyruvate kinase
PL Phospholipid
PNH Paroxysmal nocturnal hemoglobinuria
PLL Prolymphocytic leukemia
PPP Pentose phosphate pathway
PPP Platelet-poor plasma
PRCA Pure red cell aplasia
PT Prothrombin time
PTT Partial thromboplastin time
PV Polycythemia vera
RA Refractory anemia
RAEB Refractory anemia with excess blasts
RAEBIT Refractory anemia with excess blasts in transformation
RARS Refractory anemia with ringed sideroblasts
RCM Red cell mass
RDW Red cell distribution width
RES Reticuloendothelial system
RF Radio frequency
r-HuEPO Recombinant human erythropoietin
RPI Reticulocyte production index
SLE Systemic lupus erythematosus
sO$_2$ Arterial blood oxygen saturation
TC Transcobalamins
TdT Terminal deoxynucleotidyl transferase
TF Tissue factor
TFPI Tissue factor pathway inhibitor
TIBC Total iron binding capacity, serum
TPA Tissue plasminogen activator
TTP Thrombotic thrombocytopenic purpura
vWF von Willebrand factor
WIC white [cell] impedance counting method
WOC white [cell] optical counting method
ZPP Zinc protoporphyrin

Index

Page numbers followed by *f* indicate figures; those followed by *t* indicate tables.

A

Abbott Laboratories instruments, 533–536, 534–535f, 535t
Abetalipoproteinemia, 92, 129t, 133f, 241–242, 242t, 264–265
ABO blood group, 243, 722
  hemolytic disease of the newborn and, 283
  hemolytic transfusion reactions and, 284–285
Abruptio placentae, 652
Abscess, deep or occult, 360
Absolute reticulocyte count (ARC), 115–116, 117t
Absorbance, 107, 523
Acanthocytes, 92, 92f, 94f
Acanthocytosis, hereditary. *See* Abetalipoproteinemia
Accreditation of laboratory, 588–589, 596
Accuracy, of analytic method, 566–567, 567f
AccuStasis instruments, 737
Acetanilid, 83
Achlorhydria, 178t, 179–180
Achromat, 38
Achylia gastrica, 160
Acid-base balance, hemoglobin in, 81
Acid elution slide test, for hemoglobin F, 220, 236–237
"Acidophilic," 30
Acidosis, metabolic, 294
Acid phosphatase, 314
Acid phosphatase stain, 394–395, 476, 477t
ACL 3000 instrument, 746
Acquired immune hemolytic anemia (AIHA), 280–291
Acrocyanosis, 286
ACT. *See* Activated clotting time
ACTH, 150f, 353, 353t
Actin, 64, 64f, 252, 253f, 257, 309, 693, 695
Actin-binding protein, 695
α-Actinin, 695
Activated clotting time (ACT), 637–638
Activated protein C (APC), 675, 676f, 677
Activated protein C resistance (APCR), 675, 676t, 678
ADCC. *See* Antibody-dependent cell-mediated cytolysis
Addison disease, 150–151
Adenosine, 603t
Adenosine deaminase inhibitor, 484
Adenosylcobalamin, 156, 156f
ADP, 695, 699, 700f, 711–712
ADPase, 603t
ADP response test, 709t
Adrenal abnormalities, 150–151
Aerospray Hematology Slide Stainer, 32
Afibrinogenemia, 618t, 668, 709t, 710, 723t
Afibrinogenesis, 722t
Agammaglobulinemia, sex-linked, 369
Agarose plasma gel technique, 643

Agglutination, of erythrocytes, 88, 88f
Aggregometry, 710–713, 711–713f, 744–745
Agnogenic myeloid metaplasia (AMM), 93, 142f, 428, 431, 437–438, 455, 456t, 463–465, 718t, Color Plate 35-4
  clinical presentation in, 463
  course of disease, 465
  differential diagnosis of, 463–464, 465t
  effect of treatment on laboratory results, 464–465
  laboratory findings in, 463, 469t
Agranulocytosis, 348t
AIDS, 368, 496, 664. *See also* HIV infection
AIHA. *See* Acquired immune hemolytic anemia
Air drying, 27, 30f, 33–34
Albinism, partial, 366
Alcohol, 70, 723t
Alcohol-induced sideroblastic anemia, 185
Alcoholism, 89, 89f, 92, 97–98, 162t, 183t, 185, 299t, 718t, 720, 722t, 729–730
Alder-Reilly anomaly, 365, 368, 371t, Color Plate 26-2
Aleukemia leukemia, 428
Aleukemic reticuloendotheliosis. *See* Hairy cell leukemia
ALG. *See* Antilymphocyte globulin
Algorithm, 299
Alkali denaturation test, for hemoglobin F, 196, 200–201
Alkaline phosphatase, 309
  neutrophil, 360, 395, 395t
Alkaline phosphatase stain, 395, 395t, Color Plates 29-1 to 29-2
ALL. *See* Lymphoblastic leukemia, acute
Allele, 52
Allergic interstitial nephritis, 413
Allergic purpura, 609
Allergic rhinitis, 413
Allergy, 312, 342–343, 353, 353t, 512
Alloantibody, 280
Alloantigen, 722
Allogeneic stem cell transplantation, 386–388
Alloimmune hemolytic anemia, 281t, 283–285
Alloimmune thrombocytopenia purpura, neonatal, 722–723
Allopurinol, 461
Alpha granules, 463, 694f, 695–696, 695t, 696f, 699, 728–729
Alpha-naphthyl esterase stain, 396, Color Plate 29-4
Alternate-site testing. *See* Point of care testing
Alveolar hypoventilation, 134–135, 134t
Alveolar macrophages, 67, 242, 412
Amegakaryocytic thrombocytopenia (AMT), 718–719

Amegakaryocytic thrombocytopenic purpura, 436
Amidopyrine, 349
δ-Aminolevulinic acid, 176f
δ-Aminolevulinic acid dehydratase. *See* Porphobilinogen synthase
δ-Aminolevulinic acid synthase, deficiency of, 183–185
AML. *See* Nonlymphocytic leukemia, acute
AMM. *See* Agnogenic myeloid metaplasia
AMMoL. *See* Nonlymphocytic leukemia, acute, M4
Amodiaquine, 140t
Amplitude of light wave, 36
Amsacrine (m-AMSA), 451, 451t
AMT. *See* Amegakaryocytic thrombocytopenia
Amyloidosis, 508–509, 607t, 609
  primary, 508
  secondary, 508
ANA. *See* Antinuclear antibody
Anagrelide, 467–468
Analytic method, 564
  accuracy of, 566–567, 567f
  calibration of, 567
  correlation between two methods, 573–575
  evaluation and selection of, 564–566, 565t
  feasibility of, 565, 565t
  precision of, 565–568, 567f
  reliability of, 565, 565t
  reasonableness of test results, 592, 595
Analytic reliability, 565, 565t
Analytic variation
  random, 565–566
  systematic, 566
Anaphase, 51
Ancillary testing. *See* Point of care testing
Androgen, 70t, 145, 151
Anemia, 68, 125. *See also specific types of anemia*
  of abnormal globin development, 126t, 217–237
  of abnormal iron metabolism, 126t, 175–188
  of abnormal nuclear development, 126t, 155–171
  absolute versus relative, 126, 126f
  of blood loss, 126t, 129–130t, 131, 133f, 293–296
  of bone marrow failure, 126t, 139–148
  case studies of, 136–137, 151–152, 171, 187–188, 213, 296
  cause of, 299t
  classification of, 126, 126t
    combined morphologic and physiologic, 131, 132–133f
    etiologic, 127, 128–129t